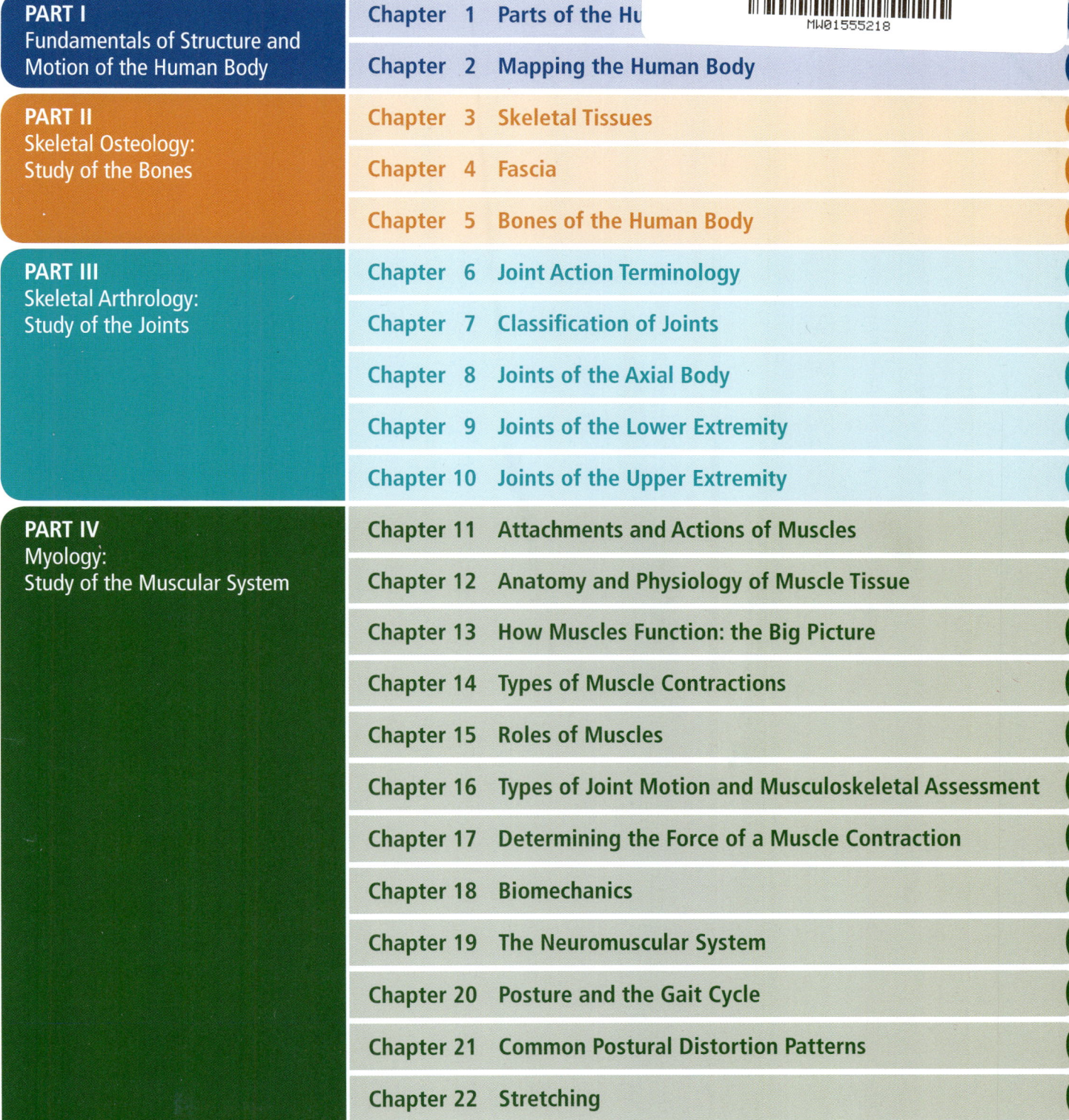

PART I Fundamentals of Structure and Motion of the Human Body	Chapter 1	Parts of the Human Body
	Chapter 2	Mapping the Human Body
PART II Skeletal Osteology: Study of the Bones	Chapter 3	Skeletal Tissues
	Chapter 4	Fascia
	Chapter 5	Bones of the Human Body
PART III Skeletal Arthrology: Study of the Joints	Chapter 6	Joint Action Terminology
	Chapter 7	Classification of Joints
	Chapter 8	Joints of the Axial Body
	Chapter 9	Joints of the Lower Extremity
	Chapter 10	Joints of the Upper Extremity
PART IV Myology: Study of the Muscular System	Chapter 11	Attachments and Actions of Muscles
	Chapter 12	Anatomy and Physiology of Muscle Tissue
	Chapter 13	How Muscles Function: the Big Picture
	Chapter 14	Types of Muscle Contractions
	Chapter 15	Roles of Muscles
	Chapter 16	Types of Joint Motion and Musculoskeletal Assessment
	Chapter 17	Determining the Force of a Muscle Contraction
	Chapter 18	Biomechanics
	Chapter 19	The Neuromuscular System
	Chapter 20	Posture and the Gait Cycle
	Chapter 21	Common Postural Distortion Patterns
	Chapter 22	Stretching
	Chapter 23	Principles of Strengthening Exercise

Kinesiology

The Skeletal System and Muscle Function

Joseph E. Muscolino, DC

Instructor, Purchase College, State University of New York
Purchase, New York
Owner, The Art and Science of Kinesiology
Stamford, Connecticut
www.learnmuscles.com

3rd Edition

ELSEVIER

ELSEVIER

3251 Riverport Lane
St. Louis, Missouri 63043

KINESIOLOGY: THE SKELETAL SYSTEM
AND MUSCLE FUNCTION, THIRD EDITION

ISBN: 978-0-323-39620-2

Copyright © 2017 by Elsevier, Inc. All rights reserved.

No part of this publication may be reproduced or transmitted in any form or by any means, electronic or mechanical, including photocopying, recording, or any information storage and retrieval system, without permission in writing from the publisher. Details on how to seek permission, further information about the Publisher's permissions policies and our arrangements with organizations such as the Copyright Clearance Center and the Copyright Licensing Agency, can be found at our website: www.elsevier.com/permissions.

This book and the individual contributions contained in it are protected under copyright by the Publisher (other than as may be noted herein).

Notices

Knowledge and best practice in this field are constantly changing. As new research and experience broaden our understanding, changes in research methods, professional practices, or medical treatment may become necessary.

Practitioners and researchers must always rely on their own experience and knowledge in evaluating and using any information, methods, compounds, or experiments described herein. In using such information or methods they should be mindful of their own safety and the safety of others, including parties for whom they have a professional responsibility.

With respect to any drug or pharmaceutical products identified, readers are advised to check the most current information provided (i) on procedures featured or (ii) by the manufacturer of each product to be administered, to verify the recommended dose or formula, the method and duration of administration, and contraindications. It is the responsibility of practitioners, relying on their own experience and knowledge of their patients, to make diagnoses, to determine dosages and the best treatment for each individual patient, and to take all appropriate safety precautions.

To the fullest extent of the law, neither the Publisher nor the authors, contributors, or editors, assume any liability for any injury and/or damage to persons or property as a matter of products liability, negligence or otherwise, or from any use or operation of any methods, products, instructions, or ideas contained in the material herein.

Previous editions copyrighted 2011 and 2006.

Library of Congress Cataloging-in-Publication Data

Names: Muscolino, Joseph E., author
Title: Kinesiology : the skeletal system and muscle function / Joseph E. Muscolino.
Description: 3rd edition. | St. Louis : Elsevier Inc., [2017] | Includes
  bibliographical references and index.
Identifiers: LCCN 2016022344 | ISBN 9780323396202 (pbk. : alk. paper)
Subjects: | MESH: Kinesiology, Applied | Musculoskeletal System | Biochemical
  Phenomena
Classification: LCC QP303 | NLM WE 103 | DDC 612.7/6—dc23
LC record available at https://lccn.loc.gov/2016022344

Content Strategist: Brandi Graham
Content Development Manager: Ellen Wurm-Cutter
Associate Content Development Specialist: Erin Garner
Publishing Services Manager: Julie Eddy
Book Production Specialist: Celeste Clingan
Design Direction: Julia Dummitt

Printed in China

Last digit is the print number: 9 8 7 6 5 4 3 2 1

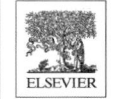
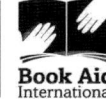

Reviewers

Sandra K. Anderson, BA, LMT, ABT, NCTMB
Co-Owner and Practitioner, Tucson Touch Therapies
Treatment Center and Education Center
Tucson, Arizona

Eva Beaulieu, MEd, ATC, LAT
Assistant Athletic Trainer
Georgia College & State University
Milledgeville, Georgia

Vincent Carvelli, BS, RTS2
President, Co-Founder, and Senior Biomechanics
Instructor, Academy of Applied Personal Training
  Education (AAPTE)
East Meadow, New York
Continuing Education Specialist, American Council on
  Exercise (ACE)
Career and Technical Education Teacher, Joseph M.
  Barry Career and Technical Education Center
Westbury, New York
Fellow, National Board of Fitness Examiners (NBFE)

Michael Choothesa, BA, CPT-AFAA
Fairfield, Connecticut

Jonathan Passmore
Investment Professional
Fairfield, Connecticut

Michael P. Reiman, PT, DPT, OCS, SCS, ATC, FAAOMPT, CSCS
Assistant Professor
Wichita State University, Physical Therapy Department
Wichita, Kansas

Pamela Shelline, LMT
Director
Massage Therapy Academy
Saint George, Utah

Third Edition Forewords

RALPH STEPHENS

It has always amazed me how education can take the most fascinating subject on the planet, the study of our own human bodies, and make it arguably the most boring, dreaded subject taught in the training of healthcare providers. That is why I am so excited about the third edition of *Kinesiology*, by my friend and colleague Joseph E. Muscolino, DC. Joe has been teaching anatomy, physiology, kinesiology, as well as hands-on manual and movement therapy techniques for over 30 years and obviously realizes the shortcomings of most anatomy textbooks and programs. Most anatomical education is taught in static, two-dimensional formats. Students memorize text and pictures, then regurgitate them back on tests and forget most of it within a few weeks. This is so sad, primarily because it negatively impacts the quality of care and treatment the public receives.

People are seeking ever-faster resolution of their pain and stress. As we learn more about how the nervous system interacts with the contractile connective tissues and how precise movements, applied as stimuli, can reset the tonus of muscles almost instantly, it has become as important to know what movements a particular muscle performs in the body as where it is. It takes both to be an effective therapist and especially to accurately stimulate the nervous system to bring about the most rapid and complete resets of dysfunctional tissues.

The patients we see are living, moving, and very dynamic organisms. Life is movement; one could define death as a "lack of movement." In *Kinesiology*, Joe has put the "life" back into the teaching and study of anatomy and physiology by combining it with the study of movement. In real life, anatomy is not separate from movement. For an exciting, memorable learning experience that can be translated into therapeutic effectiveness, they should be taught and learned together. It is the association of the movement each muscle causes and each joint allows (kinesiology) that brings anatomy alive, making it memorable and applicable to a student of any healing art. Life is 3-dimensional. Learning anatomy in a way that makes it real, meaningful, and applicable to therapeutic situations requires it to be taught in 3D.

Joe has done an impressive job of bringing anatomy off the 2-dimensional page and into 3-dimensional reality. Richly illustrated with a combination of colorful illustrations and photographs that bring the text alive, this new edition is easy to read, efficient to reference, and pleasing to the eye. More than 150 videos are included on the accompanying Evolve website, providing more than 2 hours of enhanced visual-spatial learning. Further resources are provided online including—An Interactive Muscle Program, A Stretching Program for patients, a Body Systems Quick Guide, Bony Landmark Palpation Identification Exercises, and more!—making this text a dynamic, ongoing educational resource that will serve readers not only in school but also well into their career.

As valuable as soft-tissue manual therapies can be, they are a fairly static and passive way of addressing the body, and are not very effective at elongating tissue and creating strength balance across joints. *Kinesiology* has brilliant chapters on both stretching and strengthening. This is an exciting addition to both anatomical and clinical education, as it gives practical application to the study of both musculoskeletal anatomy and movement. The answer to most patients' soft-tissue pain complaints is found in anatomy and kinesiology. This book will be an invaluable tool for the manual and movement soft-tissue therapist/physician/trainer looking for the anatomical answers.

Furthermore, in this third edition, three chapters have been added, all of which are exciting additions to this study of the body.

Chapter 4, *Fascia*, brings to the study of kinesiology the latest information on this all-pervading tissue. Co-written by Thomas Myers, Rolfer, and the author of *Anatomy Trains*, this fascinating chapter provides a wealth of easily understood information and insight into this mysterious tissue that is the focus of so much research and attention lately.

The new Chapter 18, *Biomechanics*, offers the reader an introduction to the topic of biomechanics, which is the study of how forces affect the human body. Both kinematics and kinetics are covered. This topic is of special importance for movement trainers/instructors/therapists who are studying kinesiology in university settings, and is presented to empower them to be able to understand biomechanical principles to optimize the client's needs in order to maximize performance and minimize injury.

The new Chapter 21, *Common Postural Distortion Patterns*, has now made that study much easier and quicker, giving students the awareness to help people that few therapists ever achieve. Having these patterns for reference will make the sometimes-difficult assessment of postural distortion and its role in a patient's pain complaints relatively simple. When you can get people out of pain, you will always be busy, as you will never run out of people in pain. This text gives you a solid anatomical foundation for developing a successful clinical practice.

The better you know anatomy, physiology and kinesiology the better therapist you are. It is a life-long study, pursued by serious therapists who care about helping people get out of pain and dysfunction. This book is the best starting point I have seen to date for the most important educational journey a therapist undertakes. It is written with precision, scientific accuracy, and a lot of heart. May this book guide you to better serve humanity through the power of knowledge, compassion, and manual and movement therapy.

Ralph Stephens, LMT, NCBTMB
Ralph Stephens Seminars
Coralville, Iowa

SEAN GALLAGHER

Dr. Muscolino has provided an up-to-date, comprehensive, and integrative review of osteology, arthrology, myology, movement, and special tests that allow any student to gain a unique understanding of the body in front of you when teaching, treating, or evaluating. By being able to organize and search for the tests as well as the anatomy and other body systems related to these tests in a way that allows students as well as practitioners to review for the clinical setting is a great resource. Having a book that allows you to systematically learn the anatomy, myology and body systems, and clinically relevant tests is what is demanded in today's learning environment for physical therapists who are required to have a broad-based systems understanding of the body. Dr. Muscolino's approach in this book makes learning the material not only comprehensive but also interesting at the same time. Allowing the student to make the connections through the boxes and the online materials while studying will help reinforce the learning process.

The use of boxes to highlight special considerations as well as spotlight specific areas of study or interest is a great learning tool for anyone new to this information as well as those who have a clinical need to review. To be able to gain a better understanding of the material presented, the boxes reinforce the dynamic relationships that every therapist needs to gain to truly understand how to put all the different parts together. This book and how it is organized helps students better grasp underlying complexities of the body that are often not clearly understood when learning only the anatomy or the biomechanics or the neuromuscular system as separate entities. The integrative learning style that Dr. Muscolino has presented in this book will provide anyone who uses all that it has to offer a pathway to becoming a practitioner that understands the complexities of the human body and how to scientifically as well as clinically develop a plan of action to address their particular needs.

The companion Evolve site contains over 150 videos that provide the student with an excellent review of common terms of movement and joint function providing an extra benefit in visual learning that is so integral in understanding the dynamic body. Having this material available online as a supplement to the book is especially beneficial for students as well as new or even seasoned physical therapists who need to review a muscle, special test, or concept with which a patient presents that they have not seen in a while and thus can benefit from a review that is easily accessible.

Kinesiology: The Skeletal System and Muscle Function should be in every student of movement, bodywork, and manual therapy's special category of books to keep a lifetime as it will be the go-to reference when they have anatomical or kinesiological questions they need to answer when working with their clients and patients.

Sean P. Gallagher, BFA, PT, CPI, CFP, EMT, MS
Performing Arts Physical Therapy
New York, New York

Second Edition Foreword

The many different styles of massage therapy and bodywork have become an integral component of addressing musculoskeletal pain and injury conditions. The public's expectations place a high demand on the knowledge base of these practitioners. Consequently, the professional development of massage and bodywork therapists must accommodate the changing requirements of the profession. In the first edition of this text, author Joe Muscolino made an excellent contribution to the professional literature to aid today's soft-tissue therapist. In this new edition of *Kinesiology: The Skeletal System and Muscle Function*, updates and improvements have taken this text to the next level and significantly improved an already excellent resource.

Kinesiology is a critical component of the knowledge and skills necessary for today's soft-tissue therapist. By definition kinesiology is the study of anatomy (structure), neuromuscular physiology (function), and biomechanics (the mechanics of movement related to living systems). Competence in these principles is required even for those practitioners who work in an environment where massage or movement therapy is used only for relaxation or stress reduction. The need to understand proper movement can arise in the most basic soft-tissue treatment.

The requirements for knowing the principles of kinesiology are even greater for those practitioners who actively choose to address soft-tissue pain and injury conditions. Treatment of any soft-tissue disorder begins with a comprehensive assessment of the problem. Accurate assessment is not possible without an understanding of how the body moves under normal circumstances and what may impair its movement in pathology. Joe Muscolino has continually set high standards for helping prepare practitioners of soft-tissue therapy. The improvements in this new edition build on the established foundation that is crucial for today's clinician.

Over the years of teaching orthopedic assessment and treatment to soft-tissue therapists, I have found many students deficient in their understanding of kinesiology. Similarly, students express frustration about understanding how to apply basic kinesiology principles in their practice. Although they receive some training in their initial coursework, traditional approaches to teaching kinesiology often provide little benefit to students. Overwhelmingly, basic courses in kinesiology prove to be insufficient and fail to connect the student with the skills necessary for professional success.

Learning muscle attachments and concentric actions tends to be the focus of most kinesiology curricula and is often turned into an exercise of rote memorization. Yet, there is significantly more to this important subject than these topics. Eccentric actions, force loads, angle of pull, axis of rotation, synergistic muscles, and other concepts are necessary for understanding human movement. These principles, in turn, are prerequisites for effective therapeutic treatment. An adequate understanding of kinesiology requires more than a curriculum plan that emphasizes memorization. A competent education in kinesiology requires a foundation in the functional application of its principles.

Joe Muscolino's scientific background and years of experience as an educator teaching anatomy, pathology, and kinesiology make him uniquely qualified to tackle a project of this scope. His skill, talent, and demonstrated expertise are evidenced in this work and are of great benefit to the soft-tissue professions. During the years I've known Joe as a professional colleague, we have repeatedly engaged in animated discussions about how to raise the quality of training and improve educational resources available in the profession.

I was thoroughly impressed with the content and presentation of the first edition of this text. In this new edition, the author has responded to the needs of students and educators by including new sections on strength training and stretching. These topics are of great importance to manual therapy practitioners and are often not present in this detail in many other resources. Also included is new and updated information on the role of fascia in movement, stability and posture. Many clinicians are increasingly aware of the importance of fascia, and these new findings help us understand this ubiquitous tissue even better. Finally, a new section on understanding how to read a research paper has been added to this edition. This section introduces the student/practitioner to the importance of research in the manual therapy professions, and then explains how to read and understand a research article. Research literacy is an increasingly important skill in the manual therapy profession, and this section facilitates that process.

The educational landscape is changing at a dramatic pace and one of the most powerful changes driving this transformation is the development and use of enhanced multimedia resources. The Elsevier Evolve site is a wealth of teaching and learning materials for students and users of this text. Numerous activities have been designed to aid the student in both comprehension of basic concepts as well as developing high order thinking skills that are essential in clinical practice.

When this book first came out it was clear that it excelled as both a comprehensive resource for the practicing professional and an excellent guide for students new to the field. This updated edition has broken new ground and set the bar high as a comprehensive resource and learning tool for professionals in multiple disciplines.

Whitney Lowe, LMT
Orthopedic Massage Education & Research Institute
Sisters, Oregon

Preface

The term *kinesiology* literally means *the study of motion*. Because motion of the body is created by the forces of muscle contractions pulling on bones and moving body parts at joints, kinesiology involves the study of the musculoskeletal system. Because muscle functioning is controlled by the nervous system, kinesiology might be better described as study of the neuromusculosketetal system. And because the importance of fascia is better understood and accepted, perhaps the best description might be study of the neuro-myo-fascio-skeletal system!

There are three keys to healthy motion: (1) flexibility of soft tissues to allow motion, (2) strength of musculature to create motion and stability, and (3) neural control from the nervous system. This book provides the readers/students with necessary information to apply this knowledge and to help their patients/clients in the health and fitness fields.

Kinesiology: The Skeletal System and Muscle Function, third edition, is unique in that it is written for the allied health fields of manual and movement therapies, and rehabilitation and fitness training. These fields include massage therapy, physical therapy, occupational therapy, yoga, Pilates, fitness and athletic training, Feldenkrais technique, Alexander technique, chiropractic, osteopathy, naturopathy, and exercise physiology. Information is presented in a manner that explains the fundamental basis for movement of the human body as it pertains to working with clients in these fields. Clinical applications are located throughout the text's narrative and in special lightbulb and spotlight boxes to explain relevant concepts.

CONCEPTUAL APPROACH

The purpose of this book is to explain the concepts of kinesiology in a clear, simple, and straightforward manner, without dumbing down the material. The presentation of the subject matter of this book encourages the reader or student to think critically instead of memorize. This is achieved through a clear and orderly layout of the information. My belief is that no subject matter is difficult to learn if the big picture is first presented, and then the smaller pieces are presented in context to the big picture. An analogy is a jigsaw puzzle, wherein each piece of the puzzle represents a piece of information that must be learned. When all the pieces of the puzzle first come cascading out of the box, the idea of learning them and fitting them together can seem overwhelming; and indeed it is a daunting task if we do not first look at the big picture on the front of the box. However, if the big picture is first explained and understood, then our ability to learn and place into context all the small pieces is facilitated. This approach makes the job of being a student of kinesiology much easier!

ORGANIZATION

Generally, the information within this book is laid out in the order that the musculoskeletal system is usually covered. Terminology is usually needed before bones can be discussed. Bones then need to be studied before the joints can be learned. Finally, once the terminology, bones, and joints have been learned, the muscular system can be explored. However, depending on the curriculum of your particular school, you might need to access the information in a different order and jump around within this book. The compartmentalized layout of the sections of this book easily allows for this freedom.

- Scattered throughout the text of this book are lightbulb 💡 and spotlight 🔦 icons. These icons alert the reader to additional information on the subject matter being presented. A 💡 contains an interesting fact or short amount of additional information; a 🔦 contains a greater amount of information. In most cases, these illuminating boxes immediately follow the text statements that explain the concept.
- At the beginning of each chapter is a list of learning objectives. Refer to these objectives as you read each chapter of the book.
- After the learning objectives is an overview of the information of the chapter. I strongly suggest that you read this overview so that you have a big picture idea of what the chapter covers before delving into the details.
- Immediately after the overview is a list of key terms for the chapter, with the proper pronunciation included where necessary. These key terms are also in bold blue type when they first appear in the text. A complete glossary of all key terms from the book is located on the Evolve website that accompanies this book.
- After the key terms is a list of word origins. These origins explore word roots (prefixes, suffixes, and so forth) that are commonly used in the field of kinesiology. Learning a word root once can enable you to make sense of tens or hundreds of other terms without having to look them up!

Kinesiology, The Skeletal System and Muscle Function is divided into four parts:

- **Part I** covers essential terminology that is used in kinesiology. Terminology that is unambiguous is necessary to allow for clear communication, which is especially important when dealing with clients in the health, athletic training, and rehabilitation fields.
- **Part II** covers the fascial and skeletal systems. This part explores the makeup of skeletal and fascial tissues and also contains a photographic atlas of all bones and bony landmarks, as well as joints, of the human body.
- **Part III** contains a detailed study of the joints of the body. The first two chapters explain the structure and function of joints in general. The next three chapters provide a thorough regional examination of all joints of the body.
- **Part IV** examines how muscles function. After covering the anatomy and physiology of muscle tissue, the larger kinesiologic concepts of muscle function are addressed. A big picture idea of what defines muscle contraction is first explained. From this point, various topics such as types of muscle contractions, roles of muscles, types of joint motions, musculoskeletal assessment, control by the nervous system, posture, the gait cycle, postural distortion patterns, stretching, and strength fitness training are covered. A thor-

ough illustrated atlas of all the skeletal muscles of the body, along with their attachments and major actions, is also given.

DISTINCTIVE FEATURES

There are many features that distinguish this book:
- Clear and ordered presentation of the content
- Simple and clear verbiage that makes learning concepts easy
- Full-color illustrations that visually display the concepts that are being explained so that the student can see what is happening
- Light-bulb and spotlight boxes that discuss interesting applications of the content, including pathologic conditions and clinical scenarios
- Open bullets next to each piece of information allow the student to check off what has been or needs to be learned and allows the instructor to assign clearly the material that the students are responsible to learn
- The Evolve companion site includes video clips that show and explain all joint movements of the body and the major concepts of kinesiology

NEW TO THIS EDITION

Every feature of the second edition has been preserved. In addition, the third edition has many new features:
- A greatly expanded chapter containing a thorough illustrated atlas of all the skeletal muscles of the body along with their attachments and major standard and reverse actions
- A comprehensive chapter on fascial tissue, co-authored by Tom Myers.
- An entire chapter on biomechanics.
- An entire chapter on postural distortion patterns in the body
- Evidence-based references for the entire book.

EVOLVE RESOURCES

- Video clips demonstrating all joint actions of the body are located on the Evolve site. This includes:
  - Kinesiology videos that explain key concepts of kinesiology such as anatomic position, planes, axes, how to name joint actions, and the concept of reverse actions. The videos also demonstrate and describe all the major joint actions of the human body, beginning with actions of the axial body, followed by actions of the lower extremity and upper extremity
  - Palpation demonstration videos
  - Bonus clip on teaching muscle palpation
- Bony landmark identification exercises reinforce your knowledge.
- Answers to review questions in the textbook
- Drag-and-drop labeling exercises aid in your review of the material as you drag the name of the structure and drop it into the correct position on illustrations.
- Crossword puzzles help reinforce muscle names and terminology through fun, interactive activities!
- Glossary of terms and word origins. All terms from the book are defined and explained, along with word origins, on the Evolve site.
- Additional strengthening exercise photographs demonstrate key strengthening exercises on Evolve.
- Stretching Customization allows you to create customized stretching instructions with images for clients to use at home.
- *Musculoskeletal Anatomy Flashcards* provide students with 257 full-color cards that will test their knowledge of muscles, muscle location, pronunciations, attachments, actions, and innervation information.
- Interactive muscle program
- Body systems quick guide
- Audio files for self study
- Radiographs
  - Study these radiographs for real-world application of material in the book.

INSTRUCTOR RESOURCES

For instructors, TEACH lesson plans and PowerPoints cover the book in 50-minute lectures, with learning outcomes, discussion topics, and critical thinking questions. There is also an instructor's manual that provides step-by-step approaches to leading the class through learning the content, as well as kinesthetic in-class activities. Further, a complete image collection that contains every figure in the book, and a test bank in ExamView containing 1,000 questions, are provided.

RELATED PUBLICATIONS

This book has been written to stand on its own. However, it can also complement and be used in conjunction with *The Muscular System Manual, The Skeletal Muscles of the Human Body*, fourth edition (Elsevier 2017). *The Muscular System Manual* is a thorough and clearly presented atlas of the skeletal muscles of the human body that covers all aspects of muscle function. These two textbooks, along with *Musculoskeletal Anatomy Coloring Book*, third edition (Elsevier 2018), and *Flashcards for Bones, Joints, and Actions of the Human Body*, second edition (Elsevier 2011), give the student a complete set of resources to study and thoroughly learn all aspects of kinesiology.

For more direct clinical assessment and treatment techniques, look also for *The Muscle and Bone Palpation Manual, With Trigger Points, Referral Patterns, and Stretching*, second edition (Elsevier 2016), *Flashcards for Palpation, Trigger Points, and Referral Patterns* (Elsevier 2009), and *Mosby's Trigger Point Flip Chart, with Referral Patterns and Stretching* (Elsevier 2009). For additional information about these products, visit http://joeknows.elsevier.com.

Even though kinesiology can be viewed as the science of studying the biomechanics of body movement (and the human body certainly is a marvel of biomechanical engineering), kinesiology can also be seen as the study of an art form. Movement is more than simply lifting a glass or walking across a room; movement is the means by which we live our lives and express ourselves. Therefore science and art are part of the study of kinesiology. Whether you are just beginning your exploration of kinesiology, or you are an experienced student looking to expand your knowledge, I hope that *Kinesiology: The Skeletal System and Muscle Function*, third edition, proves to be a helpful and friendly guide. Even more importantly, I hope that it also facilitates an enjoyment and excitement as you come to better understand and appreciate the wonder and beauty of human movement!

Joseph E. Muscolino, DC
February 2016

Acknowledgments

Usually only one name is listed on the front of a book, and that is the author's. This practice can give the reader the misconception that the author is the only person responsible for what lies in his or her hands. However, many people who work behind the scenes and are invisible to the reader have contributed to the effort. The Acknowledgments section of a book is the author's opportunity to both directly thank these people and acknowledge them to the readers.

First, I would like to thank William Courtland. William, now an instructor and author himself, was the student who 15 years ago first recommended that I should write a kinesiology textbook. William, thanks for giving me the initial spark of inspiration to write.

Because kinesiology is the study of movement, the illustrations in this book are just as important, if not more important, than the written text. I am lucky to have had a brilliant team of illustrators and photographers. Jeannie Robertson illustrated the bulk of the figures in this book. Jeannie is able to portray three-dimensional movements of the body with sharp, accurate, simple, and clear full-color illustrations. Tiziana Cipriani contributed a tremendous number of beautiful drawings to this book, including perhaps my two favorites, Figures 13-13*A* and 13-13*B*. Jean Luciano, my principle illustrator for the first edition of *The Muscular System Manual*, also stepped in to help with a few beautiful illustrations. And in this third edition, many beautiful illustrations have been added by Giovanni Rimasti and Jodie Bernard of Lightbox Visuals in Canada. Yanik Chauvin is the photographer who took the photos that appear in Chapters 8, 9, 10, 11, and 22, as well as a few others. Yanik is extremely talented, as well as being one of the easiest people with whom to work. Frank Forney is an illustrator who came to this project via Electronic Publishing Services (EPS). Frank drew the computer drawings of the bones that were overlaid on Yanik's photos in Chapters 8, 9, and 10. Frank proved to be an extremely able and invaluable asset to the artwork team. For Chapter 11, the newly expanded illustrated atlas of muscles chapter, Giovanni Rimasti, Frank Forney, and Dave Carlson, provided computer-drawn images of the bones and muscles overlaid on Yanik's photos. These illustrations are astoundingly beautiful! Last but not least is Dr. David Eliot of Touro University College of Osteopathic Medicine, who provided the bone photographs that are found in Chapter 5. Dr. Eliot is a PhD anatomist whose knowledge of the musculoskeletal system is as vast as his photographs are beautiful. I was lucky to have him as a contributor to this book.

I would also like to thank the models for Yanik's photographs: Audrey Van Herck, Kiyoko Gotanda, Gamaliel Martinez Fonseca, Patrick Tremblay, and Simona Cipriani. The beauty and poise of their bodies was invaluable toward expressing the kinesiologic concepts of movement in the photographs for this book.

I must thank the authors of the other kinesiology textbooks that are presently in print. I like to think that we all stand on the shoulders of those who have come before us. Each kinesiology textbook is unique and has contributed to the field of kinesiology, as well as my knowledge base. I would particularly like to thank Donald Neumann, PT, PhD of Marquette University. His book, *Kinesiology of the Musculoskeletal System*, in my opinion, is the best book ever written on joint mechanics. I once told Don Neumann that if I could have written just one book, I wish it would have been his.

Writing a book is not only the exercise of stating facts but also the art of how to present these facts. In other words, a good writer should be a good teacher. Toward that end, I would like to thank all my present and past students for helping me become a better teacher.

For the act of actually turning this project into a book, I must thank the entire Elsevier team in St. Louis who spent tremendous hours on this project, particularly Shelly Stringer, Brandi Graham, Celeste Clingan, Erin Garner, and Teresa Exley. Thank you for making the birth of this book as painless as possible.

Finally, to echo my dedication, I would like to thank my entire family, who makes it all worthwhile!

About the Author

Dr. Joseph E. Muscolino has been teaching musculoskeletal and visceral anatomy and physiology, kinesiology, neurology, and pathology courses for more than 30 years. He has also been instrumental in course manual development and has assisted with curriculum development. He has published:

- *The Muscular System Manual*, fourth edition
- *The Muscle and Bone Palpation Manual*, second edition
- *Musculoskeletal Anatomy Coloring Book*, second edition
- *Know the Body – Muscle, Bone, and Palpation Essentials*
- *Know the Body Workbook – Muscle, Bone, and Palpation Essentials*
- *Musculoskeletal Anatomy Flashcards*, second edition
- *Flashcards for Bones, Joints, and Actions of the Human Body*, second edition
- *Flashcards for Palpation, Trigger Points, and Referral Patterns*
- *Mosby's Trigger Point Flip Chart, with Referral Patterns and Stretching*
- *Advanced Treatment Techniques for the Manual Therapist: Neck*
- *Manual Therapy for the Low Back and Pelvis – A Clinical Orthopedic Approach*

He has also published more than 70 articles in the *Massage Therapy Journal, Journal of Bodywork and Movement Therapies, Massage and Bodywork Magazine, Massage Magazine, Massage Today, Pilates Style*, and numerous other overseas journals in the world of manual therapy. And he has developed and created 15 DVDs on manual and movement therapy assessment and treatment techniques for therapists, instructors, and trainers.

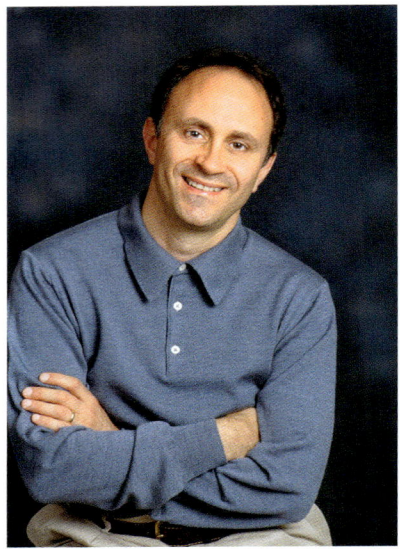

Dr. Muscolino runs continuing education workshops on topics such as body mechanics for deep tissue massage, intermediate and advanced stretching techniques, joint mobilization, kinesiology, and cadaver lab workshops. He offers a Certification in Clinical Orthopedic Manual Therapy (COMT) both within the United States and around the world. He is approved by the National Certification Board for Therapeutic Massage and Bodywork (NCBTMB) as a provider of continuing education, and grants continuing education credit (CEUs) for massage therapists toward certification renewal. Dr. Muscolino also served as a subject matter expert and member of the NCBTMB's Continuing Education and Exam Committees.

Dr. Muscolino holds a Bachelor of Arts degree in biology from the State University of New York at Binghamton, Harpur College. He attained his Doctor of Chiropractic degree from Western States Chiropractic College in Portland, Oregon, and is licensed in Connecticut, New York, and California. He has been in private practice in Connecticut for more than 30 years, currently practicing in Stamford, CT at *Synergy Health and Fitness*, and incorporates soft-tissue work into his chiropractic practice for all his patients.

If you would like further information regarding *Kinesiology: The Skeletal System and Muscle Function*, third edition, or any of Dr. Muscolino's other Elsevier publications, or if you are an instructor and would like information regarding the many supportive materials such as PowerPoint slides, test banks of questions, or instructor's manuals, please visit http://www.us.elsevierhealth.com. For questions regarding his other publications, DVDs, or his COMT Certification program, you can contact Dr. Muscolino directly at his web site: http://www. learnmuscles.com.

Contents

PART I
Fundamentals of Structure and Motion of the Human Body, 1

Chapter 1   Parts of the Human Body, 1
1.1   Major Divisions of the Human Body, 2
1.2   Major Body Parts, 3
1.3   Joints Between Body Parts, 5
1.4   Movement of a Body Part Relative to an Adjacent Body Part, 6
1.5   Movement within a Body Part, 7
1.6   True Movement of a Body Part Versus "Going Along for the Ride", 8
1.7   Regions of the Body, 9

Chapter 2   Mapping the Human Body, 11
2.1   Anatomic Position, 13
2.2   Location Terminology, 13
2.3   Anterior/Posterior, 14
2.4   Medial/Lateral, 15
2.5   Superior/Inferior and Proximal/Distal, 16
2.6   Superficial/Deep, 17
2.7   Location Terminology Illustration, 18
2.8   Planes, 19
2.9   Motion of the Human Body within Planes, 20
2.10   Axes, 22
2.11   Planes and Their Corresponding Axes, 23
2.12   Visualizing the Axes—Door Hinge Pin Analogy, 24
2.13   Visualizing the Axes—Pinwheel Analogy, 26

PART II
Skeletal Osteology: Study of the Bones, 29

Chapter 3   Skeletal Tissues, 29
3.1   Classification of Bones by Shape, 31
3.2   Parts of a Long Bone, 32
3.3   Functions of Bones, 33
3.4   Bone as a Connective Tissue, 35
3.5   Compact and Spongy Bone, 36
3.6   Bone Development and Growth, 37
3.7   Fontanels, 39
3.8   Fracture Healing, 40
3.9   Effects of Physical Stress on Bone, 41
3.10   Cartilage Tissue, 43

Chapter 4   Fascia, 47
4.1   Fascia, 48
4.2   The Fascial Web, 52
4.3   Fascial Response to Physical Stress, 55
4.4   Tendons and Ligaments, 57
4.5   Bursae and Tendon Sheaths, 58
4.6   Properties of Fascial Connective Tissues, 60

Chapter 5   Bones of the Human Body, 63
5.1   Bones of the Head, 71
5.2   Bones of the Spine (and Hyoid), 85
5.3   Bones of the Ribcage and Sternum, 103
5.4   Entire Lower Extremity, 107
5.5   Bones of the Pelvis and Hip Joint, 108
5.6   Bones of the Thigh and Knee Joint, 113
5.7   Bones of the Leg and Ankle Joint, 117
5.8   Bones of the Foot, 122
5.9   Entire Upper Extremity, 127
5.10   Bones of the Shoulder Girdle and Shoulder Joint, 128
5.11   Bones of the Arm and Elbow Joint, 133
5.12   Bones of the Forearm, Wrist Joint, and Hand, 137

PART III
Skeletal Arthrology: Study of the Joints, 150

Chapter 6   Joint Action Terminology, 150
6.1   Overview of Joint Function, 152
6.2   Axial and Nonaxial Motion, 152
6.3   Nonaxial/Gliding Motion, 153
6.4   Rectilinear and Curvilinear Nonaxial Motion, 154
6.5   Axial/Circular Motion, 154
6.6   Axial Motion and the Axis of Movement, 155
6.7   Roll and Spin Axial Movements, 156
6.8   Roll, Glide, and Spin Movements Compared, 156
6.9   Naming Joint Actions—Completely, 157
6.10   Joint Action Terminology Pairs, 158
6.11   Flexion/Extension, 159
6.12   Abduction/Adduction, 160
6.13   Right Lateral Flexion/Left Lateral Flexion, 161
6.14   Lateral Rotation/Medial Rotation, 162
6.15   Right Rotation/Left Rotation, 162
6.16   Plantarflexion/Dorsiflexion, 163
6.17   Eversion/Inversion, 164
6.18   Pronation/Supination, 164
6.19   Protraction/Retraction, 165
6.20   Elevation/Depression, 166
6.21   Upward Rotation/Downward Rotation, 167
6.22   Anterior Tilt/Posterior Tilt, 168
6.23   Opposition/Reposition, 169
6.24   Right Lateral Deviation/Left Lateral Deviation, 169
6.25   Horizontal Flexion/Horizontal Extension, 170
6.26   Hyperextension, 171
6.27   Circumduction, 172
6.28   Naming Oblique Plane Movements, 172
6.29   Reverse Actions, 174
6.30   Vectors, 175

Chapter 7 Classification of Joints, 179

- 7.1 Anatomy of a Joint, 181
- 7.2 Physiology of a Joint, 181
- 7.3 Joint Mobility Versus Joint Stability, 182
- 7.4 Joints and Shock Absorption, 183
- 7.5 Weight-Bearing Joints, 184
- 7.6 Joint Classification, 185
- 7.7 Fibrous Joints, 186
- 7.8 Cartilaginous Joints, 187
- 7.9 Synovial Joints, 188
- 7.10 Uniaxial Synovial Joints, 191
- 7.11 Biaxial Synovial Joints, 192
- 7.12 Triaxial Synovial Joints, 195
- 7.13 Nonaxial Synovial Joints, 197
- 7.14 Menisci and Articular Discs, 198

Chapter 8 Joints of the Axial Body, 202

- 8.1 Suture Joints of the Skull, 204
- 8.2 Temporomandibular Joint (TMJ), 205
- 8.3 Spine, 210
- 8.4 Spinal Joints, 213
- 8.5 Atlanto-Occipital and Atlantoaxial Joints, 221
- 8.6 Cervical Spine (The Neck), 226
- 8.7 Thoracic Spine (The Thorax), 230
- 8.8 Rib Joints of the Thorax, 231
- 8.9 Lumbar Spine (The Abdomen), 235
- 8.10 Thoracolumbar Spine (The Trunk), 237
- 8.11 Thoracolumbar Fascia and Abdominal Aponeurosis, 239

Chapter 9 Joints of the Lower Extremity, 244

- 9.1 Introduction to the Pelvis and Pelvic Movement, 247
- 9.2 Intrapelvic Motion (Symphysis Pubis and Sacroiliac Joints), 248
- 9.3 Movement of the Pelvis at the Lumbosacral Joint, 251
- 9.4 Movement of the Pelvis at the Hip Joints, 253
- 9.5 Movement of the Pelvis at the Lumbosacral and Hip Joints, 255
- 9.6 Relationship of Pelvic/Spinal Movements at the Lumbosacral Joint, 257
- 9.7 Relationship of Pelvic/Thigh Movements at the Hip Joint, 259
- 9.8 Effect of Pelvic Posture on Spinal Posture, 263
- 9.9 Hip Joint, 264
- 9.10 Angulations of the Femur, 269
- 9.11 Femoropelvic Rhythm, 271
- 9.12 Overview of the Knee Joint Complex, 272
- 9.13 Tibiofemoral (Knee) Joint, 273
- 9.14 Patellofemoral Joint, 279
- 9.15 Angulations of the Knee Joint, 280
- 9.16 Tibiofibular Joints, 283
- 9.17 Overview of the Ankle/Foot Region, 284
- 9.18 Talocrural (Ankle) Joint, 287
- 9.19 Subtalar Tarsal Joint, 293
- 9.20 Transverse Tarsal Joint, 296
- 9.21 Tarsometatarsal (TMT) Joints, 297
- 9.22 Intermetatarsal (IMT) Joints, 298
- 9.23 Metatarsophalangeal (MTP) Joints, 299
- 9.24 Interphalangeal (IP) Joints of the Foot, 301

Chapter 10 Joints of the Upper Extremity, 305

- 10.1 Shoulder Joint Complex, 308
- 10.2 Glenohumeral Joint, 309
- 10.3 Scapulocostal (ScC) Joint, 314
- 10.4 Sternoclavicular (SC) Joint, 316
- 10.5 Acromioclavicular (AC) Joint, 319
- 10.6 Scapulohumeral Rhythm, 321
- 10.7 Elbow Joint Complex, 324
- 10.8 Elbow Joint, 324
- 10.9 Radioulnar Joints, 327
- 10.10 Overview of the Wrist/Hand Region, 330
- 10.11 Wrist Joint Complex, 334
- 10.12 Carpometacarpal Joints, 339
- 10.13 Saddle (Carpometacarpal) Joint of the Thumb, 342
- 10.14 Intermetacarpal Joints, 346
- 10.15 Metacarpophalangeal (MCP) Joints, 348
- 10.16 Interphalangeal (IP) Joints of the Hand, 351

PART IV
Myology: Study of the Muscular System, 357

Chapter 11 Attachments and Actions of Muscles, 357

- 11.1 Overview of the Skeletal Muscles of the Body, 362
- 11.2 Muscles of the Shoulder Girdle, 364
- 11.3 Muscles of the Glenohumeral Joint, 367
- 11.4 Muscles of the Elbow and Radioulnar Joints, 372
- 11.5 Muscles of the Wrist Joint, 377
- 11.6 Extrinsic Muscles of the Finger Joints, 380
- 11.7 Intrinsic Muscles of the Finger Joints, 385
- 11.8 Muscles of the Spinal Joints, 391
- 11.9 Muscles of the Ribcage Joints, 410
- 11.10 Muscles of the Temporomandibular Joints, 414
- 11.11 Muscles of Facial Expression, 420
- 11.12 Muscles of the Hip Joint, 430
- 11.13 Muscles of the Knee Joint, 439
- 11.14 Muscles of the Ankle and Subtalar Joints, 444
- 11.15 Extrinsic Muscles of the Toe Joints, 448
- 11.16 Intrinsic Muscles of the Toe Joints, 450

Chapter 12 Anatomy and Physiology of Muscle Tissue, 457

- 12.1 Skeletal Muscle, 459
- 12.2 Tissue Components of a Skeletal Muscle, 460
- 12.3 Skeletal Muscle Cells, 461
- 12.4 Muscular Fascia, 462
- 12.5 Microanatomy of Muscle Fiber/Sarcomere Structure, 463
- 12.6 Sliding Filament Mechanism, 464
- 12.7 Energy Source for the Sliding Filament Mechanism, 466
- 12.8 Nervous System Control of Muscle Contraction, 467
- 12.9 Motor Unit, 469
- 12.10 All-or-None–Response Law, 470
- 12.11 Sarcomere Structure in More Detail, 471
- 12.12 Sliding Filament Mechanism in More Detail, 474
- 12.13 Red and White Muscle Fibers, 476
- 12.14 Myofascial Meridians and Tensegrity, 477

Chapter 13 How Muscles Function: the Big Picture, 488

- 13.1 "Big Picture" of Muscle Structure and Function, 489
- 13.2 What Happens When a Muscle Contracts and Shortens?, 490
- 13.3 Five-Step Approach to Learning Muscles, 492
- 13.4 Rubber Band Exercise, 493
- 13.5 Lines of Pull of a Muscle, 494

- 13.6 Functional Group Approach to Learning Muscle Actions, 496
- 13.7 Determining Functional Groups, 498
- 13.8 Off-Axis Attachment Method for Determining Rotation Actions, 500
- 13.9 Transferring the Force of a Muscle's Contraction to Another Joint, 501
- 13.10 Muscle Actions That Change, 503

Chapter 14 Types of Muscle Contractions, 507
- 14.1 Overview of the Types of Muscle Contractions, 508
- 14.2 Concentric, Eccentric, and Isometric Contraction Examples, 510
- 14.3 Relating Muscle Contraction and the Sliding Filament Mechanism, 511
- 14.4 Concentric Contractions in More Detail, 513
- 14.5 Eccentric Contractions in More Detail, 516
- 14.6 Isometric Contractions in More Detail, 519
- 14.7 Movement Versus Stabilization, 520

Chapter 15 Roles of Muscles, 523
- 15.1 Mover Muscles, 525
- 15.2 Antagonist Muscles, 527
- 15.3 Determining the "Muscle that is Working", 529
- 15.4 Stopping Unwanted Actions of the "Muscle that is Working", 531
- 15.5 Fixator/Stabilizer Muscles, 532
- 15.6 Concept of Fixation and Core Stabilization, 535
- 15.7 Neutralizer Muscles, 537
- 15.8 Step-by-Step Method for Determining Fixators and Neutralizers, 539
- 15.9 Support Muscles, 541
- 15.10 Synergists, 543
- 15.11 Coordinating Muscle Roles, 544
- 15.12 Coupled Actions, 547

Chapter 16 Types of Joint Motion and Musculoskeletal Assessment, 551
- 16.1 Active Versus Passive Range of Motion, 552
- 16.2 Resisted Motion/Manual Resistance, 555
- 16.3 Musculoskeletal Assessment: Muscle or Joint?, 556
- 16.4 Muscle Palpation, 558
- 16.5 Do We Treat Movers or Antagonists?, 560
- 16.6 Do We Treat Signs or Symptoms?, 561
- 16.7 Understanding Research, 563

Chapter 17 Determining the Force of a Muscle Contraction, 568
- 17.1 Partial Contraction of a Muscle, 570
- 17.2 Muscle Fiber Architecture, 571
- 17.3 Active Tension Versus Passive Tension, 574
- 17.4 Active Insufficiency, 574
- 17.5 Length-Tension and Force-Velocity Relationship Curves, 576
- 17.6 Leverage of a Muscle, 578
- 17.7 Leverage of a Muscle—More Detail, 580
- 17.8 Classes of Levers, 581
- 17.9 Leverage of Resistance Forces, 583

Chapter 18 Biomechanics, 588
- 18.1 Introduction to Biomechanics, 590
- 18.2 A Brief Introduction to Forces, 592
- 18.3 Basic Principles in Mechanics, 595
- 18.4 Describing Human Movement—Analyzing Kinematics, 597
- 18.5 Describing the Forces of Human Movement—Analyzing Kinetics, 602

Chapter 19 The Neuromuscular System, 609
- 19.1 Overview of the Nervous System, 611
- 19.2 Voluntary Movement Versus Reflex Movement, 615
- 19.3 Reciprocal Inhibition, 618
- 19.4 Overview of Proprioception, 619
- 19.5 Fascial/Joint Proprioceptors, 621
- 19.6 Muscle Spindles, 622
- 19.7 Golgi Tendon Organs, 625
- 19.8 Inner Ear Proprioceptors, 627
- 19.9 Other Musculoskeletal Reflexes, 630
- 19.10 Pain-Spasm-Pain Cycle, 633
- 19.11 Gate Theory, 635

Chapter 20 Posture and the Gait Cycle, 639
- 20.1 Importance of "Good Posture", 640
- 20.2 Ideal Standing Plumb Line Posture, 641
- 20.3 Analyzing Plumb Line Postural Distortions, 642
- 20.4 Secondary Postural Distortions and Postural Distortion Patterns, 644
- 20.5 General Principles of Compensation Within the Body, 646
- 20.6 Limitations of Standing Ideal Plumb Line Posture, 647
- 20.7 Gait Cycle, 648
- 20.8 Muscular Activity During the Gait Cycle, 650

Chapter 21 Common Postural Distortion Patterns, 657
- 21.1 Lower Crossed Syndrome, 659
- 21.2 Rounded Low Back/Pelvis, 662
- 21.3 Upper Crossed Syndrome, 663
- 21.4 Flat Back, 665
- 21.5 Elevated/Depressed Pelvis, 667
- 21.6 Scoliosis, 668
- 21.7 Elevated Shoulder Girdle, 669
- 21.8 Pelvic/Spinal Rotational Distortion, 670
- 21.9 Overpronation, 671
- 21.10 Rigid High Arch, 673
- 21.11 Hallux Valgus, 674
- 21.12 Hammertoes, 675
- 21.13 Morton's Foot, 676
- 21.14 Genu Valgum/Genu Varum, 676
- 21.15 Genu Recurvatum, 677
- 21.16 Pigeon-Toe/Toe-in, 678
- 21.17 Cubitus Valgus, 680

Chapter 22 Stretching, 683
- 22.1 Introduction, 684
- 22.2 Basic Stretching Techniques: Static Stretching Versus Dynamic Stretching, 688
- 22.3 Advanced Stretching Techniques: Pin and Stretch Technique, 690
- 22.4 Advanced Stretching Techniques: Contract Relax and Agonist Contract Stretching Techniques, 691

Chapter 23 Principles of Strengthening Exercise, 697
- 23.1 Reasons for Exercise, 699
- 23.2 Types of Exercise, 701
- 23.3 Types of Resistance, 703
- 23.4 Execution of Exercise, 713
- 23.5 Exercise Technique, 718
- 23.6 Program Design, 722

Index, 731

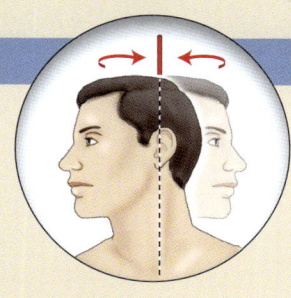

PART I
Fundamentals of Structure and Motion of the Human Body

CHAPTER 1
Parts of the Human Body

CHAPTER OUTLINE

Section 1.1 Major Divisions of the Human Body
Section 1.2 Major Body Parts
Section 1.3 Joints between Body Parts
Section 1.4 Movement of a Body Part Relative to an Adjacent Body Part
Section 1.5 Movement within a Body Part
Section 1.6 True Movement of a Body Part versus "Going along for the Ride"
Section 1.7 Regions of the Body

CHAPTER OBJECTIVES

After completing this chapter, the student should be able to perform the following:

1. Define the key terms of this chapter and state the meanings of the word origins of this chapter.
2. List the major divisions of the body.
3. List and locate the 11 major parts of the body.
4. Describe the concept of and give an example of movement of a body part.
5. List the aspects of and give an example of fully naming a movement of the body.
6. Describe the concept of and give an example of movement of smaller body parts located within larger (major) body parts.
7. Explain the difference between and give an example of true movement of a body part compared with "going along for the ride."
8. List and locate the major regions of the body.

OVERVIEW

The human body is composed of 11 major parts that are located within the axial and appendicular portions of the body. Some of these major body parts have smaller body parts within them. Separating two adjacent body parts from each other is a joint. True movement of a body part involves movement of that body part relative to another body part at the joint that is located between them.

KEY TERMS

Abdominal (ab-DOM-i-nal)
Antebrachial (AN-tee-BRAKE-ee-al)
Antecubital (an-tee-KYU-bi-tal)
Anterior view (an-TEER-ee-or)
Appendicular (ap-en-DIK-u-lar)
Arm
Axial (AK-see-al)
Axillary (AK-sil-err-ee)
Body part

Brachial (BRAKE-ee-al)
Carpal (KAR-pal)
Cervical (SER-vi-kal)
Cranial (KRAY-nee-al)
Crural (KROO-ral)
Cubital (KYU-bi-tal)
Digital (DIJ-i-tal)
Facial
Femoral (FEM-o-ral)

Foot
Forearm
Gluteal (GLOO-tee-al)
"Going along for the ride"
Hand
Head
Inguinal (ING-gwi-nal)
Interscapular (IN-ter-skap-u-lar)
Joint
Lateral view (LAT-er-al)
Leg
Lower extremity (eks-TREM-i-tee)
Lumbar (LUM-bar)
Mandibular (man-DIB-u-lar)
Neck
Palmar (PAL-mar)

Patellar (pa-TEL-ar)
Pectoral (PEK-to-ral)
Pelvis
Plantar (PLAN-tar)
Popliteal (pop-LIT-ee-al)
Posterior view (pos-TEER-ee-or)
Pubic (PYU-bik)
Sacral (SAY-kral)
Scapular (SKAP-u-lar)
Shoulder girdle
Supraclavicular (SUE-pra-kla-VIK-u-lar)
Sural (SOO-ral)
Thigh
Thoracic (tho-RAS-ik)
Trunk
Upper extremity (eks-TREM-i-tee)

WORD ORIGINS

- Ante—From Latin *ante*, meaning *before, in front of*
- Append—From Latin *appendo*, meaning *to hang something onto something*
- Ax—From Latin *axis*, meaning *a straight line*
- Fore—From Old English *fore*, meaning *before, in front of*
- Inter—From Latin *inter*, meaning *between*
- Lat—From Latin *latus*, meaning *side*
- Post—From Latin *post*, meaning *behind, in the rear, after*
- Supra—From Latin *supra*, meaning *on the upper side, above*

SECTION 1.1 MAJOR DIVISIONS OF THE HUMAN BODY

- The human body can be divided into two major sections (Figure 1-1):
  - The **axial** body
  - The **appendicular** body[1]
- When we learn how to name the location of a structure of the body or a point on the body (see Chapter 2), it will be crucial that we understand the difference between the axial body and the appendicular body.

AXIAL BODY

- The axial body is the central core axis of the body and contains the following body parts:
  - Head
  - Neck
  - Trunk

APPENDICULAR BODY

- The appendicular body is made up of appendages that are "added onto" the axial body.
- The appendicular body can be divided into the right and left upper extremities and the right and left lower extremities.

- An **upper extremity** contains the following body parts:
  - **Shoulder girdle** (scapula and clavicle)
  - Arm
  - Forearm
  - Hand[2]
- A **lower extremity** contains the following body parts:
  - **Pelvis** (pelvic girdle)
  - Thigh
  - Leg
  - Foot[2]
- The pelvis is often considered to be part of the axial body. In actuality, it is a transitional body part of both the axial body and the appendicular body[3]; the sacrum and coccyx are axial body bones and the pelvic bones are appendicular body bones. For symmetry, we will consider the pelvis to be part of the lower extremity (therefore the appendicular body), because the shoulder girdle is part of the upper extremity. Note: The word *girdle* is used because the pelvic and shoulder girdles resemble a girdle in that they encircle the body as a girdle does (actually, the shoulder girdle does not completely encircle the body because the two scapulae do not meet in back).

CHAPTER 1 Parts of the Human Body

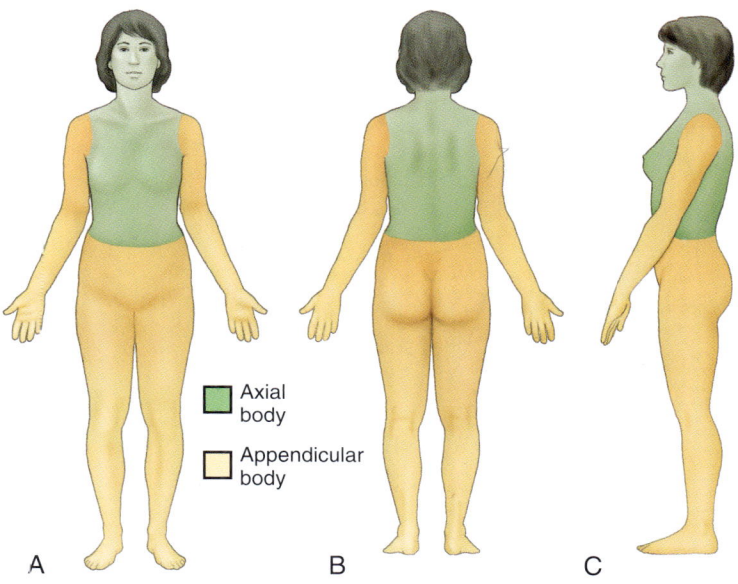

FIGURE 1-1 The major divisions of the human body: the axial body and the appendicular body. **A,** Anterior view. **B,** Posterior view. **C,** Lateral view.

SECTION 1.2 MAJOR BODY PARTS

- A **body part** is a part of the body that can move independently of another body part that is next to it.
- Generally it is the presence of a bone (sometimes more than one bone) within a body part that defines the body part.
- For example, the humerus defines the arm; the radius and ulna define the forearm.
- The human body has 11 major body parts (Figure 1-2):
  - Head ⎫
  - Neck ⎬ Axial body
  - Trunk ⎭
  - Pelvis ⎫
  - Thigh ⎪
  - Leg   ⎬ Lower extremity ⎫
  - Foot   ⎭   ⎪
  - Shoulder girdle ⎫   ⎬ Appendicular body
  - Arm   ⎬ Upper ⎪
  - Forearm   ⎪ extremity ⎭
  - Hand   ⎭

- It is important to distinguish the thigh from the leg. The thigh is between the hip joint and the knee joint, whereas the leg is between the knee joint and the ankle joint.[4] In our terminology, the thigh is not part of the leg.
- It is important to distinguish the arm from the forearm. The arm is between the shoulder joint and the elbow joint, whereas the forearm is between the elbow joint and the wrist joint. In our terminology, the forearm is not part of the arm.
- The shoulder girdle contains the scapulae and the clavicles.[4]
  - Most sources include the sternum as part of the shoulder girdle.
  - The shoulder girdle is also known as the *pectoral girdle*.
- The pelvis as a body part includes the pelvic girdle of bones.
  - The pelvic girdle contains the two pelvic bones, the sacrum, and the coccyx.[4]

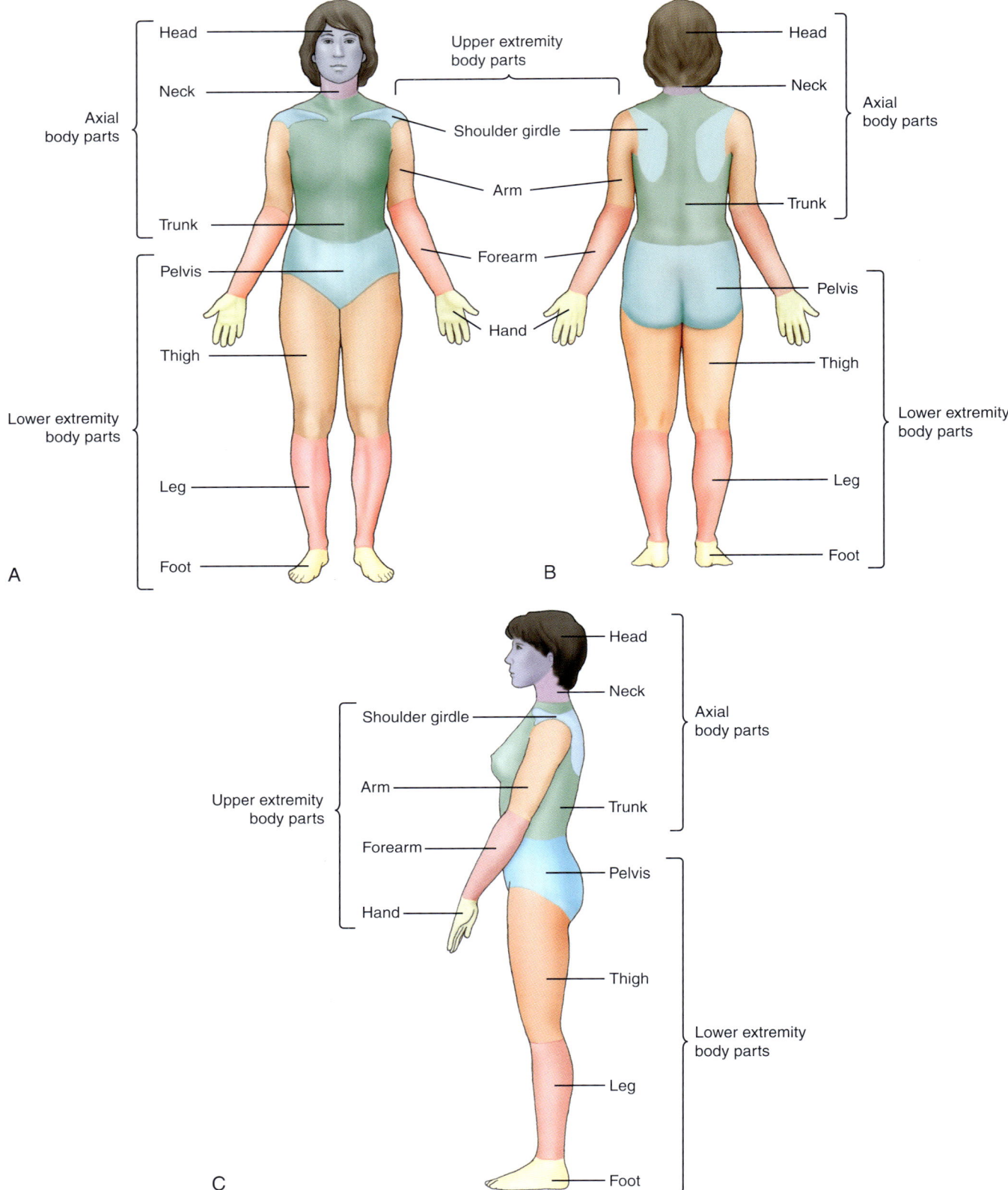

FIGURE 1-2 The 11 major parts of the human body. **A,** Anterior view. **B,** Posterior view. **C,** Lateral view. Note: The body parts indicated in this figure are key terms of this chapter.

SECTION 1.3 JOINTS BETWEEN BODY PARTS

- What separates one body part from the body part next to it is the presence of a **joint** between the bones of the body parts. A joint is located between two adjacent body parts (Figure 1-3).[3]
- When we say that a body part moves, our general rule will be that the body part moves relative to an adjacent body part.
- This movement occurs at the joint that is located between these two body parts (Figure 1-4).

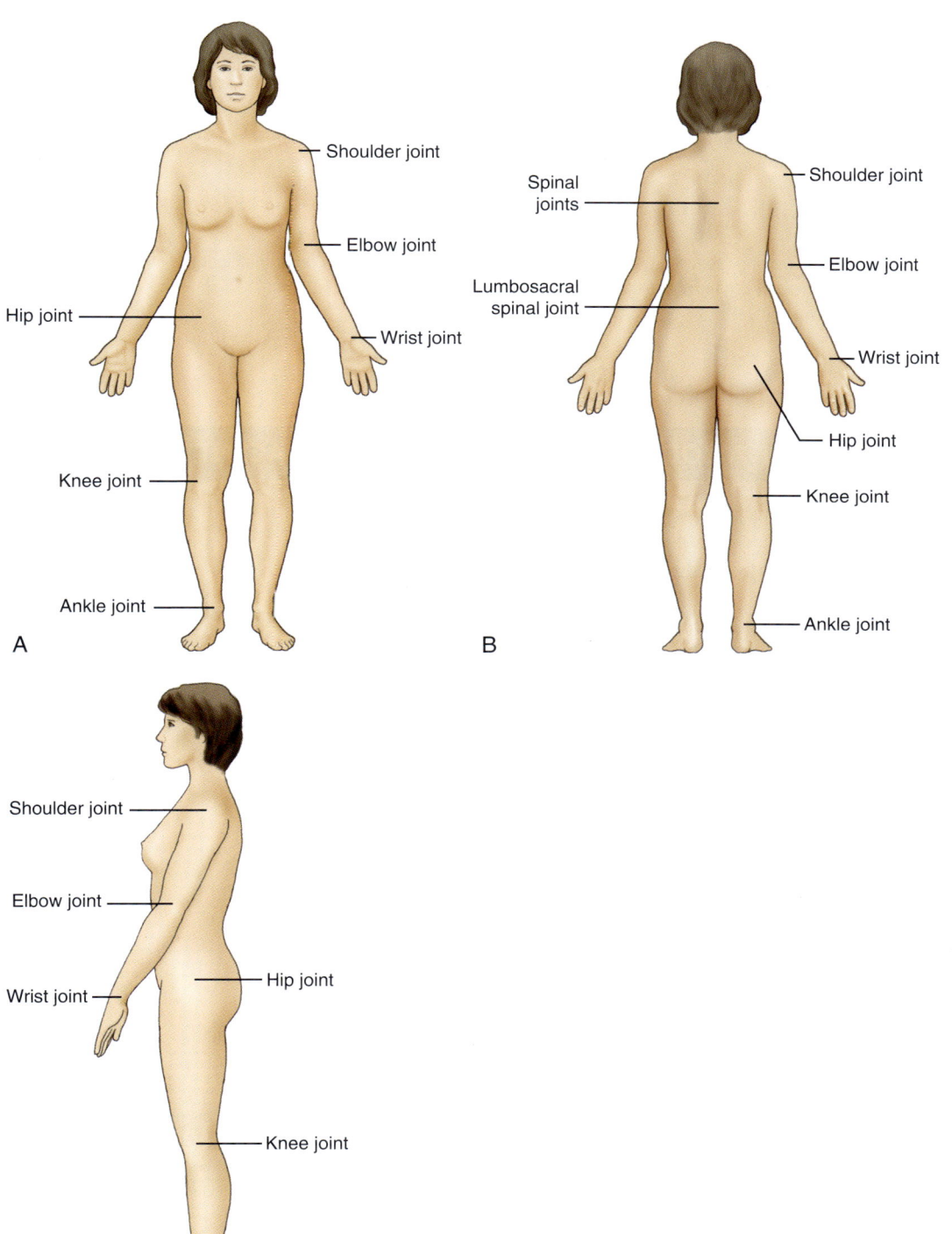

FIGURE 1-3 Illustration of the concept of a joint being located between two adjacent body parts. It is the presence of a joint that separates one body part from another body part. **A,** Anterior view. **B,** Posterior view. **C,** Lateral view.

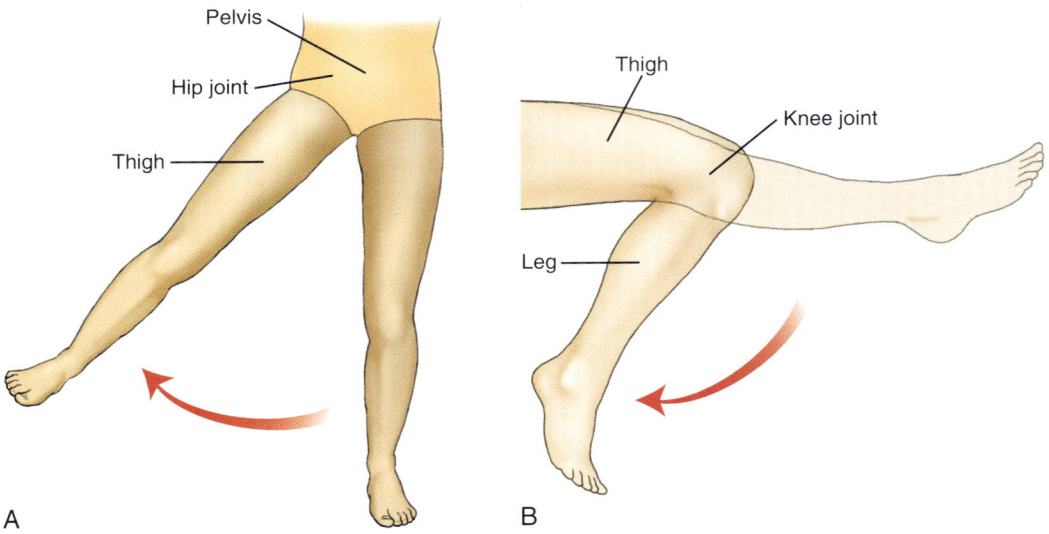

FIGURE 1-4 **A,** The thigh moving (abducting) relative to the pelvis. This motion is occurring at the hip joint, which is located between them. **B,** Leg moving (flexing) relative to the thigh. This motion is occurring at the knee joint, which is located between them.

SECTION 1.4   MOVEMENT OF A BODY PART RELATIVE TO AN ADJACENT BODY PART

- When movement of our body occurs, we see the following:
  - It is a body part that is moving.
  - That movement is occurring at a joint that is located between that body part and an adjacent body part.[5]
- To name this movement properly and fully, two things must be stated:
  1. The name of the body part that is moving
  2. The joint where the movement is occurring[5]
- Most texts describe a movement of the body by stating only the body part that is moving or by stating only the joint where the motion is occurring. However, to be complete and to fully describe and understand what is happening, both aspects should be stated. By doing this every time you describe a movement of the body, you will gain a better visual picture and understanding of the movement that is occurring.
- Figures 1-5, 1-6, and 1-7 show examples of movements of body parts relative to adjacent body parts.

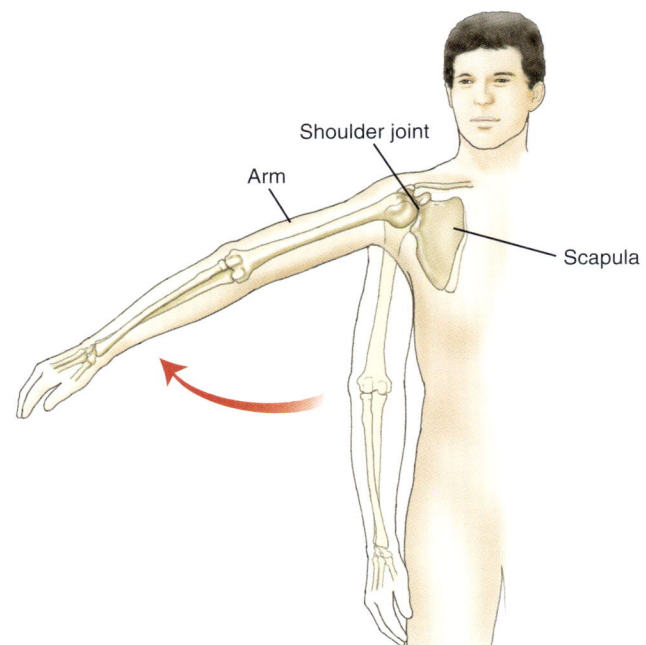

FIGURE 1-5 Illustration of a body movement. The body part that is moving is the arm, and the joint where this movement is occurring is the shoulder joint. We say that the arm is moving (abducting) at the shoulder joint. This motion of the arm occurs relative to the body part that is next to it (i.e., the shoulder girdle; more specifically, the scapula of the shoulder girdle).

CHAPTER 1 Parts of the Human Body

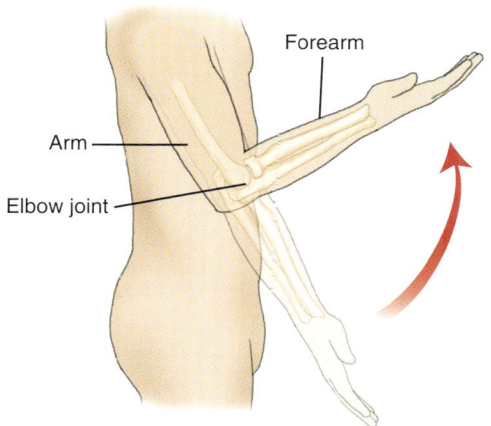

FIGURE 1-6 Illustration of a body movement. The body part that is moving is the forearm, and the joint where this movement is occurring is the elbow joint. We say that the forearm is moving (flexing) at the elbow joint. This motion of the forearm occurs relative to the body part that is next to it (i.e., the arm).

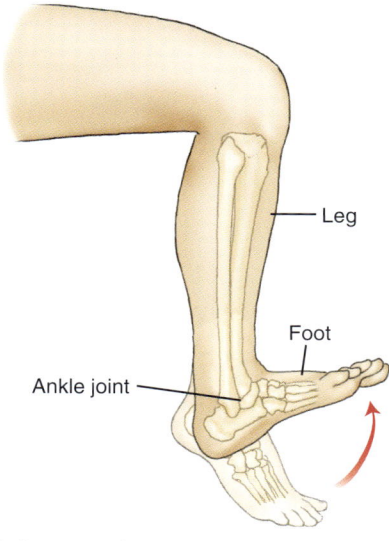

FIGURE 1-7 Illustration of a body movement. The body part that is moving is the foot, and the joint where this movement is occurring is the ankle joint. We say that the foot is moving (dorsiflexing) at the ankle joint. This motion of the foot occurs relative to the body part that is next to it (i.e., the leg).

SECTION 1.5 MOVEMENT WITHIN A BODY PART

- We have seen that when a major body part moves, the movement occurs at the joint that is located between that body part and an adjacent body part.
- Because that joint is located between two different major body parts, when one body part moves relative to another body part, it can be said that the movement occurs *between* body parts.
- However, sometimes movement can occur *within* a major body part.
- This can occur whenever the major body part has two or more smaller body parts (i.e., bones) located within it. When this situation exists, movement can occur at the joint that is located between these smaller body parts (i.e., bones) within the major body part.[5]
- The simplest example of this is the hand. The hand is considered to be a major body part, and motion of the hand is described as occurring between it and the forearm at the wrist joint (Figure 1-8, *A*). However, the hand has other body parts, the fingers, within it. Each finger is a body part in its own right, because a finger can move relative to the palm of the hand (Figure 1-8, *B*). Furthermore, each finger has three

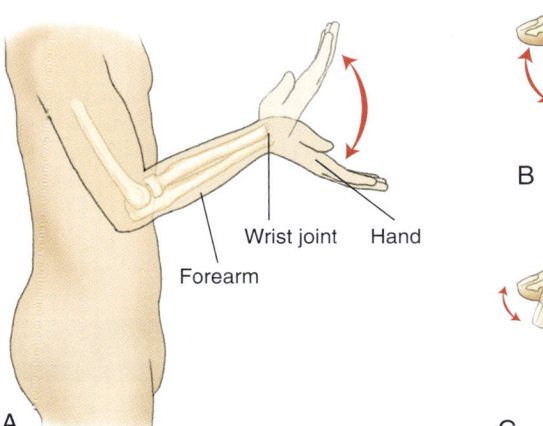
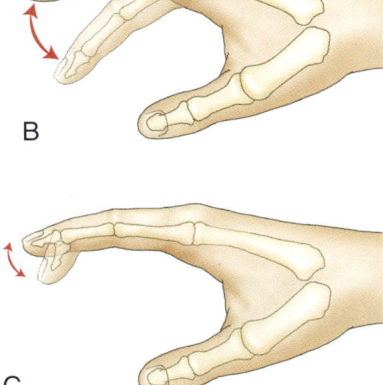

FIGURE 1-8 A, Lateral view showing the hand moving relative to the forearm at the wrist joint. **B,** Depiction of motion within the hand. This is a lateral view in which we see a finger moving relative to the palm of the hand at the joint that is located between them. **C,** Illustration of movement of one part of a finger relative to another part of the finger at the joint that is located between them. Note: **B** and **C** both illustrate the concept of movement occurring within a major body part because smaller body parts are within it.

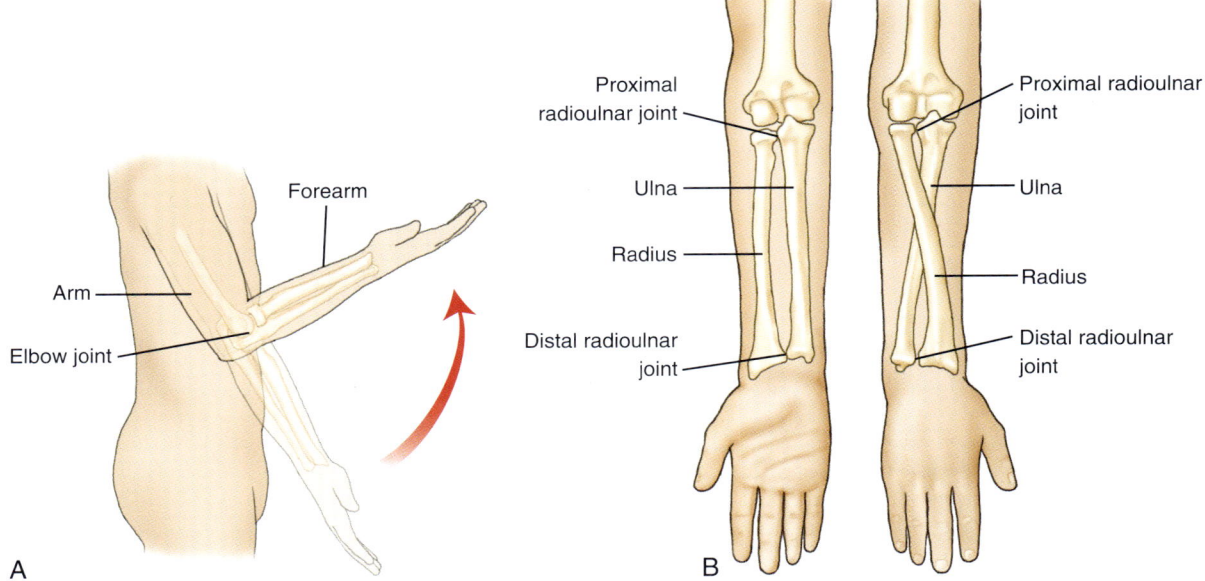

FIGURE 1-9 **A,** Lateral view showing the forearm moving (flexing) relative to the arm at the elbow joint. **B,** Movement of one of the bones (i.e., the radius) within the forearm, relative to the other bone (i.e., the ulna) of the forearm; this motion occurs at the radioulnar joints located between the two bones.

separate parts (i.e., bones) within it, and each of these parts can move independently as well (Figure 1-8, *C*).
- A second example is the forearm. The forearm is usually described as moving relative to the arm at the elbow joint (Figure 1-9, *A*). However, the forearm has two bones within it, and joints are located between these two bones. Motion of one of these bones can occur relative to the other (Figure 1-9, *B*). In this case each one of the two bones would be considered to be a separate, smaller body part.
- A third, more complicated example is the cervical spine. The cervical spine has seven vertebrae within it. The neck may be described as moving relative to the trunk that is beneath it (Figure 1-10, *A*). However, each one of the seven vertebrae can move independently. Therefore motion can occur between vertebrae within the neck at the joints located between the vertebrae (Figure 1-10, *B*).

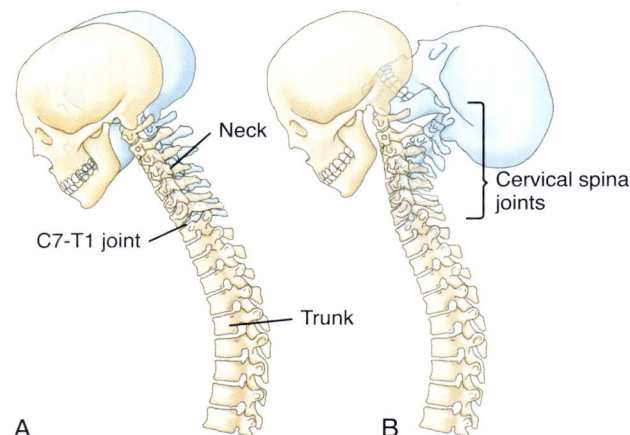

FIGURE 1-10 **A,** Lateral view of the neck showing the neck moving relative to the trunk at the spinal joint between them (C7-T1). **B,** Motion within the neck that is occurring between several individual vertebrae of the neck. This motion occurs at the spinal joints located between these bones.

SECTION 1.6 TRUE MOVEMENT OF A BODY PART VERSUS "GOING ALONG FOR THE RIDE"

- In lay terms, when we say that a body part has moved, it does not always mean that true movement of that body part has occurred (according to the terminology that is used in the musculoskeletal field for describing joint movements).
- A distinction must be made between *true movement of a body part* and what we will call "**going along for the ride**."
- For true movement of a body part to occur, the body part must move relative to an adjacent body part (or the body part must have movement occur within it).
- For example, in Figure 1-11 we see that a person is moving the right upper extremity.

- In lay terms, we might say that the person's right hand is moving because it is changing its position in space.
- However, in our terminology the right hand is not moving, because the position of the hand relative to the forearm is not changing (i.e., the right hand is not moving relative to the forearm [and motion is not occurring within the hand]).
- The movement that is occurring in Figure 1-11 is flexion of the forearm at the elbow joint. It is the forearm that is moving relative to the arm at the elbow joint.
- The hand is not moving in this scenario. We could say that the hand is merely "going along for the ride."
- Figure 1-12 depicts true movement of the hand relative to the forearm.

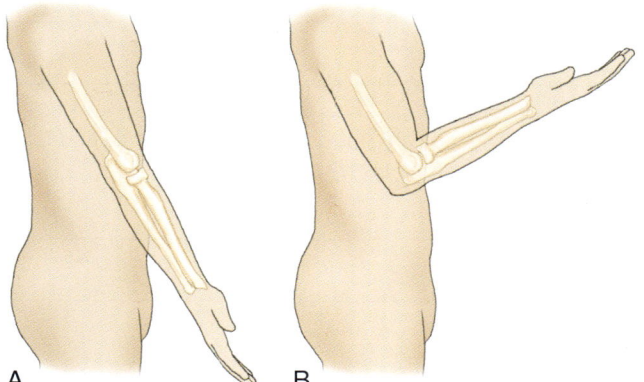

FIGURE 1-11 A and **B,** Illustration of the concept that the forearm is moving (because its position relative to the arm is changing). The motion that is occurring here is flexion of the forearm at the elbow joint. The hand is not moving, because its position relative to the forearm is not changing; the hand is merely "going along for the ride."

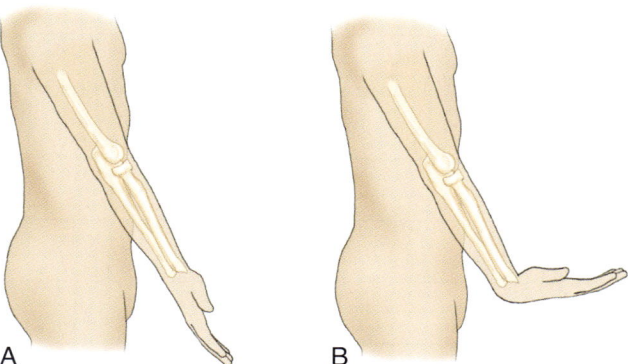

FIGURE 1-12 Illustration of true movement of the hand, because the position of the hand is changing relative to the forearm. This movement is called flexion of the hand at the wrist joint. **A,** Neutral (anatomic) position. **B,** Flexed position.

SECTION 1.7 REGIONS OF THE BODY

- Within the human body, areas or regions exist that are given names. Sometimes these regions are located within a body part; sometimes they are located across two or more body parts.

Following are illustrations that show the various regions of the body (Figure 1-13).[6]

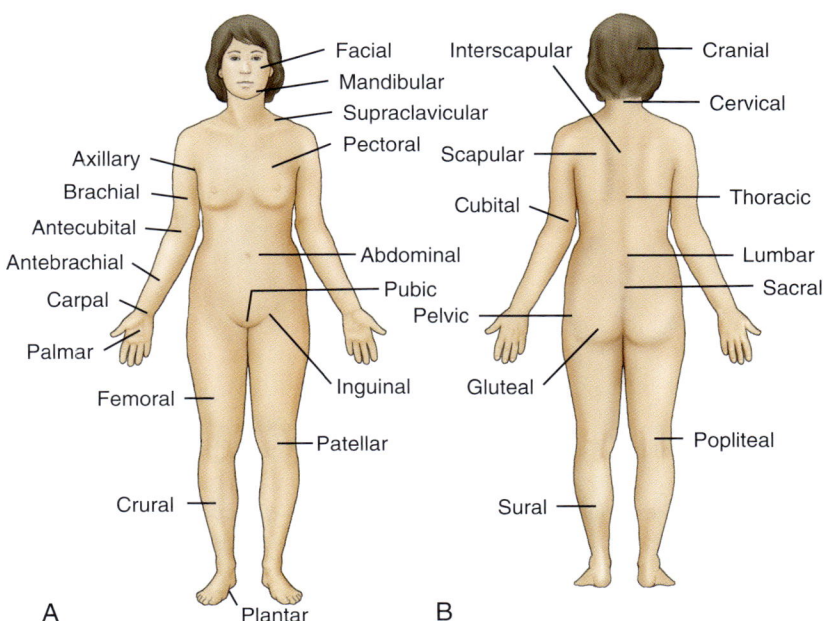

FIGURE 1-13 A, Anterior view of the body illustrating its major regions. **B,** Posterior view of the body illustrating its major regions. Note: The body regions indicated in this figure are key terms of this chapter.

REVIEW QUESTIONS

Answers to the following review questions appear on the Evolve website accompanying this book at: http://evolve.elsevier.com/Muscolino/kinesiology/.

1. What are the two major divisions of the human body?

2. What are the 11 major body parts of the human body?

3. What defines a body part?

4. What is the difference between the thigh and the leg?

5. What is the difference between the arm and the forearm?

6. What is the difference between the trunk and the pelvis?

7. What two things are stated to describe properly and fully a movement of the body?

8. How can movement occur within a body part?

9. What is the difference between *true movement* and "going along for the ride"?

10. Name five regions of the human body.

REFERENCES

1. Thibodeau GA, Paton KT: Anatomy & physiology, ed 5, St Louis, 2003, Mosby.
2. Watkins J: Structure and function of the musculoskeletal system, Champaign, Ill, 1999, Human Kinetics.
3. Neumann DA: Kinesiology of the musculoskeletal system: Foundations for physical rehabilitation, ed 3, St Louis, 2017, Elsevier.
4. Drake RL, Vogl W, Mitchell AWM: Gray's anatomy for students, Philadelphia, 2005, Churchill Livingstone.
5. Hamilton N, Weimar W, Luttgens K: Kinesiology: Scientific basis of human motion, ed 12, New York, 2012, McGraw Hill.
6. Dail NW, Agnew TA, Floyd RT: Kinesiology for manual therapies, New York, 2011, McGraw Hill.

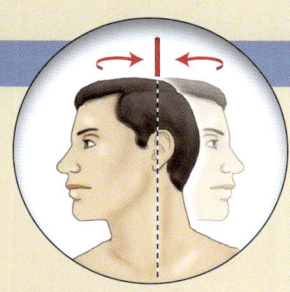

CHAPTER 2
Mapping the Human Body

CHAPTER OUTLINE

Section 2.1	Anatomic Position	Section 2.8	Planes
Section 2.2	Location Terminology	Section 2.9	Motion of the Human Body within Planes
Section 2.3	Anterior/Posterior	Section 2.10	Axes
Section 2.4	Medial/Lateral	Section 2.11	Planes and Their Corresponding Axes
Section 2.5	Superior/Inferior and Proximal/Distal	Section 2.12	Visualizing the Axes—Door Hinge Pin Analogy
Section 2.6	Superficial/Deep		
Section 2.7	Location Terminology Illustration	Section 2.13	Visualizing the Axes—Pinwheel Analogy

CHAPTER OBJECTIVES

After completing this chapter, the student should be able to perform the following:

1. Define the key terms of this chapter and state the meanings of the word origins of this chapter.
2. Describe and explain the importance of anatomic position.
3. Explain how location terminology can be used to map the body.
4. List and apply the following pairs of terms that describe relative location on the human body: anterior/posterior, medial/lateral, superior/inferior, proximal/distal, and superficial/deep.
5. List and apply the following additional pairs of terms that describe relative location on the human body: ventral/dorsal, volar/dorsal, radial/ulnar, tibial/fibular, plantar/dorsal, and palmar/dorsal.
6. List and describe the three cardinal planes and explain the concept of an oblique plane.
7. Explain how motion occurs within a plane, and give an example of motion occurring in each of the three cardinal planes and in an oblique plane.
8. Define what an axis is, and explain how motion can occur relative to an axis.
9. Do the following related to planes and their corresponding axes:
    ○ List the axes that correspond to each of the three cardinal planes.
    ○ Determine the axis for an oblique plane.
    ○ Give an example of motion occurring within each of the three cardinal planes and around each of the three cardinal axes.
10. Draw an analogy between the hinge pin of a door and the pin of a pinwheel to the axis of movement for each of the three cardinal planes.

Indicates a video demonstration is available for this concept.

OVERVIEW

The field of kinesiology uses directional terms of relative location to describe and communicate the location of a structure of the body or a point on the body. These terms are similar to geographic directional terms such as *north* and *south*, and *east* and *west*. However, instead of mapping the Earth, we use our terms to map the human body. We also need to map the space around the human body by describing the three dimensions or *planes* of space. Understanding the orientation of the planes is extremely important in the field of kinesiology because when the body moves, motion of body parts occurs within these planes. The concept of an axis is then explored, because most body movements are axial movements that occur within a plane and around an axis.

Putting the information that was learned in Chapter 1 together with the information that is presented in Chapter 2, the student will have a clear and fundamental understanding of body movement. That is, when motion of the human body occurs, a body part moves relative to an adjacent body part at the joint that is located between them, and this motion occurs within a plane; and if this motion is an axial movement, then it occurs around an axis. After the bones are studied in more detail in Chapters 3 and 5, the exact terms that are used to describe these movements of body parts are covered in Chapter 6.

KEY TERMS

Anatomic position (an-a-TOM-ik)
Angular movement
Anterior (an-TEER-ee-or)
Anteroposterior axis (an-TEER-o-pos-TEER-ee-or)
Axial movement (AK-see-al)
Axis, pl. axes (AK-sis, AK-seez)
Axis of rotation
Cardinal axis (KAR-di-nal)
Cardinal plane
Circular movement
Coronal plane (ko-RO-nal)
Deep
Distal
Dorsal (DOOR-sal)
Fibular (FIB-u-lar)
Frontal-horizontal axis
Frontal plane
Horizontal plane
Inferior (in-FEER-ee-or)
Lateral
Mechanical axis

Medial (MEE-dee-al)
Mediolateral axis (MEE-dee-o-LAT-er-al)
Midsagittal plane (MID-SAJ-i-tal)
Oblique axis (o-BLEEK)
Oblique plane
Plane
Posterior (pos-TEER-ee-or)
Proximal (PROK-si-mal)
Radial (RAY-dee-al)
Rotary movement
Sagittal-horizontal axis (SAJ-i-tal)
Sagittal plane
Superficial
Superior (sue-PEER-ee-or)
Superoinferior axis (sue-PEER-o-in-FEER-ee-or)
Tibial (TI-bee-al)
Transverse plane
Ulnar (UL-nar)
Ventral (VEN-tral)
Vertical axis
Volar (VO-lar)

WORD ORIGINS

- Ana—From Latin *ana*, meaning *up*
- Dors—From Latin *dorsum*, meaning *the back*
- Infer—From Latin *inferus*, meaning *below, lower*
- Medial—From Latin *medialis*, meaning *middle*
- Oblique—From Latin *obliquus*, meaning *slanting*
- Rota—From Latin *rota*, meaning *wheel*
- Super—From Latin *superus*, meaning *higher, situated above*
- Tome—From Latin *tomus*, meaning *a cutting*
- Trans—From Latin *trans*, meaning *across, to the other side of*
- Ventr—From Latin *venter*, meaning *belly, stomach*

CHAPTER 2 Mapping the Human Body

SECTION 2.1 ANATOMIC POSITION

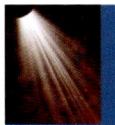

- Although the human body can assume an infinite number of positions, one position is used as the reference position for mapping the body. This position is used to name the location of body parts, structures, and points on the body and is called **anatomic position**.[1] In anatomic position the person is standing erect, facing forward, with the arms at the sides, the palms facing forward, and the fingers and thumbs extended (Figure 2-1).[2]

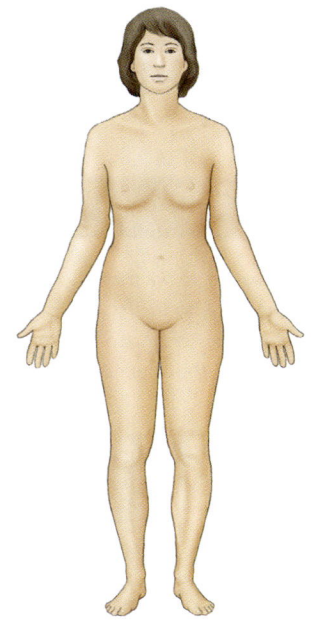

FIGURE 2-1 Anterior view of anatomic position. Anatomic position is the position assumed when a person stands erect, facing forward, with the arms at the sides, the palms facing forward, and the fingers and thumbs extended. Anatomic position is important because it is used as a reference position for naming locations on the human body.

SECTION 2.2 LOCATION TERMINOLOGY

NAMING LOCATIONS ON THE HUMAN BODY

- Whenever we want to describe the location of a structure of the human body or the location of a specific point on the human body, we always do so in reference to anatomic position.
- Describing a location on the human body involves the use of specific directional terms that describe the location of one structure or point on the body relative to another structure or point on the body (Box 2-1).
- The reason for specific terminologies like this to exist is that they help us to avoid the ambiguities of lay language. An example of a lay term that is ambiguous and can create confusion and poor communication when describing a location on the human body is the word *under*. *Under* can mean *inferior*, or it can mean *deep*. Similarly, the word *above* can mean both *superior* and *superficial*. Therefore embracing and using these terms is extremely important in the health field, where someone's health is dependent on clear communication.
- These terms always come in pairs; the terms of each pair are opposite to each other.
- These pairs of terms are similar to the terms *north/south, east/west,* and *up/down*. However, our terms specifically relate to directions on the human body.

> **BOX 2-1** **Spotlight on Describing Specific Locations**
>
> It is important to emphasize that location terminology is relative. A structure of the human body that is said to be anterior is so named because it is anterior relative to another structure that is more posterior. However, that same anterior structure may be posterior to a third structure that is more anterior than it is. For example, the sternum is anterior to the spine. However, the sternum is posterior to the skin that lies over it. Therefore, depending on which structure we are comparing it with, the sternum may be described as anterior or posterior.

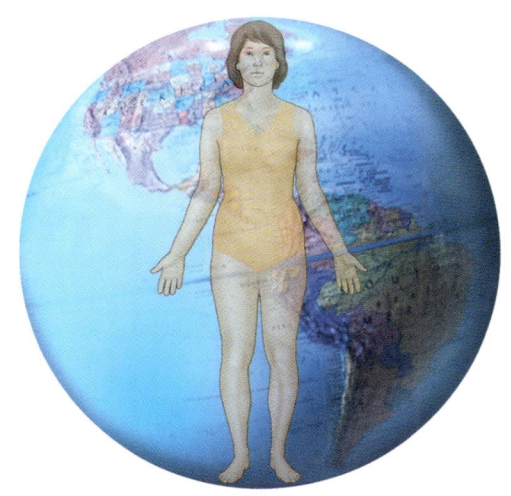

- In essence, we are mapping the human body and using specific terminology to describe points on this map. In the following sections are the pairs of directional terms for naming the relative location of structures or points on the human body.
- Once these pairs of terms for relative location have been learned, they may be combined to describe a structure or point's location. For example, a point on the body may be both anterior and medial to another point. When these terms are combined, it is customary to drop the end of the first term and combine the two terms together with the letter *o* (e.g., *anterior* and *medial* become *anteromedial*). It is also common practice for the terms *anterior* and *posterior* to come first.

SECTION 2.3 ANTERIOR/POSTERIOR

- **Anterior**—Means *farther to the front*
- **Posterior**—Means *farther to the back*
  - The terms *anterior/posterior* can be used for the entire body (i.e., for the axial and the appendicular body parts).

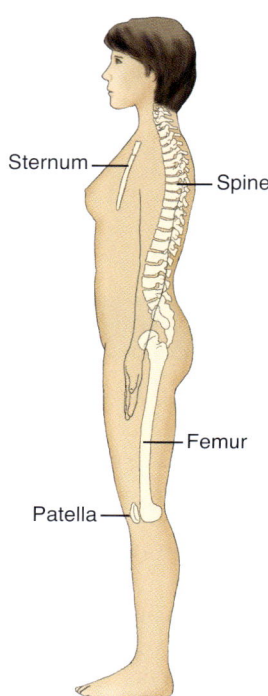

FIGURE 2-2 Lateral view of a person in anatomic position. The sternum is anterior to the spine; conversely, the spine is posterior to the sternum. The patella is anterior to the femur; conversely, the femur is posterior to the patella.

Examples: The sternum is anterior to the spine.
The spine is posterior to the sternum (Figure 2-2).
Examples: The patella is anterior to the femur.
The femur is posterior to the patella (see Figure 2-2).
Notes:
- The terms *ventral/dorsal* are often used synonymously with *anterior/posterior*.
  - **Ventral** essentially means *anterior*.
  - **Dorsal** essentially means *posterior* (Box 2-2).
- The term **volar** is occasionally used in place of anterior for the hand region (*dorsal* is usually used as the opposite term in the pair).[3]

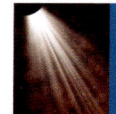

BOX 2-2 Spotlight on Ventral/Dorsal

Each body part has a soft, fleshy surface and a harder, firmer surface. The term *ventral* actually refers to the belly or the softer surface of a body part; the term *dorsal* refers to the back or the harder, firmer surface of a body part. These terms derive evolutionarily from the ventral and dorsal surfaces of a fish. The ventral surfaces of the entire upper extremity and axial body are located anteriorly; the ventral surface of the thigh is medial/posteromedial; the ventral surface of the leg is posterior; and the ventral surface of the foot is the inferior, plantar surface. The dorsal surfaces are on the opposite side of the ventral surfaces.

SECTION 2.4 MEDIAL/LATERAL

- **Medial**—Means *closer to an imaginary line that divides the body into left and right halves* (Figure 2-3). (Note: This imaginary line that divides the body into left and right halves is the *midsagittal plane*; see Section 2.8.)
- **Lateral**—Means *farther from an imaginary line that divides the body into left and right halves* (i.e., more to the left side or the right side).
  - The terms *medial/lateral* can be used for the entire body (i.e., for the axial and the appendicular body parts).

  Examples: The sternum is medial to the humerus.
  The humerus is lateral to the sternum (see Figure 2-3).

Examples: The little finger is medial to the thumb.
The thumb is lateral to the little finger (see Figure 2-3).

Notes:
- In the forearm and hand, the terms *ulnar/radial* can be used instead of *medial/lateral*. **Ulnar** means *closer to the ulna*, which is more medial. **Radial** means *closer to the radius*, which is more lateral.
- In the leg, the terms *tibial/fibular* can be used instead of *medial/lateral*. **Tibial** means *closer to the tibia*, which is more medial. **Fibular** means *closer to the fibula*, which is more lateral.[3]

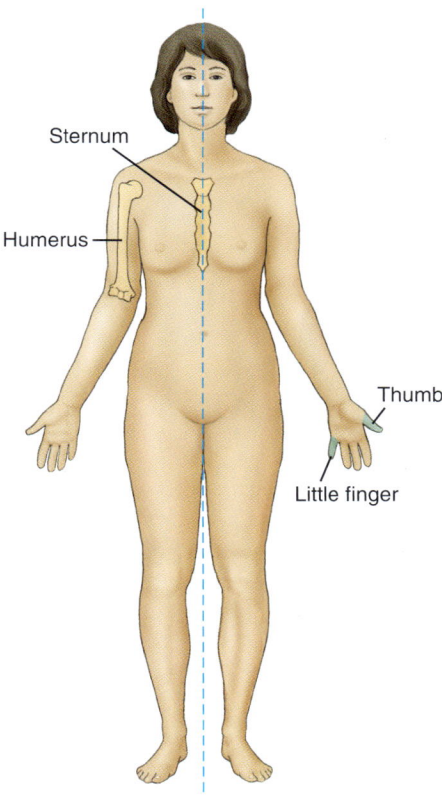

FIGURE 2-3 Anterior view of a person in anatomic position. The midline of the body, which is most medial in location, is represented by the vertical dashed line that divides the body into left and right halves. The sternum is medial to the humerus; conversely, the humerus is lateral to the sternum. The little finger is medial to the thumb; conversely, the thumb is lateral to the little finger.

SECTION 2.5 SUPERIOR/INFERIOR AND PROXIMAL/DISTAL

- **Superior**—Means *above*
- **Inferior**—Means *below*
  - The terms *superior/inferior* are used for the axial body parts only.

Examples: The head is superior to the trunk.
            The trunk is inferior to the head (Figure 2-4, *A*).

Examples: The sternum is superior to the umbilicus.
            The umbilicus is inferior to the sternum (see Figure 2-4, *A*).

Note:

- Although most sources apply these terms only to the axial body, some sources use these terms for the appendicular body as well.
- **Proximal**—Means *closer* (i.e., greater proximity) *to the axial body*
- **Distal**—Means *farther* (i.e., more distant) *from the axial body*
  - The terms *proximal/distal* are used for the appendicular body parts only.[3]

Examples: The arm is proximal to the forearm.
            The forearm is distal to the arm (Figure 2-4, *B*).

Examples: The thigh is proximal to the leg.
            The leg is distal to the thigh (see Figure 2-4, *B*).

Note regarding the use of superior/inferior versus proximal/distal:

- Given that the terms *superior/inferior* are used on the axial body and are not used on the appendicular body, and the terms *proximal/distal* are used on the appendicular body and are not used on the axial body, a dilemma arises when we look to compare the relative location of a point that is on an extremity with a point that is on the axial body. For example, the psoas major muscle attaches from the trunk to the thigh. How would one describe its attachments? It is convention to use either one pair of terms or the other but not to mix the two pairs of terms. In other words, you could describe the attachments of this muscle as being *superior and inferior*, or you could describe them as being *proximal and distal*. Do not mix these terms and describe the attachments as superior and distal, or proximal and inferior. The terms *proximal/distal* are more commonly used.

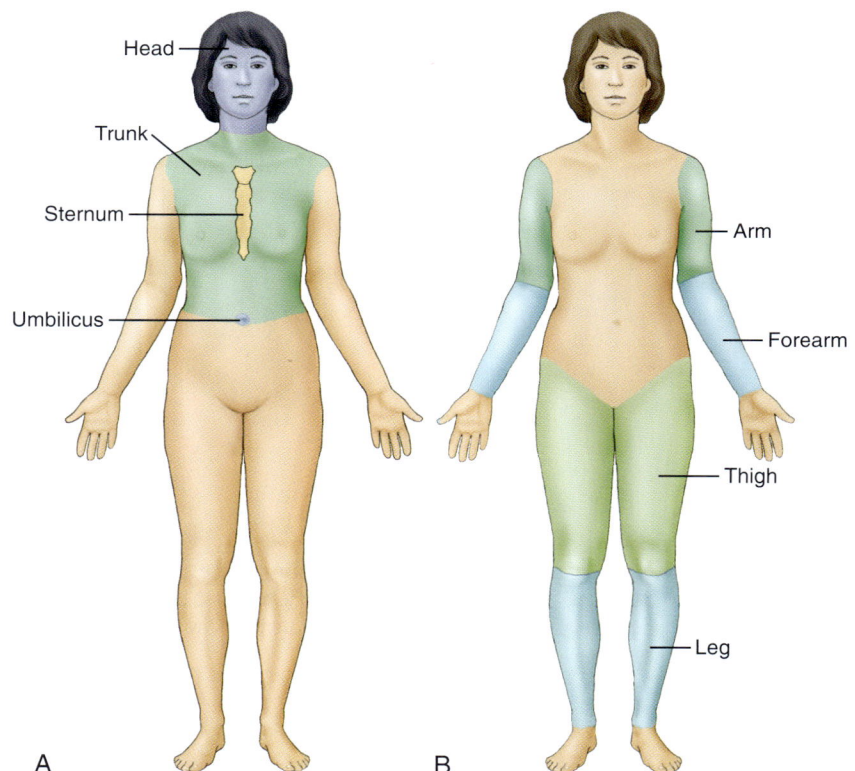

FIGURE 2-4 Anterior views of a person in anatomic position. **A,** The head is superior to the trunk; conversely, the trunk is inferior to the head. In addition, the sternum is superior to the umbilicus; conversely, the umbilicus is inferior to the sternum. **B,** The arm is proximal to the forearm; conversely, the forearm is distal to the arm. In addition, the thigh is proximal to the leg; conversely, the leg is distal to the thigh.

SECTION 2.6 SUPERFICIAL/DEEP

- **Superficial**—Means *closer to the surface of the body*
- **Deep**—Means *farther from the surface of the body* (i.e., more internal or deep)
  - The terms *superficial/deep* can be used for the entire body (i.e., for the axial and the appendicular body parts).[3]

Examples: The anterior abdominal wall muscles are superficial to the intestines.
The intestines are deep to the anterior abdominal wall muscles (Figure 2-5).

Examples: The biceps brachii muscle is superficial to the humerus (arm bone).
The humerus is deep to the biceps brachii muscle (see Figure 2-5).

Note:
- Whenever designating a structure of the human body as superficial or deep, it is important to state the perspective from which one is looking at the body. This is important because one structure may be deep to another structure from one perspective but not deep to it from another perspective. An example is the brachialis muscle of the arm. The brachialis is usually thought of as deep to the biceps brachii muscle because from the anterior perspective the brachialis is deep to it. As a result, many bodyworkers do not realize that the brachialis is superficial (deep only to the skin) and easily accessible and palpable laterally and medially. Furthermore, the deeper a structure is from one perspective of the body, the more superficial it is from the other perspective. An example is the dorsal interossei pedis muscles of the feet. These muscles are considered to be in the deepest plantar layer of musculature of the feet, and viewed from the plantar perspective they are located deep to the plantar interossei muscles. However, from the dorsal perspective, they are superficial to the plantar interossei muscles; and indeed, the dorsal interossei pedis muscles are more accessible and palpable from the dorsal side.

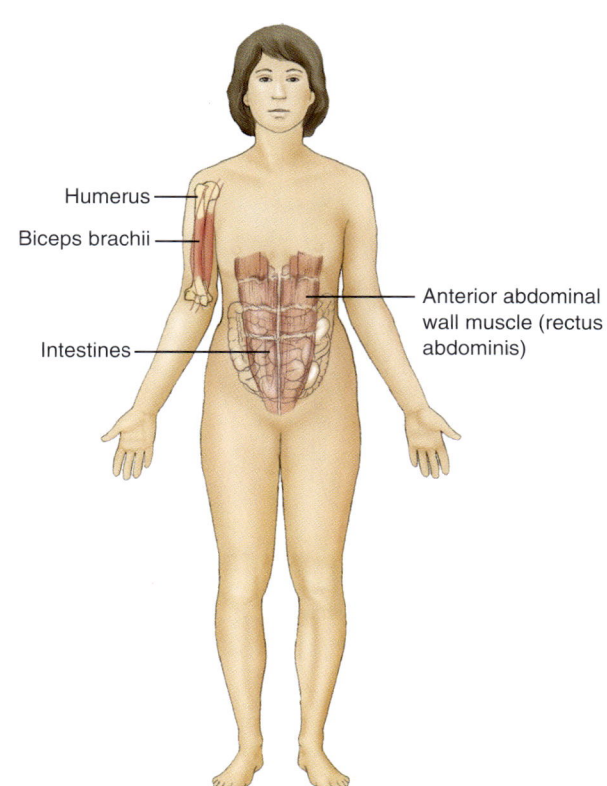

FIGURE 2-5 Anterior view of a person in anatomic position. The anterior perspective shows that the rectus abdominis muscle of the anterior abdominal wall is superficial to the intestines (located within the abdominopelvic cavity); conversely, the intestines are deep to the rectus abdominis muscle. From the anterior perspective, the biceps brachii muscle is superficial to the humerus; conversely, the humerus is deep to the biceps brachii muscle.

SECTION 2.7   LOCATION TERMINOLOGY ILLUSTRATION

Figure 2-6 is an anterior view of a person, illustrating the terms of relative location as they pertain to the body.

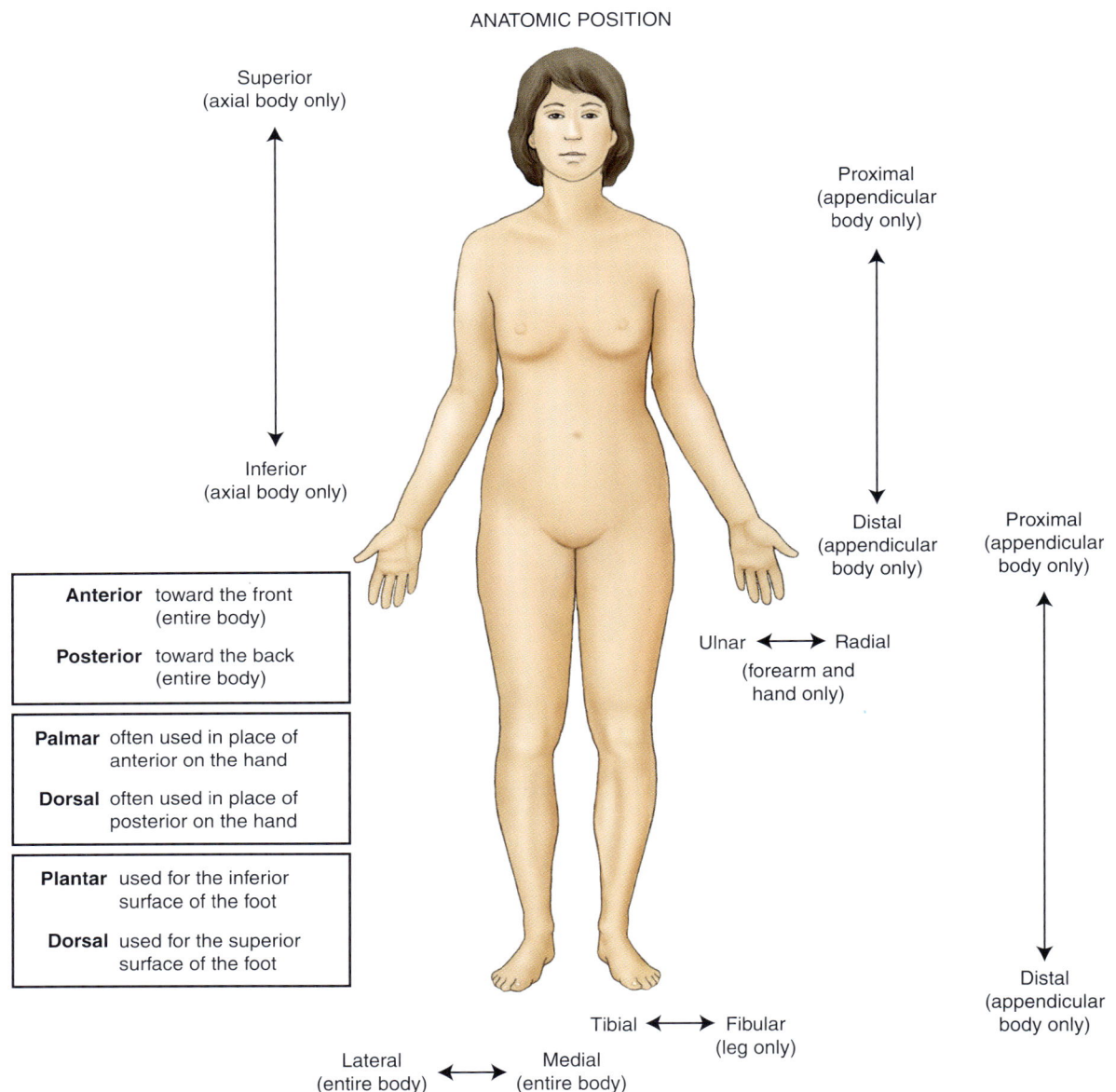

FIGURE 2-6 Various directional terms of location relative to anatomic position.

SECTION 2.8 PLANES

All too often, planes are presented in textbooks with an illustration and a one-line definition for each one. Consequently, students often memorize them with a weak understanding of what they really are and their importance. Because a clear and thorough understanding of planes greatly facilitates learning and understanding the motions caused by muscular contractions, the following is presented.

- We have already mapped the human body to describe the location of structures and/or points of the body.
- However, when we want to describe motion of the human body, we need to describe or map the space through which motion occurs.
- As we all know, space is three-dimensional (3-D); therefore to map space we need to describe its three dimensions.
- We describe each one of these dimensions with a **plane**. Because three dimensions exist, three types of planes exist.
- The word *plane* actually means *a flat surface*. Each of the planes is a flat surface that cuts through space, describing a dimension of space.
- The three major types of planes are called *sagittal, frontal,* and *transverse* (Figure 2-7).[4]
- The human body or a part of the body can move in each of these three dimensions or planes:
  - A body part can move in an anterior to posterior (or posterior to anterior) direction. This direction describes the **sagittal plane**.[4]
  - A body part can move in a left to right (or right to left) direction; this could also be described as a medial to lateral (or lateral to medial) direction of movement. This direction describes the **frontal plane**.[4]
  - A body part can stay in place and spin (i.e., rotate). This direction describes the **transverse plane**.[4]

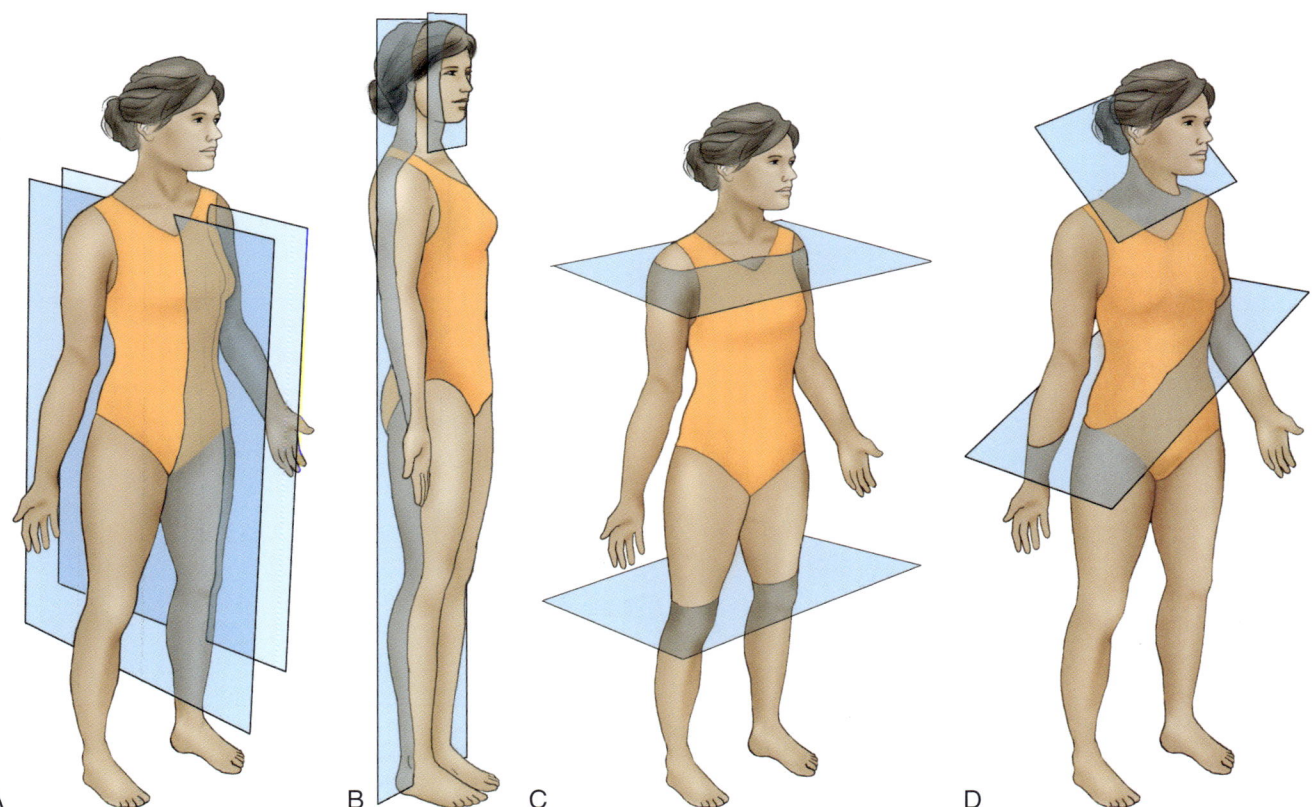

FIGURE 2-7 Anterolateral views of the body, illustrating the four types of planes: sagittal, frontal, transverse, and oblique. **A,** Two examples of sagittal planes; a sagittal plane divides the body into left and right portions. **B,** Two examples of frontal planes; a frontal plane divides the body into anterior and posterior portions. **C,** Two examples of transverse planes; a transverse plane divides the body into upper (superior and/or proximal) and lower (inferior and/or distal) portions. **D,** Two examples of oblique planes; an oblique plane is a plane that is not exactly sagittal, frontal, or transverse (i.e., it has components of two or three cardinal planes). The upper oblique plane has frontal and transverse components; the lower oblique plane has sagittal and transverse components.

- These three major planes are called **cardinal planes** and are defined as follows:
  - A sagittal plane divides the body into left and right portions.
  - The sagittal plane that is located down the center of the body and divides the body wall into equal left and right halves is called the **midsagittal plane**.
  - A frontal plane divides the body into anterior and posterior portions.
  - A transverse plane divides the body into (upper) superior/proximal and (lower) inferior/distal portions.
- Please note the following:
  - These three cardinal planes are defined relative to anatomic position. (This is not to say that motion of the human body can be initiated only from anatomic position. It only means that these three cardinal planes were originally defined with the body parts in anatomic position.)
  - Any plane that is not purely sagittal, frontal, or transverse (i.e., has components of two or three of the cardinal planes) is called an **oblique plane**.[4]
  - The sagittal and frontal planes are oriented vertically; the transverse plane is oriented horizontally.
  - An infinite number of sagittal, frontal, transverse, and oblique planes are possible.
  - The frontal plane is also commonly called the **coronal plane**.
  - The transverse plane is also commonly called the **horizontal plane**.

SECTION 2.9   MOTION OF THE HUMAN BODY WITHIN PLANES

- Because an understanding of the planes is an important part of understanding movements of the body, motion of the human body in each of the three planes should be examined. Figure 2-8, *A* to *D,* illustrates motion of the body in the sagittal, frontal, and transverse planes, as well as in an oblique plane, respectively. Figure 2-8, *E* to *H,* illustrates additional examples of motions within planes. (For a detailed discussion of the names of these motions, please see Chapter 6, Sections 6.11 through 6.25.)

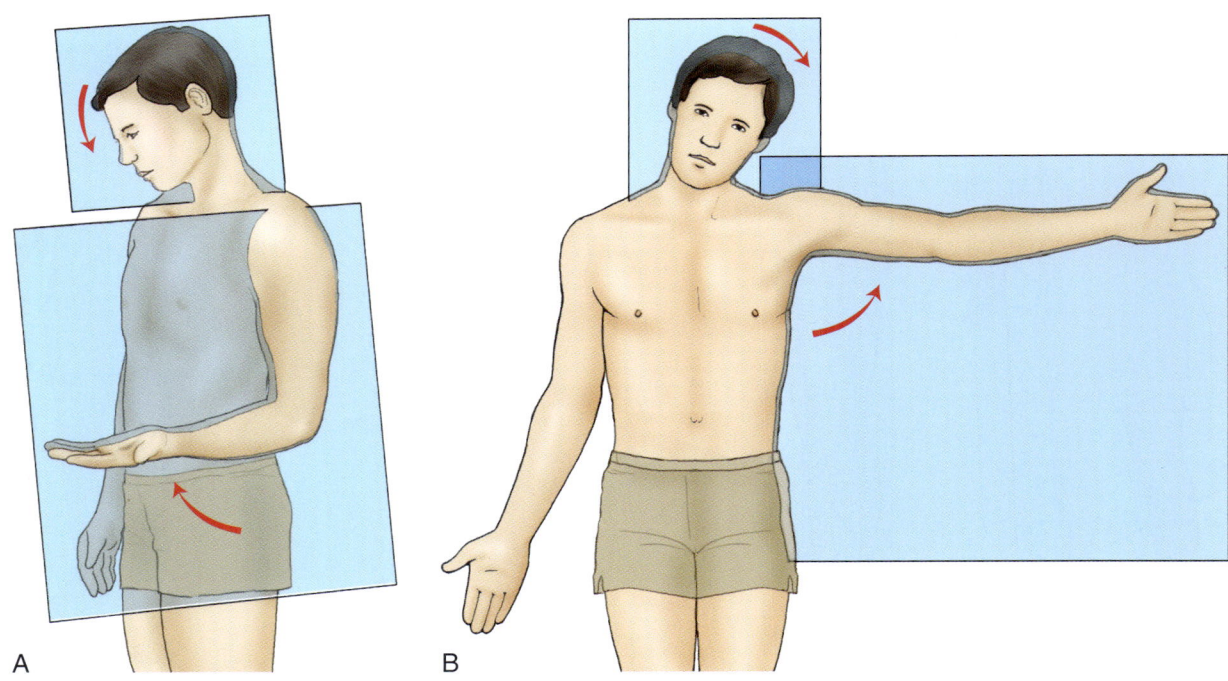

FIGURE 2-8   A, Anterolateral view illustrates two examples of the concept of motion of a body part within a sagittal plane. The head and neck are flexing (moving anteriorly) at the spinal joints, and the left forearm is flexing (moving anteriorly) at the elbow joint. **B,** Anterior view illustrates two examples of the concept of motion of a body part within a frontal plane. The head and neck are left laterally flexing (bending to the left side) at the spinal joints, and the left arm is abducting (moving laterally away from the midline) at the shoulder joint.

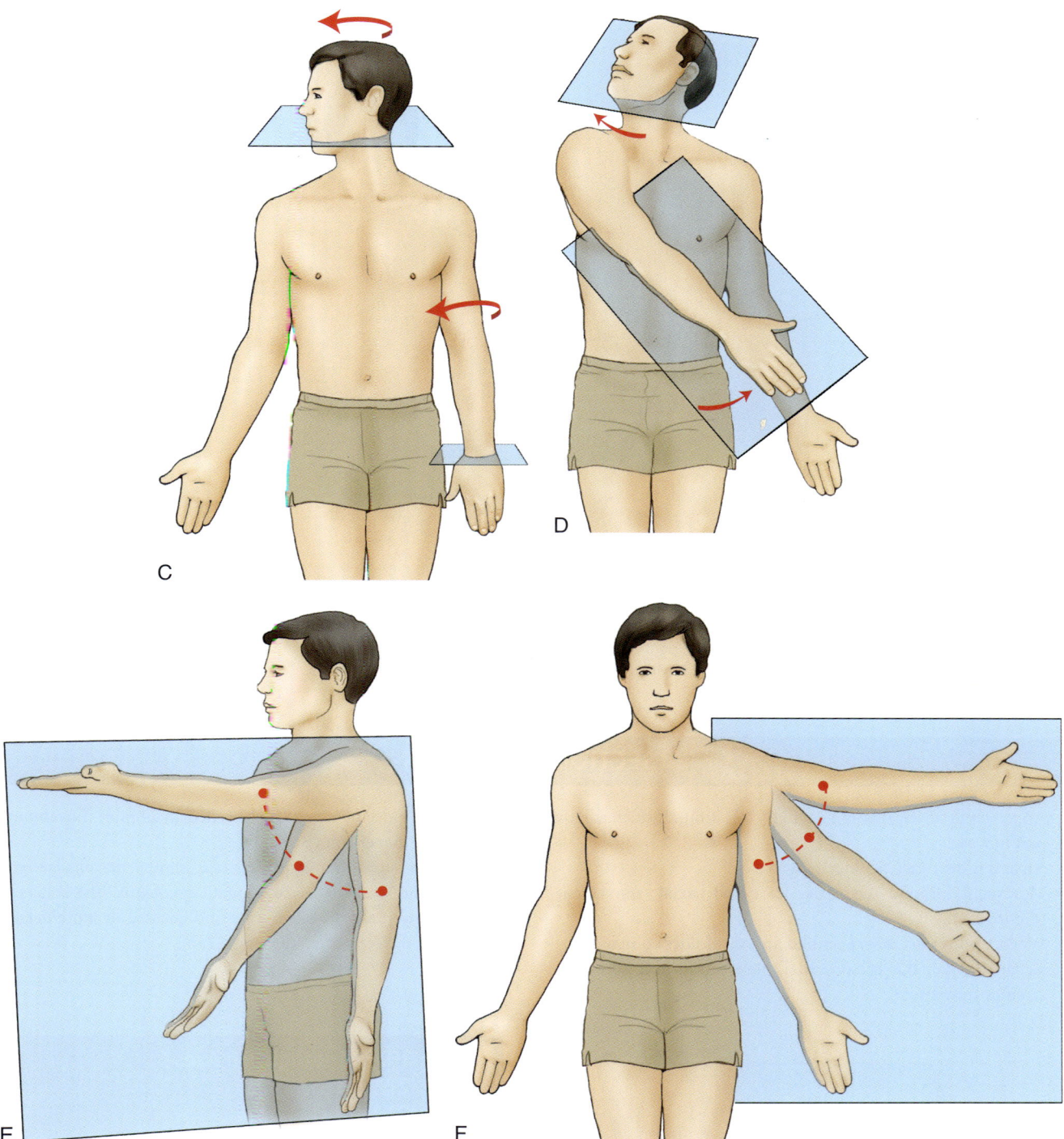

FIGURE 2-8, cont'd **C,** Anterior view illustrates two examples of the concept of motion of a body part within a transverse plane. The head and neck are rotating to the right (twisting/turning to the right) at the spinal joints; and the left arm is medially rotating (rotating toward the midline) at the shoulder joint. **D,** Anterior view illustrates two examples of the concept of motion of a body part within an oblique plane (i.e., a plane that has components of two or three of the cardinal planes). The head and neck are doing a combination of sagittal, frontal, and transverse plane movements (at the spinal joints). These movements are extension (moving posteriorly) in the sagittal plane, left lateral flexion (bending to the left side) in the frontal plane, and right rotation (twisting/turning to the right) in the transverse plane. The right arm is also doing a combination of sagittal, frontal, and transverse plane movements (at the shoulder joint). These movements are flexion (moving anteriorly) in the sagittal plane, adduction (moving medially toward the midline) in the frontal plane, and medial rotation (rotating toward the midline) in the transverse plane. *E to H,* Motion of the arm at the shoulder joint within each of the three cardinal planes and an oblique plane. A point has been drawn on the arm; the arc that is created by the movement of this point has also been drawn (in each case, the arc of motion of this point is within the plane of motion that the body part is moving within, illustrating that motion of a body part occurs within a plane). **E,** An anterolateral view illustrates the left arm flexing (moving anteriorly) at the shoulder joint within a sagittal plane. **F,** Anterior view illustrates the left arm abducting (moving laterally away from the midline) at the shoulder joint within a frontal plane.

Continued

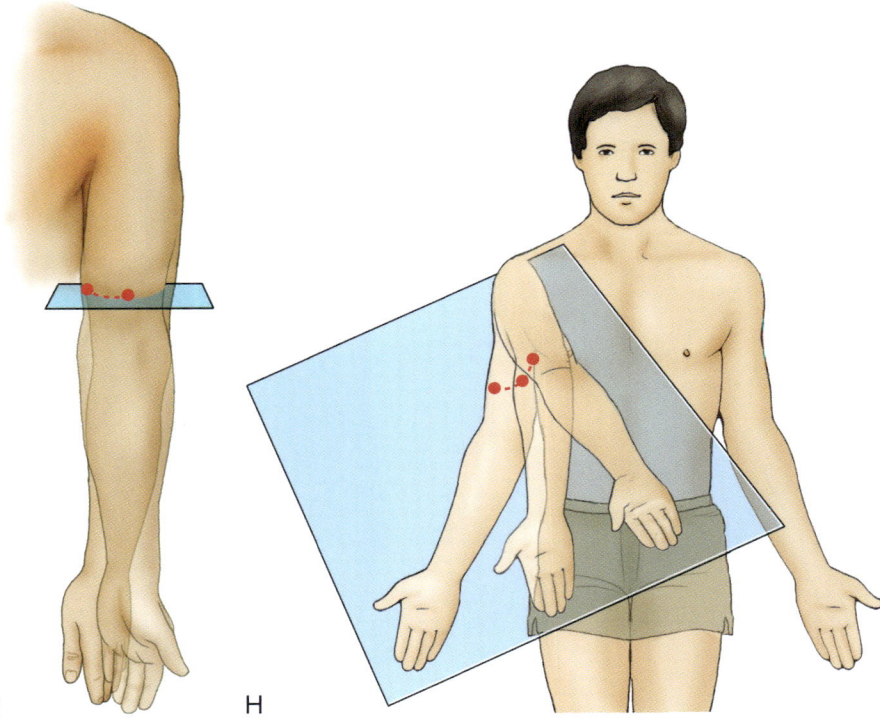

G H

FIGURE 2-8, cont'd G, Anterior view illustrates the left arm laterally rotating (rotating away from the midline) at the shoulder joint within a transverse plane. **H,** Anterior view illustrates the right arm making a motion that is a combination of flexion (moving anteriorly) and adduction (moving toward the midline) at the shoulder joint within an oblique plane.

2-5

SECTION 2.10 AXES

- An **axis** (plural: axes) is an imaginary line around which a body part moves.
- An axis is often called a **mechanical axis**.[5]
- Movement around an axis is called **axial movement** (Figure 2-9).
- When a body part moves around an axis, it does so in a circular fashion. For this reason, axial movement is also known as **circular movement**.

- An axial movement can also be called an **angular movement** or a **rotary movement** (Box 2-3).[5]
- The terms *axial movement, circular movement, angular movement,* and *rotary movement* are all synonyms. The concept of axial movement is visited again and covered in more detail in Chapter 6, Sections 6.5 through 6.7.

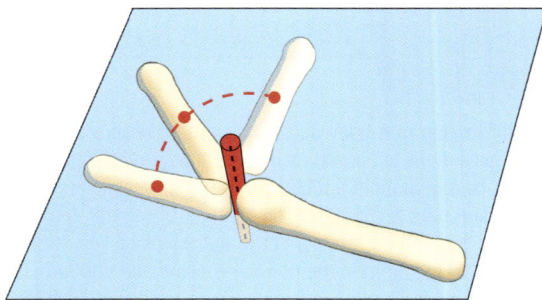

FIGURE 2-9 An axis is an imaginary line around which motion occurs. This figure illustrates the motion of a bone within a plane and around an axis; the axis is drawn in as a red tube. This type of movement is known as an axial movement. A point has been drawn on the bone, and the arc that is transcribed by the motion of this point can be seen to move in a circular path.

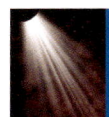 **BOX 2-3 Spotlight on Axes**

Because a body part is often described as rotating around the axis, an axial movement can also be called a rotary movement, or even rotation. Indeed, an axis is often referred to as an axis of rotation. However, referring to axial movements as rotary or rotation movements can be confusing because certain axial movements actually have the word rotation within their name (spin axial movements such as right rotation, left rotation, lateral rotation, medial rotation), whereas other types of axial movement (roll axial movements such as flexion, extension, abduction, adduction) do not. Therefore it is easy to confuse these different types of axial movements with each other. Axial movements (and in particular spin and roll axial movements) are discussed in Chapter 6, Sections 6.7 and 6.8.

SECTION 2.11 PLANES AND THEIR CORRESPONDING AXES

- When motion of a body part occurs, it can be described as occurring within a plane.
  - If the motion is axial, it can be further described as moving around an axis.
  - Therefore for each one of the three cardinal planes of the body, a corresponding cardinal axis exists; hence three cardinal axes exist (Figure 2-10, *A* to *C*).[6]
  - For every motion that occurs within an oblique plane, a corresponding oblique axis exists (Figure 2-10, *D*). Therefore an infinite number of oblique axes exist, one for each possible oblique plane.
- Naming an axis is straightforward; simply describe its orientation.
  - The three cardinal axes are the mediolateral, anteroposterior, and superoinferior (vertical) axes (see Figure 2-10, *A* to *C*).
- Please note that an axis around which motion occurs is always perpendicular to the plane in which the motion is occurring.
- An axial movement of a body part is one in which the body part moves within a plane and around an axis.

MEDIOLATERAL AXIS

- A **mediolateral axis** is a line that runs from medial to lateral (or lateral to medial [i.e., left to right or right to left]) in direction (see Figure 2-10, *A*).
- Movements that occur in the sagittal plane move around a mediolateral axis.
- The mediolateral axis is also known as the **frontal-horizontal axis** because it runs horizontally and is located within the frontal plane.[6]

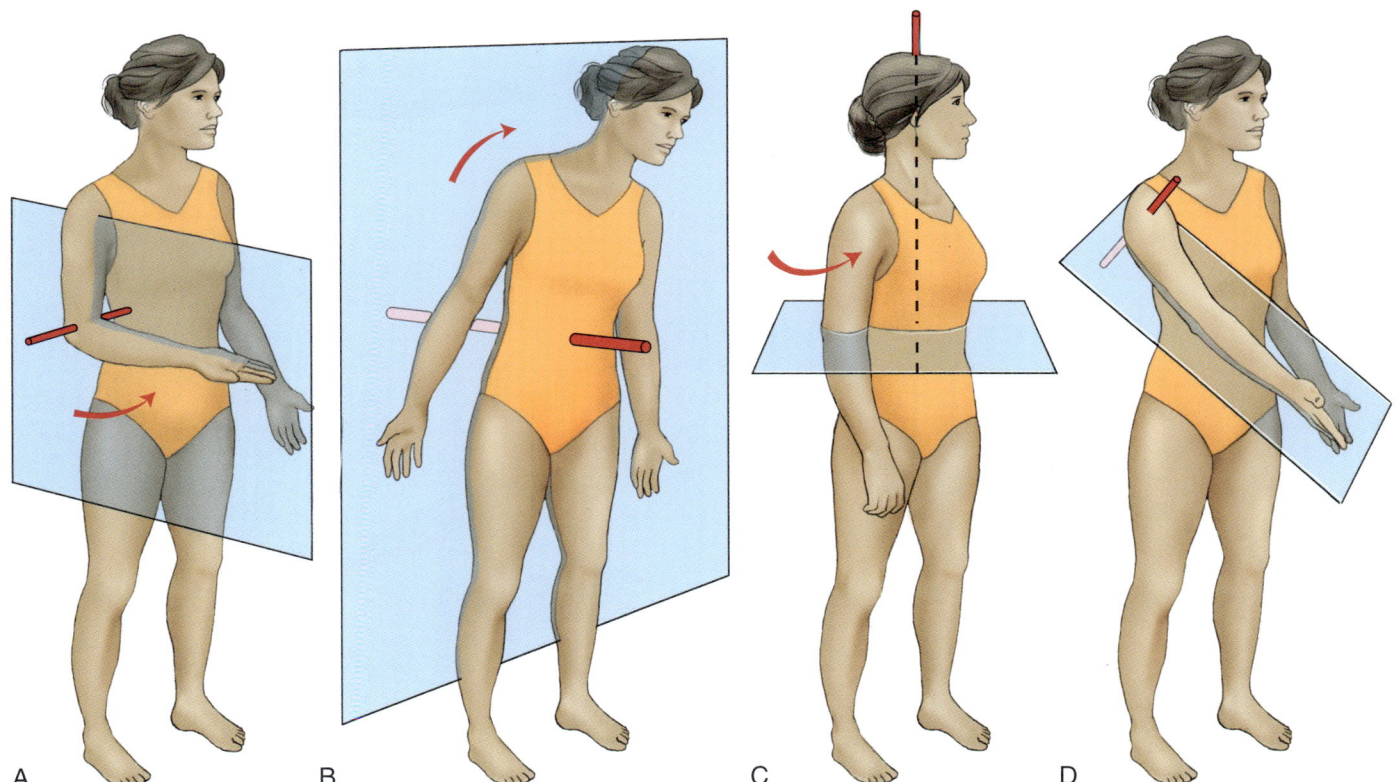

FIGURE 2-10 Anterolateral views that illustrate the corresponding axes for the three cardinal planes and an oblique plane; the axes are shown as red tubes. Note that an axis always runs perpendicular to the plane in which the motion is occurring. **A,** Motion occurring in the sagittal plane; because this motion is occurring around an axis that is running horizontally in a medial to lateral orientation, it is called the mediolateral axis. **B,** Motion occurring in the frontal plane; because this motion is occurring around an axis that is running horizontally in an anterior to posterior orientation, it is called the anteroposterior axis. **C,** Motion occurring in the transverse plane; because this motion is occurring around an axis that is running vertically in a superior to inferior orientation, it is called the superoinferior axis, or, more simply, the vertical axis. **D,** Motion occurring in an oblique plane; this motion is occurring around an axis that is running perpendicular to that plane (i.e., it is the oblique axis for this oblique plane).

ANTEROPOSTERIOR AXIS

- An **anteroposterior axis** is a line that runs anterior to posterior (or posterior to anterior) in direction (see Figure 2-10, *B*).
- Movements that occur in the frontal plane move around an anteroposterior axis.
- The anteroposterior axis is also known as the **sagittal-horizontal axis** because it runs horizontally and is located within the sagittal plane.[6]

SUPEROINFERIOR AXIS

- A **superoinferior axis** is a line that runs from superior to inferior (or inferior to superior) in direction (see Figure 2-10, *C*).
- Movements that occur in a transverse plane move around a superoinferior axis.
- The superoinferior axis is more commonly referred to as the **vertical axis** because it runs vertically. (This text will use the term *vertical axis* because it is an easier term for the reader/student to visualize.)[6]

SECTION 2.12 VISUALIZING THE AXES—DOOR HINGE PIN ANALOGY

- To help visualize an axis for motion, the following visual analogy may be helpful. An axis may be thought of as the hinge pin of a door. Just as a body part's motion occurs around its axis, a door's motion occurs around its hinge pin, which is its axis for motion (Figure 2-11).

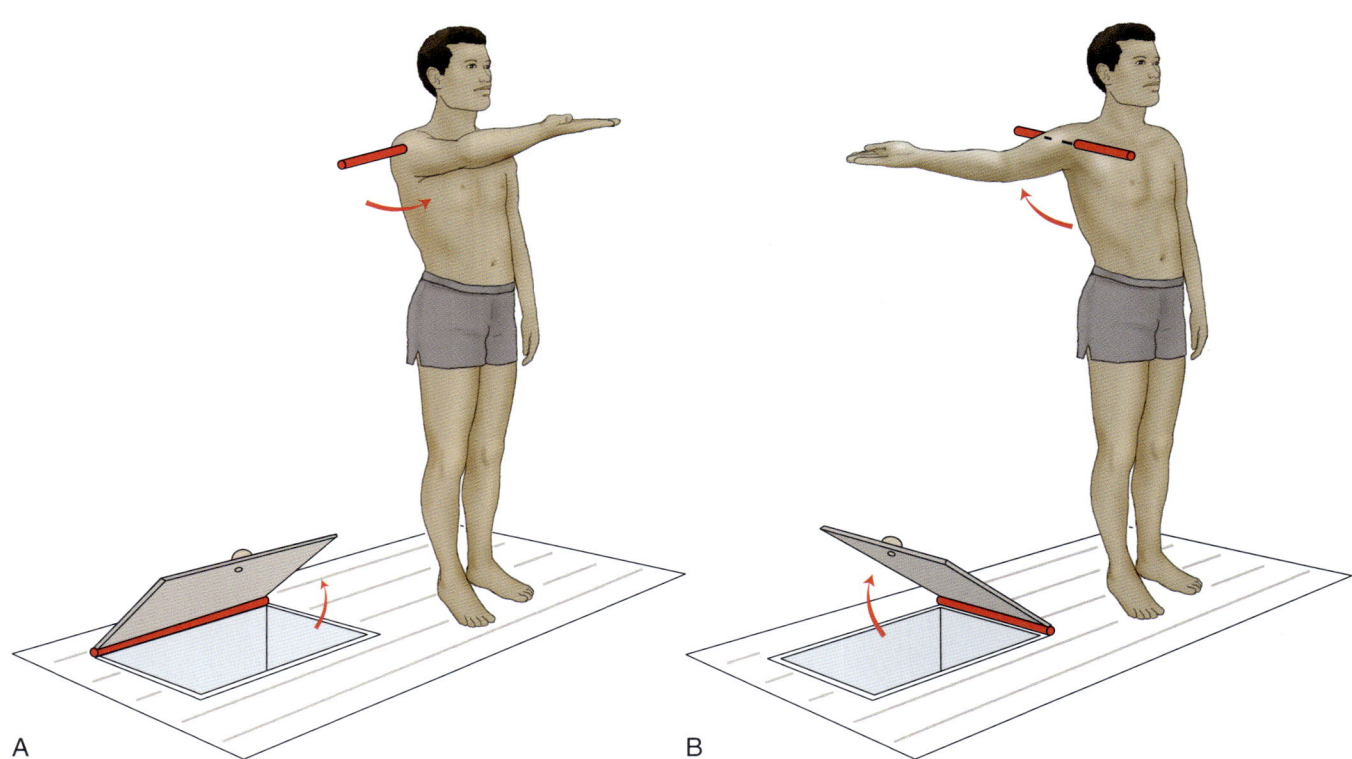

FIGURE 2-11 Anterolateral views that compare the axes of motion for movement of the arm with the axes of motion for a door that is moving (i.e., opening); the axes are drawn in as red tubes. **A,** A trap door in a floor that is moving. The person standing next to the door is moving the arm in the same manner in which the trap door is opening. These movements are occurring in the sagittal plane. If we look at the orientation of the hinge pin of the door, which is its axis of motion, we will see that it is medial to lateral in orientation. Note that the axis for the motion of the person's arm is also medial to lateral in orientation. Hence the axis for sagittal plane motion is mediolateral. **B,** A trap door in a floor that is moving (i.e., opening). The person standing next to the door is moving the arm in the same manner in which the trap door is opening. These movements are occurring in the frontal plane. If we look at the orientation of the hinge pin of the door, which is its axis of motion, we will see that it is anterior to posterior in orientation. Note that the axis for the motion of the person's arm is also anterior to posterior in orientation. Hence the axis for frontal plane motion is anteroposterior.

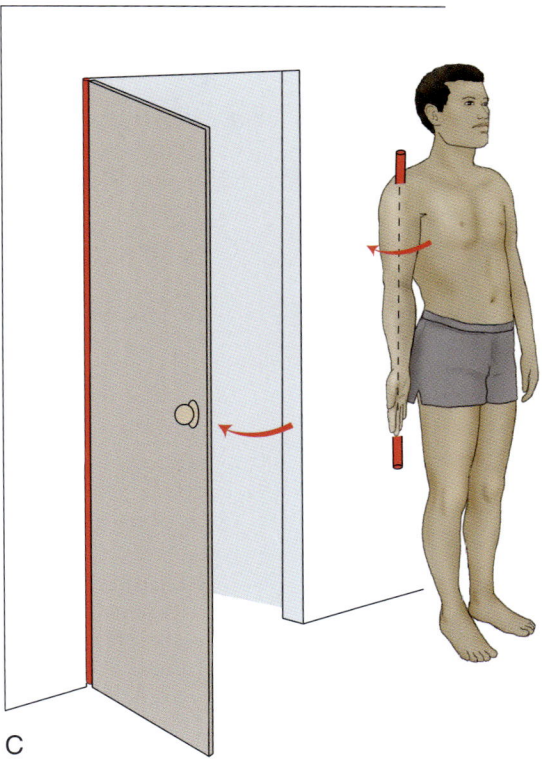

FIGURE 2-11, cont'd C, A door that is moving (i.e., opening). The person standing next to the door is moving the arm in the same manner in which the door is opening. These movements are occurring in the transverse plane. If we look at the orientation of the hinge pin of the door, which is its axis of motion, we will see that it is superior to inferior in orientation (i.e., it is vertical). Note that the axis for the motion of the person's arm is also superior to inferior in orientation. Hence the axis for transverse plane motion is vertical.

SECTION 2.13 VISUALIZING THE AXES—PINWHEEL ANALOGY

- Another visual analogy that may be helpful for determining the axis of motion is a pinwheel. When a child blows on a pinwheel, its wheel spins in a plane, and the pin is the axis around which the wheel spins. If you orient the motion of the wheel in any one of the three cardinal planes, then naming the orientation of the pin of the pinwheel will name the axis for that plane's motion (Figure 2-12, A to C).

- The face of a clock is another good example of motion within a plane and around an axis. The hands of the clock move within the plane of the face of the clock. The pin that fastens the arms to the clock face is the axis around which the hands move. If the clock is oriented to be in the sagittal, frontal, or transverse plane relative to your body, then describing the orientation of the pin in each case illustrates the axis.

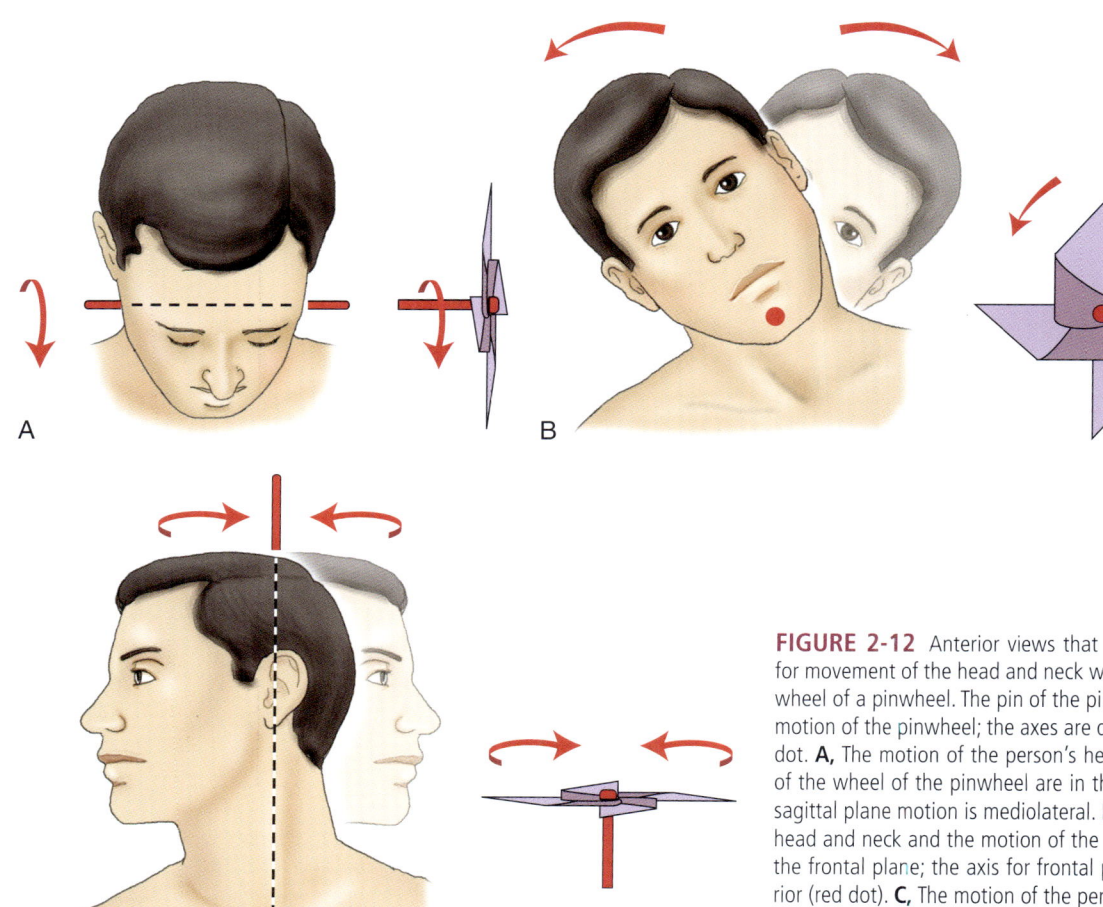

FIGURE 2-12 Anterior views that compare the axes of motion for movement of the head and neck with the axes of motion for the wheel of a pinwheel. The pin of the pinwheel represents the axis of motion of the pinwheel; the axes are drawn in as red tubes or a red dot. **A,** The motion of the person's head and neck and the motion of the wheel of the pinwheel are in the sagittal plane; the axis for sagittal plane motion is mediolateral. **B,** The motion of the person's head and neck and the motion of the wheel of the pinwheel are in the frontal plane; the axis for frontal plane motion is anteroposterior (red dot). **C,** The motion of the person's head and neck and the motion of the wheel of the pinwheel are in the transverse plane; the axis for transverse plane motion is vertical.

REVIEW QUESTIONS

evolve Answers to the following review questions appear on the Evolve website accompanying this book at: http://evolve.elsevier.com/Muscolino/kinesiology/.

1. What is the position of the body when it is in anatomic position?

2. What is the importance of anatomic position?

3. What are the five major pairs of directional terms for naming the location of a structure of the body or a point on the body?

4. In what parts of the body can each of the pairs of directional terms of location be used?

5. If point A is located farther toward the front of the body than point B is, then how do we describe the location of point A? Point B?

6. If point A is located closer to the midline of the body than point B is, then how do we describe the location of point A? Point B?

7. If point A is located on the axial body closer to the top of the body than point B is, then how do we describe the location of point A? Point B?

8. If point A is located on the appendicular body closer to the axial body than point B is, then how do we describe the location of point A? Point B?

9. If point A is located both farther toward the front and farther toward the midline of the body than point B is, then how do we describe the location of point A? Point B?

10. If point A is located closer to the surface of the body than point B is, then how do we describe the location of point A? Point B?

11. What is a plane, and what is the importance of understanding the concept of planes?

12. What are the four types of planes?

13. What is an axis, and what is the importance of understanding the concept of axes?

14. What are the corresponding axes for each of the three cardinal planes?

15. What is the relationship between axial motion and planes and axes?

16. Regarding axial motion, how is the hinge pin of a door or the pin of a pinwheel analogous to the axis?

REFERENCES

1. Thibodeau GA, Patton KT: Anatomy & physiology, ed 5, St Louis, 2003, Mosby.
2. Palastanga N, Field D, Soames R: Anatomy and human movement, ed 4, Oxford, 2002, Butterworth-Heinemann.
3. Dail NW, Agnew TA, Floyd RT: Kinesiology for manual therapies, New York, 2011, McGraw Hill.
4. Oatis CA: Kinesiology: The mechanics and pathomechanics of human movement, Philadelphia, 2004, Lippincott Williams & Wilkins.
5. Neumann DA: Kinesiology of the musculoskeletal system: Foundations for physical rehabilitation, ed 3, St Louis, 2017, Elsevier.
6. Levangie PK, Norkin CC: Joint structure and function: A comprehensive analysis, ed 5, Philadelphia, 2011, FA Davis.

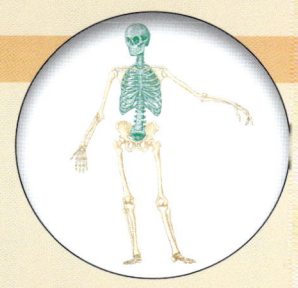

PART II

Skeletal Osteology: Study of the Bones

CHAPTER 3
Skeletal Tissues

CHAPTER OUTLINE

Section 3.1	Classification of Bones by Shape	Section 3.6	Bone Development and Growth
Section 3.2	Parts of a Long Bone	Section 3.7	Fontanels
Section 3.3	Functions of Bones	Section 3.8	Fracture Healing
Section 3.4	Bone as a Connective Tissue	Section 3.9	Effects of Physical Stress on Bone
Section 3.5	Compact and Spongy Bone	Section 3.10	Cartilage Tissue

CHAPTER OBJECTIVES

After completing this chapter, the student should be able to perform the following:

1. Define the key terms of this chapter and state the meanings of the word origins of this chapter.
2. Do the following related to classification of bones by shape:
   - List the four major classifications of bones by shape, and give an example of each one.
   - Place sesamoid bones into their major category of bones by shape, and give an example of a sesamoid bone.
   - Explain the concept of a supernumerary bone, and give an example of a supernumerary bone.
3. List and describe the major structural parts of a long bone.
4. List and describe the five major functions of bones.
5. List and describe the components of bone as a connective tissue.
6. Describe, compare, and contrast the structure of compact and spongy bone.
7. Describe, compare, and contrast the two methods of bone development and growth: endochondral ossification and intramembranous ossification.
8. Do the following related to fontanels:
   - Explain the purpose of the fontanels of the infant's skull.
   - Name, locate, and state the closure time of the major fontanels of the infant's skull.
9. Describe the steps by which a fractured bone heals.
10. Do the following related to Wolff's Law and the effects of physical stress on bone:
    - State and explain the meaning and importance of Wolff's law to the human skeleton and the fields of bodywork and exercise.
    - Explain the relationship of the piezoelectric effect to Wolff's law.
    - Explain the relationship between Wolff's law and degenerative joint disease (DJD) (also known as osteoarthritis [OA]).
11. Do the following related to cartilage tissue:
    - List and describe the components of cartilage as a connective tissue.
    - Compare and contrast the three types of cartilage tissue.

OVERVIEW

Many tissues contribute to the structure and function of the skeletal system; chief among them is bone tissue. The first sections of this chapter examine bone tissue macrostructure, microstructure, functions, and physiology. The last section of this chapter covers cartilage tissue. Chapter 4 then covers fascial tissue in detail.

KEY TERMS

Anterior fontanel (an-TEER-ee-or FON-ta-nel)
Anterolateral fontanel (AN-teer-o-LAT-er-al)
Articular cartilage (ar-TIK-you-lar KAR-ti-lij)
Articular surface
Bone marrow
Bone spur
Bony callus
Calcitonin (KAL-si-TO-nin)
Callus
Canaliculus, pl. canaliculi (KAN-a-LIK-you-lus, KAN-a-LK-you-lie)
Cancellous bone (KAN-se-lus)
Cartilage (KAR-ti-lij)
Chondroblast (KON-dro-blast)
Chondrocyte (KON-dro-site)
Chondroitin sulfate (kon-DROY-tin SUL-fate)
Compact bone
Connective tissue
Cortex (KOR-teks)
Cortical surface (KOR-ti-kal)
Cytoplasmic processes (SI-to-PLAZ-mik)
Degenerative joint disease
Diaphysis, pl. diaphyses (die-AF-i-sis, die-AF-i-seez)
Elastic cartilage
Elastin fibers (ee-LAS-tin)
Endochondral ossification (en-do-KON-dral OS-si-fi-KAY-shun)
Endosteum (en-DOS-tee-um)
Epiphysial disc (e-PIF-i-zee-al)
Epiphysial line
Epiphysis, pl. epiphyses (e-PIF-i-sis, e-PIF-i-seez)
Fibrocartilage (FI-bro-KAR-ti-lij)
Flat bones
Fontanel (FON-ta-NEL)
Frontal fontanel
Ground substance
Glucosamine (glue-KOS-a-meen)
Growth plate
Haversian canal (ha-VER-zhun)
Hematoma (HEEM-a-TOME-a)
Hematopoiesis (heem-AT-o-poy-E-sis)
Hyaline cartilage (HI-a-lin KAR-ti-lij)
Hydroxyapatite crystals (hi-DROK-see-AP-a-TIGHT)
Intramembranous ossification (in-tra-MEM-bran-us OS-si-fi-KAY-shun)

Irregular bones
Kinesiology (ki-NEE-see-OL-o-gee)
Lacuna, pl. lacunae (la-KOO-na, la-KOO-nee)
Lever
Long bones
Mastoid fontanel (MAS-toyd FON-ta-NEL)
Matrix (MAY-triks)
Medullary cavity (MEJ-you-LAR-ree)
Membrane (MEM-brain)
OA
Occipital fontanel (ok-SIP-i-tal FON-ta-NEL)
Ossification center (OS-si-fi-KAY-shun)
Osteoarthritis (OS-tee-o-ar-THRI-tis)
Osteoblast (OS-tee-o-BLAST)
Osteoclast (OS-tee-o-KLAST)
Osteocyte (OS-tee-o-SITE)
Osteoid tissue (OS-tee-OYD)
Osteon (OS-tee-on)
Osteonic canal (OS-tee-ON-ik)
Parathyroid hormone (PAR-a-THI-royd)
Perichondrium (per-ee-KON-dree-um)
Periosteum (per-ee-OS-tee-um)
Periostitis (PER-ee-ost-EYE-tis)
Posterior fontanel (pos-TEER-ee-or FON-ta-nel)
Posterolateral fontanel (POS-teer-o-LAT-er-al)
Primary ossification center
Radiograph (RAY-dee-o-graf)
Red bone marrow
Round bones
Secondary ossification centers
Sesamoid bones (SES-a-moyd)
Short bones
Sphenoid fontanel (SFEE-noyd FON-ta-NEL)
Spongy bone
Subchondral bone
Supernumerary bones (soo-per-NOO-mer-air-ee)
Tendinitis (ten-di-NI-tis)
Trabecula, pl. trabeculae (tra-BEK-you-la, tra-BEK-you-lee)
Volkmann's canal (FOK-mahns)
Wolff's law (WOLF or VULF)
Wormian bones (WERM-ee-an)
Yellow bone marrow

WORD ORIGINS

- A (an)—From Latin *a*, meaning *not, without*
- Arthr—From Greek *arthron*, meaning *a joint*
- Articular—From Latin *articulus*, meaning *a joint*
- Blastic—From Greek *blastos*, meaning *to bud, to build, to grow*
- Chondr—From Greek *chondros*, meaning *cartilage*
- Clastic—From Greek *klastos*, meaning *to break up into pieces*
- Cortical—From Latin *cortex*, meaning *outer portion of an organ, bark of a tree*
- Cyte—From Greek *kyton*, meaning *a hollow, cell*
- Endo—From Greek *endon*, meaning *within, inner*

- Epi—From Greek *epi*, meaning *on, upon*
- Extra—From Latin *extra*, meaning *outside*
- Graph—From Greek *grapho*, meaning *to write*
- Hem, hemato—From Greek *haima*, meaning *blood*
- Hyaline—From Greek *hyalos*, meaning *glass*
- Intra—From Latin *intra*, meaning *within, inner*
- Itis—From Greek *itis*, meaning *inflammation*
- Kines—From Greek *kinesis*, meaning *movement, motion*
- Medulla—From Latin *medulla*, meaning *inner portion, marrow*
- Myo—From Greek *mys*, meaning *muscle*
- Num—From Latin *numerus*, meaning *number*
- Oid—From Greek *eidos*, meaning *resembling, appearance*
- Ology—From Greek *logos*, meaning *study of, discourse, word*
- Os, ossi—From Latin *os*, meaning *bone*
- Ost, osteo—From Greek *osteon*, meaning *bone*
- Peri—From Greek *peri*, meaning *around*
- Physi, physio—From Greek *physis*, meaning *body, nature*
- Piezo—From Greek *piesis*, meaning *pressure*
- Poiesis—From Greek *poiesis*, meaning *production, making*
- Tens—From Latin *tensio*, meaning *a stretching*

SECTION 3.1 CLASSIFICATION OF BONES BY SHAPE

- Structurally, bones can be divided into four major categories based on their shape (Figure 3-1).
- These four major classifications by shape are[1]:
  - Long bones
  - Short bones
  - Flat bones
  - Irregular bones
- These classifications can be useful when discussing the structure and function of bones. However, it should be kept in mind that all classification systems are at least somewhat arbitrary, and not every bone fits perfectly into one category; sometimes the classification of a bone may be difficult because it has attributes of two or more categories.
- **Long bones** are long (i.e., they have a longitudinal axis to them). This longitudinal axis is the shaft of the bone. At each end of the shaft of a long bone is an expanded portion that forms a joint (articulates) with another bone.[2] (See Section 3.2 for the anatomy of a long bone in more detail.)
  - Examples of long bones are humerus, femur, radius, ulna, tibia, fibula, metacarpals, metatarsals, and phalanges. Even though some of the phalanges are quite short in length, they still have a longitudinal axis (i.e., a length to them) with expanded ends; therefore they qualify as long bones.
- **Short bones** are short (i.e., they are approximately as wide as they are long, and they are often described as being cube shaped).[2]
  - Examples of short bones are the carpals of the wrist.
  - Tarsal bones of the ankle region are also considered to be short bones. An exception is the calcaneus (see Section 5.8, Figures 5-53 to 5-57), which is considered to be an irregular bone, not a short bone.
- **Flat bones** are flat; that is, they are broad and thin, with either a flat or perhaps a curved surface.
  - Examples of flat bones are the ribs, sternum, cranial bones of the skull, and scapula (Box 3-1).

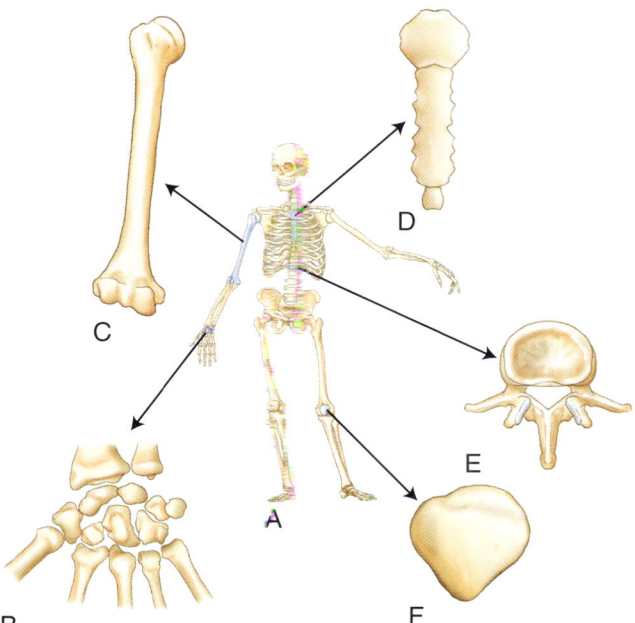

FIGURE 3-1 The four major classifications (shapes) of bones, as well as a sesamoid bone. **A,** Anterior view of the full human skeleton. **B,** The carpals (wrist bones), which are examples of short bones. **C,** A humerus, which is an example of a long bone. **D,** A sternum, which is an example of a flat bone. **E,** A vertebra, which is an example of an irregular bone. **F,** A patella (i.e., kneecap), which is an example of a sesamoid bone (a type of irregular bone).

 BOX 3-1

Given that the scapula has a spine, and acromion and coracoid processes, an argument could be made that it is an irregular bone. However, most sources place it as a flat bone.

- **Irregular bones** are irregular in shape (i.e., they do not neatly fall into any of the three preceding categories). They are neither clearly long, nor short, nor flat.[2]
  - Examples of irregular bones are the vertebrae of the spine, the facial bones of the skull, and sesamoid bones.

- Sesamoid bones are so named because they are shaped like a sesame seed—in other words, they are round. Because sesamoid bones are round in shape, they are also known as round bones. Some sources consider sesamoid bones to be a separate fifth category of bones.
- The number of sesamoid bones in the human body varies from one individual to another. The only sesamoid bones that are consistently found in all people are the two patellae (kneecaps).
- Additional bones: The number of bones in the human skeleton is usually said to be 206. This number can vary slightly from individual to individual. Whenever a person has more than the usual number of 206 bones,[3] these additional bones are called supernumerary bones. The following are examples of supernumerary bones:
  - Additional sesamoid bones (other than the two patellae) are considered to be supernumerary bones. Sesamoid bones are also usually present at the thumb and big toe. Many individuals have additional sesamoids beyond the patellae and the sesamoids of the thumb and big toe; these are usually located at other fingers.
- Wormian bones are small bones that are sometimes found in the suture joints between cranial bones of the skull.[2]
- Note: Occasionally, individuals have additional anomalous bones such as a sixth lumbar vertebra or cervical ribs.

SECTION 3.2 PARTS OF A LONG BONE

- As Section 3.1 demonstrates, no one *typical* bone exists in the human skeleton; great differences in size and shape exist among bones. Even though differences exist among the various bones, it is valuable to examine the parts of a long bone (Figure 3-2) to gain a better understanding of the typical structure of bones in general.

PARTS OF A LONG BONE

Diaphysis:
- The diaphysis[4] is the shaft of a long bone; its shape is that of a hollow cylindrical tube.
- The purpose of the diaphysis is to be a rigid tube that can withstand strong forces without bending or breaking; it must accomplish this without being excessively heavy.
- The diaphysis is composed of compact bone tissue with a thin layer of spongy bone tissue lining its inside surface. For more information on compact and spongy bone tissue, see Section 3.5.
- Located within the diaphysis at its center is the medullary cavity, which contains bone marrow.

Epiphysis:
- An epiphysis[4] (plural: epiphyses) is the expanded end of a long bone found at each end of the diaphysis. Hence, each long bone has two epiphyses.
- The purpose of an epiphysis is to articulate (form a joint) with another bone.
- By expanding, the epiphysis widens out, allowing for a larger joint surface, thus increasing the stability of the joint.
- The epiphysis is composed of spongy bone with a thin layer of compact bone tissue around the periphery.
- The spaces of spongy bone within the epiphysis contain red marrow.
- The articular surface of the epiphysis is covered with articular cartilage.

Articular Cartilage:
- Articular cartilage[4] covers the articular surfaces (i.e., joint surfaces) of a bone.

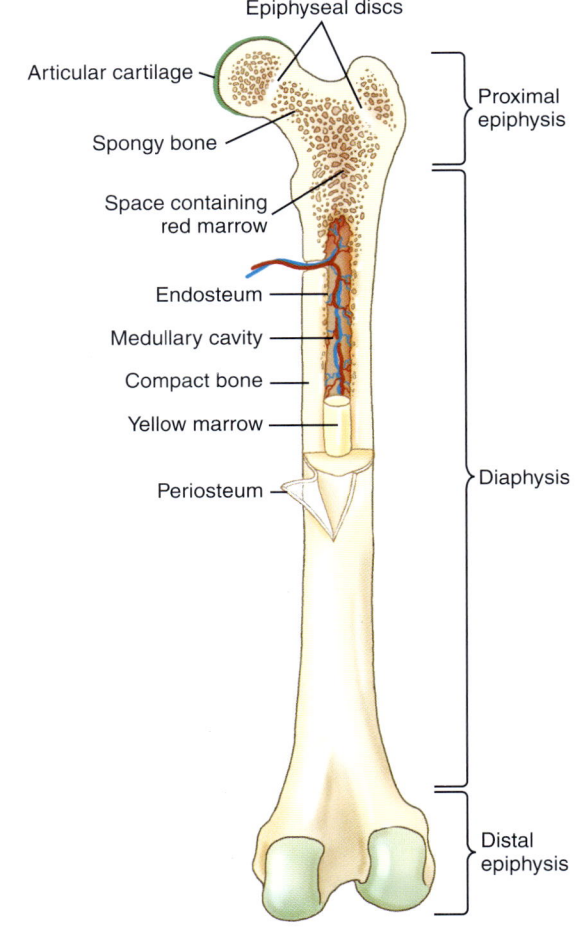

FIGURE 3-2 This is a view of a long bone (i.e., the femur) with the proximal portion opened up to expose the interior of the bone. The major structural components of a long bone are the diaphysis (i.e., the shaft) and the expanded ends (i.e., the epiphyses). Periosteum lines the entire outer surface of the bone, except the articular surfaces (i.e., joint surfaces), which are covered with articular cartilage. The inside of the diaphysis is primarily composed of compact bony tissue and also houses the medullary cavity, in which bone marrow is found. The epiphyses are primarily composed of spongy bone tissue.

- Articular cartilage is a softer tissue than bone, and its purpose is to provide cushioning and shock absorption for the joint.
- Articular cartilage is composed of hyaline cartilage. For more details on hyaline cartilage, see Section 3.10.
- It is worth noting that articular cartilage has a very poor blood supply; therefore it does not heal well after it has been damaged (Box 3-2).

BOX 3-2

The process of degenerative joint disease (DJD) (or **osteoarthritis [OA]**) involves degeneration of the articular cartilage at a joint.

Periosteum:

- **Periosteum**[4] surrounds the entire bone, except for the articular surfaces, which are covered with articular cartilage.
- Periosteum is a thin dense fibrous membrane.
- Periosteum has many purposes:
  - To provide a site of attachment for ligaments and for tendons of muscles. Fibers of ligaments and tendons literally interlace into the periosteal fibers of bone, thereby firmly anchoring the ligaments and tendons to the bone.
  - To house cells that are important in forming and repairing bone tissue.
  - To house the blood vessels that provide vascular supply to the bone.
- The periosteum of bone is highly innervated with nerve fibers and very pain sensitive when bruised (Box 3-3).

BOX 3-3

The fact that periosteum is pain sensitive is clear to anyone who has ever banged their shin against a coffee table. The shin is the anterior shaft of the tibia where very little soft tissue exists between the skin and the bone to cushion the blow to the periosteum. Any trauma that causes inflammation of the periosteum is technically called **periostitis** but is often known in lay terms as a bone bruise.

Medullary Cavity:

- The **medullary cavity**[4] is a tubelike cavity located within the diaphysis of a long bone.
- The medullary cavity houses a soft tissue known as **bone marrow** (red marrow and/or yellow bone marrow). For more details on bone marrow, see Section 3.3.

Endosteum:

- The **endosteum**[4] is a thin membrane that lines the inner surface of the bone within the medullary cavity.
- The endosteum (like the periosteum) contains cells that are important in forming and repairing bone.

Other Components of a Bone:

- All bones are highly metabolic organs that require a rich blood supply. Therefore they are well supplied with arteries and veins.
- Bones are also well innervated with sensory neurons (i.e., nerve cells). The periosteum of bones is particularly well innervated with sensory neurons.

SECTION 3.3   FUNCTIONS OF BONES

- Bones serve many functions in our body; the five major functions of bones are listed at the end of this paragraph.[5] Of these five major functions, the first two, structural support of the body and providing levers for body movements, are the two most important functions for bodyworkers, trainers, and students of kinesiology.
  - Structural support of the body
  - Provide levers for body movements
  - Protection of underlying structures
  - Blood cell formation
  - Storage reservoir for calcium

STRUCTURAL SUPPORT OF THE BODY:

- Bones create a skeletal structure that provides a rigid framework for the body. Using this framework, many tissues of the body literally attach to bones of the skeleton.[5]
  - For example, the brain is attached by soft tissue (i.e., meninges) to the cranial bones, and the internal visceral organs of the abdominopelvic cavity are literally suspended from the spine by soft tissue ligaments (Figure 3-3).
- Furthermore, the skeleton bears the weight of the tissues of the body and transfers this weight through the lower extremities to the ground (see Figure 3-3).
- The study of posture is largely concerned with understanding the manner in which bones create an effective and healthy skeletal support structure for the tissues of the body. The topic of posture is covered in more detail in Chapters 20 and 21.

PROVIDE LEVERS FOR BODY MOVEMENTS:

- The bones of the body are somewhat rigid elements that define the parts of the body.
- For example, the arm is defined by the presence of the humerus; the forearm is defined by the presence of the radius and ulna.
- By providing a rigid element within the body part, the bone of a body part provides a site to which muscles can attach. The force of a muscle contraction can then create movement of the bone and consequently movement of the body part within which the bone is located.[6]
- In this manner, a bone is a **lever** for movement of a body part[6] (Figure 3-4). This function of bones—providing levers for

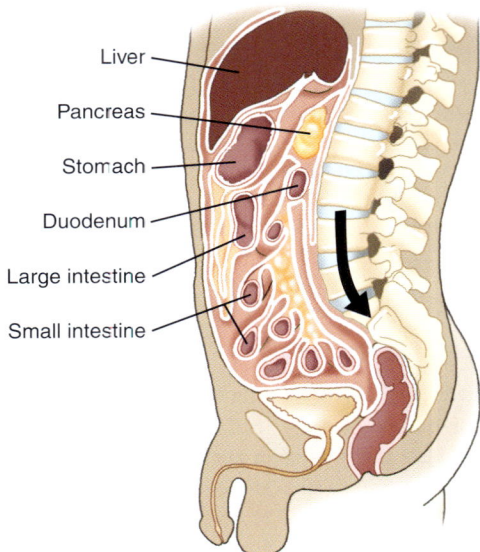

FIGURE 3-3 Bones create a skeletal structure that provides a rigid framework for the body. This rigid framework supports the internal organs, as can be seen in this illustration in which the internal organs of the abdominopelvic cavity literally hang from, and are thereby supported by, the spine. Furthermore, this rigid structure provides a weight-bearing structure through which the weight of the body parts that are located superiorly passes. The arrow drawn over the lower aspect of the spinal column represents the force of the weight of the body traveling through the spine.

PROTECTION OF UNDERLYING STRUCTURES:

○ Physical damage to our body from traumas such as falls, motor vehicle accidents, and sports injuries is always a danger. Some tissues and organs of our body are particularly sensitive to trauma, are critical to life, and need to be protected. Because bone tissue is rigid, it is ideal for providing protection to these underlying structures. For example:[7]
  ○ The brain is safely encased within the cranial cavity, fully surrounded by the bones of the cranium (Figure 3-5, *A*).
  ○ The spinal cord is located within the spinal canal, surrounded by the bony vertebrae.
  ○ The heart and lungs are located within the thoracic cavity, protected by the sternum and rib cage.

BLOOD CELL FORMATION:

○ Bones house **red bone marrow** (also known as *red marrow*), the soft connective tissue that makes blood cells[5] (Figure 3-5, *B*).
○ This process of blood cell production is called **hematopoiesis**.
○ It is important to point out that red marrow produces all types of blood cells: red blood cells, white blood cells, and platelets.
○ Red marrow is located within the medullary cavity of long bones and the spaces of spongy bone tissue.
○ In children, red marrow is found in most every bone of the body. However, as a person ages, the red bone marrow is gradually replaced with **yellow bone marrow**[2] (also known as

muscles to move parts of the body—is key to the study of kinesiology. **Kinesiology** literally means the study of movement. Because movement occurs by the forces of muscle contractions acting on bony levers, kinesiology is the study of the function of the musculoskeletal system. (For more information on levers, see Sections 17.6 to 17.8.)

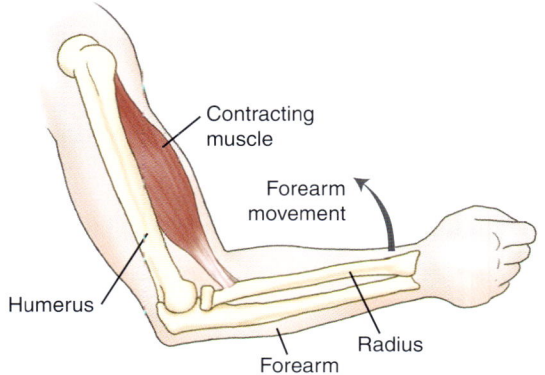

FIGURE 3-4 A bone provides a rigid lever by which a muscle can move a body part. The muscle pictured here attaches from the humerus of the arm to the radius of the forearm. This muscle is contracting, exerting an upward pull on the radius, causing the radius to move toward the humerus. Because the radius is rigid, when it moves the entire forearm moves. (Note: The muscle here does not represent an actual muscle in the human body. It is drawn only to illustrate the concept of how levers work.)

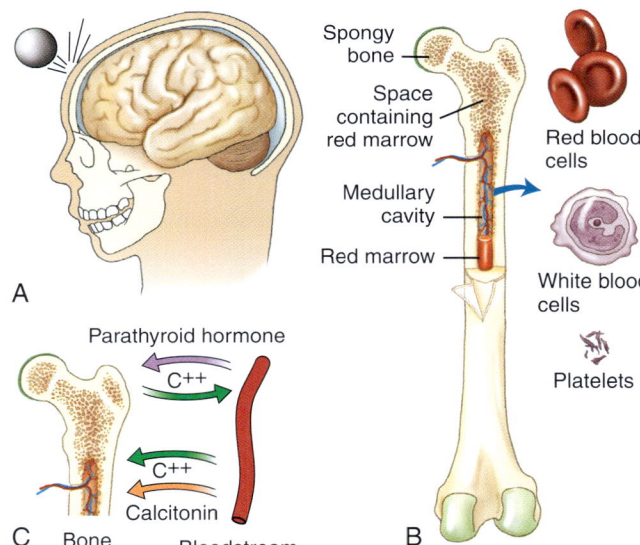

FIGURE 3-5 Three additional functions of bones. **A,** Bones protect underlying structures of the body. A hard object is seen hitting the head. The brain, located within the cranial cavity, is largely protected from the force of this blow by the bones of the skull. **B,** Hematopoiesis (i.e., the formation of blood cells). The red bone marrow seen in the medullary cavity of this long bone functions to create red blood cells, white blood cells, and platelets. **C,** Bones act as a reservoir or bank for blood levels of calcium. When the blood level of calcium is low, the body secretes parathyroid hormone, which causes the release of calcium from the bones into the bloodstream. When the blood level of calcium is high, the body secretes the hormone calcitonin, which causes excess calcium from the bloodstream to be deposited back into the bones.

yellow marrow); yellow marrow is essentially fat cells and therefore is not active in hemopoiesis.
- In an adult, red marrow is found primarily in the spongy bone tissue of the axial skeleton (skull, sternum, ribs, clavicles, vertebrae), and in the pelvis and the medullary cavities of the humerus and femur.[5]

STORAGE RESERVOIR FOR CALCIUM:

- Calcium is a mineral that is critical to the functioning of the human body.
  - Calcium is necessary for the conduction of impulses in the nervous system, the contraction of muscles, and the clotting of blood.[8-9]
- Because calcium is necessary for life, it is vital for the body to maintain proper levels of calcium in the bloodstream.
- When dietary intake of calcium is insufficient to meet the needs of the body, calcium can be taken from the bones to increase the blood level of calcium[9]; when dietary intake of calcium exceeds the need by the body, calcium in the bloodstream can be deposited back into the bones.
- The hormone **parathyroid hormone** (from the parathyroid glands) is responsible for withdrawing calcium from the bones; the hormone **calcitonin** (from the thyroid gland) is responsible for depositing calcium back into the bones.[10]
- The type of bone cell that causes the release of calcium from the bones into the bloodstream is an osteoclast; the type of bone cell that causes the deposition of calcium from the bloodstream back into bones is an osteoblast. (For more information on bone cells, see Section 3.4.)
- In this manner the bones act as a *reservoir* or *bank* from which calcium can be withdrawn and deposited, thereby maintaining proper blood levels of calcium for the body to function[5] (see Figure 3-5, *C*).

SECTION 3.4 BONE AS A CONNECTIVE TISSUE

- Bone is a type of **connective tissue**. As such, it is composed of bone cells and **matrix**[11] (Box 3-4).

BOX 3-4

Four major tissues exist in the human body: (1) nervous tissue (carries electrical impulses), (2) muscular tissue (contracts), (3) epithelial tissue (lines body surfaces open to a space or cavity), and (4) connective tissue (the most diverse of the four groups, generally considered to connect aspects of the body).

The matrix of a connective tissue is defined as everything other than the cells and is often divided into the fiber component and the ground substance component. With regard to bone tissue, the fibers are collagen fibers and make up a portion of the organic matrix of bone; the remainder of the matrix (both organic and inorganic) is the **ground substance**.

- The matrix of bone is often divided into its organic gel-like component and its inorganic rigid component.

BONE CELLS:

- Three types of bone cells exist:[4]
  - **Osteoblasts**: Osteoblasts build up bone tissue by secreting matrix tissue of the bone.
  - **Osteocytes**: Once osteoblasts are fully surrounded by the matrix of bone and lie within small chambers within the bony matrix, they are called *osteocytes*.
  - These small chambers are called *lacunae* (singular: lacuna). (For more information on lacunae, see Section 3.5.)
  - **Osteoclasts**: Osteoclasts break down bone tissue by breaking down the matrix tissue of the bone.
- It is important to realize that bone is a dynamic living tissue that has a balance of osteoblastic and osteoclastic activity occurring. This is true when a bone is growing, when it is repairing after an injury, and when calcium is being withdrawn and deposited into bone to maintain proper blood levels of calcium (which occurs throughout our entire life).

ORGANIC MATRIX:

- The gel-like organic matrix of bone adds to the resiliency of bone. Certainly bones are more rigid than soft tissues of the body, but the organic gel-like component of bone matrix that is present in living bone gives it much more resiliency than the dried up fossilized bones that we see in a museum and often think of when we think of bones.
- The organic component of matrix is composed of collagen fibers and the gel-like osteoid tissue.[4]
- This gel-like **osteoid tissue** contains large molecules called **proteoglycans**. Proteoglycans are protein/polysaccharide molecules that are composed primarily of glucosamine and chondroitin sulfate molecules. Their major purpose is to trap fluid so that bone tissue does not become too dry and brittle.[12] The composition of a living healthy bone is approximately 25% water. (For more information on proteoglycans, see Section 3.10.)
- Within this gel-like proteoglycan mix, collagen fibers are created and deposited by fibroblastic cells.
- **Collagen fibers** primarily add to a bone's tensile strength[4] (its ability to withstand pulling forces) (Box 3-5).

BOX 3-5

Vitamin C is necessary for the production of collagen, and if its intake in the diet is insufficient, a condition called scurvy occurs. Hundreds of years ago, sailors at sea would often come down with this disease because of the lack of fresh foods containing vitamin C on long sea journeys. The British were the first to realize that if they took a certain fresh food on board their ships, their sailors would not get scurvy. The fresh food that they carried with them was limes. For this reason, people from Britain have long been known as limeys.

INORGANIC MATRIX:

- The inorganic component of matrix is composed of the mineral content of bone (i.e., the calcium-phosphate salts of bone).
- These calcium-phosphate salts are also known as **hydroxyapatite crystals**.[4]
- The calcium-phosphate salts give bone its rigidity.

SECTION 3.5 COMPACT AND SPONGY BONE

- The manner in which the components of bone tissue (cells and matrix) are organized can vary. Two different arrangements of bone tissue exist[4] (Figure 3-6):
  - **Compact bone** has a compact ordered arrangement of bone tissue.
  - **Spongy bone** has an arrangement of bone tissue that is less compact, containing irregular spaces, that gives this tissue the appearance of a sponge.
  - Spongy bone is also known as **cancellous bone**.

COMPACT BONE:

- As stated, compact bone has a very ordered, tightly packed arrangement of the bony tissue.[4]
- Compact bone is primarily found in the shafts of long bones, where it provides rigidity to the shaft. Compact bone also lines the outer surface of the epiphyses of long bones and the outer surface of all other bones (i.e., short, flat, and irregular bones) (Box 3-6).

> **BOX 3-6**
>
> The outer surface of a bone is known as its **cortex** or **cortical surface**. When a physician looks at a **radiograph** (i.e., x-ray) of a bone, he or she examines the cortical surface for any break in the margin that would indicate a fracture—in other words, a broken bone.

- Compact bone is composed of structural units that are cylindric in shape called osteons[4] (Figure 3-7).
- Each **osteon** is composed of a central osteonic canal in which a blood vessel is located. **Osteonic canals** are also known as **Haversian canals**.[12]
- **Volkmann's canals** (also known as *perforating canals*) connect the blood vessel from one osteonic canal to the blood vessel of an adjacent osteonic canal.[4]
- Bloods vessels provide the nourishment necessary for all living cells, including bone cells (i.e., osteocytes). Therefore osteocytes arrange themselves around the osteonic canal in concentric circles. This arrangement of osteocytes around the osteonic canal is what creates the cylindric shape of an osteon.
- Compact bone is composed of multiple small osteons. This allows for all osteocytes to be close to their blood supply to get their nourishment via diffusion from the blood vessels located within the osteonic canals.
- Each osteocyte is located within a small chamber, surrounded by the matrix of bone. This small chamber is called a **lacuna** (plural: **lacunae**)[12] (Figure 3-8).
- Very small canals called **canaliculi** (singular: **canaliculus**) connect one lacuna to another lacuna. Osteocytes send small cytoplasmic processes through these canaliculi to communicate with adjacent osteocytes in other lacunae.[4] As a result of these processes, bone cells can communicate very well with one another, and bone tissue is very responsive to changes in its environment.

SPONGY BONE:

- As stated, spongy bone has many irregular spaces that give it the appearance of a sponge (see Figure 3-6). These spaces allow for a lighter weight while still providing adequate rigidity to the bone.
- Spongy bone is primarily found in the epiphyses of long bones and the center of all other bones (i.e., short, flat, and irregular bones).[4]
- A small amount of spongy bone is also found within the shafts of long bones (see Figure 3-7, *B*).
- Because spongy bone has many spaces within it that allow for diffusion of nutrients from the blood supply, no need exists for osteonic canals and the ordered arrangement of osteocytes in

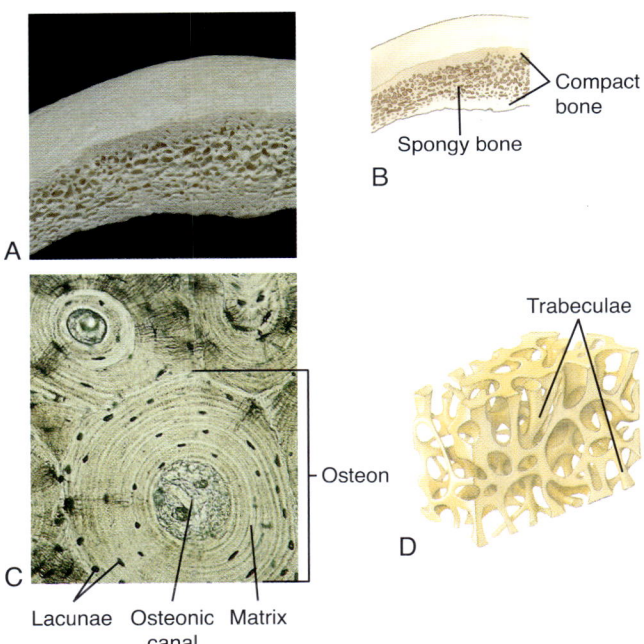

FIGURE 3-6 The two types of bone tissue: compact and spongy. **A and B,** Photograph and drawing of a cross-section of a cranial bone showing the spongy bone tissue in the middle and the compact bone tissue on both sides of the spongy bone. **C,** An enlargement that shows the osteons of compact bone. **D,** An enlargement that shows the trabeculae of spongy bone. (*C* and *D*, from Patton KT, Thibodeau GA: *Anatomy and physiology*, ed 9, St Louis, 2016, Elsevier.)

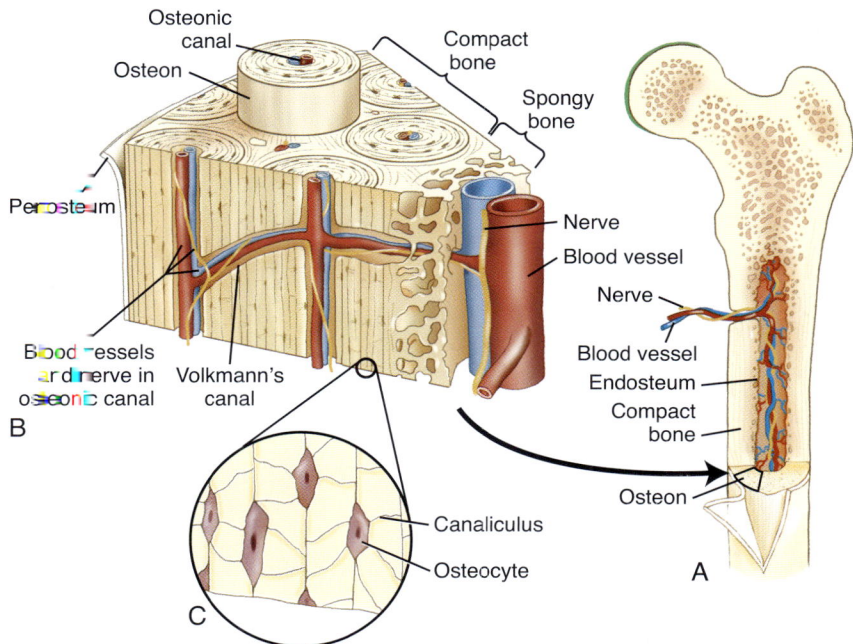

FIGURE 3-7 A, Section of a long bone illustrating the interior of the bone. **B,** Enlargement of a pie-shaped wedge of the shaft of the long bone displaying the osteons of the compact bone, as well as the spongy bone located in the interior of the shaft. **C,** Further enlargement of the compact bony tissue showing the osteocytes (located within the lacunae) that communicate with one another via the canaliculi that connect the lacunae to one another.

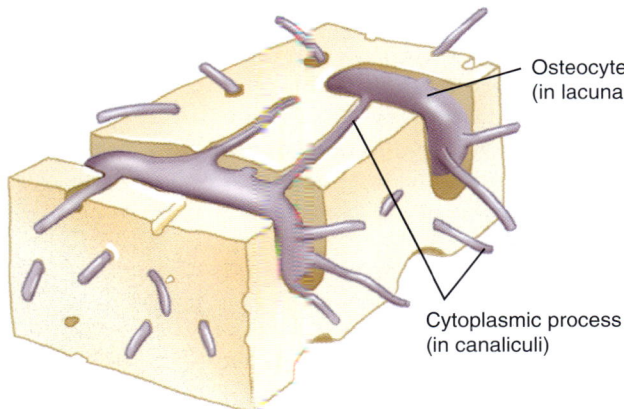

FIGURE 3-8 Illustration of the concept of osteocytes being located within lacunae and the cytoplasmic processes of the osteocytes communicating with other osteocytes via the canaliculi.

- lacunae around the blood vessel in the osteonic canal. Therefore no need exists for the ordered arrangement of osteons.
- Spongy bone consists of a latticework of bars and plates of bony tissue called **trabeculae**[4] (singular: trabecula). Between these plates are the spaces of spongy bone (see Figure 3-6, *D*).
- When we say that these spaces are irregular, it may give the impression that spongy bone is very haphazard in its arrangement, which is not true. There is a pattern to spongy bone. The trabeculae of spongy bone are arranged in a fashion that allows them to best deal with the compressive forces of weight bearing (Box 3-7).

 BOX 3-7

The pattern of trabeculae of spongy bone is usually apparent on a radiograph (i.e., x-ray).

SECTION 3.6 BONE DEVELOPMENT AND GROWTH

- When the skeleton begins to form in utero, it is not calcified. Rather, it is composed of cartilage and fibrous structures shaped like the bones of the skeleton. These cartilage and fibrous structures gradually calcify as the child grows (both in utero and after birth) and act as models for development of the mature skeleton.

- The skeleton forms by two major methods[1]: (1) **endochondral ossification** and (2) **intramembranous ossification**.

ENDOCHONDRAL OSSIFICATION:

- Endochondral ossification, as its name implies, is ossification that occurs within a cartilage model (*chondral* means cartilage).[1]

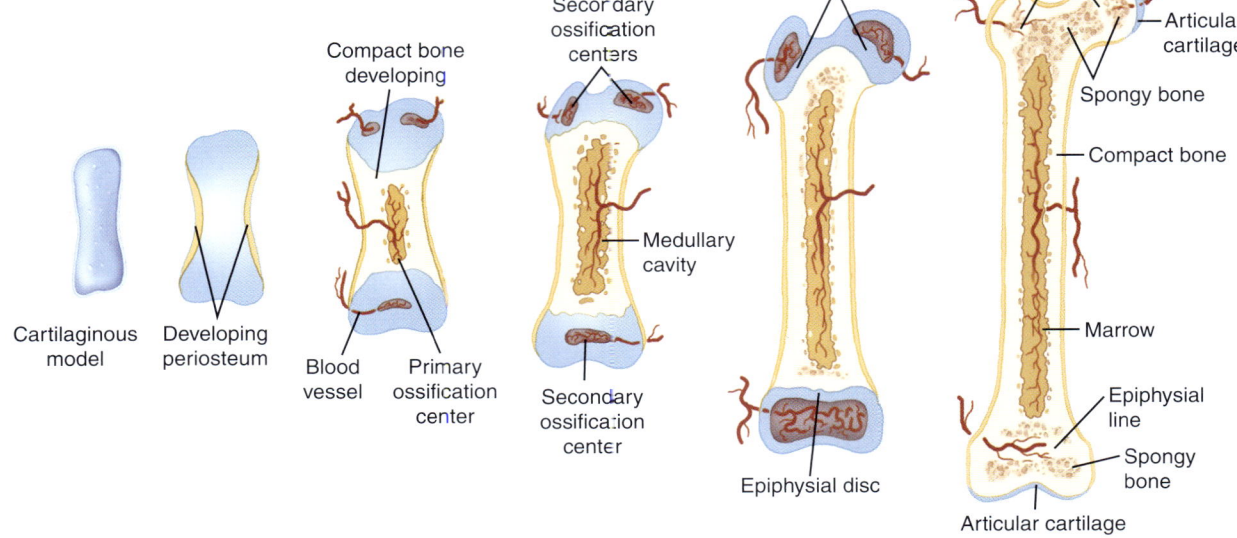

FIGURE 3-9 The steps of endochondral ossification. Beginning with a cartilaginous model, periosteum forms around the bone; then primary and secondary ossification centers develop in the diaphysis and epiphyses, respectively, and epiphysial discs are located between them. These ossification centers grow toward each other while the epiphysial discs continue to elongate the cartilage model by producing cartilage tissue. When the ossification centers meet, bone growth stops.

- Most bones of the human body develop by endochondral ossification. The steps of endochondral ossification for a long bone are as follows (Figure 3-9):
  - The cartilage model of a bone exists.
  - The cartilage model develops its periosteal lining, which surrounds the diaphysis.
  - The cartilage in the diaphysis gradually breaks down and is replaced with bone tissue by osteoblasts from the periosteum. A region of developing bone tissue is called an **ossification center**. This first region of developing bone in the diaphysis is called the **primary ossification center**.[1]
  - The primary ossification center gradually grows toward the epiphyses, replacing cartilage with bone.
  - **Secondary ossification centers** appear in the epiphyses of the long bone and grow toward the primary ossification center, replacing cartilage with bone.[1]
  - The region between the primary and secondary ossification centers still contains cartilage cells that are producing cartilage tissue, continuing to increase the length of the cartilage model of bone. This region of cartilage growth is called the **epiphysial disc**. Because the epiphysial disc is the region where the model for the future mature bone grows, it is known in lay terms as the **growth plate**.[1]
  - Meanwhile, in the center of the diaphysis, osteoclasts are breaking down the bone tissue, creating the medullary cavity.
  - As the epiphysial disc continues to lengthen the bone by laying down cartilage, the ossification centers keep growing by replacing the cartilage of the epiphysial disc with bone tissue.
  - The pace of the growth of the ossification centers is slightly faster than the growth of new cartilage within the epiphysial disc. When the ossification centers finally meet, having replaced all the cartilage tissue of the epiphysial disc, bone growth stops and the bone is mature. This occurs at approximately age 18, when a person is said to stop growing.
  - Although the length of a long bone stops growing at approximately age 18, long bones can continue to thicken into the future by deposition of bone tissue by osteoblasts of the periosteum (and breakdown of bone tissue by osteoclasts of the endosteum).
  - A remnant of the epiphysial disc is visible on a radiograph (i.e., x-ray) and is called the **epiphysial line** (Box 3-8).

 BOX 3-8

By looking at a radiograph (i.e., x-ray), a physician can determine if a person has finished growing or if much potential for growth remains, based on how large the epiphysial disc is (i.e., how close the ossification centers are to meeting each other, stopping bone growth).

INTRAMEMBRANOUS OSSIFICATION:

- Intramembranous ossification, as its name implies, is ossification that occurs within a **membrane** (i.e., a thin sheet or layer of soft tissue); this membrane is composed of fibrous tissue.[1]
- Flat bones of the skull develop by intramembranous ossification. The steps of intramembranous ossification for a flat bone are outlined here:
  - The fibrous membrane model of a bone exists.
  - Regions of osteoblasts develop within the fibrous membrane and begin to lay down bony matrix around themselves,

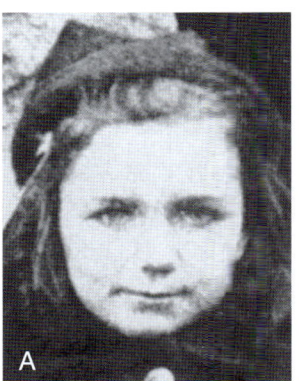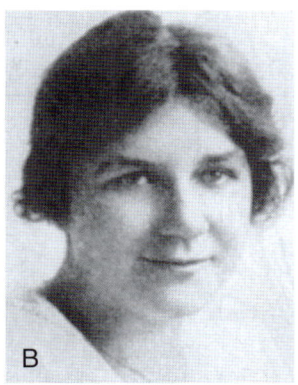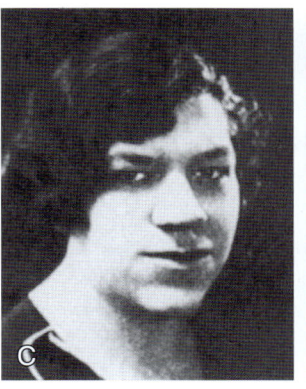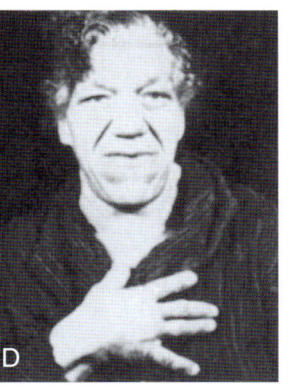

FIGURE 3-10 Four photographs of a woman with an endocrine disorder called acromegaly (an oversecretion of growth hormone in adulthood). In these four photographs from ages 9 years **(A)**, 16 years **(B)**, 33 years **(C)**, and 52 years **(D)**, the changes in facial features because of the continued intramembranous growth of her facial bones are shown. Although this example is extreme as a result of the condition, it illustrates the concept of continued intramembranous growth in adulthood that everyone experiences (to a much smaller degree). *(From Hole JW Jr: Hole's human anatomy and physiology, ed 4, Dubuque, Iowa, 1987, William C Brown.)*

- creating spongy bone. These regions of osteoblasts are known as *ossification centers*.[1]
- A periosteum arises around the membrane and begins to lay down compact bone on both sides of the developing spongy bone within the membrane.
- The bone is ossified when the entire fibrous membrane has been replaced with bony tissue.
- Continued growth of flat bones can and does continue into the future by osteoblasts of the periosteum and results in thickening of the flat bones as a person ages. This can usually be seen in the faces of elderly people (Figure 3-10).

SECTION 3.7   FONTANELS

- A **fontanel** is a soft spot on an infant's skull.[1]
- These fontanels are soft because they are areas of the primitive fibrous membrane of the skull.[4]
- These regions of fibrous membrane still exist in an infant because the process of intramembranous ossification is not yet complete (see Section 3.6).
- These fontanels are helpful because they allow some movement of the bones of the infant's head (permitting the head to compress to some degree), which allows it to more easily fit through the birth canal during labor. This is helpful to the mother and the child.
- Six major fontanels are found in a child's skull; all of these exist where the parietal bones meet other bones of the skull[7] (Figure 3-11 and Box 3-9).

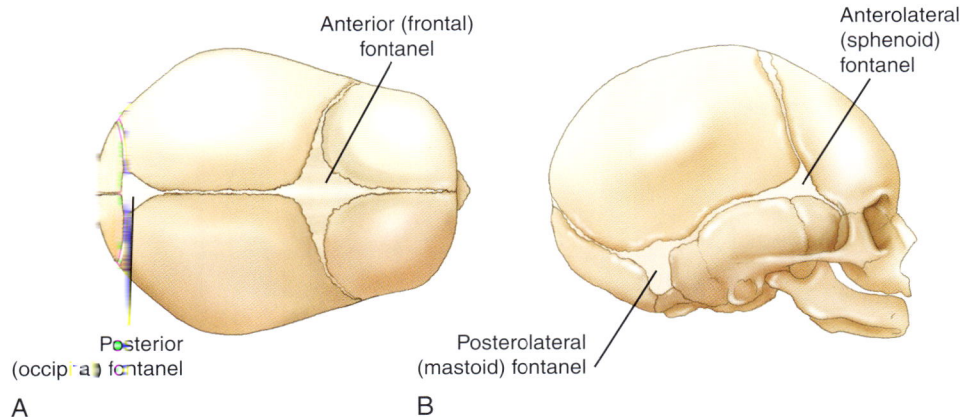

FIGURE 3-11 A, Superior view of an infant's skull; the anterior fontanel is shown between the parietal and frontal bones, and the posterior fontanel is shown between the parietal and occipital bones. **B,** Lateral view of an infant's skull; the anterolateral fontanel appears among the parietal, frontal, temporal, and sphenoid bones, and the posterolateral fontanel appears among the parietal, occipital, and temporal bones. (Note: See Section 5.1, Figures 5-3 to 5-9 for views of the skull with labels.)

BOX 3-9

The presence of soft spots (i.e., fontanels) means that a manual therapist must exercise caution when working on the head during infant and child massage.

- **Anterior fontanel**: The anterior fontanel is located at the juncture of the two parietal bones and the frontal bone.
  - The anterior fontanel closes at approximately 1 to 2 years of age.
  - The anterior fontanel is also known as the **frontal fontanel**.
- **Posterior fontanel**: The posterior fontanel is located at the juncture of the two parietal bones and the occipital bone.
  - The posterior fontanel closes at approximately 6 months of age.
  - The posterior fontanel is also known as the **occipital fontanel**.
- **Anterolateral fontanels** (paired left and right): The anterolateral fontanels are located at the juncture of the parietal, frontal, temporal, and sphenoid bones.
  - The anterolateral fontanels close at approximately 6 months of age.
  - The anterolateral fontanels are also known as the **sphenoid fontanels**.
- **Posterolateral fontanels** (paired left and right): The posterolateral fontanels are located at the juncture of the parietal, occipital, and temporal bones.
  - The posterolateral fontanels close at approximately 1 year of age.
  - The posterolateral fontanels are also known as the **mastoid fontanels**.

SECTION 3.8 FRACTURE HEALING

- A fractured bone is a broken bone, and a broken bone is a fractured bone; these two terms are synonyms.[4]
- A *fracture* (i.e., broken bone) is defined as a break in the continuity of a bone.
- Fractures are usually diagnosed by radiographic examination.
- When looking at a radiograph (i.e., x-ray) of a bone, the physician pays special attention to the cortical (outer) margin of the bone. If any discontinuity is seen in the cortical margin of a bone, it is diagnosed as fractured.
- Assuming that the two ends of a fractured bone are well aligned, fracture healing is accomplished by the following steps (Figure 3-12):
  - When a bone is fractured, blood vessels will also be broken. This causes bleeding in the region and results in a blood clot, which is called a **hematoma**.[4]
- Dead fragments of bone are resorbed by the action of osteoclasts.
- As the hematoma itself is gradually resorbed, fibrocartilage is deposited in the fracture site. This fibrocartilaginous tissue temporarily holds the two broken ends together and is called a **callus**.[4]
- This fibrocartilaginous callus then calcifies, resulting in the formation of a **bony callus**.
- Because the bony callus usually results in more bone tissue than was previously present, osteoclasts remodel the bone by resorbing the excessive tissue of the bony callus.
- The remodeling process is usually not 100% perfect, and a slight bony callus is usually present for the remainder of the person's lifetime, often palpable as a bump at the location of the break. However, the fracture is healed and the bone is structurally healthy.

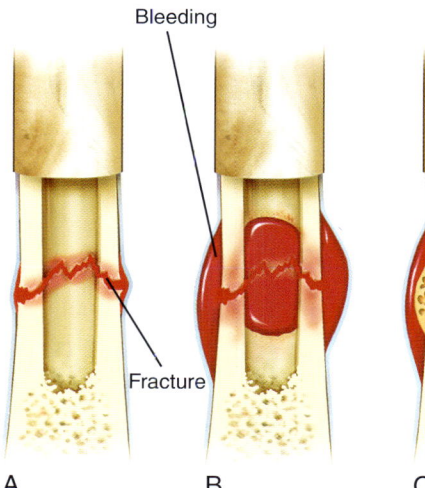
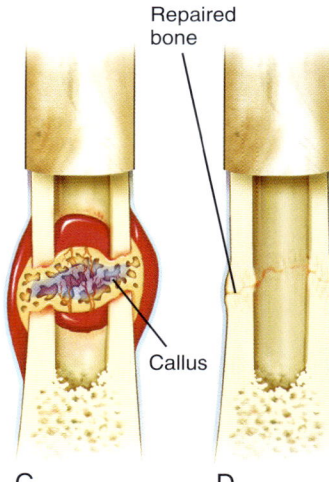

FIGURE 3-12 The steps that take place during repair of a fractured (i.e., broken) bone. **A,** Fracture of the femur. **B,** Hematoma has formed. **C,** Callus has formed; this callus is initially composed of fibrocartilaginous tissue and then later calcifies to create a bony callus. **D,** Bone repair is complete. A remnant of the bony callus is still evident and would likely be palpable as a bump at the site of the fracture. *(From Patton KT, Thibodeau GA: Anatomy and physiology, ed 9, St Louis, 2016, Mosby.)*

SECTION 3.9   EFFECTS OF PHYSICAL STRESS ON BONE

- Bone is a dynamic living tissue that responds to the physical demands placed on it. Bone tissue follows **Wolff's law**, which states, "Calcium is laid down in response to stress." Thus according to Wolff's law[12]:
  - If increased physical stress is placed on a bone, then the bone responds by gaining bony matrix and thickening.
  - If decreased physical stress is placed on a bone, then the bone responds by losing bony matrix and thinning.
  - All living tissue must be maintained with a nutrient supply provided by the cardiovascular system. Therefore increased mass of living tissue places a greater demand and stress on the heart. Furthermore, greater mass of tissue requires greater force by the muscles to be able to move our body through space; this places a greater demand and stress on our muscular system, necessitating larger and stronger muscles, which in turn requires more nutrition to be supplied by the cardiovascular system, and so forth. Therefore if any tissue of the body is unneeded, it is in the body's best interest to shed it—hence the wisdom of "use it or lose it."
- The beauty of the principle of Wolff's law is that bone can adapt to the demands that are placed on it.
  - If a bone has a great deal of stress placed on it, it will become thicker and stronger so that it will be able to deal with this stress and remain healthy.
  - Imagine the demands placed on the feet of a marathon runner and the need to respond to those demands by thickening the bones of the lower extremities.
  - On the other hand, if a bone has little stress placed on it, the bone does not need to maintain a large amount of matrix and it can afford to lose the unneeded bone mass ("use it or lose it").
  - Imagine a sedentary office worker who sits at a desk for the entire workday and never exercises; how necessary is it for the lower extremity bones of this sedentary individual to be as developed and massive as the bones of the marathon runner (Box 3-10)?

BOX 3-10

When astronauts are seen in their weightless environment in space, they are often seen exercising. This is necessary to keep their bones well mineralized, because being in a weightless environment for as little as a few days to a few weeks can cause significant loss of bone mass.

WOLFF'S LAW AND THE PIEZOELECTRIC EFFECT:

- Wolff's law is explained by the piezoelectric effect.[13]
- When pressure is placed on a tissue, a slight electric charge results in that tissue; this is known as the **piezoelectric effect**.[13] (Note: *Piezo* means *press are*.)
- The importance of the piezoelectric effect is that although osteoblasts can lay down bone in any tissue that they please, osteoclasts are unable to resorb (break down) bone in piezoelectrically charged tissue.
- The result is that a greater bone mass results in the regions of bone that are under greater pressure (i.e., greater patterns of physical stress).[13]
- Therefore Wolff's law, via the piezoelectric effect, explains how and why the trabeculae of spongy bone are laid down along the lines of stress (Figure 3-13). Furthermore, these principles also explain how it is that bones can literally remodel and change their shape in response to the forces placed on them.
- Wolff's law via the piezoelectric effect also explains why it is so important to begin movement as soon as it is safely possible after injury or surgery. Even more universally, Wolff's law explains why movement and exercise are so vital to a healthy skeleton—let alone the rest of our body!

WOLFF'S LAW "GONE BAD":

- Unfortunately, too much of a good thing can occur. When excessive stress is placed on a bone (which often occurs at the joint surfaces of a bone), excessive calcium may be deposited in that bone.[12] As the bone tissue becomes denser and denser, the body starts to place calcium along the outer margins of the bone.
- This can result in what is known as a **bone spur**,[12] and the condition that results is called **degenerative joint disease (DJD)** or **osteoarthritis (OA)** (Figure 3-14, Box 3-11).

BOX 3-11

Degenerative joint disease (DJD) (or osteoarthritis [OA]) is characterized by the breakdown of articular cartilage and the presence of bone spurs on the subchondral bone (the bone located immediately under the articular cartilage).

- Although DJD is a condition of the bones and joints, its cause is excessive physical stress that is placed on these structures (Box 3-12).

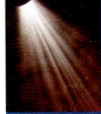

BOX 3-12   Spotlight on Degenerative Joint Disease

When muscles are chronically tight, they continually pull on their bony attachments. This constant pull creates a stress on the bones and joints, which can contribute to the progression of the arthritic changes of degenerative joint disease (DJD). Furthermore, the pain of tight muscles is very often (but not always) a major part of what is blamed as being the pain of DJD. Therefore evaluating the client's lifestyle, the tightness of the musculature, and the stresses placed on the bones by tight muscles is essential for all manual and movement therapists, instructors, and trainers.

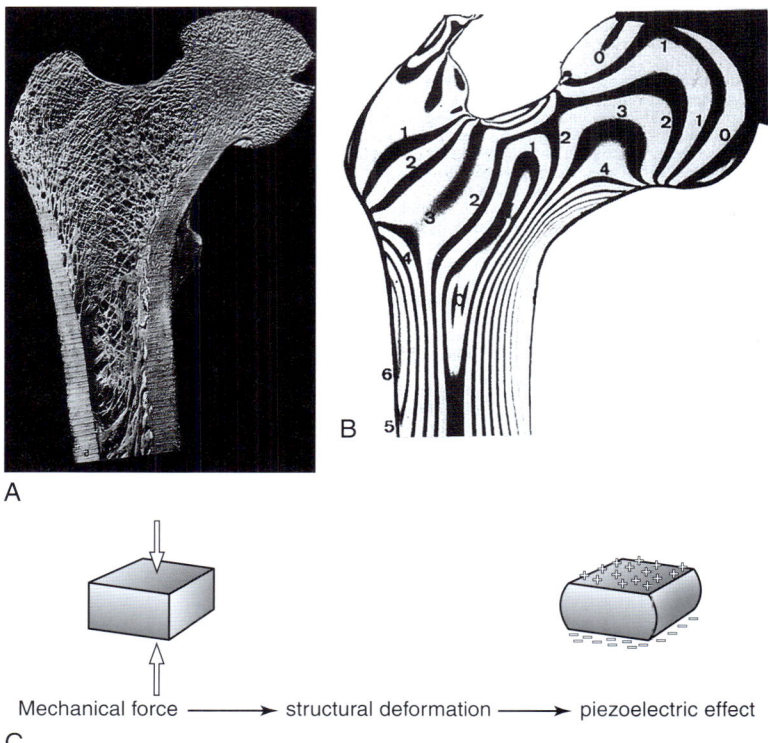

FIGURE 3-13 A, Section of the proximal femur showing the trabecular pattern of the spongy bone. **B,** Lines of stress through the proximal femur appear when the stress of weight bearing is placed on it. The trabeculae of spongy bone will align themselves along these lines of stress as a result of the piezoelectric effect. **C,** Piezoelectric effect (i.e., an electrical charge occurs in a tissue when it is subjected to a mechanical force [a stress] such as weight bearing). *(A and B, from Williams PL, editor: Gray's anatomy: the anatomical basis of clinical practice, ed 38, Edinburgh, 1995, Churchill Livingstone. C, modified from Buchwald H, Varco RL, editors: Metabolic surgery. New York, 1978, Grune & Stratton.)*

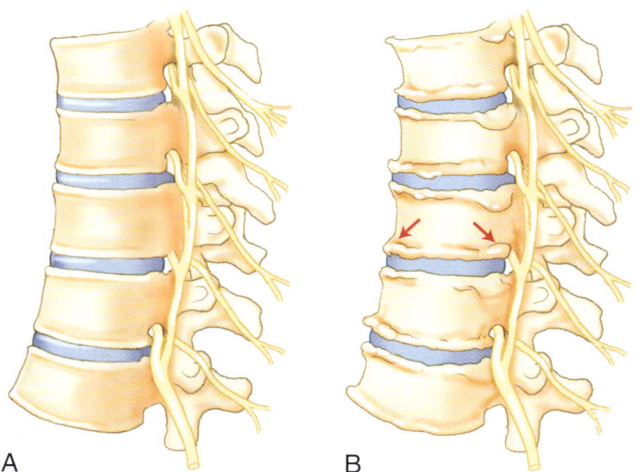

FIGURE 3-14 A, Lateral view of the vertebral column. The contours of the bodies of the vertebrae are smooth, clean, and healthy. **B,** Same view of the vertebral column is shown, this time with the presence of bone spurs (two of the bone spurs are indicated by arrows) at the margins of the vertebrae. The presence of bone spurs is indicative of degenerative joint disease (DJD) (or osteoarthritis [OA]).

SECTION 3.10   CARTILAGE TISSUE

- **Cartilage** is a type of tissue that is particularly important to the musculoskeletal system. Some of the roles of cartilage within the musculoskeletal system include the following:
  - Cartilage unites the bones of *cartilaginous joints*.[1]
  - Cartilage caps the joint (articular) surfaces of bones of synovial joints.[1]
  - Intra-articular discs that are located within many synovial joints are composed of cartilage. (For more information on cartilaginous joints, synovial joints, and intra-articular discs, see Sections 7.8, 7.9, and 7.14.)
  - Cartilage provides the framework for developing bones during the process of endochondral ossification[4] (see Section 3.6).
- Although classified as a *soft tissue*, cartilage is fairly dense and firm; it has attributes of being both partly rigid and partly flexible.
- Cartilage has a very poor blood supply and therefore has a very poor ability to heal after injury.[4]
- Most of the blood supply to cartilage comes via diffusion from blood vessels that are located in the **perichondrium**, a fibrous connective tissue that covers cartilage (Box 3-13).

BOX 3-13

Articular cartilage has no perichondrium, so its nutrient supply must come from diffusion from the synovial fluid of the joint. For this reason, articular cartilage is particularly bad at healing after an injury or damage.

- Cartilage tissue, like bone tissue, is a type of connective tissue. As such, it is composed of cartilage cells and matrix.[1]
  - The matrix of cartilage is a firm gel with fibers embedded within it.
  - Three types of cartilage exist: (1) **hyaline cartilage**, (2) **fibrocartilage**, and (3) **elastic cartilage**.

CARTILAGE CELLS:

- Two types of cartilage cells exist[1]:
  - **Chondroblasts**: Chondroblasts build up cartilage tissue by secreting the matrix tissue of the cartilage.
  - **Chondrocytes**: Once chondroblasts are mature and fully surrounded by the matrix of cartilage, they are called *chondrocytes*.
  - As in bone tissue, the cells of cartilage are said to be located within lacunae.

MATRIX:

- By definition, the components of the matrix of a connective tissue can be divided into fibers and ground substance.

Matrix Fibers:

- The fibers of cartilage are collagen and/or elastin fibers.[1]
  - Collagen fibers add to the tensile strength of cartilage.
  - **Elastin fibers** add to the elastic nature of elastic cartilage.

Matrix Ground Substance:

- The ground substance of cartilage in which the fibers are embedded is a firm gel-like organic matrix that is composed of proteoglycan molecules.[1]
- Proteoglycans are protein/polysaccharide substances that are composed primarily of glucosamine and chondroitin sulfate molecules.
- Proteoglycan molecules have feathery shapes that resemble a bottle brush in appearance.
- Proteoglycan molecules trap and hold water in the spaces that are located within and among them (Box 3-14).[1]

BOX 3-14

Chondroitin sulfate and glucosamine are nutritional supplements used in the treatment of osteoarthritis (degenerative joint disease). Chondroitin sulfate is a proteoglycan, and glucosamine is a building block of proteoglycans. Proteoglycans are found in the matrix of most all connective tissues, including cartilage. Taking these substances as nutritional supplements has recently become very popular because proteoglycans keep the connective tissue matrix of articular cartilage well hydrated (and therefore thicker and softer), so joints are better able to absorb shock without degeneration and damage.

TYPES OF CARTILAGE:

- Each one of the three types of cartilage has a slightly different structural makeup and therefore is best suited for a specific role in the body (Figure 3-15).

Hyaline Cartilage:

- Hyaline cartilage is the most common type of cartilage and resembles *milky glass* in appearance.[1]
- Hyaline cartilage is often called *articular cartilage* because it is the type of cartilage that caps the articular surfaces of the bones of synovial joints.
- Its role in capping the articular surfaces of bones is to absorb compressive shock that occurs to the joint.
- In addition to forming the articular cartilage of the joint surfaces of bones, hyaline cartilage is also found in the epiphysial plate of growing bones, forms the soft part of the nose, and is located within the rings of the respiratory passage.

Fibrocartilage:

- Fibrocartilage, as its name implies, contains a greater density of fibrous collagen fibers,[1] and therefore a lesser amount of the chondroitin sulfate ground substance.
- For this reason, fibrocartilage is the toughest form of cartilaginous tissue and is ideally suited for roles that require a great deal of tensile strength (ability to withstand being pulled and stretched).
  - Fibrocartilage is the type of cartilage that forms the union of most cartilaginous joints.
  - Examples of cartilaginous joints include the disc joints of the spine and the symphysis pubis joint of the pelvis.[12]
- Fibrocartilage is also the type of cartilage of which intra-articular discs are made.
  - Intra-articular discs are found in the sternoclavicular, wrist, and knee joints.[1]

Elastic Cartilage:

- In addition to collagen fibers, elastic cartilage also contains elastin fibers.[1]
- Therefore elastic cartilage is best suited for structures that require the firmness of cartilage but also require a great degree of elasticity.[1]
  - Elastic cartilage gives form to the external ear.
  - In addition to giving form to the ear, elastic cartilage also gives form to the epiglottis (which covers the trachea when food is swallowed) and the eustachian tube (which connects the throat to the middle ear cavity).[1]

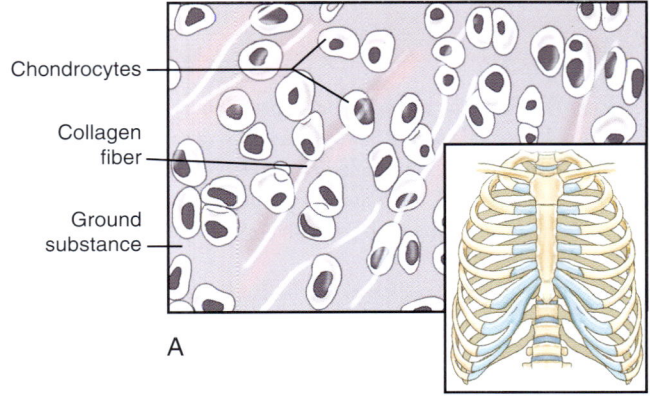

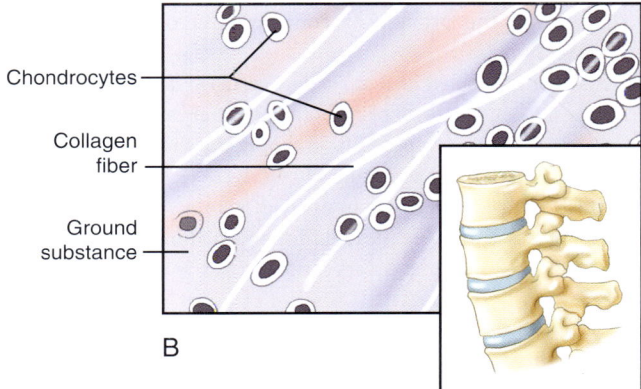

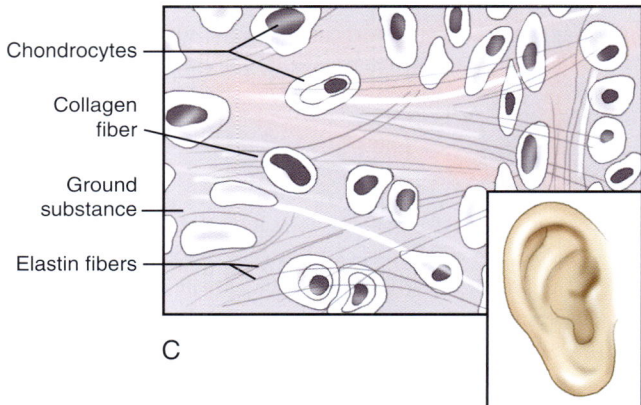

FIGURE 3-15 A, *Milky-glass* tissue composition of hyaline cartilage, the most common cartilage tissue in the body; inset shows the cartilages of the ribs (examples of hyaline cartilage). **B,** Tissue composition of fibrocartilage, containing a greater density of collagen fibers; inset shows intervertebral discs (examples of fibrocartilage). **C,** Tissue composition of elastic cartilage, containing elastin fibers in addition to collagen fibers; inset shows the ear (example of elastic cartilage).

REVIEW QUESTIONS

evolve *Answers to the following review questions appear on the Evolve website accompanying this book at:* http://evolve.elsevier.com/Muscolino/kinesiology/.

1. What are the four major classifications of bones by shape?

2. Give an example of each one of the four major classifications of bones by shape.

3. Name and describe the major structural components of a long bone.

4. What are the five major functions of bones?

5. Which function of bones is most important to the study of musculoskeletal movement and the field of kinesiology?

6. What are the two major components of bone as a connective tissue?

7. What are the functions of osteoblasts and osteoclasts?

8. Compare and contrast compact and spongy bone.

9. Where is compact bone found?

10. Where is spongy bone found?

11. Compare and contrast the two different methods of bone growth (endochondral and intramembranous ossification).

12. What is the importance of fontanels to bodywork?

13. What are the four major fontanels? Where are they located? When does each one close?

14. What are the steps involved in fracture healing?

15. What is Wolff's law, and how does the piezoelectric effect explain it?

16. How do tight muscles relate to Wolff's law, the development of DJD, and the role of a manual or movement therapist or trainer when working on a client who has DJD?

17. What are the three major types of cartilage tissue?

REFERENCES

1. Watkins J: Structure and function of the musculoskeletal system, Champaign, Ill, 1999, Human Kinetics.
2. Thibodeau GA, Patton KT: Anatomy & physiology, ed 5, St Louis, 2002, Mosby.
3. Hall SJ: Basic biomechanics, ed 6, New York, 2012, McGraw Hill.
4. White TD, Folkens PA: Human osteology, ed 22, San Diego, 2000, Academic Press.
5. McGinnis PM: Biomechanics of sport and exercise, ed 2, Champaign, Ill, 2005, Human Kinetics.
6. Harman E: Biomechanics of resistance exercise. In Baechle TR, Earle RE, editors: Essentials of strength training and conditioning, ed 3, Champaign, Ill, 2008, Human Kinetics.
7. Netter FH: Atlas of human anatomy, ed 3, Teterboro, 2004, Icon Learning Systems.
8. Lieber, RL: Skeletal muscle, structure, function, and plasticity: the physiological basis of rehabilitation, ed 2, Baltimore, 2002, Lippincott Williams & Wilkins.
9. McArdle WD, Katch FI, Katch VL: Essentials of exercise physiology, Media, 1994, Williams & Wilkins.
10. Palastonga N, Field D, Soares R: Anatomy and human movement: Structure and function, ed 4, Oxford, 2002, Butterworth-Heinmann.
11. Ratamess NA: Adaptations to anaerobic training programs. In Baechle TR, Earle RE, editors: Essentials of strength training and conditioning, ed 3, Champaign, Ill, 2008, Human Kinetics.
12. Neumann DA: Kinesiology of the musculoskeletal system: Foundations for physical rehabilitation, ed 3, St Louis, 2017, Elsevier.
13. Enoka RM: Neuromechanics of human movement, ed 3, Champaign, Ill, 2002, Human Kinetics.

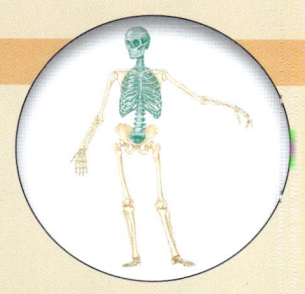

CHAPTER 4
Fascia

Co-authored by Thomas Myers and Joseph Muscolino

CHAPTER OUTLINE

Section 4.1	Fascia	Section 4.4	Tendons and Ligaments
Section 4.2	The Fascial Web	Section 4.5	Bursae and Tendon Sheaths
Section 4.3	Fascial Response to Physical Stress	Section 4.6	Properties of Fascial Connective Tissues

CHAPTER OBJECTIVES

After completing this chapter, the student should be able to perform the following:

1. Define the key terms of this chapter and state the meanings of the word origins of this chapter.
2. Compare and contrast fibrous fascia and loose fascia.
3. Describe the structure and function of the fascial web.
4. Describe the two major responses of fascia to physical stress.
5. Do the following related to tendons and ligaments:
   ○ Compare and contrast the structure and function of tendons and ligaments.
   ○ Explain why tendons and ligaments do not heal well when injured.
6. Compare and contrast the structure and function of bursae and tendon sheaths.
7. Do the following related to properties of fascial connective tissues:
   ○ Compare and contrast the concepts of elasticity and plasticity.
   ○ Relate the concepts of creep, thixotropy, and hysteresis to the fields of manual and movement therapy.

OVERVIEW

Many tissues contribute to the structure and function of the skeletal system. Chapter 3 covered bone tissue and cartilage. This chapter examines fascia tissue in detail. The beginning sections examine fascial tissue macrostructure, microstructure, functions, and physiology. The later sections of this chapter then cover specific fascial macrostructures such as tendon, ligament, bursa, and tendon sheath. The last section then covers the general properties that apply to all fascial/connective tissues.

KEY TERMS

Adipocytes (a-DIP-o-sites)
Alpha–smooth muscle actin (AL-fa)
Anatomy train
Aponeurosis, pl. aponeuroses (AP-o-noo-RO-sis, AP-o-noo-RO-seez)
Areolar fascia (AIR-ee-o-lar)
Bursa, pl. bursae (BER-sa, BER-ee)
Bursitis (ber-SIGH-tis)
Cell-to-cell web
Chondroitin sulfate (kon-DROY-tin SUL-fate)
Contractility
Creep (KREEP)
Deep fascia (FASH-a)
Dense fascia (FASH-a)
Elasticity
Elastin fibers (ee-LAS-tin)

Extracellular matrix
Extracellular-to-intracellular web
Fascia (FASH-a)
Fascial net (FASH-al)
Fascial web
Fibroblast (FI-bro-blast)
Fibronectin molecules (FI-bro-NECK-tin)
Fibrous fascia (FI-brus FASH-a)
Focal adhesion molecules
Gel state (JEL)
Glucosamine (glue-KOS-a-meen)
Hysteresis (his-ter-E-sis)
Integrin molecules (in-TEG-rin)
Langer's lines (LANG-ers)
Ligament (LIG-a-ment)
Loose fascia

Macrophages (MA-kro-fazsh-is)
Mast cells
Myofascial meridian (MY-o-FASH-al)
Myofibroblast (MY-o-FI-bro-blast)
Plasticity (plas-TIS-i-tee)
Protomyofibroblast (PRO-to-MY-o-FI-bro-blast)
Reticular fibers (re-TIK-you-lar)
Retinaculum, pl. retinacula (ret-i-NAK-you-lum, ret-i-NAK-you-la)
Sol state (SOLE)
Sprain
Strain
Stretch

Subcutaneous fascia (SUB-cue-TANE-ee-us FASH-a)
Synovial tendon sheath (si-NO-vee-al)
Tendinitis (ten-di-NI-tis)
Tendon
Tendon sheath
Tenosynovitis (TEN-o-sin-o-VI-tis)
Tensile (TEN-sile)
Tensile strength
Thixotropy (thik-SOT-tro-pee)
Viscoelasticity (VIS-ko-ee-las-TIS-i-tee)
Viscoplasticity (VIS-ko-plas-TIS-i-tee)
Weight bearing

WORD ORIGINS

- A (an)—From Latin *a*, meaning *not, without*
- Adip—From Latin *adeps*, meaning *fat*
- Fascia—From Latin *fascia*, meaning *bandage, band*
- Fibr, fibro—From Latin *fibra*, meaning *fiber*
- Itis—From Greek *itis*, meaning *inflammation*
- Myo—From Greek *mys*, meaning *muscle*
- Ology—From Greek *logos*, meaning *study of, discourse, word*
- Piezo—From Greek *piesis*, meaning *pressure*
- Proto—From Greek *protos*, meaning *first*
- Tens—From Latin *tensio*, meaning *a stretching*

SECTION 4.1 FASCIA

FASCIA DEFINED:

- As described in Section 3.4, connective tissue is the most diverse of the four major types of tissues, protecting and providing functioning form for the softer muscle, nerve, and epithelial tissues. Ever since individual cells began to coalesce into multicellular organisms some billion years ago, connective tissues have taken on the job of secreting a wide range of bio-materials with which they surround all these other specialized tissues to give them a strong but pliable substrate and to give us a shape that can deal with the endogenous and exogenous forces our movement and gravity create.
- The resulting building blocks of our shape serve many purposes from the cornea of the eye to the dentin in the teeth to the valves of the heart, running from bone and cartilage, the previously described "hard" varieties, to the viscous fluids of fat, blood, and lymph. In between, in the kinesiological sphere, which is the subject of this book, are a number of soft fibrous connective tissues popularly known as **fascia** (plural: fasciae).
- Medically defined, **fascia** includes only sheets of fibrous tissue that can be separately dissected, such as the subcutaneous fascia, Scarpa's fascia, the plantar fascia, the fascia latae, et al.[1] For the purposes of this chapter, we expand the definition to include all the collagenous soft-tissues that perform a structural role, stretching this classical definition in order to emphasize that all these tissues work together as a system.[2] Our method of anatomy—the scalpel—emphasizes separations, but histological examination shows that—except in the synovial joint spaces—there is no clear separation between the various named soft-tissue layers and structures, which are continuous from skin to bone.[3] Therefore all the collagenous soft tissues can be seen to act within a single system—our biomechanical regulatory system. For lack of a better word, *fascia* fills this semantic gap.
- We are well aware—as we tackle a problem in the median nerve, for example—that we are working within the body-wide nervous system. Viewing the brachial artery, we understand it as embedded within the entire circulatory system. When someone shows up with plantar fasciitis, however, therapists tend to view (and treat) this condition as if it were a failure of an isolated structure within the foot. We appropriate the word *fascia* to emphasize the systemic nature of the "fibrous body"—a third interactive and self-regulating system of shape and biomechanics. In actuality, the controlling factor for plantar fasciitis may well exist at some distance from the problem—commonly residing in the leg or even in the pelvis or neck.[4]
- Thus our appropriation of the word *fascia* for this subset of soft connective tissues does not conform to the anatomical tradition. Other inclusive terms, however, lead to other problems. *Connective tissue* itself includes the blood and immune cells outside the structural function we emphasize here.[5] *Extracellular matrix* includes all these building materials, but it also includes a lot of other exudates not involved in maintaining posture and movement and excludes the fibroblasts and other cells that create, repair, and remodel these materials to suit the forces we place upon them with our activities.[6] Until a better term is agreed upon for our system of biomechanical autoregulation, we will follow other writers and researchers in using the term *fascia* to designate this system.
- Well-named, connective tissues are all connected to each other, connect and enclose all the other body tissues, and in this way connect all the branches of medicine.[7] In fact, however, these

sheets and bags also separate structures from each other, directing specific flow of fluids and transfer of forces. By forming tightly woven sacs, our fascia is able to support the two-thirds of us that is water up off the surface of the earth. Nearly every organ—the brain, the heart, the liver, the kidney, and each and every muscle—is contained in fascial sacs that at once contain each organ within its confines as well as allowing (or not, if it is adhesed) a lubricated movement between each organ and adjacent structures.[8]

TYPES OF FASCIA:

- The term *fascia* derives from the Latin meaning *bandage* or *bundle*, in that it wraps around and bundles (i.e., connects) structures (Box 4-1). The word reminds us of the Aesop's fable of the farmer who came across his three sons fighting over their inheritance. The farmer picked up three sticks and broke each easily over his knee. He took another three sticks and bundled them together to demonstrate that they could not be broken as long as they remained united. The Romans adapted this story into a symbol of their power, the *fasces*, which was a bundle of rods bound around an ex, an outward representation of the strength through unity—later appropriated in a negative way into the concept of Fascism. (Tired of being called "fascists," those of us advocating for the new understanding of *fascia* explored in these pages prefer the term *afascianado*.[9])

BOX 4-1

The terms fascia and fascism share the same Latin word root origin, fascia, which means bandage. Fascial tissue is so named because like a bandage, it wraps around and connects structures. Fascism derives from the Latin word fasces, which was a bundle of rods tied (bandaged) around an axe, and was an ancient Roman symbol of authority. The symbolism of the fasces represented strength through unity because whereas a single rod is easily broken, a bundle is difficult to break.

- In a similar way, no one element of our fascial system is strong, but bundled together from microscopic elements into macroscopic structures, they can be stronger than steel of comparable weight, yet pliable, elastic, efficient, and adjustable—a nearly miraculous example of what Walter Cannon called "the wisdom of the body."[10]
- While the system is everywhere continuous from one structure to another and strict boundaries are difficult to define, it is still a useful exercise to distinguish the components of fascia and the generalized types of structures they create. For example, fasciae are often named, and therefore subdivided, based on the region of the body where they are located. By this naming system, fasciae are usually divided into myofascial, arthrofascial, visceral, and subcutaneous fascial tissues.
  - Myofascial tissue concerns itself with the fascia of the musculature.
  - Arthrofascial tissue is the intrinsic fascial tissue of joints. It includes the fibrous joint capsule and ligaments.
  - Visceral fascial tissue is involved with the internal visceral organs of the body cavities.
  - Subcutaneous fascial tissue is the fascia located immediately deep to the skin.
- Fasciae are often further divided into two main structural types, **fibrous fascia** and **loose fascia**.
  - Fibrous fascia is often called **deep fascia**, which includes many types of **dense fascia**.
  - Loose fascia is often called **areolar fascia**, including the **subcutaneous fascia** just beneath your skin.
- Fibrous fascia is composed primarily of tough collagen fibers. It inhabits the bone and cartilage already discussed, as well as the ligaments, periostea, tendons, aponeuroses, and membranous coverings of muscle tissue that bind muscles to bones and other structures, as well as connect and ensheath muscle fibers. These examples of fibrous fascia are often called *muscular fascia* (Box 4-2) or *myofascia*. Note: For more on myofascia, see Section 12.4.

BOX 4-2

Fascial collagen fibers of the peri- and endomysium of muscles fibers have a spider-webby appearance. Gil Hedley, educator and author, has coined the term *fuzz* to describe fibrous fascia.

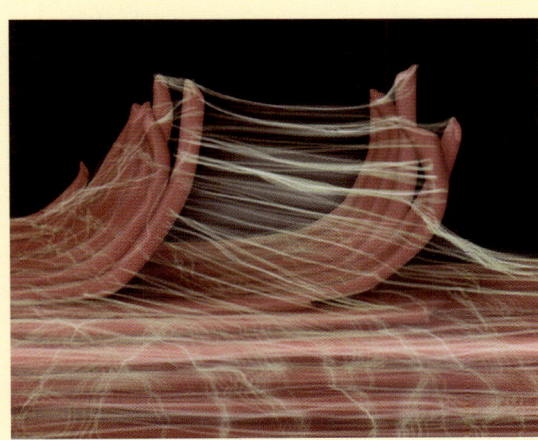

Reproduced with kind permission from Joseph E. Muscolino. Modeled from a photo by Ronald Thompson.

- Loose fascia is primarily composed of ground substance (see *Components of Fascia*, immediately following) that mixes fluid, gel, and various types of collagen and elastin fibers, more loosely woven. This amorphous fascia is found in every area of the body, including the layer directly under the skin that simultaneously acts to bind the dermis layer of the skin while allowing it to move easily in any direction. Loose fascia also allows movement in the underlying visceral organs and between skeletal muscles.
- It is worth noting that the tolerance of this tissue for movement is not limitless: areolar tissue becomes a very effective force transmitter when it reaches its elastic limit. To see this for yourself, put a finger on the opposite forearm and move the skin 1 cm in any direction; it will move easily. Now move the skin away from

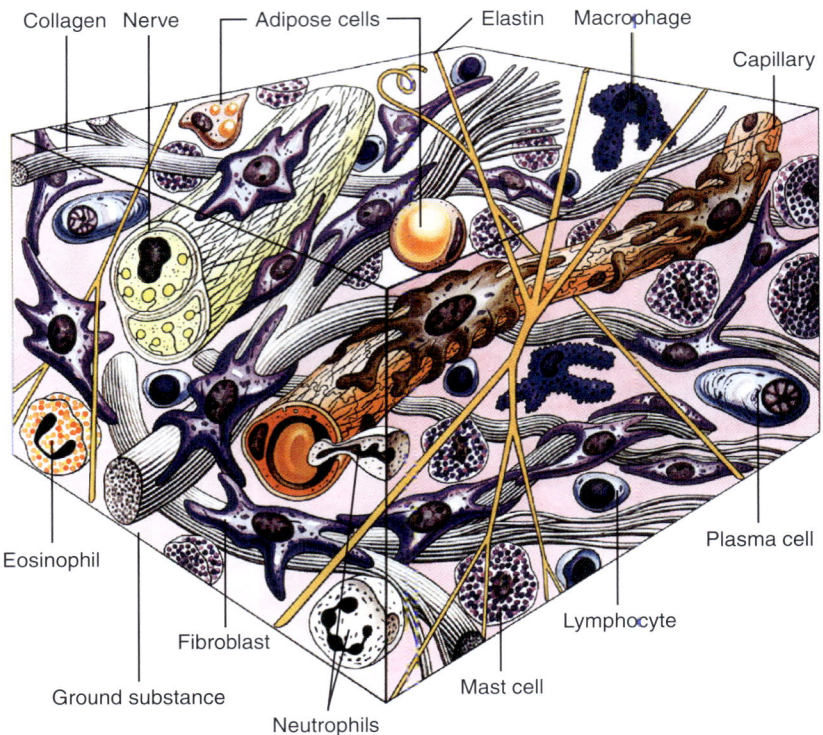

FIGURE 4-1 Fascia is composed of cells, fibers, and fluid/gel-like ground substance (with proteoglycans—not pictured). *(From Williams PL, ed:* Gray's anatomy: the anatomical basis of clinical practice, *ed 38, Edinburgh, 1995, Churchill Livingstone.)*

your wrist and toward your elbow 3 to 5 cm, and you will feel how the motion reaches a limit and suddenly you can feel the pull down to your wrist. This shows that areolar tissue, which commonly is cut away as insignificant intermuscular lubricating tissue, is in fact, a vital part of myofascial force transmission.[11]
- Although fibrous/dense fascia and loose fascia can appear quite different from each other, they share the same characteristic components and construction and actually form a continuum with each other. Dense fascia contains a greater proportion of fibers; loose fascia contains a greater proportion of fluid/gel-like ground substance. Let us now explore these components.

COMPONENTS OF FASCIA:

- Fascia, like all connective tissues, is composed of three elements: cells, fibers, and ground substance (Figure 4-1). Note: The term **extracellular matrix** (ECM) is often used to describe the fibers and ground substance of fascia, but the ECM includes other components of lymph, cytokines, and other cellular-exchange molecules that are not part of the "fibrous body" we are considering here.

Cells:

- There are many different types of cells found in fascia. **Fibroblasts** (Figure 4-2) are by far the most common, and they come in several varieties. There are also **mast cells**, **macrophages**, plasma cells and other white blood cells, and **adipocytes**.
  - Mast cells are responsible for the secretion of histamine, a chemical involved in inflammation.
  - Macrophages are phagocytic cells that engulf large substances, including invading pathogenic microorganisms.
  - Plasma and other white blood cells are involved in fighting infection.
  - Adipocytes (also known as fat cells) store fat.
  - Fibroblasts have many functions:
    - They produce the ground substance of fascia, as well as the precursors for all the fibers that are found in fascia.
    - They can also resorb, or break down, fascia by secreting enzymes (proteinases, metallurases) that cut up and recycle "old" or damaged fascial arrays.
    - They are involved in inflammation and wound healing, working to bring the edges of the wound back together.
    - They are responsive to physical stresses placed on them. When physical stress is placed on fibroblasts, especially

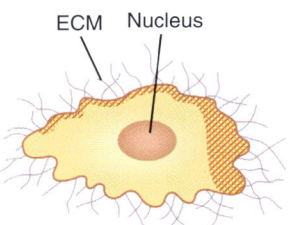

FIGURE 4-2 Fibroblast. Fibroblasts are the most common cell found in fascia. *(Modified from Tomasek J et al: Nature reviews, Molecular Cell Biology, 2002. In Myers T:* Anatomy trains, *ed 2, Edinburgh, 2009, Churchill Livingstone/Elsevier.)*

tensile (pulling) force, fibroblasts respond by lining up along the line of pull and secreting proteins to make the collagenous arrays resistive to the force.
- In relaxed tissue, the fibroblasts spread their processes within the fibrous net, rather like the dendrites of a nerve, in order to monitor and repair their area of the fascial web. Many times these processes touch processes from neighboring fibroblasts, thus forming a "syncytium" (**cell-to-cell web** continuity) similar to the more familiar neural and vascular syncytia.[12] When the fibrous network is tensed, when more forces pass through the tissue, the fibroblasts retract their "arms" toward the cell body, to prepare to respond to the greater forces by manufacturing more collagen or strengthen existing connections to meet the increased force.

Fibers:

- Fibroblasts manufacture three types of fibers that are commonly found in fascia. They are **collagen fibers**, **elastin fibers**, and **reticular fibers** (Figure 4-3). These fibers are impervious to water (hydrophobic); they are more-or-less wet all the time, like everything in the body, but they do not absorb or bind with water.
  - Elastin fibers are responsible for the property of sustained elasticity, which is the ability to return to a shortened state after being stretched for a sustained period of time. You can pull on your ear for a full minute, but the second you let it go, it will snap back to its original shape like a rubber band—the yellowish elastin fibers are responsible for this property. (Collagen fibers are also elastic, but they have the "rebound" of a steel ball bounced on a cement sidewalk—it is a short and sharp elasticity, with a high "coefficient of restitution."[13])
  - Reticular fibers are a type of collagen fiber (Type III). They are given the name *reticular fibers* because they are cross-linked to form a fine meshwork, also known as a *reticulum*. These "immature" collagen fibers are produced mostly in the embryo, though some survive into adulthood, but what their function is in the adult is not known.
  - By far the most common fiber type found in fascia is collagen. There are approximately 26 different types of collagen fibers, named Type I, Type II, Type III, Type IV, and so on. The basic molecular structure of collagen is the same for all types, with differences in the length and composition of the side-chains.

- Type I is the most common. It forms extremely strong fibrils that are inextensible, that is, they are highly resistant to tensile (pulling) forces. Therefore collagen is said to have great **tensile strength**. Because of its great tensile strength, collagen is the principal component of tendons, aponeuroses, and ligaments. Tendons and aponeuroses function to transfer pulling forces from the muscle belly to the muscle's attachment (often on bone). Ligaments function to resist pulling forces that might otherwise tear and/or dislocate the joint (and ligaments can also be reinforced by muscles in a variety of ways[14]). These tissues also demonstrate elasticity, but the stored tension must be released within a short time (within about a second)—such as when the Achilles tendon is stretched during running and "gives back" the stored energy during the push-off phase a second later.

Ground Substance:

- The term **ground substance** is used to describe the medium in which the cells and fibers of fascia are located. It can be thought of as the *background* medium. Ground substance ranges in quality from being a fluid (such as synovial fluid) to a gel (cartilage is the most "gelled" of these tissues). It is essentially a fluid solution in which many large water-loving (hydrophilic) molecules are suspended.
- The majority of these molecules are called **proteoglycans** because they have a protein and a carbohydrate component (*proteo* refers to protein; *glycan* refers to carbohydrate). A well-known proteoglycan used as a nutritional supplement is **chondroitin sulfate**. **Glucosamine**, another nutritional supplement, is a building block of proteoglycans.
- Proteoglycan molecules have a feathery shape that resembles a fern in appearance (Figure 4-4). They function to bind to and trap water in the spaces among them—in the same fashion that a small packet of Jell-O® binds a large bowl of water. By so doing, they keep the ground substance hydrated and prevent fascia from drying out and becoming brittle and also provide a shock-absorbing viscosity.[15]
- Keeping tissue hydrated creates the gel-like consistency that is characteristic of fascia, especially loose fascia. This gel-like consistency is important to lubricate fascial planes and its viscosity absorbs and dissipates forces that are placed on it, especially quick compression forces. In dehydrated fascia, the "ferns"

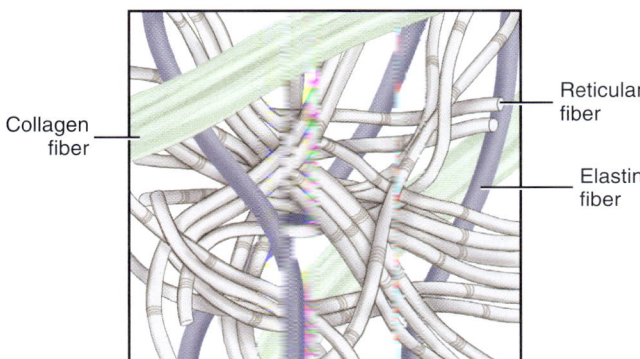

FIGURE 4-3 Collagen, elastin, and reticular fibers of fascial tissue.

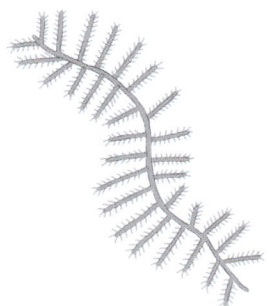

FIGURE 4-4 Proteoglycan molecules of fascial ground substance resemble a bottle brush in appearance. They function to bind and trap water in the ground substance, thereby keeping the ground substance well hydrated.

- of the proteoglycans curl up, inhibiting "glide" and perfusion/hydration through the neighboring cells.
- Ground substance is also important for creating the fluid medium that is necessary for the transfer of nutrients and other substances between arterial, venous, and lymphatic capillary networks and cells. All the tissues of the body must dance between the viscosity required to stay together in a coherent shape and the hydration required for perfusion to and from the cells.
- Thicker gel-like consistency in the ground substance is not all pathological—it forms a sticky thicket to impede the passage and isolate pathogenic microorganisms that might cause infection.
- As previously stated, the distinction between fibrous fascia and loose fascia is one of degrees of the relative proportions of fibers and ground substance. In fact, some sources consider cartilage and bone tissues to be essentially more rigid forms of fascia, given that they are constructed in a similar way.

SECTION 4.2   THE FASCIAL WEB

FASCIAL WEB:

- From a larger design viewpoint, the various fasciae of the body interweave into one another to create a **fascial web** or **fascial net** (Figure 4-5, Box 4-3).

Anatomy of the Fascial Web:

- The fascial web suspends and supports the entire body. Indeed, if all the cells could be magically rendered invisible, the collagenous system would form a perfect three-dimensional model of the body. Other than the fascial system, this claim can be made for only the arteriovenous (cardiovascular) and nervous

BOX 4-3

The collagen fibers of the dermis and aponeurotic sheets of deep fibrous fascia have a discernible direction, like grain in wood. The directional lines of these fibers are called **Langer's lines** (see accompanying illustration). An application of this knowledge is that when a CORE myofascial therapist performs spreading strokes, they are applied in accordance with Langer's lines.

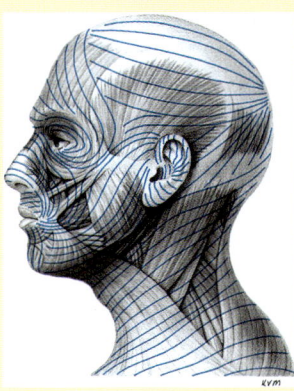

Modeled from Standring S, ed: *Gray's anatomy: the anatomical basis of clinical practice,* ed 38, Edinburgh, 1995, Churchill Livingstone.

systems. This web not only connects each of the regions of the body to one another, it also connects external with internal structures from just under epithelium of the skin deep into the bones, organs, and brain. This fascial web so permeates the body as to be part of the immediate environment of every cell. Given the mechanical protein connections that cross the membrane to connect to the cytoskeleton, tugging on the web can even affect the functioning of the cells (see below).

Physiology of the Fascial Web:

- The functions of the fascial web are many. As stated, on a local level the ground substance of the web provides a fluid/gel medium through which nutrients, enzymes, cytokines, and neuropeptides perfuse to the cells, and carbon dioxide, waste, and messenger molecules pass back from each cell to the bloodstream. In addition, the sticky gel-like consistency of the ground substance provides an ideal setting in which the immune system's "policemen" of white blood cells and phagocytic macrophages

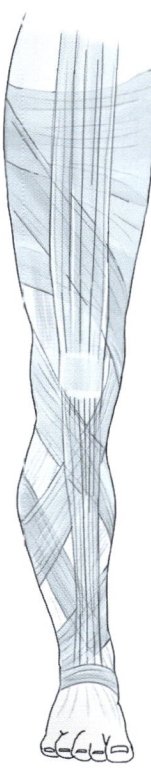

FIGURE 4-5 The fascia of the thigh seamlessly weaves into the fascia of the leg, which weaves into the fascia of the foot. In a similar fashion, lower extremity fascia weaves into the fascia of the axial body, which also weaves into the fascia of the upper extremity. Although it is possible to speak of the many fasciae of the body, it is perhaps more accurate to speak of a singular fascial web that envelops the entire body. *(From Paoletti S:* The fasciae: anatomy, dysfunction and treatment, *Seattle, 2006, Eastland Press.)*

lie in wait to resist infection by pathogenic microorganisms if the skin barrier is broken.
○ Now let's turn our attention to the *body-wide* functions of the fascial web. The two major body-wide functions are creating a "skeletal" framework and transmitting tension forces throughout the body.

Skeletal Framework:
○ The fascial web is a necessary complement to the skeletal framework; together, the web and framework truly connect and support all parts of the body. Not only does this network form the *immediate environment of each* of the cells, most cells are firmly "Velcro®-ed" to the net with up to thousands of tiny adhesive bonds. (The "free swimming" red blood cells (erythrocytes) are the exceptions, but even they can be "caught up" in these connections, for repair, recycling, or in pathological or toxic conditions.) Contrary to our common conception, cells do not simply float within the body but are instead held in place by several hundred types of these adhesive molecules.[16] Thus all cells are connected biomechanically to one another, and the messages of mechanics—tension and compression and their relatives, shear, bending, and torsion—that run through the fascial net are also transmitted to the cells (Figure 4-6).
○ At this intimate level, the fascial web continues even more deeply to create an **extracellular–intracellular web**, connecting the fascia outside of the cells to the internal cytoskeleton framework within the cells (Figure 4-7). These connections are made via internal cytoskeletal contractile actin filaments and compression-resistant microtubules attached to the cell's membrane via larger internal **focal adhesion molecules**. These focal adhesion molecules then attach to **integrin molecules** (or other molecules in this adhesive clan) that traverse the cell membrane to then connect to **fibronectin molecules** (or other mucus-like ground substance molecules) just outside the cell. These fibronectin molecules are attached in turn to collagen fibers in the fascial web. Thus the fascial web is truly an intimate connecting network that communicates externally and internally with every cell of the body from the DNA to the coordination of organismic movement!

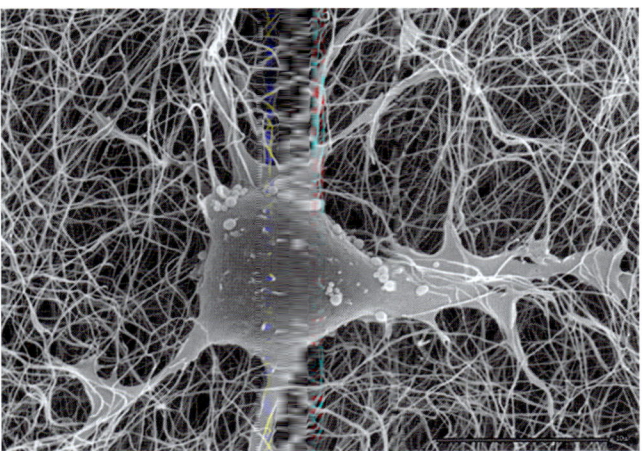

FIGURE 4-6 The fascial web extends down to the cellular level, creating a fine meshwork of intercellular fibers that attach to and connect every cell. *(From Jiang H, Grinnell F: Cell-matrix entanglement and mechanical anchorage of fibroblasts in three-dimensional collagen matrices, Molecular Biology of the Cell 16:5070-5076, 2005.)*

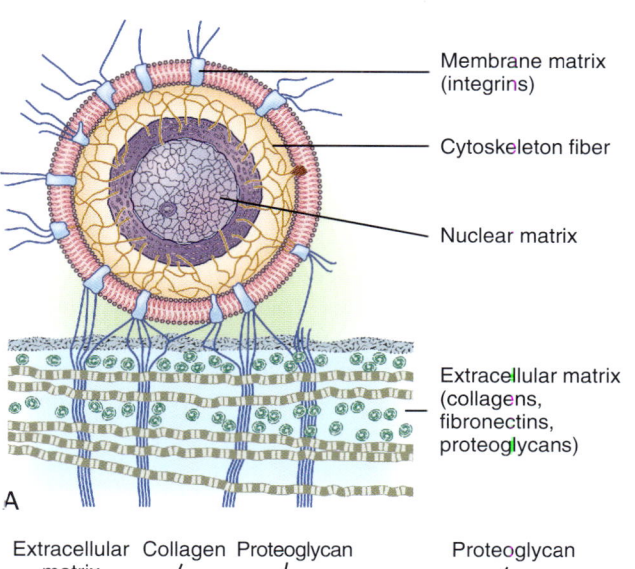
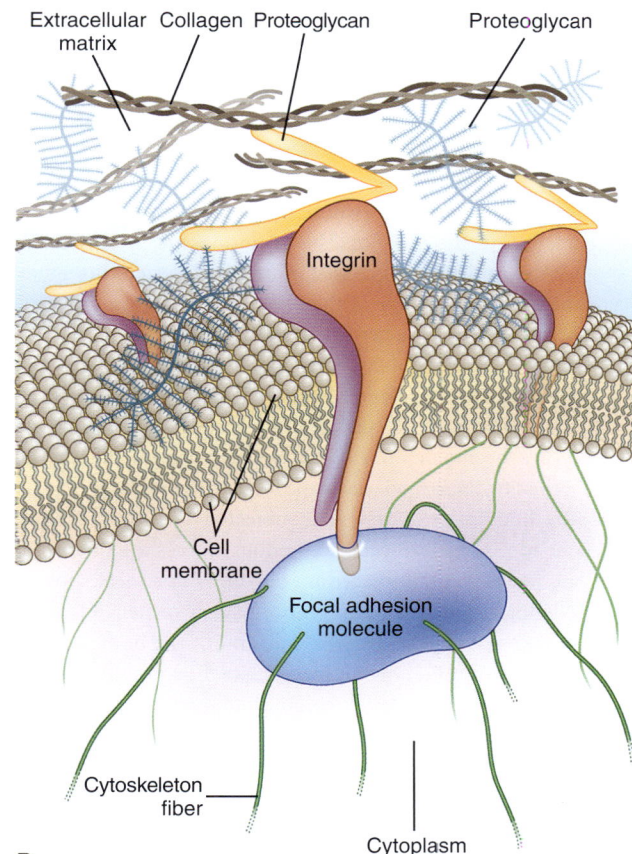

FIGURE 4-7 The fascial web of the extracellular matrix extends even more intimately to connect to the interior of cells via fibronectin molecules, integrins, focal adhesion molecules, and internal cytoskeletal (actin) fibers. **A,** Broad view. **B,** Detailed view. *(A, Reprinted from Pianta KJ, Coffey DS: Medical Hypotheses, "Cellular harmonic information transfer through a tissue tensegrity-matrix system," Jan 1991. With permission from Elsevier. B, From Tomasek J et al: Nature reviews, Molecular Cell Biology, 2002. In Myers T: Anatomy trains, ed 2, Edinburgh, 2009, Churchill Livingstone/Elsevier.)*

○ These connections have already been shown to affect cell function and even gene expression within the cell. Thus body movement—especially the organized body movement of exercise, stretching, walking, working, and sport—does more than just up the circulation to and metabolism of our cells; it can actually change how well the cells function. Cells in their "happy" mechanical environment do their job properly; cells that are overstretched or compressed sometimes cannot express their genes fully and instead spend their energy dealing with the mechanical stress. These mechanisms point to an explanation for why a program of movement can have totally unexpected health benefits to digestion, cognition, menstrual cycles, and other physiological measures not directly connected to exercise.

Transmit Tension Forces:

○ Not only does fascia function to transmit tension force locally (for example, between a muscle belly and its bony attachment, or between two bones via a ligament), it distributes and disperses forces globally. By virtue of the interconnectedness of the entire fascial web, forces are communicated throughout the entire body (see Section 12.14 on *Tensegrity*). These transmitted forces are of two types: internal and external.

  ○ Internal (endogenous) forces are created by the pressure and tension generated within the body—mostly by the contraction of the muscles. The jaw brings the teeth together with considerable force that must be dissipated throughout the head—this is one of the reasons we need a round skull. Breathing creates a series of forces that are handled by the bones, muscles, and fascia around the ventral cavity. Beyond the muscles, the visceral organs themselves are held to the body wall by fascial sacs and membranes, and in gait and sport, the momentum of the visceral organs must be absorbed by these fasciae and the biomechanical body.

  ○ The body is of course also subjected to forces from the outside. These external (exogenous) forces are often pulling forces that are placed on our body at a local spot: for example, someone pulling on our arm to help lift us up from a seated position, the collision of the body with the earth in running, or the force created by grabbing onto a pole with a hand and swinging our body around it. The application of these forces would likely cause damage to our body at the point where they were applied if the force were not resisted by the tensile force of fascia, as well as absorbed by being transferred and dissipated over more of the fascial web.

  ○ These forces—gravity chief among them—also create compressive loads through the fascial web. Jumping off a stool creates large forces on the bottoms of the feet when we land; these forces are of course handled by the skeleton in part, but these forces are also distributed to the ligaments, tendons, and other containing fascial sheets at the speed of sound.

○ Muscles create internal forces that not only act locally at their points of attachment, but via the fascial web can be transmitted to distant sites in the body. In this manner the fascia can be looked on as ropes that travel throughout the entire body, anchoring at certain attachment points and then continuing. These fascial ropes transfer the pulling forces from anchor point to anchor point throughout the body. Although the muscles are the motors of these pulling forces locally, they are transmitted at a distance by the associated myofascia and deep fascia (Figure 4-8).

○ In this way, we can see the muscles not simply as local movers but as contractile organs embedded within a body-wide fascial webbing. A **myofascial meridian** (also known as an **anatomy train**) maps traceable tracks of muscles and fascia running in more or less straight lines within the body.[17] In effect, the muscles of a myofascial meridian are connected by fibrous fascia connective tissue so that they can act together synergistically, transmitting tension and movement through the meridian by means of their contractions and thus handling both the endogenous and exogenous forces without damaging our delicate biology. (For more on myofascial meridians, see Section 12.14.)

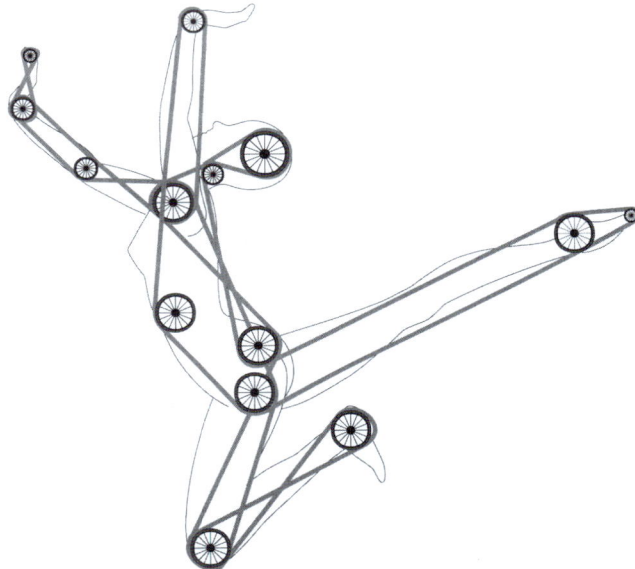

FIGURE 4-8 The myofascial web as viewed by Serge Paoletti is likened to a series of ropes that interconnect the body. Individual muscles may anchor at their attachment sites, but via the interconnected web their forces transfer beyond and travel throughout the entire body. *(From Paoletti S:* The fasciae: anatomy, dysfunction and treatment, *Seattle, 2006, Eastland Press.)*

SECTION 4.3 FASCIAL RESPONSE TO PHYSICAL STRESS

○ Fascial tissue responds to sustained physical stress placed on it by remodeling itself to deal with and resist that specific stress. This occurs via the creation and orientation of increased collagen fibers as a result of the piezoelectric effect that is produced by the physical force. Fascial tissue also responds to physical stress by the formation of cells called *myofibroblasts*.

THE PIEZOELECTRIC EFFECT:

○ When pressure or tension is placed on fascia, a slight electric charge results; this is known as the **piezoelectric effect**. *Piezo* means *pressure* (the piezoelectric effect on bone tissue was discussed in Section 3.9). This electric field causes the long polarized collagen molecules to orient themselves relative to that field (Figure 4-9). This results in the fibers being laid down along the line of force that caused the piezoelectric effect to occur, thereby reinforcing and strengthening the fascia within that line. Most often, these forces are tensile pulling forces. Therefore the reinforced fascia's increased tensile strength enables it to better resist that tension (Figure 4-10, Box 4-4).

MYOFIBROBLAST FORMATION:

○ Fascial sheets subjected to physical stress can in certain situations also increase their strength by the formation of special cells called **myofibroblasts**. The root *myo* comes from the Latin word for muscle, indicating that myofibroblasts have the ability to contract as muscle tissue does. This contractile ability is a result of the presence of **alpha-smooth muscle actin** filaments. These cells can thus be thought of as transitional between fibroblasts and smooth muscle cells.

○ The number of myofibroblasts present within a fascial tissue varies from place to place and person to person, but their activity increases based on the degree of physical stress that the fascial tissue is experiencing (and chemical stimulation as well, see below). Myofibroblasts are very active in wound healing, for instance, where the altered stress in the fascia underlying the skin stimulates the myofibroblasts to proliferate to pull the edges of the tissue back together. As greater and greater tensile forces are placed on the fascia, more and more myofibroblasts develop from the normal fibroblasts of the fascial tissue (Figure 4-11). The process gradually

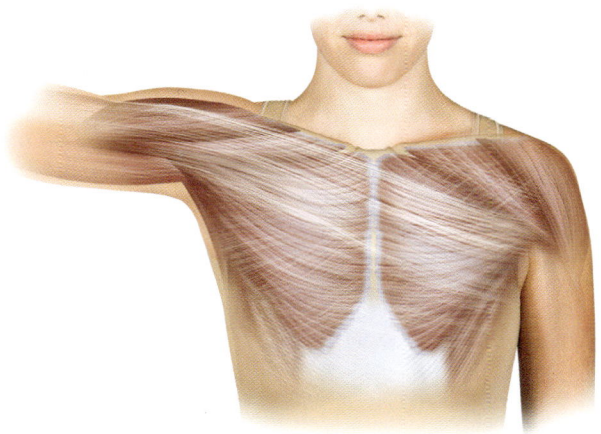

FIGURE 4-10 Superficial pectoral fascia of the sternal region of the trunk is seen. The fascia from the top right to bottom left (from our perspective: top left to bottom right) is clearly denser than the fascia that runs from the top left to the bottom right (from our perspective: top right to bottom left). This likely indicates that this individual experienced greater physical stresses through the right arm, perhaps from being right-handed. (Reproduced with kind permission from Joseph E. Muscolino. Modeled from a photo by Ronald Thompson.)

transforms a normal fibroblast into a **protomyofibroblast** and then into a fully mature myofibroblast. Myofibroblasts develop increased alpha–smooth muscle actin filaments that attach into focal adhesion molecules, which attach through the membrane into the fibers of the ground substance (extracellular matrix), and thereby into the fascial web. These myofibroblasts can then create an active pulling force that counters and opposes the pulling force that the fascial tissue is experiencing. In large sheets such as the thoracolumbar fascia or crural fascia, the combined effect of the myofibroblasts can cause significant contraction or stiffening of the fascia.

○ It is important to understand that myofibroblast contraction does not occur with anything like the speed of voluntary skeletal muscular contraction. Instead, it builds up slowly over a period of 15 to 30 minutes and fades over hours. Given this, it seems that the purpose of fascial contraction is to stiffen tissues in response to long-standing or oft-repeated postural tensile forces.

○ Fascial tissues with high concentrations of myofibroblasts have been found to have sufficiently strong force to affect

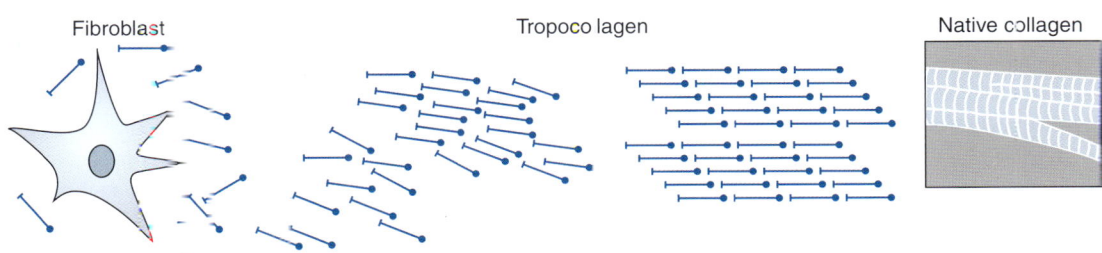

FIGURE 4-9 Collagen fibers secreted into the ground substance of fascial tissue align themselves along the line of physical stress that is placed on the tissue. Fascial tissue is most responsive to tensile lines of force. (Redrawn from Juhan D. Job's body: a handbook for bodywork, ed 3. Barrytown, NY, 2002, Station Hill Press.)

BOX 4-4

The fact that fascia is laid down along the line of tension within a tissue shows the remarkable adaptability of the human body to model itself to accommodate the forces placed on it. This concept becomes extremely important for clients who have had surgery. The fascial healing process involves the formation of collagen fibers to bind and close the wound. If movement is engaged across the site of the surgical incision, then the collagen that is laid down to heal the incision will be appropriately oriented along the lines of tension that the tissue site normally encounters (of course, the degree of motion must be mild and appropriate to the healing process postsurgery; excessive motion would prevent the incision from healing at all). This is the goal of the passive motion exercises that are usually instituted by physical therapists to aid in the client's rehabilitation after surgery. If no rehabilitation program is instituted—in other words, if the client is not given passive motion exercises and instead immobilizes the region—then the collagen fibers that bind the incision site will be laid down in a disorganized willy-nilly, felt-like fashion (see accompanying photograph). This increases the likelihood of excessive scarring as well as the likelihood that the scar tissue that is laid down will not be appropriately organized to deal with the lines of tension of that tissue. This could have long-term effects for that client far into the future. For this reason, appropriate and immediate physical therapy rehabilitation after surgery is crucial.

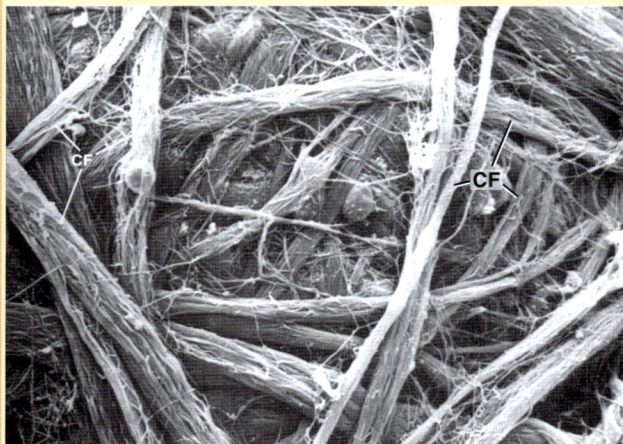

Copyright, Kessel RG and Kardon RH: *Tissues and organs: a text-atlas of scanning electron microscopy*, San Francisco, 1979, W.H. Freeman.

- Interestingly, the contraction of fascial myofibroblasts, unlike skeletal muscle fiber contraction, is not under direct neural control. Rather, they seem to contract in response to tensile forces that are placed on the tissue and also in response to certain chemical compounds such as nitric oxide, oxytocin, and growth factors that are present in the tissue (Box 4-5).

BOX 4-5

Interestingly, once a fascial tissue has transitioned to contain sufficient numbers of myofibroblasts to allow for contraction, a number of factors have been found that can actually cause the contraction to occur. Physical stress to the area is one. The presence of certain cytokines (protein factors released by cells that have the ability to signal/direct the activity of other cells, in this case, the myofibroblasts) is another. Interestingly, these cytokines are often present during inflammatory states. Hence inflammatory conditions would likely increase fascial tone. The sympathetic branch of the autonomic nervous system (ANS) of the central nervous system (CNS) has also been found to have the ability to modulate fascial contraction by its effect upon the release of the appropriate cytokines. The ANS can also cause the pH of the area to lower, which has also been found to increase fascial tone. However, when we describe the CNS as having the ability to cause fascial contraction, it is important to make the distinction between CNS activation of muscle contraction and ANS/CNS activation of fascial contraction. Muscle tone is controlled by direct connections with alpha motor neurons and is relatively instantaneous. Fascial tissue has no direct neural connections; when the appropriate factors are present for fascial contraction (mechanical strain, cytokines, lowered pH), fascial tissue typically requires anywhere from 5-30 minutes to contract.

- While present in larger numbers in wound healing, uninjured fascial tissues—especially large sheets such as the thoracolumbar fascia of the back, the plantar fascia of the foot, and the fascia latae of the thigh—have more recently been found to contain significant numbers of myofibroblasts. In cases where an overt physical trauma is absent, these myofibroblasts have developed in response to the accumulation of pulling tensile forces placed on these tissues (Box 4-6). Lower myofibroblast concentrations, although not sufficiently strong to affect musculoskeletal dynamics, have been found to exert sufficient isometric contraction pulling force to maintain their tissue integrity in the face of the tensile forces they are experiencing. Myofibroblasts in the crural fascia surrounding the lower leg, for instance, get active when there is an accumulation of lymph (say, from sitting too long in an airplane), thus squeezing the lower leg, reducing swelling, and aiding in the return of the lymph fluid to the heart.

musculoskeletal mechanics—that is, their active pulling forces are strong enough to contribute to increased stabilization in the fascial sheets. The field of kinesiology needs to consider contractile forces within the fascia when evaluating the musculoskeletal system. Albeit far weaker in degree and much slower in time than our skeletal muscular contraction forces, these fascial contraction forces are significant enough to change the dynamics of force distribution.

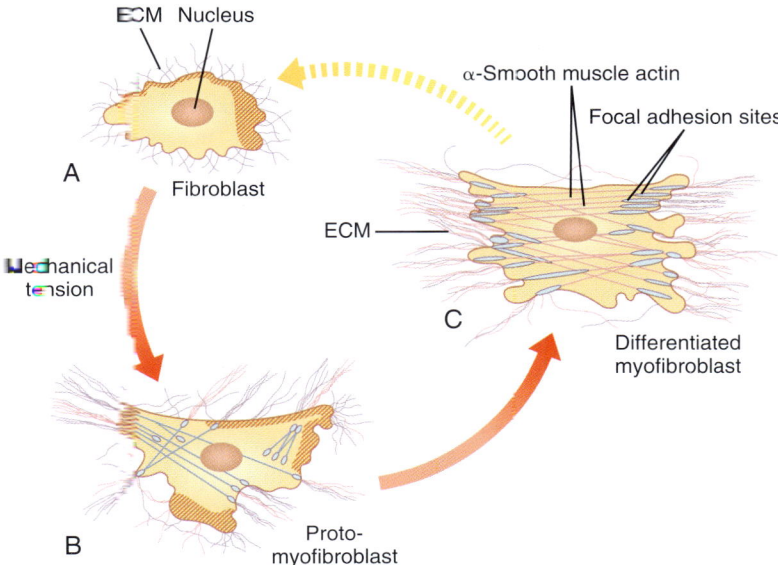

FIGURE 4-11 In response to physical stress, especially tensile pulling forces, fibroblasts in fascial tissue can transform into protomyofibroblasts and then fully mature myofibroblasts, which have the ability to contract. *ECM*, Extracellular matrix (i.e., the fiber/ground substance mix). (*Modified from Tomasek J et al: Nature reviews, Molecular Cell Biology, 2002. In Myers T: Anatomy trains, ed 2, Edinburgh, 2009, Churchill Livingstone/Elsevier.*)

BOX 4-6

The application of myofibroblastic development to musculoskeletal pathology may be very important. This knowledge points to the ability of fascial scar tissue to exert contractile forces that are helpful in closing and binding together wounded tissue. However, it also points to the possibility that if myofibroblastic contractile activity is excessive compared with the demands placed on the fascial tissue within which it is located, it may create an unhealthy—perhaps even destructive—effect on fascial and other nearby tissues. This would most likely occur in uninjured tissues that are experiencing chronic tensile stresses, such as chronically tight and taut tissues (e.g., tight muscles and taut ligaments). In these pathologically contracted fascial tissues, manual and movement therapies may be particularly valuable and effective, helping to change the stress loads that are placed on the fascia, thereby minimizing myofibroblastic development.

SECTION 4.4 TENDONS AND LIGAMENTS

- A **tendon** connects a muscle to a bone. More exactly, the fascia around and through the muscle continues into the tendon, so that there is no separation between the two. The muscle tissue simply "runs out" at the myotendinous junction, and the fascia continues. What was spun in a net around the muscle tissue (similar to an onion bag) is now simply more tightly wound within itself to make the tendon connection to the attachment.
- By definition, a tendon's shape is round and cordlike. If the shape of a tendon is broad and flat, the tendon is termed an **aponeurosis** (plural: aponeuroses). Tendons and aponeuroses are identical in their tissue makeup; they merely differ in shape.
- A **ligament** connects a bone to a bone.
  - Within the context of the musculoskeletal system, a ligament is defined as connecting a bone to a bone. However, the actual definition of a ligament is broader in that a ligament can attach any two structures (except a muscle and bone) to each other.
  - Ligaments have long been considered to be a parallel system to the muscles, a passive structure until the bones are pulled into a configuration where the ligament is tightened to prevent the bones from going "too far" and damaging the bones, tendon, or joint. In practice, most ligaments are tightened by nearby muscles and thus actively participate in joint stabilization through the entire range of movement.[18] This is very obvious in the rotator cuff, for example, where the tendons of the muscles blend totally with the ligamentous capsule. Similar reinforcement of the ligaments by nearby muscles is, in fact, happening all over the body. Only a few ligaments are "true" ligaments, independent of muscle tension; the cruciate ligaments of the knee and the odontoid ligament in the spine are examples.
- A tendon functions to transmit the pulling force of a muscle to its bony attachment, creating movement.
- A ligament functions to create stability at a joint by holding the bones of the joint together to prevent excess or damaging movement. (For a fuller discussion of the mobility and stability of a joint, see Section 7.3.)
- Both tendons and ligaments are types of dense fibrous connective tissue, composed of many collagen fibers packed tightly

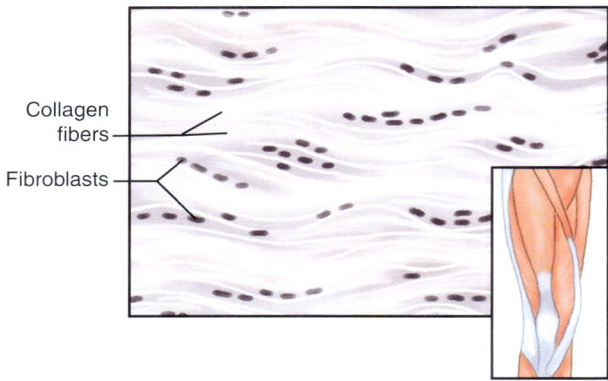

FIGURE 4-12 Tissue composition of tendons and ligaments (examples of which are shown in the inset). Tendons and ligaments are dense fibrous connective tissue, made up almost entirely of collagen fibers with occasional scattered fibroblast cells.

together and glued with a minimum of highly viscous ground substance (Figure 4-12).
- Very few cells are present; the cells that are present are primarily fibroblasts. Fibroblasts create the fibrillar threads of collagen (Box 4-7).
- A few elastin fibers are present in tendons; ligaments vary more widely in the proportions of elastin and collagen fibers depending on the location and demand. Consider any of your distal finger joints: try moving the bones from side to side—they are very resistant to that movement because that portion of the ligamentous capsule is highly collagenous. If you flex and extend the same joint, it will move easily, and those portions of the ligamentous capsule will have larger percentages of elastin fibers, to keep the capsule pulled away from being trapped between the bones of the joint, which would be very painful and counterproductive.
- Being made up nearly entirely of collagen fibers gives tendons and ligaments extremely strong tensile force (the ability to withstand strong pulling forces without damage or injury).
- This strong tensile force is needed in two situations:
  - It is needed by a tendon when the muscle to which it is attached contracts and pulls on it (e.g., concentric contraction).
  - It is needed by tendons and ligaments when they are stretched and pulled (eccentric loading), because the joint that they cross is moved in the opposite direction, perhaps as a result of contraction and shortening of the muscles on the opposite side of the joint (resulting in movement of the bones of the joint in the opposite direction).
- Having collagen fibers tightly packed together leaves little space for blood vessels; therefore tendons and ligaments have a poor blood supply and do not heal quickly after an injury (Box 4-8).
- Because tearing a tendon causes inflammation, it is called **tendinitis** (also spelled *tendonitis*).
- By definition, tearing of a ligament is called a sprain.
- Tearing of the fibrous capsule of a (synovial) joint is also termed a *sprain*, because the fibrous capsule is ligamentous tissue.
- In contrast, tearing of a muscle is called a **strain**.

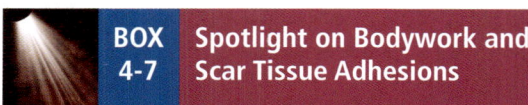

BOX 4-7 Spotlight on Bodywork and Scar Tissue Adhesions

Scar tissue adhesions are made up of fibrin threads of collagen that are created by fibroblasts. Scar tissue adhesions help heal wounded tissues by binding them together. However, they may also be oversecreted by the body, resulting in the loss of normal and healthy mobility of the tissues. The ground substance in scar tissue can also alter (depending on genetics) to include rubbery keloid proteins that make scars harder to mobilize. Much of the value of manual therapy, movement, and exercise is to break up patterns of excessive scar tissue adhesions.

 BOX 4-8

Except in extraordinary circumstances, biology has determined that it is usually better to break a bone than it is to tear (sprain) a ligament (or rupture a tendon), because bones have a greater blood supply and therefore heal better after an injury. Although bones usually return to 100% function after an injury, ligament tears rarely if ever heal fully and some instability of the joint remains. Ironically, after an injury people will often be heard to say something like, "Thank goodness I didn't break the bone. It's just a sprain."

SECTION 4.5   BURSAE AND TENDON SHEATHS

- Bursae (singular: bursa) and tendon sheaths are located in regions of the body where the friction between two structures against each other needs to be minimized and lubricated.
- This is necessary because friction causes the buildup of heat, and excessive heat can cause damage and inflame the tissues (Box 4-9).
- A **bursa** is a flattened sac of synovial membrane that contains a film of synovial fluid within it. (For more information on synovial membranes and synovial fluid, see Section 7.9.)
- A bursa is usually an independent structure. However, it may be continuous with the synovial membrane of a synovial joint. One example is the suprapatellar bursa of the knee joint (see Section 7.9, Figure 7-11, *C*.), which is sometimes separate and sometimes continuous with the knee capsule.
- Bursae are often found between a tendon and an adjacent joint structure, usually a bone.
- Bursae are found in many areas of the body including the shoulder joint and the ankle joint (Figure 4-13, *A* to *C*).
- A **tendon sheath** can be thought of as a sheath-like bursa that envelops a tendon.
  - Though filled with synovial-like liquid, the space in the sheath also contains fibers that create microvacuoles (bubble-like structures) that allow the limited number of capillaries to traverse the space from the outside of the sheath to the tendon. In other words, unlike regular bursae, the sheath and the tendon are continuous.

BOX 4-9

If the ability of a bursa to minimize friction is overcome and the bursa itself becomes inflamed, the condition is called **bursitis**. The most well-known bursitis occurs to the subacromial bursa at the shoulder joint. However, bursitis can occur at almost any joint of the body. If the ability of a tendon sheath to minimize friction is overcome and the tendon sheath itself becomes inflamed, the condition is called **tenosynovitis**. A common form of this condition occurs at the tendon sheath that envelops the abductor pollicis longus and extensor pollicis brevis tendons. With excessive movement of the thumb, these tendons rub against the styloid process at the radius, resulting in a form of tenosynovitis known as de Quervain's tenosynovitis (or de Quervain's disease).

- Bursae and tendon sheaths are similar in tissue structure; they differ in shape.
- Because tendon sheaths are constructed of synovial membrane tissue, they are also known as **synovial tendon sheaths**.
- Tendon sheaths are commonly found in the wrists and ankles, where long tendons rub against an adjacent structure such as a bone or a retinaculum (Figure 4-13, C and D).
- A **retinaculum** (plural: retinacula) is a thin sheet of fibrous connective tissue that holds down and stabilizes (i.e., retains) a structure. Retinacula are commonly found retaining the tendons of muscles that cross into the hands or the feet. To minimize friction between the tendons and these retinacula, tendon sheaths are located in these regions (see Figure 4-13, C). (For more information on retinacula, see Section 8.17.)

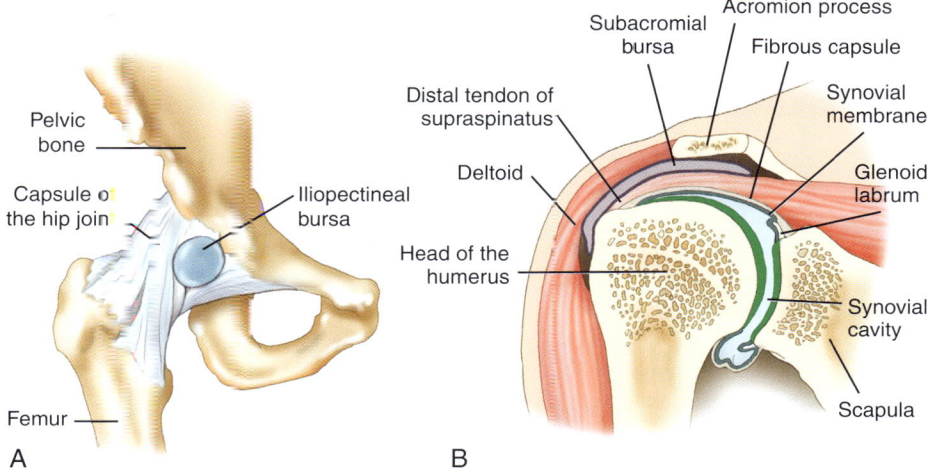

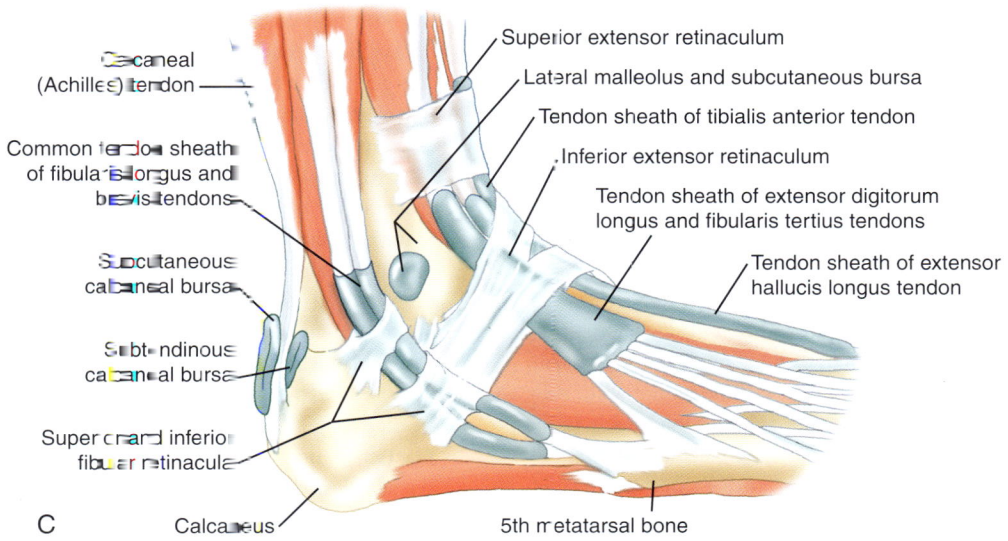

FIGURE 4-13 **A,** Anterior view with a bursa shown overlying the hip joint. This bursa helps to reduce friction between the capsule of the hip joint and the overlying iliopsoas and pectineus muscles. **B,** Anterior view of a cross-section of a shoulder joint. The subacromial bursa is located between the supraspinatus portion of the rotator cuff tendon inferiorly and the acromion process of the scapula and the deltoid muscle superiorly. The subacromial bursa functions to minimize friction between these structures, thereby maintaining the health of the rotator cuff tendon. **C,** Lateral view of the ankle joint region. A number of bursae and tendon sheaths are seen. Specifically the tendon sheaths function to minimize friction between the tendons that enter the foot and their adjacent structures, including the underlying bones and the overlying retinacula.

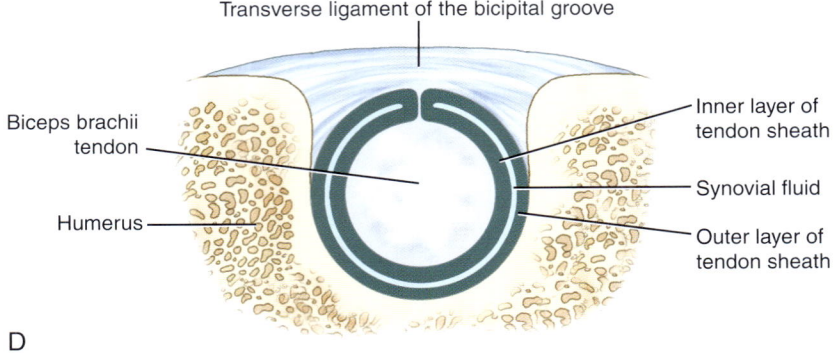

FIGURE 4-13, cont'd D, Cross-section through the humerus (i.e., bone of the arm) showing a tendon sheath encasing the biceps brachii muscle's long head tendon as it runs within the bicipital groove of the humerus.

SECTION 4.6   PROPERTIES OF FASCIAL CONNECTIVE TISSUES

- To fully understand the nature of fascial connective tissue and to be able to better deliver therapeutic manual therapy and guide clients in movement and exercise, it is helpful to understand the properties that these tissues possess. Following are terms that describe properties of skeletal connective tissues. The degree to which each individual tissue possesses each of the following properties varies.
- **Stretch**: The ability of a tissue to stretch is simply its ability to become longer without injury or damage. Certainly all *soft* connective tissues of the body are (and need to be) able to lengthen and stretch with various body movements. Because tight (taut) tissues are generally unable to stretch without damage, a major focus of manual therapy and stretching exercises is to gradually stretch and loosen these tight (taut) tissues.
- **Contractility**: The ability to contract is the ability to actively shorten.
  - It has classically been stated that this property is unique to muscular tissue and that musculoskeletal connective tissue—in other words, fascia—does not possess this ability. However, new research has shown that fascia contains a type of cell called a myofibroblast, which generates contraction that transfers through the connective tissues (for more on fascia and myofibroblasts, see Section 3.13).
  - The use of the terms *contraction* and *contractility* is problematic when speaking about muscle function, because although the ability to contract is the ability to shorten, not all muscle *contractions* actually result in shortening of the muscle in its entirety, even if individual sarcomeres are actually shortening within the muscles as a whole. (For further study, the topic of muscular contraction is discussed in more detail in Chapter 14.)
- **Weight bearing**: Weight bearing is the ability of a tissue of the body to bear the compressive force of the body mass that is located above it, without injury or damage. Generally the joints of the lower extremity and the axial body are weight-bearing joints. Because of the stress involved, weight-bearing joints generally demonstrate greater stability so that they are not damaged and injured.
- **Tensile strength**: The tensile strength of a connective tissue is its ability to withstand a distending (lengthening) force without injury or damage. Collagen fibers, the main component of connective tissues, have great tensile strength.
  - The ability to stretch and tensile ability are very similar. The difference is that the *stretchability* of a tissue is defined by how long it can become. The *tensile strength* of a tissue is defined by how much distension force the tissue can withstand without tearing.
- **Elasticity**: Elasticity of a connective tissue is its ability to return to its normal length after being stretched. For example, after being stretched, a rubber band is elastic because it returns to its original length. Similarly, most healthy connective tissues of the body also possess a good degree of elasticity. The presence of elastin fibers adds sustained elasticity to a connective tissue; collagen arrays also demonstrate elasticity, but the storage of that elasticity lasts only about a second.[19,20]
  - **Viscoelasticity**: The term *viscoelasticity* is a synonym for elasticity.
- **Plasticity**: *Plasticity* is a term that describes the ability of a tissue to have its shape molded or altered, and the tissue then retains that new shape. For example, after bubble gum (that has already been chewed) is stretched, it is said to be plastic because it does not return to its original shape; rather, it maintains its new shape. Plastic is named for its property of plasticity.
  - **Viscoplasticity**: The term *viscoplasticity* is a synonym for plasticity.
- **Elasticity and plasticity compared**: Understanding the concepts of elasticity and plasticity is important when working with soft tissues of the body. Whenever a soft tissue of the body has been altered or deformed in some manner because a force has been applied to it (whether it has been compressed or pulled on), the tissue has a certain elastic ability to return to its original shape; if that elasticity is exceeded, then plasticity describes the fact that the shape of the tissue will remain altered or deformed to some degree. An example is a ligament that is stretched. If it is only slightly stretched, its elastic ability allows it to return to

its original length. However, if it is stretched to a greater degree and its elastic ability is exceeded, the tissue will enter its *plastic range* and will become permanently overstretched and lax. This can result in a permanent decrease in stability of the joint where this ligament is located. Exceeding the elastic range or applying the stretch with too much speed will result in a tear or sprain.

○ **Creep**: The term *creep* describes the gradual change in shape of a tissue when it is subjected to a force that is applied to the tissue in a slow and sustained manner. The *creep* of the tissue may be temporary or permanent. If the creep is temporary, then the tissue is sufficiently elastic to return to its original form (stretch a gummy snake and watch it slowly return to near its original resting length). If the creep is permanent, then the elasticity of the tissue has been exceeded and the tissue is said to be plastic. The concept of creep may be negative, such as when a client changes the tissue shape and structure of the cruciate ligaments over time because of hyperextended knees, or it may be positive, such as when manual and movement therapy are done to change and correct a client's poor tissue shape and structure (Box 4-10).

BOX 4-10 Spotlight on Bodywork and Creep

The fact that creep of a tissue tends to occur more readily when a force is applied slowly is one reason why pressure applied during manual therapy should not be sudden and forceful; rather, the increasing depth of pressure should be done in a slow and incremental manner. This is not to say that deep pressure cannot be delivered, but rather that one should slowly sink into the muscles and fascia when applying deep pressure. Depth and speed are inversely proportional in effective manual therapy.

○ **Thixotropy**: Thixotropy describes the ability of a soft tissue of the body to change from a softer, more hydrated (i.e., liquid) **sol state** to a more rigid **gel state**. This concept is particularly important to manual and movement therapy. The matrix component of most connective tissues has a substantial ability to attain more of a sol state (because of the presence of proteoglycans which can sponge up available water), which is desirable because it allows for greater freedom of blood and nutrient flow and greater freedom of movement. Manual and movement therapy applied to body tissues can result in a change from gel to sol state (Box 4-11).

BOX 4-11

Thixo comes from the Greek word for touch, and *tropy* comes from the Greek word for change. Therefore *thixotropy* literally means to *change by touch*, illustrating the importance of massage and bodywork to this property of tissue!

○ The term *thixotropy* can be a daunting term for new students. Perhaps a better term is the one coined by Bob King, who was a distinguished educator in the field of massage and bodywork. He referred to reducing thixotropy as *rejuicification* of the tissue.
○ **Hysteresis**: Hysteresis describes the process wherein a tissue exhibits fluid loss and minute structural damage as a result of friction and heat buildup when it is worked excessively as in repetitive strain injury. Manual and movement therapy that result in hysteresis of a tissue may be any type of stroke, technique, or movement that repetitively and excessively compresses or stretches the client's tissue.

REVIEW QUESTIONS

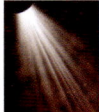 *Answers to the following review questions appear on the Evolve website accompanying this book at: http://evolve.elsevier.com/Muscolino/kinesiology/.*

1. What is the role of proteoglycan molecules in fascial tissues?

2. What is the definition of a tendon?

3. What is the definition of a ligament?

4. What is the function of fibroblasts?

5. How do myofibroblasts form in fascial tissue?

6. What is the difference between a sprain and a strain?

7. Compare and contrast a tendon with an aponeurosis.

8. Compare and contrast a bursa with a tendon sheath.

9. How does the concept of thixotropy apply to the fields of manual and movement therapy?

10. How do the properties of stretch, tensile strength, elasticity, and plasticity apply to the delivery of manual and movement therapy?

11. What is the difference between elasticity and plasticity of a tissue?

12. How does the concept of hysteresis apply to the fields of manual and movement therapy?

REFERENCES

1. Stecco C: Functional atlas of the human fascial system, Edinburgh, 2015, Elsevier.
2. Schleip R: Fascia in sport and movement. Edinburgh, 2015, Handspring Publishing.
3. Guimberteau JC: Strolling under the skin. Paris, 2004, Elsevier.
4. Myers T: Anatomy trains, ed 3, Edinburgh, 2014, Elsevier.
5. Williams P: Gray's anatomy, ed 38, New York, 1995, Churchill Livingstone.
6. Langevin HM, Huijing P: Communicating about fascia: History, pitfalls, and recommendations. IJTMB, 2(4), 3-8, 2009.
7. Snyder G: Fascia: Applied anatomy and physiology, Kirksville, MO, 1975, Kirksville College of Osteopathy.
8. Barrall JP, Mercier P: Visceral manipulation, Revised ed, Seattle, WA, 2006, Eastland Press.
9. Vleeming A: (personal conversation with Andry Vleeming in 2009), Movement, stability, and lumbopelvic pain, Edinburgh, 2007, Elsevier.
10. Cannon W: The wisdom of the body, New York, 1932, W.W. Norton & Company.
11. Huijing PA: Intra-, extra-, and intermuscular myofascial force transmission of synergists and antagonists: Effects of muscle length as well as relative position. IJTMB, 2, 1-15, 2002.
12. Myers T: Anatomy trains, ed 3, Edinburgh, 2014, Elsevier, pp 24-37.
13. Schleip R: Fascial tissues in motion: Elastic storage and recoil dynamics. In: Fascia in sport and medicine, Edinburgh, 2015, Handspring Publishing, pp 93-99.
14. Van der Wal JC: The architecture of connective tissue as parameter for proprioception—An often overlooked functional parameter as to proprioception in the locomotor apparatus. IJTMB, 2(4), 9-23, 2009.
15. Pischinger A: The extracellular matrix and ground regulation, Berkeley, CA, 2007, North Atlantic.
16. Zaidel-Bar R, Itzkovitz S, Ma'ayan A, et al: Functional atlas of the integrin adhesome. Nature Cell Biology, 9(8), 858-867, 2007.
17. Myers T: Anatomy trains, ed 3, Edinburgh, 2014, Elsevier.
18. Van der Wal JC: The architecture of connective tissue as parameter for proprioception—An often overlooked functional parameter as to proprioception in the locomotor apparatus. IJTMB, 2(4), 9-23, 2009.
19. Kawakami Y, Muraoka T, Ito S, Kanehisa H, Fukunaga T: In vivo muscle fibre behavior during countermovement exercise in humans reveals a significant role for tendon elasticity. J Physiol, 540, 635-646, 2002.
20. Fukunaga T, Kawakami Y, et al: Muscle and tendon interaction during human movements. Exercise Sport Science Review, 30(3), 106-110, 2002.

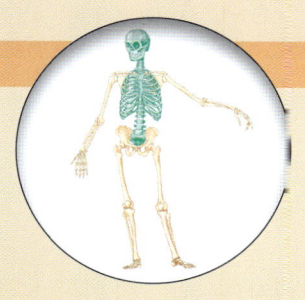

CHAPTER 5
Bones of the Human Body

CHAPTER OUTLINE

Axial Skeleton
- Section 5.1 Bones of the Head
- Section 5.2 Bones of the Spine (and Hyoid)
- Section 5.3 Bones of the Ribcage and Sternum

Appendicular Skeleton, Lower Extremity
- Section 5.4 Entire Lower Extremity
- Section 5.5 Bones of the Pelvis and Hip Joint
- Section 5.6 Bones of the Thigh and Knee Joint
- Section 5.7 Bones of the Leg and Ankle Joint
- Section 5.8 Bones of the Foot

Appendicular Skeleton, Upper Extremity
- Section 5.9 Entire Upper Extremity
- Section 5.10 Bones of the Shoulder Girdle and Shoulder Joint
- Section 5.11 Bones of the Arm and Elbow Joint
- Section 5.12 Bones of the Forearm, Wrist Joint, and Hand

CHAPTER OBJECTIVES

After completing this chapter, the student should be able to perform the following:

1. Define the key terms of this chapter and state the meanings of the word origins of this chapter.
2. List the major divisions of the skeleton.
3. Name and locate the bones, bony landmarks, and joints of the axial skeleton.
4. Name and locate the bones, bony landmarks, and joints of the lower extremity skeleton.
5. Name and locate the bones, bony landmarks, and joints of the upper extremity skeleton.

KEY TERMS

Accessory (ak-SES-or-ee)
Acetabulum (AS-i-TAB-you-um)
Acromion (a-KROM-ee-on)
Ala, pl. alae (A-la, A-lee)
Alveolar (al-VEE-o-lar)
Apex, pl. apices (A-peks, A-pi-sees)
Arch (ARCH)
Arcuate (ARE-cue-at)
Articular (are-TIK-you-lar)
Atlanto/atlas (at-LAN-to/AT-as)
Auditory (AW-di-tore-ee)
Auricular (or-IK-you-lar)
Axis (AKS-is)
Base/basilar (BASE/BAZE-i-lar)
Bicipital (bye-SIP-i-tal)
Bifid (BYE-fid)
Calcaneus, pl. calcanei (kal-KAY-nee-us, kal-KAY-nee-eye)
Canine (KAY-nine)
Capitate, capitulum (KAF-i-tate, ka-PICH-you-lum)
Carotid (ka-ROT-id)

Carpal (CAR-pull)
Cervical (SERV-i-kul)
Clavicle (KLAV-i-kul)
Coccyx, pl. coccyges (KOK-siks, KOK-si-jeez)
Concha, pl. conchae (KON-ka, KON-kee)
Condyle (KON-dial)
Conoid (CONE-oid)
Coracoid (CORE-a-koyd)
Cornu, pl. cornua (KORN-oo, KORN-oo-a)
Coronoid (CORE-o-noyd)
Costal (COST-al)
Coxal (COCK-sal)
Cranium (KRAY-nee-um)
Cribriform (KRIB-ri-form)
Crista galli (KRIS-ta GA-li)
Cuboid (KEW-boyd)
Cuneiform (kew-NEE-a-form)
Deltoid (DEL-toyd)
Dens, pl. dentes (DENS, DEN-tees)
Disc (DISK)

Dorsum sellae (DOOR-sum SELL-ee)
Epicondyle (EP-ee-KON-dial)
Ethmoid (ETH-moyd)
Facet (fa-SET)
Femur, pl. femora (FEE-mur, FEM-or-a)
Fibula (FIB-you-la)
Fovea (FOE-vee-ah)
Frontal (FRON-tal)
Glabella (gla-BELL-a)
Glenoid (GLEN-oyd)
Gluteal (GLUE-tee-al)
Hamate (HAM-ate)
Hamulus, pl. hamuli (HAM-you-lus, HAM-you-lie)
Hemifacet (HEM-ee-fa-SET)
Hiatus (hi-ATE-us)
Humerus, pl. humeri (HUME-er-us, HUME-er-eye)
Hyoid (HI-oyd)
Ilium, pl. ilia (IL-lee-um, IL-ee-a)
Incisive (in-SISE-iv)
Infraspinatus (IN-fra-spine-ATE-us)
Inion (IN-yon)
Innominate (i-NOM-i-nate)
Intercostal (IN-ter-KOST-a)
Interosseus (IN-ter-oss-ee-us)
Ischium, pl. ischia (IS-kee-um, IS-kee-a)
Jugular (JUG-you-lar)
Kyphosis (ki-FOS-is)
Lacerum (LA-ser-um)
Lacrimal (LAK-ri-mal)
Lambdoid (LAM-doyd)
Lamina, pl. laminae (LAM-i-na, LAM-i-nee)
Lingula (LING-you-la)
Lordotic (lor-DOT-ik)
Lumbar (LUM-bar)
Lunate (LOON-ate)
Magnum (MAG-num)
Malleolus, pl. malleoli (mal-EE-o-lus, mal-EE-o-lie)
Mamillary (MAM-i-lary)
Mandible (MAN-di-bul)
Manubrium, pl. manubria (ma-NOOB-ree-um, ma-NOOB-ree-a)
Mastoid (MAS-toyd)
Maxilla, pl. maxillae (MAX-i-la, MAX-i-lee)
Meatus (me-ATE-us)
Mental/menti (MEN-tal/MEN-tee)
Metacarpal (MET-a-CAR-pal)
Metatarsal (MET-a-TARS-al)
Mylohyoid (MY-low-HI-oyd)
Nasal (NAY-sul)
Navicular (na-VIK-you-lar)
Nuchal (NEW-kul)
Obturator (OB-tour-ate-or)
Occipital (ok-SIP-i-tal)
Odontoid (o-DONT-oyd)
Olecranon (o-LEK-ran-on)
Optic (OP-tik)
Palatine (PAL-a-tine)
Parietal (pa-RYE-it-al)
Patella, pl. patellae (pa-TELL-a, pa-TELL-ee)
Pedicle (PED-i-kul)
Pelvic bone (PEL-vik)
Petrous (PEE-trus)
Phalanx, pl. phalanges (FAL-anks, fa-LAN-jeez)
Pisiform (PIES-a-form)
Promontory (PROM-on-tor-ee)
Pterygoid (TER-i-goid)
Pubis, pl. pubes (PYU-bis, PYU-bees)
Radius, pl. radii (RAY-dee-us, RAY-dee-eye)
Ramus, pl. rami (RAY-mus, RAY-my)
Sacrum (SA-krum)
Sagittal (SAJ-i-tal)
Scaphoid (SKAF-oyd)
Scapula, pl. scapulae (SKAP-you-la, SKAP-you-lee)
Sciatic (sigh-AT-ik)
Sella turcica (SEL-a TER-si-ka)
Sesamoid (SES-a-moid)
Soleal (SO-lee-al)
Sphenoid (SFEE-noyd)
Spine/spinous (SPINE/SPINE-us)
Squamosal (squaw-MOS-al)
Sternum (STERN-um)
Styloid (STI-loyd)
Subscapular (SUB-SKAP-you-lar)
Subtalar (sub-TAL-ar)
Sulcus, pl. sulci (SUL-kus, SUL-ki)
Superciliary (SOO-per-CIL-ee-air-ee)
Supernumerary bone (SOO-per-noom-er-air-ee)
Supraorbital (SOO-pra-OR-bi-tal)
Supraspinatus (SOO-pra-spine-ATE-us)
Sustentaculum (sus-ten-TAK-you-lum)
Suture (SOO-cher)
Symphysis (SIM-fi-sis)
Talus, pl. tali (TA-lus, TA-lie)
Tarsal (TAR-sal)
Temporal (TEM-por-al)
Thoracic (thor-AS-ik)
Tibia, pl. tibiae (TIB-ee-a, TIB-ee-ee)
Transverse (TRANS-vers)
Trapezium (tra-PEEZ-ee-um)
Trapezoid (TRAP-i-zoyd)
Triquetrum (try-KWE-trum)
Trochanter (tro-CAN-ter)
Trochlea (TRO-klee-a)
Tubercle (TWO-ber-kul)
Tuberosity (TWO-ber-OS-i-tee)
Ulna, pl. ulnae (UL-na, UL-nee)
Uncus (UN-kus)
Vomer (VO-mer)
Wormian bones (WERM-ee-an)
Xiphoid (ZI-foyd)
Zygomatic (ZI-go-MAT-ik)

WORD ORIGINS

- Accessory—From Latin *accessorius*, meaning *supplemental*
- Acetabulum—From Latin *acetum*, meaning *vinegar*, and Latin *abulum*, meaning *small receptacle, cup*
- Acromion—From Greek *akron*, meaning tip and Greek *omos*, meaning *shoulder*
- Ala, pl. alae—From Latin *ala*, meaning *wing*
- Alveolar—From Latin *alveolus*, meaning *a concavity, a bowl*
- Apex, pl. apices—From Latin *apex*, meaning *tip*
- Arch—From Latin *arcus*, meaning *a bow*
- Arcuate—From Latin *arcuatus*, meaning *bowed, shaped like an arc*
- Articular—From Latin *articulus*, meaning *joint*
- Atlanto/atlas—From Greek *Atlas*, the Greek figure who supports the world (the first cervical vertebra supports the head)
- Auditory—From Latin *auditorius*, meaning *pertaining to the sense of hearing*
- Auricular—From Latin *auricula*, meaning *a little ear*
- Axis—From Latin *axis*, meaning *axis* (an imaginary line about which something revolves)
- Base/basilar—From Latin *basilaris*, meaning *the base of something*
- Bicipital—From Latin *bi*, meaning *two*, and Greek *kephale*, meaning *head*
- Bifid—From Latin *bis*, meaning *twice*, and Latin *findere*, meaning *to cleave*
- Calcaneus, pl. calcanei—From Latin *calcaneus*, meaning *heel bone*
- Canine—From Latin *caninus*, meaning *pertaining to a dog* (refers to proximity to canine tooth)
- Capitate, capitulum—From Latin *caput*, meaning *a small head*
- Carotid—From Greek *karoun*, meaning *to plunge into sleep or stupor* (because compression of the carotid arteries can result in unconsciousness)
- Carpal—From Greek *karpos*, meaning *wrist*
- Cervical—From Latin *cervicalis*, meaning *pertaining to the neck*
- Clavicle—From Latin *clavicula*, meaning *a small key*
- Coccyx, pl. coccyges—From Greek *kokkyx*, meaning *cuckoo bird*
- Concha—From Greek *konch*, meaning *shell*
- Condyle—From Greek *kondylos*, meaning *knuckle*
- Conoid—From Greek *konos*, meaning *cone*, and Greek *eidos*, meaning *resemblance*
- Coracoid—From Greek *korax*, meaning *raven*, and Greek *eidos*, meaning *resemblance*
- Cornu, pl. cornua—From Latin *cornu*, meaning *horn*
- Coronoid—From Greek *korone*, meaning *crown*, and Greek *eidos*, meaning *resemblance*
- Costal—From Latin *costa*, meaning *rib*
- Coxal—From Latin *coxa*, meaning *hip*
- Cranium—From Latin *cranium*, meaning *skull*
- Cribriform—From Latin *cribrum*, meaning *sieve*, and Latin *forma*, meaning *shape*
- Crista galli—From Latin *crista*, meaning *crest* or *plume*, and Latin *gallus*, meaning *rooster*
- Cuboid—From Greek *kubos*, meaning *cube*, and Greek *eidos*, meaning *resemblance*
- Cuneiform—From Latin *cuneus*, meaning *wedge*, and Latin *forma*, meaning *shape*
- Deltoid—From Latin *deltoides*, meaning *shaped like a delta* (Δ), and Greek *eidos*, meaning *resemblance*
- Dens, pl. dentes—From Latin *dens*, meaning *tooth*
- Disc—From Greek *diskos*, meaning *a flat round structure*
- Dorsum sellae—From Latin *dorsum*, meaning *back*, and Latin *sella*, meaning *saddle* (the dorsum sellae is the posterior wall of the sella turcica)
- Epicondyle—From Greek *epi*, meaning *upon*, and Greek *kondylos*, meaning *knuckle*
- Ethmoid—From Greek *ethmos*, meaning *sieve*, and Greek *eidos*, meaning *resemblance*
- Facet—From French *facette*, meaning *a small face*
- Femur, pl. femora—From Latin *femur*, meaning *thighbone*
- Fibula—From Latin *fibula*, meaning *that which clasps or clamps*
- Fovea—From Latin *fovea*, meaning *a pit*
- Frontal—From Latin *frontalis*, meaning *anterior*
- Glabella—From Latin *glaber*, meaning *smooth*
- Glenoid—From Greek *glene*, meaning *socket*, and Greek *eidos*, meaning *resemblance*
- Gluteal—From Greek *gloutos*, meaning *buttock*
- Hamate—From Latin *hamatus*, meaning *hooked*
- Hamulus, pl. hamuli—From Latin *hamulus*, meaning *a small hook*
- Hemifacet—From Greek *hemi*, meaning *half*, and French *facette*, meaning *small face*
- Hiatus—From Latin *hiatus*, meaning *an opening*
- Humerus, pl. humeri—From Latin *humerus*, meaning *shoulder*
- Hyoid—From Greek *hyoeides*, meaning *U-shaped*
- Ilium, pl. ilia—From Latin *ilium*, meaning *groin, flank*
- Incisive—From Latin *incisus*, meaning *to cut* (refers to proximity to incisor teeth)
- Infraspinatus—From Latin *infra*, meaning *beneath* (the spine of the scapula)
- Inion—From Greek *inion*, meaning *back of the neck*
- Innominate—From Latin *innominatus*, meaning *nameless, unnamed*
- Intercostal—From Latin *inter*, meaning *between*, and Latin *costa*, meaning *rib*
- Interosseus—From Latin *inter*, meaning *between*, and Latin *ossis*, meaning *bone*
- Ischium, pl. ischia—From Greek *ischion*, meaning *hip*
- Jugular—From Latin *jugularis*, meaning *neck* (refers to jugular vein)
- Kyphosis—From Greek *kyphos*, meaning *bent, humpback*
- Lacerum—From Latin *lacerare*, meaning *to tear*
- Lacrimal—From Latin *lacrimal*, meaning *tear*
- Lambdoid—From Greek letter *lambda* (l), and Greek *eidos*, meaning *resemblance*

- Lamina, pl. laminae—From Latin *lamina*, meaning *a thin flat layer or plate*
- Lingula—From Latin *lingua*, meaning *tongue*
- Lordotic—From Greek *lordosis*, meaning *a bending backward*
- Lumbar—From Latin *lumbus*, meaning *loin, low back*
- Lunate—From Latin *luna*, meaning *moon*
- Magnum—From Latin *magnum*, meaning *large*
- Malleolus, pl. malleoli—From Latin *malleolus*, meaning *little hammer*
- Mamillary—From Latin *mamma*, meaning *breast*
- Mandible—From Latin *mandere*, meaning *to chew*
- Manubrium, pl. manubria—From Latin *manubrium*, meaning *handle*
- Mastoid—From Greek *mastos*, meaning *breast*, and Greek *eidos*, meaning *resemblance*
- Maxilla, pl. maxillae—From Latin *maxilla*, meaning *jawbone* (especially the upper one)
- Meatus—From Latin *meatus*, meaning *a passage*
- Mental/menti—From Latin *mentum*, meaning *mind*
- Metacarpal—From Greek *meta*, meaning *after*, and Greek *karpos*, meaning *wrist*
- Metatarsal—From Greek *meta*, meaning *after*, and from Greek *tarsas*, referring to the *tarsal bones*
- Mylohyoid—From Greek *myle*, meaning *mill* (refers to molar teeth that grind food), and Greek *hyoeides*, meaning *U-shaped*
- Nasal—From Latin *nasus*, meaning *nose*
- Navicular—From Latin *navicula*, meaning *boat*
- Nuchal—From Latin *nucha*, meaning *back of the neck*
- Obturator—From Latin *obturare*, meaning *to stop up*
- Occipital—From Latin *occipitalis*, meaning *back of the head*
- Odontoid—From Greek *odous*, meaning *tooth*, and Greek *eidos*, meaning *resemblance*
- Olecranon—From Greek *olecranon*, meaning *elbow*
- Optic—From Greek *optikos*, meaning *pertaining to the sense of sight* (the optic foramen contains the optic nerve)
- Palatine—From Latin *palatinus*, meaning *concerning the palate*
- Parietal—From Latin *parietalis*, meaning *pertaining to the wall of a cavity*
- Patella, pl. patellae—From Latin *patella*, meaning *a plate*
- Pedicle—From Latin *pediculus*, meaning *small foot*
- Pelvic bone—From Latin *pelvis*, meaning *basin*
- Petrous—From Latin *petra*, meaning *stone*
- Phalanx, pl. phalanges—From Latin *phalanx*, meaning *a line of soldiers*
- Pisiform—From Latin *pisum*, meaning *pea*, and Latin *forma*, meaning *shape*
- Promontory—From Latin *promontorium*, meaning *a projecting process or part*
- Pterygoid—From Greek *pterygion*, meaning *wing*
- Pubis, pl. pubes—From Latin *pubes*, meaning *grown up*
- Radius, pl. radii—From Latin *radius*, meaning *rod, spoke of a wheel*
- Ramus, pl. rami—From Latin *ramus*, meaning *branch*
- Sacrum—From Latin *sacrum*, meaning *sacred*
- Sagittal—From Latin *sagittal*, meaning *arrow* (refers to a posterior/anterior direction)
- Scaphoid—From Greek *skaphe*, meaning *a skiff* or *boat*, and Greek *eidos*, meaning *resemblance*
- Scapula, pl. scapulae—From Latin *scapulae*, meaning *shoulder blades*
- Sciatic—From Latin *sciaticus*, meaning *pertaining to ischium* (i.e., hip)
- Sella turcica—From Latin *sella*, meaning *saddle*, and Latin *turcica*, meaning *Turkish*
- Sesamoid—From Greek *sesamon*, meaning *sesame seed*, and Greek *eidos*, meaning *resemblance*
- Soleal—From Latin *solea*, meaning *sole of the foot*
- Sphenoid—From Greek *sphen*, meaning *wedge*, and Greek *eidos*, meaning *resemblance*
- Spine/spinous—From Latin *spina*, meaning *thorn*
- Squamosal—From Latin *squamosus*, meaning *scaly*
- Sternum—From Greek *sternon*, meaning *chest, breastbone*
- Styloid—From Greek *stylos*, meaning *pillar* or *post*, and Greek *eidos*, meaning *resemblance*
- Subscapular—From Latin *sub*, meaning *under* (referring to the underside [i.e., the anterior side] of the scapula)
- Subtalar—From Latin *sub*, meaning *under*, and *talar*, referring to the talus
- Sulcus, pl. sulci—From Latin *sulcus*, meaning *groove*
- Superciliary—From Latin *super*, meaning *above*, and Latin *cilium*, meaning *eyebrow*
- Supraorbital—From Latin *supra*, meaning *above*, and Latin *orbis*, meaning *circle, orb*
- Supraspinatus—From Latin *supra*, meaning *above* (the spine of the scapula)
- Sustentaculum—From Latin *sustentaculum*, meaning *support*
- Suture—From Latin *sutura*, meaning *a seam*
- Symphysis—From Greek *sym*, meaning *with* or *together*, and Greek *physis*, meaning *nature, body*
- Talus, pl. tali—From Latin *talus*, meaning *ankle*
- Tarsal—From Greek *tarsos*, meaning *a broad flat surface*
- Temporal—From Latin *temporalis*, meaning *pertaining to* or *limited in time* (refers to the temple region of the head)
- Thoracic—From Greek *thorax*, meaning *chest*
- Tibia, pl. tibiae—From Latin *tibia*, meaning *the large shinbone*
- Transverse—From Latin *transversus*, meaning *lying across*
- Trapezium, trapezoid—From Greek *trapeza*, meaning *a (four-sided) table*
- Triquetrum—From Latin *triquetrus*, meaning *triangular*
- Trochanter—From Greek *trochanter*, meaning *to run*
- Trochlea—From Latin *trochlear*, meaning *pulley*
- Tubercle—From Latin *tuberculum*, or *tuber*, meaning *a small knob, swelling, tumor*
- Tuberosity—From Latin *tuberositas*, or *tuber*, meaning *a knob, swelling, tumor*
- Ulna, pl. ulnae—From Latin *ulna*, meaning *elbow*
- Uncus—From Latin *uncus*, meaning *hook*
- Vomer—From Latin *vomer*, meaning *ploughshare*
- Xiphoid—From Greek *xiphos*, meaning *sword*, and Greek *eidos*, meaning *resemblance*
- Zygomatic—From Greek *zygon*, meaning *to join, a yolk*

The following key terms are a number of general terms that are used to describe landmarks on bones. Many bony landmarks are raised aspects of a bone's surface that serve as muscle and/or ligament attachment sites.

Angle—A corner of a bone.
Articular surface—The surface of a bone that articulates with another bone (i.e., the joint surface).
Body—The main portion of a bone; the body of a long bone is the shaft.
Condyle—Rounded bump found at the end of a long bone (part of the epiphysis); usually part of a joint fitting into a fossa of an adjacent bone.
Crest—A moderately raised ridge of bone; often a site of muscle attachment.
Eminence—A raised prominent area of a bone.
Epicondyle—A small bump found on a condyle; often a site of muscle attachment.
Facet—A smooth (usually flat) surface on a bone that forms a joint with another facet or flat surface of an adjacent bone.
Fissure—A cleft or cracklike hole in a bone that allows the passage of nerves and/or vessels.
Foramen—A hole within a bone that allows the passage of a nerve and/or vessel (plural: foramina).
Fossa—A depression in a bone that often receives an articulating bone (plural: fossae).
Groove—A narrow elongated depression within a bone, often containing a tendon, nerve, or vessel.
Head—The expanded rounded end (epiphysis) of a long bone; usually separated from the body (i.e., shaft) of the bone by a neck.
Hiatus—An opening in a bone.
Impression—A shallow groove on a bone often formed by a tendon, nerve, or vessel.
Line—A mildly raised ridge of bone (usually less than a crest); often a site of muscle attachment.
Lip—A raised liplike structure that forms the border of a groove or opening.
Margin—The edge of a bone.
Meatus—A tubelike channel within a bone.
Neck—A narrowed portion of a bone that separates the head from the body (i.e., shaft) of a bone.
Notch—A V-shaped or U-shaped depression in a bone.
Process—A projection of a bone; may be involved with an articulation or may be a site of muscle attachment.
Protuberance—A bump on a bone; often the site of muscle attachment.
Ramus—A portion of bone that branches from the body of the bone (plural: rami).
Sinus—A cavity within a bone.
Spine—A thornlike, sharp, pointed process of a bone; often a site of muscle attachment.
Sulcus—A groove or elongated depression in a bone (plural: sulci).
Trochanter—A large bump on a bone (larger than a tubercle/tuberosity); usually a site of muscle attachment.
Tubercle/tuberosity—A moderately sized bump on a bone; often a site of muscle attachment. A tubercle is usually considered to be smaller than a tuberosity.

THE SKELETAL SYSTEM:

- The human skeleton is usually said to have 206 bones[1] (Box 5-1).
- This number is based on the axial skeleton having 80 bones and the appendicular skeleton having 126. The axial skeleton makes up the central vertical axis of the body and is composed of the bones of the head, neck, trunk, and the sacrum and coccyx[2] (Box 5-2).
- The appendicular skeleton is made up of the appendages that attach onto the axial skeleton (i.e., the upper and lower extremities), including the bones of the shoulder girdle (scapulae and clavicles) and the pelvic girdle (pelvic bones).[2] Figures 5-1 and 5-2 illustrate the axial and appendicular skeletons. Table 5-1 lists the bones of the human body.
- Note: Whenever a bone exists on both sides of the body, the right-sided bone is shown in this chapter.

BOX 5-1

The stated number of 206 bones in the human body is variable. Sesamoid bones in addition to the patellae usually exist, and small islets of bone located within the sutures of the skull called **wormian bones**[6] are often present. Furthermore, occasional anomalous bones may exist. Any bone beyond the usual number of 206 may be called a **supernumerary bone**.

BOX 5-2

Another way to look at the axial skeleton is to say that it is composed of the bones of the head, spinal column (the sacrum and coccyx are part of the spinal column), ribcage, and hyoid.

TABLE 5-1 Bones of Skeleton (206 Total)

Axial Skeleton (80 Bones Total)

Part of Body	Name of Bone(s)
Skull (28 bones total)	
Cranium (8 bones)	Frontal (1)
	Parietal (2)
	Temporal (2)
	Occipital (1)
	Sphenoid (1)
	Ethmoid (1)
Face (14 bones)	Nasal (2)
	Maxillary (2)
	Zygomatic (2)
	Mandible (1)
	Lacrimal (2)
	Palatine (2)
	Inferior nasal conchae (2)
	Vomer (1)
Ear bones (6 bones)	Malleus (2)
	Incus (2)
	Stapes (2)
Hyoid bone (1)	
Spinal column (26 bones total)	Cervical vertebrae (7)
	Thoracic vertebrae (12)
	Lumbar vertebrae (5)
	Sacrum (1)
	Coccyx (1)
Sternum and ribs (25 bones total)	Sternum (1)
	True ribs (14)
	False ribs (10)

Appendicular Skeleton (126 Bones Total)

Part of Body	Name of Bone(s)
Upper extremities (including shoulder girdle) (64 bones total)	Clavicle (2)
	Scapula (2)
	Humerus (2)
	Radius (2)
	Ulna (2)
	Carpals (16)
	Metacarpals (10)
	Phalanges (28)
Lower extremities (including pelvic girdle) (62 bones total)	Pelvis (2)
	Femur (2)
	Patella (2)
	Tibia (2)
	Fibula (2)
	Tarsals (14)
	Metatarsals (10)
	Phalanges (28)

From Thibodeau GA, Patton KT: Anatomy and physiology, ed 9, St Louis, 2016, Elsevier.

FULL SKELETON—ANTERIOR VIEW

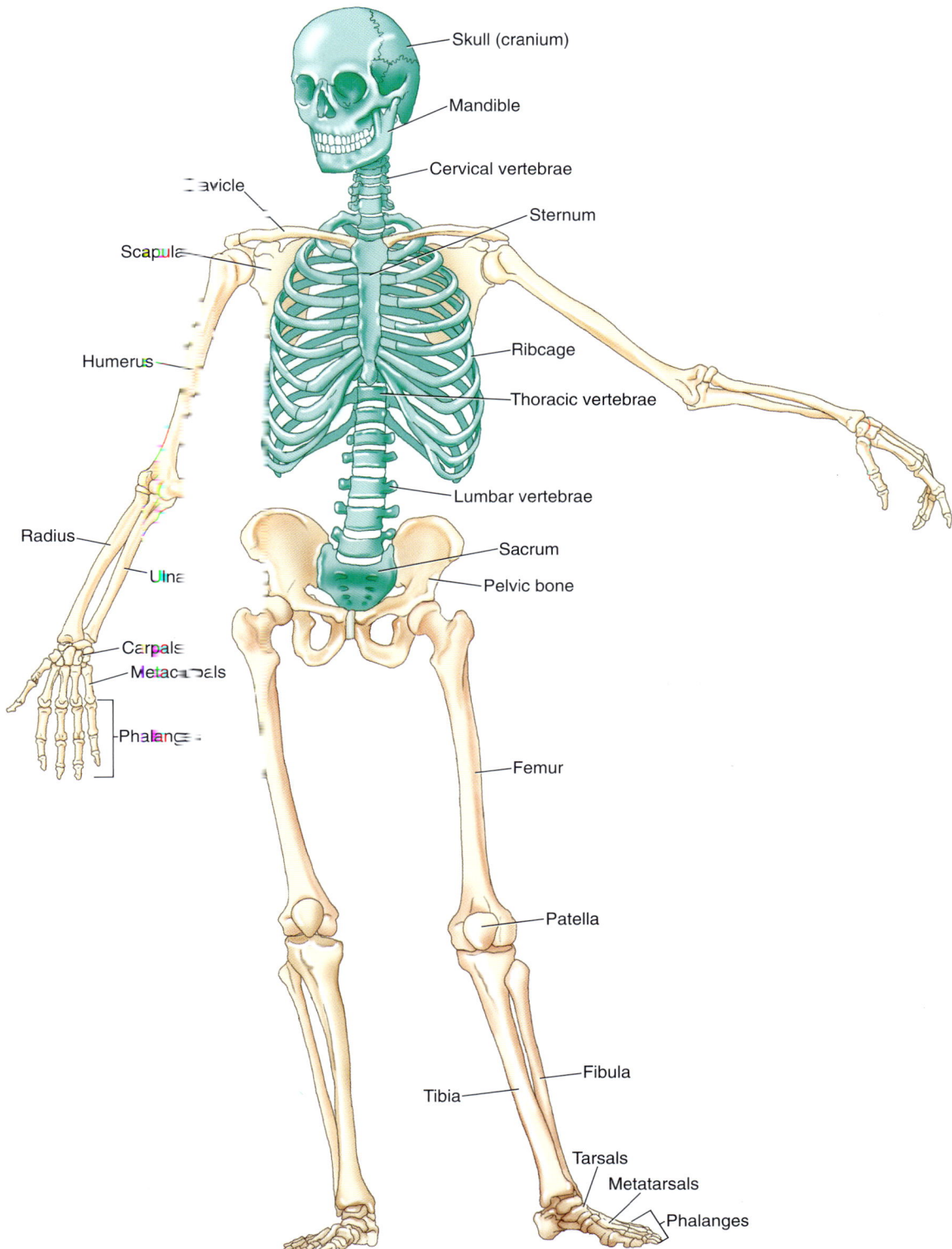

FIGURE 5-1 Bones colored beige are bones of the appendicular skeleton; bones colored green are bones of the axial skeleton.

FULL SKELETON—POSTERIOR VIEW

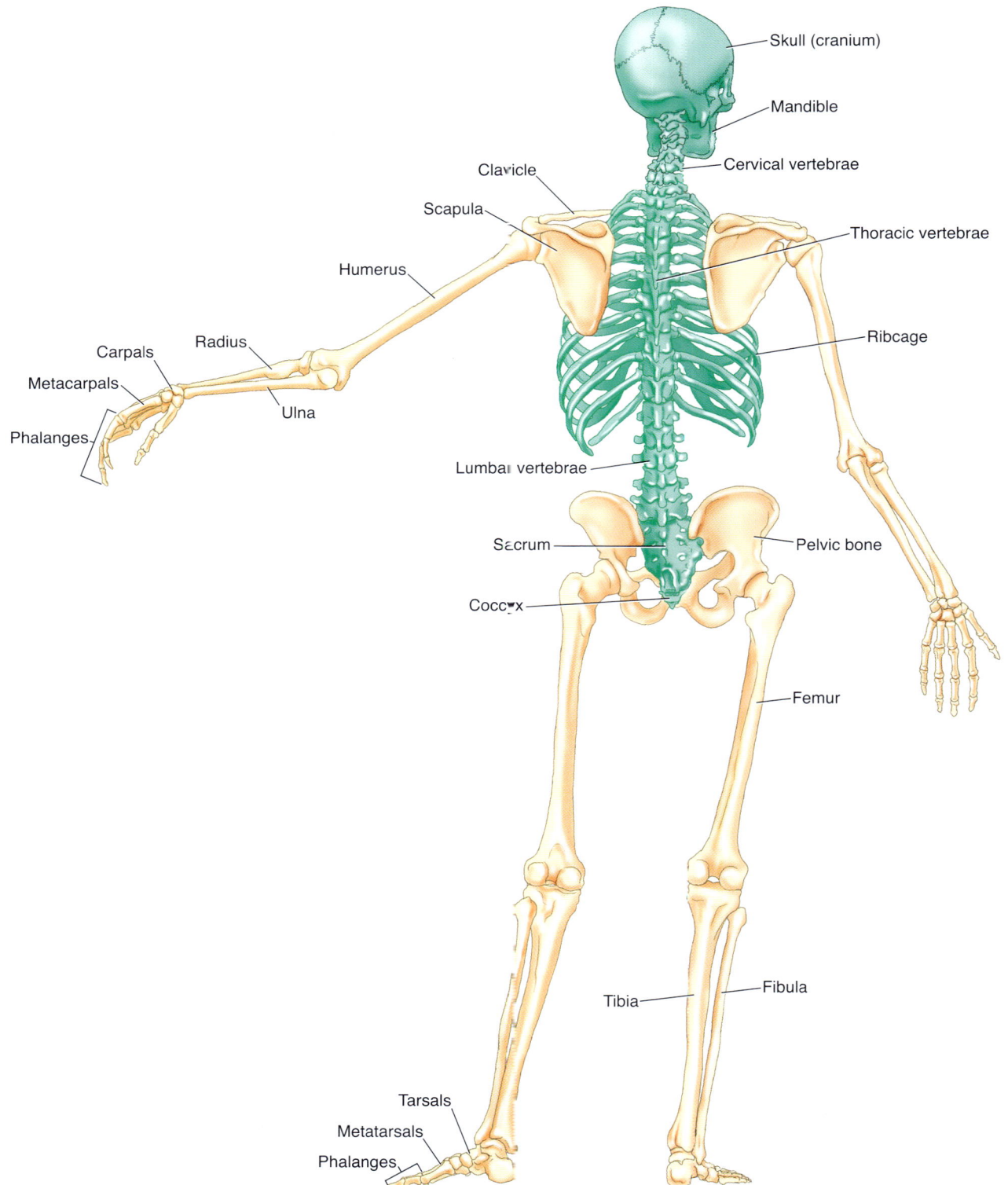

FIGURE 5-2 Bones colored beige are bones of the appendicular skeleton; bones colored green are bones of the axial skeleton.

SECTION 5.1 BONES OF THE HEAD

SKULL—ANTERIOR VIEW (COLORED)

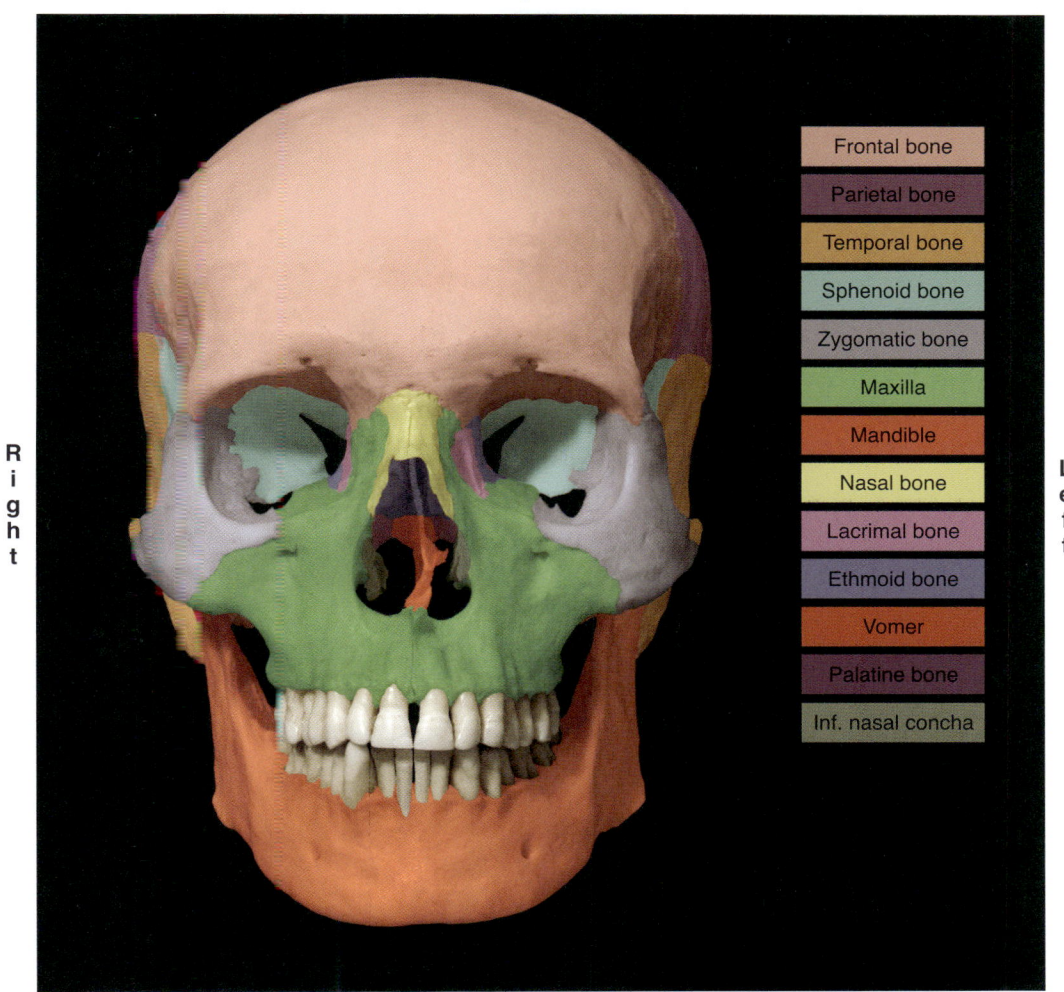

FIGURE 5-3
Frontal bone
Parietal bone
Occipital bone (not seen)
Temporal bone
Sphenoid bone
Zygomatic bone
Maxilla
Mandible
Nasal bone
Lacrimal bone
Ethmoid bone
Vomer
Palatine bone
Inferior nasal concha

NOTES
1. Embryologically, two maxillary bones (left and right) exist. However, these two bones fuse to form one maxilla[3] (an incomplete fusion results in a cleft palate). For this reason, we may speak of one maxilla (singular) or of two maxillary bones (plural).
2. The frontal, sphenoid, zygomatic, maxillary, lacrimal, and ethmoid bones all have a presence in the orbital cavity.[4]
3. The ethmoid, vomer, and inferior nasal concha are all visible in this anterior view of the nasal cavity.

SKULL—ANTERIOR VIEW

FIGURE 5-4

1. Frontal bone (#1-6)
2. Superciliary arch
3. Supraorbital margin
4. Supraorbital notch
5. Glabella
6. Orbital surface
7. Nasal bone
8. Internasal suture
9. Frontonasal suture
10. Nasomaxillary suture
11. Orbital cavity
12. Superior orbital fissure
13. Inferior orbital fissure
14. Greater wing of sphenoid
15. Lesser wing of sphenoid
16. Lacrimal bone
17. Ethmoid bone
18. Middle nasal concha (of ethmoid bone)
19. Inferior nasal concha
20. Vomer
21. Palatine bone
22. Frontozygomatic suture
23. Infraorbital margin
24. Zygomatic bone
25. Zygomaticomaxillary suture

Maxilla (#26-31):
26. Frontal process
27. Infraorbital foramen
28. Canine fossa
29. Incisive fossa (indicated by dotted line)
30. Alveolar process (indicated by dashed line)
31. Anterior nasal spine
32. Intermaxillary suture

Mandible (#33-43):
33. Body
34. Ramus
35. Angle
36. Mental foramen
37. Incisive fossa (indicated by dotted line)
38. Alveolar fossa (indicated by dashed line)
39. Symphysis menti
40. Mental tubercle
41. Oblique line (indicated by solid line)
42. Temporal bone
43. Parietal bone

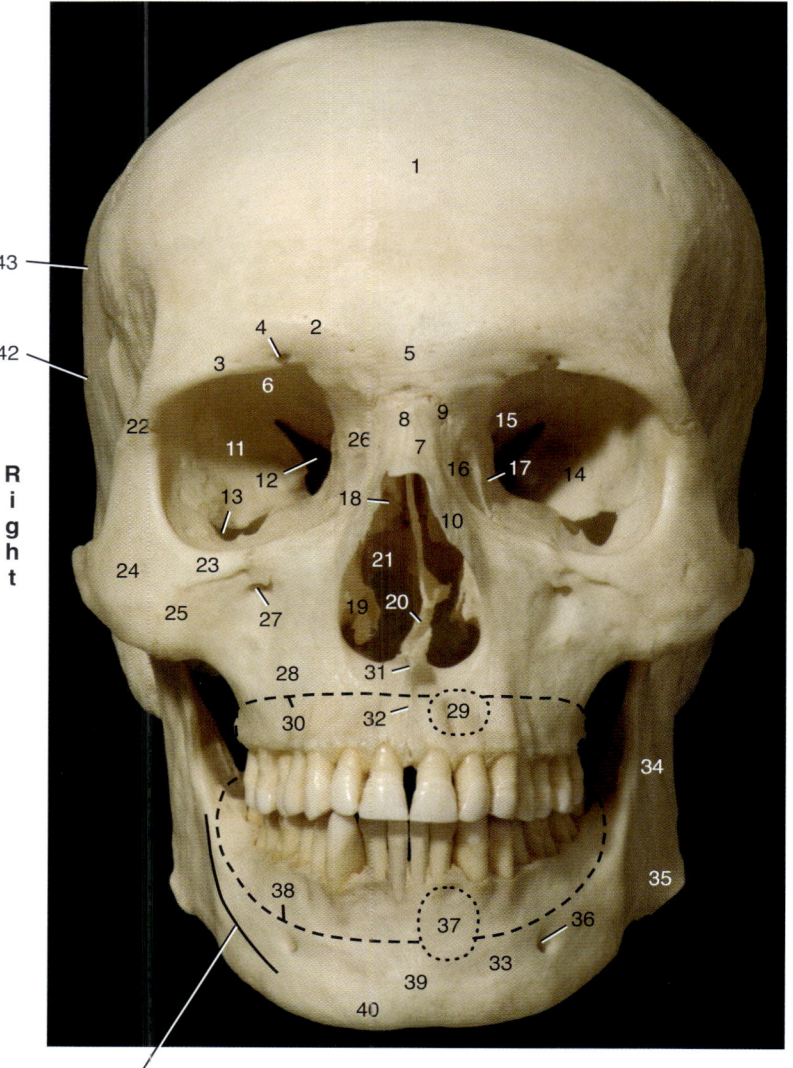

NOTES

1. The term *cranium* is usually considered to be synonymous with the term *skull*. Some sources exclude the mandible and/or other facial bones from the term cranium.[3]
2. The glabella (#5) is a smooth prominence on the frontal bone, just superior to the nose.[3]
3. The inferior nasal concha (#19) is an independent bone. The middle and superior nasal conchae are landmarks of the ethmoid bone (#17).[4]
4. The vomer (#20) and ethmoid (#17) both contribute to the nasal septum, which divides the nasal cavity into left and right nasal passages.[4]
5. The supraorbital margin (#3) is wholly located on the frontal bone; the infraorbital margin (#23) is located on the maxilla and the zygomatic bone.[4]

CHAPTER 5 Bones of the Human Body

SKULL—RIGHT LATERAL VIEW (COLORED)

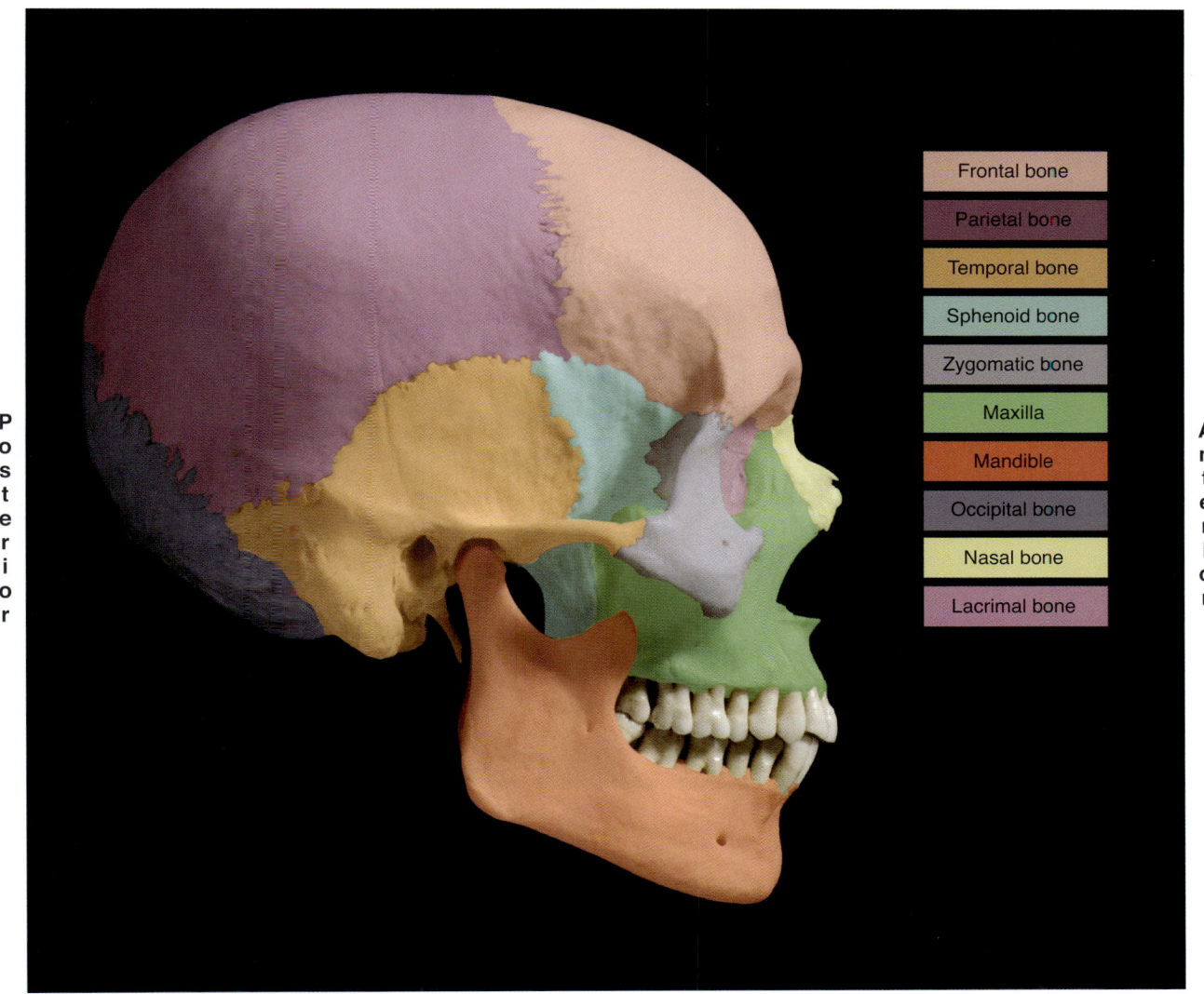

FIGURE 5-5
Frontal bone
Parietal bone
Temporal bone
Sphenoid bone
Zygomatic bone
Maxilla
Mandible
Occipital bone
Nasal bone
Lacrimal bone

NOTES
1. The occipital bone is often referred to as the occiput.
2. In this lateral view, the sphenoid bone is visible posterior to the maxilla (between the condyle and coronoid process of the mandible).

SKULL—RIGHT LATERAL VIEW

FIGURE 5-6
1. Frontal bone
2. Glabella
3. Coronal suture
4. Frontozygomatic suture
5. Superior temporal line
6. Parietal bone
7. Lambdoid suture
8. Occipital bone
9. External occipital protuberance (EOP)
10. Temporal bone (#11-14)
11. Mastoid process
12. Styloid process
13. External auditory meatus
14. Zygomatic arch
15. Squamosal suture
16. Zygomaticotemporal suture
17. Temporomandibular joint (TMJ)
18. Greater wing of sphenoid bone
19. Lateral pterygoid plate (of the pterygoid process) of the sphenoid bone
20. Zygomatic bone
21. Nasal bone
22. Maxilla
23. Anterior nasal spine
24. Frontal process of maxilla
25. Lacrimal bone

Mandible (#26-32):
26. Body
27. Angle
28. Ramus
29. Coronoid process
30. Condyle
31. Mental foramen
32. Mental tubercle

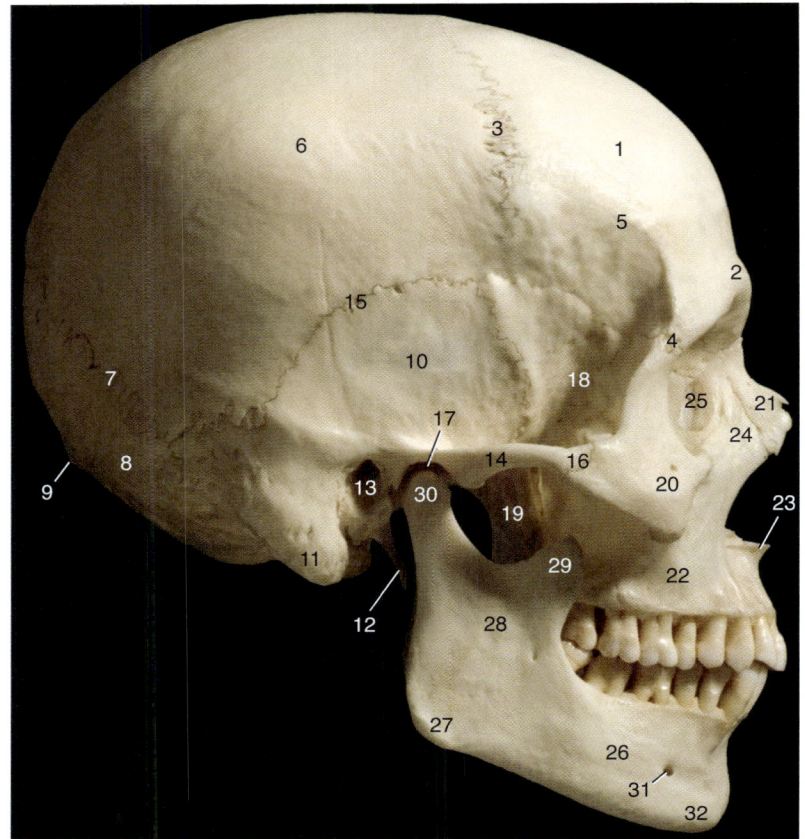

NOTES

1. The temporal fossa (the attachment site of the temporalis muscle) is a broad area of the skull that overlies the temporal, parietal, frontal, and sphenoid bones. The superior margin of the temporal fossa is the superior temporal line (#5), visible on the frontal bone.[4]
2. The external auditory meatus (#13) is the opening into the middle ear cavity, which is located within the temporal bone.[2]
3. The zygomatic arch (#14) is usually spoken of as being a landmark only of the temporal bone. However, technically the zygomatic arch is a landmark of both the temporal and zygomatic bones formed by the zygomatic process of the temporal bone and the temporal process of the zygomatic bone[4] (see Figure 5-15, C).
4. The squamosal suture (#15) is named for being next to the squamous portion (the superior aspect near the parietal bone) of the temporal bone. The squamous portion of the temporal bone is so named because it usually has a scaly appearance[3] (squamous means scaly).
5. The lateral pterygoid plate (of the pterygoid process) of the sphenoid bone (#19) is the medial attachment site of the lateral and medial pterygoid muscles. The medial pterygoid muscle attaches to its medial surface; the lateral pterygoid muscle attaches to its lateral surface[4] (#19).

CHAPTER 5 Bones of the Human Body

SKULL—POSTERIOR VIEWS

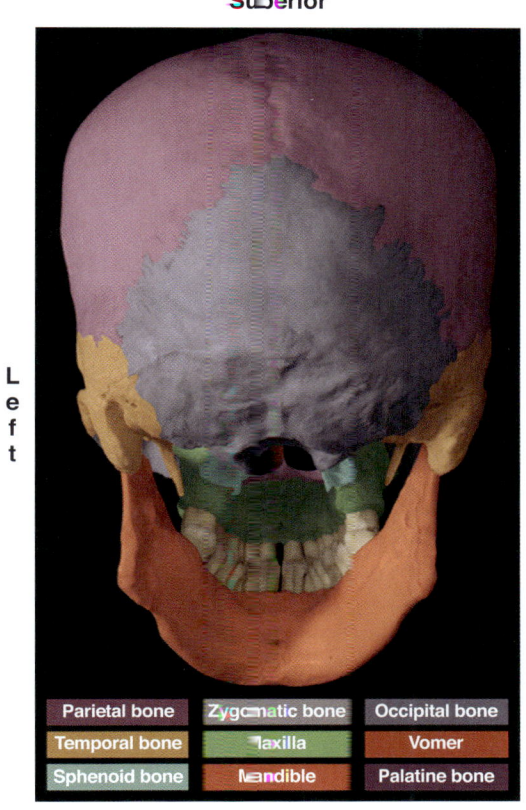

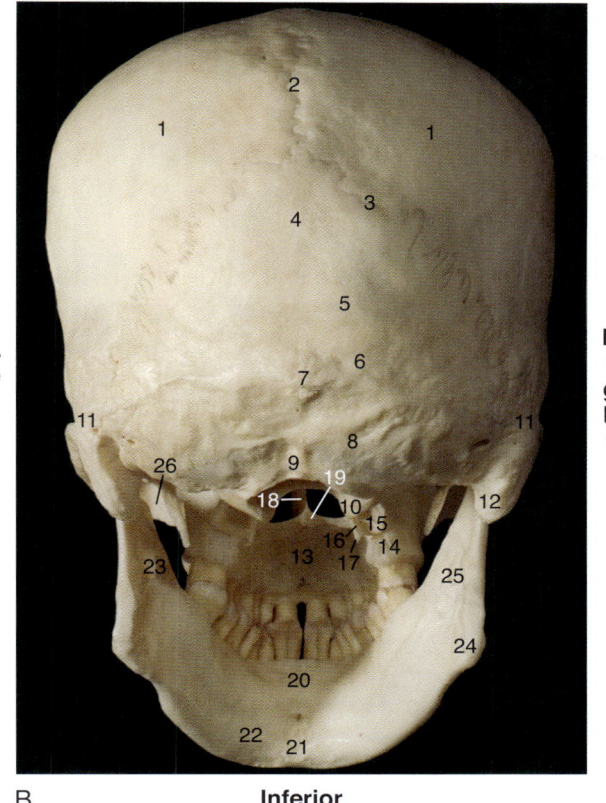

FIGURE 5-7
1. Parietal bone
2. Sagittal suture
3. Lambdoid suture

Occipital bone (#5-10):
4. Occipital bone
5. Highest nuchal line
6. Superior nuchal line
7. External occipital protuberance (EOP)
8. Inferior nuchal line
9. External occipital crest
10. Condyle
11. Temporal bone
12. Mastoid process of the temporal bone
13. Maxilla
14. Tuberosity of the maxilla

Sphenoid bone (#15-17):
15. Lateral pterygoid plate of the pterygoid process
16. Medial pterygoid plate of the pterygoid process
17. Pterygoid hamulus
18. Vomer
19. Palatine bone

Mandible (#20-25):
20. Mandible
21. Inferior and superior mental spines
22. Mylohyoid line
23. Lingula
24. Angle
25. Ramus
26. Zygomatic bone

NOTES
1. The external occipital protuberance (EOP) (#7) is also known as the inion.
2. The EOP is located in the middle of the superior nuchal line (#6) of the occiput.[4]
3. The lateral and medial pterygoid plates are landmarks of the pterygoid process of the sphenoid bone.[4]
4. The lateral pterygoid muscle attaches to the lateral surface of the lateral pterygoid plate of the sphenoid (#15); the medial pterygoid muscle attaches to the medial surface of the lateral pterygoid plate of the sphenoid.[2]

SKULL—INFERIOR VIEWS

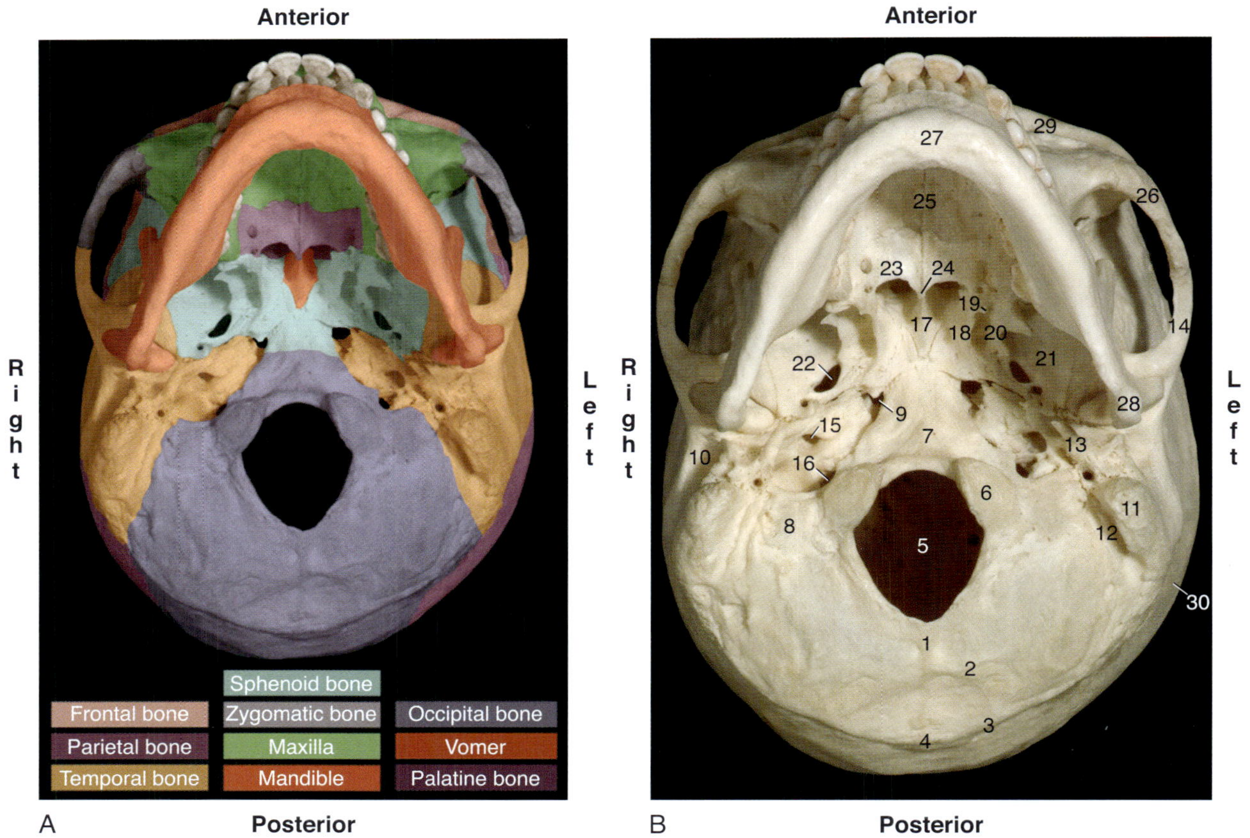

FIGURE 5-8

Occipital bone (#1-9):
1. External occipital crest
2. Inferior nuchal line
3. Superior nuchal line
4. External occipital protuberance (EOP)
5. Foramen magnum
6. Condyle
7. Basilar part
8. Jugular process
9. Foramen lacerum

Temporal bone (#10-15):
10. Temporal bone
11. Mastoid process
12. Mastoid notch
13. Styloid process
14. Zygomatic arch
15. Carotid canal
16. Jugular foramen (of the occipital bone)
17. Vomer

Sphenoid bone (#18-22):
18. Medial pterygoid plate of pterygoid process
19. Pterygoid hamulus
20. Lateral pterygoid plate of pterygoid process
21. Greater wing of sphenoid
22. Foramen ovale

23. Palatine bone
24. Posterior nasal spine of palatine bones
25. Maxilla
26. Zygomatic bone
27. Mandible
28. Angle of the mandible
29. Frontal bone
30. Parietal bone

NOTES

1. The foramen magnum (#5) is the division point between the brain and spinal cord. The brain and spinal cord are actually one structure; superior to the foramen magnum is the brain; inferior to it is the spinal cord.
2. The foramen lacerum (#9) is mostly blocked with cartilage, allowing only a small nerve, the nerve of the pterygoid canal, to pass through.[5]
3. The carotid canal (#15) provides a passageway for the internal carotid artery to enter the cranial cavity.[5]
4. The jugular foramen (#16) provides a passageway for cranial nerves (CNs) IX, X, and XI to pass from the brain to the neck. Venous blood draining from the brain to the internal jugular vein also passes through the jugular foramen.[5]
5. The foramen ovale (#22) provides a passageway for the mandibular division of the trigeminal nerve (CN V) to pass from the brain to the neck.[5]

CHAPTER 5 Bones of the Human Body

SKULL—INTERNAL VIEWS

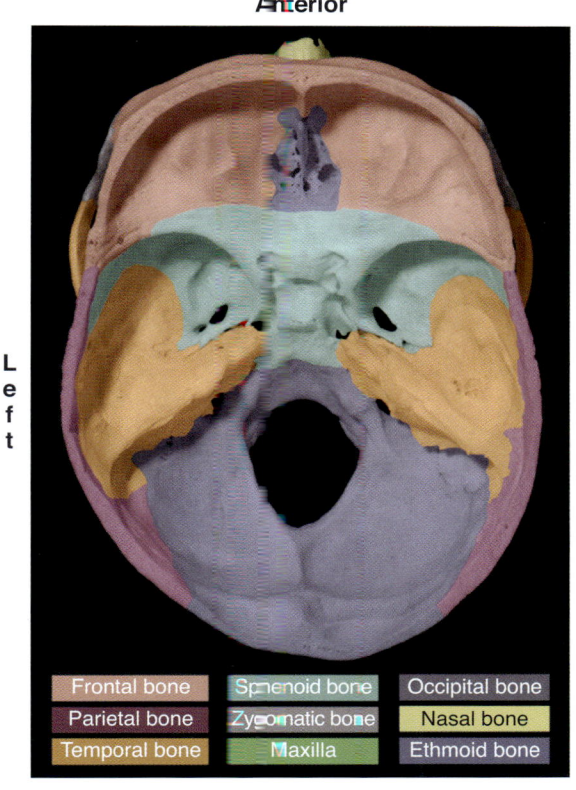

FIGURE 5-9

Occipital bone (#1-5):
1 Occipital bone
2 Internal occipital protuberance
3 Foramen magnum
4 Basilar part
5 Jugular foramen
6 Parietal bone
7 Squamous part of temporal bone
8 Petrous part of temporal bone
9 Foramen lacerum

Sphenoid bone (#10-16):
10 Sphenoid bone
11 Lesser wing
12 Greater wing
13 Sella turcica
14 Dorsum sellae
15 Foramen ovale
16 Optic foramen
17 Frontal bone (orbital part)
18 Frontal crest
19 Crista galli of ethmoid bone
20 Cribriform plate of ethmoid bone
21 Nasal bone
22 Maxilla
23 Zygomatic arch of temporal bone
24 Temporal arch of zygomatic bone

> **NOTES**
> 1. The sella turcica (#13) of the sphenoid (#10) is where the pituitary gland sits[6] (sella turcica literally means Turkish saddle).
> 2. The optic foramen (#16) allows passage of the optic nerve (cranial nerve [CN] II) from the eye to the brain.[3]
> 3. From this view, the eyeball is located deep to the orbital part of the frontal bone (#17).
> 4. The crista galli of the ethmoid (#19) is an attachment site of the falx cerebri of the dura mater, one of the meninges of the brain.[3]
> 5. Receptor cells for the sense of smell from the nasal cavity pierce the cribriform plate of the ethmoid bone (#20) to connect with the olfactory bulb (CN I) of the brain.[5]
> 6. The basilar portion of the occiput (#4) and the most posterior portion of the sphenoid (#10) are often collectively called the clivus.[4]

SKULL—SAGITTAL SECTION AND THE ORBITAL CAVITY

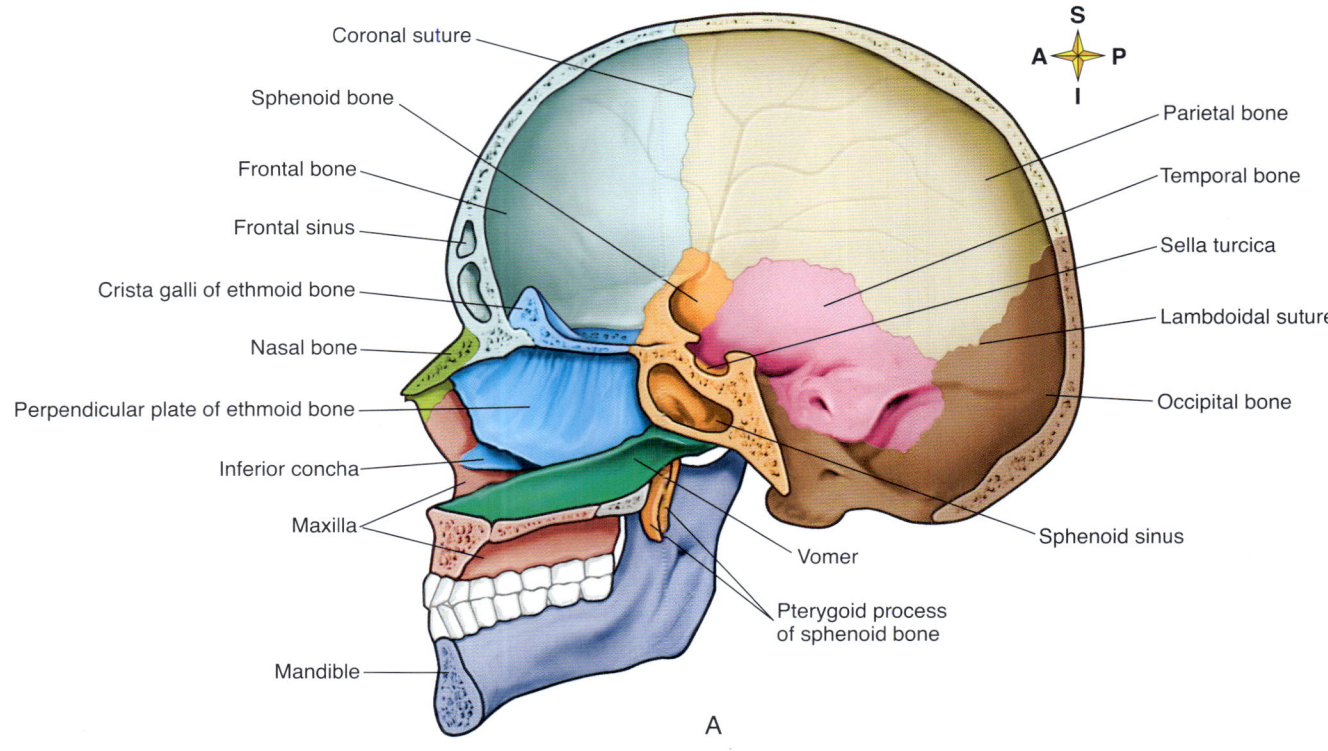

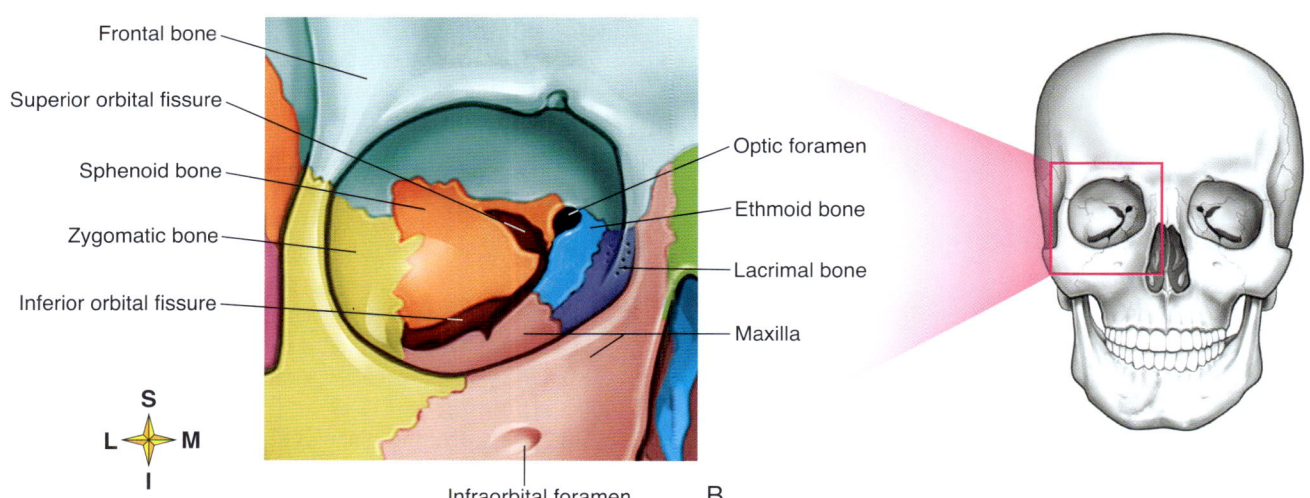

FIGURE 5-10 **A,** Right half of the skull viewed from within. **B,** Bones that form the right orbit. *(Modified from Patton KT, Thibodeau GA: Anatomy and physiology, ed 3, St Louis, 2016, Elsevier.)*

MANDIBLE

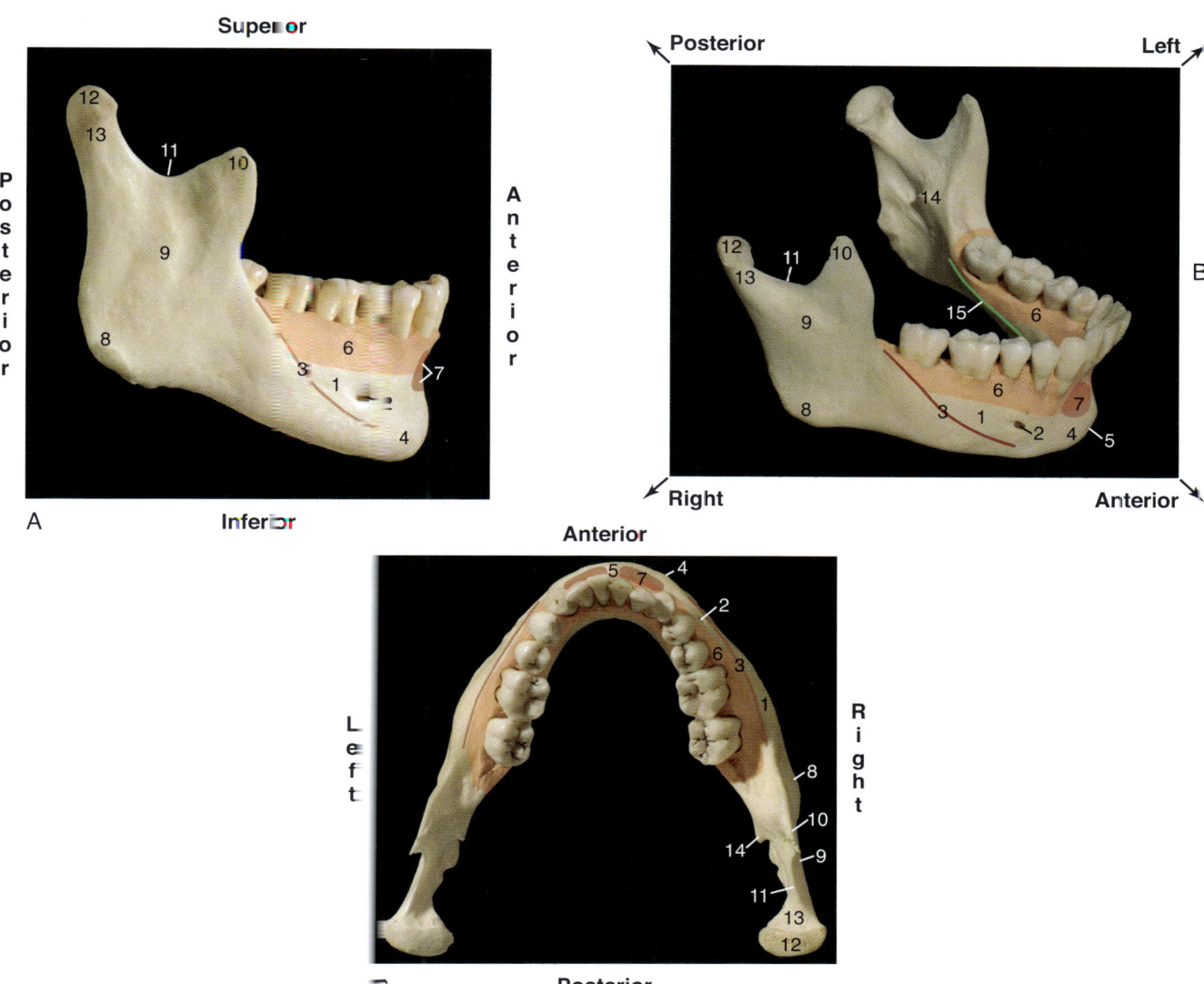

FIGURE 5-11 A, Right lateral view. B, Oblique view. C, Superior view.
1. Body
2. Mental foramen
3. Oblique line
4. Mental protuberance
5. Symphysis menti
6. Alveolar process (indicated in light pink)
7. Incisive fossa (indicated in dark pink)
8. Angle
9. Ramus
10. Coronoid process
11. Mandibular notch
12. Head of condyle
13. Neck of condyle
14. Lingula
15. Mylohyoid line

NOTES
1. The symphysis menti (#5) is where the left and right sides of the mandible fuse together.
2. The word ramus means branch. The ramus of the mandible (#9) branches from the body of the mandible.
3. The coronoid process (#10) and condyle (#13) are landmarks of the ramus of the mandible (#9).[3]
4. The condyle of the mandible (#12) articulates with the temporal bone, forming the temporomandibular joint (TMJ).[4]
5. The head of the condyle (#12) is easily palpable just anterior to the ear while the mouth is opened and closed[4] (elevating and depressing the mandible at the TMJ). Alternatively, place your palpating finger inside your ear and press anteriorly while opening and closing the mouth.
6. The mylohyoid line (#15) is the attachment site on the internal mandible of the mylohyoid muscle.[3]

PARIETAL, TEMPORAL, AND FRONTAL BONES

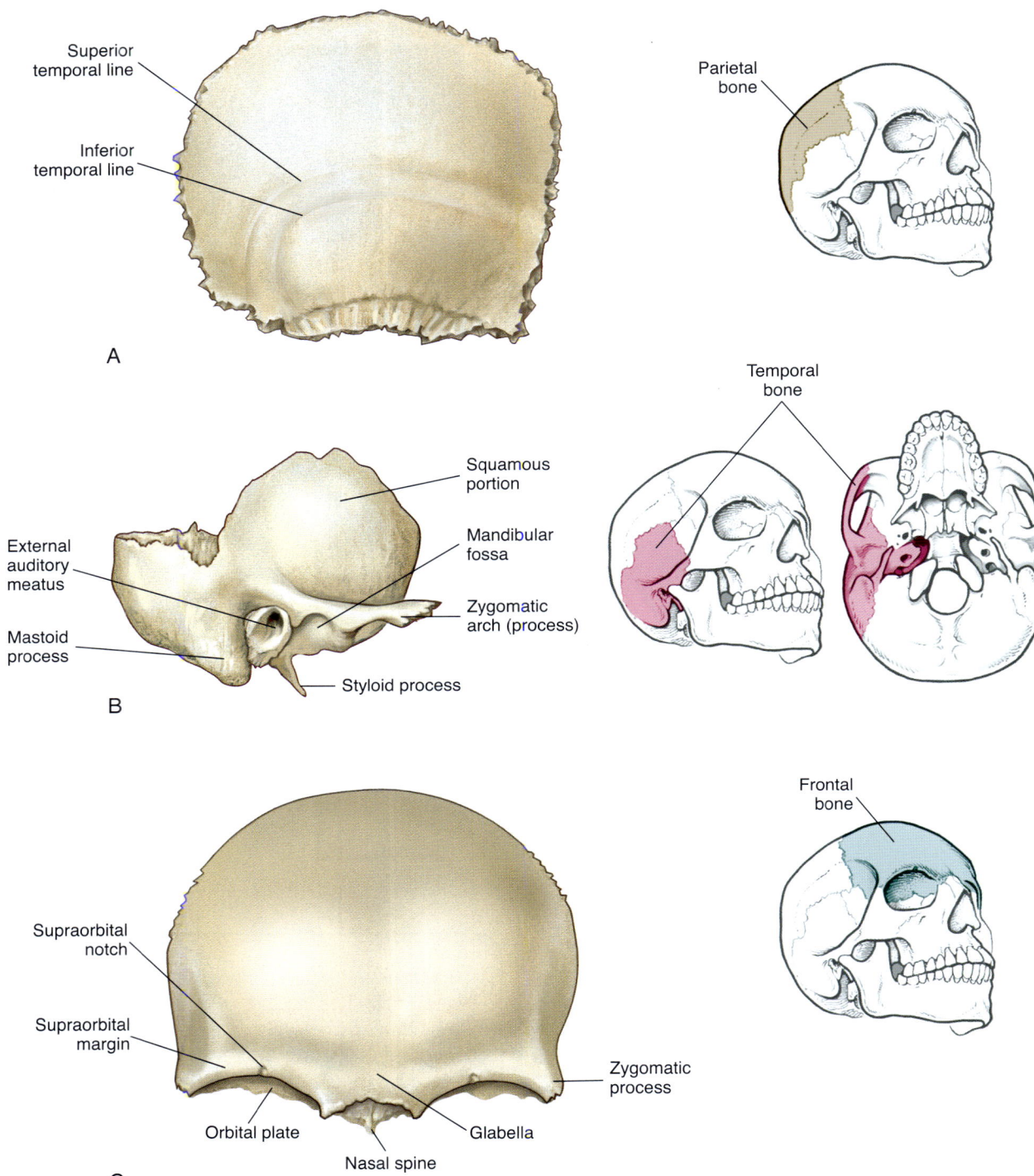

FIGURE 5-12 **A,** Lateral view at the right parietal bone. **B,** Lateral view of the right temporal bone. **C,** Anterior view of the frontal bone. *(Modified from Patton KT, Thibodeau GA: Anatomy and physiology, ed 9, St Louis, 2016, Elsevier.)*

OCCIPITAL AND SPHENOID BONES

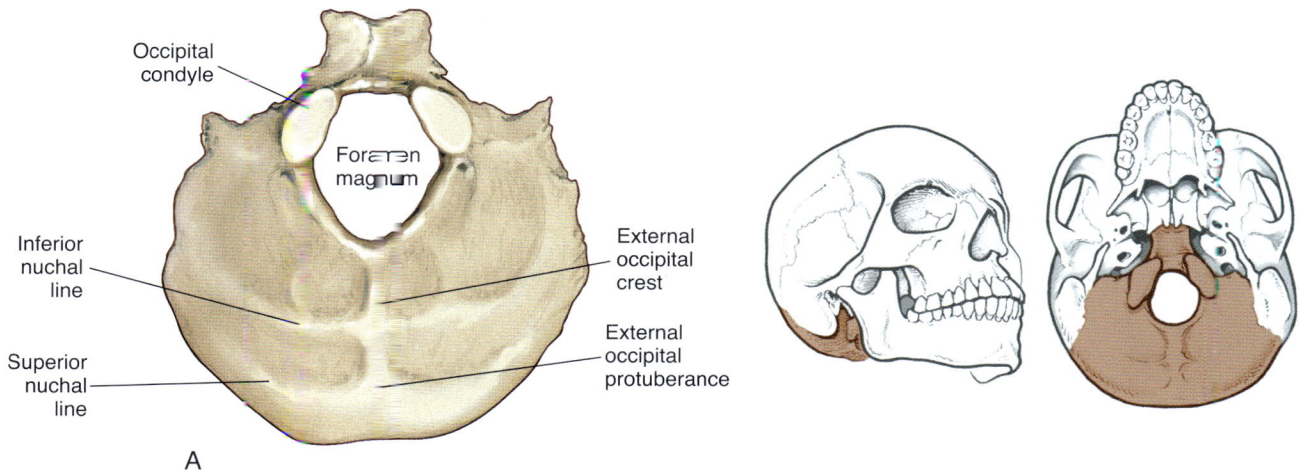
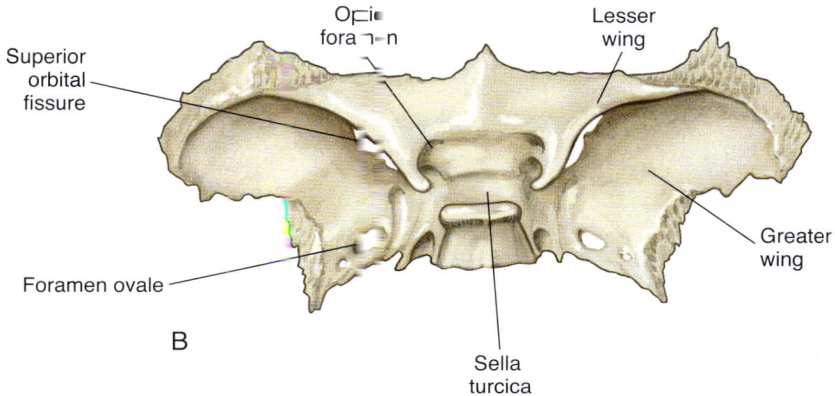
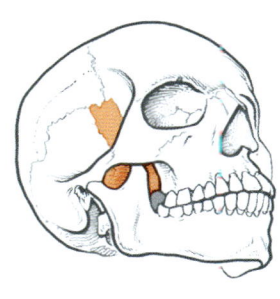
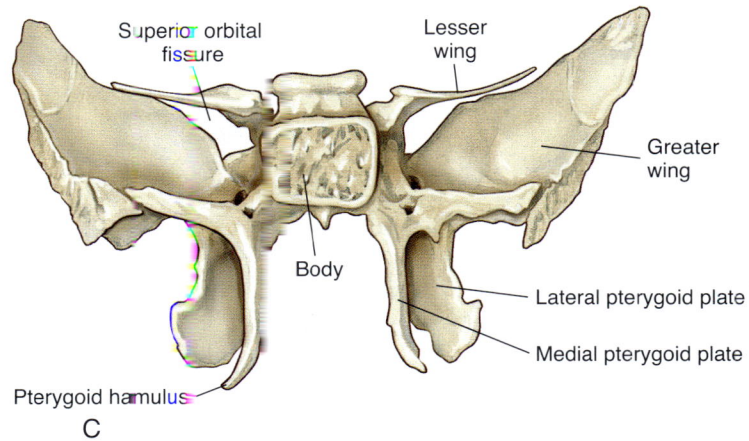
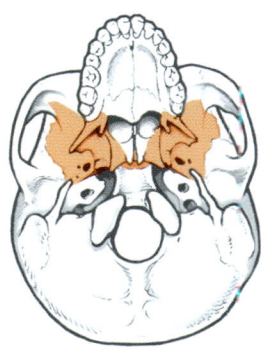

FIGURE 5-13 **A,** Inferior view of the occipital bone. **B,** Superior view of the sphenoid bone (within the cranial cavity). **C,** Posterior view of the sphenoid bone. *(Modified from Patton KT, Thibodeau GA: Anatomy and physiology, ed 9, St Louis, 2016, Elsevier.)*

ETHMOID AND VOMER

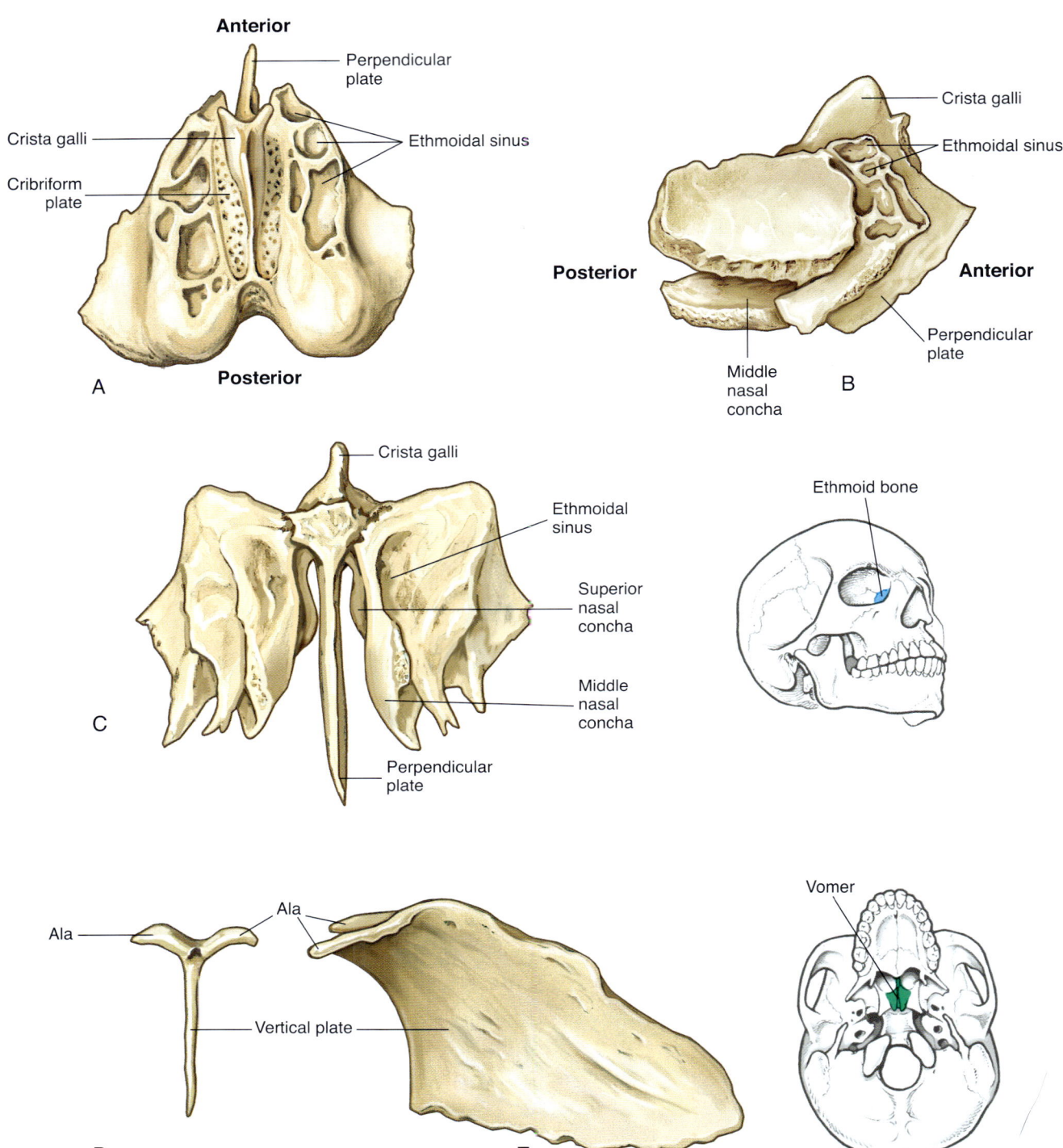

FIGURE 5-14 **A,** Superior view of the ethmoid bone. **B,** Right lateral view of the ethmoid bone. **C,** Anterior view of the ethmoid bone. **D,** Anterior view of the vomer. **E,** Right lateral view of the vomer. *(Modified from Patton KT, Thibodeau GA: Anatomy and physiology, ed 9, St Louis, 2016, Elsevier.)*

MAXILLARY AND ZYGOMATIC BONES

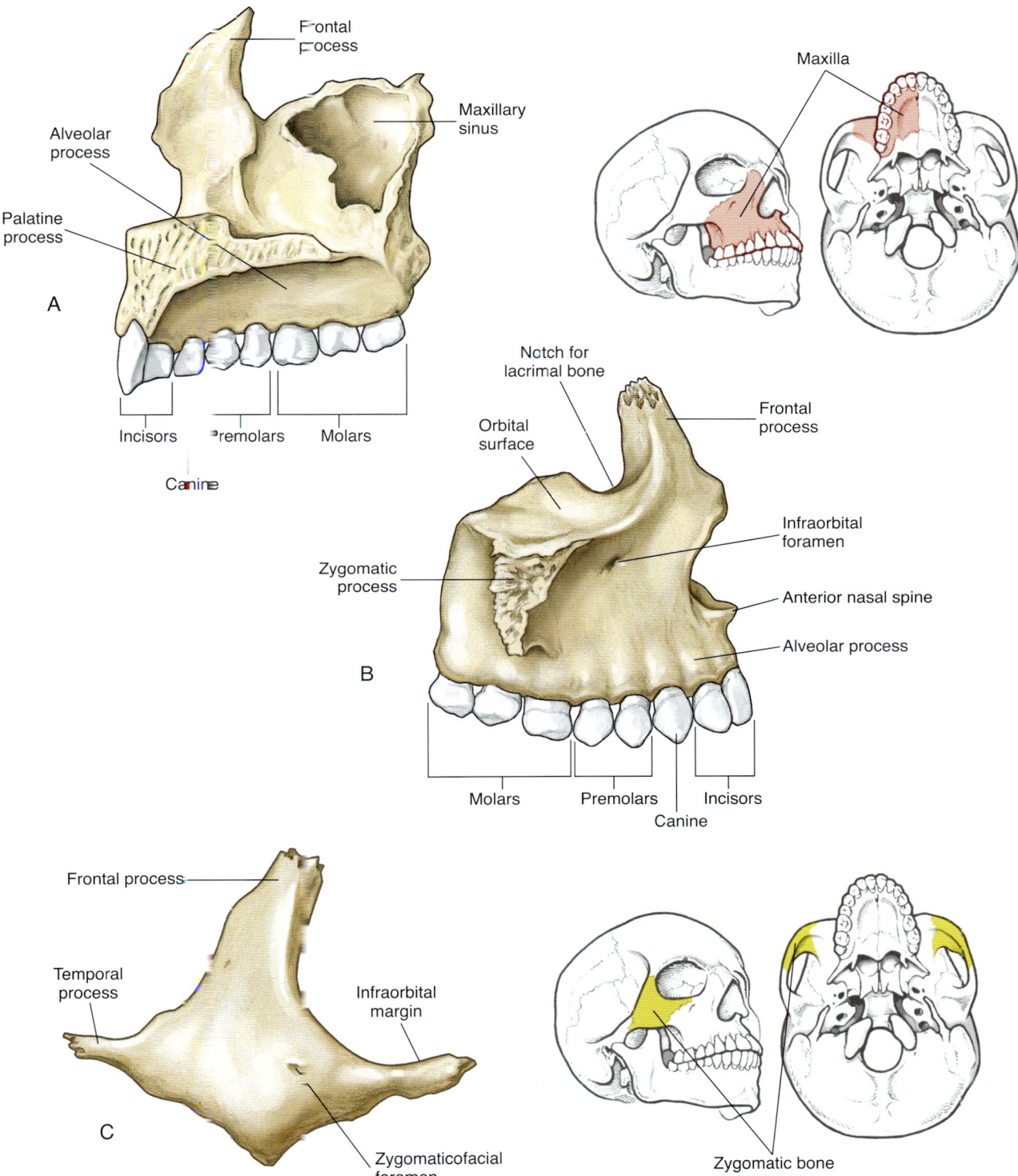

FIGURE 5-15 A, Medial view of the right maxilla. **B,** Lateral view of the right maxilla. **C,** Lateral view of the right zygomatic bone. *(Modified from Patton KT, Thibodeau GA: Anatomy and physiology, ed 9, St Louis, 2016, Elsevier.)*

PALATINE, LACRIMAL, AND NASAL BONES

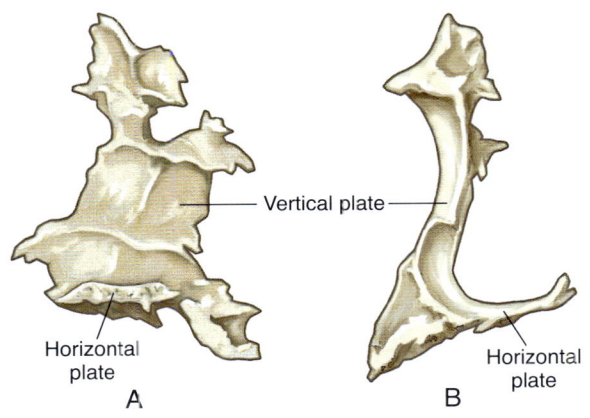
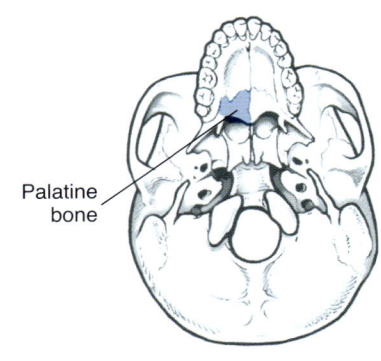

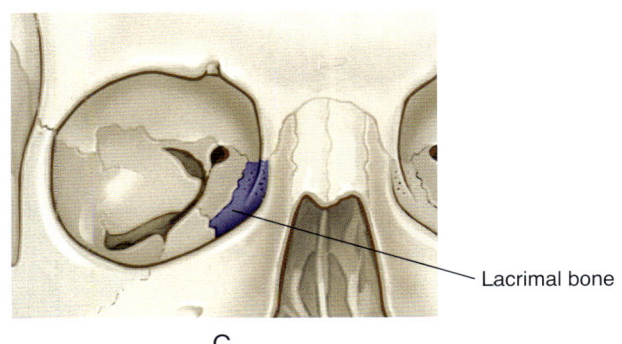
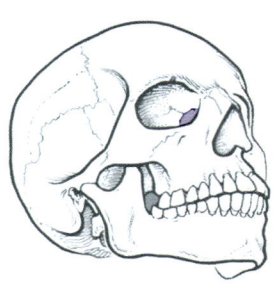

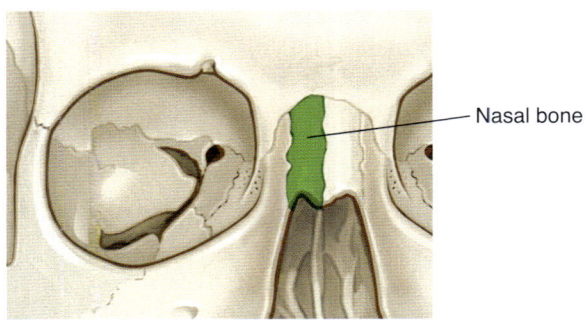
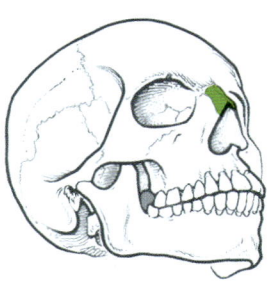

FIGURE 5-16 **A,** Medial view of the right palatine bone. **B,** Anterior view of the right palatine bone. **C,** Anterior view of the right lacrimal bone. **D,** Anterior view of the right nasal bone. *(From Patton KT, Thibodeau GA: Anatomy and physiology, ed 9, St Louis, 2016, Elsevier.)*

SECTION 5.2 BONES OF THE SPINE (AND HYOID)

SPINAL COLUMN—POSTERIOR VIEW

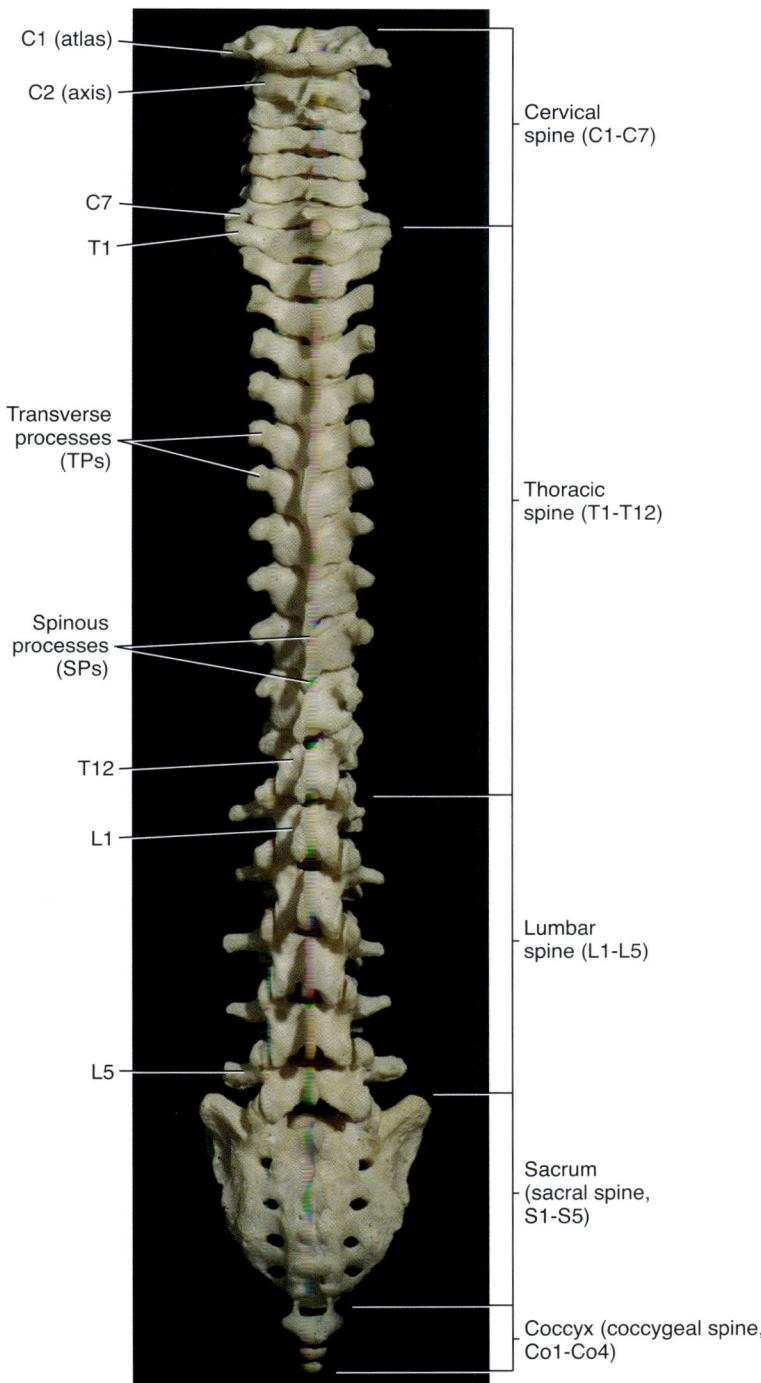

FIGURE 5-17

NOTES
1. The spine is part of the axial skeleton and is composed of five regions: the cervical, thoracic, lumbar, sacral, and coccygeal spines.
2. The spine has seven cervical vertebrae (named C1-C7), 12 thoracic vertebrae (named T1-T12), five lumbar vertebrae (named L1-L5), one sacrum (composed of five fused sacral vertebrae, named S1-S5), and one coccyx (usually composed of four rudimentary vertebrae, named Co1-Co4).[2]
3. Vertebra is singular; vertebrae is plural.
4. The spinal column is composed of 24 vertebrae, a sacrum, and a coccyx.[2]
5. The cervical spine is located within the neck.
6. The thoracic and lumbar spines are located in the trunk.
7. The thoracic spine constitutes the thorax; the lumbar spine constitutes the abdomen.
8. The thoracic spine is defined by having the ribcage attach to it; hence humans have 12 pairs of ribs and 12 thoracic vertebrae.[2]
9. The sacrum and coccyx are located within the pelvis.

SPINAL COLUMN—RIGHT LATERAL VIEW

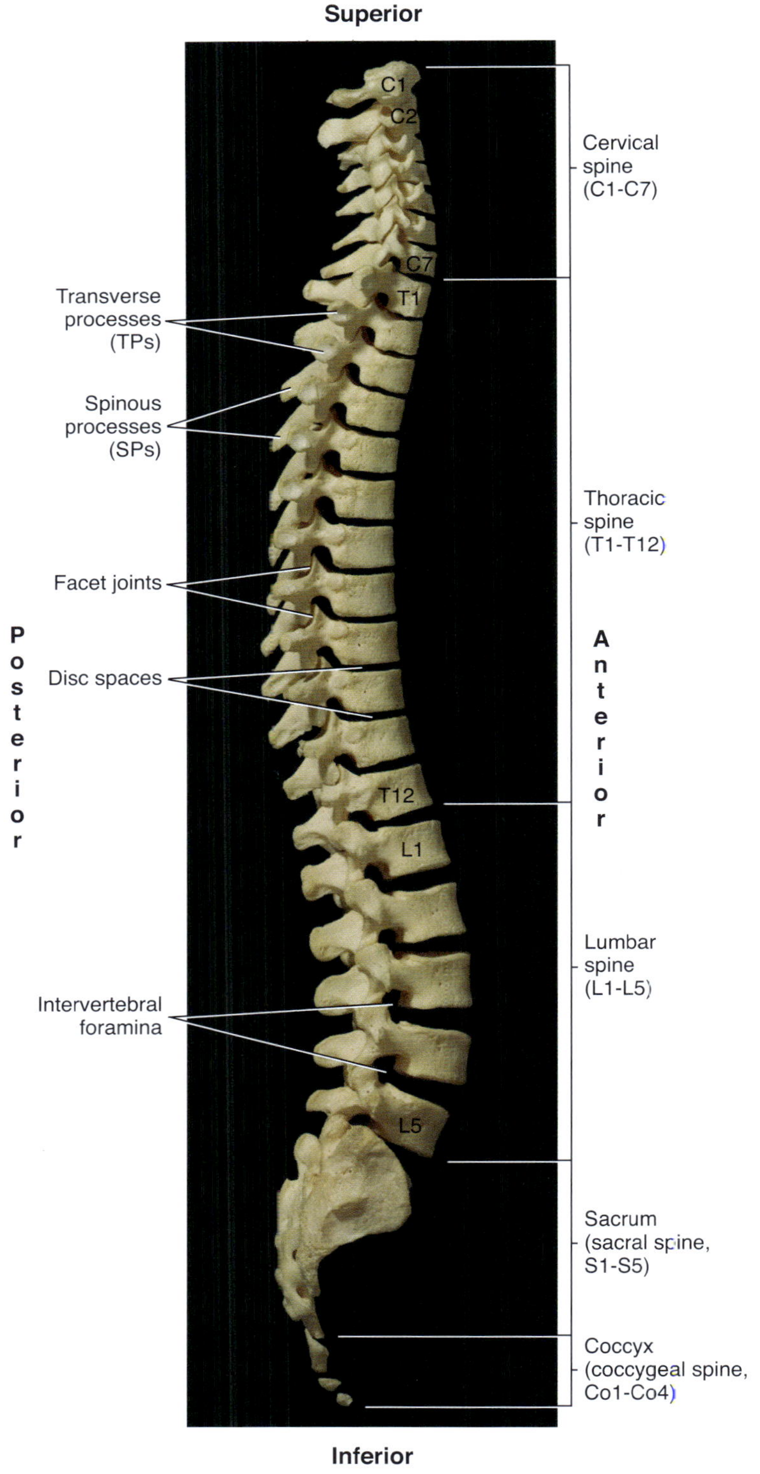

FIGURE 5-18

NOTES
1. Curves of the spine: The cervical and lumbar spines are lordotic (i.e., concave posteriorly); the thoracic and sacral (sacrococcygeal) spines are kyphotic (i.e., concave anteriorly[2]).
2. Generally, a disc joint and paired right and left facet joints are found between each two contiguous vertebrae.[7]
3. Intervertebral foramina (singular: foramen) are where spinal nerves enter/exit the spine.[7]
4. Spinous processes (SPs) project posteriorly and are usually easily palpable. (Note: The word spine means thorn; SPs are pointy like thorns.)
5. Transverse processes (TPs) project laterally in the transverse plane (hence their name).
6. Because the spine is a weight-bearing structure, the bodies of the vertebrae (the weight-bearing aspect of the spinal column) get progressively larger from superior to inferior.[7]

CERVICAL SPINE AND HYOID

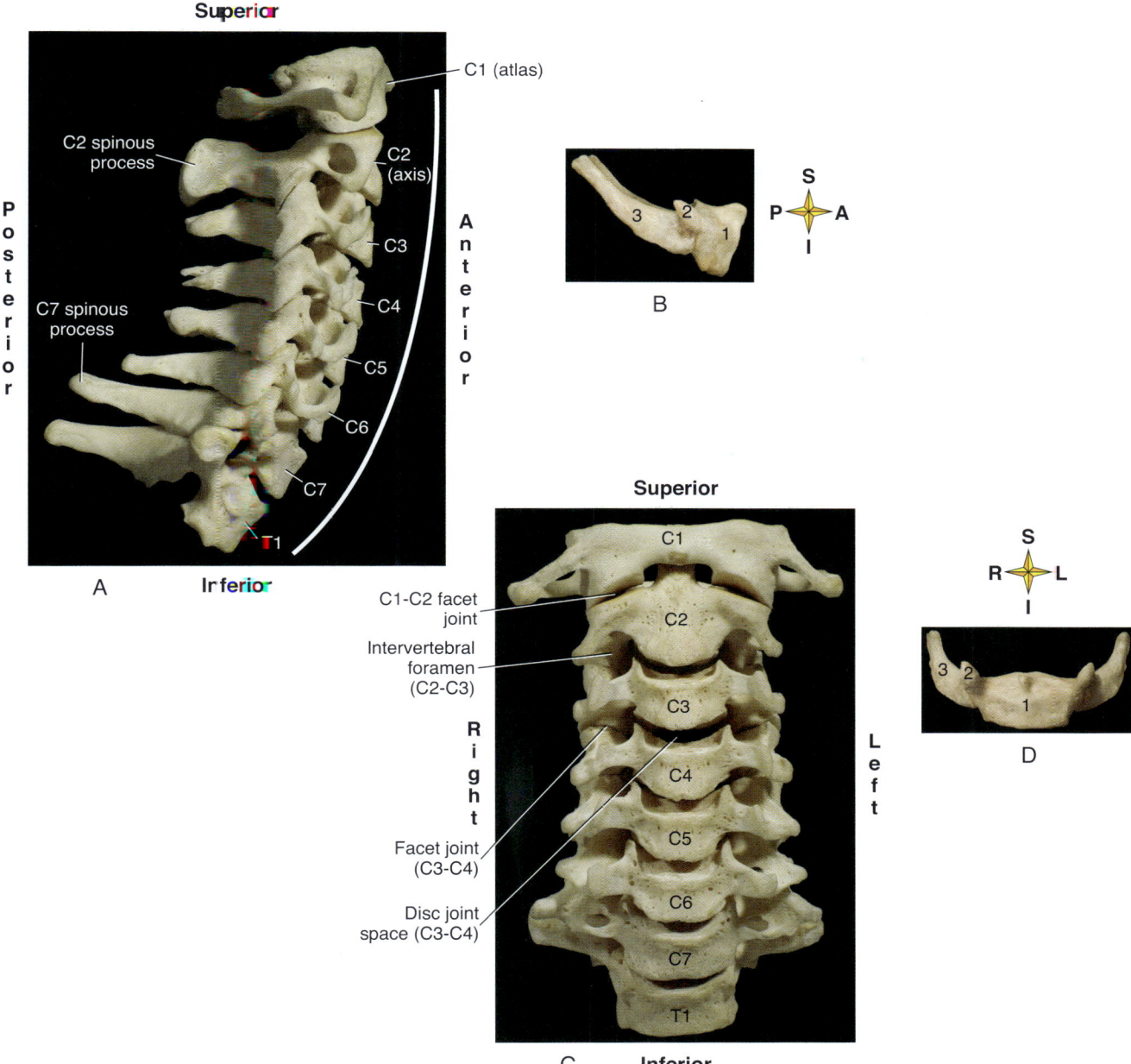

FIGURE 5-19 **A,** Right lateral view of the cervical spine. **B,** Right lateral view of the hyoid bone. **C,** Anterior view of the cervical spine. **D,** Anterior view of the hyoid bone.
1 Body
2 Lesser cornu
3 Greater cornu

NOTES
1. The hyoid is located at the level of the C3 vertebra.[2]
2. The greater cornu and lesser cornu of the hyoid are also known as the greater and lesser horns.
3. The hyoid bone serves as an attachment site for the hyoid muscle group, as well as many muscles of the tongue.[8]
4. The hyoid is the only bone in the human body that does not articulate with another bone.[8]
5. The lordotic (i.e., concave posteriorly) curve of the cervical spine is indicated by the line drawn anterior to the cervical spine.
6. The spinous processes (SPs) of C2 and C7 are very palpable and serve as excellent landmarks.[2]

CERVICAL SPINE (CONTINUED)

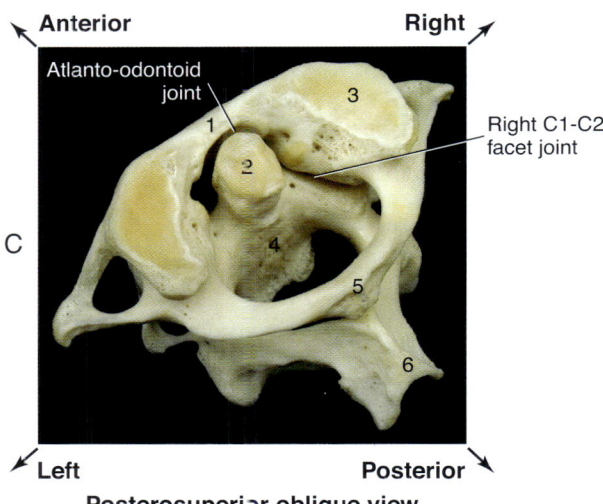

FIGURE 5-20 A, Posterior view. B, Anterolateral oblique view. C, Posterosuperior oblique view.
1 Anterior arch of C1 (atlas)
2 Dens of C2 (axis)
3 Superior articular process/facet of C1
4 Body of C2
5 Posterior tubercle of C1
6 Spinous process (SP) of C2

NOTES
1. The oblique view of the cervical spine demonstrates the intervertebral foramina well (the right C3-C4 intervertebral foramen is labeled). The intervertebral foramen is where the spinal nerve enters/exits the spinal cord.[7]
2. The posterosuperior oblique view demonstrates the atlanto-axial joint complex well (Figure 5-20, C).

ATLAS (C1)

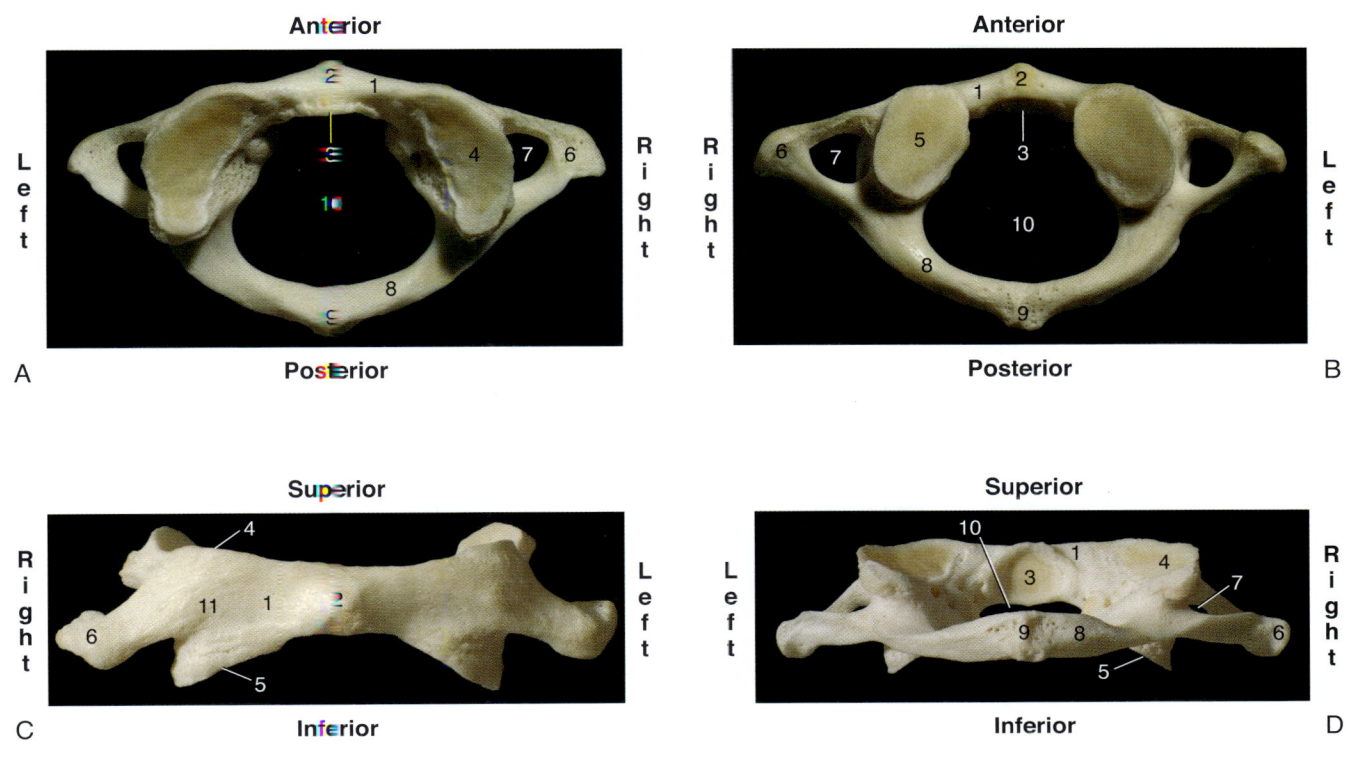

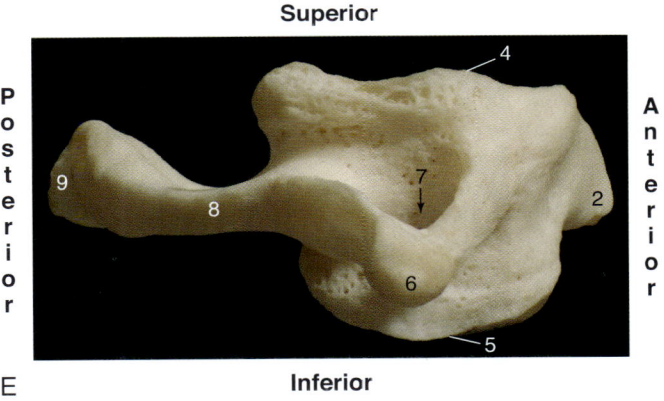

FIGURE 5-21 **A**, Superior view. **B**, Inferior view. **C**, Anterior view. **D**, Posterior view. **E**, Right lateral view.
1. Anterior arch
2. Anterior tubercle
3. Facet for dens of axis (C2)
4. Superior articular process/facet
5. Inferior articular process/facet
6. Transverse process (TP)
7. Transverse foramen
8. Posterior arch
9. Posterior tubercle
10. Vertebral foramen
11. Lateral mass

NOTES:
Unlike the other vertebrae, the atlas has no body. What would have been the body of the atlas became the dens of the axis (C2).
1. Also unique to the atlas are the anterior and posterior arches. The centers of these arches have the anterior and posterior tubercles, respectively.
2. The superior articular processes (#4) of the atlas articulate with the occipital condyles at the atlanto-occipital joint; the inferior articular processes (#5) of the atlas articulate with the superior articular processes of the axis at the atlantoaxial (C1-C2) joint.
3. The superior and inferior articular processes of the atlas create what is termed the lateral mass (labeled #11 in the anterior view).

AXIS (C2)

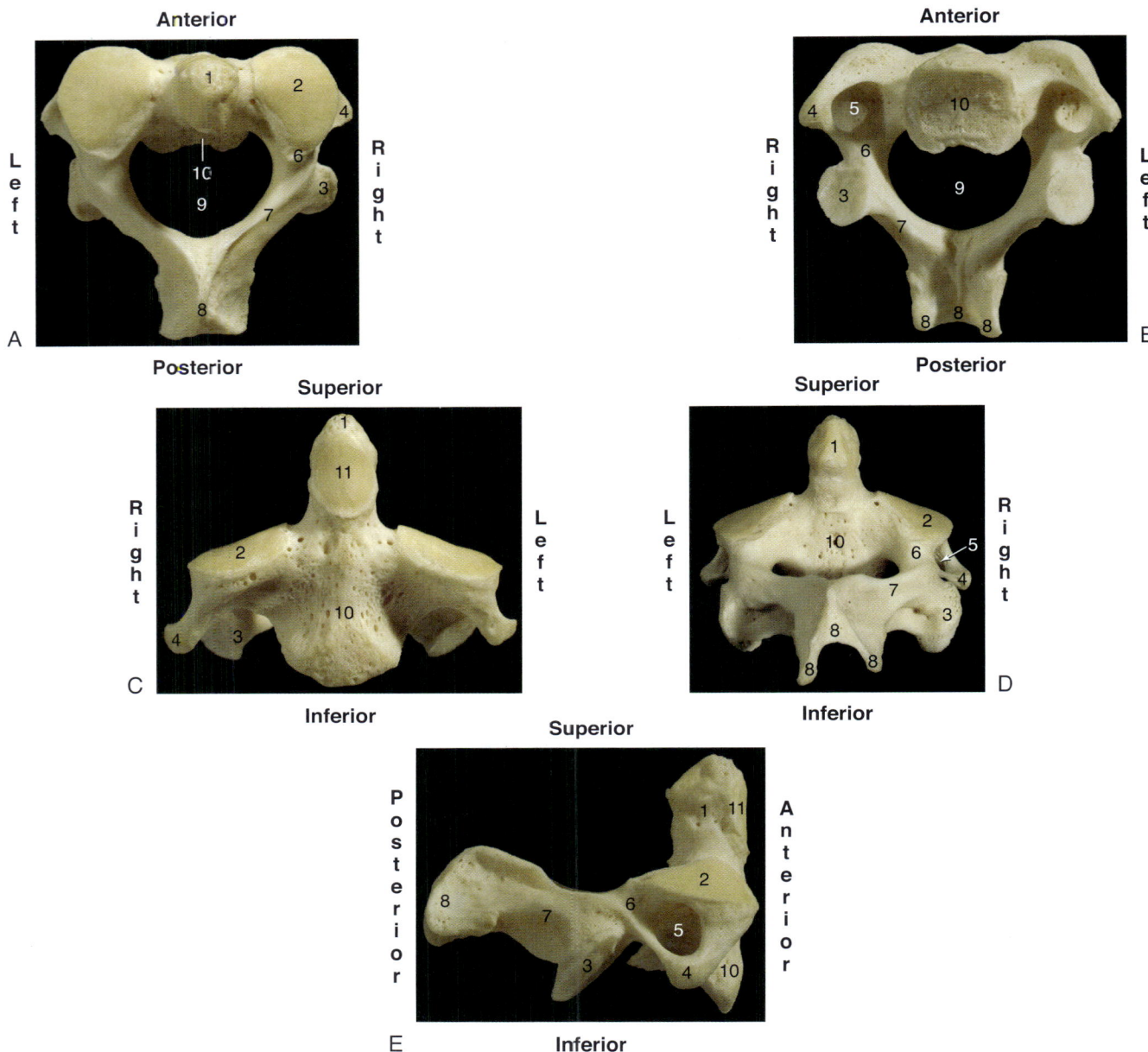

FIGURE 5-22 A, Superior view. B, Inferior view. C, Anterior view. D, Posterior view. E, Right lateral view.
1. Dens (odontoid process)
2. Superior articular process/facet
3. Inferior articular process/facet
4. Transverse process (TP)
5. Transverse foramen
6. Pedicle
7. Lamina
8. Spinous process (SP) (bifid)
9. Vertebral foramen
10. Body
11. Facet on dens

NOTES
1. The dens of the axis (#1) creates an axis of rotation for the atlas to rotate about,[2] hence the name C2 (i.e., the axis).
2. The superior articular processes of the axis (#2) articulate with the inferior articular processes of the atlas.[7]
3. The spinous process (SP) (#8) of C2 is very large and an excellent landmark when a client's posterior neck is palpated. It will be the first large structure felt midline, inferior to the skull.[5]
4. The SP of the axis is bifid. Furthermore, the two bifid points are often asymmetric in size and shape.[2]
5. The facet on the dens (#11) articulates with the anterior arch of the atlas, forming the atlanto-odontoid joint.[9]

C5 (TYPICAL CERVICAL VERTEBRA)

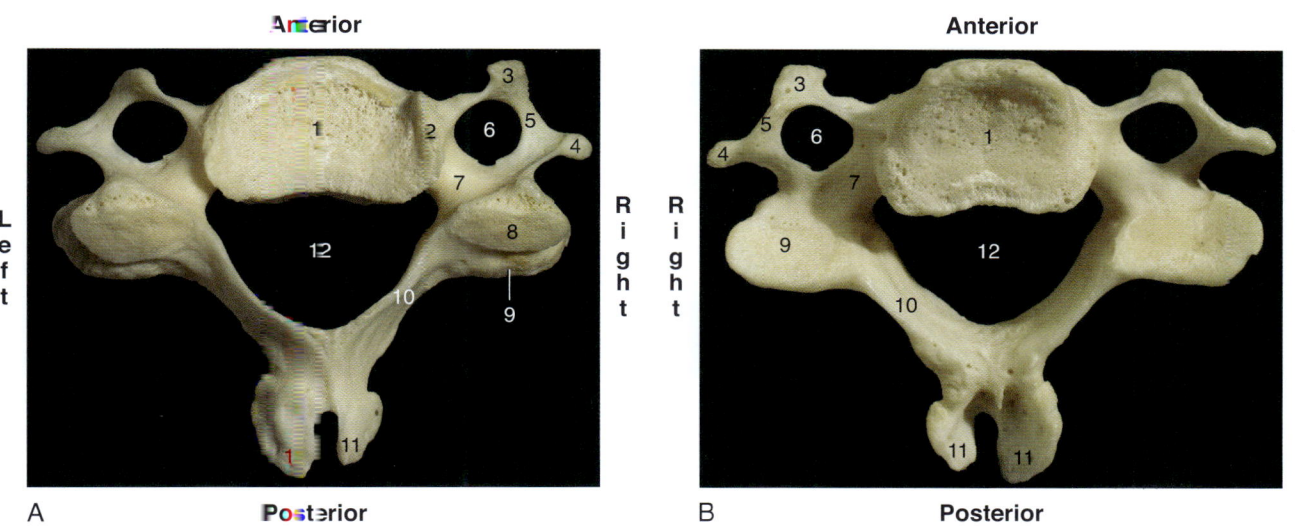

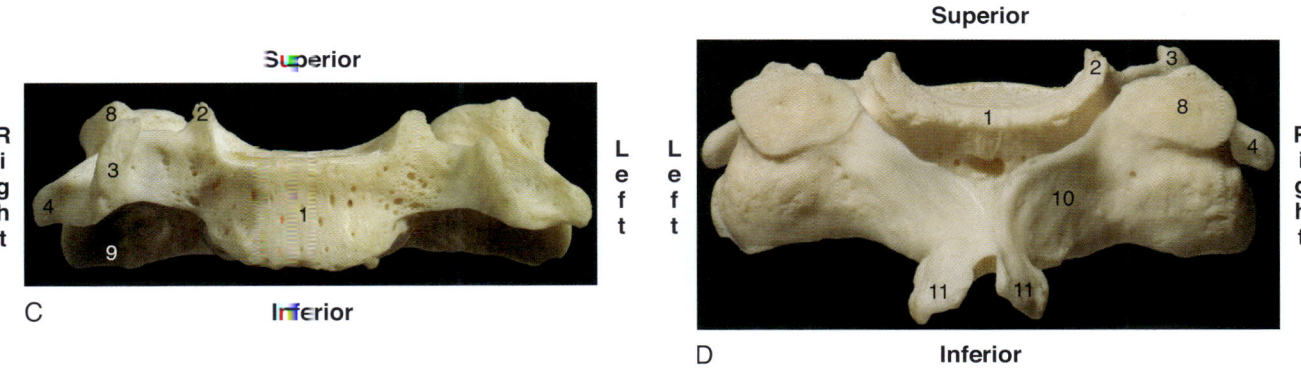

FIGURE 5-23 **A**, Superior view. **B**, Inferior view. **C**, Anterior view. **D**, Posterior view.
  1 Body
  2 Uncus of body
  3 Anterior tubercle of transverse process (TP)
  4 Posterior tubercle of TP
  5 Groove for spinal nerve (on TP)
  6 Transverse foramen
  7 Pedicle
  8 Superior articular process/facet
  9 Inferior articular process/facet
 10 Lamina
 11 Spinous process (SP) (bifid)
 12 Vertebral foramen

NOTES
1. The articular process is the entire structural landmark that projects outward from the bone; the articular facets (#8, 9) are the smooth articular surfaces located on the articular process.[2]
2. The plural of foramen is foramina.
3. The cervical vertebrae possess a number of structures that the other vertebrae do not: an uncus (#2) is located on the left and right sides of the body[2]; they have bifid (i.e., two points on their) spinous processes (SPs)[3]; their transverse processes (TPs) have an anterior and posterior tubercle[3]; and they have a foramen located within the TP[3] (hence the name transverse foramen, #6).
4. The bifid SP of a cervical vertebra is often asymmetric. This may lead one to conclude on palpatory examination that the vertebra is rotated when it is not.
5. The cervical transverse foramen allows passage up to the skull of the vertebral artery.[7]

C5 (CONTINUED) AND CERVICAL ENDPLATES

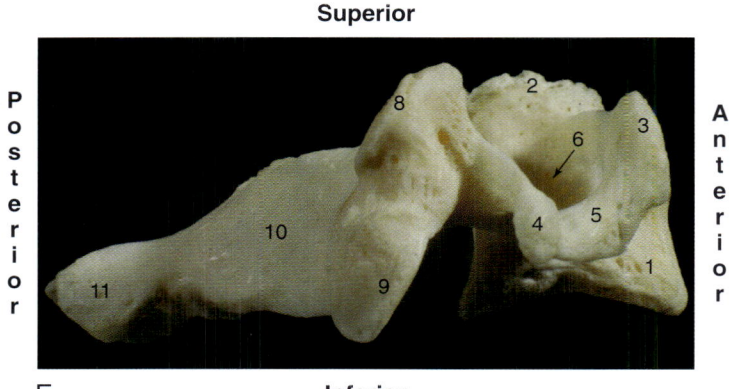

FIGURE 5-23, cont'd E, Right lateral view. F, Oblique posterior view.
1 Body
2 Uncus of body
3 Anterior tubercle of transverse process (TP)
4 Posterior tubercle of TP
5 Groove for spinal nerve (on TP)
6 Transverse foramen
7 Pedicle
8 Superior articular process/facet
9 Inferior articular process/facet
10 Lamina
11 Spinous process (SP) (bifid)
12 Vertebral foramen

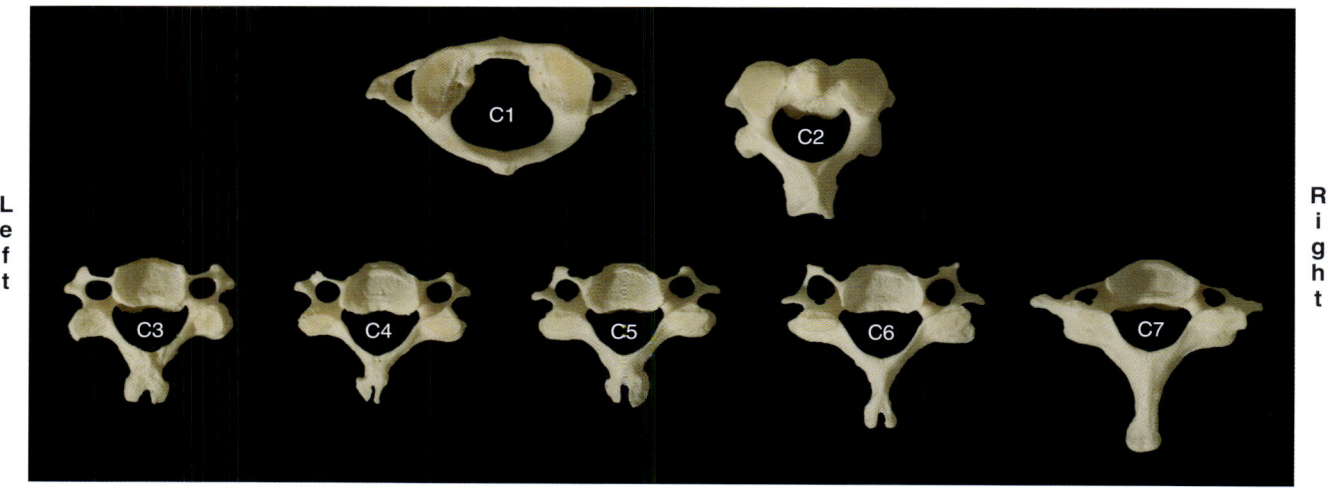

FIGURE 5-24 Superior view of all seven cervical vertebrae.

NOTES

1. Figure 5-24 shows the superior view of all seven cervical vertebrae (cervical endplate view). The differences from one cervical level to another can be seen.
2. C1 is also known as the atlas; C2 is also known as the axis.[2]
3. The anterior tubercle of the transverse process (TP) of C6 is larger than the other anterior tubercles and is known as the carotid tubercle.[8]
4. The large spinous process (SP) of C7 more closely resembles the SPs of the thoracic vertebrae than it does those of the other cervical vertebrae. This large SP gives C7 its name, the vertebra prominens.[8]

THORACIC SPINE—RIGHT LATERAL VIEW

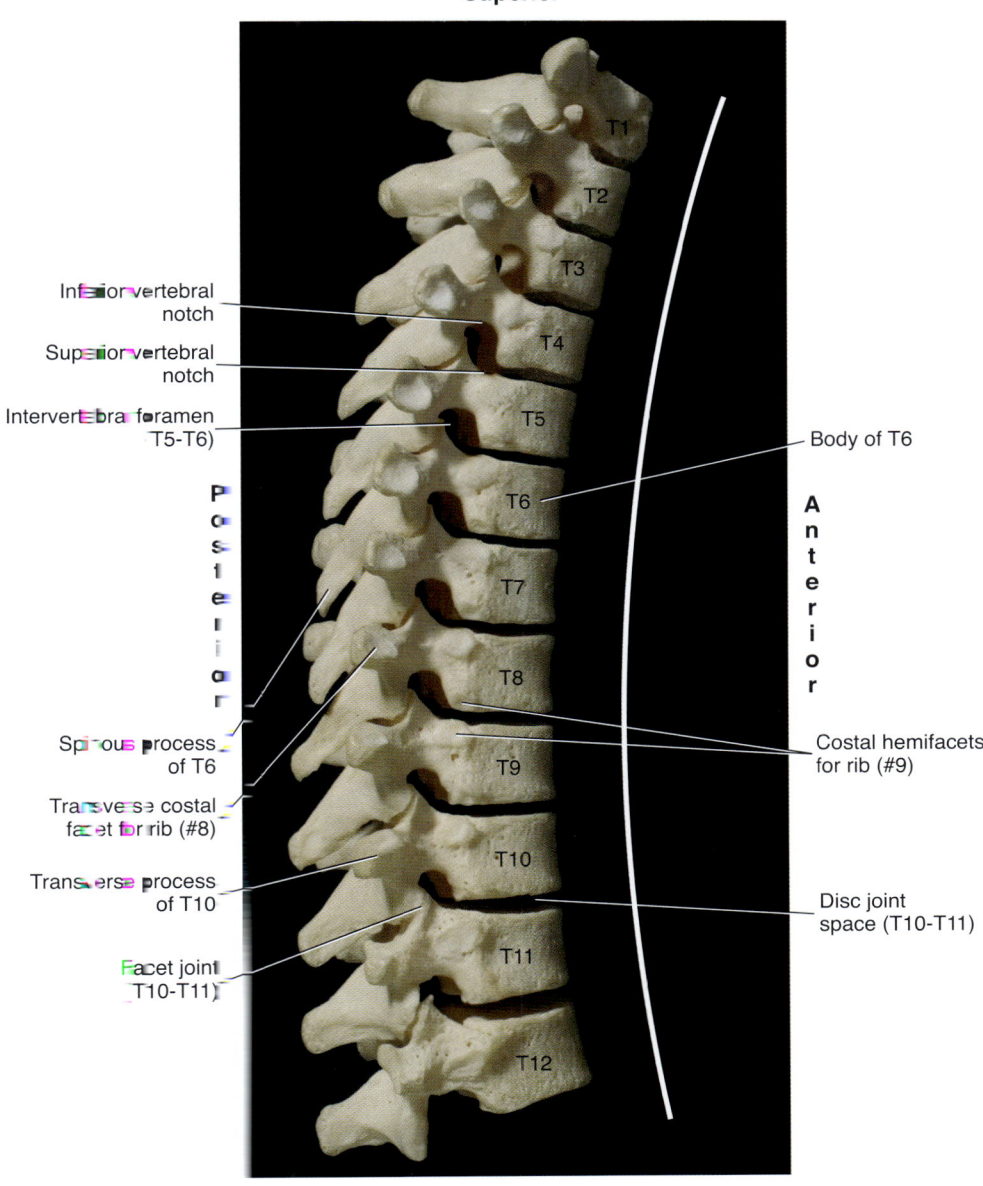

FIGURE 5-25

NOTES
1. The kyphotic (i.e., concave anteriorly) curve of the thoracic spine is indicated by the line drawn anterior to the thoracic spine.
2. The lateral view of the thoracic spine demonstrates the intervertebral foramina (well, the right T5-T6 intervertebral foramen is labeled). The intervertebral foramen is where the spinal nerve enters/exits the spinal cord.
3. The long downward-slanted orientation of the thoracic spinous processes (SPs), especially of the midthoracic spine, can be seen. The tip of a thoracic SP is at the level of the body of the vertebra below it (e.g., see the body and SP of T6, labeled).
4. The SPs of the thoracic spine are easily palpable (the word spine means thorn [i.e., a pointy projection]).
5. The vertebral body costal hemifacets for a rib (i.e., for the costovertebral joint) are labeled at the T8-T9 level. They are located on two contiguous vertebral bodies and span across the disc that is located between.[3]
6. The transverse costal facet for a rib (i.e., for the costotransverse joint) is labeled at the T8 level.
7. The gradual increase in size of the thoracic vertebral bodies from T1 to T12 can be seen.

94   PART 2   Skeletal Osteology: Study of the Bones

THORACIC SPINE—POSTERIOR VIEW

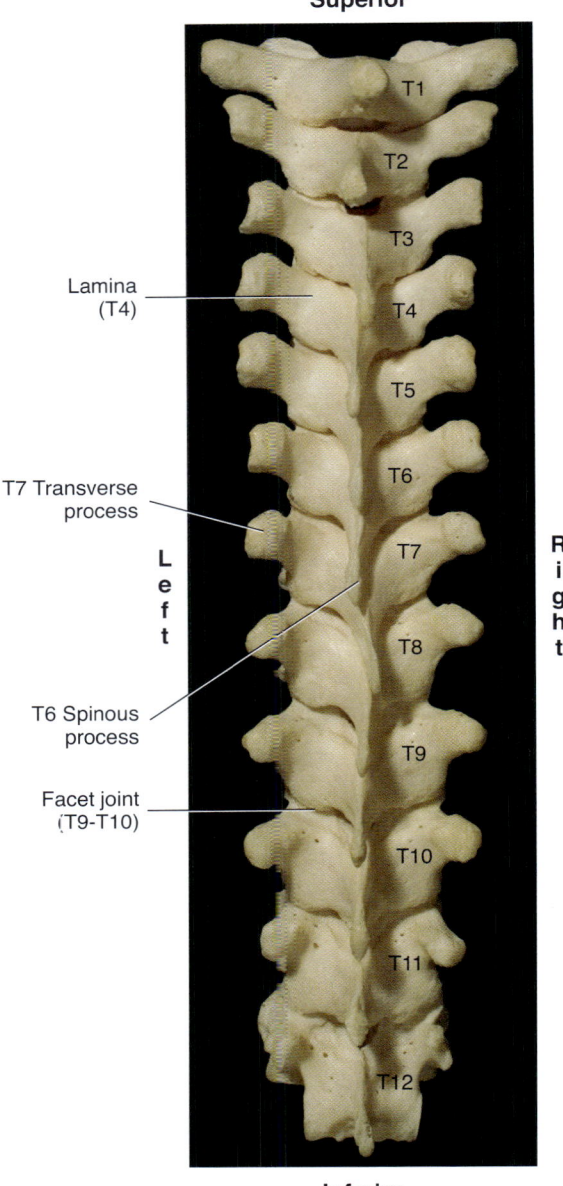

FIGURE 5-26

> **NOTES**
> 1. The differences in spinous processes (SPs) from T1 to T12 can be seen.
> 2. The SP of T6 and the transverse process (TP) of T7 are labeled, illustrating the relative location of a vertebral TP relative to the more palpable SP of the vertebra above. When palpating the thoracic spine (especially the midthoracic spine), the downward slope of the SPs should be kept in mind.
> 3. The TPs of the spine project laterally into the transverse plane, hence their name.
> 4. The crooked SP of T7 of this specimen can be seen; bones of the body often have slight asymmetries such as this. A flexible understanding of the shapes of bones is important; otherwise the crooked SP of T7 in this case could be interpreted as a rotated vertebra when in fact it is not.

CHAPTER 5 Bones of the Human Body

T5 (TYPICAL THORACIC VERTEBRA)

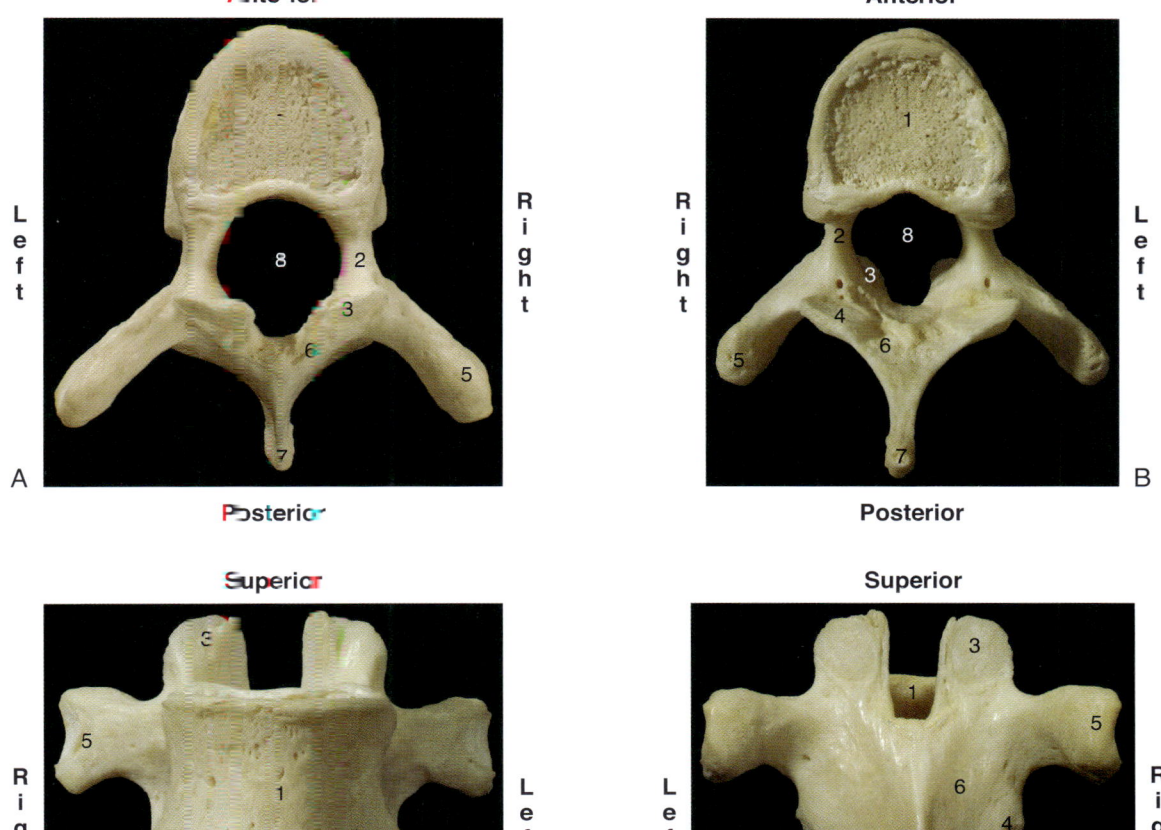

FIGURE 5-27 A, Superior view. B, Inferior view. C, Anterior view. D, Posterior view.
1. Body
2. Pedicle
3. Superior articular process/facet
4. Inferior articular process facet
5. Transverse process (TP)
6. Lamina
7. Spinous process (SP)
8. Vertebral foramen

NOTES
1. The pedicle (#2) of a vertebra is the structure that connects the body to the rest of the structures of the vertebra.[6] If one looks at the superior or inferior view of a vertebra such that the body is at the bottom of the page, the pedicles may be viewed as the feet (ped means foot) of a statue that is standing on its base or pedestal (the body of the vertebra being analogous to the base or pedestal of the statue).
2. The articular process is the entire structural landmark that projects outward from the bone; the articular facets (#3, 4) are the smooth articular surfaces located on the articular process.
3. The laminae (singular: lamina, #6) may be viewed as laminating together to form the spinous process (SP) of a vertebra.[6]
4. Plural of foramen is foramina.
5. The vertebral foramina (#8) of the spinal column create the spinal canal, though which the spinal cord runs.[3]

T5 (CONTINUED) AND THORACIC ENDPLATES

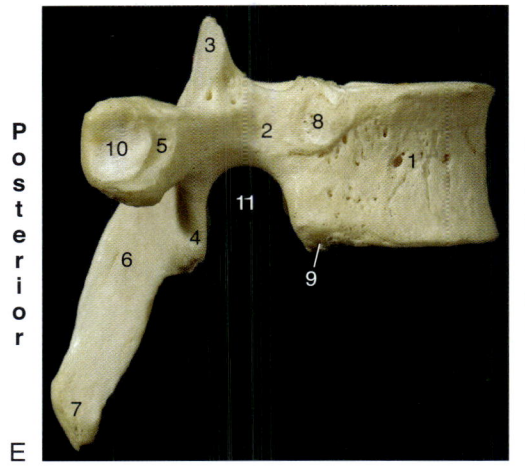

FIGURE 5-27, cont'd E, Right lateral view. F, Posterior oblique view.
1. Body
2. Pedicle
3. Superior articular process/facet
4. Inferior articular process/facet
5. Transverse process (TP)
6. Lamina
7. Spinous process (SP)
8. Superior costal hemifacet
9. Inferior costal hemifacet
10. Transverse costal facet
11. Intervertebral foramen
12. Inferior vertebral notch
13. Superior vertebral notch

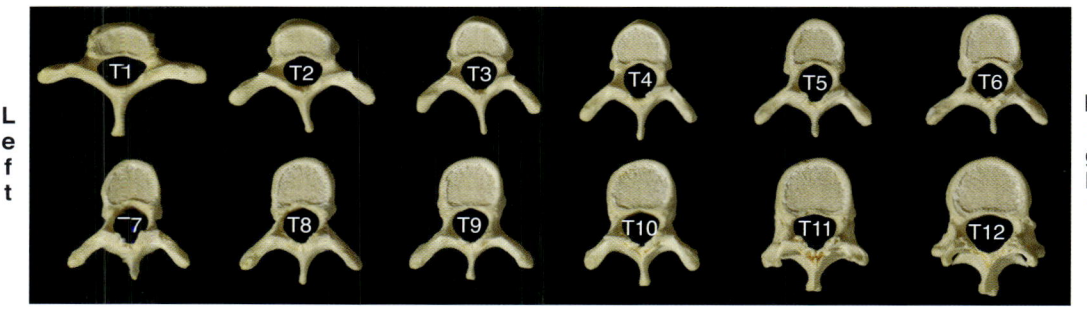

FIGURE 5-28 Superior view of all twelve thoracic vertebrae.

NOTES

1. The superior and inferior costal hemifacets (#8, 9) on the bodies are the vertebral articular surfaces for the costovertebral joint[3]; the transverse costal facet (#10) on the transverse process (TP) is the vertebral articular surface for the costotransverse joint.[3]

2. The lateral view of a thoracic vertebra is ideal for visualizing the intervertebral foramen, which is formed by the inferior vertebral notch of the superior vertebra (#12) juxtaposed next to the superior vertebral notch of the inferior vertebra (#13).

3. Costal hemifacets on the bodies of thoracic vertebrae usually create the articular surface for the costovertebral joints of ribs #2 through #10. Usually, T1, T11, and T12 have full facets for ribs #1, #11, and #12, respectively[3] (see Figure 5-25).

4. Figure 5-28 shows a superior view of all twelve thoracic vertebrae (thoracic endplate view). A gradual change in the shape of the thoracic vertebrae is seen from superior to inferior. Specifically, the change in the shape of the spinous processes (SPs) and bodies can be seen.

LUMBAR SPINE—RIGHT LATERAL VIEW

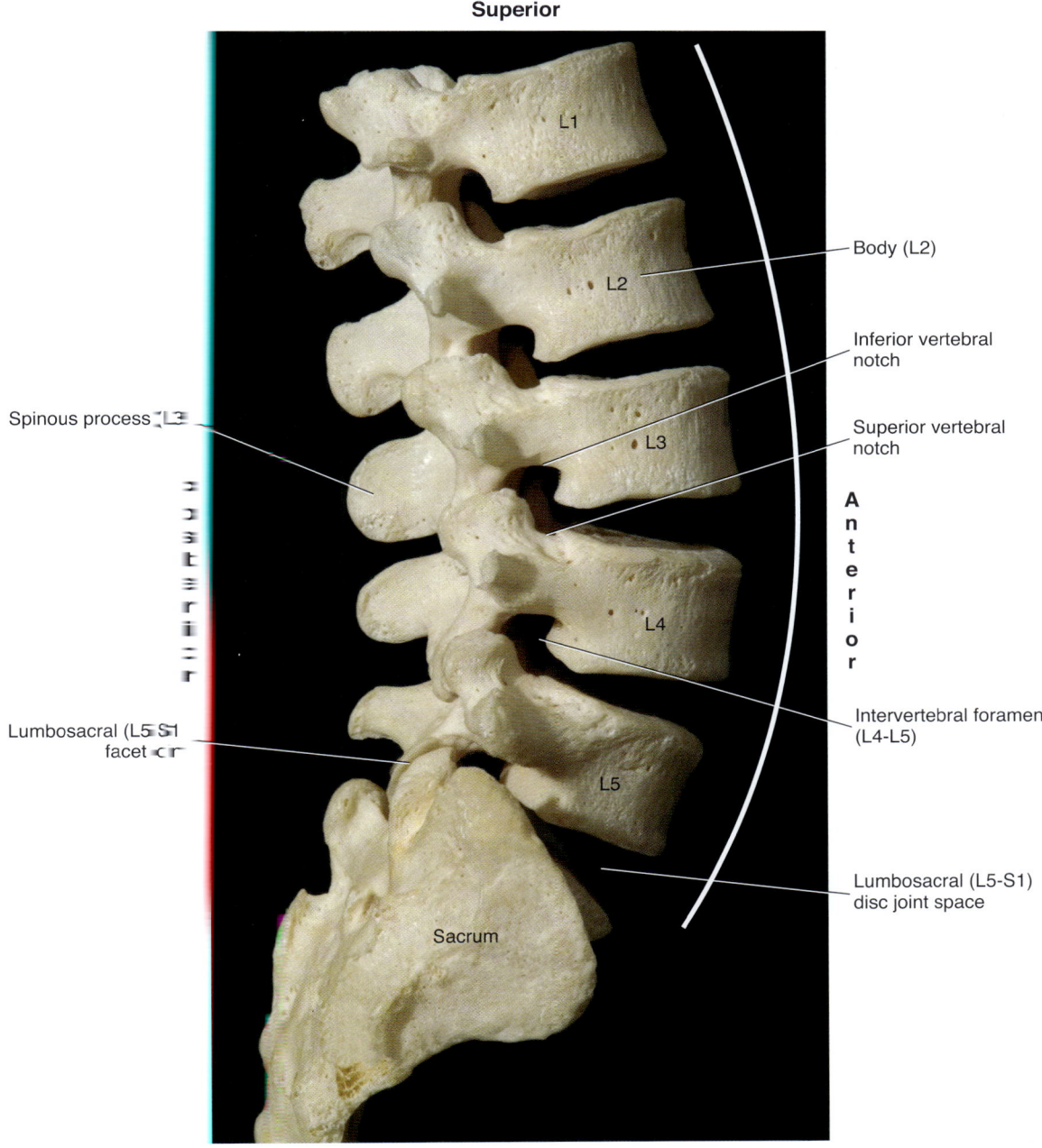

FIGURE 5-29

NOTES
1. Note the lordotic (concave posteriorly) curve of the lumbar spine (indicated by the line drawn anterior to the lumbar spine).
2. The lateral view of the lumbar spine demonstrates the intervertebral foramina (the right L4-L5 intervertebral foramen is labeled). The intervertebral foramen is where the spinal nerve enters/exits the spinal cord.
3. Note the large blunt quadrate-shaped lumbar spinous processes.[2]
4. The spinous processes of the lumbar spine may be difficult to palpate depending on the degree of the client's lordotic curve.
5. The disc joint spaces are well visualized in the lateral view.

LUMBAR SPINE—POSTERIOR VIEW

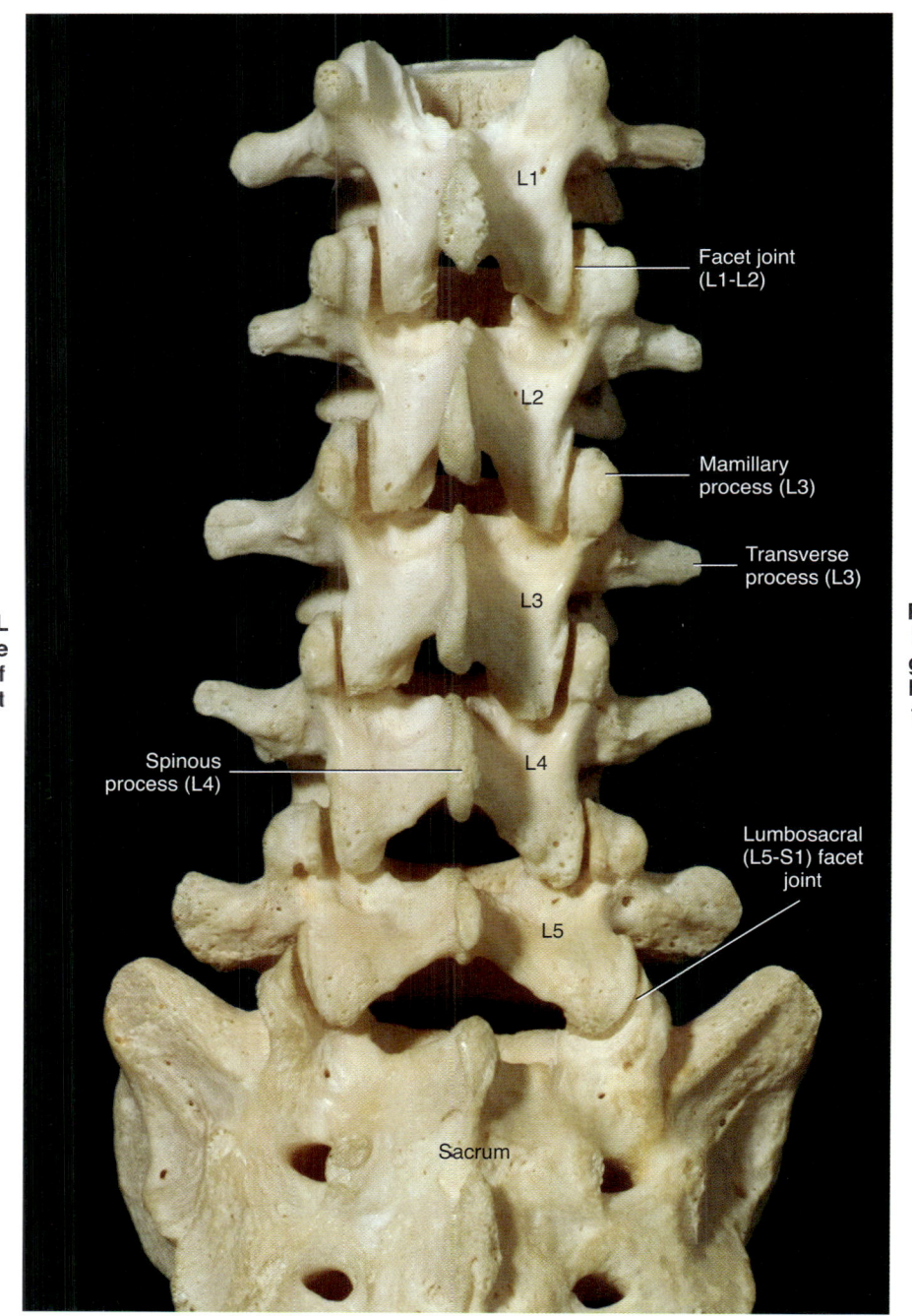

FIGURE 5-30

NOTES

1. The facet joints of the lumbar spine are well visualized in the posterior view because they are oriented in the sagittal plane.[2]
2. The lumbosacral (L5-S1) facet joints change their orientation; they are oriented more toward the frontal plane than are the other lumbar facet joints.[2]
3. The prominence of the mamillary processes of the lumbar spine can be seen.

L3 (TYPICAL LUMBAR VERTEBRA)

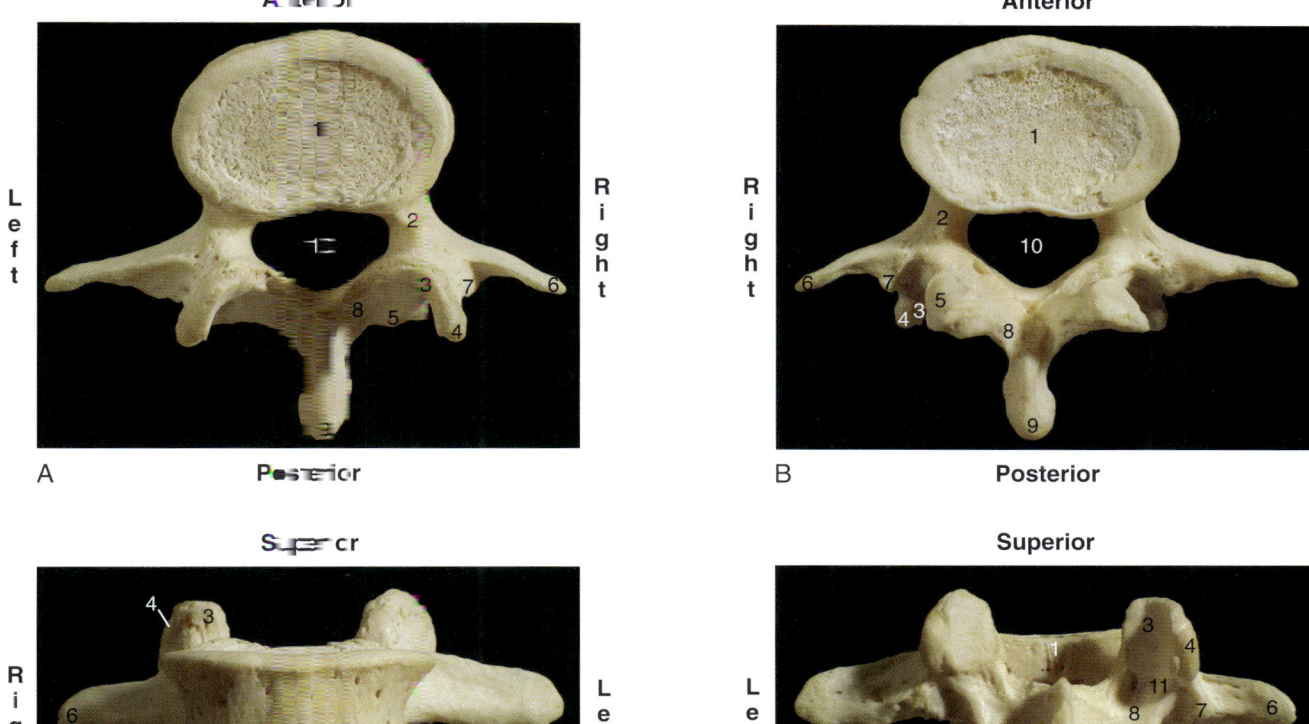

FIGURE 5-31 **A**, Superior view. **B**, Inferior view. **C**, Anterior view. **D**, Posterior view.
1. Body
2. Pedicle
3. Superior articular process facet
4. Mamillary process
5. Inferior articular process facet
6. Transverse process (TP)
7. Accessory process
8. Lamina
9. Spinous process (SP)
10. Vertebral foramen
11. Pars interarticularis

NOTES
1. The bodies of lumbar vertebrae (#1) are very large because they need to bear all the body weight from above.
2. The articular process is the entire structural landmark that projects outward from the bone; the articular facets (#3, 5) are the smooth articular surfaces located on the articular process.
3. Lumbar vertebrae are unique in that they possess two additional landmarks, mamillary, and accessory processes. The mamillary process (#4) is located on the superior articular process[4]; the accessory process (#7) is located on the transverse process.
4. Plural of foramen is foramina.

L3 (CONTINUED) AND LUMBAR ENDPLATES

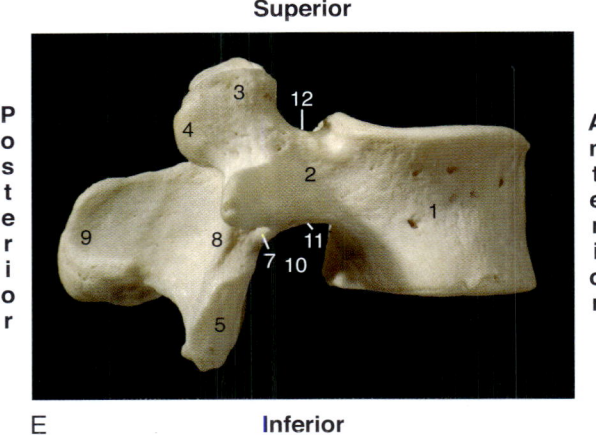

FIGURE 5-31, cont'd E, Right lateral view. F, Anterior oblique view.
1 Body
2 Pedicle
3 Superior articular process/facet
4 Mamillary process
5 Inferior articular process/facet
6 Transverse process (TP)
7 Accessory process
8 Lamina
9 Spinous process (SP)
10 Intervertebral foramen
11 Inferior vertebral notch
12 Superior vertebral notch

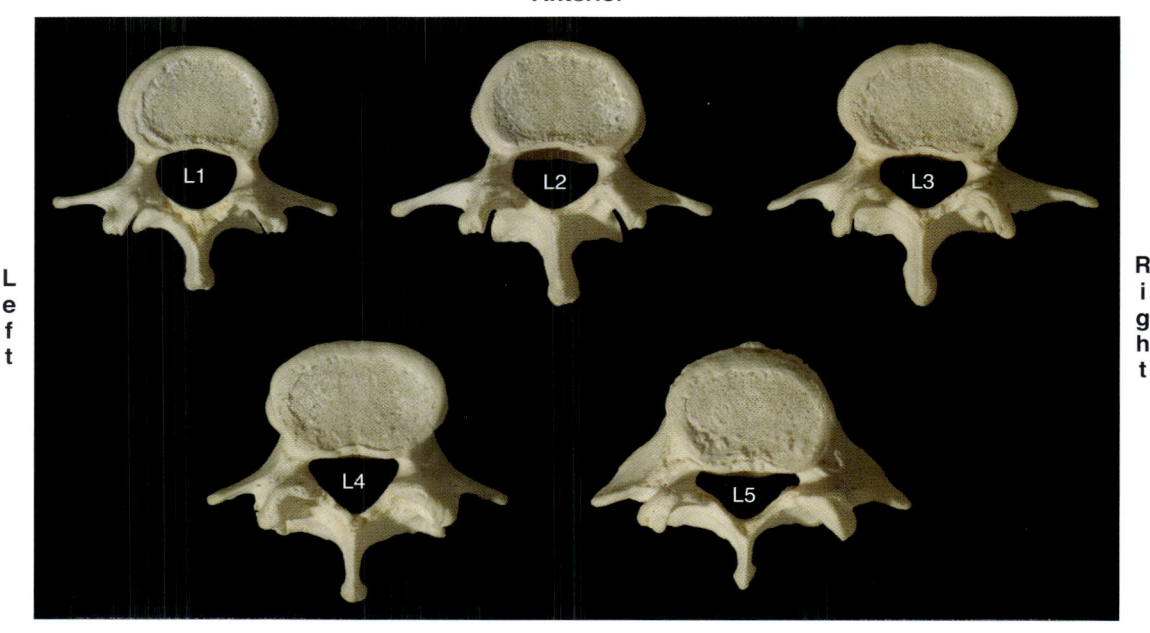

FIGURE 5-32 Superior view of all five lumbar vertebrae.

NOTES
1. Lumbar vertebrae possess large, blunt, quadrate-shaped spinous processes (SPs),[2] as evident in the lateral view.
2. Figure 5-32 shows a superior view of all five lumbar vertebrae (lumbar endplate view). The transition in shape from superior to inferior can be seen.

SACROCOCCYGEAL SPINE

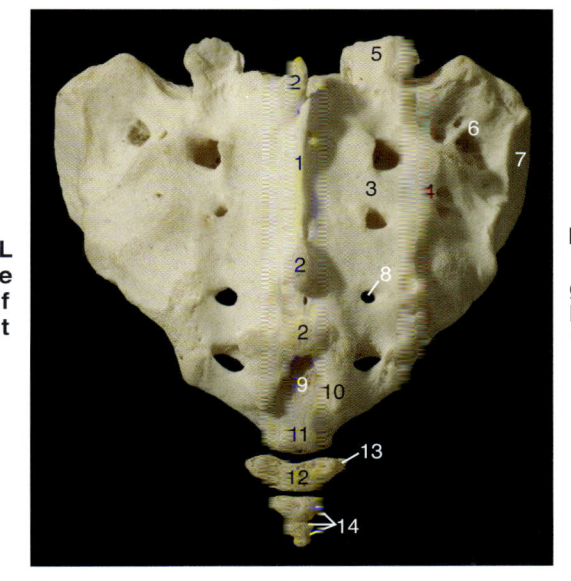

A, Inferior

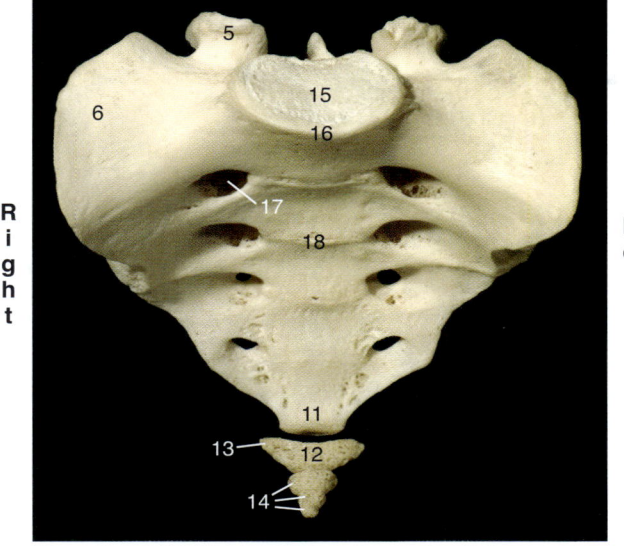

B, Inferior

FIGURE 5-33 A, Posterior view. B, Anterior view.
1. Median sacral crest
2. Tubercles along the median sacral crest
3. Intermediate sacral crest
4. Lateral sacral crest
5. Superior articular process/facet
6. Ala (wing)
7. Auricular surface (articular surface for ilium)
8. Third posterior foramen
9. Sacral hiatus
10. Sacral cornu
11. Apex
12. First coccygeal element
13. Coccygeal transverse process (TP)
14. Second to fourth coccygeal elements (fused)
15. Sacral base
16. Sacral promontory
17. First anterior foramen
18. Fusion of second and third sacral vertebrae

NOTES
1. The sacrum is formed by the fusion of five sacral vertebrae.[3]
2. The sacrum is shaped like an upside-down triangle. The sacral base (#15) is located superiorly; the sacral apex (#11) is located inferiorly.[2]
3. The medial sacral crest (#1) is the fusion of the sacral spinous processes (SPs)[3]; the intermediate sacral crest (#3) is the fusion of the articular processes[8]; the lateral sacral crest (#4) is the fusion of the transverse processes (TPs).[8]
4. The median sacral crest often has projections (remnants of SPs) that are called sacral tubercles.[7] This specimen has prominent first (asymmetric) and third sacral tubercles.
5. The superior articular processes (#5) of the sacrum articulate with the inferior articular processes of L5 (forming the lumbosacral [L5-S1] facet joints).[2]
6. The sacral ala (#6) is the winglike superolateral aspect of the sacrum (ala means wing).[3]
7. Four pairs of posterior (#8) and four pairs of anterior sacral foramina (#17) exist where sacral spinal nerves enter/exit the spinal canal.[7]
8. The sacral hiatus (#9) is the inferior opening of the sacral canal.[5]
9. The coccyx is usually composed of four rudimentary vertebrae[5]; however, the number may vary from two to five. Some sources state that the coccyx is the evolutionary remnant of a tail.

SACROCOCCYGEAL SPINE (CONTINUED)

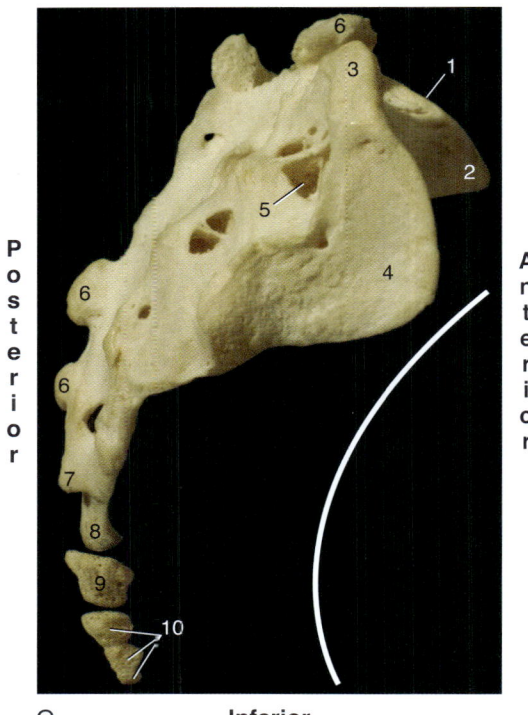

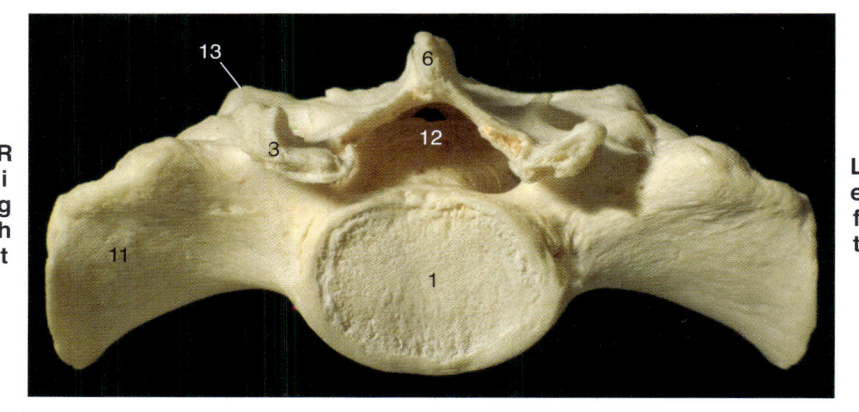

FIGURE 5-33 **C,** Right lateral view. **D,** Superior view.
1. Base
2. Promontory
3. Superior articular process
4. Auricular surface (articular surface for ilium)
5. First posterior foramen
6. (Tubercles of) median sacral crest
7. Cornu
8. Apex
9. First coccygeal element
10. Second to fourth coccygeal elements
11. Ala (wing)
12. Sacral canal
13. Lateral sacral crest

NOTES
1. The kyphotic (i.e., concave anteriorly) curve of the sacrococcygeal spine is indicated by the line drawn anterior to the sacrococcygeal spine.
2. The body of L5 sits on the base of the sacrum (#1), forming the lumbosacral (L5-S1) disc joint.[10]
3. The sacral promontory (#2) is the portion of the base of the sacrum that projects anteriorly.[7]
4. The cauda equina of nerves from the spinal cord travels through the sacral canal (#12).[7]

CHAPTER 5 Bones of the Human Body

SECTION 5.3 BONES OF THE RIBCAGE AND STERNUM

RIBCAGE—ANTERIOR VIEW

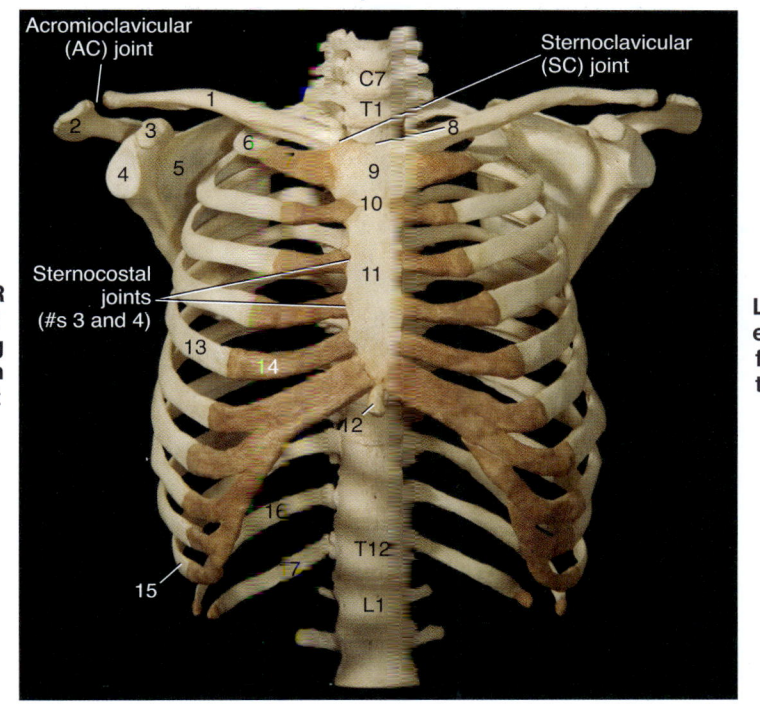

FIGURE 5-34
1. Clavicle
2. Acromion process
3. Coracoid process
4. Glenoid fossa
5. Subscapular fossa
6. First rib
7. Cartilage of first rib
8. Sternal notch
9. Manubrium of sternum
10. Sternal angle
11. Body of sternum
12. Xiphoid process of sternum
13. Fifth rib
14. Cartilage of fifth rib
15. Tenth rib
16. Eleventh rib
17. Twelfth rib
18. Clavicular notch of the manubrium
19. Notch for first costal cartilage
20. Notch for second costal cartilage
21. Notch for third costal cartilage
22. Notch for fourth costal cartilage
23. Notch for fifth costal cartilage
24. Notch for sixth costal cartilage
25. Notch for seventh costal cartilage

NOTES
1. The sternal notch (#8) is also known as the jugular notch.[3]
2. The lateral border of the sternal notch is a good landmark to palpate movement of the sternoclavicular (SC) joint.
3. The sternal angle (#10) is also known as the angle of Louis and is the joint between the manubrium and body of the sternum. It is located at the junction of the second costal cartilage with the sternum and is often palpable.[10]
4. The xiphoid process (#12) remains cartilaginous long into life[2] and is also a landmark used to locate the proper location to administer cardiopulmonary resuscitation (CPR).
5. The ribcage is composed of 12 pairs of ribs. Of these, the first seven pairs (#1-7) are called true ribs, because their costal cartilages articulate directly with the sternum. The last five pairs (#8-12) of ribs are called false ribs, because they do not articulate directly to the sternum; pairs #8-10 have their cartilage join the costal cartilage of rib #7, and ribs #11 and #12 do not articulate with the sternum at all. Because the last two pairs of false ribs do not attach to the sternum at all, they are called floating ribs.[6]
6. The attachment of a rib to the sternum via its costal cartilage is called a sternocostal joint.
7. The sternums in A and B are not the same. The differences in the shape of the manubrium and body of these two specimens can be seen.

RIBCAGE—RIGHT LATERAL VIEW

FIGURE 5-35
1. Clavicle

Scapula (#2-7):
2. Acromion process
3. Coracoid process
4. Glenoid fossa
5. Superior angle
6. Spine of scapula
7. Inferior angle
8. First rib
9. Cartilage of first rib
10. First intercostal space
11. Fifth rib
12. Fifth intercostal space
13. Sixth rib
14. Tenth rib
15. Eleventh rib
16. Twelfth rib
17. Vertebral spinous processes (SPs)

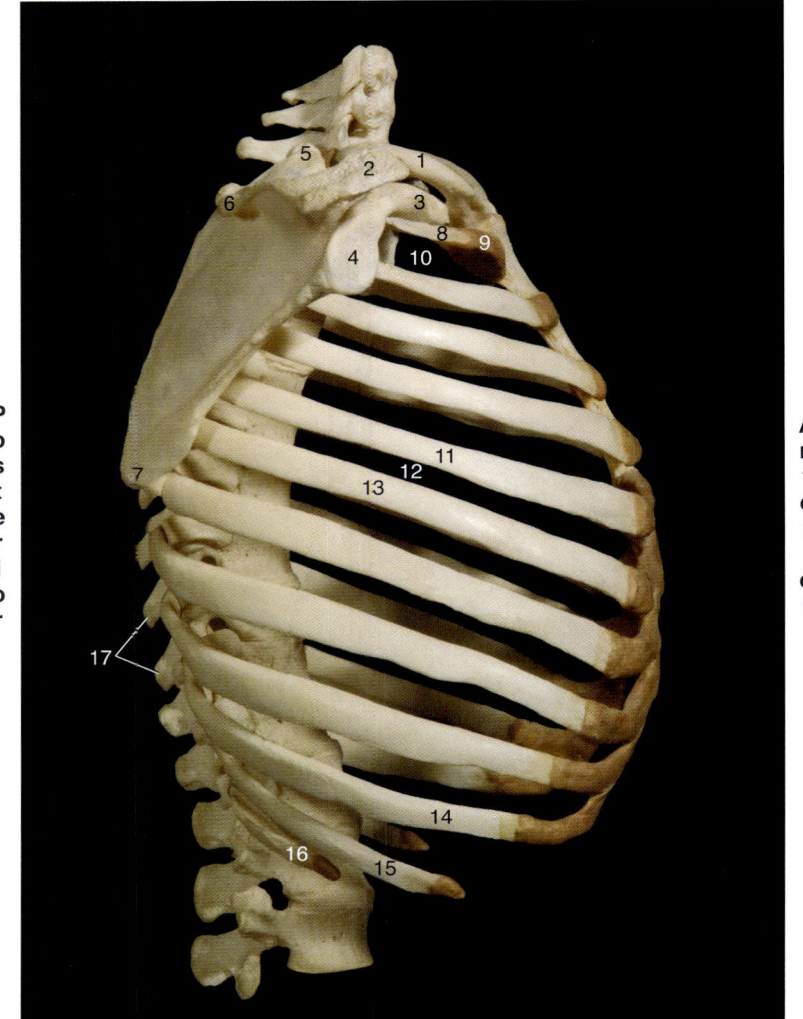

NOTES
1. The ribs articulate with the spine posteriorly and the sternum anteriorly (except for the floating ribs [#11 and #12], which do not articulate with the sternum).[6]
2. Eleven intercostal spaces are located between ribs. They are named for the rib that is located superior to the space.
3. The intercostal spaces contain intercostal muscles that often become tight in people with chronic obstructive pulmonary disorders (COPD) such as asthma, emphysema, and chronic bronchitis.[11]
4. The lateral view of the thorax nicely demonstrates the plane of the scapula, which lies neither perfectly in the frontal nor sagittal plane. The plane of the scapula is usually located approximately 35 degrees off the frontal plane toward the sagittal plane.

COSTOSPINAL JOINTS

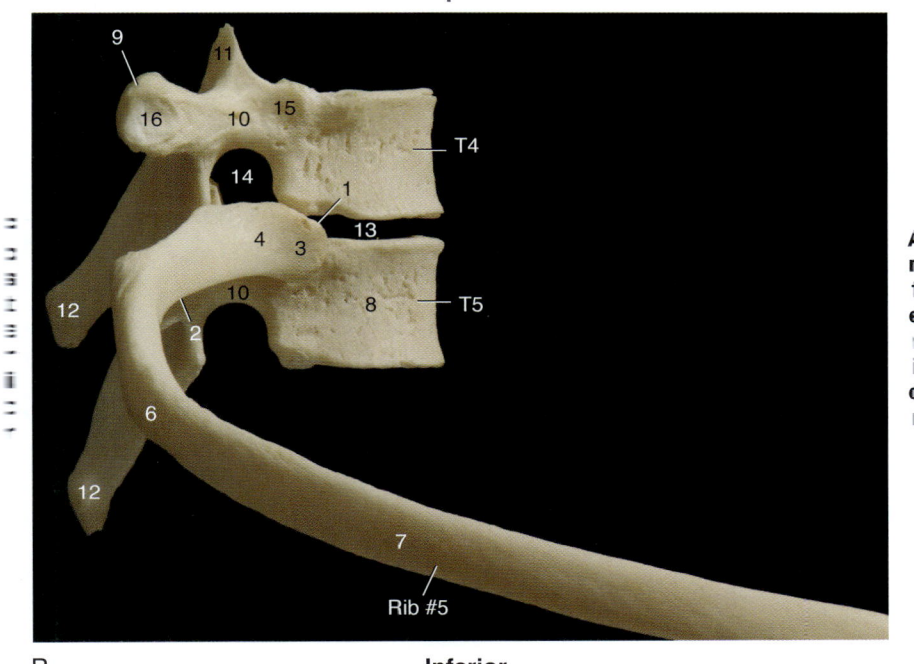

FIGURE 5-36 A, Superior view. B, Right lateral view.
1. Costovertebral joint
2. Costotransverse joint
3. Head of rib
4. Neck of rib
5. Tubercle of rib
6. Angle of rib
7. Body of rib
8. Vertebral body
9. Transverse process (TP)
10. Pedicle
11. Superior articular process/facet
12. Spinous process (SP)
13. Disc space (T4-T5)
14. Intervertebral foramen (T4-5)
15. Costal hemifacet for rib #4
16. Transverse costal facet for rib #4

NOTES[10]
1. A rib articulates with the spinal column in two places, forming two costospinal joints, the costovertebral joint (#1) and the costotransverse joint (#2).
2. The costovertebral joint is typically formed by the head of the rib articulating with the (vertebral costal hemifacets of the) bodies of two contiguous vertebrae, as well as the disc that is located between them. Usually ribs #1, #11, and #12 articulate with only one (full vertebral costal facet of a) vertebral body.
3. The costotransverse joint is formed by the tubercle of a rib articulating with the (transverse costal facet of the) transverse process of a vertebra.

RIGHT RIBS

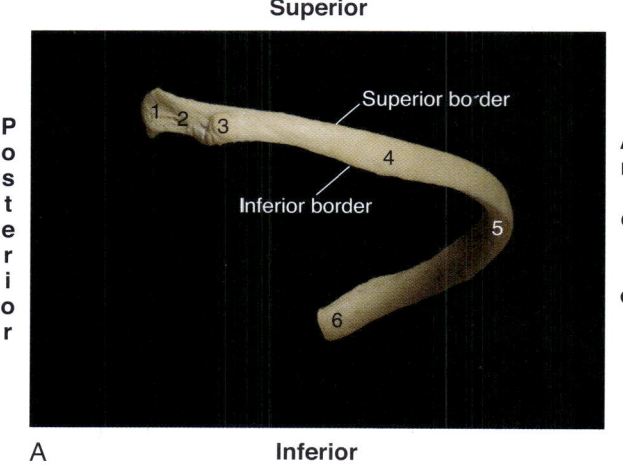
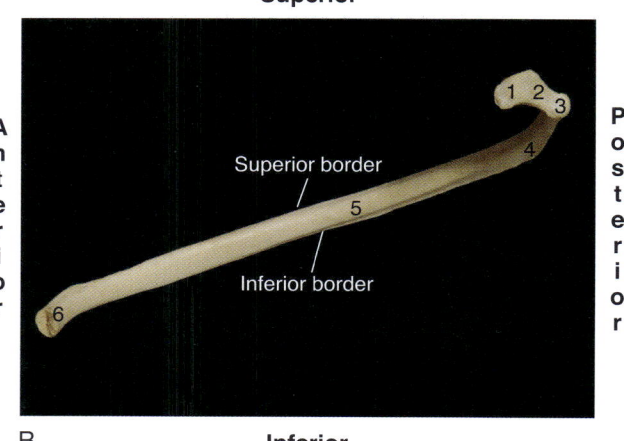

FIGURE 5-37 **A**, Posterior view. **B**, Medial view. **C**, Superior view.
1 Head
2 Neck
3 Tubercle
4 Angle
5 Body
6 Anterior end

NOTES
1. The head of the rib (#1) articulates with the vertebral body (or bodies) to form the costovertebral joint.[2]
2. The tubercle of the rib (#3) articulates with the vertebral transverse process (TP) to form the costotransverse joint.[2]
3. The anterior end of the rib meets the sternum via costal cartilage.[2]
4. The first seven pairs of ribs (#1-7) are called true ribs.[6]
5. The last five pairs of ribs (#8-12) are called false ribs.[6]
6. The last two pairs of false ribs (#11-12) are called floating ribs.[6]

CHAPTER 5 Bones of the Human Body

SECTION 5.4 ENTIRE LOWER EXTREMITY

RIGHT LOWER EXTREMITY

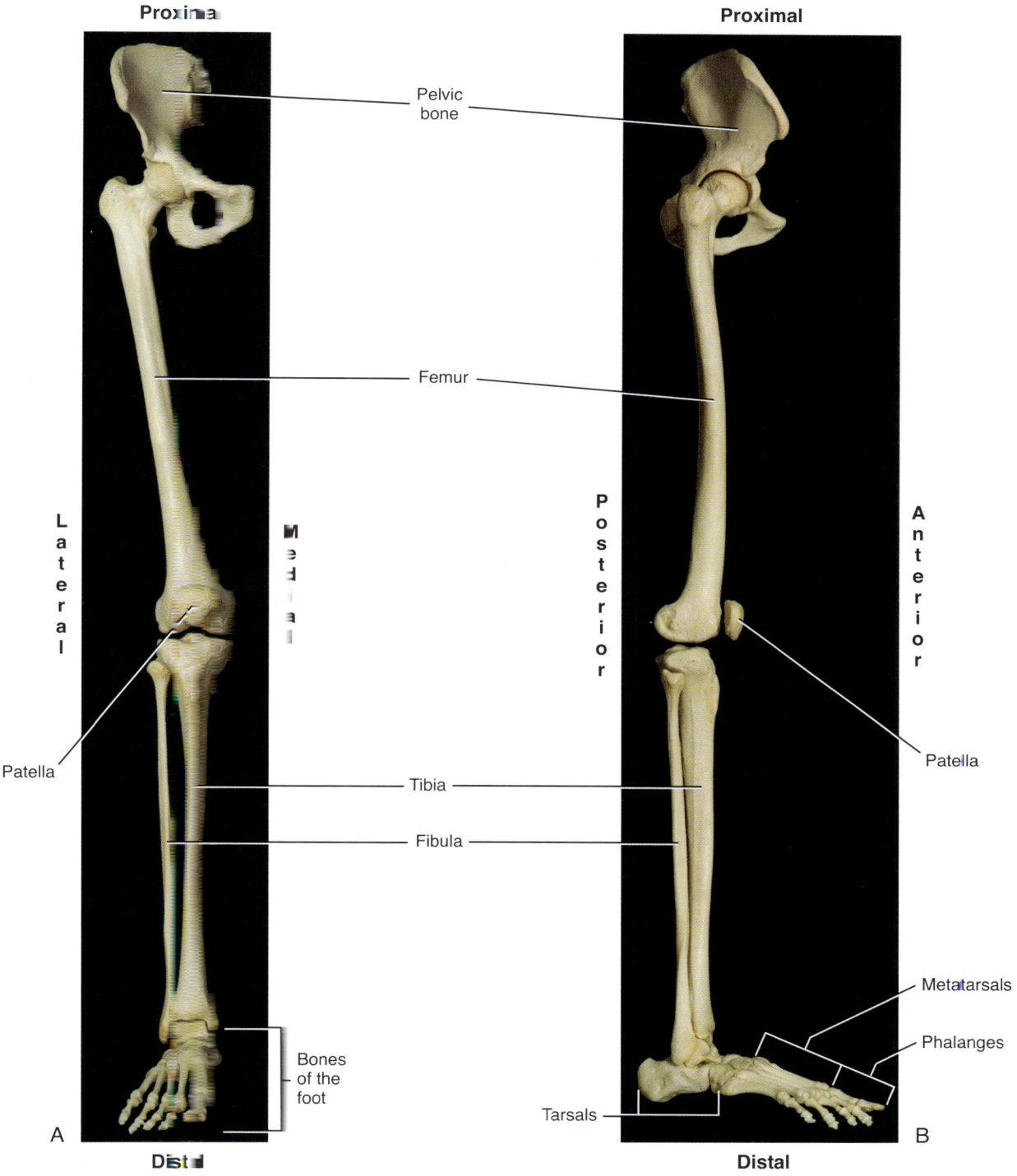

FIGURE 5-38 **A**, Anterior view. **B**, Right lateral view.

> **NOTE**
> The femur is in the thigh; the tibia and fibula are in the leg; and the tarsals, metatarsals, and phalanges are in the foot.[2]

SECTION 5.5 BONES OF THE PELVIS AND HIP JOINT

FULL PELVIS

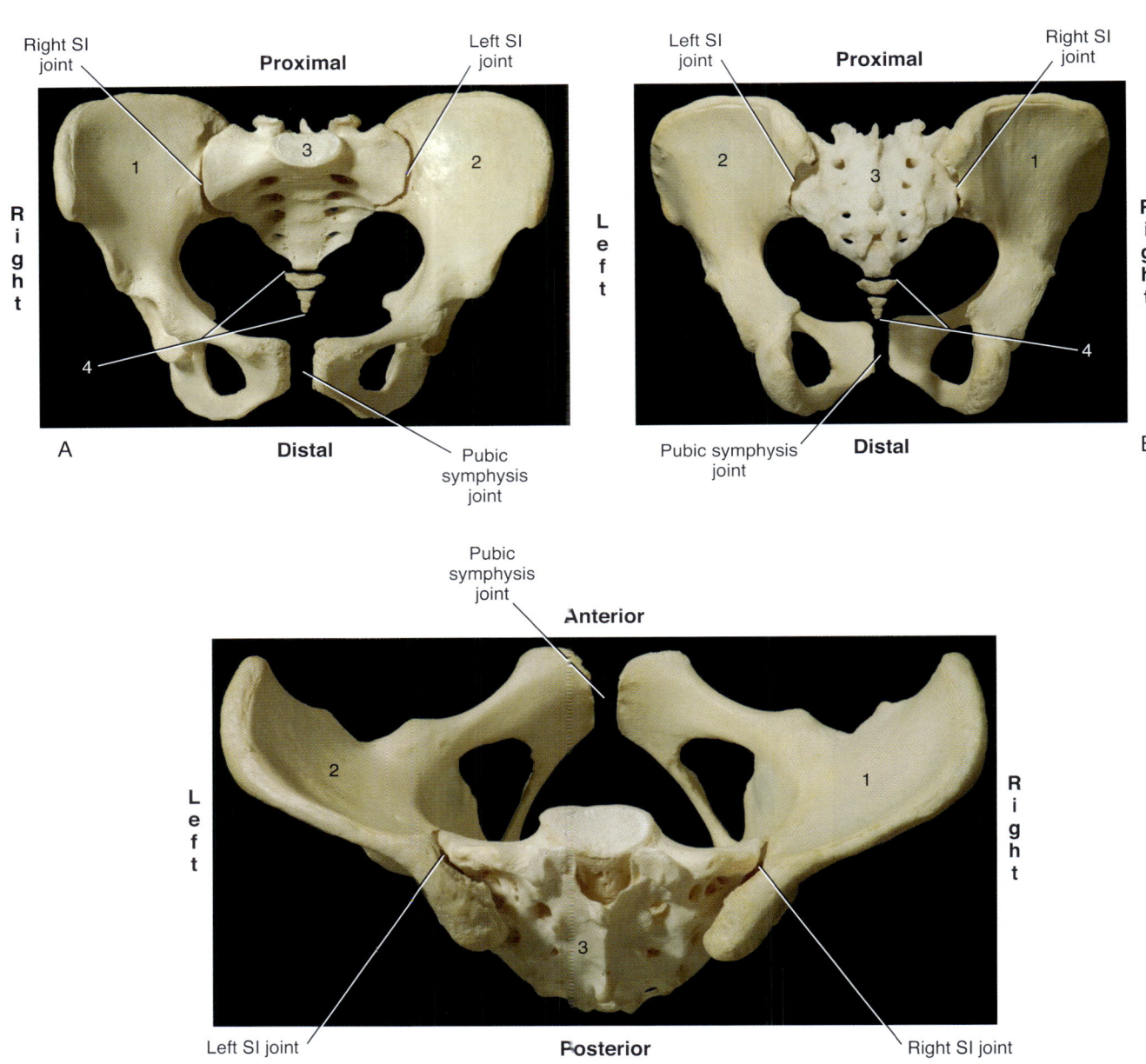

FIGURE 5-39 **A**, Anterior view. **B**, Posterior view. **C**, Superior view.
1 Right pelvic bone
2 Left pelvic bone
3 Sacrum
4 Coccyx

NOTES
1. On the pelvis, either proximal/distal or superior/inferior terminology can be used.
2. There are two sacroiliac (SI) joints, paired left and right. There is one pubic symphysis joint.[4]

CHAPTER 5   Bones of the Human Body

RIGHT PELVIC BONE—ANTERIOR VIEWS

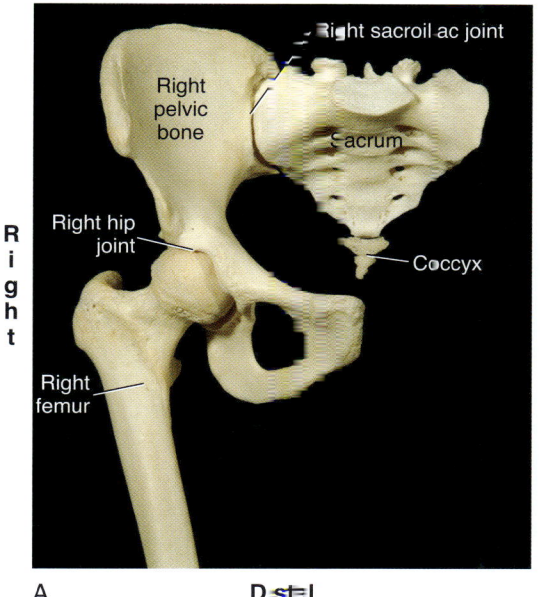

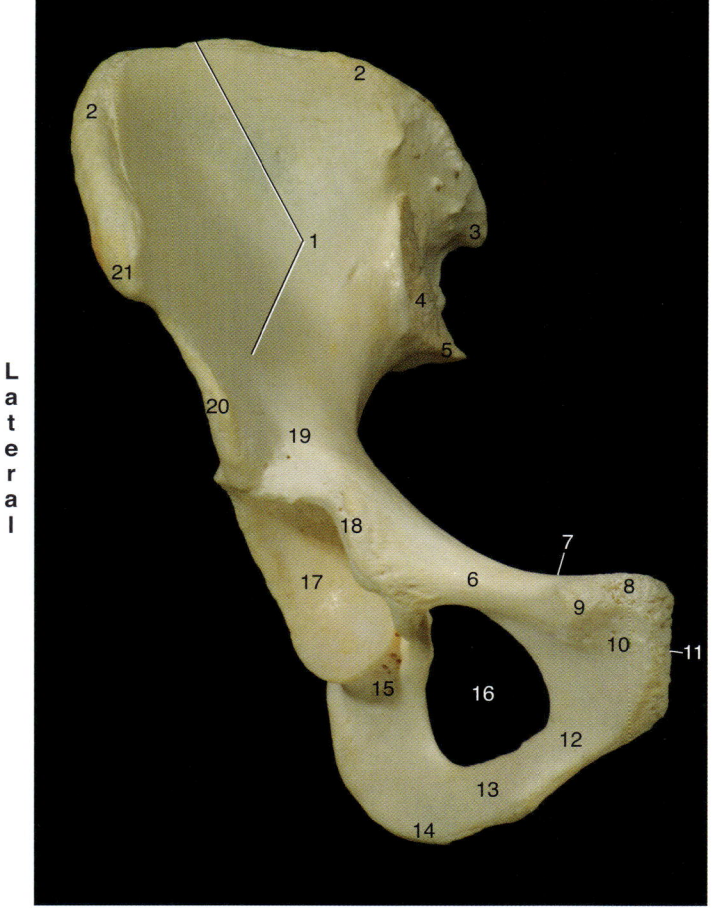

FIGURE 5-40
1. Wing of the ilium (iliac fossa on internal surface)
2. Iliac crest
3. Posterior superior iliac spine (PSIS)
4. Articular surface for sacroiliac joint
5. Posterior inferior iliac spine (PIIS)
6. Superior ramus of pubis
7. Pectineal line of pubis
8. Pubic crest
9. Pubic tubercle
10. Body of pubis
11. Articular surface for pubic symphysis
12. Inferior ramus of pubis
13. Ramus of ischium
14. Ischial tuberosity
15. Body of ischium
16. Obturator foramen
17. Acetabulum
18. Rim of acetabulum
19. Body of ilium
20. Anterior inferior iliac spine (AIIS)
21. Anterior superior iliac spine (ASIS)

NOTE
The articular surface of the ilium for the sacroiliac joint is also known as the auricular surface because it has the shape of an ear[3] (auricle means ear).

RIGHT PELVIC BONE—POSTERIOR VIEWS

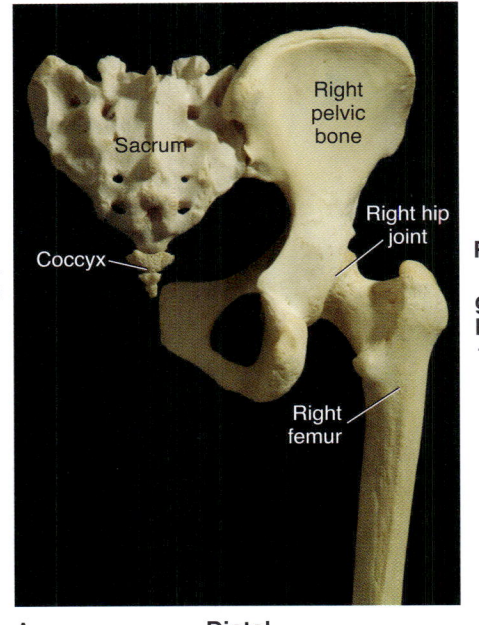

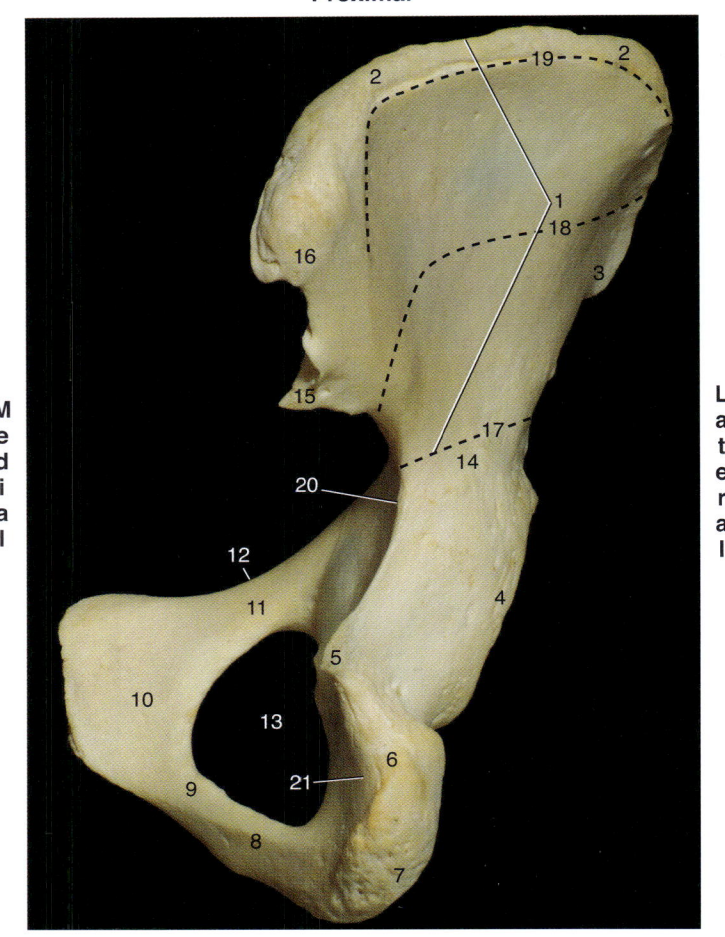

FIGURE 5-41
1. Wing of the ilium (iliac fossa on internal surface)
2. Iliac crest
3. Anterior superior iliac spine (ASIS)
4. Rim of acetabulum
5. Ischial spine
6. Body of ischium
7. Ischial tuberosity
8. Ramus of ischium
9. Inferior ramus of pubis
10. Body of pubis
11. Superior ramus of pubis
12. Pectineal line of pubis
13. Obturator foramen
14. Body of ilium
15. Posterior inferior iliac spine (PIIS)
16. Posterior superior iliac spine (PSIS)
17. Inferior gluteal line (dashed line)
18. Anterior gluteal line (dashed line)
19. Posterior gluteal line (dashed line)
20. Greater sciatic notch
21. Lesser sciatic notch

NOTE
The obturator internus and obturator externus muscles are named for their attachment relative to the obturator foramen (#13).

RIGHT PELVIC BONE—LATERAL VIEWS

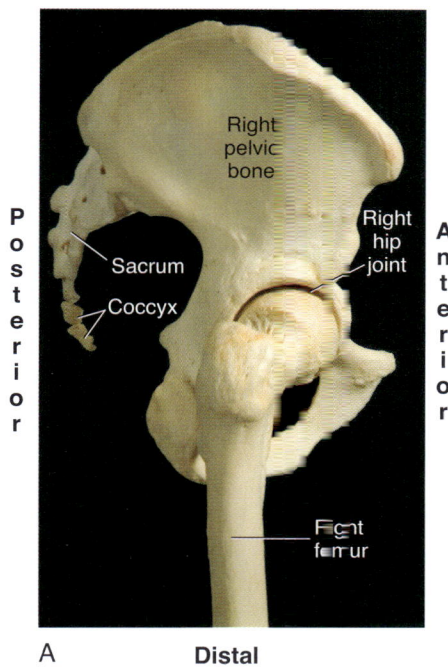

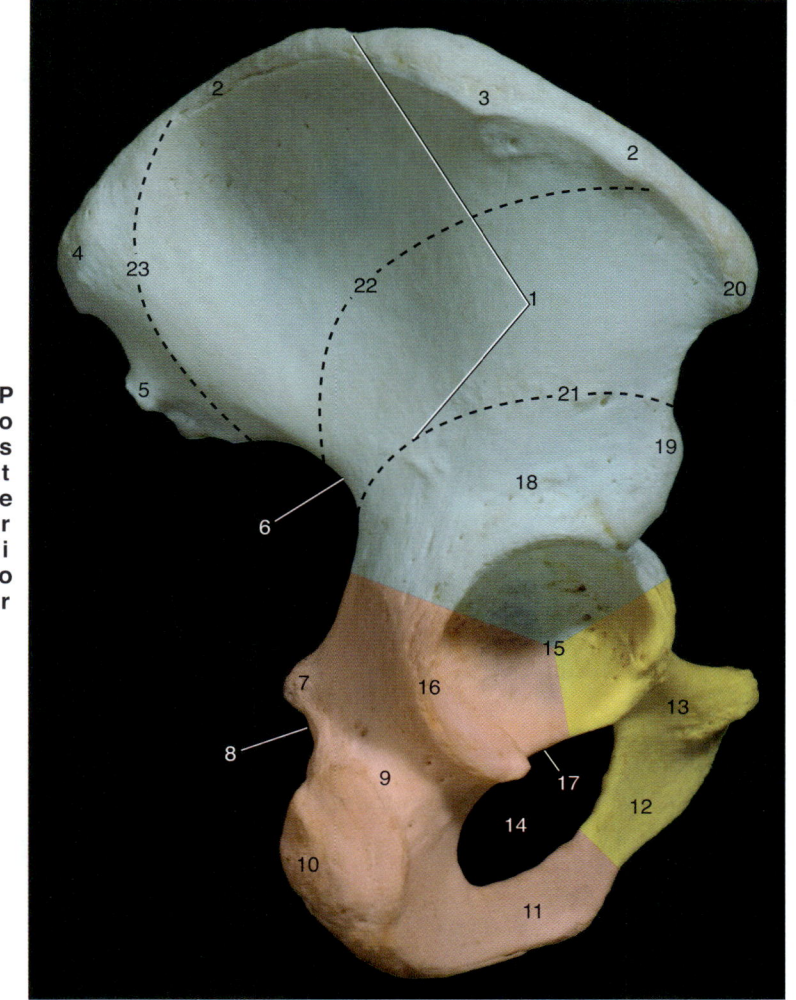

FIGURE 5-42
1. Wing of the ilium (external/gluteal surface)
2. Iliac crest
3. Tubercle of the iliac crest
4. Posterior superior iliac spine (PSIS)
5. Posterior inferior iliac spine (PIIS)
6. Greater sciatic notch
7. Ischial spine
8. Lesser sciatic notch
9. Body of ischium
10. Ischial tuberosity
11. Ramus of ischium
12. Inferior ramus of pubis
13. Body of pubis
14. Obturator foramen
15. Acetabulum
16. Rim of acetabulum
17. Notch of acetabulum
18. Body of ilium
19. Anterior inferior iliac spine (AIIS)
20. Anterior superior iliac spine (ASIS)
21. Inferior gluteal line (dashed line)
22. Anterior gluteal line (dashed line)
23. Posterior gluteal line (dashed line)

NOTES
1. The pelvic bone is also known as the coxal, hip, or innominate bone.[3]
2. The pelvic bone is formed by the union of the ilium, ischium, and pubis[4] (see colored shading: the ilium is blue, the ischium is pink, and the pubis is yellow).
3. All three bones of the pelvis (ilium, ischium, and pubis) come together in the acetabulum.[4]
4. The ramus of the ischium (#11) and inferior ramus of the pubis (#12) are often grouped together and called the ischiopubic ramus.[3]

RIGHT PELVIC BONE—MEDIAL VIEWS

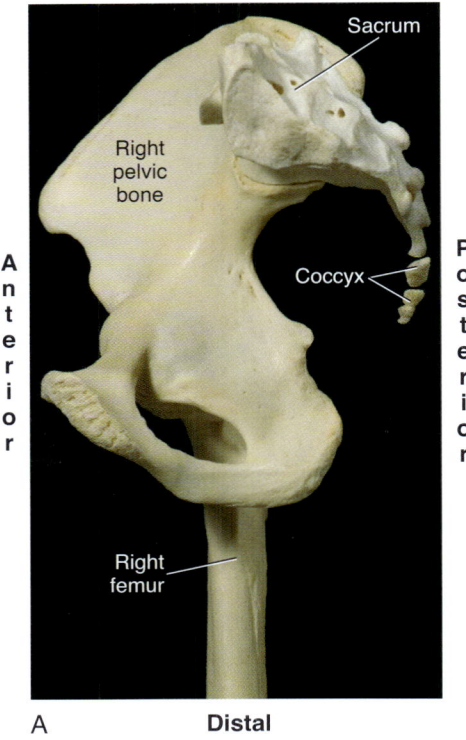

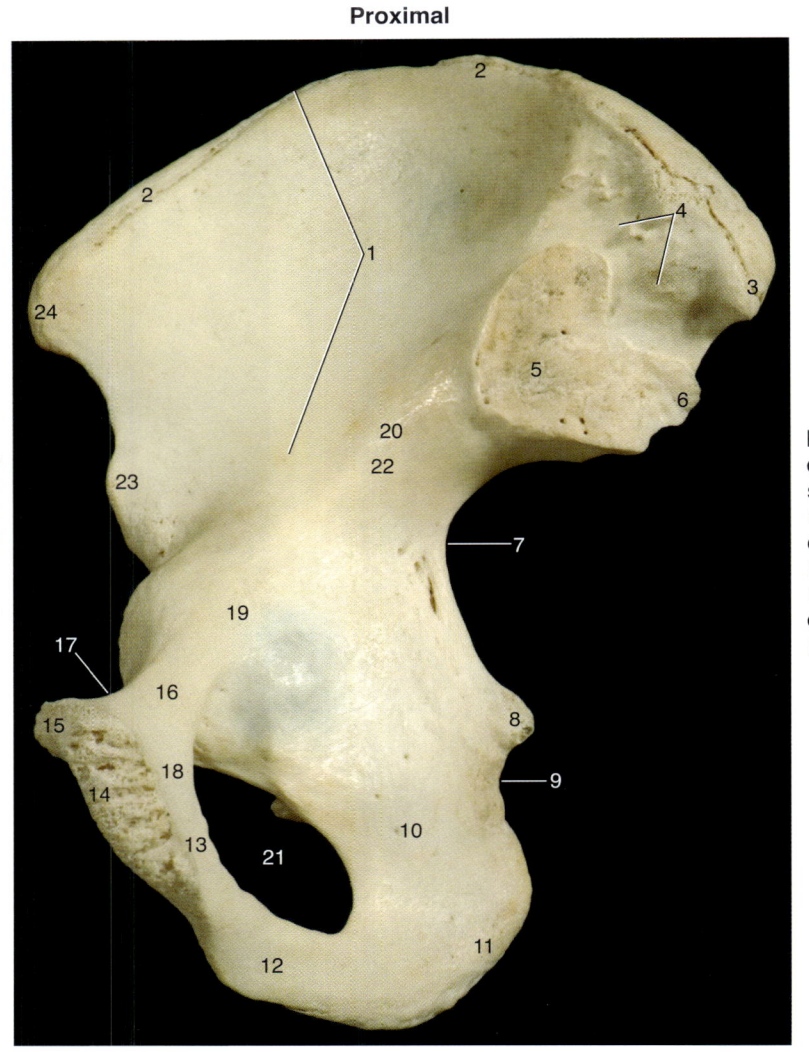

FIGURE 5-43
1. Wing of the ilium (iliac fossa on internal surface)
2. Iliac crest
3. Posterior superior iliac spine (PSIS)
4. Iliac tuberosity
5. Articular surface of ilium for sacroiliac joint
6. Posterior inferior iliac spine (PIIS)
7. Greater sciatic notch
8. Ischial spine
9. Lesser sciatic notch
10. Body of ischium
11. Ischial tuberosity
12. Ramus of ischium
13. Inferior ramus of pubis
14. Articular surface of pubis for pubis symphysis
15. Pubic tubercle
16. Superior ramus of pubis
17. Pectineal line of pubis
18. Body of pubis
19. Iliopectineal line
20. Arcuate line of the ilium
21. Obturator foramen
22. Body of ilium
23. Anterior inferior iliac spine (AIIS)
24. Anterior superior iliac spine (ASIS)

NOTE
The iliopectineal line (#19) is located on the ilium and pubis.

CHAPTER 5 Bones of the Human Body

SECTION 5.6 BONES OF THE THIGH AND KNEE JOINT

RIGHT FEMUR—ANTERIOR AND POSTERIOR VIEWS

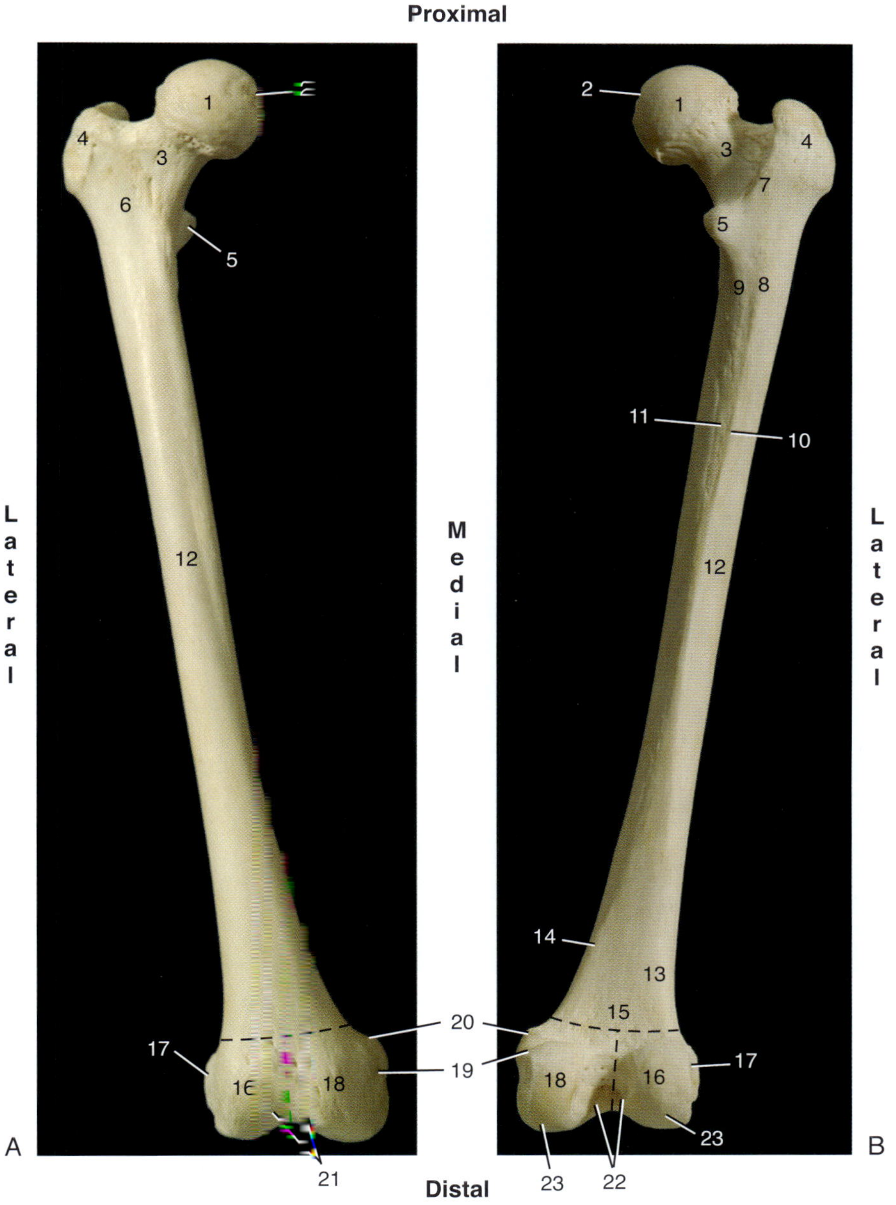

FIGURE 5-44
1. Head
2. Fovea of the head
3. Neck
4. Greater trochanter
5. Lesser trochanter
6. Intertrochanteric line
7. Intertrochanteric crest
8. Gluteal tuberosity
9. Pectineal line
10. Lateral lip of linea aspera
11. Medial lip of linea aspera
12. Body (shaft)
13. Lateral supracondylar line
14. Medial supracondylar line
15. Popliteal surface
16. Lateral condyle
17. Lateral epicondyle
18. Medial condyle
19. Medial epicondyle
20. Adductor tubercle
21. Articular surface for patellofemoral joint
22. Intercondylar fossa
23. Articular surface for knee (tibiofemoral) joint

NOTES
1. The fovea of the head of the femur (#2) is the attachment site for the ligamentum teres of the hip joint.[3]
2. The intertrochanteric line (#6) runs between the greater and lesser trochanters anteriorly; the intertrochanteric crest (#7) runs between the greater and lesser trochanters posteriorly.
3. The linea aspera (#10, 11) is an attachment site for seven muscles.[2] The linea aspera can be looked at as branching proximally to give rise to the gluteal tuberosity (#8) and pectineal line (#9), and branching distally to give rise to the lateral and medial supracondylar lines (#13, 14).
4. The gluteal tuberosity (#8) is a distal attachment of the gluteus maximus.[12]
5. The pectineal line (#9) is the distal attachment of the pectineus.[3]
6. The adductor tubercle (#20) is a distal attachment site for the adductor magnus.[3]
7. The borders of the lateral and medial condyles (#16, 18) are shown by dashed lines.

RIGHT FEMUR—LATERAL AND MEDIAL VIEWS

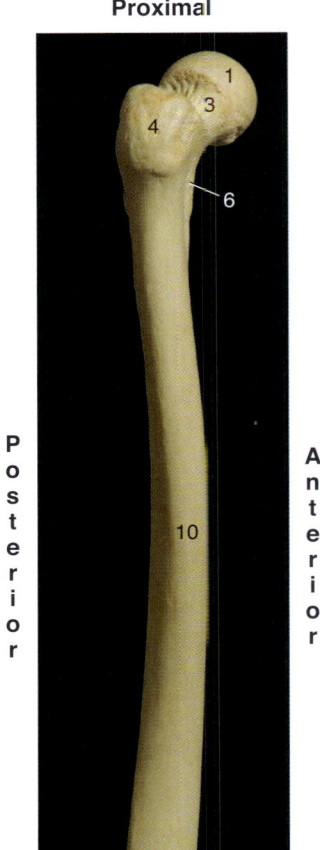
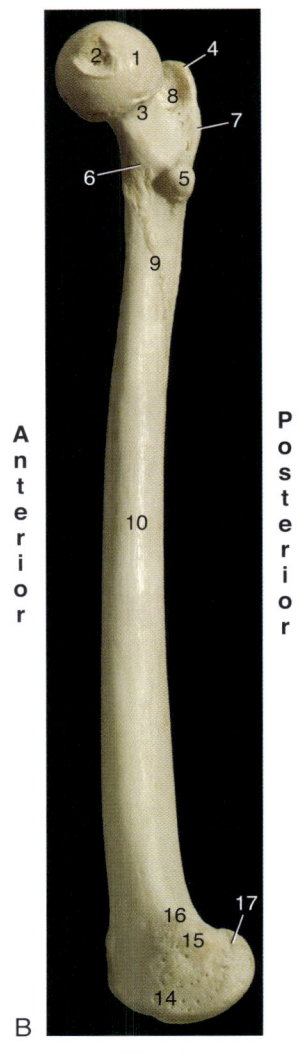

FIGURE 5-45 **A,** Lateral view. **B,** Medial view.
1. Head
2. Fovea of the head
3. Neck
4. Greater trochanter
5. Lesser trochanter
6. Intertrochanteric line
7. Intertrochanteric crest
8. Trochanteric fossa
9. Pectineal line
10. Body (shaft)
11. Lateral condyle
12. Lateral epicondyle
13. Groove for popliteus tendon
14. Medial condyle
15. Medial epicondyle
16. Adductor tubercle
17. Impression for lateral gastrocnemius

NOTES
1. The shaft of the femur, when viewed from the lateral or medial perspective, is not purely vertical; rather a bow to the shaft exists.
2. The pectineal line of the femur (#9) should not be confused with the pectineal line of the pubis (they are the distal and proximal attachments of the pectineus).
3. The femoral condyles (#11, 14) articulate with the tibia, forming the knee (i.e., tibiofemoral) joint.[3] The epicondyles (#12, 15) are the most prominent points on the condyles.

RIGHT FEMUR—PROXIMAL AND DISTAL VIEWS

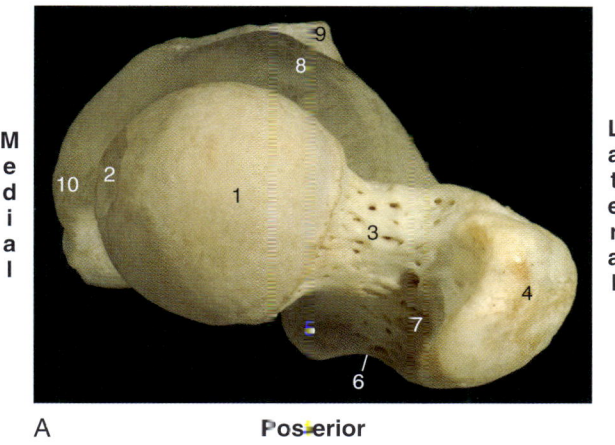

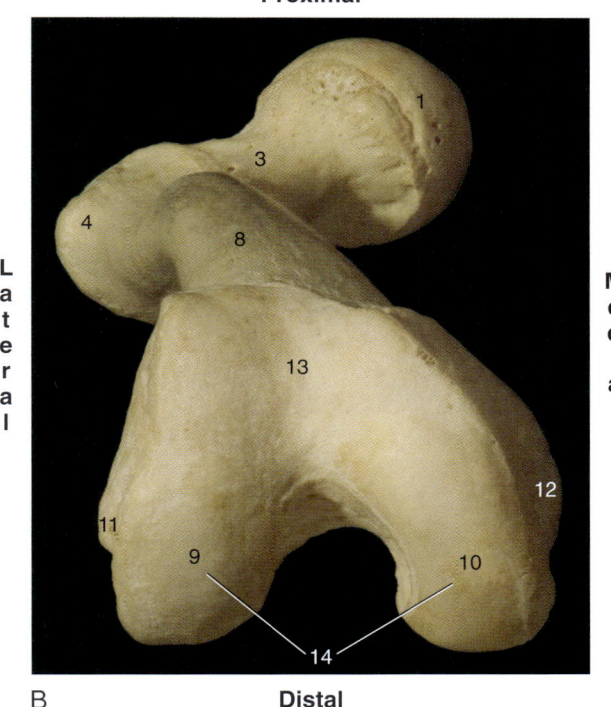

FIGURE 5-46 A, Proximal (superior) view. B, Distal (inferior) view.
1. Head
2. Fovea of the head
3. Neck
4. Greater trochanter
5. Lesser trochanter
6. Intertrochanteric crest
7. Trochanteric fossa
8. Body (shaft), anterior surface
9. Lateral condyle
10. Medial condyle
11. Lateral epicondyle
12. Medial epicondyle
13. Articular surface for patellofemoral joint
14. Articular surface for knee (tibiofemoral) joint

NOTES
1. The neck of the femur (#3) deviates anteriorly (usually approximately 15 degrees) from the greater trochanter to the head.[2] (See proximal view.)
2. The lesser trochanter (#5) is medial, and it projects somewhat posteriorly as well.
3. From a distal perspective, it is clear that the two condyles of the distal femur (#9, 10) are distinct from each other. For this reason, some speak of the knee (i.e., tibiofemoral) joint as having two aspects: a medial tibiofemoral joint and a lateral tibiofemoral joint.

RIGHT KNEE JOINT AND PATELLA

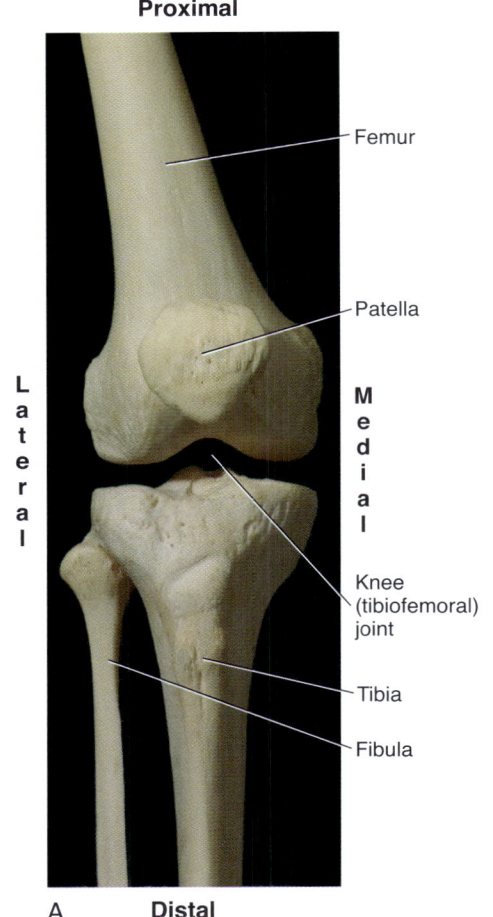

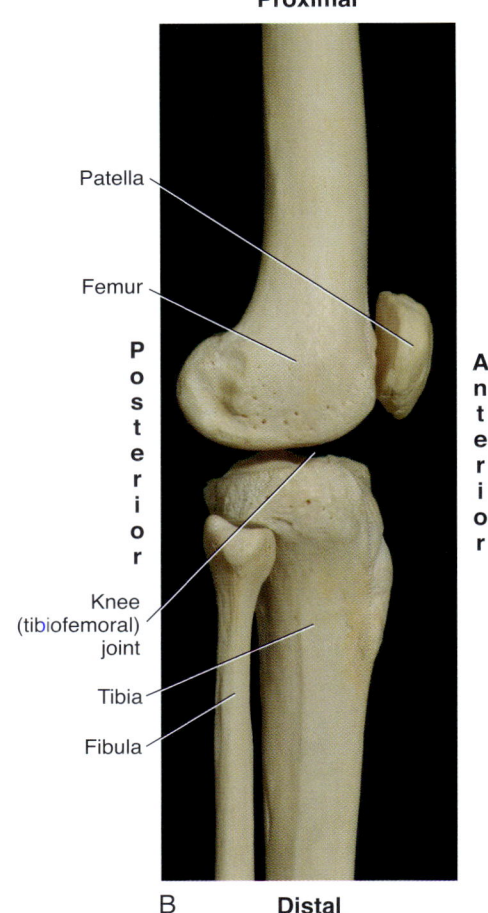

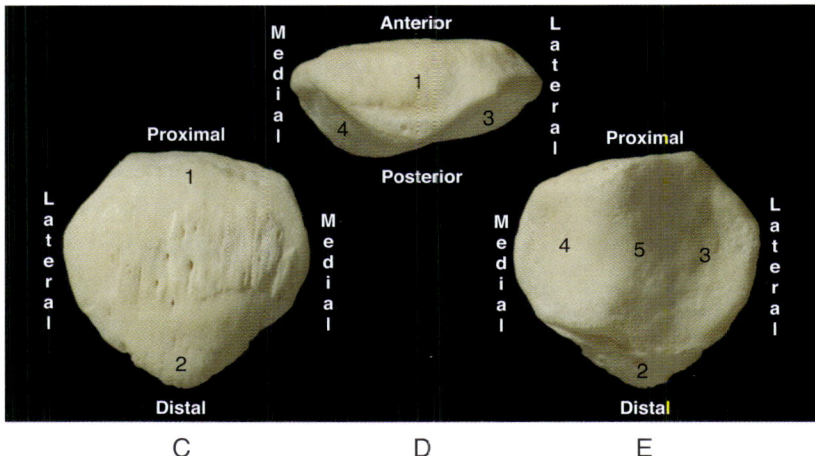

FIGURE 5-47 **A,** Anterior view. **B,** Lateral view. **C,** Anterior view. **D,** Proximal (superior) view. **E,** Posterior view.
1. Base
2. Apex
3. Facet for lateral condyle of femur
4. Facet for medial condyle of femur
5. Vertical ridge

NOTES[3]
1. The lateral facet of the posterior patella (#3) is larger than the medial facet (#4).
2. The articular surfaces of the lateral and medial facets do not extend to the apex of the patella.

SECTION 5.7 BONES OF THE LEG AND ANKLE JOINT

RIGHT TIBIA/FIBULA—ANTERIOR AND PROXIMAL VIEWS

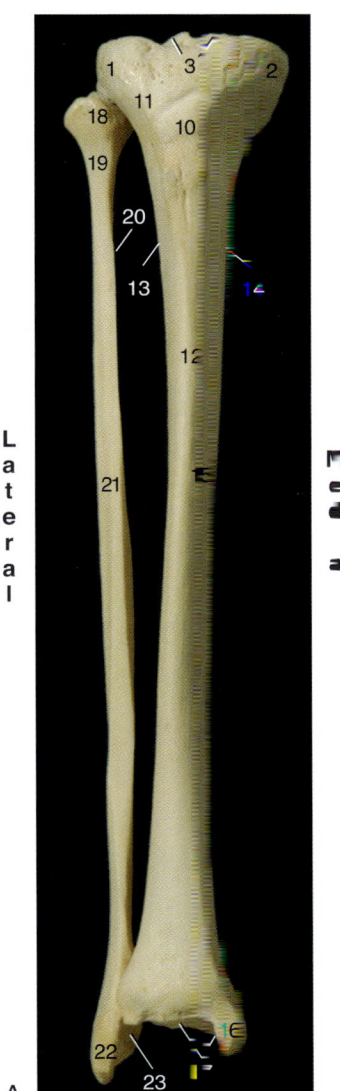
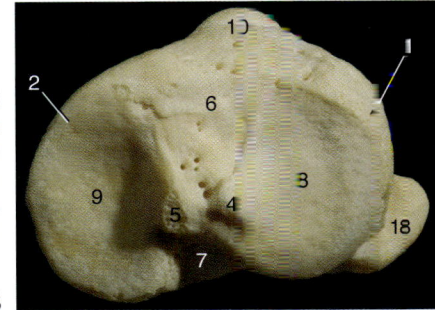

FIGURE 5-48 **A**, Anterior view. **B**, Proximal view.

Tibial landmarks:
1. Lateral condyle
2. Medial condyle
3. Intercondylar eminence
4. Lateral tubercle of intercondylar eminence
5. Medial tubercle of intercondylar eminence
6. Anterior intercondylar area
7. Posterior intercondylar area
8. Lateral facet (articular surface for knee [i.e., tibiofemoral] joint)
9. Medial facet (articular surface for knee [i.e., tibiofemoral] joint)
10. Tuberosity
11. Impression for iliotibial tract
12. Crest (i.e., anterior border)
13. Interosseus border
14. Medial border
15. Body (shaft)
16. Medial malleolus
17. Articular surface for ankle joint

Fibular landmarks:
18. Head
19. Neck
20. Interosseus border
21. Body (shaft)
22. Lateral malleolus
23. Articular surface for ankle joint

> **NOTES**
> 1. The entire proximal surface of the tibia is often referred to as the tibial plateau.[3]
> 2. The impression on the tibia for the iliotibial tract (#11) is often referred to as Gerdy's tubercle.[4]
> 3. The body (i.e., shaft) of the tibia has three borders: anterior (the crest), medial, and interosseus.
> 4. The anterior intercondylar area of the tibia (#6) is the attachment site of the anterior cruciate ligament; the posterior intercondylar area of the tibia (#7) is the attachment site of the posterior cruciate ligament.[3]
> 5. At the knee joint, the lateral facet of the tibia accepts the lateral condyle of the femur, forming the lateral tibiofemoral joint of the knee joint; the medial facet of the tibia accepts the medial condyle of the femur, forming the medial tibiofemoral joint of the knee joint.[12]

RIGHT TIBIA/FIBULA—POSTERIOR AND DISTAL VIEWS

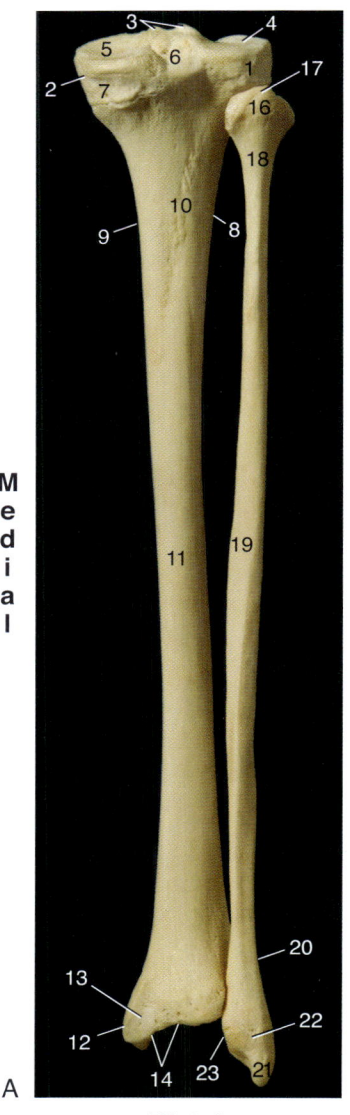

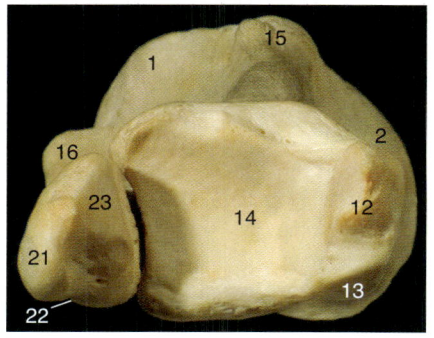

FIGURE 5-49
Tibial landmarks:
1. Lateral condyle
2. Medial condyle
3. Intercondylar eminence
4. Lateral facet (articular surface for knee [i.e., tibiofemoral] joint)
5. Medial facet (articular surface for knee [i.e., tibiofemoral] joint)
6. Posterior intercondylar area
7. Groove for semimembranosus muscle
8. Interosseus border
9. Medial border
10. Soleal line
11. Body (shaft)
12. Medial malleolus
13. Groove for tibialis posterior
14. Articular surfaces for ankle joint
15. Tuberosity

Fibular landmarks:
16. Head
17. Apex of head
18. Neck
19. Body (shaft)
20. Lateral surface
21. Lateral malleolus
22. Groove for fibularis brevis muscle
23. Articular surface for ankle joint

NOTES
1. The apex of the fibular head (#17) is also known as the styloid process of the fibula.[3]
2. The soleal line of the tibia (#10) is part of the proximal attachment of the soleus muscle.[3]
3. The groove for the fibularis brevis (#22) is created by the distal tendon of the fibularis brevis muscle as it passes posterior to the lateral malleolus to enter the foot.[3]
4. The lateral malleolus of the fibula (#21) extends further distally than the medial malleolus of the tibia. This configuration results in a range of motion of the foot that involves less eversion than inversion.[2]

RIGHT TIBIA/FIBULA—LATERAL VIEWS

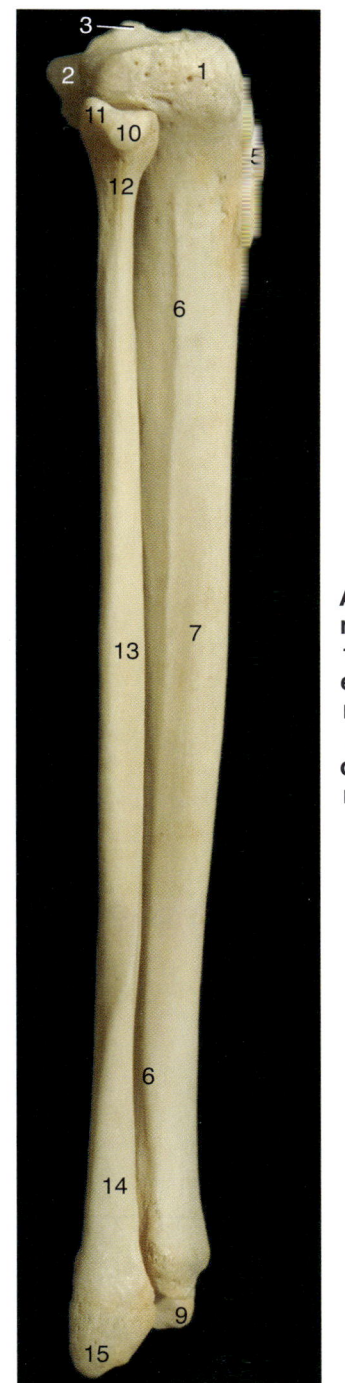
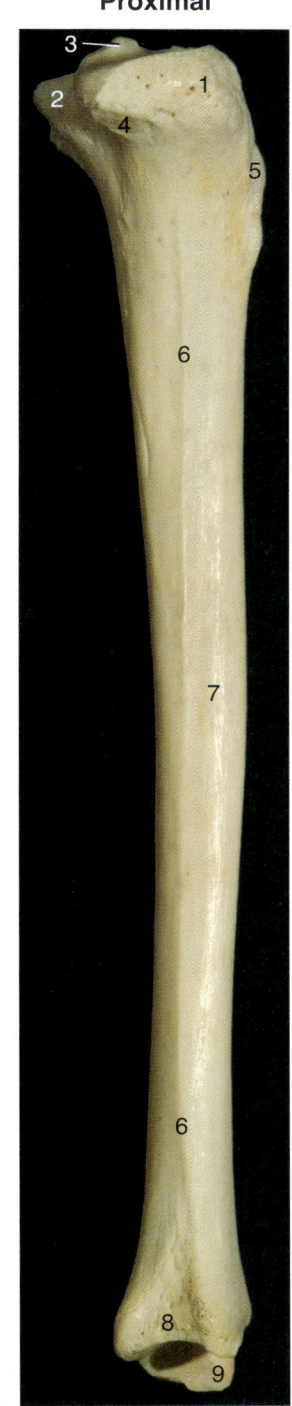

FIGURE 5-50 **A,** Lateral view of the tibia and fibula articulated. **B,** Lateral view of just the tibia.

Tibial landmarks:
1. Lateral condyle
2. Medial condyle
3. Intercondylar eminence
4. Articular facet for proximal tibiofibular joint
5. Tuberosity
6. Interosseus border
7. Body (shaft)
8. Fibular notch
9. Medial malleolus

Fibular landmarks:
10. Head
11. Apex of head
12. Neck
13. Body (shaft)
14. Triangular subcutaneous area
15. Lateral malleolus

NOTES[5]

1. The interosseus border on the lateral tibia (#6) is the site of attachment for the interosseus membrane of the leg.
2. The triangular subcutaneous area (#14) is a triangular area of the distal lateral shaft of the fibula that is palpable through the skin.
3. The articular facet for the proximal tibiofemoral joint (#4) on the lateral proximal tibia accepts the head of the fibula.
4. The fibular notch on the lateral distal tibia (#8) accepts the distal fibula, forming the distal tibiofibular joint.

RIGHT TIBIA/FIBULA—MEDIAL VIEWS

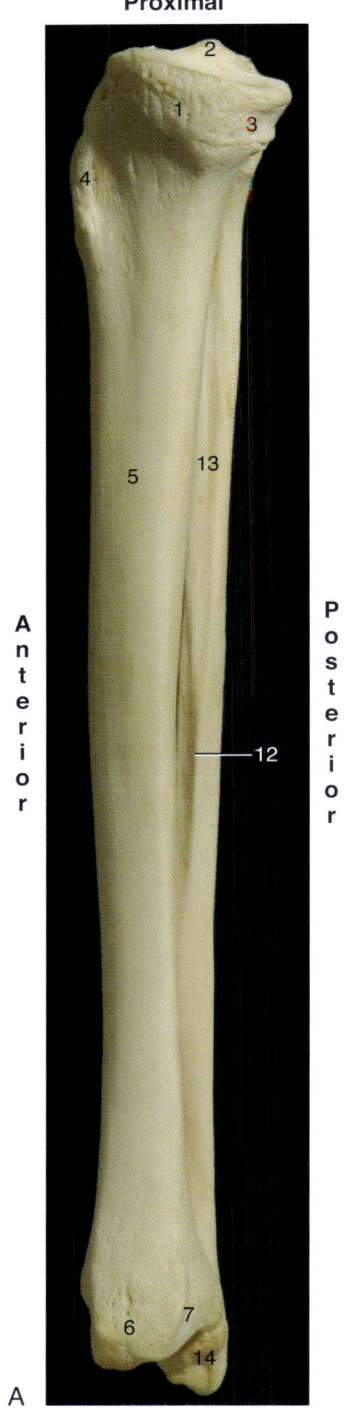

FIGURE 5-51 **A,** Medial view of the tibia and fibula articulated. **B,** Medial view of just the fibula.

Tibial landmarks:
1. Medial condyle
2. Intercondylar eminence
3. Groove for semimembranosus muscle
4. Tuberosity
5. Body (shaft)
6. Medial malleolus
7. Groove for tibialis posterior muscle

Fibular landmarks:
8. Head
9. Apex of head
10. Articular surface for proximal tibiofibular joint
11. Neck
12. Interosseus border
13. Body (shaft)
14. Lateral malleolus
15. Articular surface for ankle joint

NOTES
1. The interosseus border on the medial fibula (#12) is the site of attachment for the interosseus membrane of the leg.[5]
2. The medial view of the tibia demonstrates the groove for the semimembranosus muscle (#3) proximally and the groove for the tibialis posterior muscle (#7) distally.

RIGHT ANKLE JOINT

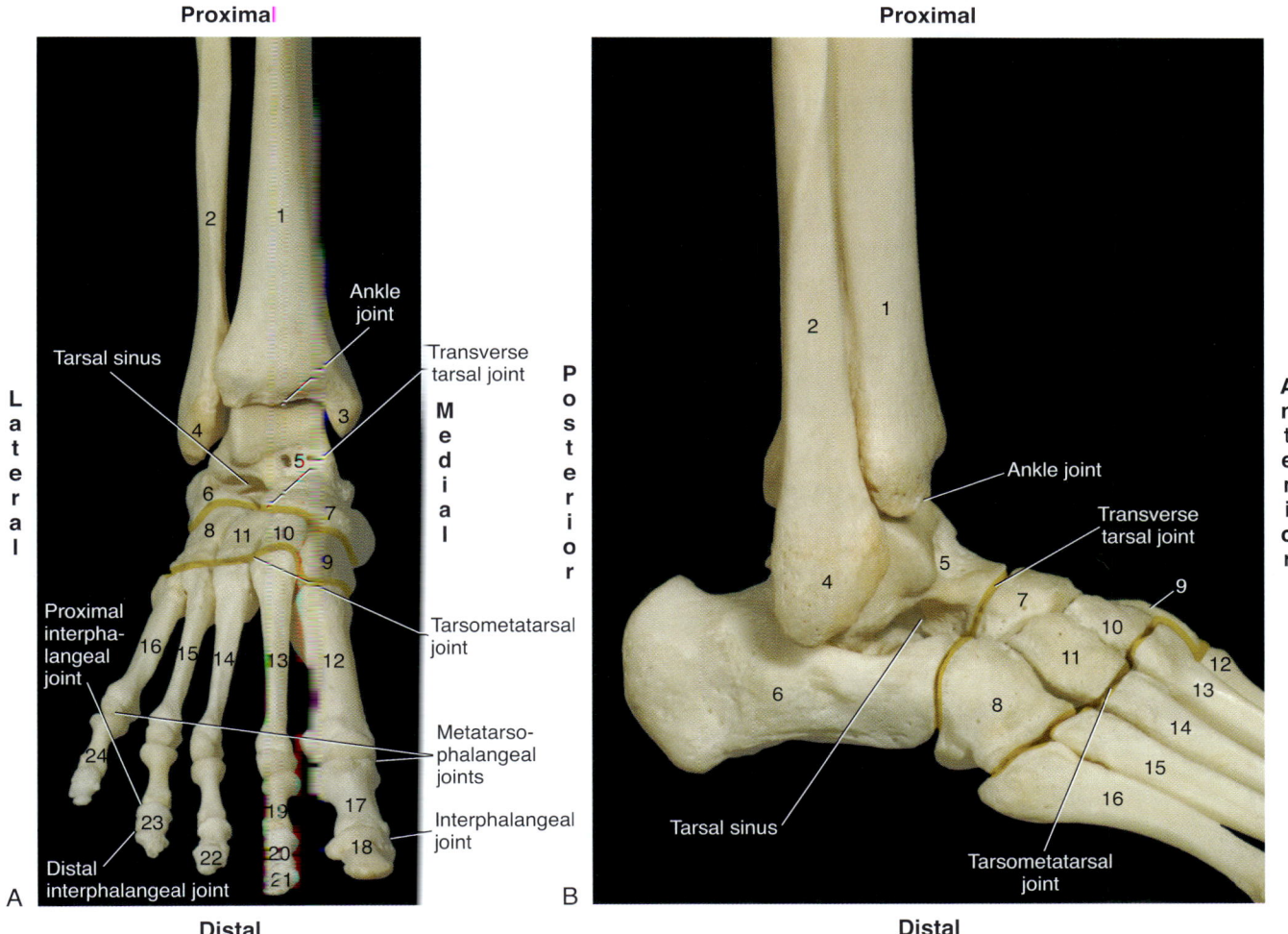

FIGURE 5-52 A, Anterior view. B, Lateral view.
1. Tibia
2. Fibula
3. Medial malleolus (of tibia)
4. Lateral malleolus (of fibula)
5. Talus
6. Calcaneus
7. Navicular
8. Cuboid
9. First cuneiform
10. Second cuneiform
11. Third cuneiform
12. First metatarsal
13. Second metatarsal
14. Third metatarsal
15. Fourth metatarsal
16. Fifth metatarsal
17. Proximal phalanx of big toe
18. Distal phalanx of big toe
19. Proximal phalanx of second toe
20. Middle phalanx of second toe
21. Distal phalanx of second toe
22. Distal phalanx of third toe
23. Middle phalanx of fourth toe
24. Proximal phalanx of little toe (i.e., fifth toe)

> **NOTES**
> 1. The ankle joint is formed by the talus (#5) being held between the malleoli of the tibia and fibula (#3, 4).[6] The ankle joint is also known as the talocrural joint.[3]
> 2. The subtalar joint is located between the talus and calcaneus (i.e., under the talus). The subtalar joint is located between tarsal bones; hence it is a tarsal joint.[10]
> 3. The transverse tarsal joint is composed of the talonavicular joint and the calcaneocuboid joint.[10]
> 4. The tarsometatarsal joint is located between the cuneiforms and cuboid proximally (posteriorly), and the metatarsals distally (anteriorly).[10]

SECTION 5.8 BONES OF THE FOOT

RIGHT SUBTALAR JOINT

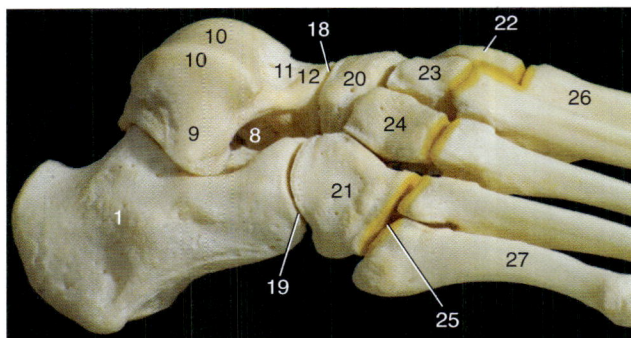
A, Lateral view

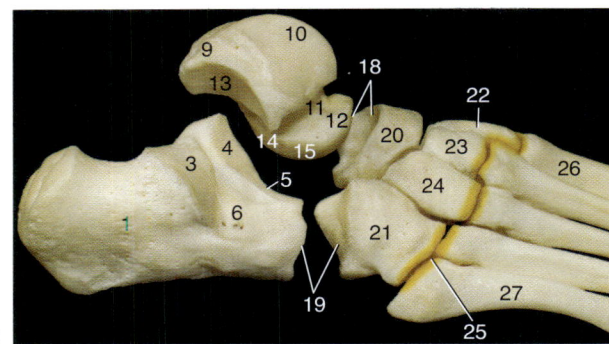
B, Lateral view, subtalar joint open

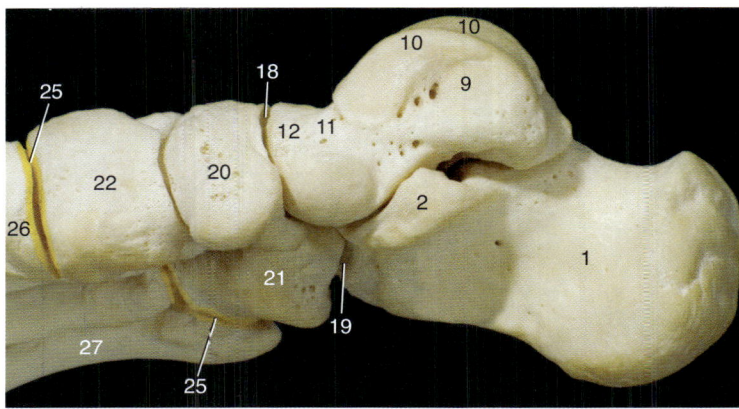
C, Medial view

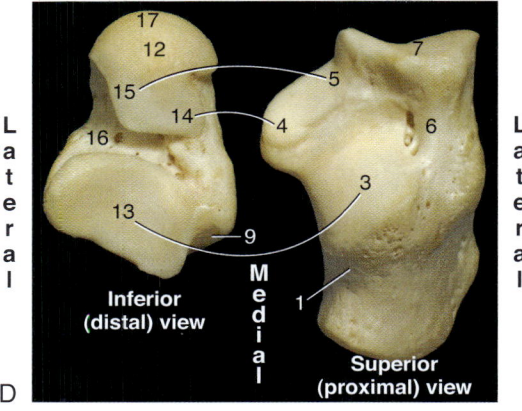
D, Subtalar joint, articular surfaces

FIGURE 5-53 A, Right lateral view. B, Right lateral view, subtalar joint open. C, Medial view. D, Subtalar joint, articular surfaces.

1 Calcaneus (#1-7)
2 Sustentaculum tali
3 Calcaneal posterior facet (of subtalar joint)
4 Calcaneal middle facet (of subtalar joint)
5 Calcaneal anterior facet (of subtalar joint)
6 Sulcus (of calcaneus)
7 Articular surface for calcaneocuboid joint (of transverse tarsal joint)
8 Tarsal sinus
9 Talus (#9-17)
10 Articular surface for ankle joint
11 Neck of talus
12 Head of talus
13 Talar posterior facet (of subtalar joint)
14 Talar middle facet (of subtalar joint)
15 Talar anterior facet (of subtalar joint)
16 Sulcus (of talus)
17 Articular surface for talonavicular joint (of transverse tarsal joint)
18 Talonavicular joint (of transverse tarsal joint)
19 Calcaneocuboid joint (of transverse tarsal joint)
20 Navicular
21 Cuboid
22 First cuneiform
23 Second cuneiform
24 Third cuneiform
25 Tarsometatarsal joint
26 First metatarsal
27 Fifth metatarsal

NOTES[10]

1. The subtalar joint between the talus (#9) and calcaneus (#1) is composed of three articular surfaces: posterior, middle, and anterior. The posterior articulation is formed by the posterior facets of each bone; the middle articulation is formed by the middle facets of each bone; the anterior articulation is formed by the anterior facets of each bone.
2. The posterior aspect of the subtalar joint is the largest of the three.
3. The tarsal sinus (#8) is formed by the sulcus of the calcaneus and the sulcus of the talus.
4. The transverse tarsal joint is formed by the talonavicular and calcaneocuboid joints (#18, 19).

RIGHT FOOT—DORSAL VIEW

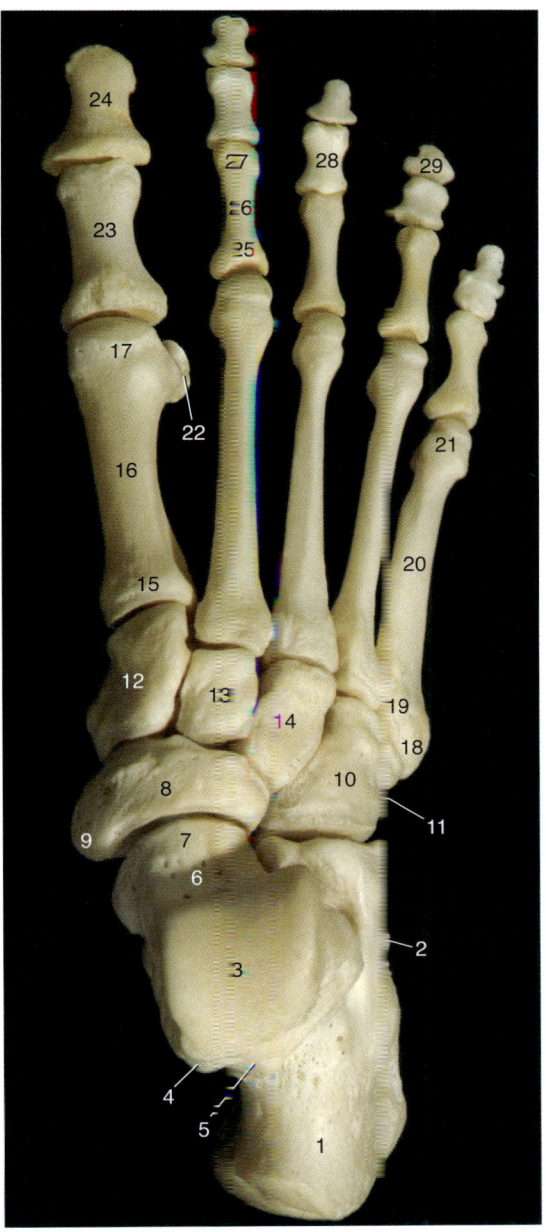

FIGURE 5-54
1. Calcaneus
2. Fibular trochlea of calcaneus
3. Articular surface of talus for ankle joint
4. Medial tubercle of talus
5. Lateral tubercle of talus
6. Neck of talus
7. Head of talus
8. Navicular
9. Navicular tuberosity
10. Cuboid
11. Groove for fibularis longus
12. First cuneiform
13. Second cuneiform
14. Third cuneiform
15. Base of first metatarsal
16. Body (shaft) of first metatarsal
17. Head of first metatarsal
18. Tuberosity of base of fifth metatarsal
19. Base of fifth metatarsal
20. Body (shaft) of fifth metatarsal
21. Head of fifth metatarsal
22. Sesamoid bone of big toe
23. Proximal phalanx of big toe
24. Distal phalanx of big toe
25. Base of proximal phalanx of second toe
26. Body (shaft) of proximal phalanx of second toe
27. Head of proximal phalanx of second toe
28. Middle phalanx of third toe
29. Distal phalanx of fourth toe

NOTES
1. The word phalanx is singular only; plural of phalanx is phalanges.
2. The articular surface of the talus for the ankle joint (#3) is called the trochlea of the talus.[2]
3. The first, second, and third cuneiforms (#12, 13, 14) are also known as the medial, intermediate, and lateral cuneiforms, respectively.[3]
4. The first cuneiform articulates with the first metatarsal; the second cuneiform articulates with the second metatarsal; the third cuneiform articulates with the third metatarsal; and the cuboid articulates with the fourth and fifth metatarsals.[8]
5. All metatarsals and phalanges have a base proximally, a body (i.e., shaft) in the middle, and a head distally.[12]
6. The middle and distal phalanges of the little toe in this specimen have fused together.

RIGHT FOOT—PLANTAR VIEW

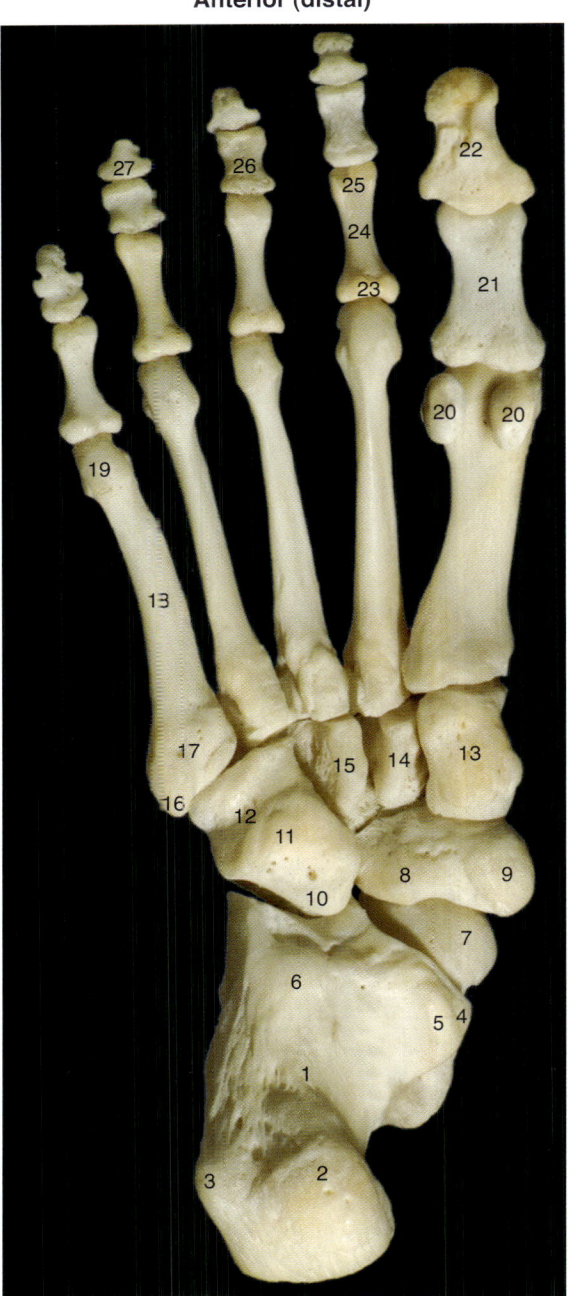

Anterior (distal)

Posterior (proximal)

Lateral

Medial

FIGURE 5-55
1. Calcaneus
2. Medial process of calcaneal tuberosity
3. Lateral process of calcaneal tuberosity
4. Sustentaculum tali of calcaneus
5. Groove for distal tendon of flexor hallucis longus muscle (on sustentaculum tali)
6. Anterior tubercle of calcaneus
7. Head of talus
8. Navicular
9. Navicular tuberosity
10. Cuboid
11. Tuberosity of cuboid
12. Groove for distal tendon of fibularis longus muscle
13. First cuneiform
14. Second cuneiform
15. Third cuneiform
16. Tuberosity of base of fifth metatarsal
17. Base of fifth metatarsal
18. Body (shaft) of fifth metatarsal
19. Head of fifth metatarsal
20. Sesamoid bone of big toe
21. Proximal phalanx of big toe
22. Distal phalanx of big toe
23. Base of proximal phalanx of second toe
24. Body (shaft) of proximal phalanx of second toe
25. Head of proximal phalanx of second toe
26. Middle phalanx of third toe
27. Distal phalanx of fourth toe

NOTES
1. On the calcaneal tuberosity, the medial process (#2) is much larger than the lateral process (#3).
2. The base of the fifth metatarsal bone has a large palpable tuberosity (#16).[5]
3. The big toe usually has two sesamoid bones (#20).[13]
4. The groove for the distal tendon of the fibularis longus tendon (#12) is clearly visible on the plantar surface of the cuboid, demonstrating its passage deep in the plantar foot.[5]
5. The middle and distal phalanges of the little toe have fused together in this specimen.

CHAPTER 5 Bones of the Human Body

RIGHT FOOT—MEDIAL VIEW

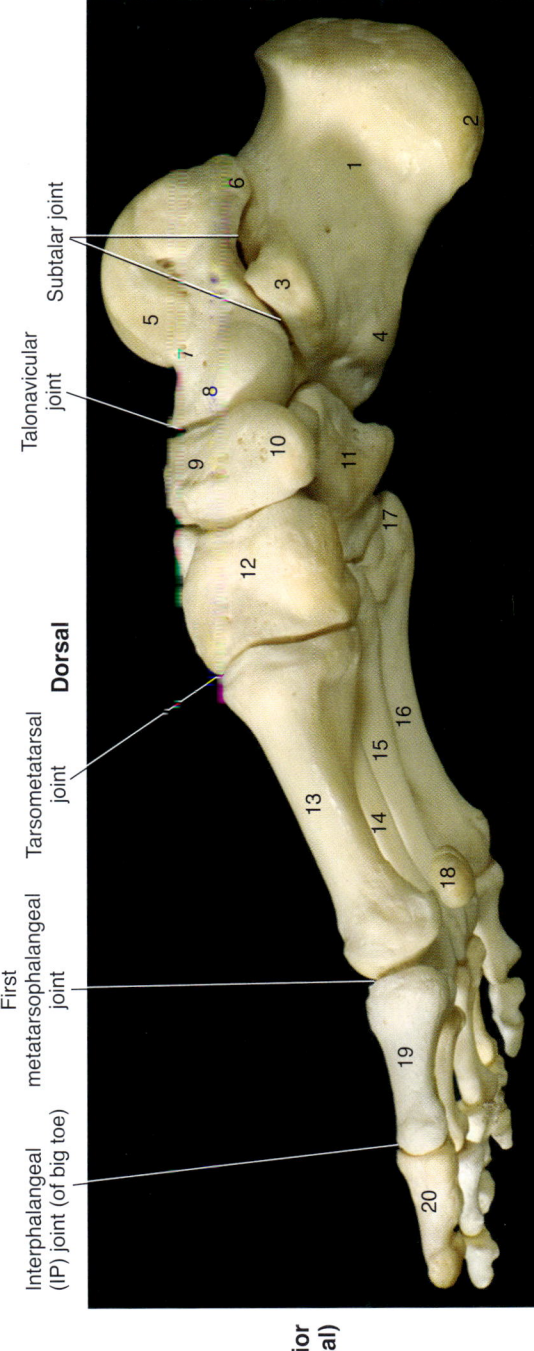

FIGURE 5-56
1. Calcaneus (medial surface)
2. Medial process of calcaneal tuberosity
3. Sustentaculum tali of calcaneus
4. Anterior tubercle of calcaneus
5. Articular surface of talus for (medial malleolus of) ankle joint
6. Medial tubercle of talus
7. Neck of talus
8. Head of talus
9. Navicular
10. Navicular tuberosity
11. Cuboid
12. First cuneiform
13. First metatarsal
14. Third metatarsal
15. Fourth metatarsal
16. Fifth metatarsal
17. Tuberosity of base of fifth metatarsal
18. Sesamoid bone of big toe
19. Proximal phalanx of big toe
20. Distal phalanx of big toe

NOTES
1. The sustentaculum tali of the calcaneus (#3) forms a ledge on which the talus sits.[3]
2. On the medial side of the foot, the sustentaculum tali (#3) of the calcaneus and the navicular tuberosity (#10) are easily palpable landmarks.[13]
3. The second metatarsal is not visible in this view.
4. The subtalar joint is located between the talus and the calcaneus.[10]
5. The talonavicular joint (of the transverse tarsal joint) is located between the talus and the navicular.[10]
6. The arch (i.e., medial longitudinal arch) of the foot is apparent in a medial view.

RIGHT FOOT—LATERAL VIEW

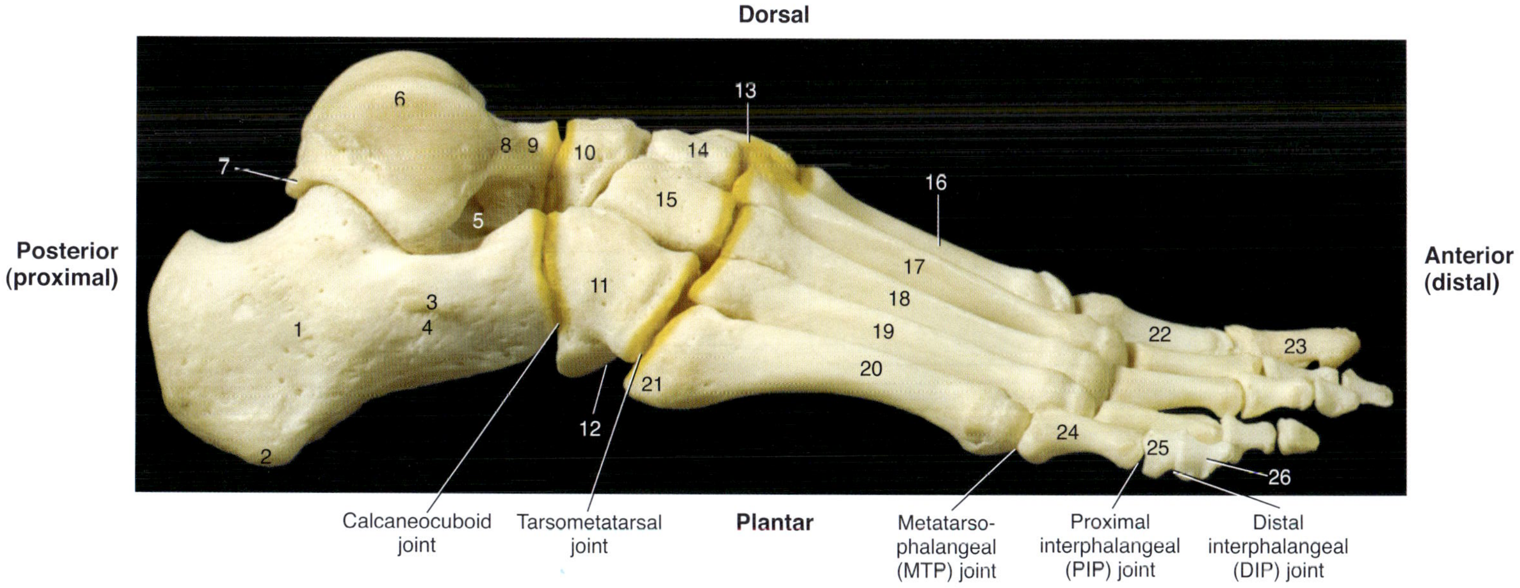

FIGURE 5-57

1. Calcaneus (lateral surface)
2. Lateral process of calcaneal tuberosity
3. Fibular trochlea
4. Groove for distal tendon of fibularis longus muscle
5. Tarsal sinus
6. Articular surface of talus for (lateral malleolus of) ankle joint
7. Lateral tubercle of talus
8. Neck of talus
9. Head of talus
10. Navicular
11. Cuboid
12. Groove for distal tendon of fibularis longus muscle
13. First cuneiform
14. Second cuneiform
15. Third cuneiform
16. First metatarsal
17. Second metatarsal
18. Third metatarsal
19. Fourth metatarsal
20. Fifth metatarsal
21. Tuberosity of base of fifth metatarsal
22. Proximal phalanx of big toe
23. Distal phalanx of big toe
24. Proximal phalanx of little toe
25. Middle phalanx of little toe
26. Distal phalanx of little toe

NOTES

1. The tuberosity of the base of the fifth metatarsal (#21) is easily palpable on the lateral side of the foot.[13]
2. The subtalar joint is located between the talus and the calcaneus.[10]
3. The tarsal sinus (#5) is a space located between the talus and calcaneus.[10]
4. The calcaneocuboid joint of the transverse tarsal joint is located between the calcaneus and the cuboid.[10]
5. The middle and distal phalanges of the little toe are fused together in this specimen.

SECTION 5.9 ENTIRE UPPER EXTREMITY

RIGHT UPPER EXTREMITY

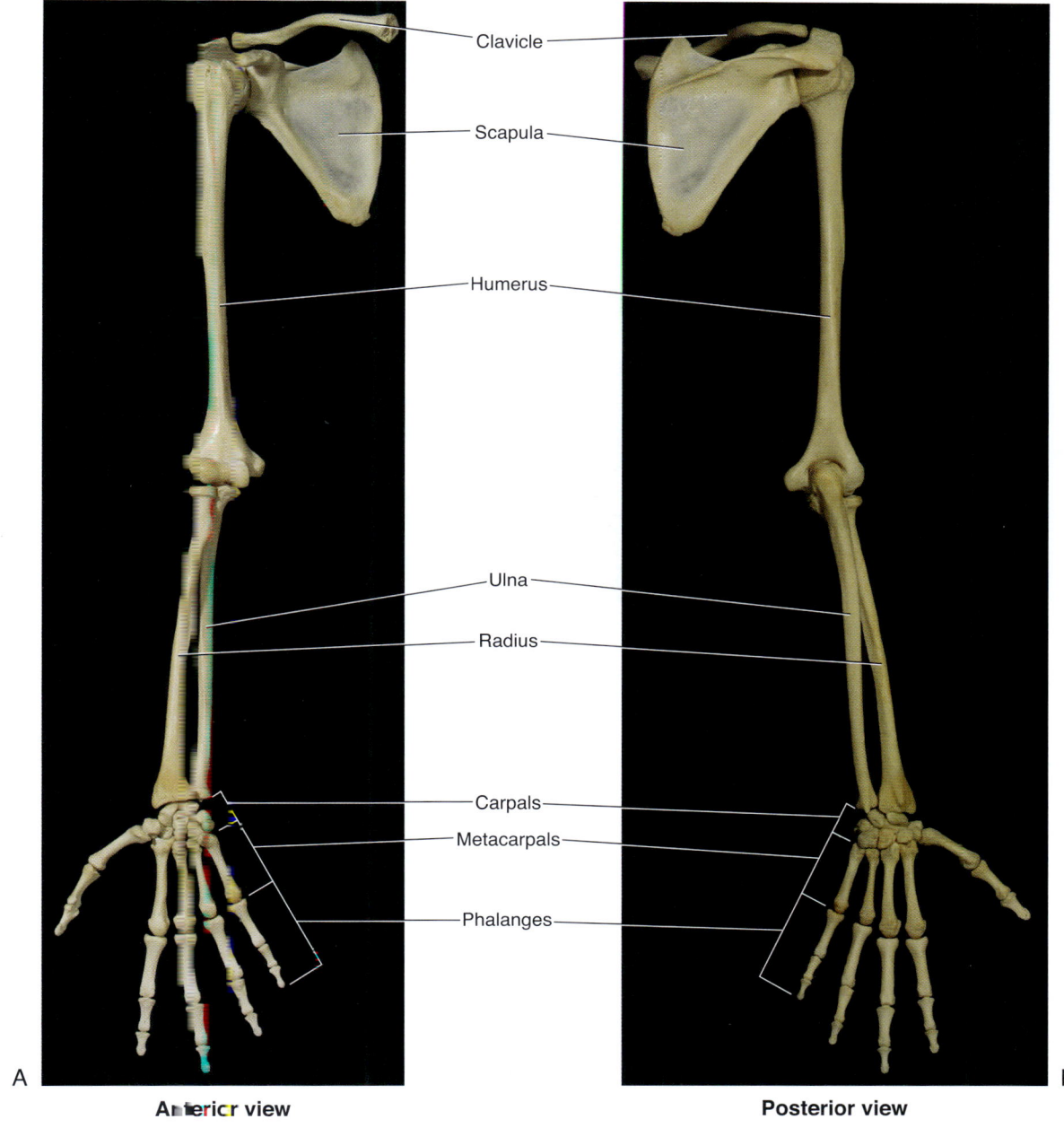

FIGURE 5-58 **A,** Anterior view. **B,** Posterior view.

NOTES[2]
1. The upper extremity is composed of the bones of the shoulder girdle, arm, forearm, and hand.
2. The shoulder girdle is composed of the scapula and clavicle, and the arm contains the humerus.
3. The forearm contains the radius, which is lateral, and the ulna, which is medial.
4. The hand contains eight carpals, five metacarpals, and 14 phalanges.

SECTION 5.10 BONES OF THE SHOULDER GIRDLE AND SHOULDER JOINT

RIGHT SHOULDER JOINT

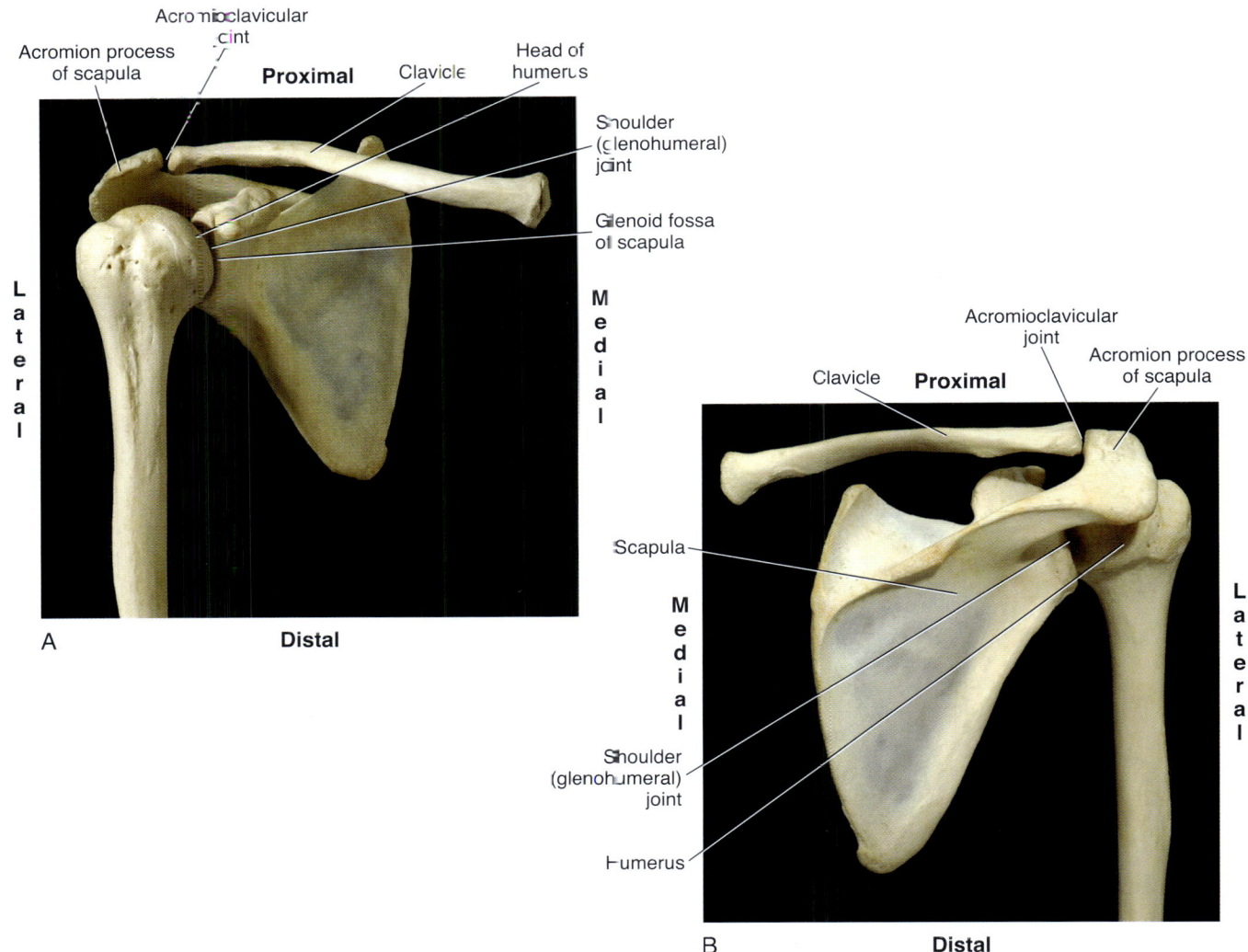

FIGURE 5-59 **A,** Anterior view. **B,** Posterior view.

NOTES[9]
1. The shoulder joint is formed by the head of the humerus articulating with the glenoid fossa of the scapula. It is also known as the glenohumeral joint.
2. Even though the glenohumeral joint is a ball-and-socket joint, the glenoid fossa (i.e., the socket) is shallow.
3. The acromioclavicular (AC) joint is formed by the acromion process of the scapula articulating with the lateral end of the clavicle.

RIGHT SCAPULA—POSTERIOR AND DORSAL VIEWS

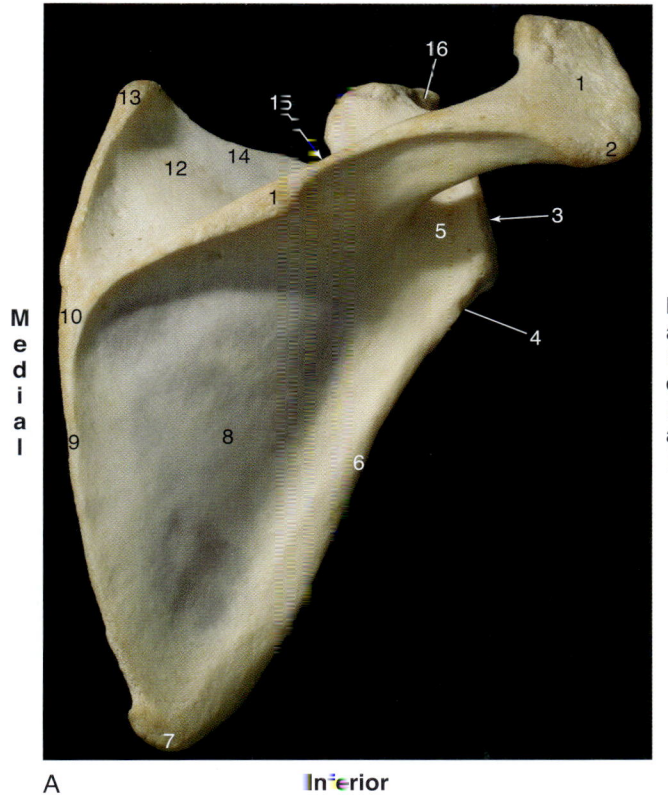

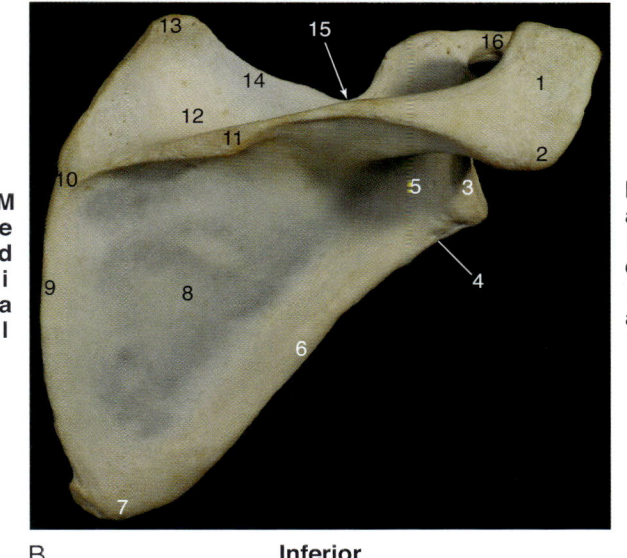

FIGURE 5-60 **A,** Posterior view. **B,** Dorsal view.
1. Acromion process
2. Acromial angle
3. Glenoid fossa
4. Infraglenoid tubercle
5. Neck
6. Lateral border
7. Inferior angle
8. Infraspinous fossa
9. Medial border
10. Root of the spine
11. Spine
12. Supraspinous fossa
13. Superior angle
14. Superior border
15. Suprascapular notch
16. Coracoid process

NOTES
1. A is a pure posterior view of the scapula as it sits on the body; B is a view of the dorsal surface of the scapula itself. The difference in these two perspectives can be seen.
2. The medial border (#9) is also known as the vertebral border.[13]
3. The lateral border (#6) is also known as the axillary border.[13]
4. The supraspinous and infraspinous fossae (#12, 8) are proximal attachment sites of the supraspinatus and infraspinatus muscles.[4]
5. The infraglenoid tubercle (#4) and the suprascapular notch (#15) are not well developed on this scapula and therefore not well visualized.[13]

RIGHT SCAPULA—ANTERIOR AND SUBSCAPULAR VIEWS

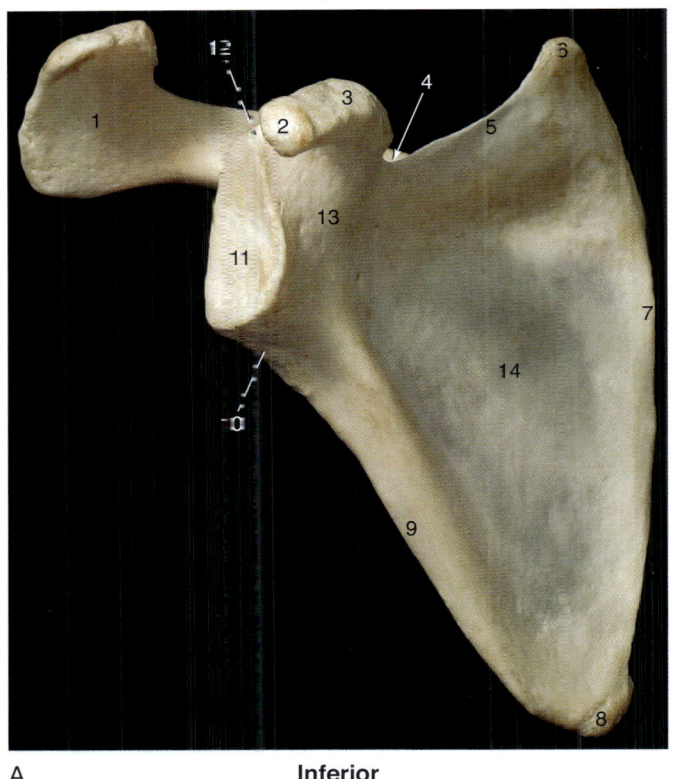
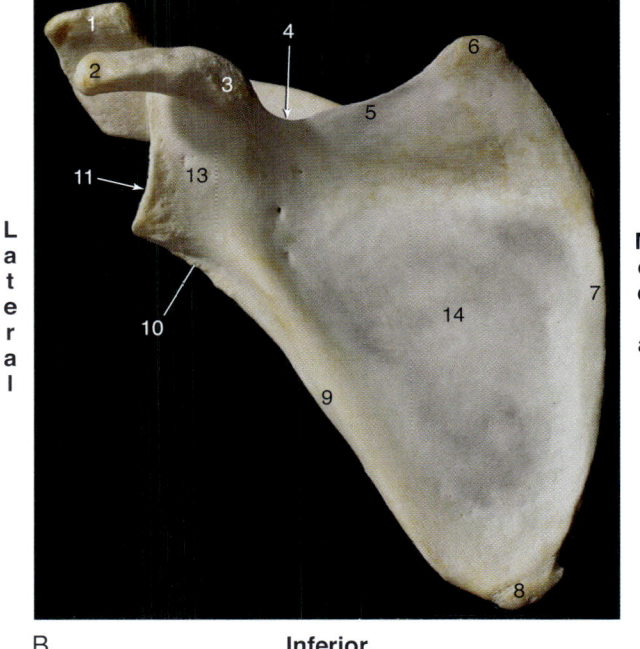

FIGURE 5-61 **A,** Anterior view. **B,** Subscapular view.
1. Acromion process
2. Apex of coracoid process
3. Base of coracoid process
4. Suprascapular notch
5. Superior border
6. Superior angle
7. Medial border
8. Inferior angle
9. Lateral border
10. Infraglenoid tubercle
11. Glenoid fossa
12. Supraglenoid tubercle
13. Neck
14. Subscapular fossa

NOTES
1. A is a pure anterior view of the scapula as it sits on the body; B is a view of the subscapular (i.e., costal) surface of the scapula itself. The differences in these two perspectives can be seen.
2. The coracoid process (#2, 3) projects anteriorly; it also points laterally.[4]
3. The subscapular fossa (#14) is the proximal attachment site of the subscapularis muscle.[4]
4. The supraglenoid tubercle (#12) is not well developed on this scapula and therefore not well visualized.

RIGHT SCAPULA—LATERAL AND SUPERIOR VIEWS

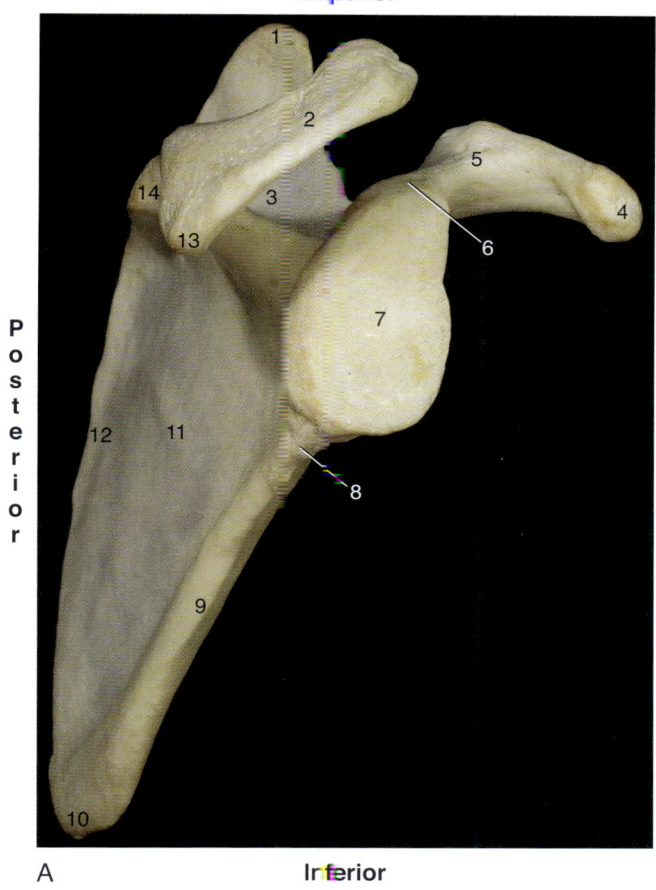

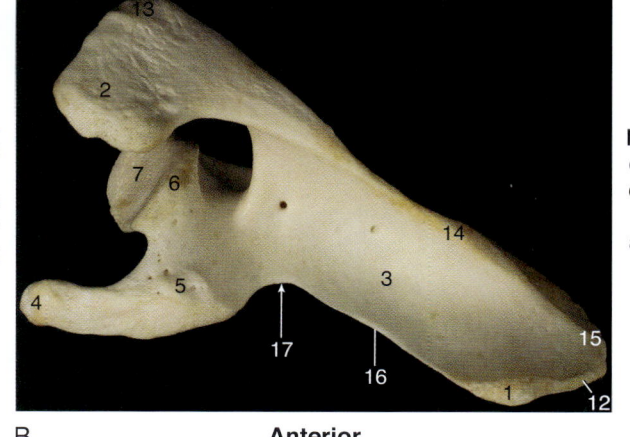

FIGURE 5-62 A, Lateral view. B, Superior view.
1. Superior angle
2. Acromion process
3. Supraspinous fossa
4. Apex of coracoid process
5. Base of coracoid process
6. Supraglenoid tubercle
7. Glenoid fossa
8. Infraglenoid tubercle
9. Lateral border
10. Inferior angle
11. Infraspinous fossa
12. Medial border
13. Acromial angle
14. Spine
15. Root of the spine
16. Superior border
17. Suprascapular notch

NOTES:
1. The supraglenoid tubercle (#6) is the proximal attachment site of the long head of the biceps brachii muscle.
2. The infraglenoid tubercle (#8) is the proximal attachment site of the long head of the triceps brachii muscle.

RIGHT CLAVICLE

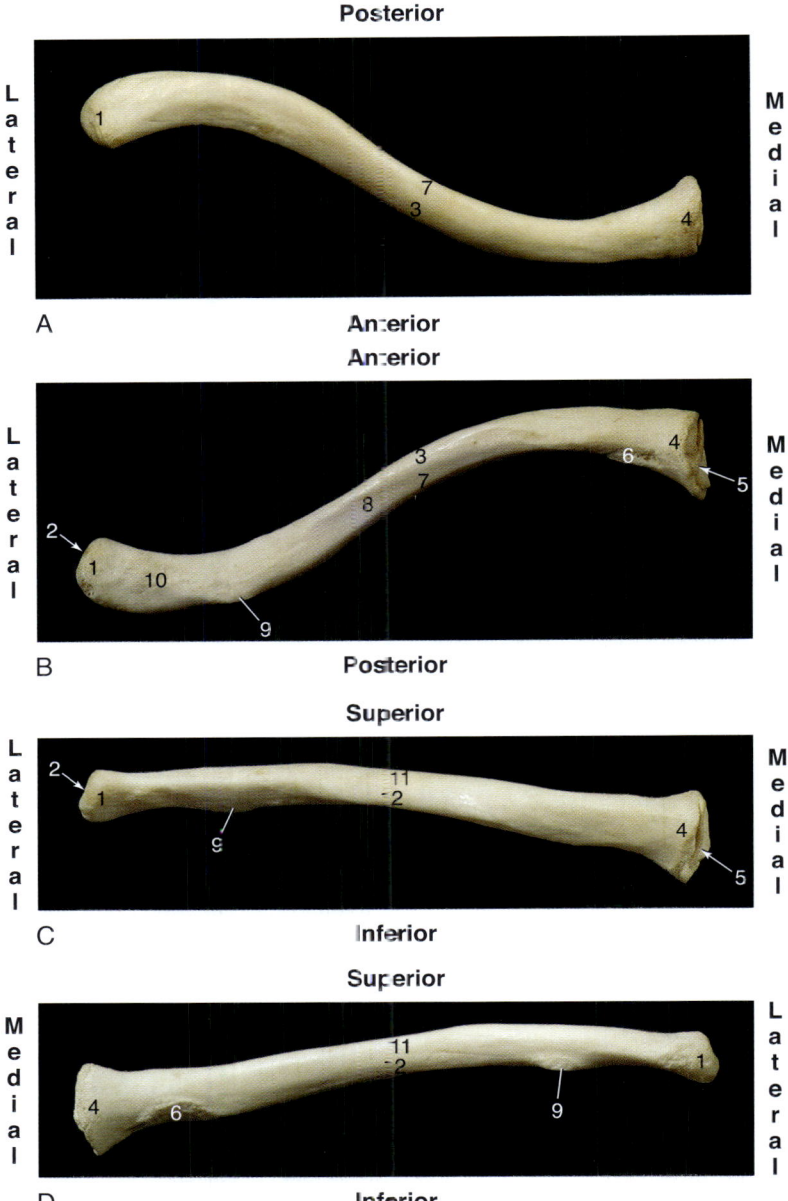

FIGURE 5-63 A, Superior view. B, Inferior view. C, Anterior view. D, Posterior view.
1 Acromial end
2 Articular surface for acromioclavicular (AC) joint
3 Anterior border
4 Sternal end
5 Articular surface for sternoclavicular joint
6 Costal tubercle
7 Posterior border
8 Subclavian groove
9 Conoid tubercle
10 Trapezoid line
11 Superior border
12 Inferior border

NOTES[5]
1. The acromial end is the lateral (distal) end.
2. The sternal end is the medial (proximal) end.
3. The sternal end of the clavicle is more bulbous, whereas the acromial end is flatter.
4. The medial ⅔ of the clavicle is convex anteriorly; the lateral ⅓ is concave anteriorly.
5. The conoid tubercle (#9) is the attachment site of the conoid ligament of the coracoclavicular ligament.
6. The trapezoid line (#10) is the attachment site of the trapezoid ligament of the coracoclavicular ligament.
7. The costal tubercle (#6) is the attachment site of the costoclavicular ligament.

CHAPTER 5 Bones of the Human Body

SECTION 5.11 BONES OF THE ARM AND ELBOW JOINT

RIGHT HUMERUS—ANTERIOR AND POSTERIOR VIEWS

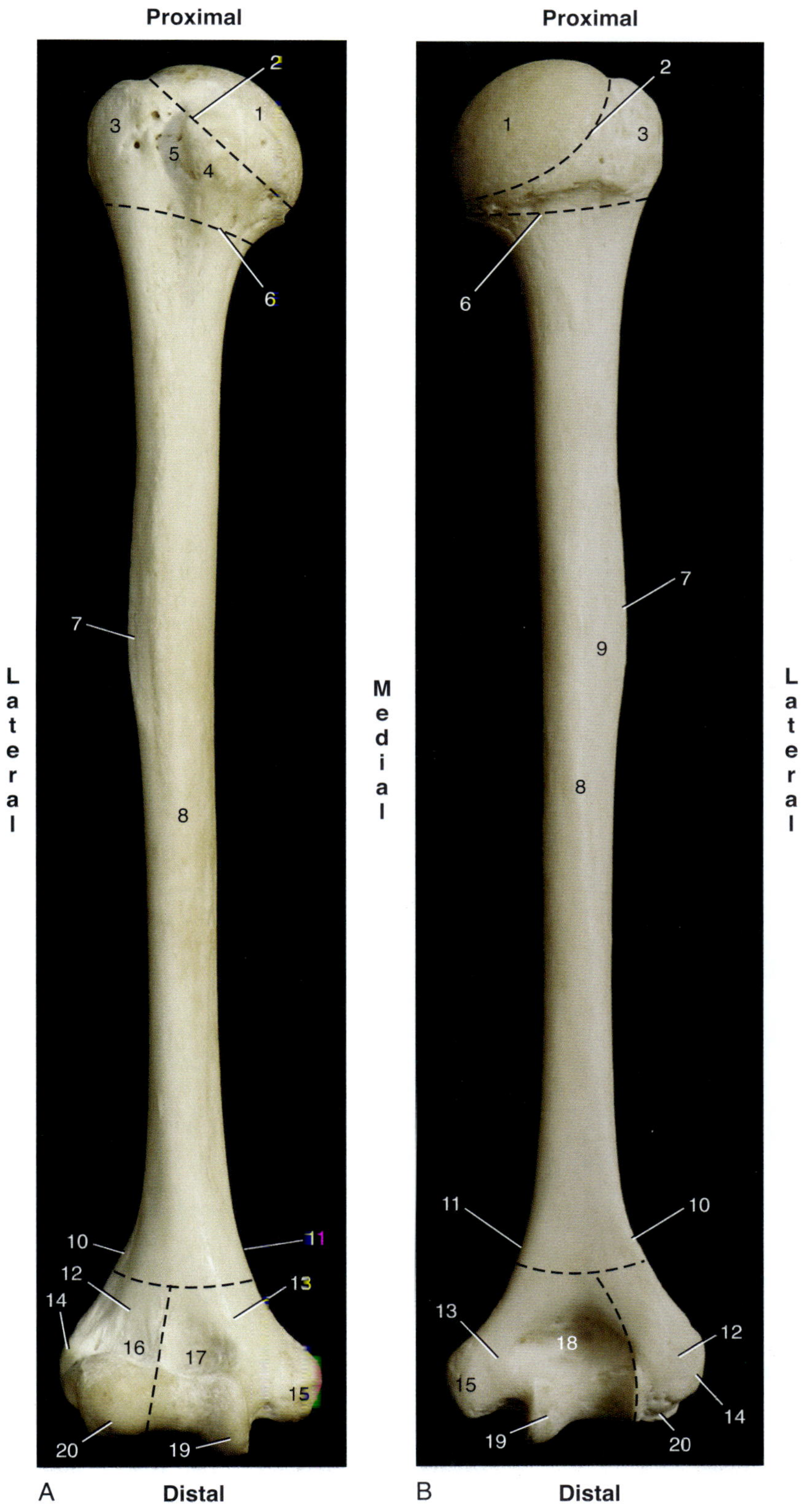

FIGURE 5-64 **A**, Anterior view. **B**, Posterior view.
1. Head
2. Anatomic neck
3. Greater tubercle
4. Lesser tubercle
5. Bicipital groove
6. Surgical neck
7. Deltoid tuberosity
8. Body (shaft)
9. Groove for radial nerve
10. Lateral supracondylar ridge
11. Medial supracondylar ridge
12. Lateral condyle
13. Medial condyle
14. Lateral epicondyle
15. Medial epicondyle
16. Radial fossa
17. Coronoid fossa
18. Olecranon fossa
19. Trochlea
20. Capitulum

NOTES
1. Proximally, the anatomic and surgical necks are indicated by dashed lines (#2, 6); distally, the borders of the lateral and medial condyles are indicated by dashed lines (#12, 13).
2. The radial and coronoid fossae (#16, 17) accept the head of the radius and the coronoid process of the ulna, respectively, when the elbow joint is flexed; the olecranon fossa accepts the olecranon process of the ulna when the elbow joint is extended.[2]
3. The bicipital groove (#5) (so named because the biceps brachii long head tendon runs through it) is also known as the intertubercular groove (so named because it is located between the greater and lesser tubercles).[5]
4. The groove for the radial nerve (#9) is also known as the spiral groove.[5]

RIGHT HUMERUS—LATERAL AND MEDIAL VIEWS

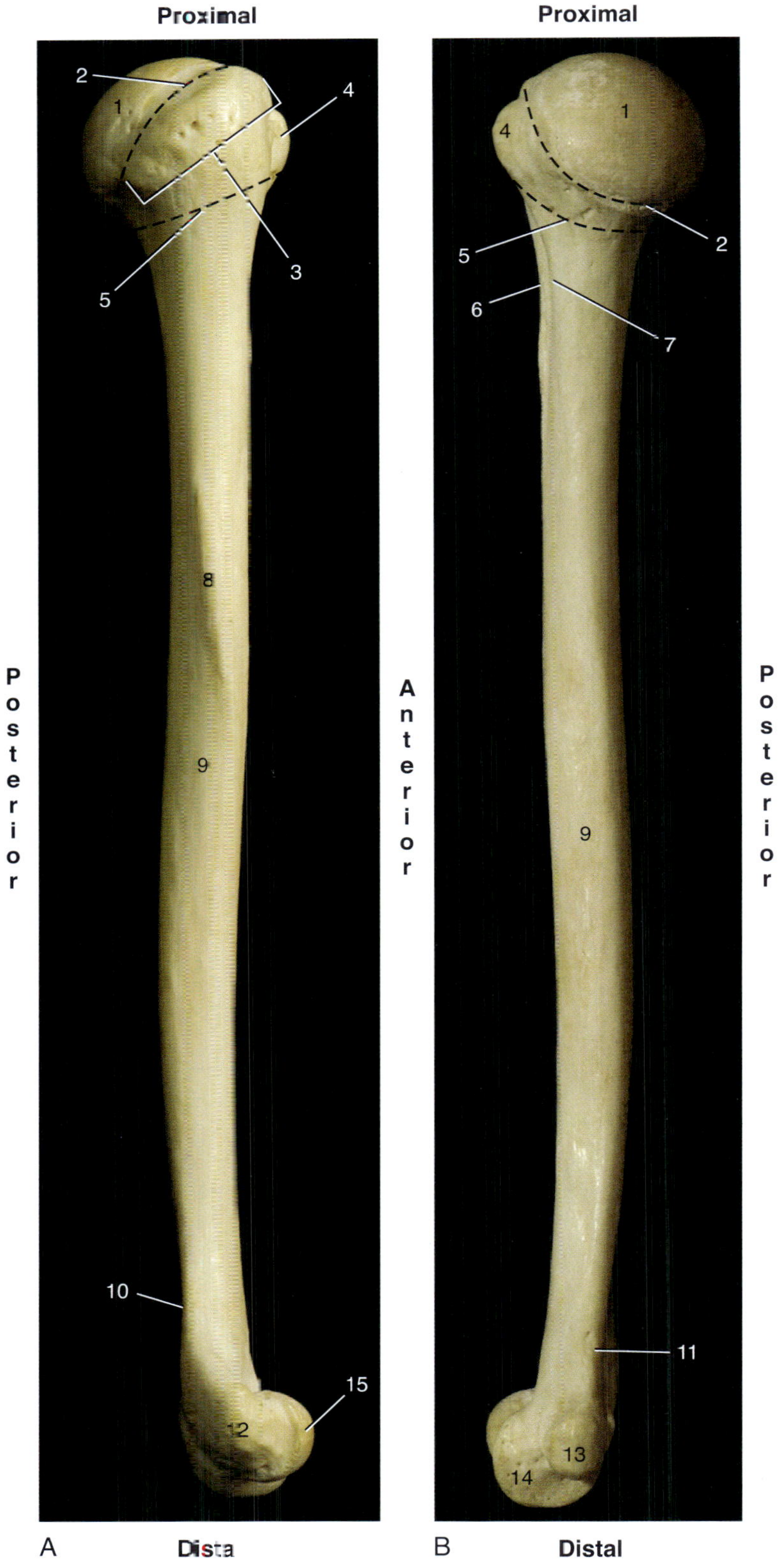

FIGURE 5-65 **A**, Lateral view. **B**, Medial view.
1. Head
2. Anatomic neck
3. Greater tubercle
4. Lesser tubercle
5. Surgical neck
6. Lateral lip of bicipital groove
7. Medial lip of bicipital groove
8. Deltoid tuberosity
9. Body (shaft)
10. Lateral supracondylar ridge
11. Medial supracondylar ridge
12. Lateral epicondyle
13. Medial epicondyle
14. Trochlea
15. Capitulum

NOTES
1. The anatomic and surgical necks (#2, 5) are indicated by dashed lines.
2. The lateral epicondyle (#12) and capitulum (#15) are landmarks on the lateral condyle; the medial epicondyle (#13) and trochlea (#14) are landmarks on the medial condyle.[3]
3. The lateral and medial epicondyles are the most prominent points on the lateral and medial condyles, respectively.[3]
4. The medial epicondyle (#13) is the attachment site of the common flexor tendon of many of the anterior forearm muscles; the lateral epicondyle (#12) is the attachment site of the common extensor tendon of many of the posterior forearm muscles.[2]
5. The deltoid tuberosity (#8) is the distal attachment site of the deltoid muscle.[2]

RIGHT HUMERUS—PROXIMAL AND DISTAL VIEWS

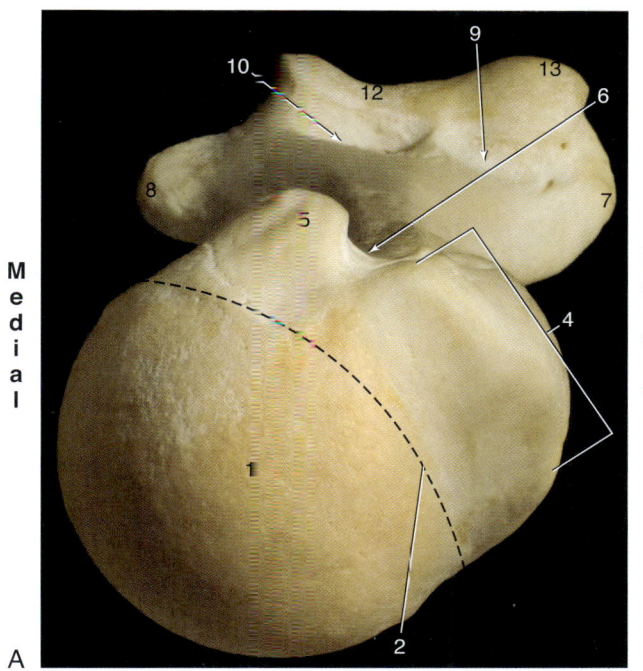

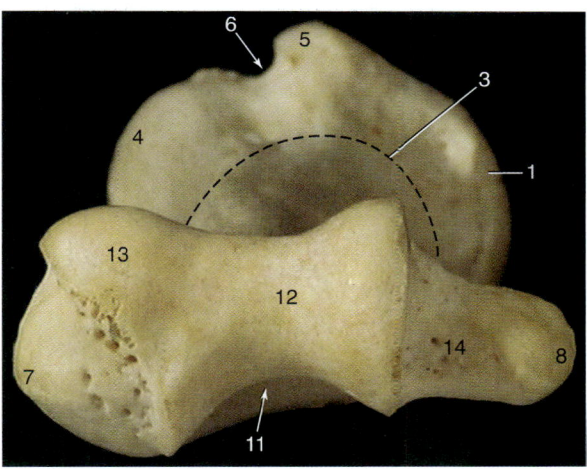

FIGURE 5-66 **A,** Proximal (superior) view. **B,** Distal (inferior) view.
1. Head
2. Anatomic neck
3. Surgical neck
4. Greater tubercle
5. Lesser tubercle
6. Bicipital groove
7. Lateral epicondyle
8. Medial epicondyle
9. Radial fossa
10. Coronoid fossa
11. Olecranon fossa
12. Trochlea
13. Capitulum
14. Groove for ulnar nerve

NOTES
1. The anatomic and surgical necks (#2, 3) are indicated by dashed lines.
2. The ulnar nerve runs in a groove (#14) that is located between the medial epicondyle and trochlea of the humerus[4] (it can easily be palpated at this location). The ulnar nerve at this site is often referred to as the "funny bone."

RIGHT ELBOW JOINT

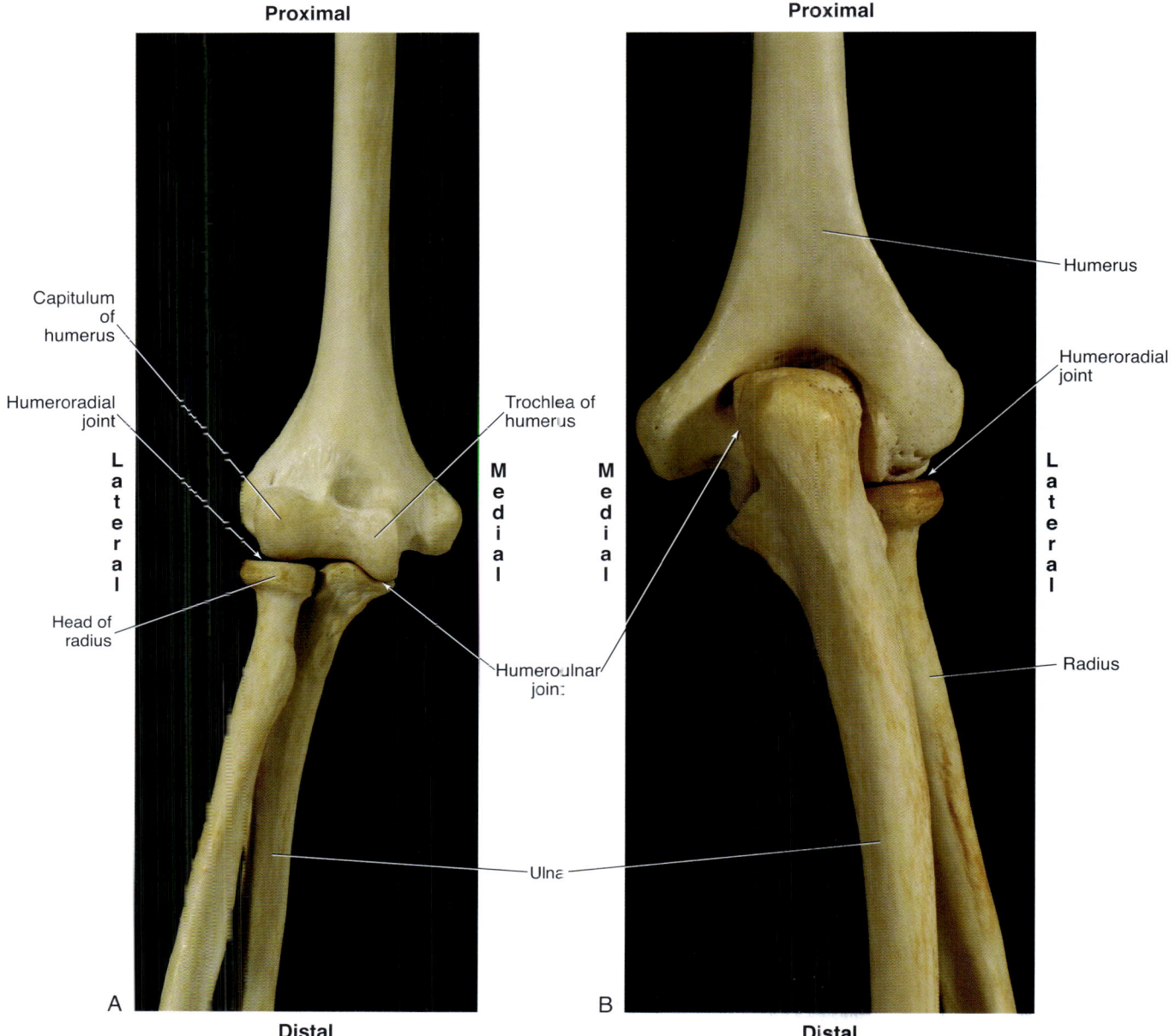

FIGURE 5-67 **A,** Anterior view. **B,** Posterior view.

NOTES
1. The elbow joint is composed of the humeroulnar and humeroradial joints.[2]
2. The major articulation of the elbow joint is the humeroulnar joint, where the trochlea of the humerus articulates with the trochlear notch of the ulna[10] (see Figure 5-68).
3. The humeroradial articulation is not very important functionally to movement at the elbow joint; the humeroradial articulation is formed between the capitulum of the humerus and the head of the radius.
4. The proximal radioulnar joint between the head of the radius and the radial notch of the ulna is anatomically within the same joint capsule as the elbow joint. However, functionally it is distinct from the elbow joint.[10]

SECTION 5.12 BONES OF THE FOREARM, WRIST JOINT, AND HAND

RIGHT RADIUS/ULNA—ANTERIOR VIEW

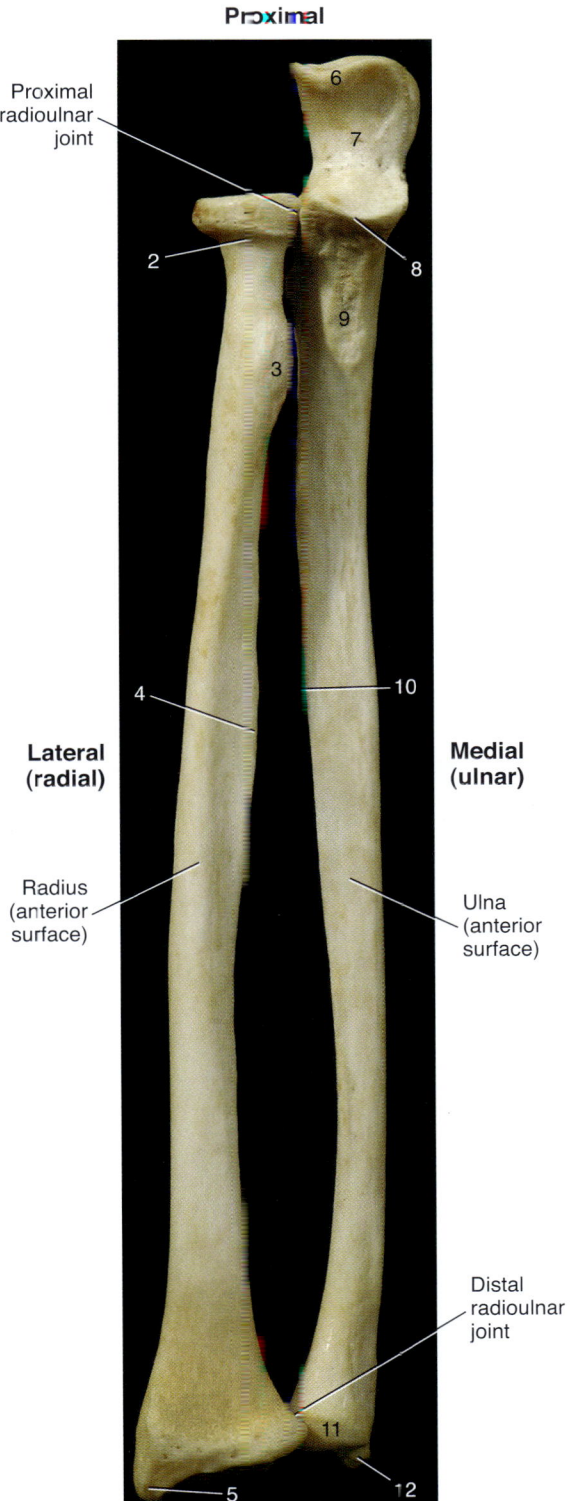

FIGURE 5-68
Landmarks of the radius:
1. Head
2. Neck
3. Tuberosity
4. Interosseus crest
5. Styloid process

Landmarks of the ulna:
6. Olecranon process
7. Trochlear notch
8. Coronoid process
9. Tuberosity
10. Interosseus crest
11. Head
12. Styloid process

NOTES
1. The radius and ulna articulate with each other both proximally (at the proximal radioulnar joint) and distally (at the distal radioulnar joint).[14]
2. The interosseous crests of the radius and ulna (#4, 10) are the attachment sites of the interosseus membrane of the forearm[3] (this interosseus membrane uniting the radius and ulna creates the middle radioulnar joint).
3. The styloid process of the radius (#5) projects laterally; the styloid process of the ulna (#12) projects posteriorly.[4]

RIGHT RADIUS/ULNA—POSTERIOR VIEW

FIGURE 5-69
Landmarks of the radius:
1. Head
2. Neck
3. Interosseus crest
4. Dorsal tubercle
5. Styloid process

Landmarks of the ulna:
6. Olecranon process
7. Coronoid process
8. Supinator crest
9. Interosseus crest
10. Head
11. Styloid process

NOTES
1. The dorsal tubercle of the radius (#4) is also known as Lister's tubercle.
2. The distal tendons of the extensors carpi radialis longus and brevis muscles pass between the dorsal tubercle (#4) and styloid process (#5) of the radius.[3]
3. The distal tendons of the extensor digitorum, extensor indicis, and extensor pollicis longus muscles pass medial to the dorsal tubercle (#4) of the radius.[13]
4. The distal tendon of the extensor carpi ulnaris muscle is located within a groove located between the styloid process (#11) and head (#10) of the ulna.[4]

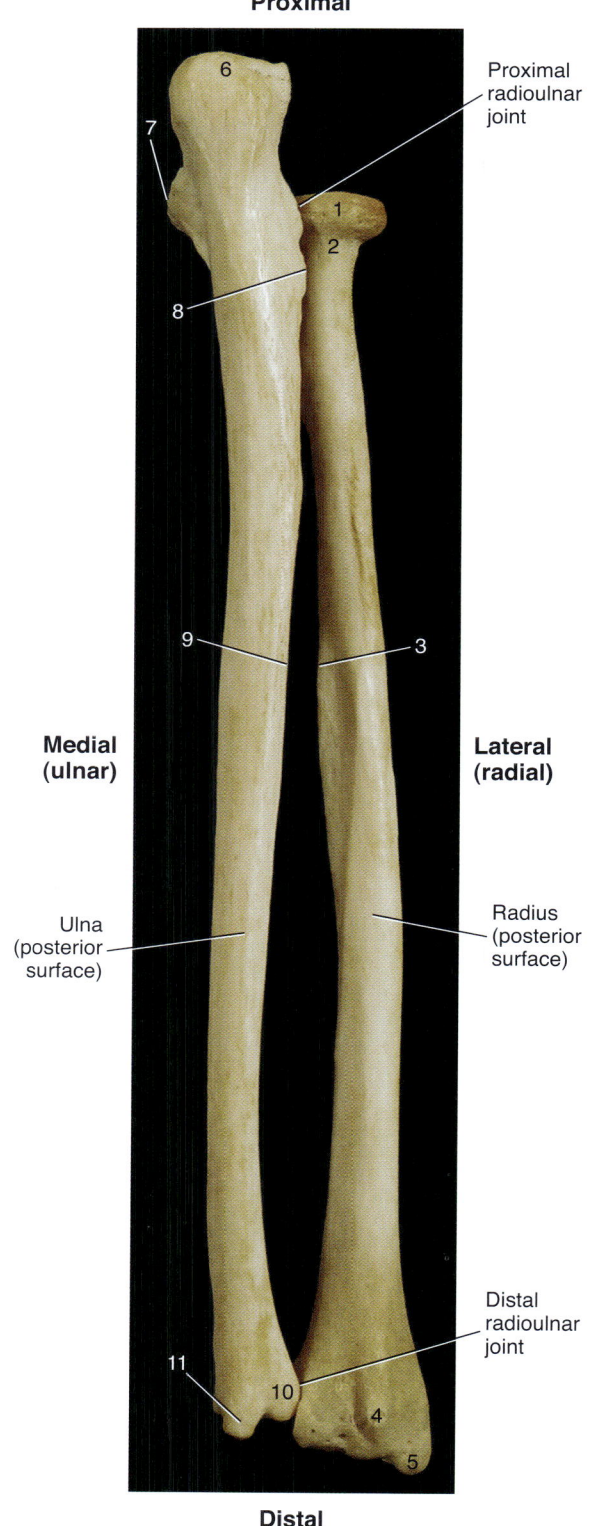

RIGHT RADIUS/ULNA—LATERAL VIEWS

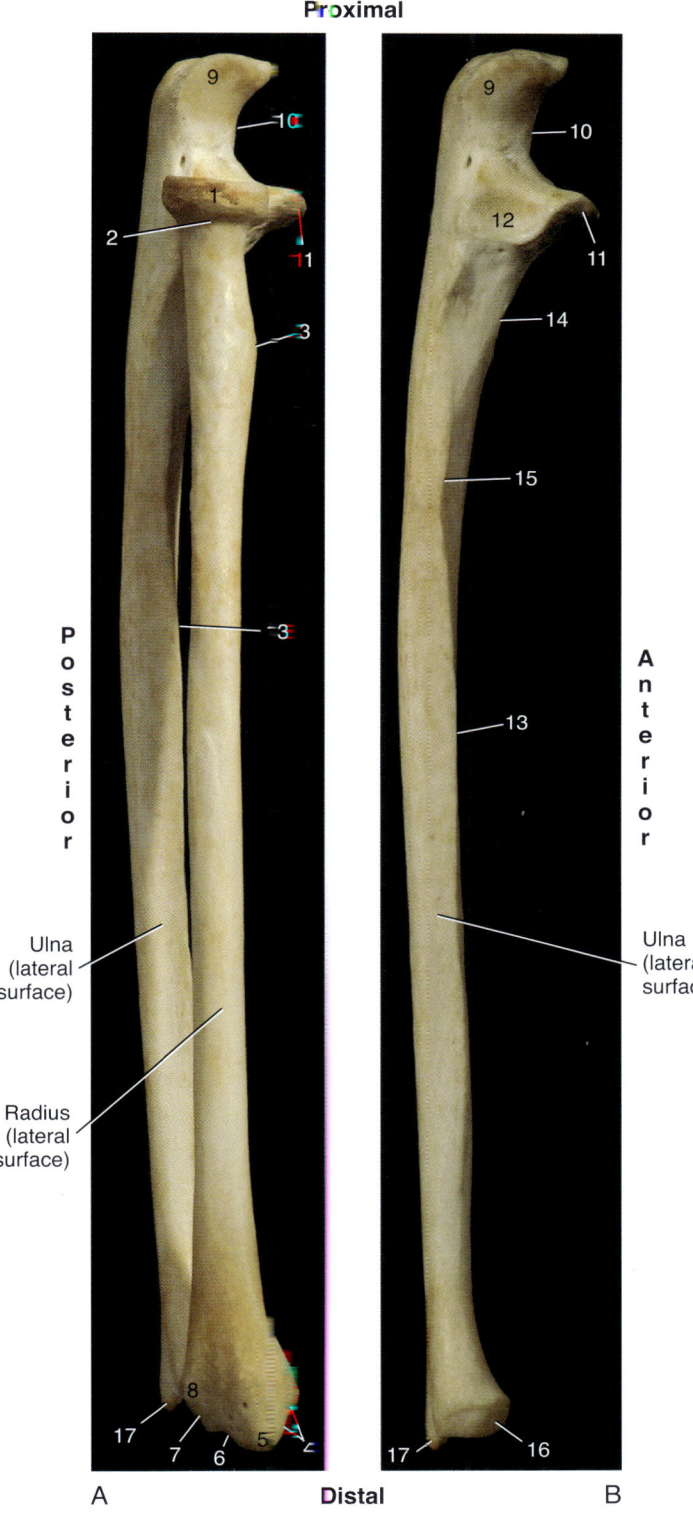

FIGURE 5-70 **A,** Lateral view of the radius and ulna articulated. **B,** Lateral view of just the ulna.

Landmarks of the radius:
1. Head
2. Neck
3. Radial tuberosity
4. Grooves for the abductor pollicis longus and extensor pollicis brevis
5. Styloid process
6. Groove for the extensor carpi radialis longus
7. Groove for the extensor carpi radialis brevis
8. Dorsal tubercle

Landmarks of the ulna:
9. Olecranon process
10. Trochlear notch
11. Coronoid process
12. Radial notch
13. Interosseus crest
14. Tuberosity
15. Supinator crest
16. Head
17. Styloid process

NOTES
1. The head of the radius articulates with the ulna at the radial notch (#12).[3]
2. The lateral view of the ulna (B) nicely demonstrates the interosseous crest of the ulna (#13).
3. The grooves for the abductor pollicis longus and extensor pollicis brevis distal tendons (#4) are located just anterior to the styloid process of the radius (#5).
4. The tuberosity of the ulna (#14) is not well developed on this ulna and therefore is not well visualized.

RIGHT RADIUS/ULNA—MEDIAL VIEWS

FIGURE 5-71 A, Medial view of the radius and ulna articulated. **B,** Medial view of just the radius.

Landmarks of the radius:
1. Head
2. Neck
3. Tuberosity
4. Interosseus crest
5. Ulnar notch
6. Styloid process

Landmarks of the ulna:
7. Olecranon process
8. Trochlear notch
9. Coronoid process
10. Tuberosity
11. Head
12. Styloid process

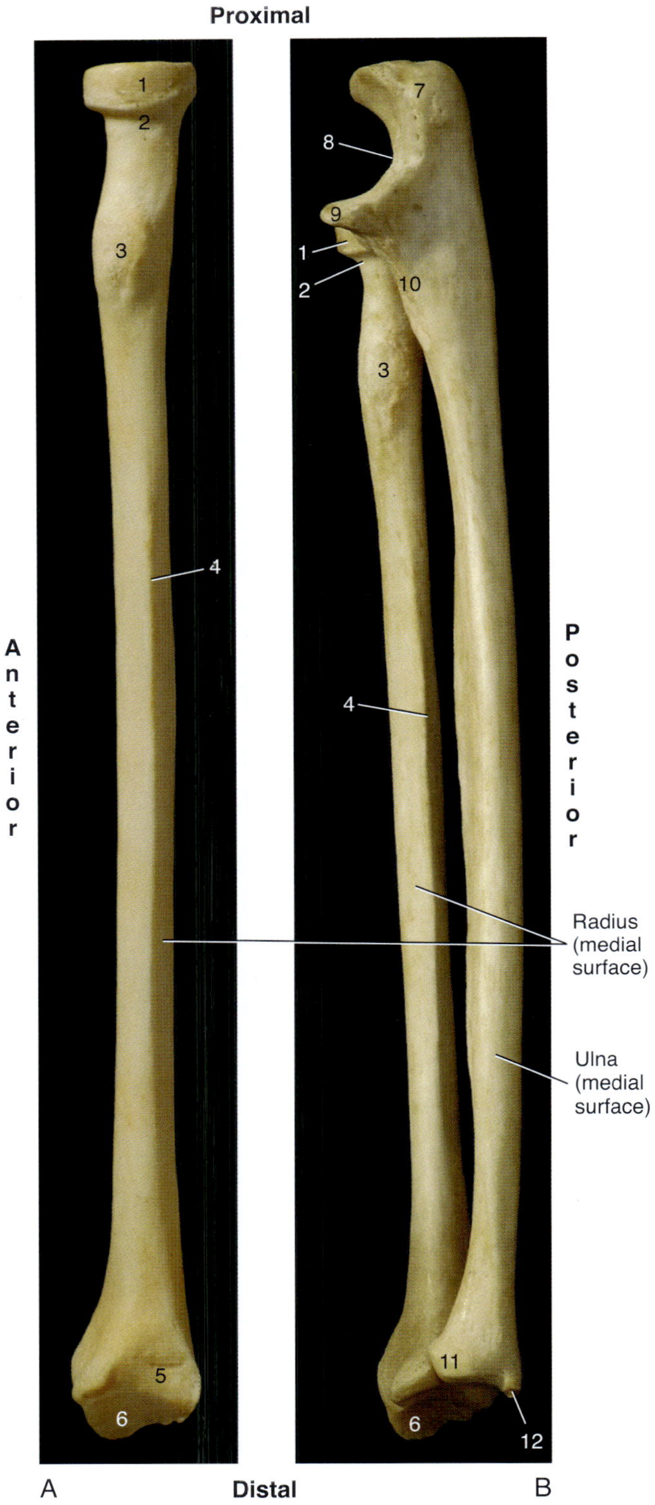

NOTES
1. The distal end of the ulna articulates with the radius at the ulnar notch (#5) of the radius.[3]
2. The medial view of the radius (B) nicely demonstrates the interosseous crest of the radius (#4).

RIGHT RADIUS/ULNA—PRONATED

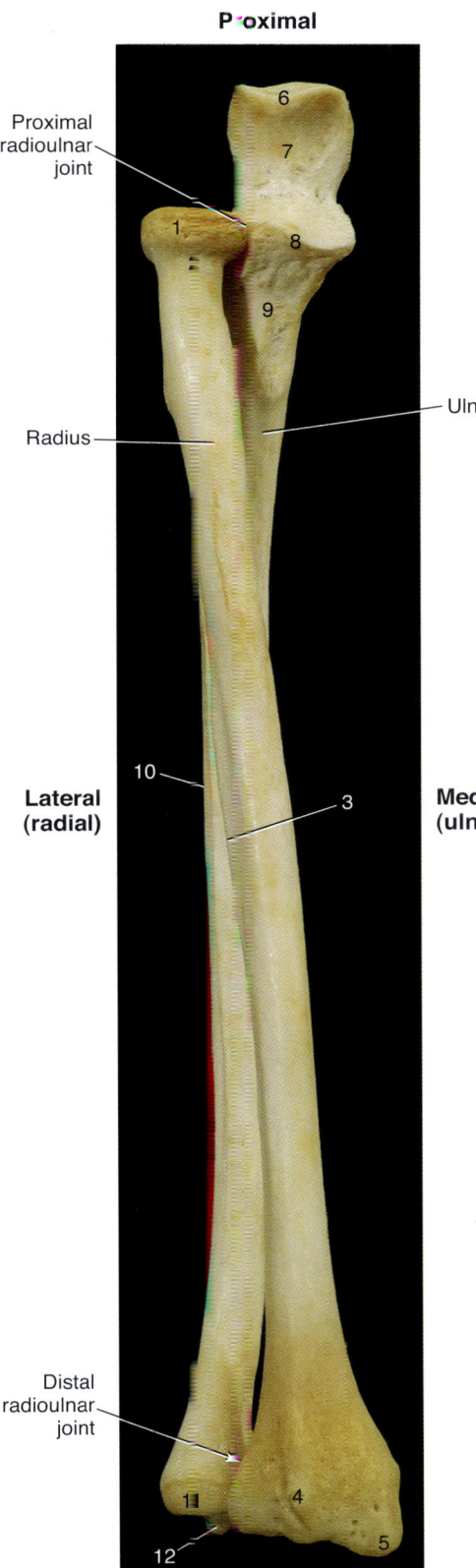

FIGURE 5-72
Landmarks of the radius:
1. Head
2. Neck
3. Interosseus crest
4. Dorsal tubercle
5. Styloid process

Landmarks of the ulna:
6. Olecranon process
7. Trochlear notch
8. Coronoid process
9. Tuberosity
10. Interosseus crest
11. Head
12. Styloid process

> **NOTES:**
> 1. Pronation of the forearm bones causes the bones to cross each other from the anterior perspective.
> 2. Pronation and supination of the forearm occur at the radioulnar joints and usually involve a mobile radius moving around a fixed ulna. The head of the radius rotates relative to the ulna, and the distal radius swings around the distal ulna (from this anterior perspective, we see the posterior surface of the distal radius).

RIGHT RADIUS/ULNA—PROXIMAL AND DISTAL VIEWS

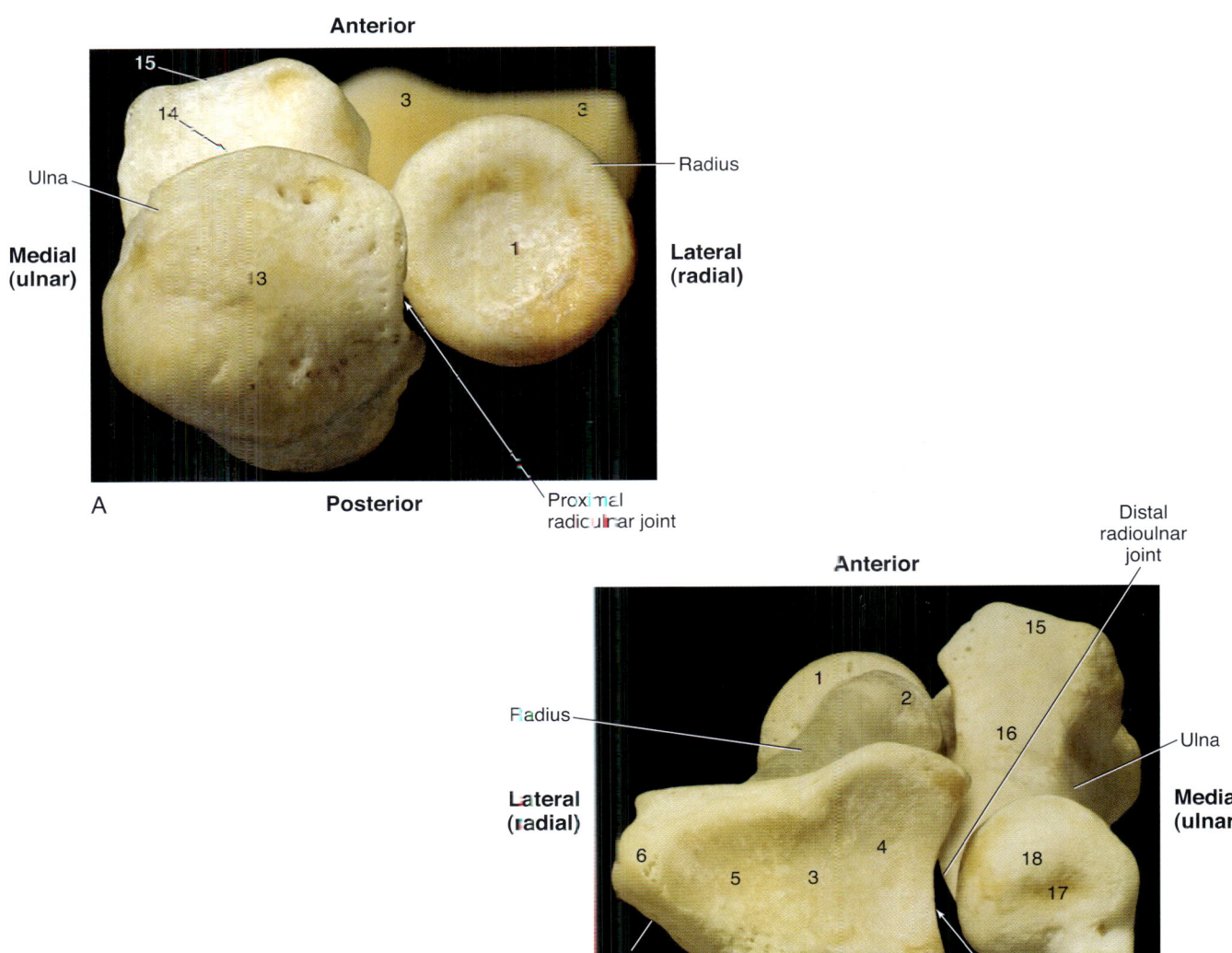

FIGURE 5-73 **A,** Proximal (superior) view of the radius and ulna articulated. **B,** Distal (inferior) view of the radius and ulna articulated.

Landmarks of the radius:
1 Head
2 Tuberosity
3 Distal end of the radius
4 Articular surface for lunate
5 Articular surface for scaphoid
6 Styloid process
7 Groove for extensor carpi radialis longus tendon
8 Groove for extensor carpi radialis brevis tendon
9 Dorsal tubercle
10 Groove for extensor pollicis longus tendon
11 Groove for extensor digitorum and extensor indicis tendons
12 Ulnar notch

Landmarks of the ulna:
13 Olecranon process
14 Trochlear notch
15 Coronoid process
16 Tuberosity
17 Distal end of the ulna
18 Head
19 Styloid process

NOTES[3]
1. The head of the radius (#1) has a concavity at its proximal end to accept the capitulum of the humerus (at the humeroradial joint).
2. The distal end of the ulna (#17) articulates with the radius at the ulnar notch of the radius (at the distal radioulnar joint).

RIGHT CARPAL BONES (SEPARATED)—ANTERIOR VIEW

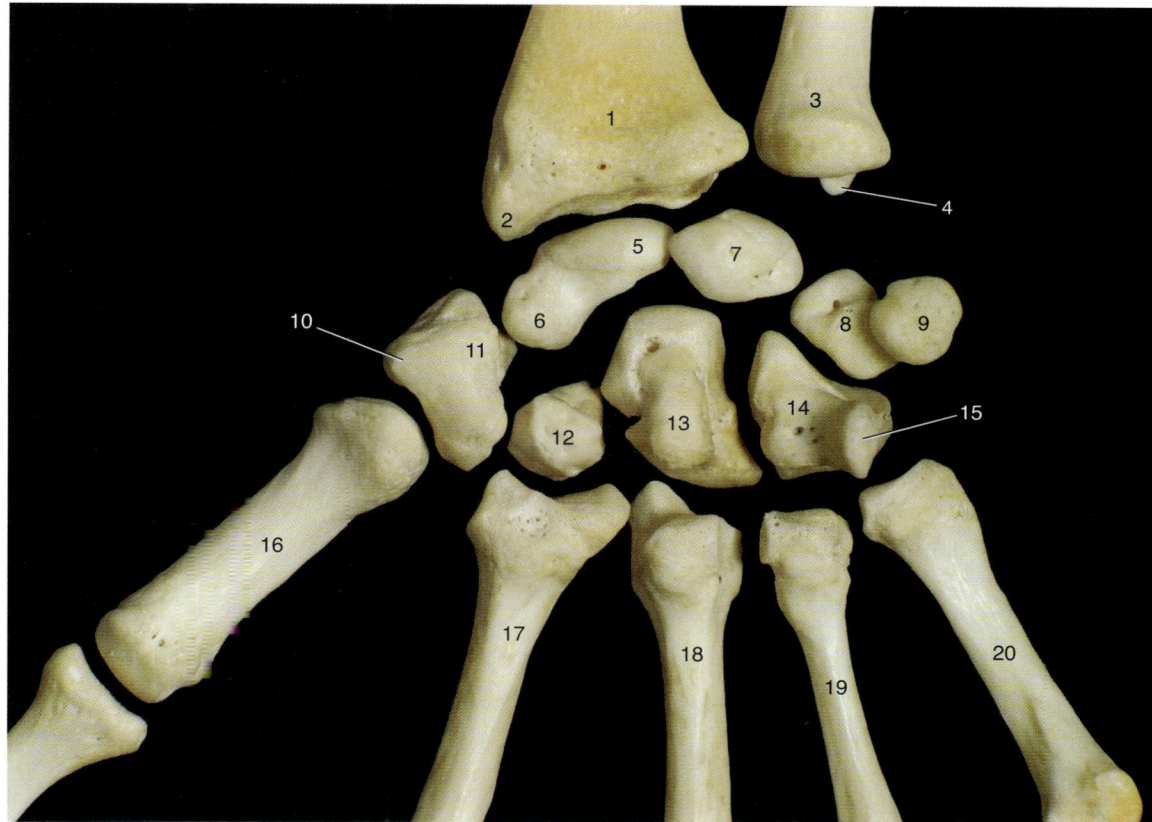

FIGURE 5-74
1. Radius
2. Styloid process of radius
3. Ulna
4. Styloid process of ulna
5. Scaphoid
6. Tubercle of scaphoid
7. Lunate
8. Triquetrum
9. Pisiform
10. Trapezium
11. Tubercle of trapezium
12. Trapezoid
13. Capitate
14. Hamate
15. Hook of hamate
16. First metacarpal (of thumb)
17. Second metacarpal (of index finger)
18. Third metacarpal (of middle finger)
19. Fourth metacarpal (of ring finger)
20. Fifth metacarpal (of little finger)

NOTES
1. Eight carpal bones are arranged in two rows: proximal and distal. The proximal row (radial to ulnar) is composed of the scaphoid, lunate, triquetrum, and pisiform (#5, 7, 8, 9); the distal row (radial to ulnar) is composed of the trapezium, trapezoid, capitate, and hamate (#10, 12, 13, 14).[2]
2. A mnemonic can be used to learn the names of the carpal bones. From proximal row to distal row (always radial to ulnar), it is: Some Lovers Try Positions That They Can't Handle.
3. The flexor retinaculum, which forms the ceiling of the carpal tunnel, attaches to the tubercles of the scaphoid and trapezium (#6, 11) on the radial side and the hook of the hamate (#15) and pisiform (#9) on the ulnar side.[13]
4. The pisiform (#9) is a sesamoid bone (explaining why humans have eight carpal bones and seven tarsal bones).[3]
5. The metacarpal bones are numbered 1 to 5 (numbering begins on the radial [i.e., thumb] side).[3]

RIGHT CARPAL BONES (SEPARATED)—POSTERIOR VIEW

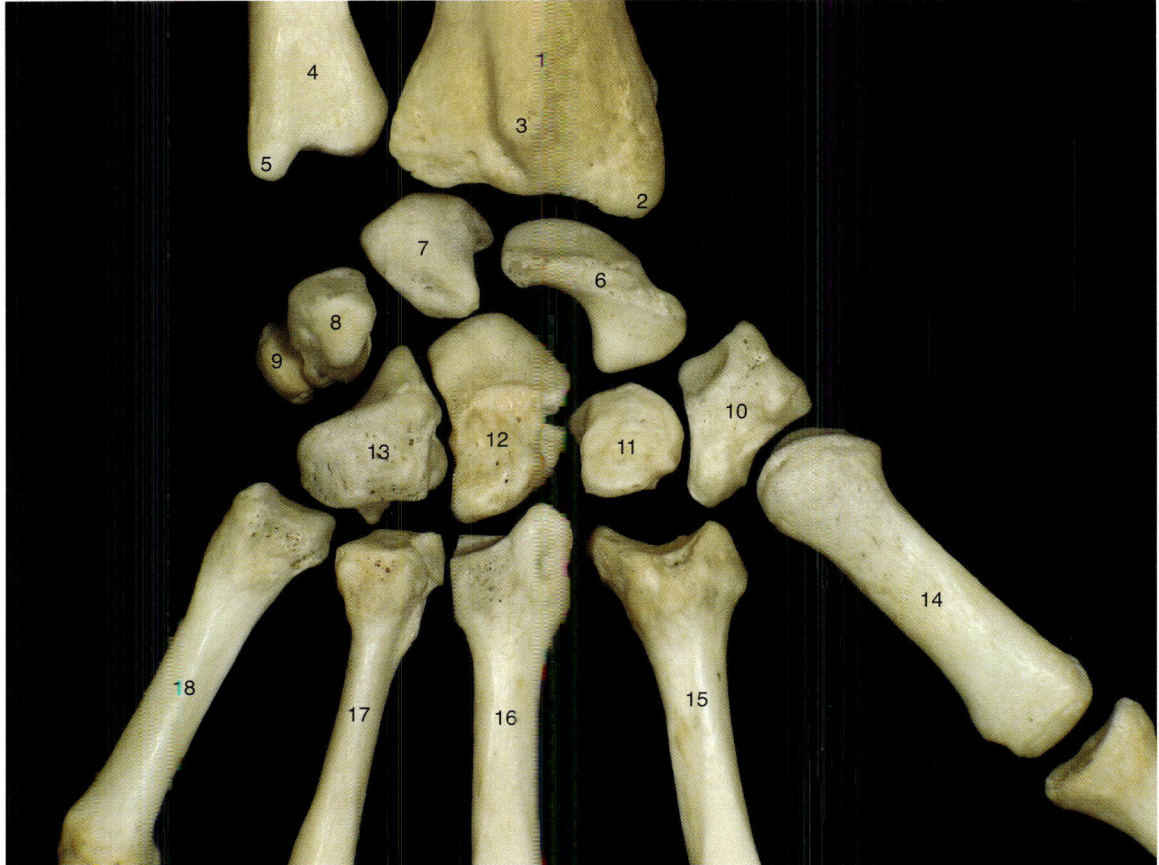

FIGURE 5-75
1. Radius
2. Styloid process of radius
3. Dorsal tubercle of radius
4. Ulna
5. Styloid process of ulna
6. Scaphoid
7. Lunate
8. Triquetrum
9. Pisiform
10. Trapezium
11. Trapezoid
12. Capitate
13. Hamate
14. First metacarpal (of thumb)
15. Second metacarpal (of index finger)
16. Third metacarpal (of middle finger)
17. Fourth metacarpal (of ring finger)
18. Fifth metacarpal (of little finger)

NOTES
1. The trapezium (#10) articulates with the first metacarpal (of the thumb); the trapezoid (#11) articulates with the second metacarpal (of the index finger); the capitate (#12) articulates with the third metacarpal (of the middle finger); and the hamate (#13) articulates with the fourth and fifth metacarpals (of the ring and little fingers).[3]
2. The joint between the trapezium and first metacarpal (of the thumb) is the first carpometacarpal joint, also known as the saddle joint of the thumb.
3. At the wrist region, it is the radius that articulates with the carpal bones, not the ulna; the wrist joint is often referred to as the radiocarpal joint.[13]
4. The scaphoid (#6) is the most commonly fractured carpal bone.[10] The lunate (#7) is the most commonly dislocated carpal bone.[13]

RIGHT WRIST/HAND—ANTERIOR VIEW

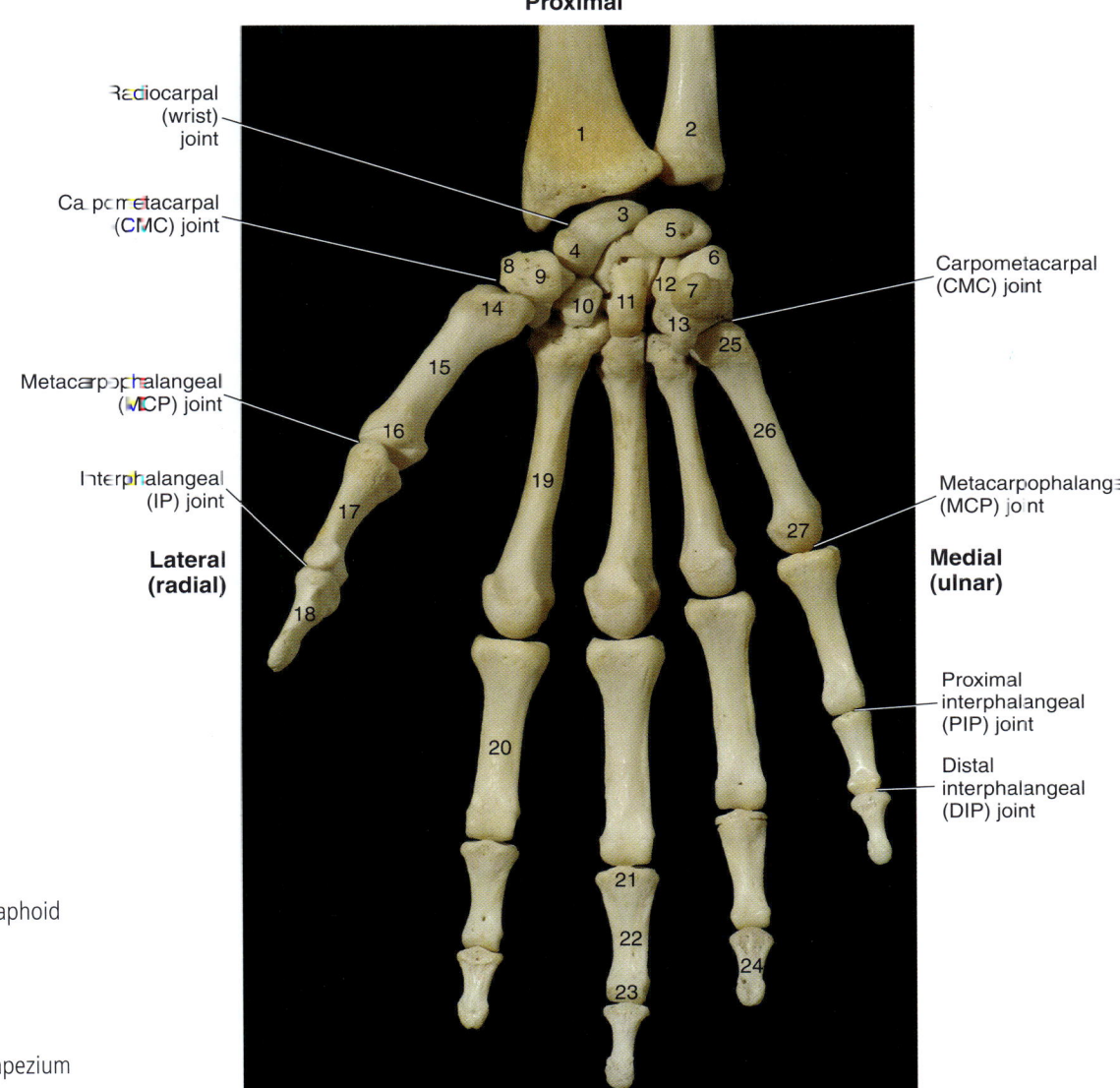

FIGURE 5-76
1. Radius
2. Ulna
3. Scaphoid
4. Tubercle of scaphoid
5. Lunate
6. Triquetrum
7. Pisiform
8. Trapezium
9. Tubercle of trapezium
10. Trapezoid
11. Capitate
12. Hamate
13. Hook of hamate
14. Base of first metacarpal (of thumb)
15. Body (shaft) of first metacarpal (of thumb)
16. Head of first metacarpal (of thumb)
17. Proximal phalanx of thumb
18. Distal phalanx of thumb
19. Second metacarpal (of index finger)
20. Proximal phalanx of index finger
21. Base of middle phalanx of middle finger
22. Body (shaft) of middle phalanx of middle finger
23. Head of middle phalanx of middle finger
24. Distal phalanx of ring finger
25. Base of fifth metacarpal (of little finger)
26. Body (shaft) of fifth metacarpal (of little finger)
27. Head of fifth metacarpal of little finger

NOTES
1. The thumb has two phalanges—proximal and distal; the other four fingers each have three phalanges—proximal, middle, and distal.[4]
2. All metacarpals and phalanges have the following landmarks: a base proximally, a body (shaft) in the middle, and a head distally.[10]
3. The length of a metacarpal of a ray is equal to the length of the proximal and middle phalanges of that ray added together; the length of a proximal phalanx of a ray is equal to the length of the middle and distal phalanges of that ray added together.

146 PART 2 Skeletal Osteology: Study of the Bones

RIGHT WRIST/HAND—POSTERIOR VIEW

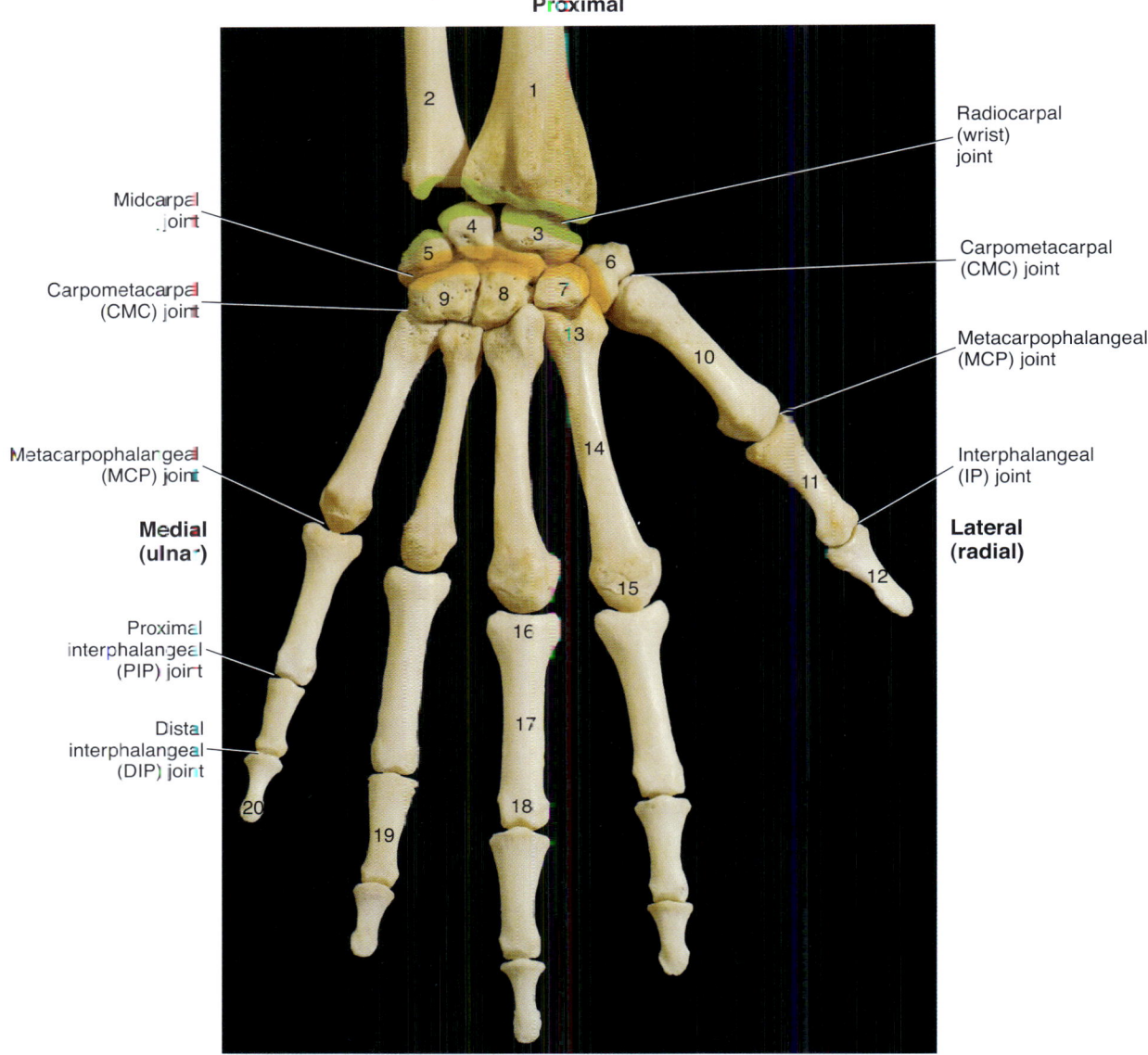

FIGURE 5-77
1. Radius
2. Ulna
3. Scaphoid
4. Lunate
5. Triquetrum
6. Trapezium
7. Trapezoid
8. Capitate
9. Hamate
10. First metacarpal (of thumb)
11. Proximal phalanx of thumb
12. Distal phalanx of thumb
13. Base of metacarpal of index finger
14. Body (shaft) of metacarpal of index finger
15. Head of metacarpal of index finger
16. Base of proximal phalanx of middle finger
17. Body (shaft) of proximal phalanx of middle finger
18. Head of proximal phalanx of middle finger
19. Middle phalanx of ring finger
20. Distal phalanx of little finger

NOTES
1. The wrist joint is composed of the radiocarpal and midcarpal joints.[13]
2. The radiocarpal joint is located between the radius and the proximal row of carpal bones. The midcarpal joint is located between the proximal and distal rows of carpal bones.[2] In Figure 5-77, the radiocarpal joint is indicated in green and the midcarpal joint is indicated in orange.

CHAPTER 5 Bones of the Human Body

RIGHT WRIST/HAND—MEDIAL VIEW

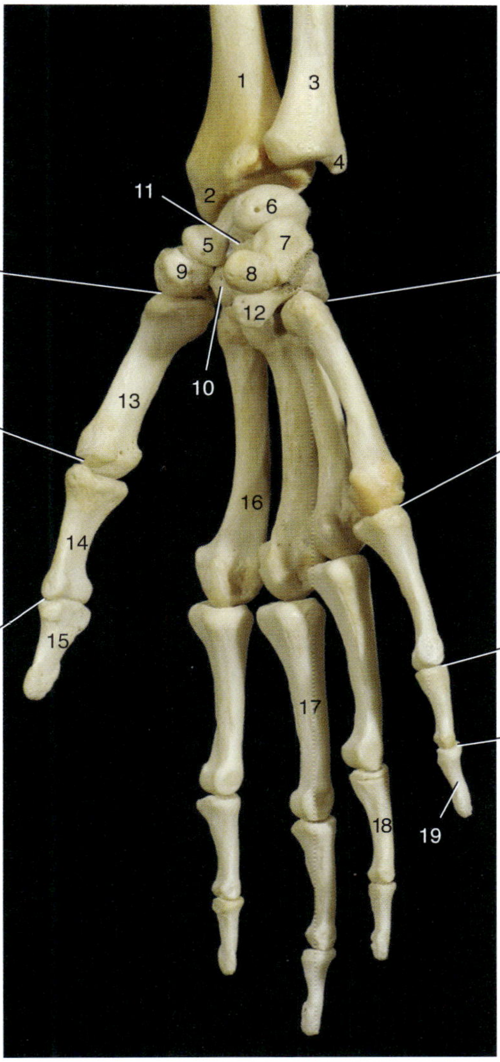

FIGURE 5-78
1. Radius
2. Styloid process of the radius
3. Ulna
4. Styloid process of the ulna
5. Scaphoid
6. Lunate
7. Triquetrum
8. Pisiform
9. Trapezium
10. Trapezoid
11. Capitate
12. Hamate
13. First metacarpal (of thumb)
14. Proximal phalanx of thumb
15. Distal phalanx of thumb
16. Metacarpal of index finger
17. Proximal phalanx of middle finger
18. Middle phalanx of ring finger
19. Distal phalanx of little finger

NOTES:
1. The thumb has only two phalanges, hence only one interphalangeal joint.
2. The other fingers have three phalanges, hence two interphalangeal joints—a proximal interphalangeal joint and a distal interphalangeal joint.
3. An interphalangeal joint is often abbreviated as an IP joint.
4. The proximal interphalangeal joint is often abbreviated as the PIP joint.
5. The distal interphalangeal joint is often abbreviated as the DIP joint.
6. The carpometacarpal joint is often abbreviated as the CMC joint.
7. The metacarpophalangeal joint is often abbreviated as the MCP joint.

RIGHT WRIST/HAND (FLEXED) AND CARPAL TUNNEL

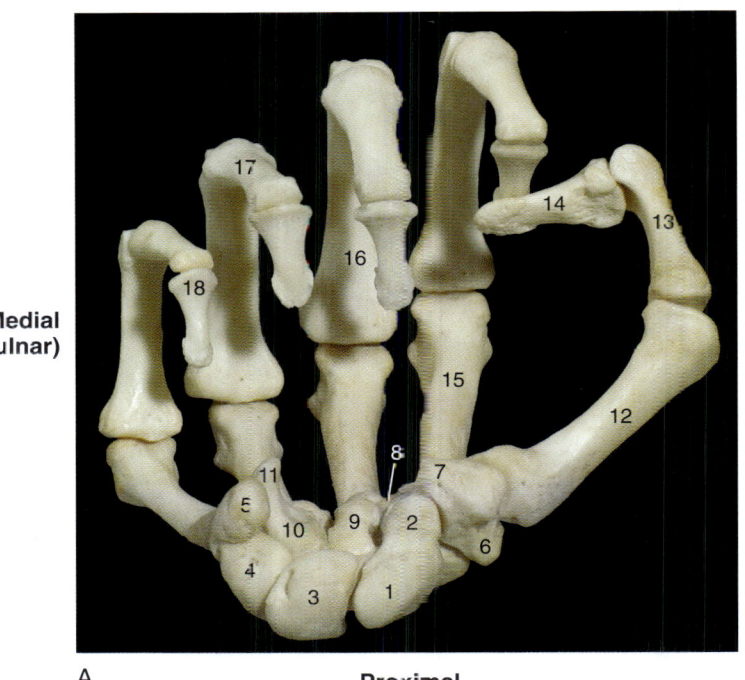

FIGURE 5-79 **A,** Proximal view of right wrist and hand with fingers flexed. **B,** Proximal view of right carpal tunnel.

1. Scaphoid
2. Tubercle of scaphoid
3. Lunate
4. Triquetrum
5. Pisiform
6. Trapezium
7. Tubercle of trapezium
8. Trapezoid
9. Capitate
10. Hamate
11. Hook of hamate
12. First metacarpal (of thumb)
13. Proximal phalanx of thumb
14. Distal phalanx of thumb
15. Second metacarpal (of index finger)
16. Proximal phalanx of middle finger
17. Middle phalanx of ring finger
18. Distal phalanx of little finger

NOTES
1. In figure A, the hand is shown with flexion of the fingers at the metacarpophalangeal and interphalangeal joints.
2. Figure B is a proximal to distal view demonstrating the tunnel that is formed by the carpal bones known as the carpal tunnel.
3. The flexor retinaculum encloses and forms the ceiling of the carpal tunnel by attaching to the tubercles of the scaphoid and trapezium (#2, 7) on the radial side and the pisiform (#5) and hook of the hamate (#11) on the ulnar side.[13]

REFERENCES

1. Hall SJ: Basic biomechanics, ed 6, New York, 2012, McGraw Hill.
2. Neumann DA: Kinesiology of the musculoskeletal system: Foundations for physical rehabilitation, ed 3, St Louis, 2017, Elsevier.
3. Palastanga N, Field D, Soames R: Anatomy and human movement: Structure and function, ed 4, Oxford, 2002, Butterworth-Heinmann.
4. Netter FH: Atlas of human anatomy, ed 3, Teterboro, 2003, Icon Learning Systems.
5. Patton KT, Thibodeau GA: Anatomy & physiology, ed 9, St Louis, 2016, Elsevier.
6. White TD, Folnens PA: Human osteology, ed 2, San Diego, 2000, Academic Press.
7. Cramer GD, Darby SA: Basic and clinical anatomy of the spine, spinal cord, and ANS, St Louis, 1995, Mosby.
8. Drake RL, Vogl AW, Mitchell AWM, et al: Gray's atlas of anatomy, Philadelphia, 2008, Churchill Livingstone Elsevier.
9. Levangie PK, Norkin CC: Joint structure and function: A comprehensive analysis, ed 5, Philadelphia, 2011, FA Davis.
10. Oatic CA: Kinesiology: The mechanics and pathomechanics of human movement, Philadelphia, 2004, Lippincott Williams & Wilkins.
11. Werner R: A massage therapist's guide to pathology, ed 4, Philadelphia, 2004, Lippincott Williams & Wilkins.
12. Drake RL, Vogl W, Mitchell AWM: Gray's anatomy for students, Philadelphia, 2005, Churchill Livingstone.
13. Smith LK, Weiss EL, Lehmkuhl LO: Brunstrom's clinical kinesiology, ed 5, Philadelphia, 1996, FA Davis.
14. Hamill J, Knutzen KM: Biomechanical basis of human movement, ed 12, Baltimore, 2003, Lippincott Williams & Wilkins

PART III

Skeletal Arthrology: Study of the Joints

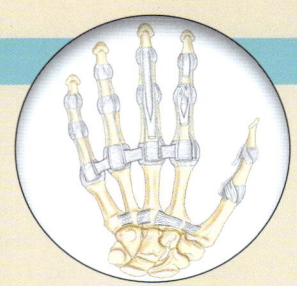

CHAPTER 6

Joint Action Terminology

CHAPTER OUTLINE

Section 6.1	Overview of Joint Function	Section 6.16	Plantarflexion/Dorsiflexion
Section 6.2	Axial and Nonaxial Motion	Section 6.17	Eversion/Inversion
Section 6.3	Nonaxial/Gliding Motion	Section 6.18	Pronation/Supination
Section 6.4	Rectilinear and Curvilinear Nonaxial Motion	Section 6.19	Protraction/Retraction
Section 6.5	Axial/Circular Motion	Section 6.20	Elevation/Depression
Section 6.6	Axial Motion and the Axis of Movement	Section 6.21	Upward Rotation/Downward Rotation
Section 6.7	Roll and Spin Axial Movements	Section 6.22	Anterior Tilt/Posterior Tilt
Section 6.8	Roll, Glide, and Spin Movements Compared	Section 6.23	Opposition/Reposition
		Section 6.24	Right Lateral Deviation/Left Lateral Deviation
Section 6.9	Naming Joint Actions—Completely		
Section 6.10	Joint Action Terminology Pairs	Section 6.25	Horizontal Flexion/Horizontal Extension
Section 6.11	Flexion/Extension	Section 6.26	Hyperextension
Section 6.12	Abduction/Adduction	Section 6.27	Circumduction
Section 6.13	Right Lateral Flexion/Left Lateral Flexion	Section 6.28	Naming Oblique Plane Movements
Section 6.14	Lateral Rotation/Medial Rotation	Section 6.29	Reverse Actions
Section 6.15	Right Rotation/Left Rotation	Section 6.30	Vectors

CHAPTER OBJECTIVES

After completing this chapter, the student should be able to perform the following:

1. Define the key terms of this chapter and state the meanings of the word origins of this chapter.
2. Do the following related to joint function:
   - Explain the function of joints, muscles, and ligaments/joint capsules.
   - Describe the relationship between joint mobility and joint stability.
3. Compare and contrast the characteristics of axial motion and nonaxial motion.
4. Describe, compare, and contrast rectilinear and curvilinear motion.
5. Explain the relationship between axial/circular motion and the axis of movement.
6. Describe roll and spin axial movements.
7. Explain the relationship of roll, spin, and glide movements.
8. Describe how to completely name joint actions.
9. Define joint action terms, and show examples of each one.
10. Explain the two uses of the term hyperextension.
11. Demonstrate and state the component actions of circumduction.
12. Explain how oblique plane movements are broken down into their component cardinal plane actions.
13. Explain the concept of a reverse action, and demonstrate examples of reverse actions.

 Indicates a video demonstration is available for this concept.

14. Do the following related to vectors:
    ○ Explain how drawing a vector can help us learn the actions of the muscle.
    ○ Draw a vector that represents the line of pull of a muscle; and if the muscle's line of pull is oblique, resolve that vector into its component cardinal plane vectors.

OVERVIEW

Chapter 2 began the discussion of motion in the body. Chapter 6 now continues that discussion. The larger picture of joint function is addressed, axial and nonaxial motions are examined in detail, and the fundamental types of joint movement, (i.e., roll, glide, and spin) are covered. Joint action terminology pairs that describe cardinal plane actions are then presented so that the student is conversant with the language necessary to fully and accurately describe cardinal plane actions of the human body. Finally, oblique plane movement is covered and the concept of breaking an oblique plane movement into its cardinal plane component actions is explained. A strong learning tool to help accomplish this is presented: that is, placing an arrow (vector) along the direction of the fibers of the muscle, from one attachment of the muscle to its other attachment. This gives us a visual sense of the overall line of pull of the muscle. Resolving this vector into its component vectors then offers us a visual way to figure out the cardinal plane lines of pull and therefore the cardinal plane actions of the muscle.

One other topic, crucial to the understanding of musculoskeletal function, is presented and explored in this chapter; that topic is reverse actions. For too long, students of kinesiology have memorized muscle actions with the flawed belief that one attachment, the origin, always stays fixed, and the other attachment, the insertion, always moves. The concept of reverse actions explains how to look at a muscle's actions in a fundamentally simpler and more accurate way.

From here, Chapter 7 presents a classification of joints of the body, and Chapters 8 to 10 then regionally examine the joints of the body in much more detail.

KEY TERMS

Abduction (ab-DUK-shun)
Action
Adduction (ad-DUK-shun)
Angular motion
Anterior tilt (an-TEER-ee-or)
Axial motion (AK-see-al)
Circular motion
Circumduction (SIR-kum-DUK-shun)
Contralateral rotation (CON-tra-LAT-e-ral)
Curvilinear motion (KERV-i-LIN-ee-ar)
Depression
Dorsiflexion (door-see-FLEK-shun)
Downward rotation
Elevation
Eversion (ee-VER-shun)
Extension (ek-STEN-shun)
Flexion (FLEK-shun)
Gliding motion
Hiking the hip
Horizontal abduction (ab-DUK-shun)
Horizontal adduction (ad-DUK-shun)
Horizontal extension (ek-STEN-shun)
Horizontal flexion (FLEK-shun)
Hyperextension (HI-per-ek-STEN-shun)
Inversion (in-VER-shun)
Ipsilateral rotation (IP-see-LAT-er-al)
Joint action
Lateral deviation
Lateral flexion (FLEK-shun)
Lateral rotation
Lateral tilt

Left lateral deviation
Left lateral flexion (FLEK-shun)
Left rotation
Linear motion
Medial rotation (MEE-dee-al)
Nonaxial motion (NON-AK-see-al)
Oblique plane movements (o-BLEEK)
Opposition (OP-po-ZI-shun)
Plantarflexion (PLAN-tar-FLEK-shun)
Posterior tilt (pos-TEER-ee-or)
Pronation (pro-NAY-shun)
Protraction (pro-TRAK-shun)
Rectilinear motion (REK-ti-LIN-ee-or)
Reposition (REE-po-ZI-shun)
Resolve a vector (VEK-tor)
Retraction (ree-TRAK-shun)
Reverse action
Right lateral deviation
Right lateral flexion (FLEK-shun)
Right rotation
Rocking movement
Rolling movement
Rotary motion
Scaption (SKAP-shun)
Sliding motion
Spinning movement
Supination (SUE-pin-A-shun)
Translation
Upward rotation
Vector (VEK-tor)

WORD ORIGINS

- Abduct—From Latin *abductus*, meaning *to lead away*
- Adduct—From Latin *adductus*, meaning *to draw toward*
- Circum—From Latin *circum*, meaning *circle*
- Contra—From Latin *contra*, meaning *opposed* or *against*
- Curv—From Latin *curvus*, meaning *bent, curved*
- Exten—From Latin *ex*, meaning *out*, and *tendere*, meaning *to stretch*
- Flex—From Latin *flexus*, meaning *bent*
- Hyper—From Greek *hyper*, meaning *above, over*
- Ipsi—From Latin *ipse*, meaning *same*
- Lateral—From Latin *latus*, meaning *side*
- Linea—From Latin *linea*, meaning *a linen thread, a line*
- Oppos—From Latin *opponere*, meaning *to place against*
- Pelvis—From Latin *pelvis*, meaning *basin*
- Rect—From Latin *rectus*, meaning *straight, right*
- Repos—From Latin *reponere*, meaning *to replace*

SECTION 6.1 OVERVIEW OF JOINT FUNCTION

- Following is a simplified overview of joint function (For more information on joint function, see Section 6.2.):
  - The primary function of a joint is to allow movement. This is the reason why a joint exists in the first place.
  - The movement that occurs at a joint is created by muscles. The role of a muscle contraction is actually to create a force on the bones of a joint; that force can create movement at the joint. However, the force of the muscle contraction can also stop or modify movement. (For more information on muscle function, see Chapters 11 to 20)
- Ligaments and joint capsules function to limit excessive movement at a joint.
  - Therefore, the following general rules can be stated:
  - Joints *allow* movement.
  - Muscles can *create* movement.
  - Ligaments/joint capsules *limit* movement.
- In addition to allowing movement to occur, joints have three characteristics:

- Weight bearing: Many joints of the body are weight-bearing joints—that is, they bear the weight of the body parts located above them. Almost every joint of the lower extremity and all the spinal joints of the axial body are weight-bearing joints. As a rule, weight-bearing joints need to be very stable to support the weight that is borne through them.
- Shock absorption: Joints can function to absorb shock. This is especially important for weight-bearing joints. The primary means by which a joint absorbs shock is the cushioning effect of the fluid within the joint cavity.
- Stability: Even though the primary function of a joint is to allow motion to occur, excessive motion would create an unstable joint. Therefore a joint must be sufficiently stable so that it does not lose its integrity and become injured or dislocated.
  - Each joint of the body finds a balance between mobility and stability.
  - Mobility and stability are antagonistic properties: A more mobile joint is less stable; a more stable joint is less mobile.

SECTION 6.2 AXIAL AND NONAXIAL MOTION

When a body part moves at a joint, it may undergo two basic types of motion: (1) **axial motion** and (2) **nonaxial motion** (Figure 6-1).

AXIAL MOTION:

- Axial motion is motion of a body part that occurs about or around an axis.[1]
- This type of motion is also known as **circular motion** because the body part moves along a circular path around the axis (in such a manner that a point drawn anywhere on the body part would transcribe a circular path around the axis).
- With axial motion not every point on the body part moves the same amount.[1] A point closer to the axis moves less (and would transcribe a smaller circle) than a point farther from the axis (which would transcribe a larger circle) (Figure 6-2, *A*).
- In other words, with axial motion the body part moves in a circular path around the axis in such a manner that one aspect of the body part moves more than another aspect of the body part (see Figure 6-1, *A*).

NONAXIAL MOTION:

- Nonaxial motion is motion of a body part that does not occur about or around an axis.[2]
- This type of motion is also known as a **gliding motion** because the body part glides along another body part.
- With nonaxial motion, every aspect of the body part moves/ glides the same amount. In other words, every point on the body part moves in a linear path exactly the same amount in the same direction at the same time as every other point on the body part (Figure 6-2, *B*).[2]
- With nonaxial motion the body part does not move around an axis but instead glides as a whole in a linear direction (see Figure 6-1, *B*).
- In essence, a nonaxial gliding motion is when the entire body part moves as a whole and moves in one direction; an axial circular motion is a circular motion around an axis wherein one aspect of the body part moves more than another aspect of the body part. (For more information on axial motion, see Sections 6.5 through 6.7. For more information on nonaxial motion, see Sections 6.3 and 6.4.)

CHAPTER 6 Joint Action Terminology

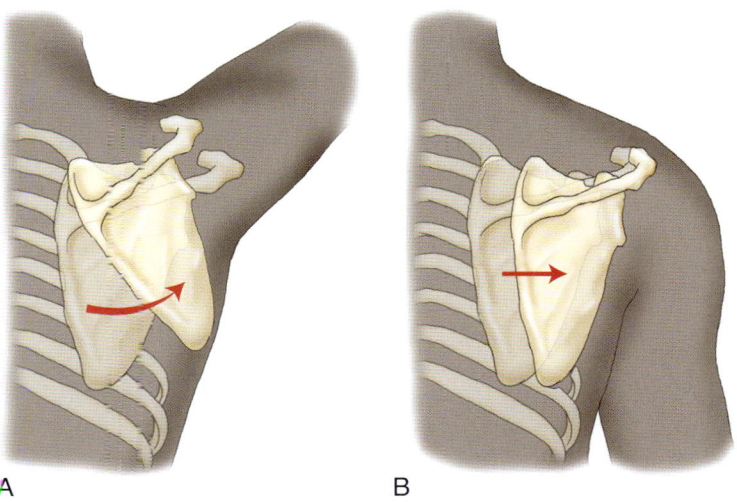

FIGURE 6-1 A, The scapula upwardly rotating, which is an example of axial/circular motion. **B,** The scapula protracting, which is an example of nonaxial/gliding motion.

SECTION 6.3 NONAXIAL/GLIDING MOTION

NONAXIAL MOTION

- Nonaxial motion is motion of a body part that does not occur around an axis, hence the name *nonaxial* motion.
- Nonaxial motion involves a gliding motion (also known as **sliding motion**) because the bone that moves is said to *glide* (or *slide*) along the other bone of the joint.
- Nonaxial movement of a body part is also known as **translation** of the body part because the entire body part moves the same exact amount[1]; therefore the entire body part can be looked at as changing its location or *translating* its location from one position to another.
- Nonaxial motion is also known as **linear motion** of a body part because every point on the body part moves in the same linear path, the exact same amount as every other point on the body part[2] (see Figure 6-2, *B*).
- All of these synonyms for nonaxial motion are used commonly in the field of kinesiology, so it is useful to be familiar with all of them. Furthermore, each one of them is helpful in visually describing a nonaxial motion.
- In other words, with nonaxial motion the body part does not move around an axis. Instead the entire body part translates its location and glides/slides as a whole in a linear direction along the other bone of the joint.
- Even though linear nonaxial motion does not occur around an axis, it can be described as moving within a plane. It may even be described as occurring within two planes.

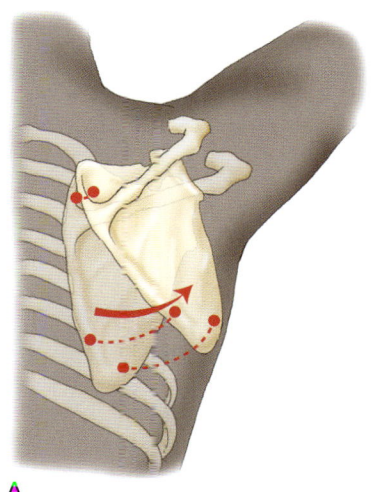 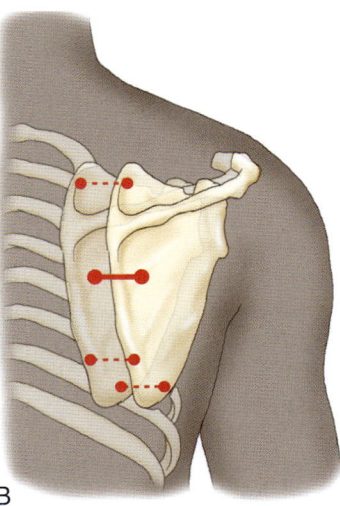

FIGURE 6-2 A, With axial motion, one point on the scapula moves more than another point. **B,** With nonaxial motion, each point moves the same as every other point.

Figure 6-2, *B* shows a nonaxial motion of the scapula (in this case the scapula is protracting). If we pick any point along the scapula and draw a line to demonstrate the path of movement that this point undergoes, we see that this line is identical to the line drawn for the movement of every other point on the scapula. All of these lines would be identical to one another. Therefore one line can be drawn to demonstrate the motion of the entire scapula. This means the entire scapula moves as a whole, the same amount in the same direction at the same time. Because this motion does not occur around an axis, it is called *nonaxial*. Because one line can be drawn to demonstrate this motion, it can also be called *linear motion*.

Figure 6-3 shows other examples of nonaxial linear motion.

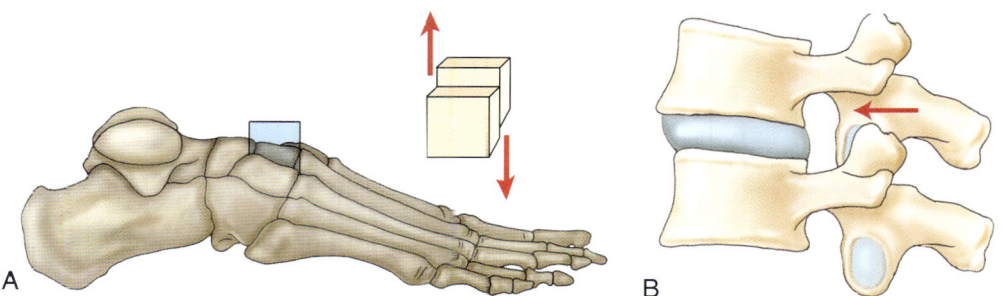

FIGURE 6-3 A, Nonaxial motion of one tarsal bone of the ankle along an adjacent tarsal bone. **B,** Nonaxial motion of one vertebra along another vertebra at the facet joints of the spine.

SECTION 6.4 RECTILINEAR AND CURVILINEAR NONAXIAL MOTION

- Two different types of nonaxial linear motion exist: (1) rectilinear and (2) curvilinear.[3] Figure 6-4 illustrates these two different types.
- In Figure 6-4, *A*, a person is skiing. The person's entire body is moving in a straight line. Because *rect* means *straight*, motion such as this is termed **rectilinear motion**.[3]
- Figure 6-4, *B* illustrates the same skier jumping through the air. Now the person's entire body is moving along a curved line. Because *curv* means *curved*, motion such as this is termed **curvilinear motion**.[3]

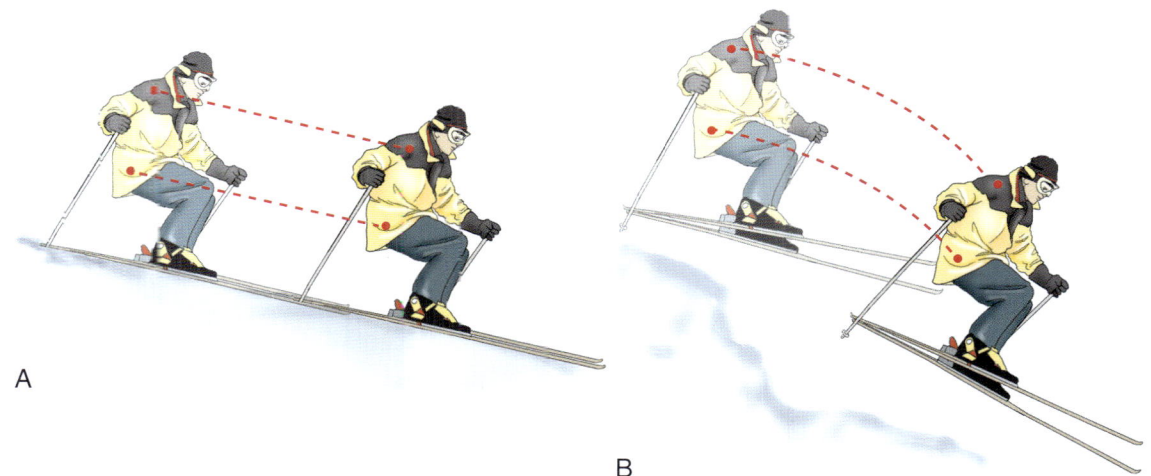

FIGURE 6-4 Person skiing and demonstrating two different types of nonaxial linear motion of the entire body. **A,** Rectilinear motion. **B,** Curvilinear motion.

SECTION 6.5 AXIAL/CIRCULAR MOTION

AXIAL MOTION:

- Axial motion is motion of a body part that occurs around or about an axis, hence the name *axial* motion.
- Axial motion is also known as *circular motion* because the body part moves along a circular path around the axis (in such a manner that a point drawn anywhere on the body part would transcribe a circular path around the axis).
- When moving in this circular path, not every point on the body part moves an equal amount; points closer to the axis move less than points farther from the axis (see Figure 6-2, *A*). However, every point on the body part does move along a circular path

through the same angle in the same direction (at the same time) as every other point on the body part. Because the direction of motion for every point on the body part is through the same angle, axial motion is also called **angular motion**.[2]

❍ One other synonym for axial motion is **rotary motion**[2] (i.e., rotation motion) because the body part moves in a rotary fashion around the axis.

❍ As with nonaxial motion, many synonyms for axial motion exist. Because all of them are used, it is necessary to be familiar with all of them. Furthermore, each one of them is useful in its own way toward visually describing axial motion. The one synonym for axial motion that should be used with caution (at least for the beginning student of kinesiology) is *rotary/rotation motion*. Use of the word *rotary* or *rotation* in this context can be confusing, because when we start to name the pairs of directional terms used to describe axial motions at joints, the word *rotation* is used again, but it is used to describe a certain type of axial movement, which is a spinning rotation of the bone around its long axis. For example, *medial rotation* is a term that uses the word *rotation* to describe a long-axis spinning rotation; yet *flexion* is a term to describe a rotary motion that does not involve spinning of the bone around its long axis, and *in this context* we do not say that flexion is rotation (even though as an axial movement it can be described as a *rotary* or *rotation movement*). (For more details, see the section on spin and roll axial movements in this chapter [Section 6.7].)

Figure 6-5 illustrates axial/circular motion of the forearm (in this case the forearm is flexing). We see that every point on the forearm moves along its own circular path; the line of this path for one point along the forearm will not be the same as for any other point along the forearm (i.e., the amount of movement will be different for each point). Therefore this type of motion is not linear. However, the angle that each point on the forearm moves through is the same, hence axial motion is also known as *angular motion*.

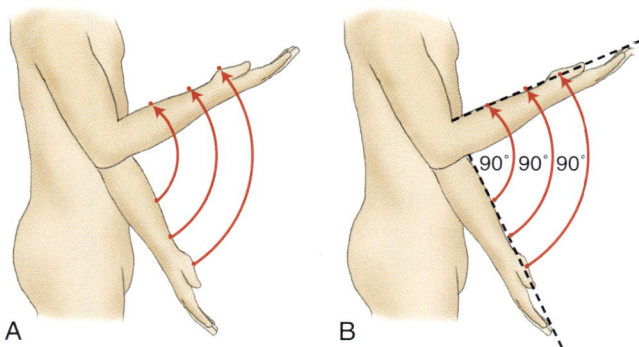

FIGURE 6-5 A, Flexion of the forearm at the elbow joint (a type of axial/circular motion). The paths of movement of three points along the forearm have been drawn. **B,** Same axial/circular movement as depicted in **A**. Angles have been drawn between the forearm and the arm for the three points that were considered in **A**. The angle formed by the motion of each point of the forearm is identical; therefore axial motion is also called angular motion.

SECTION 6.6 AXIAL MOTION AND THE AXIS OF MOVEMENT

❍ With axial motion the body part moves along a circular path. If we place a point at the center of this circular path, we will have the point around which the body part moves.

❍ If we now draw a line through this center point that is perpendicular to the plane in which the movement is occurring, we will have the axis of movement for this axial motion.

❍ As described in Section 6.5, motion of the body part may be described as rotary, because the body part is rotating around the axis; therefore an axis of movement is often called an *axis of rotation*. For reasons explained in Section 6.5, beginning kinesiology students might want to avoid use of the term *axis of rotation* and instead use the simpler term *axis of movement*. (For more on axes, see Sections 2.10 through 2.13.)

❍ Every axial movement moves around an axis.

❍ Conversely, an axis is an imaginary line in space around which axial motions occur.[2]

Figure 6-6 illustrates two examples of axial movements and shows the axis for each movement.

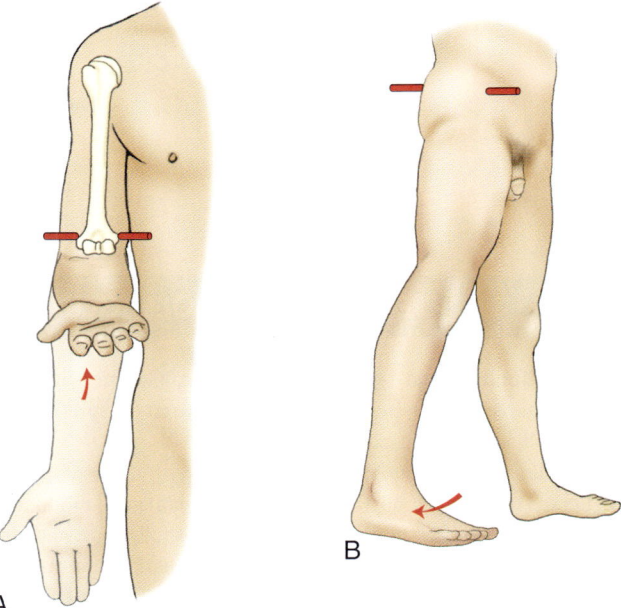

FIGURE 6-6 A, Flexion of the forearm at the elbow joint with the axis of movement drawn; axis is mediolateral (i.e., medial-lateral) in orientation. **B,** Abduction of the thigh at the hip joint with the axis of movement drawn; axis is anteroposterior (i.e., anterior-posterior) in orientation. Axes of movement are always perpendicular to the plane in which the motion is occurring.

SECTION 6.7 ROLL AND SPIN AXIAL MOVEMENTS

Axial movements can be broadly divided into two categories:
- One category is when the body part changes its position in space and one end of the bone moves more than the other end of the bone.
  - This type of axial movement is called a **rolling movement**.
  - A rolling movement can also be called a **rocking movement**[3] ("rock and roll").
  - Figure 6-7, *A* illustrates flexion, an example of a rolling movement of the body.
- An oblique plane movement of the humerus/arm at the shoulder joint in the plane of the scapula is shown here as an example of a roll axial movement. It is an axial motion because the humerus moves around an axis (located at the shoulder joint), and the humerus is not spinning, but rather the head of the humerus is rolling within the socket (i.e., glenoid fossa of the scapula) of the shoulder joint to create this motion.[3] However, as will be explained in Section 6.8, this movement also incorporates some nonaxial glide motion so that the head of the humerus does not dislocate by rolling right out of the shoulder joint socket. This concept is true for all roll movements: roll and glide movements couple together. (See Section 6.8 for a better understanding of the relationship between roll and glide movements.)
- The other category is when the body part does not change its position in space; rather it rotates or spins, staying in the same location.[4]
  - This type of axial movement is called a **spinning movement**.
  - Spinning movements are generally thought of as long-axis *rotation movements*.
  - Figure 6-7, *B* illustrates an example of a spin movement of the body. The humerus is moving within an oblique plane that is perpendicular to the plane of the scapula.

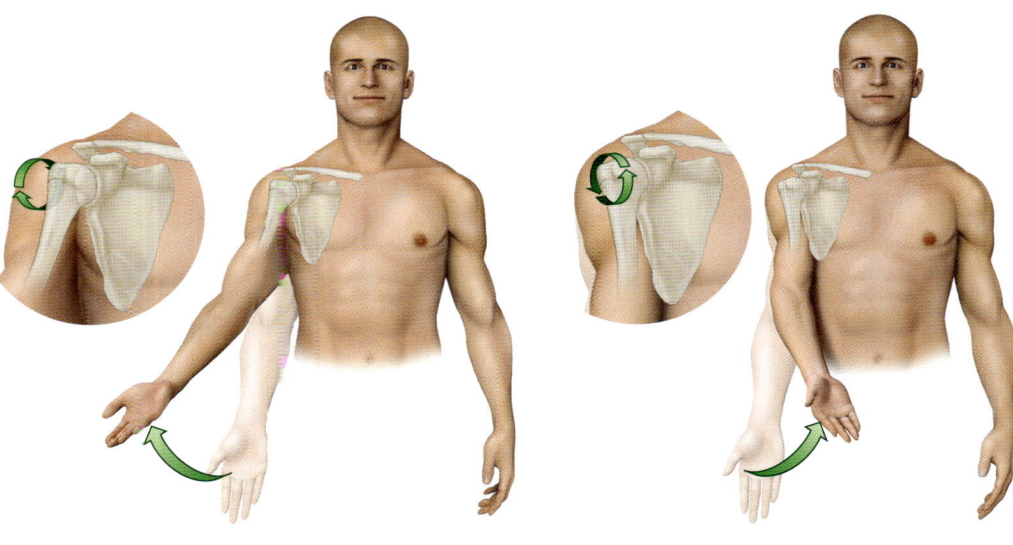

FIGURE 6-7 A, Roll movement. This particular motion is an oblique plane movement of the humerus/arm at the shoulder joint within the plane of the scapula. **B**, Spin movement. This particular motion is an oblique plane movement of the humerus at the shoulder joint within the plane that is perpendicular to the plane of the scapula such that the humeral head spins relative to the glenoid fossa. *(Courtesy Joseph E. Muscolino.)*

SECTION 6.8 ROLL, GLIDE, AND SPIN MOVEMENTS COMPARED

- Three fundamental types of movement can occur when one bone moves on another[4]: (1) roll, (2) glide, and (3) spin.
  - Roll and spin are axial movements.
  - Glide is a linear nonaxial movement.
- Figure 6-8 depicts all three of these fundamental motions at the joint level. The fundamental motions of roll, glide, and spin shown in Figure 6-8 depict the convex-shaped bone as moving on the concave-shaped bone. It is also possible for the concave-shaped bone to move along the convex-shaped bone.
- Figure 6-9 draws an analogy for these movements to movements of a car tire.
- It is important to realize that these fundamental motions do not always occur independently of each other. As a rule, rolling and gliding motions must couple together or the bone that is rolling will dislocate by rolling off the other bone of the joint. For this reason, motions of flexion, extension, abduction, adduction, right lateral flexion, and left lateral flexion are actually made up of a combination of axial roll and nonaxial glide motions.
- When the convex-shaped bone moves relative to the concave-shaped bone, the roll occurs in one direction and the glide occurs in the opposite direction. However, when the concave-shaped bone moves relative to the convex-shaped bone, the roll occurs in one direction and the glide occurs in the same direction.
- A spinning motion can occur independently. However, it is possible for a motion of the body to incorporate a spinning movement along with a rolling/gliding motion (e.g., when a person simultaneously flexes and laterally rotates the arm at the shoulder joint [both motions depicted in Figure 6-7]).

CHAPTER 6 Joint Action Terminology

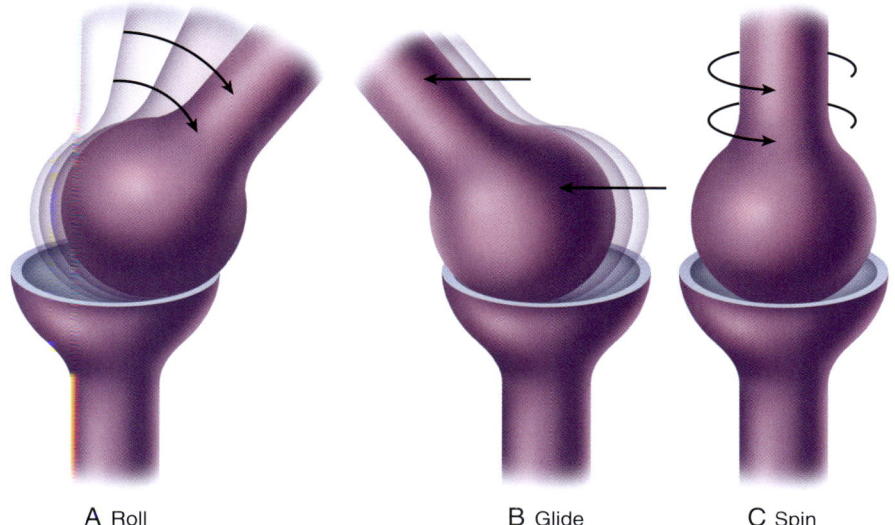

A Roll   B Glide   C Spin

FIGURE 6-8 A, Rolling of one bone on another; roll is an axial movement. **B,** Gliding of one bone on another; glide is a nonaxial movement. **C,** Spinning of one bone on another; spin is an axial movement. This figure shows the fundamental motions of roll, glide, and spin by showing the convex-shaped bone moving on the concave-shaped bone.

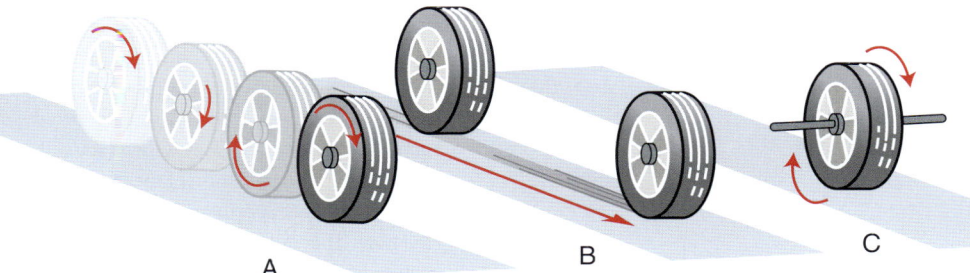

A   B   C

FIGURE 6-9 To better visualize the fundamental joint motions of roll, glide, and spin, an analogy can be made to a car tire. **A,** Tire that is rolling along the ground. **B,** Tire that is gliding/sliding (skidding) along the ground. **C,** Tire that is spinning without changing location.

SECTION 6.9 NAMING JOINT ACTIONS—COMPLETELY

- When we want to name a specific cardinal plane movement of the body, we will refer to it as an **action**.
- Because movement of a body part occurs at a joint, the term **joint action** is synonymous with action.
- It is worth noting that most of the commonly thought-of actions of the human body are axial (i.e., circular) movements (i.e., the body part that moves at a joint moves in a circular path around the axis of movement).
- Generally the axis of movement is a line that runs through the joint.[3]
- When we describe these movements that occur, we will use terms that indicate the direction that the body part has moved. These terms come in pairs, and the terms of each pair are the opposites of each other.
- Joint action terminology pairs are similar to the pairs of terms that are used to describe a location on the body (see Chapter 2 for more details). The difference is that the terms described in Chapter 2 were used to describe a static location on the body, whereas these movement terms are used to describe the direction that a body part is moving during an action that is occurring at a joint.
- Once we know these terms, we will then use three steps to describe an action that occurs:
  1. We will use the directional term describing the direction of the action.
  2. We will then state which body part moved during this action.
  3. We will then state at which joint the action occurred.
- For example, the action that is occurring in Figure 6-10 would be described the following way: Flexion of the right forearm at the elbow joint. This tells us three things:
  1. The direction of the action: flexion
  2. The body part that is moving: the right forearm
  3. At which joint the action is occurring: the right elbow joint

- The reader should note that most people and most textbooks do not specify the body part that is moving *and* the joint at which the movement is occurring. For example, the action illustrated in Figure 6-10 is usually referred to as either *flexion of the elbow joint* (and the term *forearm* is left out) or as *flexion of the forearm* (and the term *elbow joint* is left out).
- However, naming an action either of these ways can lead to confusion. For example, if we try to describe pronation of the forearm, we can say that the forearm pronated, but we cannot say that the elbow joint pronated because pronation of the forearm does not occur at the elbow joint, it occurs at the radioulnar joints. Therefore in this instance, elbow joint and forearm are not synonymous with each other.
- Furthermore, flexion of the elbow joint does not necessarily mean that the forearm moved; the arm can also flex at the elbow joint. In addition, flexion of the forearm does not necessarily mean that the elbow joint flexed; the forearm can also flex at the wrist joint.
- Just as forearm and elbow joint are not synonymous with each other because the forearm can also move at the radioulnar joints, confusion can also occur with movements of the foot. The foot can move at the ankle joint, but it can also move at the subtalar joint instead.
- The arm flexing at the elbow joint and the forearm flexing at the wrist joint are examples of what is called a *reverse action*.[5] For example, the arm can move at the elbow joint if the forearm is fixed; this motion occurs during a pull-up, as well as whenever we grab a banister or other object and pull ourselves toward it. Movement of the forearm at the wrist joint is not as common but can occur when the hand is fixed. (For more information on reverse actions, see Section 6.29).
- The advantage to being more complete in naming joint actions is that it requires us to clearly see exactly what is happening with each action of the body that occurs. Therefore to be most clear and eliminate the chance of possible vagueness and confusion, both the body part and the joint at which motion is occurring should be specified.
- A bone can also be named as doing the moving, instead of the body part that the bone is within. Most of the time, naming the bone is interchangeable with naming the body part. For example, flexion of the humerus at the shoulder joint is interchangeable with flexion of the arm at the shoulder joint, because it is the humerus that moves when the arm moves. Sometimes naming the bone instead of the body part can actually be advantageous, because it more specifically describes what is actually moving. For example, with pronation/supination of the forearm, it is usually the radius of the forearm that is primarily either pronating or supinating about the ulna. Therefore stating pronation of the radius instead of pronation of the forearm can actually create a clearer visual picture.

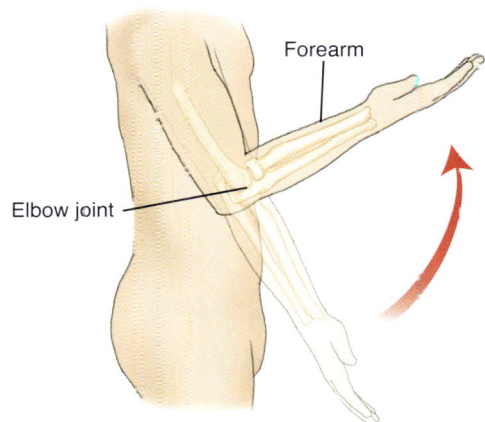

FIGURE 6-10 Flexion of the right forearm at the elbow joint.

SECTION 6.10 JOINT ACTION TERMINOLOGY PAIRS

Following are the terms that are used to describe joint actions:
- These terms come in pairs; each term of a pair is the opposite of the other term of the pair.
- It is important to remember that these terms do not describe the static location that a body part and/or a joint is in; rather they describe the direction in which a body part is moving at a joint. In other words, motion should be occurring for these terms to be used.
- Even though these terms are meant to describe movement, there are times when they are used to help describe a static position. For example, it might be said that the client's arm is *in a position of flexion* at the shoulder joint. This is said because relative to anatomic position, the arm is flexed at the shoulder joint. However, this type of use of these motion terms to describe a static position can sometimes lead to confusion. For example, the client with the arm in flexion may have previously been in a position of further flexion, and then the client extended to get to that lesser position of flexion; not every motion begins from anatomic position.

In other words, knowing a static position does not tell us what joint action was done by the client to get into that position. In addition, because it is more often joint action movement that causes injury and not the static position that a joint is in, it is best to use these terms to describe an actual motion that is occurring.
- Five major pairs of directional terms are used throughout most of the body:
  1. Flexion/extension
  2. Abduction/adduction
  3. Right lateral flexion/left lateral flexion
  4. Lateral rotation/medial rotation
  5. Right rotation/left rotation

The following pairs of directional terms are used for certain actions at specific joints of the body.[7]
- Plantarflexion/dorsiflexion
- Eversion/inversion
- Pronation/supination
- Protraction/retraction

- Elevation/depression
- Upward rotation/downward rotation
- Anterior tilt/posterior tilt
- Opposition/reposition
- Lateral deviation to the right/lateral deviation to the left
- Horizontal flexion/horizontal extension
- A few additional terms are used when describing joint actions/motions of the body.
- Hyperextension
- Circumduction

SECTION 6.11 FLEXION/EXTENSION

- **Flexion** is defined as a movement at a joint so that the ventral (soft) surfaces of the two body parts at that joint come closer together[8] (Box 6-1).

> **BOX 6-1**
>
> The word ventral derives from the word belly. The ventral surface of a body part has come to mean the soft "underbelly" aspect of the body part. Generally it is the anterior surface, but in the lower extremity the ventral surface shifts to the posterior surface (and is the plantar surface of the foot). The opposite of ventral is dorsal. Evolutionarily, these terms derive from the ventral and dorsal surfaces of a fish.

- **Extension** is the opposite of flexion (i.e., the dorsal [harder] surfaces of the body parts come closer together).
- See Figure 6-11 for examples of flexion and extension.
- Flexion and extension are movements that occur in the sagittal plane.[5]
- Flexion and extension are axial movements that occur around a mediolateral axis.[9]

- Flexion and extension are terms that can be used for the entire body (i.e., the body parts of the axial skeleton and the body parts of the appendicular skeleton).
- Flexion of a body part involves an anterior movement of that body part; extension of a body part involves a posterior movement of that body part.
  - The exception to this rule is at the knee joint and farther distally, where flexion is a posterior movement of the body part and extension is an anterior movement.
  - Another exception is flexion and extension of the thumb at the saddle joint. These motions are unusual in that they occur within the frontal plane. See Section 10.13 for more details regarding movement of the thumb.
- Generally, flexion involves a *bending* at a joint, whereas extension involves a joint straightening out.
  - The word *flexion* comes from the Latin word meaning *to bend.*
  - The word *extension* comes from the Latin word meaning *to straighten out.*
- An easy way to remember flexion is to think of the fetal position. When a person goes to sleep in the fetal position, most or all of the joints are in flexion.

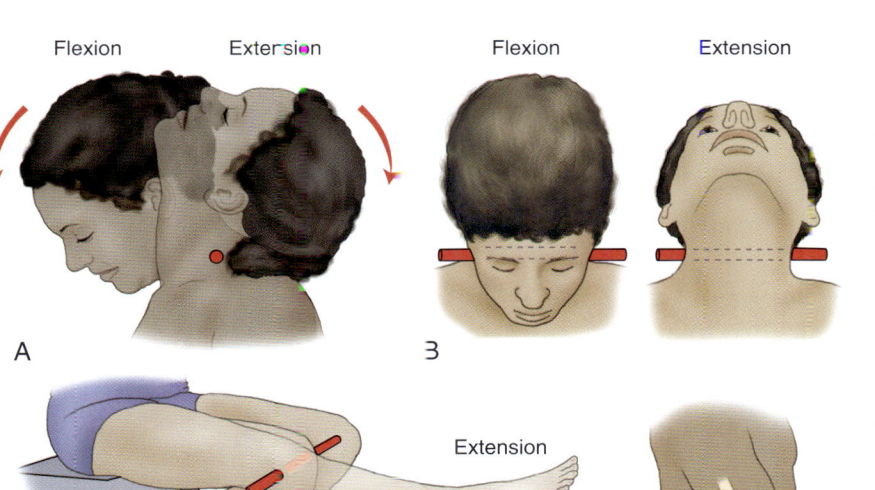
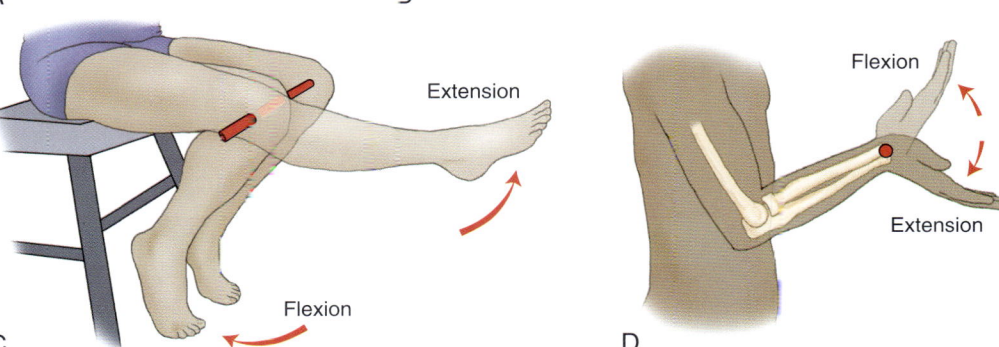
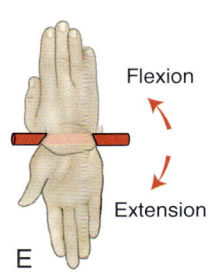

FIGURE 6-11 Examples of flexion and extension. **A** and **B,** Flexion and extension of the head and neck at the spinal joints. **C,** Flexion and extension of the leg at the knee joint. **D** and **E,** Flexion and extension of the hand at the wrist joint. (Note: In the illustrations, the red tube or red dot represents the axis of movement.)

SECTION 6.12 ABDUCTION/ADDUCTION

- **Abduction** is defined as a movement at a joint that brings a body part away from the midline of the body.[8] To *abduct* is to take away (Box 6-2).

BOX 6-2

The fingers and toes do not abduct/adduct relative to the midline of the body. The reference line about which abduction/adduction of the fingers occurs is an imaginary line through the middle finger; the reference line about which abduction/adduction of the toes occurs is an imaginary line through the second toe. Movement of a finger away from the middle finger and movement of a toe away from the second toe is abduction; movement toward these reference lines is adduction. Frontal plane movements of the middle finger itself are termed radial and ulnar abduction; similar movements of the second toe are termed fibular and tibial abduction. Another exception to this rule is abduction/adduction of the thumb (See Section 10.13 for more details regarding movements of the thumb.)

- The midline of the body is an imaginary line that divides the body into two equal left and right halves.
- **Adduction** is the opposite of abduction; in other words, the body part moves closer toward the midline (it is *added* to the midline).
  See Figure 6-12 for examples of abduction and adduction.
- Abduction and adduction are movements that occur in the frontal plane.[9]
- Abduction and adduction are axial movements that occur around an anteroposterior axis.[9]
- Abduction of a body part involves a lateral movement of that body part; adduction of a body part involves a medial movement of that body part.
- *Abduction* and *adduction* are terms that can be used for the body parts of the appendicular skeleton only (i.e., the upper and lower extremities).
  - An exception to these rules is abduction/adduction of the thumb. (See Section 10.13 for more details.)

FIGURE 6-12 Examples of abduction and adduction. **A** and **B**, Abduction and adduction of the thigh at the hip joint. **C** and **D**, Abduction and adduction of the arm at the shoulder joint. **E** and **F**, Abduction and adduction of the hand at the wrist joint. (Note: In the illustrations, the red tube or red dot represents the axis of movement.)

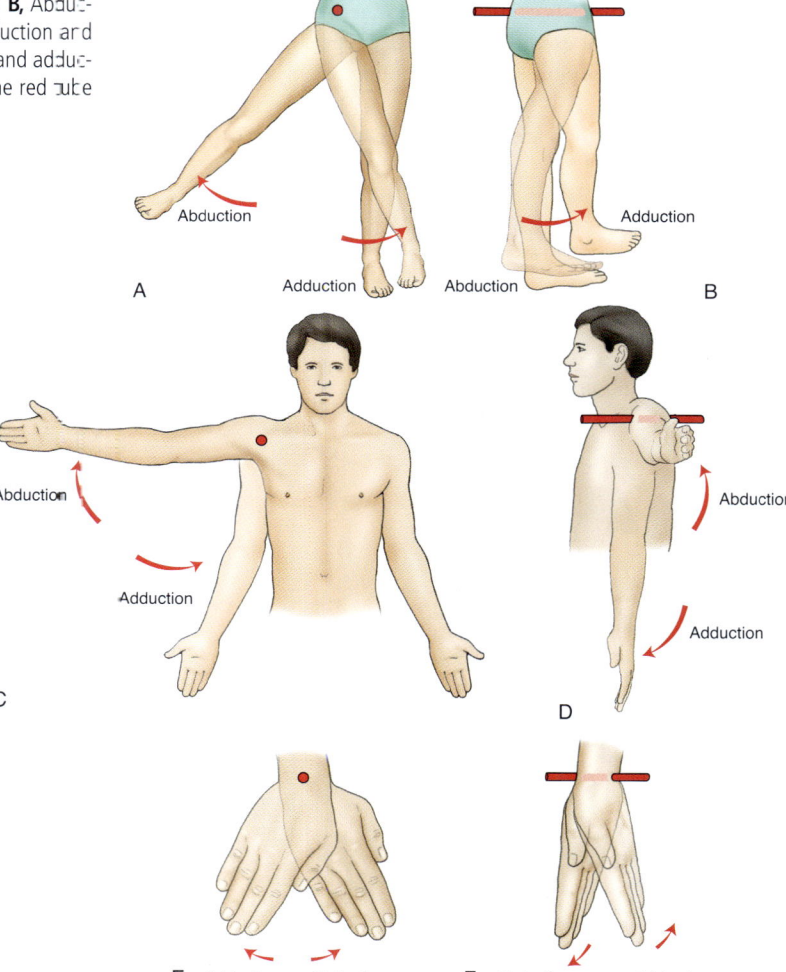

SECTION 6.13 RIGHT LATERAL FLEXION/LEFT LATERAL FLEXION

- **Right lateral flexion** is defined as a movement at a joint that bends a body part to the right side.[9]
- **Left lateral flexion** is the opposite of right lateral flexion; in other words, the body part bends to the left side.
  See Figure 6-13 for examples of right lateral flexion and left lateral flexion.
- Right lateral flexion and left lateral flexion are movements that occur in the frontal plane.[9]
- Right lateral flexion and left lateral flexion are axial movements that occur around an anteroposterior axis.[6]
- Right lateral flexion of a body part involves a lateral movement of that body part to the right; left lateral flexion of a body part involves a lateral movement of that body part to the left.
- Right lateral flexion and left lateral flexion are terms that can be used for the body parts of the axial skeleton only (i.e., the head, neck, and trunk).
- **Lateral flexion** is often called *side bending*.
- When we describe a muscle as laterally flexing a body part, we usually do not specify whether it is lateral flexion to the right or left because a muscle that laterally flexes can only do so to the same side of the body where it is located. Therefore, all muscle joint actions of lateral flexion are same-sided lateral flexion (i.e., ipsilateral lateral flexion).
- Note: Lateral flexion should not be confused with flexion, although the word *flexion* is contained within the term *lateral flexion*. Flexion is a sagittal plane movement, and lateral flexion is a frontal plane movement.

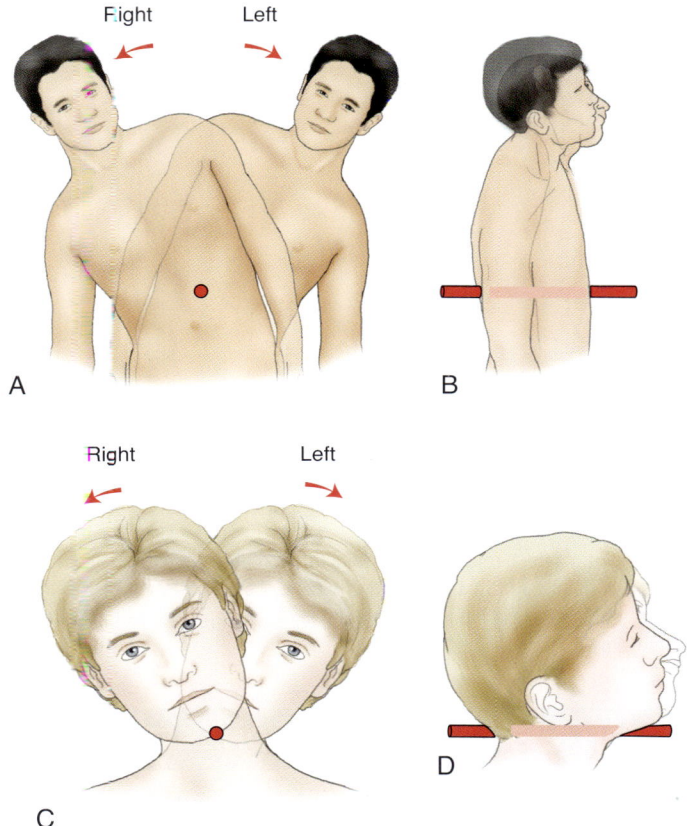

FIGURE 6-13 Examples of right and left lateral flexion. **A** and **B**, Anterior and lateral views (respectively) of right and left lateral flexion of the trunk at the spinal joints. **C** and **D**, Anterior and lateral views (respectively) of right and left lateral flexion of the neck at the spinal joints. (Note: In the illustrations, the red tube or red dot represents the axis of movement.)

SECTION 6.14 LATERAL ROTATION/MEDIAL ROTATION

- **Lateral rotation** is defined as a movement at a joint wherein the anterior surface of the body part rotates away from the midline of the body.[8]
- **Medial rotation** is the opposite of lateral rotation; in other words, the anterior surface of the body part rotates toward the midline of the body.
  See Figure 6-14 for examples of lateral rotation and medial rotation.
- Lateral rotation and medial rotation are movements that occur in the transverse plane.[9]
- Lateral rotation and medial rotation are axial movements that occur around a vertical axis.[9]
- Lateral rotation and medial rotation of a body part involve a rotation (i.e., spin) of the body part around the longitudinal axis that runs through the length of the bone of the body part. When this rotation occurs, the body part does not actually change its physical location in space; rather it stays in the same location and spins or rotates around its own axis.
- *Lateral rotation* and *medial rotation* are terms that can be used for the body parts of the appendicular skeleton only (i.e., the upper and lower extremities only).
  - Lateral rotation is often referred to as external rotation; medial rotation is often referred to as internal rotation.

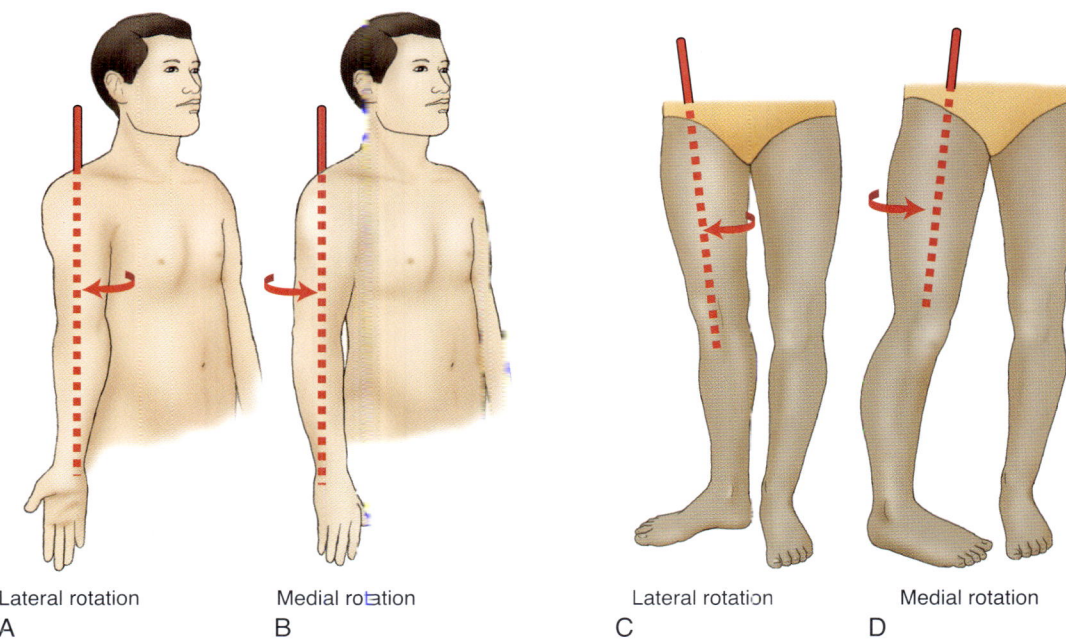

Lateral rotation   Medial rotation   Lateral rotation   Medial rotation
A   B   C   D

FIGURE 6-14 Examples of lateral rotation and medial rotation. **A,** Lateral rotation of the arm at the shoulder joint. **B,** Medial rotation of the arm at the shoulder joint. **C,** Lateral rotation of the thigh at the hip joint. **D,** Medial rotation of the thigh at the hip joint. (Note: In all illustrations the red tube and the dashed line represent the axis of movement.)

SECTION 6.15 RIGHT ROTATION/LEFT ROTATION

- **Right rotation** is defined as a movement at a joint wherein the anterior surface of the body part rotates to the right.[8]
- **Left rotation** is the opposite of right rotation; in other words, the anterior surface of the body part rotates to the left.
  See Figure 6-15 for examples of right rotation and left rotation.
- Right rotation and left rotation are movements that occur in the transverse plane.[9]
- Right rotation and left rotation are axial movements that occur around a vertical axis.[9]
- Right rotation and left rotation of a body part involve a rotation (i.e., spin) of the body part around the longitudinal axis that runs through the length of the bone(s) of the body part. When this rotation occurs, the body part does not actually change its physical location in space; rather it stays in the same location and spins or rotates around its own axis.
- *Right rotation* and *left rotation* are terms that can be used for the body parts of the axial skeleton only (i.e., the head, neck, and trunk).
  - An exception is the pelvis, which is described as rotating to the right and the left. (Note: The pelvis is a transitional body part containing elements of the axial and appendicular skeleton.)

Note:
- Two terms are often used when describing the actions of muscles that can rotate an axial body part within the transverse plane. These terms are *ipsilateral rotation* and *contralateral rotation*.

CHAPTER 6 Joint Action Terminology

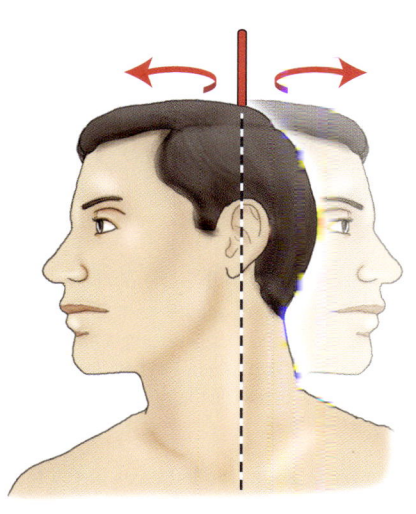
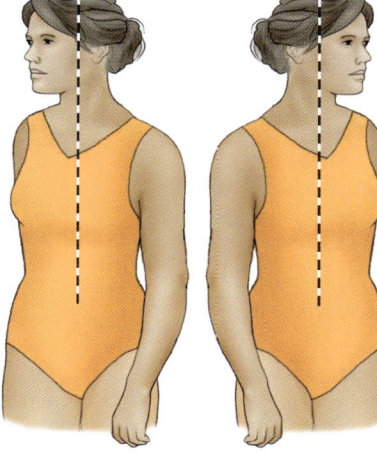

Right rotation   Left rotation   Right rotation   Left rotation
A   B   C

FIGURE 6-15 Examples of right rotation and left rotation. **A,** Right and left rotation of the head and neck at the spinal joints. **B,** Right rotation of the trunk at the spinal joints. **C,** Left rotation of the trunk at the spinal joints. (Note: In all illustrations the red tube and the dashed line represent the axis of movement.)

○ The terms *ipsilateral rotation* and *contralateral rotation* do not define joint actions; rather they indicate whether a muscle rotates an axial body part (or the pelvis) toward the same side of the body as where it is located, or toward the opposite side of the body from where it is located.

○ A muscle does **ipsilateral rotation** if it rotates an axial body part (or the pelvis) toward the same side of the body as where it is located.[10] For example, the splenius capitis muscle is an ipsilateral rotator because the right splenius capitis rotates the head and neck to the right, and the left splenius capitis rotates the head and neck to the left.

○ A muscle does **contralateral rotation** if it rotates an axial body part (or the pelvis) toward the opposite side of the body from where it is located.[10] For example, the sternocleidomastoid muscle is a contralateral rotator because the right sternocleidomastoid rotates the head and neck to the left, and the left sternocleidomastoid rotates the head and neck to the right.

SECTION 6.16 PLANTARFLEXION/DORSIFLEXION

○ **Plantarflexion** is defined as the movement at the ankle joint wherein the foot moves inferiorly, toward the plantar surface of the foot.[9]

○ The plantar surface of the foot is the surface that you plant on the ground (i.e., the inferior surface). The dorsal surface is the opposite side of the foot (i.e., the superior surface).

○ **Dorsiflexion** is the opposite of plantarflexion; in other words, the foot moves superiorly toward its dorsal surface (Box 6-3). See Figure 6-16 for an example of plantarflexion and dorsiflexion.

○ Plantarflexion and dorsiflexion are movements that occur in the sagittal plane.[9]

○ Plantarflexion and dorsiflexion are axial movements that occur around a mediolateral axis.[9]

○ *Plantarflexion* and *dorsiflexion* are terms that are used for the foot moving at the ankle joint.

BOX 6-3

Plantarflexion and dorsiflexion are terms that are used in place of flexion and extension. Because the foot is positioned at a 90-degree angle to the rest of the body, movements appear to be inferior and superior instead of anterior and posterior; for this reason, plantarflexion and dorsiflexion are used (instead of flexion and extension) to eliminate the possibility of confusion. When the terms flexion and extension are used to describe sagittal plane actions of the foot, controversy exists over which term is which. Some sources say that dorsiflexion is flexion, because dorsiflexion is bending of the ankle joint and the word flexion means to bend. Others sources state that plantarflexion is flexion for two reasons:
  Flexion is a posterior movement from the knee joint and further distal, and plantarflexion is a posterior movement.
  Flexion is usually an approximation of two ventral (i.e., soft) surfaces of adjacent body parts, and plantarflexion accomplishes this.
  (Note: Dorsiflexion and plantarflexion can also occur to a small degree at the subtalar and transverse tarsal joints of the foot.)

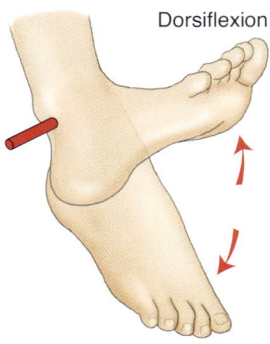

FIGURE 6-16 Plantarflexion and dorsiflexion of the foot at the ankle joint. (The red tube represents the axis of movement.)

SECTION 6.17 EVERSION/INVERSION

- **Eversion** is defined as the movement between tarsal bones wherein the plantar surface of the foot turns away from the midline of the body.[9]
- **Inversion** is the opposite of eversion; in other words, the plantar surface of the foot turns toward the midline of the body.
- *Inversion* can be thought of as turning the foot inward, toward the midline of the body. Therefore eversion would be turning the foot outward, away from the midline of the body.
  See Figure 6-17 for an example of eversion and inversion.
- Eversion and inversion are movements that occur in the frontal plane.[9]
- Eversion and inversion are axial movements that occur around an anteroposterior axis.[9]

- *Eversion* and *inversion* are terms that are used to describe the motion of the foot between tarsal bones. These movements do not occur at the ankle joint (Box 6-4).

BOX 6-4

Eversion is an action that is one component of another term, *pronation*, used to describe a broader movement of the foot; inversion is an action that is one component of another term, *supination*, used to describe a broader movement of the foot. (For more details on this, see Section 9.19.)

- Eversion and inversion occur about the long axis of the foot (i.e., anteroposterior axis). Because rotation actions of a body part occur about the long axis of the body part, this means that eversion and inversion may be thought of as lateral and medial rotation of the foot (although this is not technically correct). Rotations usually occur about a long axis that is vertical, but because the position of the foot is set at a 90-degree angle to the rest of the body, its long axis is anteroposterior (i.e., horizontal).
- The principal tarsal joint is the subtalar joint. For this reason, eversion and inversion are often said to occur at the subtalar joint. For more information on the tarsal joints of the foot, see Sections 9.19 and 9.20.
- Eversion of a body part involves a lateral movement of that body part; inversion of a body part involves a medial movement of that body part.

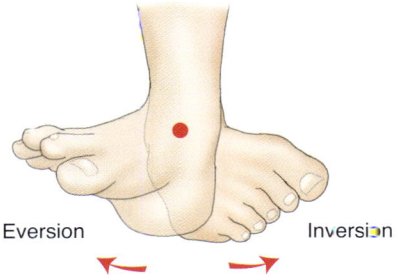

FIGURE 6-17 Eversion and inversion of the foot at the tarsal joints (i.e., the subtalar joint). (The red dot represents the axis of movement.)

SECTION 6.18 PRONATION/SUPINATION

- **Pronation** is defined as the movement of the forearm wherein the radius crosses over the ulna.[9]
- **Supination** is the opposite of pronation; in other words, the radius uncrosses to return to a position parallel to the ulna.
- Pronation and supination of the forearm are often referred to as *pronation* and *supination of the radius,* because it is the radius that usually does the vast majority of the moving. The ulna does actually move a small amount. This can be felt if you palpate the distal end of the ulna while doing pronation and supination of the forearm.
- Note: If the hand (and therefore the radius) is fixed, it is the ulna that moves relative to the radius during pronation and supination movements of the forearm; this scenario would be an example of a (closed-chain) reverse action.
  See Figure 6-18 for examples of pronation and supination.
- Pronation and supination are movements that occur in the transverse plane.[9]
- Pronation and supination are axial movements that occur around a vertical axis.[9]
- *Pronation* and *supination* are terms that are used for the radius moving at the radioulnar joints.
- The axis for pronation and supination of the forearm is a longitudinal axis that runs approximately from the head of the radius through the styloid process of the ulna (see Figure 6-18).

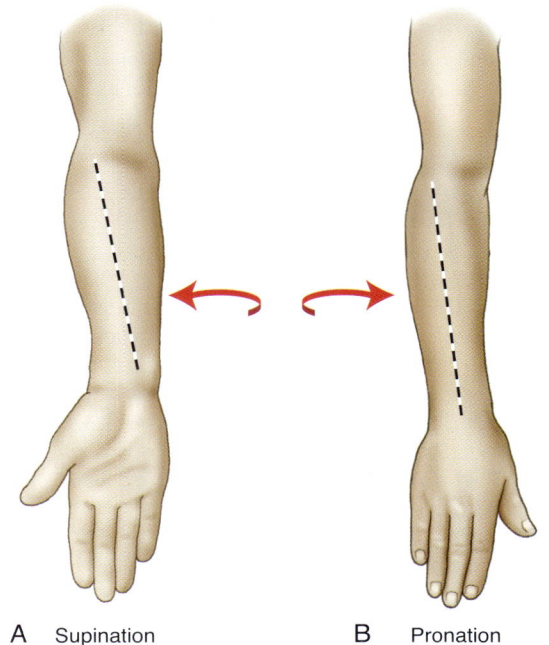

A Supination   B Pronation

FIGURE 6-18 Supination and pronation of the right forearm at the radioulnar joints. (The dashed line represents the axis of movement.)

- Pronation of the forearm involves two separate motions. The proximal radius medially rotates at the proximal radioulnar joint, and the distal radius moves around the distal end of the ulna.
- In anatomic position, our forearms are fully supinated.
- Pronation and supination result in an altered position of the distal radius. Because the hand articulates primarily with the radius, pronation and supination of the forearm result in the hand changing positions. Therefore the practical effect of pronation and supination of the forearm is that they allow us to be able to place the hand in a greater number of positions. Pronation results in the palm of the hand facing posteriorly; supination results in the palm of the hand facing anteriorly.
- This altered position of the hand is a result of motion at the radioulnar joints; it does not occur at the wrist joint (i.e., radiocarpal joint).
- To avoid confusing pronation/supination of the forearm at the radioulnar joints with medial rotation/lateral rotation of the arm at the shoulder joint, first flex the forearm at the elbow joint to 90 degrees and then perform pronation and supination of the forearm and then medial and lateral rotation of the arm at the shoulder joint. The resultant body positions will be markedly different from each other.
- The terms *pronation* and *supination* are also used to describe certain broad movements of the foot. (See Section 9.19 for more details.)

SECTION 6.19   PROTRACTION/RETRACTION

- **Protraction** is defined as a movement at a joint that brings a body part anteriorly.[5]
- **Retraction** is the opposite of protraction; in other words, the body part moves posteriorly (*retraction* literally means *to take it back*, hence a posterior movement).
See Figure 6-19 for examples of protraction and retraction.
- Protraction and retraction are movements that are usually considered to occur in the sagittal plane.[5]
- Protraction and retraction can be axial or nonaxial movements depending on the body part. (When the motion is axial, the movement occurs around an axis; when the motion is nonaxial, there is no axis around which the motion occurs.)
- *Protraction* and *retraction* are terms that can be used for the mandible, scapula, and clavicle (Box 6-5).

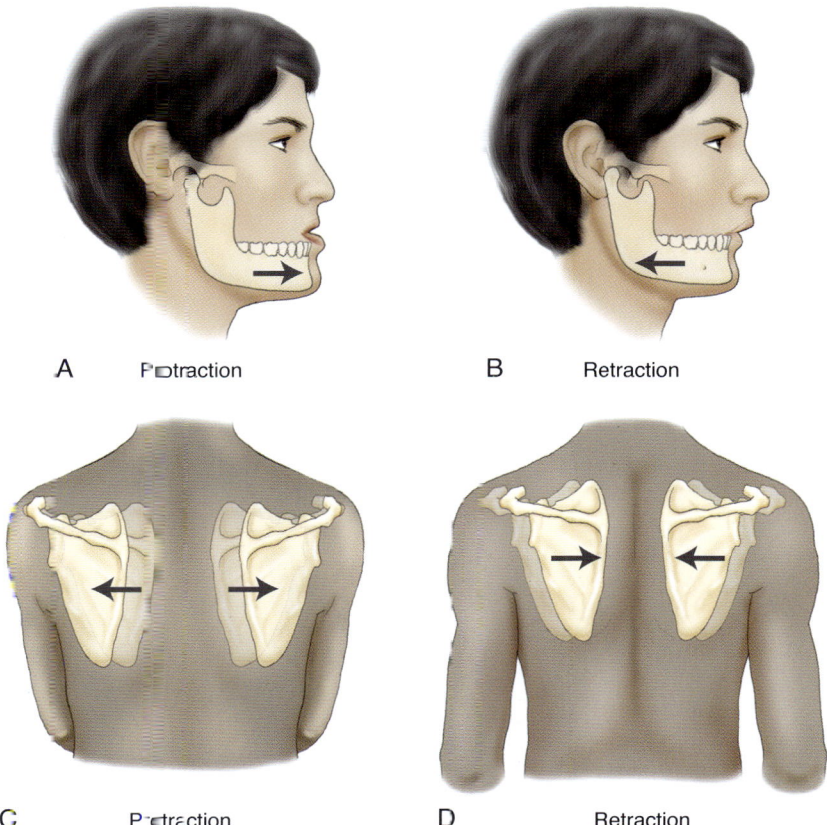

FIGURE 6-19 Examples of protraction and retraction. **A** and **B**, Protraction and retraction, respectively, of the mandible at the temporomandibular joints (TMJs). **C** and **D**, Protraction and retraction, respectively, of the scapula at the scapulocostal joint.

BOX 6-5

The named actions of protraction and retraction can be axial or nonaxial movements, depending on the body part that is moving. Protraction and retraction of the scapula and mandible are nonaxial movements; protraction and retraction of the clavicle are axial movements. (For more information on how these body parts move, see Sections 10.3, 8.2, and 10.4, respectively.)

The tongue and lips may also be said to protract and retract.

Protraction and retraction of the scapula are sometimes referred to as abduction and adduction of the scapula. The terms protraction and retraction refer to sagittal plane movements, whereas abduction and adduction refer to frontal plane movements. The reason for this seeming contradiction in terms is that the scapula lies in a plane that is approximately midway between the sagittal and frontal planes. When the scapula moves in this plane, its movement has a component in both of these planes; hence certain sources choose to describe the motion as sagittal plane movement and others choose to describe the motion as frontal plane movement. When scapular movement is viewed from the anterior or lateral perspectives, the anterior-posterior motion of protraction and retraction is more visible and seems to better describe the scapular movement that is occurring. However, when scapular movement is viewed from the posterior perspective, the lateral-medial motion of abduction and adduction away from and toward the midline is more visible and seems to better describe the scapular movement that is occurring. We will use protraction/retraction in this textbook, but we will also reference abduction and adduction. To eliminate this problem, some sources use the term **scaption** to describe the plane of the scapula.

SECTION 6.20 ELEVATION/DEPRESSION

- **Elevation** is defined as a movement at a joint that brings a body part superiorly[7] (*elevate* literally means *to bring up*).
- **Depression** is the opposite of elevation; in other words, the body part moves inferiorly (*depress* literally means *to bring down*). See Figure 6-20 for examples of elevation and depression.
- Elevation and depression are movements that occur in a vertical plane[9] (i.e., sagittal or frontal).
- Elevation and depression can be axial or nonaxial movements depending on the body part. (When the motion is axial, the movement occurs around an axis; when the motion is nonaxial, there is no axis around which the motion occurs.)
- An example of nonaxial elevation and depression would be the scapula. An example of axial elevation and depression would be the mandible. (For more information on how these body parts move, see Sections 10.3 and 8.2, respectively.)
- *Elevation* and *depression* are terms that can be used for the mandible, scapula, clavicle, and pelvis (Box 6-6).

FIGURE 6-20 Examples of elevation and depression. **A** and **B**, Depression and elevation, respectively, of the mandible at the temporomandibular joints (TMJs) (red dot represents the axis of movement of the mandible). **C** and **D**, Depression and elevation, respectively, of the scapula at the scapulocostal joint.

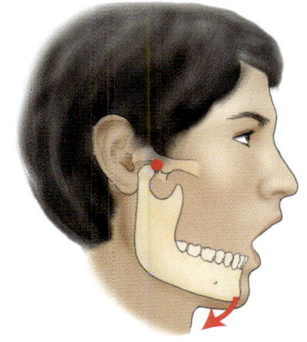
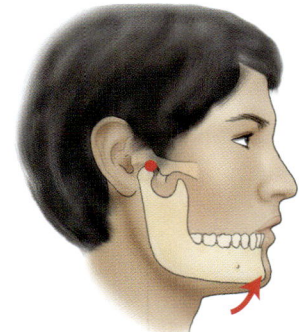

A Depression   B Elevation

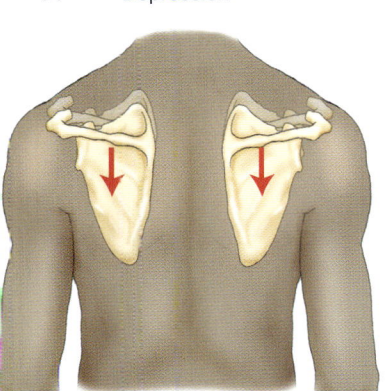
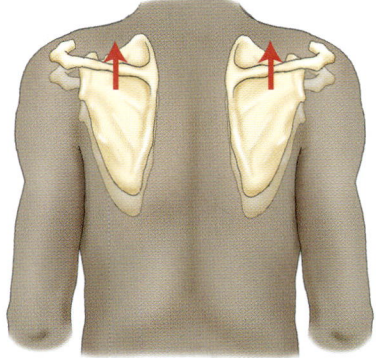

C Depression   D Elevation

BOX 6-6

Sometimes the term elevation is used more generally to describe movement of a long bone when its distal end elevates. For example, from anatomic position, flexion of the arm is sometimes referred to as elevation, because the distal end moves to a position that is higher. Although technically not incorrect, this use of the term elevation is less precise and therefore less desirable. The term depression is sometimes used in a similar manner.

Depression of the pelvis is also known as **lateral tilt** of the pelvis; elevation of the pelvis is also sometimes referred to as **hiking the hip**. (Note: Use of the term hiking the hip is not recommended; it can be confusing because hip movements are often thought of as thigh movements at the hip joint.) (For more information on the pelvis, see Sections 9.1 through 9.8.)

SECTION 6.21 UPWARD ROTATION/DOWNWARD ROTATION

Upward rotation and **downward rotation** are terms that may be used to describe movement of the scapula and the clavicle[7] (Box 6-7).

SCAPULA (FIGURE 6-21, A):

- Upward rotation is defined as a movement of the scapula wherein the scapula rotates in such a manner that the glenoid fossa orients superiorly.
- Downward rotation is the opposite of upward rotation; in other words, the scapula rotates to orient the glenoid fossa inferiorly.
- Upward rotation and downward rotation of the scapula are axial movements that occur in a vertical plane about an anteroposterior axis.
- The importance of upward rotation of the scapula is to orient the glenoid fossa superiorly. This allows the arm to further flex and/or abduct relative to the trunk.

BOX 6-7

The actual plane that the scapula moves within is the plane of the scapula, sometimes called the scaption plane, which lies between the frontal and sagittal planes.

According to usual terminology, an action of a body part is the motion of that body part relative to the body part that is directly next to it, with the motion occurring at the joint that is located between them. However, when actions of the arm or the shoulder joint are spoken of, the entire range of motion of the arm relative to the trunk (not the scapula) is often considered. This lumps the actions of the humerus with the actions of the scapula and clavicle (i.e., the shoulder girdle). Therefore the total motion of the humerus moving at the glenohumeral joint and the shoulder girdle moving at its joints are often considered. Similarly, motion of the thigh or the hip joint often includes the motion of the pelvic girdle.

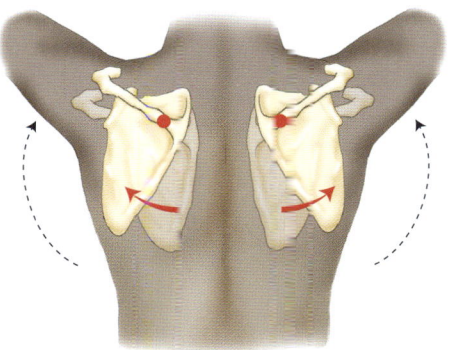

A   Upward rotation

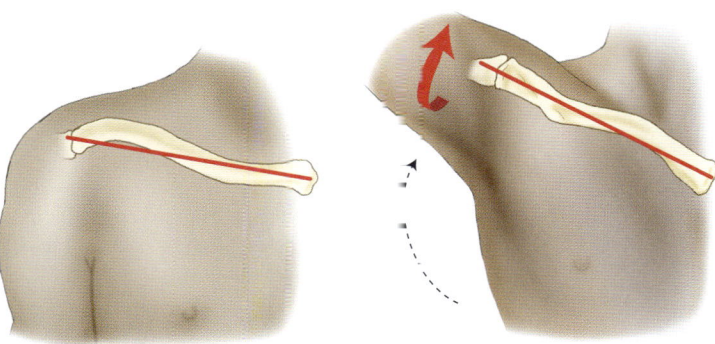

B Anatomic position   C   Upward rotation

FIGURE 6-21 Examples of upward rotation and downward rotation. **A,** Upward rotation of the scapula at the scapulocostal joint from anatomic position (downward rotation of the scapula would be returning to anatomic position). The red dot represents the location of the axis of movement. **B,** Clavicle in anatomic position. **C,** Upward rotation of the clavicle at the sternoclavicular joint (downward rotation of the clavicle would be returning to anatomic position). The red line in **B** and **C** represents the axis of movement.

CLAVICLE (FIGURE 6-21, B AND C):

- Upward rotation may also be used to describe the rotation of the clavicle in which the inferior surface comes to face anteriorly.
- Being the opposite action, downward rotation returns the inferior surface (now facing anteriorly) back to face inferiorly again.
- If one were to look at the right clavicle from the (right) lateral side, upward rotation would be a counterclockwise motion of the clavicle; downward rotation would be a clockwise motion of the clavicle.
- Viewing the left clavicle from the left side, upward rotation would be a clockwise motion and downward rotation would be a counterclockwise motion.
- Upward rotation and downward rotation of the clavicle are axial movements that occur in a sagittal plane around an axis that is approximately mediolateral in orientation.
- Because of the curve in the distal clavicle, when the clavicle upwardly rotates, the distal end elevates. Therefore one important aspect of upward rotation of the clavicle is to help elevate the shoulder girdle as a whole to facilitate further flexion and/or abduction of the arm relative to the trunk. (For more detailed information on the role of the clavicle [and scapula] in motion of the upper extremity, see Section 10.6.)

SECTION 6.22   ANTERIOR TILT/POSTERIOR TILT

- *Anterior tilt* and *posterior tilt* are terms that may be used to describe movement of the pelvis.
- Unfortunately, many terminology systems exist for naming movements of the pelvis. Because *anterior tilt* and *posterior tilt* are the most common and easiest terms to use when describing sagittal plane movements of the pelvis, this book will use these terms.
- Anterior tilt is defined as the movement of the pelvis wherein the superior aspect of the pelvis tilts anteriorly[3] (Figure 6-22, *A*).
- Posterior tilt is defined as the movement of the pelvis wherein the superior aspect of the pelvis tilts posteriorly (Figure 6-22, *B*).
- Anterior tilt and posterior tilt are movements that occur in the sagittal plane.
- Anterior tilt and posterior tilt are axial movements that occur around a mediolateral axis.
- *Anterior tilt* and *posterior tilt* are terms that are used for the pelvis moving at the lumbosacral and/or the hip joints. The majority of pelvic motion occurs at the hip joints.
- The postural position of anterior/posterior tilt of the pelvis is extremely important because the spine sits on the pelvis; if the amount of anterior/posterior tilt of the pelvis changes, the curves of the spine must change (i.e., increase or decrease) to compensate. (For more information on the effect of the pelvis on the posture of the spine, see Section 9.8.)
- The word *pelvis* is derived from the Latin word for basin. If one thinks of the pelvis as a basin filled with water, then the word *tilt* refers to where the water would spill out when the pelvis tilts (Figure 6-23).
  - Note: The terms *right lateral tilt* and *left lateral tilt* are sometimes used to describe movements of the pelvis in the frontal plane. This book will use the term *depression of the pelvis* (see Sections 9.3 through 9.5) in place of *lateral tilt of the pelvis*.

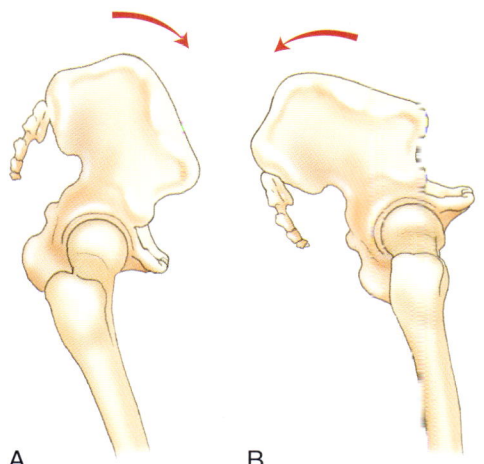

FIGURE 6-22 A, Anterior tilt of the pelvis. **B,** Posterior tilt of the pelvis. Motions are shown as occurring at the hip joint.

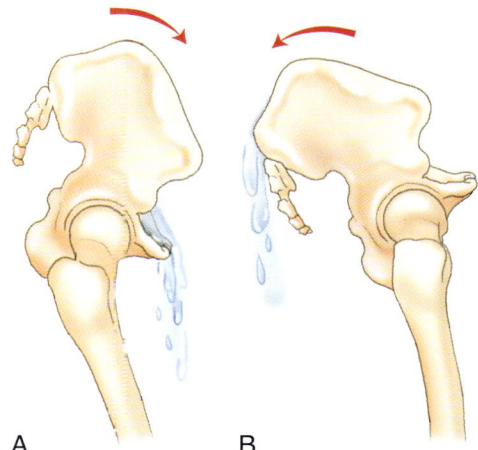

FIGURE 6-23 Water spilling out of the pelvis based on the tilt of the pelvis. To learn the tilt actions of the pelvis, it can be helpful to think of the pelvis as a basin that holds water. Whichever way that the pelvis tilts, water will spill out in that direction.

SECTION 6.23 OPPOSITION/REPOSITION

- **Opposition** is defined as the movement of the thumb wherein the pad of the thumb meets the pad of another finger[3] (Figure 6-24, *A*).
- **Reposition** is the opposite of opposition; in other words, the thumb returns to its starting position (usually anatomic position) (Figure 6-24, *B*).
- Opposition is not a specific action; it is a combination of three actions.
  - Opposition is a combination of abduction, flexion, and medial rotation of the metacarpal of the thumb at the saddle joint of the thumb (first carpometacarpal joint).[11]
- Reposition is not a specific action; it is a combination of three actions.
  - Reposition is a combination of extension, lateral rotation, and adduction of the metacarpal of the thumb at the saddle joint of the thumb (first carpometacarpal joint) (Box 6-8).

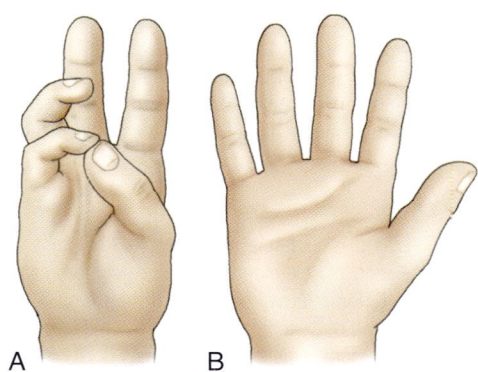

FIGURE 6-24 **A**, Opposition of the thumb at the saddle (first carpometacarpal) joint. **B**, Reposition of the thumb at the saddle joint.

COMPONENTS OF OPPOSITION/REPOSITION:

- Flexion and extension of the thumb occur in the frontal plane around an anteroposterior axis. With flexion and extension, the thumb moves parallel to the palm of the hand.[3]
- Abduction and adduction of the thumb occur in the sagittal plane around a mediolateral axis. With abduction and adduction, the thumb moves perpendicular to the palm of the hand.[3]
- Medial rotation and lateral rotation of the thumb occur in the transverse plane around a vertical axis.[3]
  - The exact components of opposition (and therefore reposition) can vary depending on the motion of the finger to which the thumb is being opposed. If that finger remains in anatomic position, then the thumb abducts from anatomic position and then may actually adduct posteriorly to meet the pad of that finger. However, if the other finger flexes, then the thumb need only abduct. Also, the amount of thumb flexion that occurs varies based upon which finger the thumb is opposing to meet; it flexes more to meet the little finger and less to meet the index finger. (For more information on movement of the thumb, see Section 10.13.)
- The terms *opposition* and *reposition* are also used to describe movements of the little finger. (For more information on movement of the little finger, see Section 10.12.)

BOX 6-8

The cardinal plane component actions of opposition and reposition of the thumb are unusual in that flexion/extension and abduction/adduction do not occur in their usual planes; flexion and extension of the thumb occur in the frontal plane instead of the sagittal plane, and abduction and adduction of the thumb occur in the sagittal plane instead of the frontal plane. The reason for this is that the thumb rotated embryologically so that it can be opposed to the other fingers for grasping objects. This can be seen if you look at the orientation of the thumb pad when the thumb is in anatomic or resting position. You will see that the thumb pad primarily faces medially, whereas the pads of the other fingers face anteriorly. Therefore because of this embryologic rotation, flexion/extension and abduction/adduction are named as occurring in planes that are 90 degrees different from the planes within which they usually occur.

SECTION 6.24 RIGHT LATERAL DEVIATION/LEFT LATERAL DEVIATION

- **Right lateral deviation** is defined as a movement at a joint that brings a body part to the right.[3]
- **Left lateral deviation** is the opposite of right lateral deviation; in other words, the body part moves to the left.
- Right lateral deviation and left lateral deviation are movements that could be considered to occur in the transverse, or perhaps the frontal plane.[9]
- **Lateral deviation** (to the right or left) can be an axial or nonaxial movement depending on the body part. (When the motion is axial, the movement occurs around an axis; when the motion is nonaxial, there is no axis around which the motion occurs.)
- *Right lateral deviation* and *left lateral deviation* are terms that are used for the mandible and the trunk (Figure 6-25, Box 6-9).
- Lateral deviation of the trunk is an axial movement. Lateral deviation of the mandible at the temporomandibular joints (TMJs) is a linear nonaxial movement.

BOX 6-9

Lateral deviation of the trunk occurs as the reverse action of a muscle that crosses the glenohumeral and scapulocostal joints from the arm to the trunk (e.g., the pectoralis major or the latissimus dorsi). When the arm stays fixed and the muscle contracts, the trunk moves toward the fixed arm. This movement can occur at the scapulocostal joint if the scapula is fixed to the humerus; in this case the trunk moves relative to the fixed scapula and arm. Alternatively, it can occur at the shoulder joint (i.e., glenohumeral joint); in this case the trunk and scapula move as a unit relative to the fixed humerus. (For more on reverse actions of the trunk at the shoulder joint, see illustrations in Section 8.10.)

FIGURE 6-25 Examples of lateral deviation (to the right or left). **A,** Left lateral deviation of the mandible at the temporomandibular joints (TMJs). **B** and **C,** Right lateral deviation of the trunk. In this scenario the hand is holding onto an immovable object and is fixed; when muscles such as the pectoralis major and latissimus dorsi contract, the trunk is laterally deviated to the right, toward the right arm. (Note: The arm has also flexed at the elbow joint.)

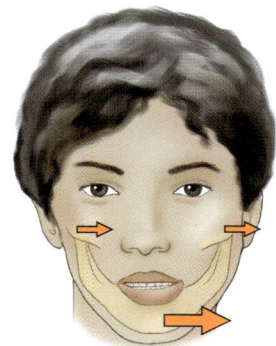

A   Left lateral deviation

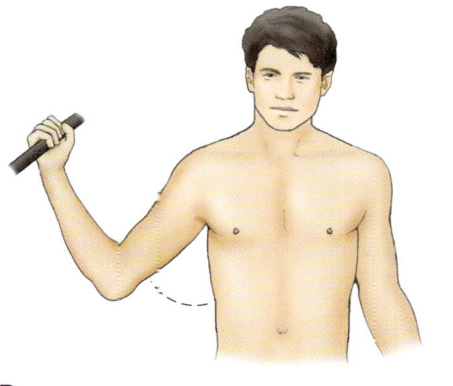

B   Neutral position

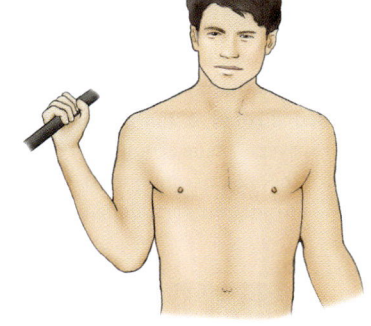

C   Right lateral deviation

SECTION 6.25 HORIZONTAL FLEXION/HORIZONTAL EXTENSION

- **Horizontal flexion** is defined as a horizontal movement in an anterior direction of the arm at the shoulder joint or thigh at the hip joint.[7]
- **Horizontal extension** is the opposite of horizontal flexion; in other words, a horizontal movement in a posterior direction of the arm or thigh.

See Figure 6-26 for an example of horizontal flexion and horizontal extension.

- Horizontal flexion and horizontal extension are movements that occur once the arm or thigh is first abducted 90 degrees.
  - Horizontal flexion is also known as **horizontal adduction**; horizontal extension is also known as **horizontal abduction**.

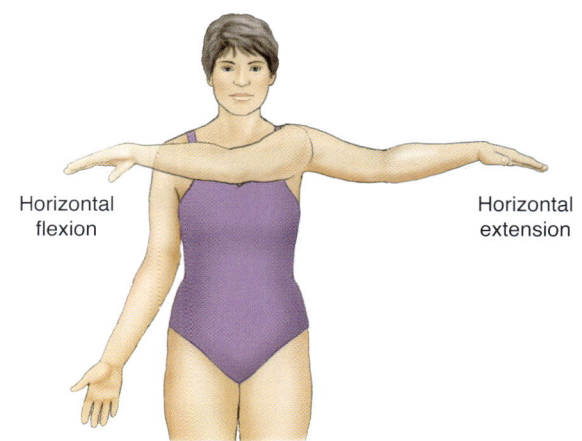

Horizontal flexion   Horizontal extension

FIGURE 6-26 Horizontal flexion and horizontal extension of a person's left arm at the shoulder joint.

- Horizontal flexion and horizontal extension occur in the transverse plane.
- Horizontal flexion and horizontal extension are axial movements that occur around a vertical axis.
- The terms *horizontal flexion* and *extension* are useful terms created to describe horizontal movements of the arm and/or thigh that commonly occur in many sporting activities (e.g., a baseball swing, or tennis forehand or backhand), as well as activities of daily life[7] (e.g., reaching across your body to move an object or perhaps dusting a bookshelf).

SECTION 6.26 HYPEREXTENSION

6-3

- **Hyperextension** is a term that can be used in two different ways:
  - To denote movement that is beyond what is considered to be a normal or healthy range of motion[9]
  - To describe normal, healthy extension beyond anatomic position[10]
- The prefix *hyper* is used to denote a greater than normal or a greater than healthy amount of something. Therefore hyperextension should theoretically mean an amount of extension of a body part at a joint that is greater than the normal amount or greater than the healthy amount of extension that the joint normally permits. That is the way in which the term hyperextension will be used in this book.
- It should be kept in mind that "normal" and "healthy" are not necessarily the same thing. For example, it is normal for an elderly person in our society to have arteriosclerosis; however, the presence of this condition would not be considered healthy.

- Whether or not hyperextension describes a healthy or unhealthy condition depends on the individual. For example, dancers or contortionists who have extremely flexible muscles and ligaments can hyperextend their joints; this hyperextension would certainly be beyond normal movement, hence the term *hyperextension,* but would not be unhealthy for these individuals. Another person might extend a body part at a joint much less than a dancer or contortionist would, and this movement might result in a sprain and/or strain; this hyperextension having caused tissue damage would be considered to be unhealthy.
- Given this reasoning, terms such as *hyperflexion* and *hyperabduction* could also be used in a similar manner to describe any movement that is greater than the normal or healthy amount that the joint normally permits.
- However, another use of the term *hyperextension* exists. Hyperextension is often used to describe only the particular phase of extension wherein a body part extends beyond anatomic position. In this terminology system, the term *extension* is then reserved for the phase of motion wherein a body part that is first flexed, then extends back toward anatomic position (Figure 6-27). We will not be using this meaning for the term *hyperextension;* however, given how often the term is used in this manner, it is important that a student of kinesiology be familiar with it (Box 6-10).

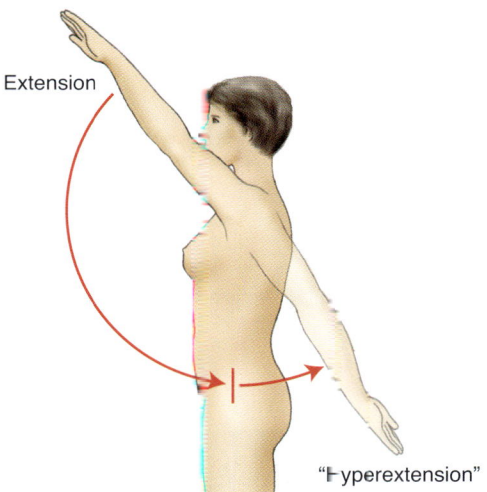

FIGURE 6-27 Woman extending her arm (that was first flexed) at the shoulder joint toward anatomic position; she then "hyperextends" her arm beyond anatomic position. (Note: This book does not adopt this use of the term hyperextension.)

 BOX 6-10

Although use of the term hyperextension to denote extension beyond anatomic position is fairly common, it is not recommended for two reasons:
1. It is inconsistent with the normal use of the prefix hyper (extending beyond anatomic position is not excessive or unhealthy).
2. It is not symmetric; no other joint action beyond anatomic position is given the prefix hyper (e.g., flexion beyond anatomic position is not called hyperflexion, abduction beyond anatomic position is not called hyperabduction, and so forth).

SECTION 6.27 CIRCUMDUCTION

- **Circumduction** is a term that is often used when describing joint actions. However, circumduction is not an action; rather it is a combination of actions of a body part that occur sequentially at a joint.[13]
- Circumduction of an appendicular body part involves the frontal and sagittal plane actions of adduction, extension, abduction, and flexion (not necessarily in that order).
- Circumduction of an axial body part involves the frontal and sagittal plane actions of right lateral flexion, extension, left lateral flexion, and flexion (not necessarily in that order).
- A good example of circumduction is shown in Figure 6-28. The arm is seen to first adduct, then extend, then abduct, and then flex (at the shoulder joint). If each of these four joint actions is performed individually, one after the other, the distal end of the upper extremity will carve out a square, and it will be clear that four separate actions occurred (Figure 6-28, *A*). However, if the same actions are performed, but now the corners of the square are "rounded out," the movement of the upper extremity will now carve out a circle (Figure 6-28, *B* and *C*).
- Many people erroneously believe that circumduction is or involves some form of rotation. However, no rotation occurs. In Figure 6-28, *B* the adductors first adduct the arm, then the extensors extend it, then the abductors abduct it, and finally the flexors flex it. In this example, it can be seen that circumduction of the arm involves no rotation.
- The term *circumduction* is used regardless of the sequence of the movements (i.e., using Figure 6-28 as our example); it does not matter if the order is adduction, extension, abduction, and then flexion, or if the order is the opposite (i.e., extension, adduction, flexion, and then abduction). In other words, whether the circle is clockwise or counterclockwise in direction, a circle formed by a sequence of four joint actions is called *circumduction*.
- The arm, thigh, hand, foot, head, neck, trunk, and pelvis can all circumduct.

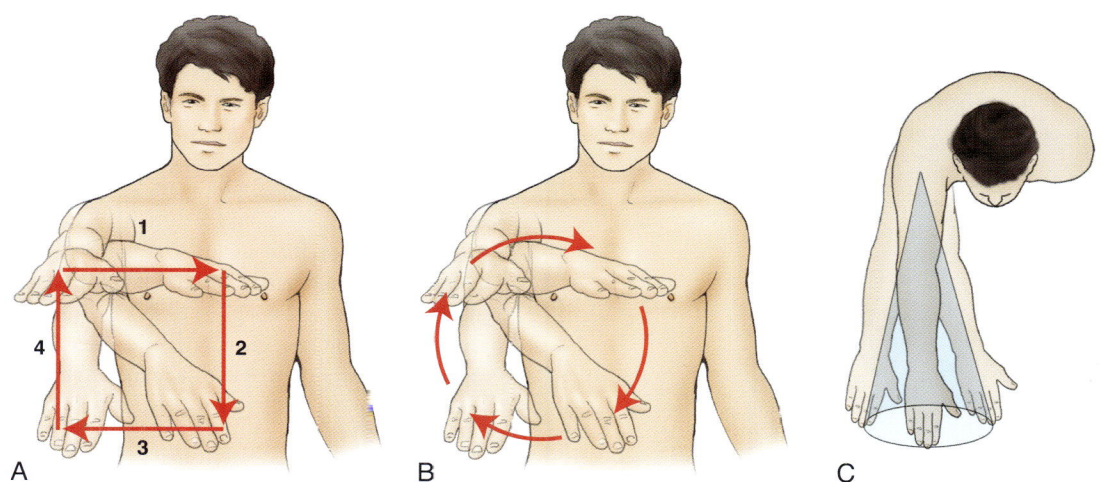

FIGURE 6-28 Circumduction of the arm at the shoulder joint. **A,** Four separate component joint actions of circumduction carving out a square. **B** and **C,** Circumduction as it typically looks, carving out a circle (**B** is an anterior view; **C** is a superior view).

SECTION 6.28 NAMING OBLIQUE PLANE MOVEMENTS

- An **oblique plane movement** occurs within an oblique plane.
- An oblique plane is a plane that is not purely sagittal, frontal, or transverse (i.e., an oblique plane is a combination of two or three cardinal planes).[7]
- Naming a joint action that occurs purely in a cardinal plane is simple. We simply name the action that occurred using one of the terms for movement that we have just learned. There is one joint action term that exists for each cardinal plane movement because these joint action terms are defined with respect to cardinal planes.
- However, our body's motions do not always occur within pure cardinal planes; we often move within oblique planes.[3] When describing a movement that occurs within an oblique plane, it is a little more challenging because it is necessary to break the one oblique plane movement down into the components that can be described by cardinal plane movement terms.
- For example, Figure 6-29 shows a person moving the arm in an oblique plane. This motion is occurring in only one direction; however, that direction is a combination of sagittal plane flexion and frontal plane abduction. We do not have one specific term to describe this one movement; instead we must describe it with two terms by saying that the person has flexed and adducted the arm at the shoulder joint. By our description that includes these

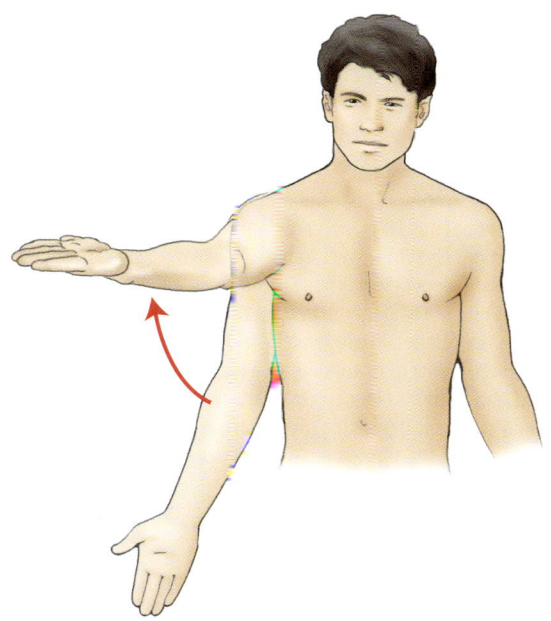

FIGURE 6-29 Movement that is within an oblique plane that is between the sagittal and frontal planes. This one movement is described as flexion and abduction of the arm at the shoulder joint (or abduction and flexion of the arm at the shoulder joint; the order does not matter).

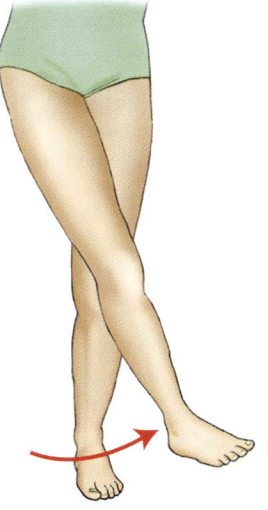

FIGURE 6-31 Movement occurring within an oblique plane. This oblique plane is a combination of all three cardinal planes; therefore the movement that is occurring has component actions in all three cardinal planes. The person is flexing, adducting, and medially rotating the right thigh at the hip joint (the order in which these three actions are listed is not important).

two terms, it may seem as if the person made two separate movements. In reality, the person made only one movement. However, for us to describe that one movement, we have to break that one oblique movement into two separate cardinal plane actions.

- The order in which we say these two components is not important. We can say that the person flexed and adducted the arm at the shoulder joint, or we can say that the person adducted and flexed the arm at the shoulder joint.
- An analogy can be made to geographic directions on a map. If a person is walking northwest, he or she is walking in one direction. In geographic terms, we can state this in one term, *northwest,* which gives the reader the sense that the person is, in fact, walking in one direction (Figure 6-30). However, in kinesiology terminology, we do not combine our joint action terms into one-word combinations as we do in geographic terminology. In the case of Figure 6-29, we cannot say that the person is "flexoabducting" or "abductoflexing." Instead we say that the person flexed *and* abducted (or abducted and flexed). It is important to realize that the person only moved the arm in one oblique direction, but we describe this one oblique movement by breaking it up into its two pure cardinal plane action components.
- Whenever a person moves a body part in an oblique plane that is a combination of two or three cardinal planes, we must separate that one oblique movement into its two or three pure cardinal plane movements. Figure 6-31 illustrates another example of this concept.

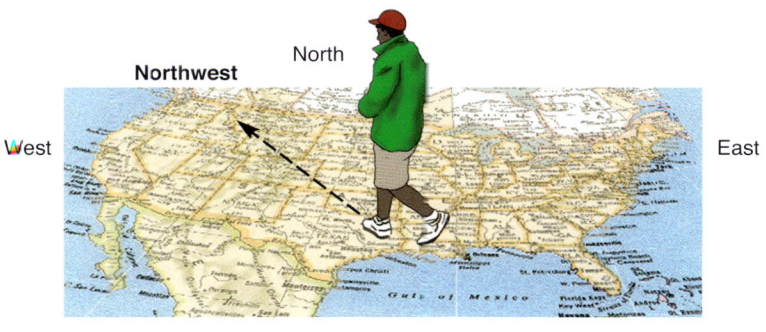

FIGURE 6-30 Person walking in a northwesterly direction. In geographic terms, this movement is described as northwest, instead of saying that the person is walking north and west (or west and north).

SECTION 6.29 REVERSE ACTIONS

- A *reverse action* is when a muscle contracts and the attachment that is usually considered to be more fixed—often termed, the *origin*—moves, and the attachment that is usually considered to be more mobile—often termed, the *insertion*—stays fixed[8] (Box 6-11).
- As explained in Chapter 11 (see Section 13.2), whenever a muscle contracts and shortens, it can move either attachment A toward attachment B, or attachment B toward attachment A, or it can move both attachments A and B toward each other. Generally speaking, one of the attachments, call it *attachment A*, will usually do the moving. This is because this attachment, attachment A, weighs less and therefore moves more easily than attachment B (conversely, attachment B is usually heavier and therefore more fixed and will not move as easily). When origin/insertion terminology is used, this attachment that usually moves is called the *insertion*, and the other attachment that usually does not move is called the *origin*.
- In Figure 6-32, *A* we see the brachialis, which is a flexor of the elbow joint (the brachialis crosses the elbow joint anteriorly, attaching from the arm to the forearm).
- When the brachialis contracts, it usually moves the forearm, not the arm, at the elbow joint, because the forearm is lighter (i.e., less fixed) than the arm. Figure 6-32, *B* illustrates the forearm moving when the brachialis contracts; this action is called *flexion of the forearm at the elbow joint*.

BOX 6-11

It is interesting to note that the mover action of a muscle that is considered to be its usual standard action is not always its most common mover action. Generally it is assumed that the distal attachment of a muscle of the appendicular body is the more movable attachment (i.e., the insertion). In the upper extremity, this is generally true. However, in the lower extremity we are usually in a weight-bearing position such as standing, walking, or running in which the feet are planted on the ground and therefore more fixed than the more proximal attachment. During the gait cycle (walking), for example, our feet are planted on the ground 60% of the time. Therefore reverse mover actions in the lower extremity actually occur more often than the standard mover actions that most students memorize in their beginning kinesiology classes!

- However, in certain circumstances, such as doing a pull-up, the forearm might be more fixed than the arm, and the arm may do the moving instead. Figure 6-32, *C* illustrates the arm moving at the elbow joint when the brachialis contracts; this action is called *flexion of the arm at elbow joint*. When the brachialis moves the arm instead of the forearm, it can be called the *reverse action* because it is the opposite action from the standard mover action that usually occurs (i.e., the arm is moving instead of the forearm). In origin/insertion terminology the reverse

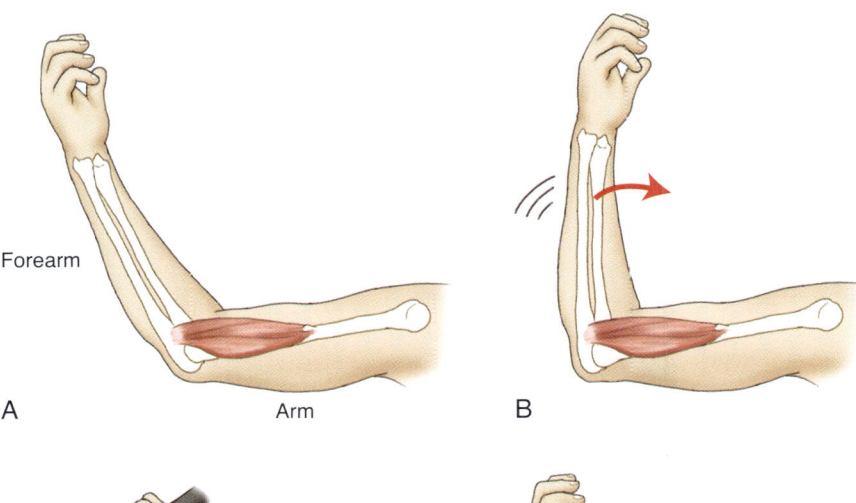

FIGURE 6-32 *A*, Medial view of the brachialis muscle. *B*, Brachialis muscle contracting and causing flexion of the forearm at the elbow joint. *C*, Brachialis muscle contracting to do a pull-up. In this scenario the hand is fixed to the pull-up bar, so the forearm (being attached to the hand) is now more fixed than the arm; therefore the arm moves instead of the forearm. The resulting action is flexion of the arm at the elbow joint. *D*, Both attachments of the brachialis are moving, so both the forearm and the arm are flexing at the elbow joint.

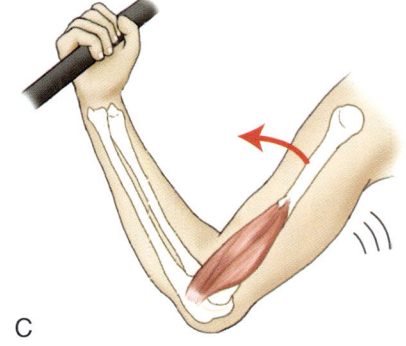
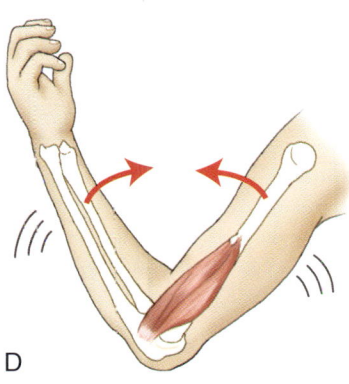

action is said to occur whenever the origin moves instead of the insertion.
- Reverse actions occur during what is described as closed-chain movements. Closed-chain movements occur when the distal segment (of the kinematic chain of elements), usually the hand or foot, is fixed against a stable surface. When the distal body part is fixed, the proximal body is more mobile and moves instead, hence, a closed-chain reverse action occurs.
- It should be emphasized that the reverse action of a muscle is always theoretically possible. Again, a muscle can always move either attachment A toward attachment B or attachment B toward attachment A.
- It is also possible for both attachment A and attachment B to move. In other words, both the standard and the reverse mover actions can occur at the same time (Figure 6-32, D).
- Understanding the concept of reverse actions of a muscle is not only fundamental to understanding how the musculoskeletal system works but also extremely important when working clinically so that we can best assess muscle contractions and how they relate to the client's postures, movement patterns, and health!

SECTION 6.30 VECTORS

- A **vector** is nothing more than an arrow drawn to represent the line of pull of a muscle.
- This vector arrow is drawn along the direction of the fibers of the muscle, from one attachment to the other attachment, and helps us visually see the action(s) of the muscle.
- A vector has two components to it. The direction that the arrowhead is pointed tells us the direction of the line of pull of the muscle; the length of the stem of the arrow tells us the magnitude of the muscle's pull (i.e., how far the muscle pulls its attachment).[1] However, in kinesiology textbooks, vectors are often not drawn to scale because it is the direction of the muscle's line of pull represented by the direction of the arrowhead that is usually of primary interest. Note: The direction that the arrowhead of a vector points can be reversed for reverse actions.
    - A very brief explanation of vectors can be helpful in understanding how to figure out a muscle's actions.
    - If the muscle's line of pull is in an oblique plane, vectors can be especially helpful for breaking down and seeing the component cardinal plane actions of that muscle.
- Figure 6-33 illustrates retraction (i.e., adduction) of the scapula at the scapulocostal joint. The direction of the line of pull of the muscle that is creating this action is shown by a vector, which is simply an arrow that is drawn pointing in the direction of the muscle's line of pull. Vectors can be drawn for all muscle lines of pull. Vectors are valuable because they help give us a visual image of the muscle's action.
- In Figure 6-34, A we see that the rhomboids' major and minor muscles also attach to and can move the scapula.
- Figure 6-34, B shows a vector that has been drawn that demonstrates the movement that the rhomboids can have on the scapula.
- In this case, as shown by the vector, the rhomboids' pull on the scapula is diagonal (i.e., oblique). Therefore when the rhomboids contract, they pull the scapula in this diagonal direction.
- Figure 6-34, C shows how this diagonal vector can be resolved into its component vectors. We see that to **resolve a vector**, we simply draw in the component vector arrows that begin at the tail of the vector arrow and end at the vector's arrowhead.[14]
- When an oblique vector is broken down into its cardinal plane component vectors, it is said to be *resolved*. When resolving a vector, note that we must start at the beginning of the tail of the arrow and end at the arrowhead. Being able to resolve a vector that represents the oblique line of pull of a muscle is extremely helpful toward seeing the component cardinal plane actions of the muscle!
- Each of these two component vectors represents the two component cardinal plane actions of this muscle. The horizontal component vector arrow shows that the rhomboids can retract (adduct) the scapula; the vertical component vector arrow shows that the rhomboids can elevate the scapula.
- Figure 6-35 illustrates another example of resolving a vector arrow to determine the actions of another muscle (the coracobrachialis muscle).

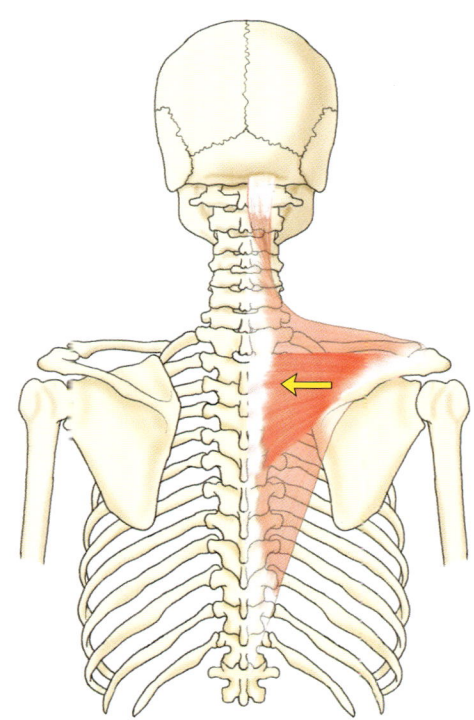

FIGURE 6-33 Fibers of a muscle (the fibers of the middle trapezius muscle) that can move the scapula (at the scapulocostal joint). Also drawn is a vector that demonstrates the line of pull of the middle trapezius. The direction in which the yellow arrow is pointing represents the muscle's line of pull; in this case it is medial. The fibers of the middle trapezius can pull the scapula medially (i.e., retract the scapula [at the scapulocostal joint]).

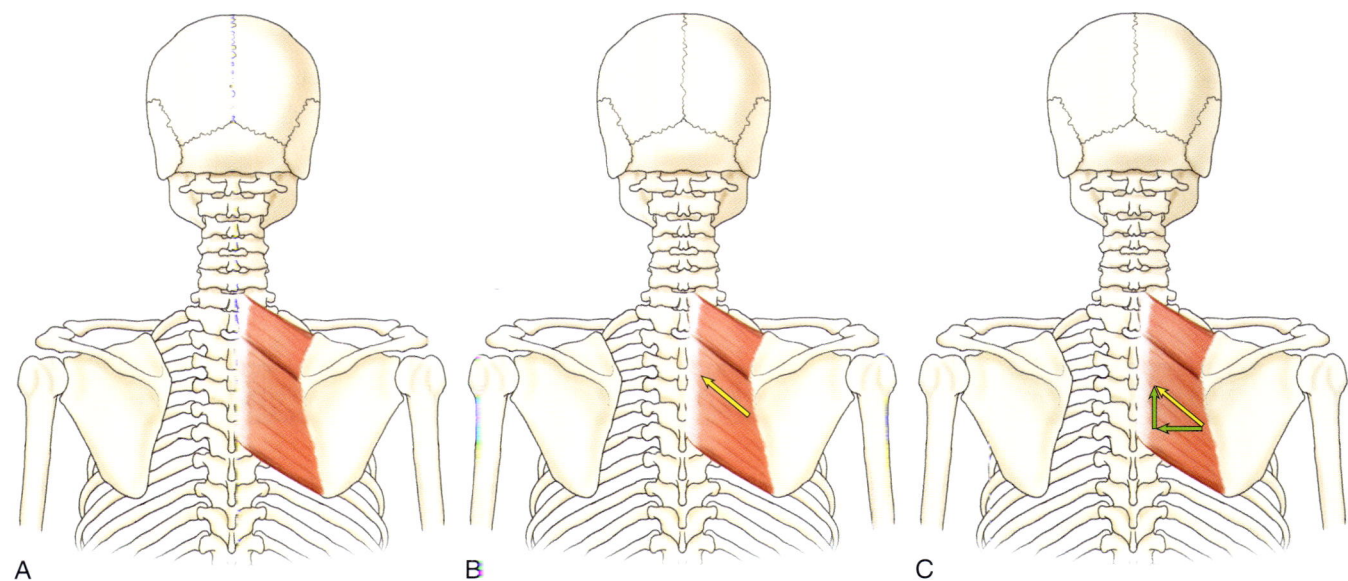

FIGURE 6-34 A, Rhomboid muscles. **B,** Vector arrow drawn in yellow represents the direction of fibers and resultant line of pull of the rhomboids on the scapula. **C,** This vector arrow of the rhomboids resolved into component green vectors that represent the cardinal plane actions of the rhomboids.

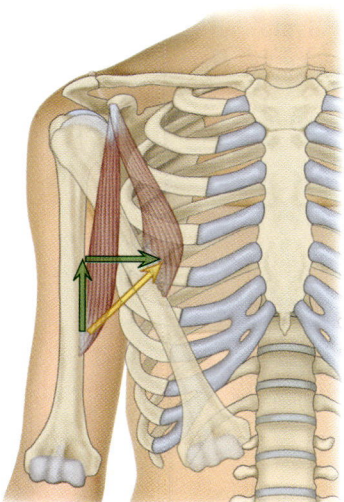

FIGURE 6-35 Vector analysis of the action(s) of the right coracobrachialis muscle. The yellow arrow represents the overall pull of the coracobrachialis on the arm at the shoulder joint. Resolving this vector, we draw in a vertical and a horizontal vector (drawn in green) that begin at the tail of the yellow arrow and end at the head of the yellow arrow. The vertical vector represents the muscle's ability to flex the arm; the horizontal vector represents the muscle's ability to adduct the arm. By resolving the vector that represents the line of pull of the coracobrachialis, we see that the coracobrachialis can both flex and adduct the arm at the shoulder joint.

REVIEW QUESTIONS

Answers to the following review questions appear on the Evolve website accompanying this book at: http://evolve.elsevier.com/Muscolino/kinesiology/.

1. What is the primary function of a joint?

2. What is the relationship between the stability and mobility of a joint?

3. What is the main function of a muscle?

4. What is the main function of a ligament?

5. What is the difference between axial and nonaxial motion?

6. Name two synonyms for axial motion.

7. What is the difference between rectilinear and curvilinear motion?

8. What is the difference between curvlinear motion and axial motion?

9. What are the three fundamental ways in which one bone can move along another bone?

10. What three things must be stated to fully name and describe a joint action?

11. What are the five major joint action terminology pairs used to describe motion?

12. What term is used to describe a movement of the scapula at the scapulocostal joint in which the glenoid fossa orients superiorly?

13. What term is used to describe an anterior movement of the mandible at the temporomandibular joints (TMJs)?

14. Within what plane does flexion generally occur?

15. What is the name of the axis for medial and lateral rotation movements?

16. What are the three component cardinal plane actions of opposition of the thumb at its saddle joint?

17. What are the two manners in which the term *hyperextension* can be used?

18. Why is circumduction not an action?

19. How do we describe the actions of a muscle with a line of pull in an oblique plane?

20. What is a reverse action?

21. What is the reverse action of flexion of the right forearm at the elbow joint?

22. What is the reverse action of flexion of the left thigh at the hip joint?

23. What is a vector?

24. How can knowledge of vectors be helpful in the study of kinesiology?

REFERENCES

1. Oatis CA: Kinesiology: The mechanics and pathomechanics of human movement, Philadelphia, 2004, Lippincott Williams & Wilkins.
2. Watkins J: Structure and function of the musculoskeletal system, Champaign, IL, 1999, Human Kinetics.
3. Neumann DA: Kinesiology of the musculoskeletal system: Foundations for physical rehabilitation, ed 3, St Louis, 2017, Elsevier.
4. Palastanga N, Field D, Soames R: Anatomy and human movement, ed 4, Oxford, 2002, Butterworth-Heinemann.
5. Muscolino JE: The muscular system manual: The skeletal muscles of the human body, ed 4, St. Louis, 2017, Elsevier.
6. McGinnis PM: Biomechanics of sport and exercise, ed 2, Champaign, IL, 2005, Human Kinetics.
7. Hammill J, Knutzen KM: Biomechanical basis of human movement, ed 2, Baltimore, 2003, Lippincott Williams & Wilkins.
8. Levangie PK, Norkin CC: Joint structure and function: A comprehensive analysis, ed 5, Philadelphia, 2001, FA Davis.
9. Hall SJ: Basic biomechanics, ed 6, New York, 2012, McGraw Hill.
10. Dail NW, Agnew TA, Floyd RT: Kinesiology for manual therapies, New York, 2011, McGraw Hill.
11. Kapandji TA: The physiology of the joints: Volume one: Upper limbs, ed 5, Edinburgh, 2002, Churchill Livingstone.
12. Dimon Jr. T: Anatomy of the moving body: A basic course in bones, muscles, and joints, Berkeley, CA, 2011, North Atlantic Books.
13. Hamilton N, Weimar W, Luttgens K: Kinesiology: Scientific basis of human motion, ed 12, New York, 2012, McGraw Hill.
14. Enoka RM: Neuromechanics of human movement, ed 3, Champaign, IL, 2002, Human Kinetics.

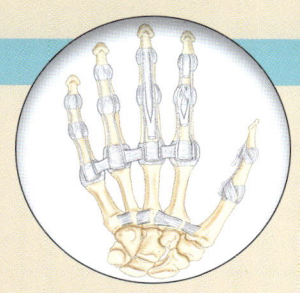

CHAPTER 7
Classification of Joints

CHAPTER OUTLINE

Section 7.1	Anatomy of a Joint	Section 7.8	Cartilaginous Joints
Section 7.2	Physiology of a Joint	Section 7.9	Synovial Joints
Section 7.3	Joint Mobility versus Joint Stability	Section 7.10	Uniaxial Synovial Joints
Section 7.4	Joints and Shock Absorption	Section 7.11	Biaxial Synovial Joints
Section 7.5	Weight-Bearing Joints	Section 7.12	Triaxial Synovial Joints
Section 7.6	Joint Classification	Section 7.13	Nonaxial Synovial Joints
Section 7.7	Fibrous Joints	Section 7.14	Menisci and Articular Discs

CHAPTER OBJECTIVES

After completing this chapter, the student should be able to perform the following:

1. Define the key terms of this chapter and state the meanings of the word origins of this chapter.
2. Describe the anatomy of a joint.
3. Describe the physiology of a joint, and explain the function of joints, muscles, and ligaments/joint capsules.
4. Describe the relationship between joint mobility and joint stability, and list the three major determinants of the mobility/stability of a joint.
5. Explain the importance of shock absorption and weight bearing to joints.
6. Do the following related to joint classification:
   ○ List and describe the three major structural categories of joints.
   ○ List and describe the three major functional categories of joints.
   ○ Explain the relationship between the structural and functional categories of joints.
   ○ List and describe the three categories of fibrous joints; give an example of each of the categories of fibrous joints.
   ○ List and describe the two categories of cartilaginous joints; give an example of each of the categories of cartilaginous joints.
7. Do the following related to synovial joints:
   ○ List the structural components of, and draw a typical synovial joint.
   ○ Discuss the roles of ligaments and muscles in a synovial joint.
   ○ List and describe the four categories of synovial joints.
   ○ Describe and give examples of the two types of uniaxial synovial joints.
   ○ Describe and give examples of the two types of biaxial synovial joints.
   ○ Describe and give examples of triaxial synovial joints.
   ○ Describe and give examples of nonaxial synovial joints.
8. Explain the purpose of menisci and articular discs, and give an example of each one.

OVERVIEW

The discussion of motion in the body began in Chapter 2 and continued in Chapter 6. Chapter 7 now deepens the exploration of motion by examining the structural and functional characteristics of joints of the body. Specifically, shock absorption, weight bearing, and the concept of mobility versus stability are addressed. This chapter then continues by laying out the classification system for all joints of the body. The three major structural categories of joints (fibrous, cartilaginous, and synovial) are each examined. A special emphasis is placed on synovial joints; their four major categories (uniaxial, biaxial, triaxial, and nonaxial) are discussed in detail. The chapter concludes with a look at the role of articular discs and menisci within joints.

KEY TERMS

Amphiarthrotic joint (amphiarthrosis, pl. amphiarthroses) (AM-fee-are-THROT-ik, AM-fee-are-THROS-is, AM-fee-are-THROS-eez)
Articular cartilage (ar-TIK-you-lar)
Articular disc
Articulation (ar-TIK-you-LAY-shun)
Ball-and-socket joint
Biaxial joint (bye-AK-see-al)
Cartilaginous joint (kar-ti-LAJ-in-us)
Closed-packed position
Compound joint
Condyloid joint (KON-di-loyd)
Congruent (kon-GREW-ent)
Degrees of freedom
Diarthrotic joint (diarthrosis, pl. diarthroses) (DIE-are-THROT-ik, DIE-are-THROS-is, DIE-are-THROS-eez)
Ellipsoid joint (ee-LIPS-oid)
Extra-articular (EKS-tra-ar-TIK-you-lar)
Fibrous joint
Functional joint
Ginglymus joint (GING-la-mus)
Gliding joints
Gomphosis, pl. gomphoses (gom-FOS-is, gom-FOS-eez)
Hinge joint
Intra-articular (IN-tra-ar-TIK-you-lar)
Irregular joints
Joint
Joint capsule (KAP-sool)
Joint cavity
Meniscus, pl. menisci (men-IS-kus, men-IS-KIY)

Mobility
Nonaxial joints (non-AKS-ee-al)
Open-packed position
Ovoid joint (O-void)
Pivot joint
Plane joint
Polyaxial joint (PA-lee-AKS-ee-al)
Saddle joint
Sellar joint (SEL-ar)
Shock absorption
Simple joint
Stability
Structural joint
Suture joint (SOO-chur)
Symphysis joint (SIM-fa-sis)
Synarthrotic joint (synarthrosis, pl. synarthroses) (SIN-are-THROT-ik, SIN-are-THROS-is, SIN-are-THROS-eez)
Synchondrosis joint, pl. synchondroses (SIN-kon-DROS-is, SIN-kon-DROS-seez)
Syndesmosis, pl. syndesmoses (SIN-des-MO-sis, SIN-des-MO-seez)
Synostosis, pl. synostoses (SIN-ost-O-sis, SIN-ost-O-seez)
Synovial cavity (sin-O-vee-al)
Synovial fluid
Synovial joint
Synovial membrane
Triaxial joint (try-AKS-see-al)
Trochoid joint (TRO-koid)
Uniaxial joint (YOU-nee-AKS-see-al)
Weight-bearing joint

WORD ORIGINS

- Amphi—From Greek *amphi*, meaning *on both sides, around*
- Bi—From Latin *bis*, meaning *two, twice*
- Cavity—From Latin *cavus*, meaning *hollow, concavity*
- Congruent—From Latin *congruere*, meaning *to come together*
- Di—From Greek *dis*, meaning *two, twice*
- Ellips—From Greek *elleipsis*, meaning *oval*
- Extra—From Latin *extra*, meaning *outside, beyond*
- Ginglymus—From Greek *ginglymos*, meaning *hinge joint*
- Intra—From Latin *intra*, meaning *within, inner*
- Meniscus—From Greek *meniskos*, meaning *crescent moon*
- Non—From Latin *non*, meaning *not, other than*
- Ovial—From Latin *ovum*, meaning *egg*
- Plane—From Latin *planus*, meaning *flat*
- Poly—From Greek *polys*, meaning *many*
- Sella—From Latin *sella*, meaning *chair, saddle*
- Stabile—From Latin *stabilis*, meaning *stationary, resistant to change* (i.e., resistant to movement)
- Sym—From Greek *syn*, meaning *together, with* (Note: *sym* is the same prefix root as *syn*; *sym* appears before words that begin with *b, p, ph,* or *m*.)
- Syn—From Greek *syn*, meaning *together, with*
- Tri—From Latin *tres*, meaning *three*
- Uni—From Latin *unus*, meaning *one*

SECTION 7.1 ANATOMY OF A JOINT

- Structurally, a **joint** is defined as a place of juncture between two or more bones.[1] At this juncture, the bones are joined to one another by soft tissue.
  - In other words, structurally, a joint is defined as a place where two or more bones are joined to one another by soft tissue.
  - A typical joint involves two bones; however, more than two bones may be involved in a joint. For example, the elbow joint incorporates three bones: the humerus, radius, and ulna. Any joint that involves three or more bones of the skeleton is called a **compound joint**. In contrast, the term **simple joint** is sometimes used to describe a joint that has only two bones.[2]
- The type of soft tissue that connects the two bones of a joint to each other determines the structural classification of the joint (Box 7-1). (For more information on the structural classification of joints, see Section 7.6.)
  - The following are the three major structural classifications of a joint[3]:
    - Fibrous
    - Cartilaginous
    - Synovial
- A joint is also known as an **articulation**.[4]
- Figure 7-1 illustrates the components of a typical joint of the body. (Note: It should be stated that there really is no typical joint of the body. As will be seen later in the chapter, many different types of joints exist, both structurally and functionally.)

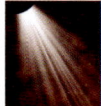

BOX 7-1 Spotlight on Structural versus Functional Joints

The definition of a joint as bones connected to each other by soft tissue is a structural definition. As explained in Section 7.2, the function of a joint is to allow movement; so functionally a joint is defined by its ability to allow movement. These structural and functional definitions usually coincide with each other (i.e., a structural joint is a functional joint and a functional joint is a structural joint). However, sometimes they do not perfectly match each other. The scapulocostal joint between the scapula and ribcage is an example of a joint that allows movement between the bones but is not a structural joint because the bones are not attached to each other by soft tissue (fibrous, cartilaginous, or synovial). For this reason, the scapulocostal joint cannot be defined as a structural joint but is considered to be a **functional joint**.[1] Another example of the difference between the structural definition of a joint and the functional definition of a joint is the knee joint. Structurally, the distal femur, proximal tibia, and patella are all connected to one another and enclosed within one joint capsule; therefore all these bones constitute one **structural joint**.[1] However, this one structural joint would be considered to be a number of separate functional joints, because the functional movement of the femur and patella and of the femur and tibia are somewhat independent of each other. Many physiologists/kinesiologists would even divide the tibiofemoral joint (between the tibia and femur) into the medial tibiofemoral joint and the lateral tibiofemoral joint because the two condyles of the femur move somewhat independently of each other on the tibia!

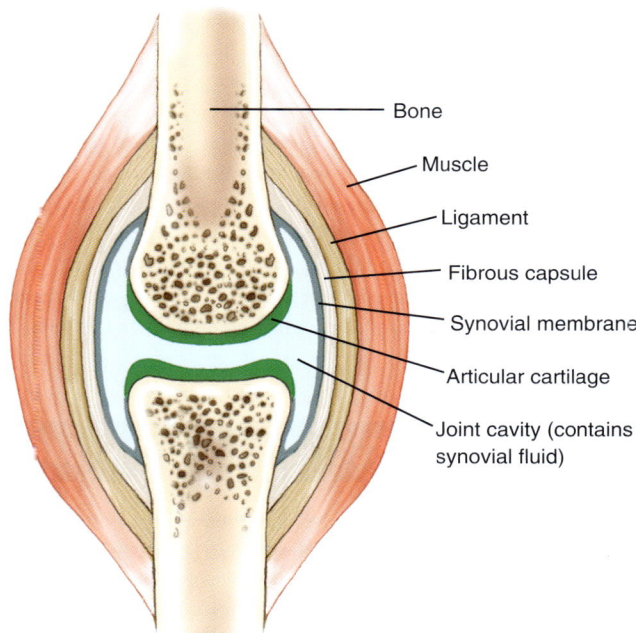

FIGURE 7-1 Typical joint (in this case a synovial joint is shown). The major features of this joint include a space between the two bones; this space is bounded by a capsule and is filled with fluid. Furthermore, ligaments connect the two bones of the joint to each other, and muscles cross this joint by attaching from one bone of the joint to the other bone of the joint.

SECTION 7.2 PHYSIOLOGY OF A JOINT

- The main function of a joint is to allow movement.
- As we have seen, a joint contains a space between the two bones. At this space, the bones can move relative to each other. Figure 7-2 illustrates motion at a joint.
- There actually are joints in the human body that do not allow movement. However, they exist because they once did allow movement in the past. An example would be the joint between a

tooth and the maxilla. When the tooth was "coming in," movement was necessary for the tooth to descend and erupt through the maxilla. However, no movement occurs between the tooth and the maxilla now. Another example that is often given is that of the suture joints of the skull. These joints once required movement to allow the passage of the baby's head through the birth canal of the mother. Once the child has been born and grows to

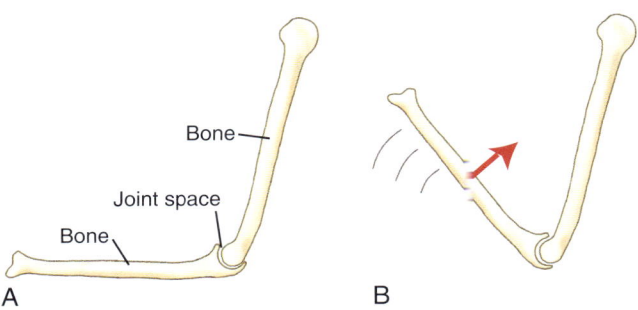

FIGURE 7-2 Illustration of how motion of one bone relative to the other bone of the joint occurs around the space of the joint.

maturity, movement is no longer needed at these suture joints and they often fuse. It must be emphasized that if no movement were needed at a certain point in the body, then there would be no need to have a joint there. Structurally, our body would be far more stable if we had a solid skeleton that was made up of one bone, with no joints located in it at all. However, we do need movement to occur, so at each location where movement is desired, a break or space exists between bones and a joint is formed. It can be useful to think of the Tin Man in the film *The Wizard of Oz*. When he was first found, it was as if he had no joints at all because the spaces of the joints were all rusted together. Then as Dorothy applied oil to each spot, the joints began to function and could once again allow movement.
- When we say that the main function of a joint is to allow movement, the word *allow* must be emphasized. A joint is a passive structure that allows movement to occur; it does not create the movement.
- As will be learned in later chapters, it is the musculature that crosses the joint that contracts to *create* the movement that occurs at a joint.
- In addition, it is the ligaments/joint capsules that connect the bones to each other to keep the bones from moving too far from each other (i.e., dislocating) and therefore *limit* the movement at a joint.

Therefore we can state the following three general rules[1] (Box 7-2):
- Joints *allow* movement.
- Muscles *create* movement.
- Ligament/joint capsules *limit* movement.

BOX 7-2

These rules, although generally true, are a bit simplistic. Muscle contractions are the primary means by which joint motion occurs. However, it is more correct to say that the role of a muscle contraction is actually to create a force on the bones of a joint. That force can create movement at the joint; however, the force of the muscle contraction can also stop or modify movement. A clinical application of this knowledge is that a tight muscle that crosses a joint will limit the motion of the joint by not allowing the bones to move. The motion that will be limited will be the movement in the opposite direction from where this tight muscle is located. For more information on this concept, see Chapter 16.

SECTION 7.3 JOINT MOBILITY VERSUS JOINT STABILITY

- By definition, a joint is mobile. However, a joint must also be sufficiently stable so that it maintains its structural integrity (i.e., it does not dislocate).
- Every joint of the body finds a balance between **mobility** and **stability**[5] (Box 7-3).

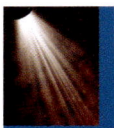

BOX 7-3 Spotlight on Closed-Packed and Open-Packed Joint Positions

Each joint of the body has a position in which it is most stable; this position is known as its **closed-packed position**.[1] The stable, closed-packed position of a joint is usually the result of a combination of the position of the bones such that they are maximally congruent (i.e., their articular surfaces best fit each other) and the ligaments are most taut. These two factors result in a position that restricts motion and therefore increases stability.[1] The **open-packed position** of a joint is effectively the opposite of the closed-packed position; it is any position of the joint wherein the combination of the congruence of the bony fit is poor and the ligaments are lax, resulting in greater mobility but poorer stability of the joint.[1]

- The more mobile a joint is, the less stable it is.
  - The price to pay for greater mobility is less stability.
  - Less stability means a joint has a greater chance for injury.
- The more stable a joint is, the less mobile it is.
  - The price to pay for greater stability is less mobility.
  - Less mobility means that a joint has a decreased ability to move and place body parts in certain positions.
- Therefore mobility and stability are antagonistic concepts; more of one means less of the other!

The following are three major factors that determine the balance of mobility and stability of a joint[5]:
- The shape of the bones of the joint
- The ligament/joint capsule complex of the joint (Note: Ligaments and joint capsules are both made up of the same fibrous material, and both act to limit motion of a joint; therefore they can be grouped together as the ligament/joint capsule complex.)
- The musculature of the joint
  - Because a muscle crosses a joint (by attaching via its tendons to the bones of the joint), the more massive a muscle is, the more stability it lends to the joint. However, this greater stability also means less mobility. For this reason, people who work out and have very large muscle mass are sometimes

referred to as being *muscle-bound*. If the baseline tone of the musculature that crosses a joint is high (i.e., the muscles are tight), stability increases even more and mobility decreases commensurately. (For more information regarding the concept of stabilization of a joint by a muscle, see Section 14.7.)
- These concepts are well illustrated by comparing the mobility/stability of the shoulder joint with that of the hip joint. The shoulder joint and hip joint are both the same type of joint—ball-and-socket joint. However, the shoulder joint is much more mobile and much less stable than the hip joint; conversely, the hip joint is much more stable and much less mobile than the shoulder joint.

Comparing these two joints with each other, we see three things:
1. The bony shape of the socket of the shoulder joint (i.e., the glenoid fossa of the scapula) is much shallower than the socket of the hip joint (i.e., the acetabulum) (Figure 7-3).
2. The ligament/joint capsule complex of the shoulder joint is much looser than the ligament/joint capsule complex of the hip joint.
3. The musculature crossing the shoulder joint is less massive than the musculature crossing the hip joint.
   - The advantage of the greater mobility of the shoulder joint is the increased motion, allowing the hand to be placed in a greater variety of positions. However, the disadvantage of the greater mobility of the shoulder joint is a higher frequency of injury.

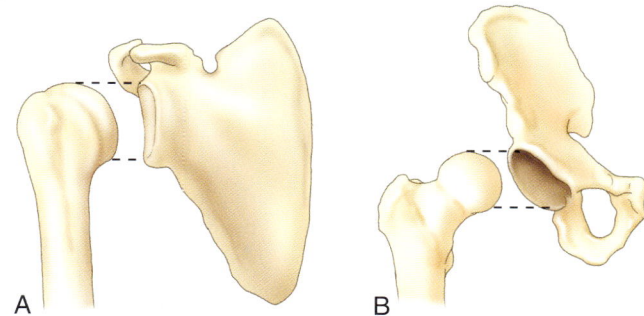

FIGURE 7-3 A, Shallow socket (glenoid fossa of the scapula) of the shoulder joint. **B,** Deep socket (acetabulum of the pelvis bone) of the hip joint. Shallowness/depth of the socket affects the relative mobility versus stability of the joint.

- The advantage of the greater stability of the hip joint is the low frequency of injury. The disadvantage of the greater stability of the hip joint is the inability to place the foot in as great a variety of positions.
- It is actually possible to have great mobility and great stability at a joint. This is accomplished via the soft tissues of the joint. If the muscles and the ligament/joint capsule tissues are loose, mobility is increased. However, if the muscles are developed and strong, stability is also increased. Dancers are an excellent example of people whose joints are both flexible and stable.

SECTION 7.4 JOINTS AND SHOCK ABSORPTION

- In addition to allowing motion to occur, a joint may also serve the purpose of **shock absorption** for the body. In addition to the soft tissue located between the bones of a joint, many joints also have fluid located in a capsule of the joint. This fluid can be very helpful toward absorbing shock waves that are transmitted through the joint.[5] (See Section 7.9 for a discussion of synovial joints, which have fluid located within a joint cavity.)
- Although all joints have the ability to absorb shock, lower extremity and spinal joints are especially important for providing shock absorption, given the forces that enter our body whenever we walk, run, or jump and hit the ground.[7] The force of our body weight hitting the ground causes an equivalent force to be transmitted up through our body.[1] The fluid located in the joints of our lower extremities and the joints of our spine can help to absorb and dampen this shock. Figure 7-4 illustrates this concept.
- Note: Our joints function to absorb and dampen shock in a similar manner to the shock absorbers of a car. A car's shock absorber is a cylinder filled with fluid. When the car hits a pothole or a bump, the fluid within the shock absorber absorbs and dampens the compression force that occurs (i.e., the shock wave that would otherwise be transmitted to the rest of the car, as well as the people sitting within the car).

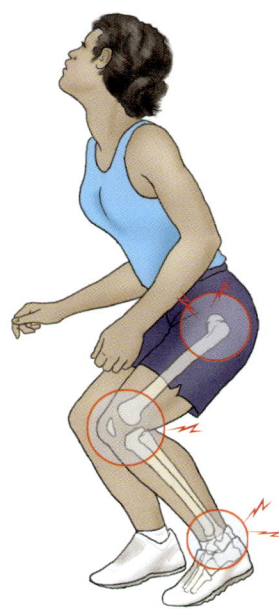

FIGURE 7-4 Joints of the lower extremity help to absorb shock when a person lands on the ground after having jumped up into the air. All weight-bearing joints, including the joints of the spine, would help with shock absorption in this scenario.

SECTION 7.5 WEIGHT-BEARING JOINTS

- Many joints of the body are **weight-bearing joints**. A joint is a weight-bearing joint if the weight of the body is borne through that joint.
- Many textbooks describe weight bearing as another function of some of the joints of our body. Although it is certainly true that many of the joints of our body have the additional function of bearing weight, bearing weight is not a reason for a joint to exist in the first place. Weight bearing places a stress on a joint that requires greater stability. By definition, a joint allows movement, which, by definition, decreases stability. If weight bearing is the goal, and stability is therefore needed, the body would be better off not even having a joint in that location. If, for example, the lower extremity did not have a knee joint, and the entire lower extremity were one bone instead of having a separate femur and tibia, the lower extremity would be much more stable and able to bear the weight of the body through it more efficiently. Having the knee joint allows for movement there and decreases the stability of the lower extremity; therefore it does not help with weight bearing. Of course, once present, the knee joint does now have the added responsibility of bearing weight. Perhaps it is better to say that it is a characteristic, not a function, of some joints that they bear weight.
- Almost all joints of the lower extremities, and the joints of the spine are weight-bearing joints[7] (Box 7-4). In addition to allowing movement, these joints must also be able to bear the weight of the body parts that are above them.

BOX 7-4

The disc joints of the spine have the major responsibility of weight bearing. The facet joints of the spine are meant primarily to guide movement. (See Section 8.4 for more details.)

- Because of the stress of bearing weight, weight-bearing joints tend to be more stable and less mobile.
- Because a greater proportion of body weight is above joints that are lower in the body, the amount of weight-bearing stress that a joint must bear is greater for the joints that are lower in the body. For example, the upper cervical vertebrae need bear only the weight of the head above them; however, the lower lumbar vertebrae must bear the entire weight of the head, neck, trunk, and upper extremities above them. The joints of the ankle and foot have the greatest combined weight of body parts above them and therefore bear the greatest weight.
- Potentially, the weight-bearing stress on the ankle and foot joints is the greatest. However, because two lower extremities exist, the weight-bearing load on them is divided by two when a person is standing on both feet. Of course, when a person is standing on only one foot, the entire weight of the body is borne through the joints of that side's lower extremity.
- Upper extremity joints (and some other miscellaneous joints) are not usually weight-bearing joints.

Figure 7-5 illustrates the weight-bearing joints of the human body.

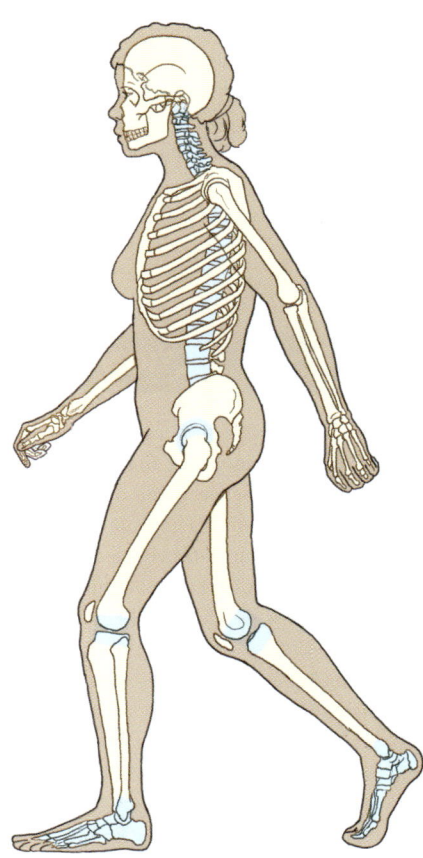

FIGURE 7-5 Weight-bearing joints of the body. Almost all joints of the lower extremities, and the spinal joints of the axial body are weight-bearing joints.

SECTION 7.6 JOINT CLASSIFICATION

- Joints may be classified based on their structure (i.e., the type of soft tissue that connects the bones to one another).
  - Structurally, joints are usually divided into three categories.
- Joints may also be classified based on their function (i.e., the degree of movement that they allow).
  - Functionally, joints are usually divided into three categories.

STRUCTURAL CLASSIFICATION OF JOINTS

- Structurally, joints can be divided into the following three categories: (1) fibrous, (2) cartilaginous, and (3) synovial[3] (Table 7-1).
  - A joint in which the bones are held together by a dense fibrous connective tissue is known as a **fibrous joint**.
  - A joint in which the bones are held together by either fibrocartilage or hyaline cartilage is known as a **cartilaginous joint**.
  - A joint in which the bones are connected by a joint capsule, which is composed of two distinct layers (an outer fibrous layer and an inner synovial layer), is known as a **synovial joint**.
  - It is worth noting that fibrous and cartilaginous joints have no joint cavity; synovial joints do enclose a joint cavity.

TABLE 7-1	Classification of Joints by Structure

- Joints without a joint cavity
  - Fibrous
  - Cartilaginous
- Joints with a joint cavity
  - Synovial

Joints without a Joint Cavity

- Fibrous: Fibrous joints are joints in which dense fibrous tissue attaches the two bones of the joint to each other.
- Cartilaginous: Cartilaginous joints are joints in which cartilaginous tissue attaches the two bones of the joint to each other.[8]

Joints with a Joint Cavity

- Synovial: Synovial joints are joints in which a joint capsule attaches the two bones of the joint to each other.[8]
  - This joint capsule has two layers: (1) an outer fibrous layer and (2) an inner synovial membrane layer.
  - This capsule encloses a synovial cavity, which has synovial fluid within it.
  - The articular ends of the bones are lined with hyaline cartilage.

FUNCTIONAL CLASSIFICATION OF JOINTS

- Functionally, joints can also be divided into three categories: (1) synarthrotic, (2) amphiarthrotic, and (3) diarthrotic[6] (Table 7-2).
  - As in all categories of classification, alternates exist. Another common classification of joints divides them into only two functional categories: (1) synarthroses, lacking a joint cavity,

TABLE 7-2	Classification of Joints by Function
Synarthrotic	Synarthrotic joints are joints that allow very little or no movement.
Amphiarthrotic	Amphiarthrotic joints are joints that allow a moderate but limited amount of movement.
Diarthrotic	Diarthrotic joints are joints that are freely moveable and allow a great deal of movement.

and (2) diarthroses, possessing a joint cavity.[7] Synarthroses are then divided into synostoses (united by bony tissue), synchondroses (united by cartilaginous tissue), and syndesmoses (united by fibrous tissue).[9] Diarthroses are synovial joints (united by a capsule enclosing a joint cavity).

- A joint that allows very little or no movement is known as a **synarthrotic joint**[9] (**synarthrosis**; plural: synarthroses).
- A joint that allows a moderate but limited amount of movement is known as an **amphiarthrotic joint**[6] (**amphiarthrosis**; plural: amphiarthroses).
- A joint that is freely moveable and allows a great deal of movement is known as a **diarthrotic joint**[9] (**diarthrosis**; plural: diarthroses).
- It is worth noting that although general agreement exists among sources as to the classification of joints into three categories based on movement, the exact delineation among these relative amounts of movement may differ at times.
- It is a major principle of anatomy and physiology that structure and function are intimately related to each other. It is often said that structure determines function. That is, the anatomy of a body part determines what the physiology of the body part will be. Relating this to the study of joints, the structure of a joint determines the motion possible at that joint.
- Therefore although joints may be divided into three categories by structure, and joints may also be divided into three categories by function (i.e., movement), it is important to realize that these three structural and these three functional categories are related to each other. They are only different categories based on whether the perspective is that of an anatomist, who looks at structure, or that of a physiologist or kinesiologist, who looks at function.
- Therefore the following general correlations can be made (Table 7-3):
  - Fibrous joints are synarthrotic joints.[7]
  - Cartilaginous joints are amphiarthrotic joints.[6]
  - Synovial joints are diarthrotic joints.[7]

TABLE 7-3	Joint Classifications
Fibrous	Synarthrotic
Cartilaginous	Amphiarthrotic
Synovial	Diarthrotic

SECTION 7.7 FIBROUS JOINTS

- Fibrous joints are joints in which the soft tissue that unites the bones is a dense fibrous connective tissue; hence a fibrous joint has no joint cavity (Table 7-4; Figure 7-6).
- Fibrous joints typically permit very little or no movement; therefore they are considered to be synarthrotic joints.

TABLE 7-4	Types of Synarthrotic Fibrous Joints
Syndesmosis	Bones united by a fibrous ligament or an aponeurosis
Suture	Bones united by a thin layer of fibrous material
Gomphosis	Peg-in-hole–shaped bones united by fibrous material

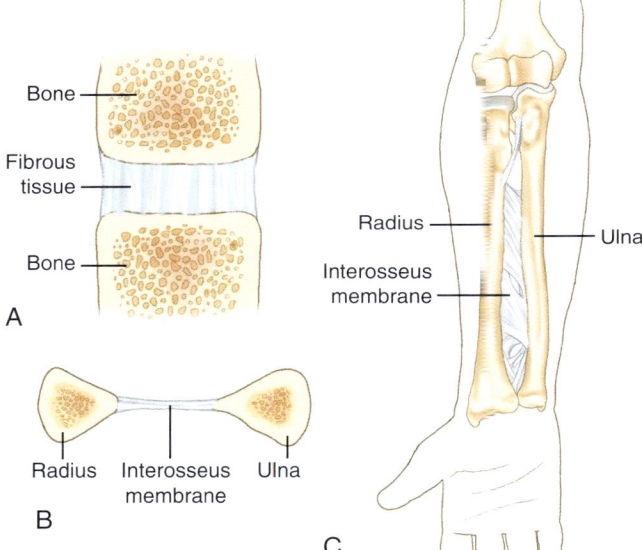

FIGURE 7-6 **A**, Fibrous tissue that unites the two bones of a fibrous joint. **B** and **C**, Cross-sectional and anterior views of the interosseus membrane of the forearm that unites the radius and ulna. Structurally, the interosseus membrane of the forearm is a fibrous syndesmosis joint.

- Three types of fibrous joints exist[5]:
  - Syndesmosis joints
  - Suture joints
  - Gomphosis joints

SYNDESMOSIS JOINTS

- In a **syndesmosis joint**, a fibrous ligament or fibrous aponeurotic membrane unites the bones of the joint.[5]
- Syndesmoses permit a small amount of movement between the two bones of the joint.
- The interosseus membrane between the radius and ulna is an example of a syndesmosis joint (see Figure 7-6, *B* and *C*).
- The interosseus membrane between the tibia and fibula is another example of a syndesmosis joint.

SUTURE JOINTS:

- In a **suture joint**, a thin layer of fibrous tissue unites the two bones of the joint.[5]
- Suture joints are found only in the skull (Figure 7-7).
- A small amount of movement is permitted at these joints early in life.
- The principal purpose of the suture joints is to allow the bones of the skull of a baby to move relative to one other to allow easier passage through the birth canal during delivery of the baby.
- Suture joints are usually considered to allow little or no movement later in life, but controversy exists regarding this (Box 7-5).

BOX 7-5

A great deal of controversy exists regarding the ability of suture joints to move. A major premise of craniosacral (also known as sacro-occipital) technique is that suture joints allow an appreciable amount of movement. Part of their technique is to manipulate the bones of the skull at the suture joints for the purpose of aiding the movement of cerebrospinal fluid. Although some degree of motion does remain at the suture joints, study of the skulls of adults shows that these joints do tend to become synostotic as we get older (a **synostosis** is a joint that has fused over with bone).

GOMPHOSIS JOINTS:

- In a **gomphosis joint**, fibrous tissue unites two bony components with surfaces that are adapted to each other like a peg in a hole[5] (Figure 7-8).
- This type of joint is found only between the teeth and the mandible, or the teeth and the maxilla.
- Gomphoses permit movement of the teeth relative to the mandible or the maxilla early in life, but in an adult no movement is permitted in a gomphosis joint.

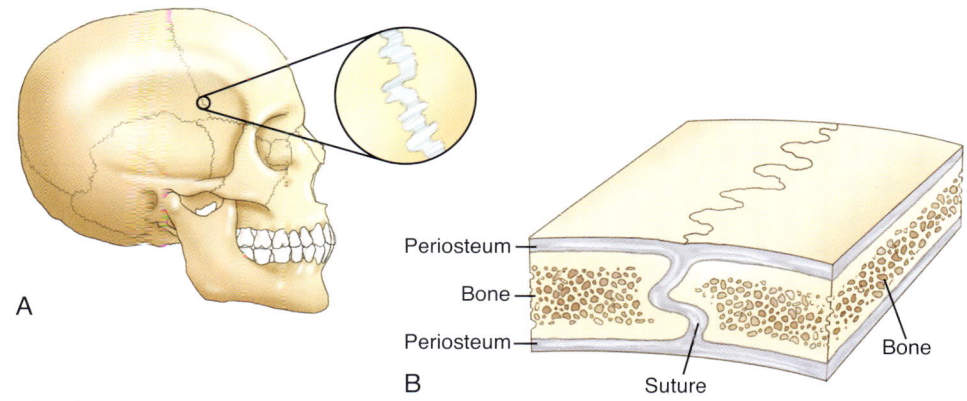

FIGURE 7-7 **A,** Lateral view that illustrates the coronal suture of the skull that is located between the frontal and parietal bones. Structurally, this joint is a fibrous suture. **B,** Cross-sectional view of the same suture joint.

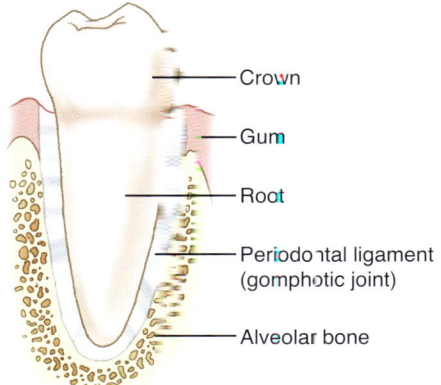

FIGURE 7-8 View of the joint between a tooth and the adjacent bone. The crown of the tooth is located above the gum line, and the root of the tooth is located below the gum line. The periodontal ligament is the fibrous tissue of the gomphotic joint. Structurally, this joint is a fibrous gomphosis joint.

SECTION 7.8 CARTILAGINOUS JOINTS

- Cartilaginous joints are joints in which the soft tissue that unites the bones is cartilaginous connective tissue (usually fibrocartilage, but occasionally hyaline cartilage); hence a cartilaginous joint has no joint cavity.[5]
- Cartilaginous joints typically permit a moderate but limited amount of movement; therefore they are considered to be amphiarthrotic joints.
- Two types of cartilaginous joints exist[6]:
  - Symphysis joints
  - Synchondrosis joints

SYMPHYSIS JOINTS

- In a **symphysis joint**, fibrocartilage in the form of a disc unites the bodies of two adjacent bones.[5] (The term *body* of a bone is usually used to refer to the largest aspect of a bone.) These fibrocartilaginous discs can be quite thick. Consequently, although not allowing the extent of motion that a diarthrotic synovial joint allows, cartilaginous joints can allow a moderate amount of motion.
- An example of a cartilaginous symphysis joint is the intervertebral disc joint of the spine (Figure 7-9, *A*).
  - Technically, an intervertebral disc joint could be considered to have a joint cavity filled with fluid. The cavity is enclosed by the fibrocartilaginous annular fibers and the fluid is the "pulpy" nucleus pulposus. (For more on intervertebral discs, see Section 8.4.)
- Another example is the symphysis pubis joint of the pelvis (Figure 7-9, *B*).

SYNCHONDROSIS JOINTS

- In a **synchondrosis joint**, hyaline cartilage unites the two bones of the joint.[5]
- An example of a cartilaginous synchondrosis joint is the cartilage (i.e., costal cartilage) that is located between a rib and the sternum (Figure 7-10, *A*).
- The growth plate (i.e., epiphysial disc) of a growing bone may also be considered to be another type of synchondrosis joint (Figure 7-10, *B*).
  - Eventually a growth plate ossifies and only a remnant, the epiphysial line, remains.[1] Many sources do not consider the epiphysial disc of a growing bone to be another type of synchondrosis joint, because the main purpose of the growth plate is growth, not movement.[1] (For more information on growth plates, see Section 3.6.)

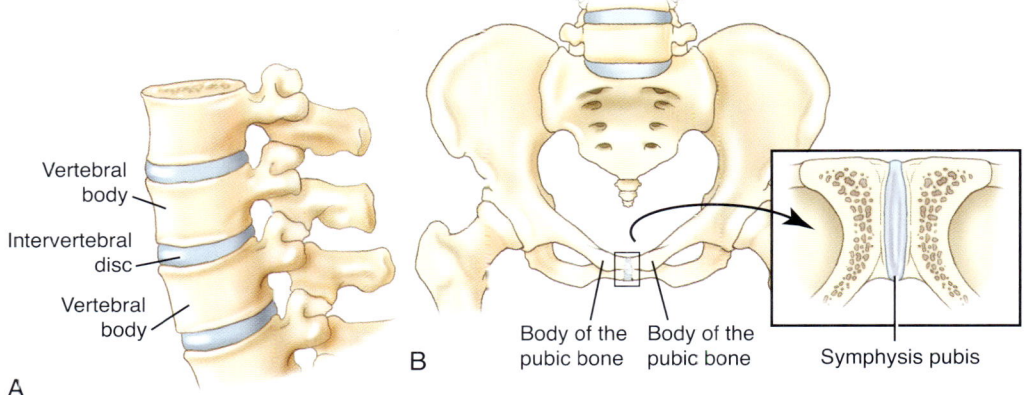

FIGURE 7-9 A, Lateral view that illustrates an intervertebral disc joint located between adjacent vertebral bodies of the spine. Structurally, this joint is a cartilaginous symphysis joint. **B,** Anterior view of the pelvis (with a close-up view in the inset box) that illustrates the symphysis pubis joint between the right and left bodies of the pubic bones of the pelvis. Structurally, this joint is a cartilaginous symphysis joint.

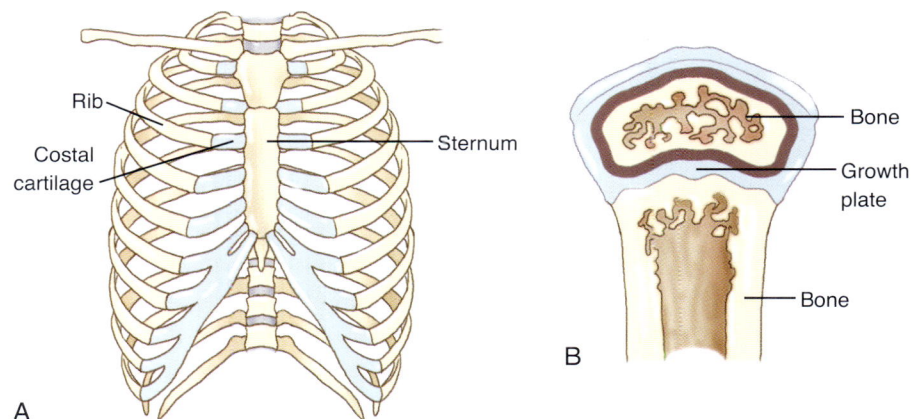

FIGURE 7-10 A, Anterior view of the ribcage. A costal cartilage is an example of a cartilaginous synchondrosis joint that unites a rib with the sternum. Structurally it is a cartilaginous synchondrosis joint. **B,** Growth plate (epiphysial disc) between the adjacent regions of bony tissue of a developing long bone. This is an example of a temporary, cartilaginous synchondrosis joint.

SECTION 7.9   SYNOVIAL JOINTS

- Structurally, synovial joints are the most complicated joints of the body.
- They are also the joints that most people think of when they think of joints. The wrist, elbow, shoulder, ankle, knee, and hip joints are a few examples of synovial joints.

COMPONENTS OF A SYNOVIAL JOINT

- The bones of a synovial joint are connected by a **joint capsule**, which encloses a **joint cavity**.[5]
- This joint capsule is composed of two distinct layers: (1) an outer fibrous layer and (2) an inner **synovial membrane** layer[5] (Table 7-5).
- The inner synovial membrane layer secretes **synovial fluid** into the joint cavity, also known as the **synovial cavity**.[6]
- Furthermore, the articular ends of the bones are capped with **articular cartilage** (i.e., hyaline cartilage).[3]
- Synovial joints are the only joints of the body that possess a joint cavity.
- By virtue of the presence of a joint cavity, synovial joints typically allow a great deal of movement; hence they are considered to be diarthrotic joints.

Figure 7-11 illustrates some examples of synovial joints.

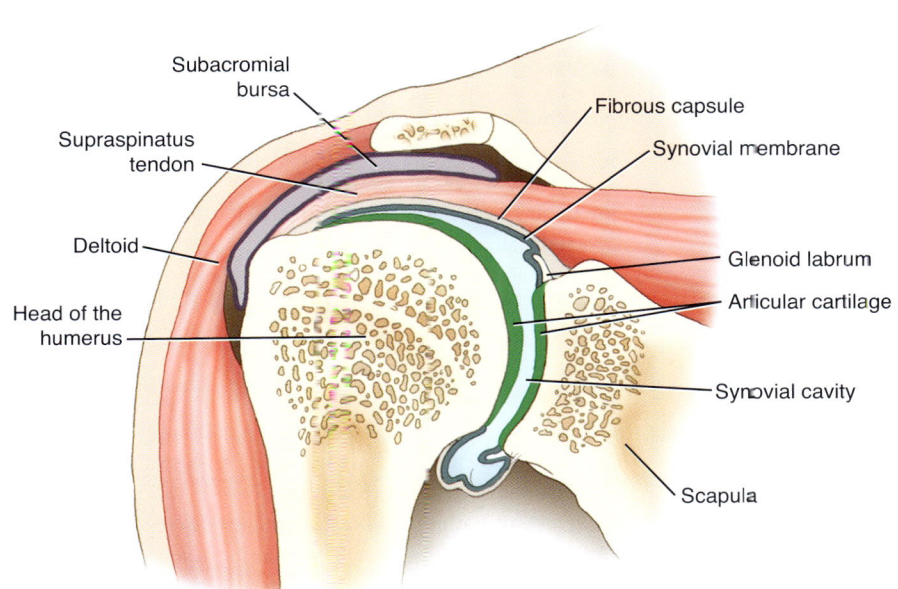
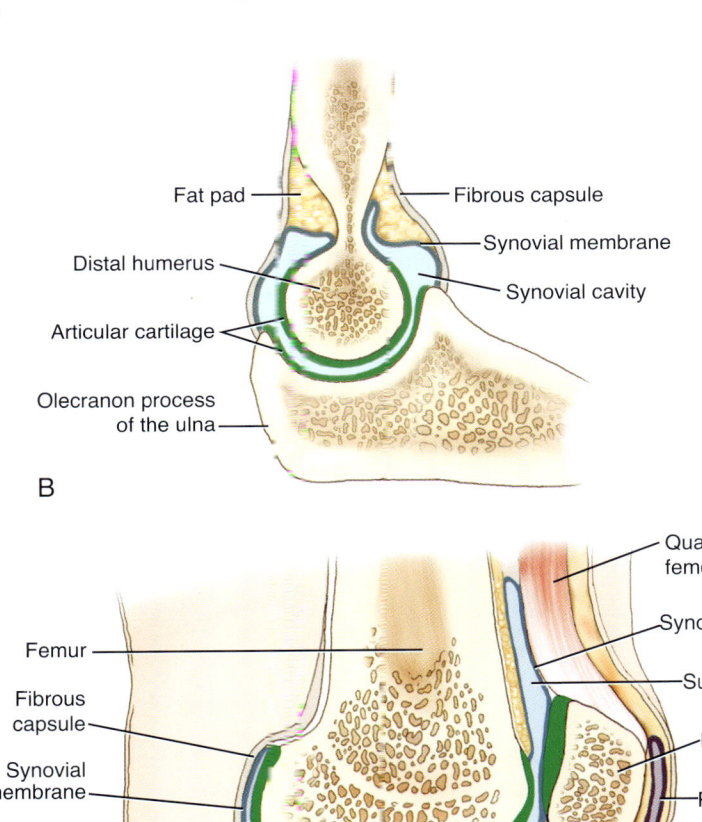

FIGURE 7-11 Examples of synovial joints. **A**, Anterior view cross-section of the shoulder joint. **B**, Lateral view cross-section of the elbow (humeroulnar) joint. **C**, Lateral view cross-section of the knee joint.

TABLE 7-5	Components of a Synovial Joint*

Outer fibrous layer of the joint capsule
Inner synovial membrane layer of the joint capsule
Synovial cavity
Synovial fluid
Articular hyaline cartilage lining the articular ends of the bones
Ligaments
Muscles

*Note: Table 7-5 lists the structures of a synovial joint. Ligaments and muscles are placed within this table even though they are usually not located within a synovial joint. Their reason for inclusion here is their role in the functioning of a synovial joint. Although ligaments and muscles do play a role in the functioning of other joints, given the tremendous motion possible at synovial joints, the role of ligaments and muscles in the functioning of synovial joints is extremely important and vital to the concepts of stability and mobility.

ROLES OF LIGAMENTS AND MUSCLES IN A SYNOVIAL JOINT

Ligaments

- By definition, a ligament is a fibrous structure (made primarily of collagen fibers) that attaches from any one structure of the body to any other structure of the body[10] (except a muscle to a bone).
- In the musculoskeletal field, a ligament is defined more narrowly as attaching from one bone to another bone.
- Therefore ligaments cross a joint, attaching the bones of a joint together.
- Evolutionarily, ligaments of a synovial joint formed as thickenings of the outer fibrous layer of the joint capsule.
  - Some ligaments gradually evolved to be completely independent from the fibrous capsule; other ligaments never fully separated and are simply named as thickenings of the fibrous capsule.
- For this reason, the term *ligamentous/joint capsule complex* is often used to describe the ligaments and the joint capsule of a joint together.
- Synovial joint ligaments are usually located outside of the joint capsule and are therefore extra-articular; however, occasionally a ligament is located within the joint cavity and is intra-articular.[2]
- Functionally, the purpose of a ligament is to limit motion at a joint.[11]

Muscles

- By definition, a muscle is a soft tissue structure that is specialized to contract.[1]
- A muscle attaches via its tendons to the two bones of a joint. Therefore a muscle connects the two bones of the joint that it crosses to each other.[1]
- Some muscles cross more than one joint and do not attach to every bone of each joint that they cross. For example, the biceps brachii crosses the shoulder and elbow joints, but it attaches proximally to the scapula, and then skips over the humerus to attach distally onto the radius.
- Muscles are nearly always extra-articular. Only a couple of examples can be found of a tendon of a muscle being located intra-articularly (i.e., within a joint cavity). The long head of the biceps brachii runs through the shoulder (i.e., glenohumeral) joint; the proximal tendon of the popliteus is located within the knee joint.[12]
- The major function of a muscle is to contract and generate a force on one or both bones of a joint. This contraction force can move one or both of the bones and create motion at the joint. (The role that muscles play in the musculoskeletal system is covered in much greater depth in Chapters 13 to 15.)

CLASSIFICATION OF SYNOVIAL JOINTS:

- Synovial joints can be divided into four categories based on the number of axes of movement that exist at the joint[4] (Box 7-6):
  1. Uniaxial joint: A uniaxial joint allows motion to occur around one axis, within one plane.
  2. Biaxial joint: A biaxial joint allows motion to occur around two axes, within two planes.
  3. Triaxial joint: A triaxial joint allows motion to occur around three axes, within three planes (a triaxial joint is also known as a polyaxial joint).
  4. Nonaxial joint: A nonaxial joint allows motion to occur within a plane, but this motion is a gliding type of motion and does not occur around an axis.

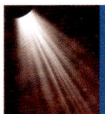

BOX 7-6　Spotlight on Degrees of Freedom

The term **degrees of freedom** is often applied to joints that permit axial motions. When a joint allows motion within one plane around one axis, it is said to possess one degree of freedom. When it allows motion in two planes around two axes, it possesses two degrees of freedom. When it allows motion in three planes around three axes, it possesses three degrees of freedom. If its only type of movement is nonaxial, then it possesses zero degrees of freedom.

SECTION 7.10 UNIAXIAL SYNOVIAL JOINTS

- A uniaxial joint allows motion to occur around one axis; this motion occurs within one plane.
- Two types of uniaxial synovial joints exist[3]:
  - Hinge joint (also known as a **ginglymus joint**)
  - Pivot joint (also known as a **trochoid joint**)

HINGE JOINTS

- A **hinge joint** is a joint in which the surface of one bone is spool-like and the surface of the other bone is concave. The spool-like surface moves within the concave surface of the other bone.[4]
- A hinge joint is similar in structure and function to the hinge of a door; hence its name.
- An example of a hinge joint is the elbow joint[5] (Figure 7-12, A).
- Another example of a hinge joint is the ankle joint (Figure 7-12, B).

PIVOT JOINTS

- A **pivot joint** is a joint in which one surface is shaped like a ring, and the other surface is shaped so that it can rotate within the ring.[3]
- A pivot joint is similar in structure and function to a doorknob.
- An example of a pivot joint is the atlantoaxial joint between the ring-shaped atlas (C1) and the odontoid process (i.e., dens) of the axis (C2) in the cervical spine[6] (Figure 7-13, A).
- Another example of a pivot joint is the proximal radioulnar joint of the forearm, in which the radial head rotates within the ring-shaped structure created by the radial notch of the ulna and the annular ligament[6] (Figure 7-13, B).

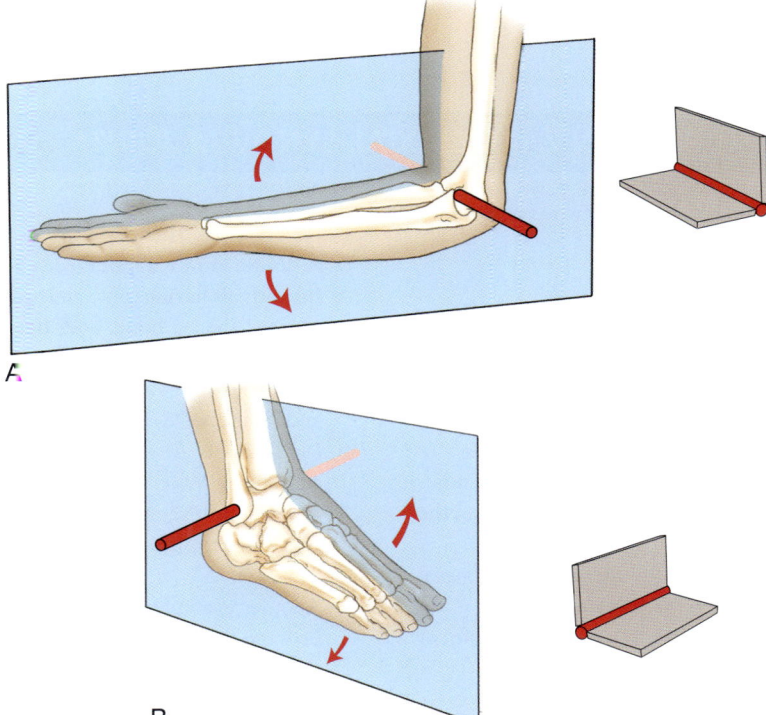

FIGURE 7-12 Uniaxial hinge synovial joints. **A,** Elbow joint (the humeroulnar joint of the elbow). The elbow joint is a uniaxial hinge joint that allows only the actions of flexion and extension to occur. These actions occur around a mediolateral axis and occur within the sagittal plane. **B,** Ankle joint. The ankle joint is a uniaxial hinge joint that allows only the actions of plantarflexion and dorsiflexion to occur. These actions occur around a mediolateral axis and occur within the sagittal plane. A hinge is drawn next to each of these joints, demonstrating the similarity in structure of these joints to a hinge. (Note: In all illustrations the red tube represents the axis of movement.)

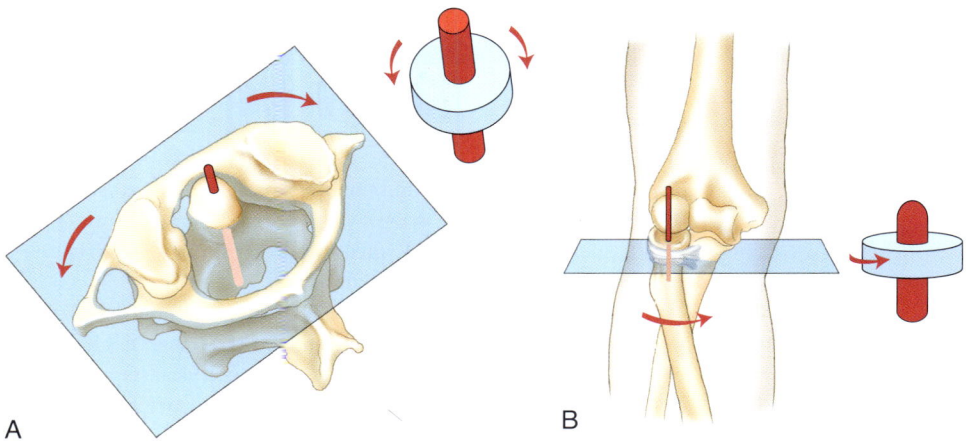

FIGURE 7-13 Uniaxial pivot synovial joints. **A,** Atlantoaxial joint (formed by the ring-shaped atlas and the odontoid process of the axis). The atlantoaxial joint is a pivot joint that allows only right rotation and left rotation to occur. These actions occur around a vertical axis and occur within the transverse plane. **B,** Proximal radioulnar joint. The proximal radioulnar joint is a pivot joint that allows only medial and lateral rotation of the head of the radius to occur (creating the actions of pronation and supination of the radius of the forearm). This movement of the radial head occurs around a vertical axis and occurs within the transverse plane. (Note: In these illustrations the red tube represents the axis of movement.)

SECTION 7.11   BIAXIAL SYNOVIAL JOINTS

- A biaxial joint allows motion to occur around two axes; this motion occurs within two planes.[8]
- Two types of biaxial synovial joints exist[6]:
  - Condyloid joint (also known as an **ovoid joint** or an **ellipsoid joint**)
  - Saddle joint (also known as a **sellar joint**)

CONDYLOID JOINTS

- In a **condyloid joint**, one bone is concave in shape and the other bone is convex (i.e., oval) in shape. The convex bone fits into the concave bone.[8]
- An example of a condyloid joint is the metacarpophalangeal (MCP) joint of the hand[6] (Figure 7-14, *A* and *B*).
- Another example of a condyloid joint is the radiocarpal joint of the wrist (Figure 7-14, *C* and *D*).

SADDLE JOINTS

- A **saddle joint** is a modified condyloid joint.[4]
- Instead of having one convex-shaped bone that fits into a concave-shaped bone, both bones of a saddle joint are shaped such that each bone has a convexity and a concavity to its surface; the convexity of one bone fits into the concavity of the other bone and vice versa.[8]
- Saddle joints are similar in structure and function to a person sitting in a Western saddle on a horse.
- The classic example of a saddle joint is the carpometacarpal (CMC) joint of the thumb[5] (Figure 7-15, *A* and *B*, and Box 7-7).
- Another example of a saddle joint is the sternoclavicular joint between the manubrium of the sternum and the medial end of the clavicle (Figure 7-15, *C* and *D*).

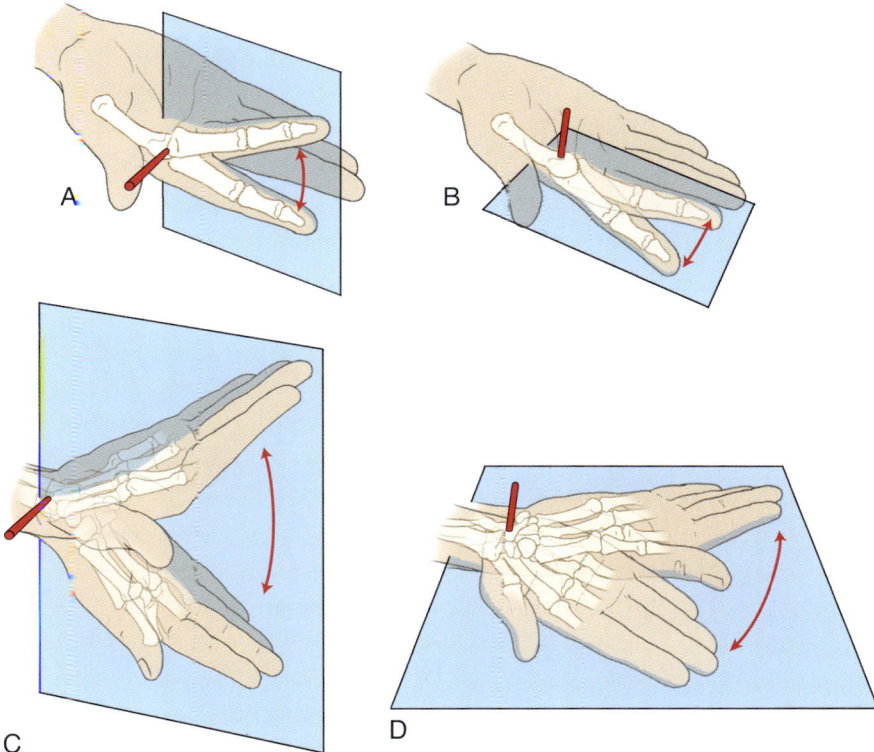

FIGURE 7-14 Biaxial condyloid synovial joints. **A,** Metacarpophalangeal (MCP) joint is a condyloid joint that allows the actions of flexion and extension to occur within the sagittal plane around a mediolateral axis. **B,** Actions of abduction and adduction occur within the frontal plane around an anteroposterior axis. **C,** Radiocarpal joint of the wrist is a condyloid joint that allows the actions of flexion and extension to occur within the sagittal plane around a mediolateral axis. **D,** Actions of abduction and adduction at the radiocarpal joint of the wrist occur within the frontal plane around an anteroposterior axis. (Note: In these illustrations the red tube represents the axis of movement.)

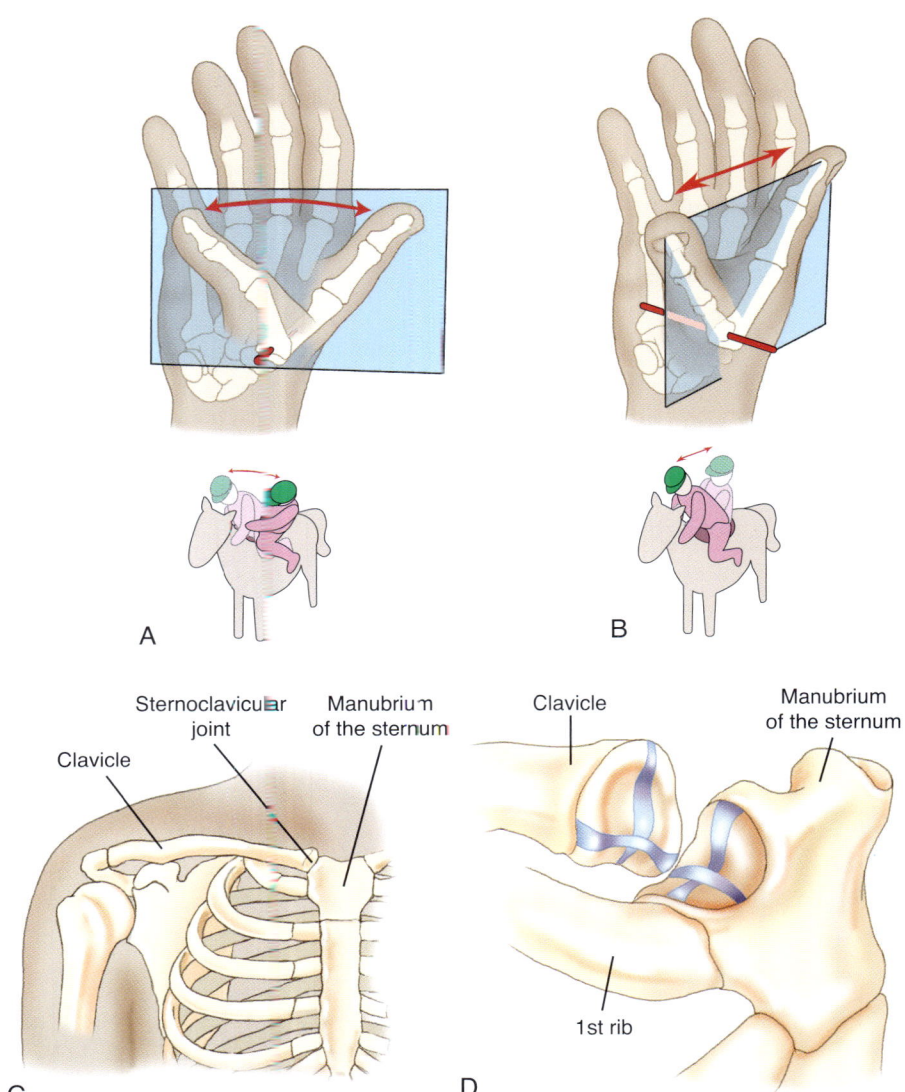

FIGURE 7-15 Biaxial saddle synovial joints. **A,** Carpometacarpal (CMC) joint is a saddle joint that allows the motions of flexion and extension to occur within the frontal plane around an anteroposterior axis. **B,** CMC joint also allows abduction and adduction to occur within the sagittal plane around a mediolateral axis. An illustration of a person sitting in a Western saddle on a horse has been placed next to each figure, demonstrating the similar structure and movement of the saddle joint of the thumb to a Western saddle. In both illustrations the red tube represents the axis of movement. **C,** Sternoclavicular joint between the manubrium of the sternum and the medial end of the clavicle **D,** Sternoclavicular joint opened up to show the saddlelike concave-convex articulating surfaces of both the manubrium and the clavicle.

BOX 7-7

Because of the orientation of the thumb, the terminology for naming its actions is unusual; flexion and extension occur in the frontal plane, and abduction and adduction occur in the sagittal plane.[1] (For more information on movements of the thumb, see Sections 6.23 and 10.13.)

The saddle joint of the thumb is an interesting joint to classify. It permits a greater degree of movement than a condyloid joint because it also allows a limited amount of rotation. With this rotation, the saddle joint of the thumb moves in all three cardinal planes; however, it is still classified as a biaxial joint because it only allows motion around two axes. Transverse plane medial rotation must couple with frontal plane flexion, and transverse plane lateral rotation must couple with frontal plane extension. Therefore only two axes of motion exist: the axis for cardinal (sagittal) plane motions of abduction/adduction and the axis for oblique (frontal/transverse) plane motions of medial rotation coupled with flexion and lateral rotation coupled with extension. (For more details, see Section 10.13.)

SECTION 7.12 TRIAXIAL SYNOVIAL JOINTS

- A triaxial joint allows motion to occur around three axes; this motion occurs within three planes.[4]
- Only one major type of triaxial synovial joint exists—the ball-and-socket joint.
- An example of a ball-and-socket joint is the hip joint[6] (Figure 7-16).
- Another example of a ball-and-socket joint is the shoulder joint[8] (Figure 7-17).

BALL-AND-SOCKET JOINTS

- In a **ball-and-socket joint**, one bone has a ball-like convex surface that fits into the concave-shaped socket of the other bone.[3]

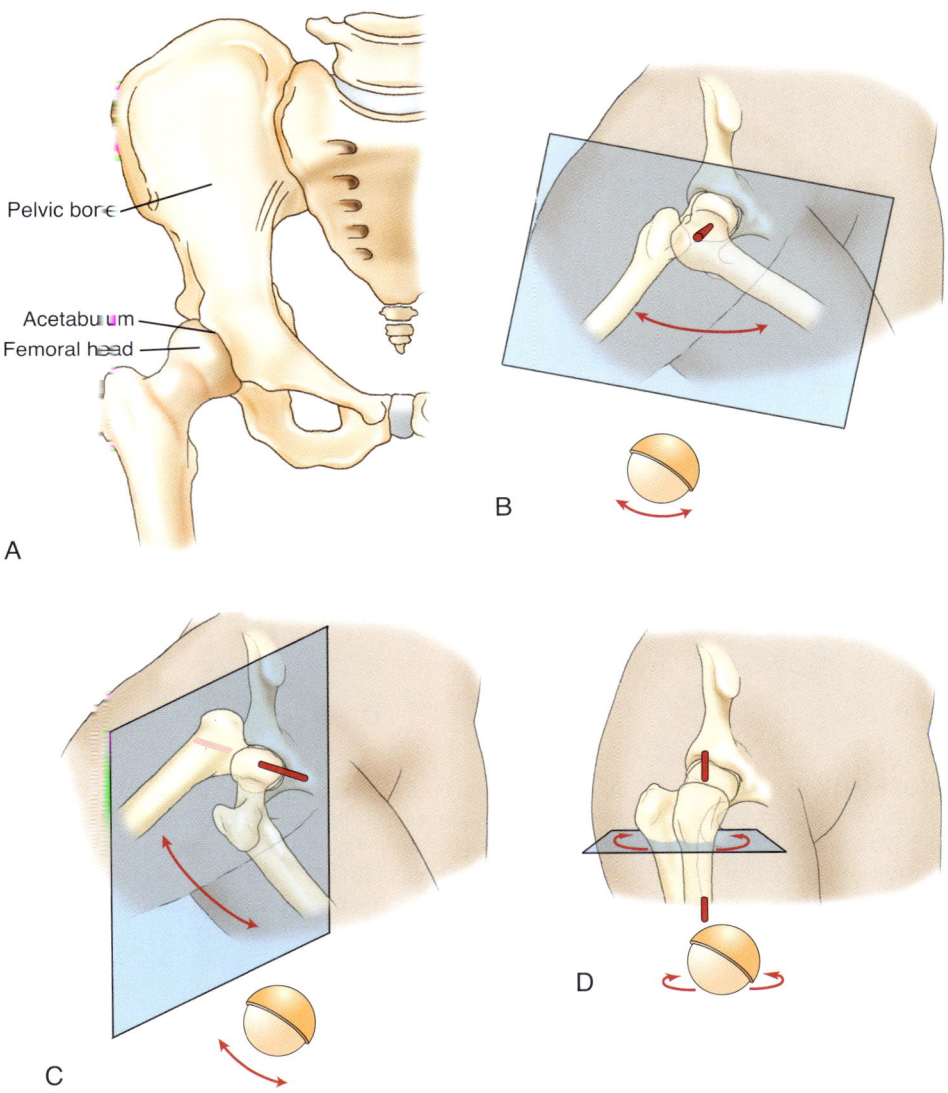

FIGURE 7-16 The hip joint. **A,** Anterior view of the ball-and-socket joint of the hip. The head of the femur, which is a convex-shaped ball, fits into the acetabulum of the pelvis, which is a concave-shaped socket. **B,** Flexion and extension of the thigh at the hip joint occur in the sagittal plane around a mediolateral axis. **C,** Abduction and adduction of the thigh at the hip joint occur in the frontal plane around an anteroposterior axis. **D,** Lateral rotation and medial rotation of the thigh at the hip joint occur in the transverse plane around a vertical axis. (Note: In these illustrations the red tube represents the axis of movement.)

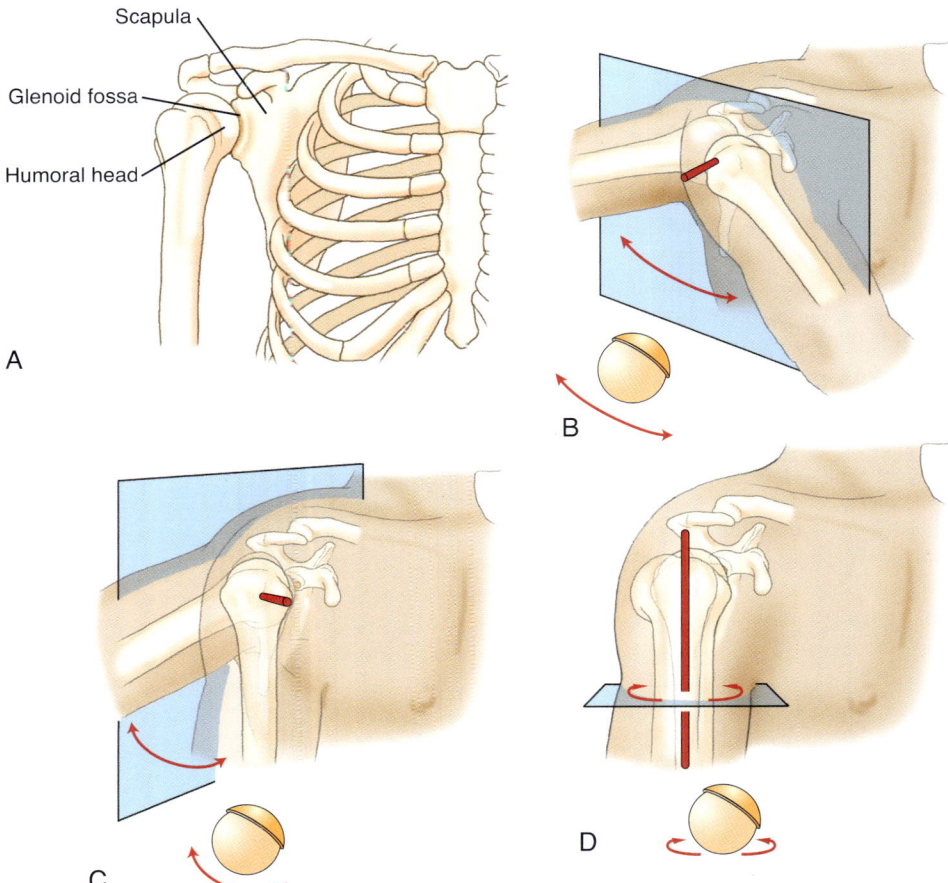

FIGURE 7-17 The shoulder joint. **A,** Anterior view of the ball-and-socket joint of the shoulder (the glenohumeral joint). Head of the humerus, which is a convex-shaped ball, fits into the glenoid fossa of the scapula, which is a concave-shaped socket. (Note: Comparing this figure with Figure 6-16, *A*, we can see that the socket of the shoulder joint is not as deep as the socket of the hip joint.) **B,** Flexion and extension of the arm at the shoulder joint occur in the sagittal plane around a mediolateral axis. **C,** Abduction and adduction of the arm at the shoulder joint occur in the frontal plane around an anteroposterior axis. **D,** Lateral rotation and medial rotation of the arm at the shoulder joint occur in the transverse plane around a vertical axis. (Note: In these illustrations the red tube represents the axis of movement.)

SECTION 7.13 NONAXIAL SYNOVIAL JOINTS

- A nonaxial joint allows motion to occur within a plane, but this motion does not occur around an axis.[2]
- The motion that occurs at a nonaxial joint is a gliding movement in which the surface of one bone merely translates (i.e., glides) along the surface of the other bone.[4] (See Sections 6.2 to 6.4 for more information on nonaxial translation motion.)
- It is important to emphasize that motion at a nonaxial joint may occur within a plane, but it does not occur around an axis; hence the name *nonaxial* joint.
- The surfaces of the bones of a nonaxial joint are usually flat or slightly curved.
- Examples of nonaxial joints are the joints found between adjacent tarsal bones[5] (i.e., intertarsal joints) (Figure 7-18).
- Another example of a nonaxial joint is a facet joint of the spine (Figure 7-19).
- A nonaxial joint is also known as a **gliding joint**, an **irregular joint**, or a **plane joint**.[13]

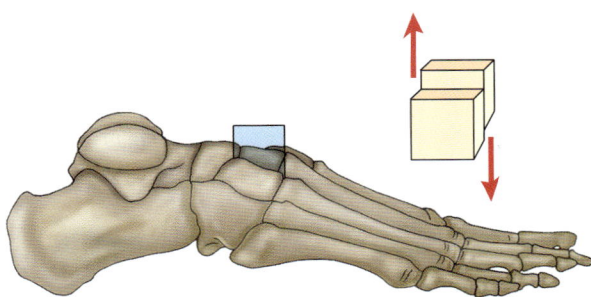

FIGURE 7-18 Joint between two adjacent tarsal bones (an intertarsal joint). The adjacent surfaces of the tarsals are approximately flat. When one tarsal bone moves relative to another, it glides along the other bone. This motion does not occur around an axis.

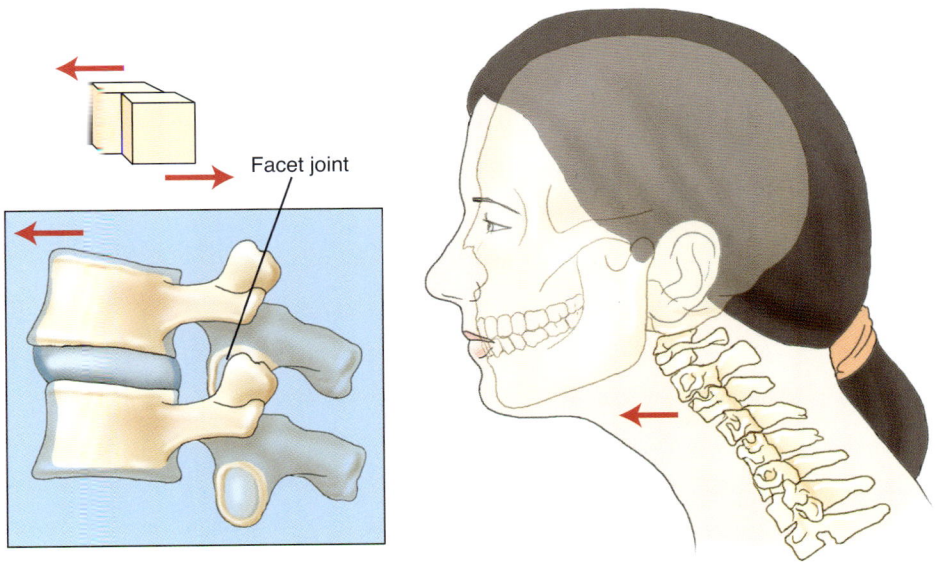

FIGURE 7-19 Facet joint of the spine. The surfaces of the superior facet (of the inferior vertebra) and the inferior facet (of the superior vertebra) are approximately flat or slightly curved. When one facet moves relative to the other, it glides along the other facet. This motion does not occur around an axis.

SECTION 7.14 MENISCI AND ARTICULAR DISCS

- Most often, the bones of a joint have opposing surfaces that are **congruent** (i.e., their surfaces match each other). However, sometimes the surfaces of the bones of a joint are not well matched. In these cases the joint will often have an additional intra-articular structure interposed between the two bones.
- These additional intra-articular structures are made of fibrocartilage and function to help maximize the congruence of the joint by helping to improve the fit of the two bones.[14]
- By improving the congruence of a joint, these structures help to do two things:
  - Maintain normal joint movements: Because of the better fit between the two bones of the joint, these structures help to improve the movement of the two bones relative to each other.[1]
  - Cushion the joint: These structures help to cushion the joint by absorbing and transmitting forces (e.g., weight bearing, shock absorption) from the bone of one body part to the bone of the next body part.[1]
- If this fibrocartilaginous structure is ring shaped, it is called an **articular disc**.
- If it is crescent shaped, it is called a **meniscus** (plural: menisci).
- Although these structures are in contact with the articular surfaces of the joints, they are not attached to the joint surfaces but rather to adjacent soft tissue of the capsule or to bone adjacent to the articular surface.[14]
- Articular discs are found in many joints of the body.
  - One example is the temporomandibular joint (TMJ), which has an articular disc located within its joint cavity[1] (Figure 7-20, A).
  - Another example is the sternoclavicular joint, which has an articular disc located within its joint cavity (Figure 7-20, B).
- Articular menisci are found between the tibia and the femur in the knee joint[4] (Figure 7-21).

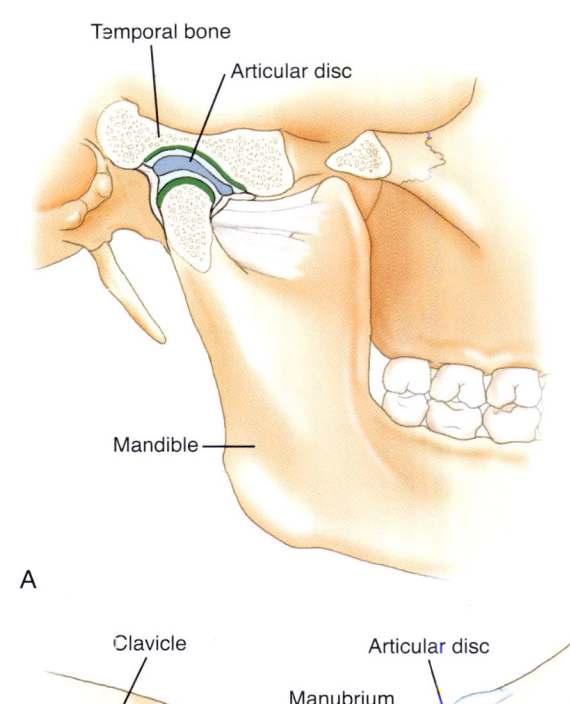

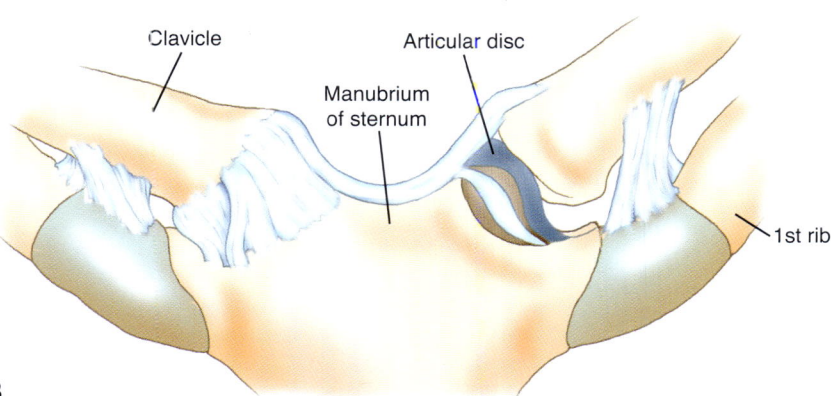

FIGURE 7-20 **A,** Lateral cross-section view of the temporomandibular joint (TMJ) illustrates the articular disc of the TMJ. **B,** Anterior view of the sternoclavicular joint illustrates the articular disc of the sternoclavicular joint. It can be seen that these articular discs help to improve the fit between the opposing articular surfaces of the joints involved, thereby helping to improve the stability and movement of the joints.

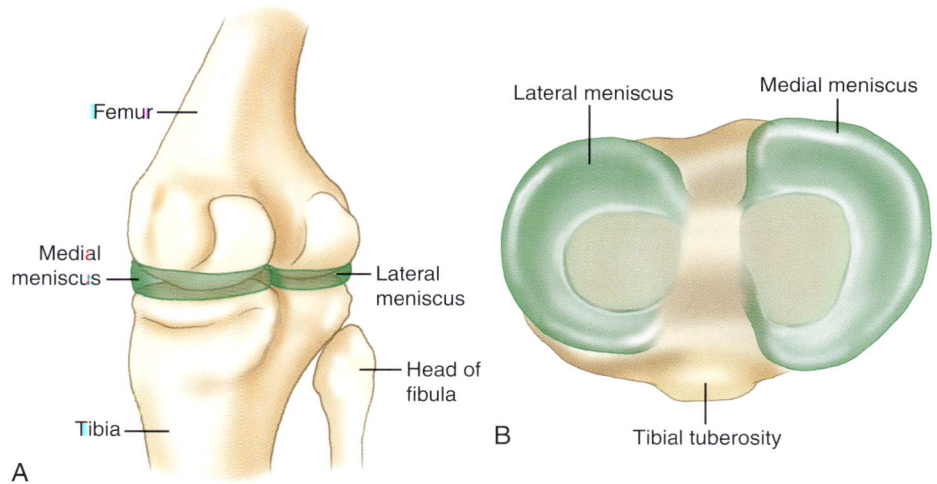

FIGURE 7-21 A, Posteromedial view of the right knee joint; it illustrates the crescent- or C-shaped fibrocartilaginous structures called menisci that are located between the tibia and femur of the knee joint. A lateral meniscus and a medial meniscus are found in each knee joint. It can be seen that these menisci help to improve the congruence (i.e., fit) between the opposing articular surfaces of the joint. **B,** Proximal (superior) view looking down on the tibia, illustrating the medial and lateral menisci of the right knee joint.

REVIEW QUESTIONS

evolve *Answers to the following review questions appear on the Evolve website accompanying this book at:* http://evolve.elsevier.com/Muscolino/kinesiology/.

1. What is the definition of a structural joint?

2. What is the definition of a functional joint?

3. What is the difference between a simple joint and a compound joint?

4. What is the main function of a joint?

5. What is the main function of a muscle?

6. What is the main function of a ligament?

7. What is the relationship between the stability and mobility of a joint?

8. If a joint is more stable, then it is less what?

9. How do joints absorb shock?

10. Where are most weight-bearing joints of the body located?

11. When joints are classified by structure, what are their three major categories?

12. Which structural category of joints possesses a joint cavity?

13. When joints are classified by function, what are their three major categories?

14. Which functional category of joints allows the most movement?

15. Name the three types of fibrous joints.

16. Name the two types of cartilaginous joints.

17. Give an example in the human body of a fibrous joint, a cartilaginous joint, and a synovial joint.

18. What are the components of a synovial joint?

19. By motion, what are the four major types of synovial joints? Give an example in the human body of each type.

20. Around how many axes does a saddle joint permit motion?

21. In reference to a joint, to what does the term *congruency* refer?

22. Name a joint that has an intra-articular disc.

23. Draw a *typical* synovial joint.

REFERENCES

1. Neumann DA: Kinesiology of the musculoskeletal system: Foundations for physical rehabilitation, ed 3, St Louis, 2017, Elsevier.
2. Hammill J, Knutzen KM: Biomechanical basis of human movement, ed 2, Baltimore, 2003, Lippincott Williams & Wilkins.
3. Palastanga N, Field D, Soames R: Anatomy and human movement, ed 4, Oxford, 2002, Butterworth-Heinemann.
4. Behnke RS: Kinetic anatomy, ed 2, Champaign, IL, 2006, Human Kinetics.
5. Levangie PK, Norkin CC: Joint structure and function: A comprehensive analysis, ed 5, Philadelphia, 2001, FA Davis.
6. Hall SJ: Basic biomechanics, ed 6, New York, 2012, McGraw Hill.
7. Hamilton N, Weimar W, Luttgens K: Kinesiology: Scientific basis of human motion, ed 12, New York, 2012, McGraw Hill.
8. Watkins J: Structure and function of the musculoskeletal system, Champaign, IL, 1999, Human Kinetics.
9. Oatis CA: Kinesiology: The mechanics and pathomechanics of human movement, Philadelphia, 2004, Lippincott Williams & Wilkins.
10. Nordin M, Frankel VH: Basic biomechanics of the musculoskeletal system, ed 3, Baltimore, 2001, Lippincott Williams & Wilkins.
11. White TD: Human osteology, ed 2, San Diego, 2000, Academic Press.
12. Muscolino JE: The muscular system manual: The skeletal muscles of the human body, ed 4, St Louis, 2017, Mosby Elsevier.
13. McGinnis PM: Biomechanics of sport and exercise, ed 2, Champaign, IL, 2005, Human Kinetics.
14. Smith LK, Weiss EL, Lehmkuhl LO: Brunstrom's clinical kinesiology, ed 5, Philadelphia, 1996, FA Davis.

CHAPTER 8
Joints of the Axial Body

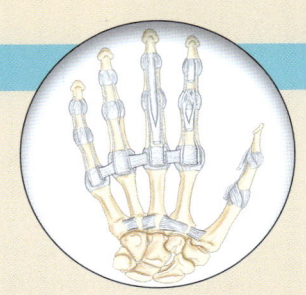

CHAPTER OUTLINE

Section 8.1	Suture Joints of the Skull	Section 8.7	Thoracic Spine (the Thorax)
Section 8.2	Temporomandibular Joint (TMJ)	Section 8.8	Rib Joints of the Thorax
Section 8.3	Spine	Section 8.9	Lumbar Spine (the Abdomen)
Section 8.4	Spinal Joints	Section 8.10	Thoracolumbar Spine (the Trunk)
Section 8.5	Atlanto-Occipital and Atlantoaxial Joints	Section 8.11	Thoracolumbar Fascia and Abdominal Aponeurosis
Section 8.6	Cervical Spine (the Neck)		

CHAPTER OBJECTIVES

After completing this chapter, the student should be able to perform the following:

1. Define the key terms of this chapter and state the meanings of the word origins of this chapter.
2. Describe the suture bones of the skull, including the relationship between cranial suture joints and childbirth.
3. Do the following related to the temporomandibular joint:
   - Discuss the bones of the temporomandibular joint.
   - Discuss the major motions allowed by the temporomandibular joint.
   - List the major ligaments of the temporomandibular joint.
   - List the major muscles of mastication, and describe their role in mastication.
   - Explain the possible relationship between TMJ dysfunction and the muscular system.
4. Do the following related to the spine:
   - Define the curves of the spine, and describe their development.
   - Describe the structure and function of the spine.
5. Do the following related to spinal joints:
   - State the major difference between the function of the disc joint and the function of the facet joints.
   - Describe the orientation of the planes of the facets in the cervical, thoracic, and lumbar regions of the spine. In addition, explain and give examples of how the plane of the facet joints determines the type of motion that occurs at that segmental level.
   - Describe the structure and function of the median and lateral joints of the spine.
6. Describe the structure and function of the atlanto-occipital and atlantoaxial joints of the cervical spine.
7. Discuss the features, functions, and major motions allowed for the cervical and thoracic spine.
8. Do the following related to rib joints of the thoracic spine:
   - List the joints at which rib motion occurs; explain how the movement of a bucket handle is used to illustrate rib motion.
   - Describe the roles of the muscles of respiration.
   - Explain the mechanism of thoracic breathing versus abdominal breathing.
   - Discuss costospinal joints in detail.
9. Describe the general structure and function of the lumbar spine.
10. Describe the structure and function of the thoracolumbar spine, the thoracolumbar fascia, and the abdominal aponeurosis.

 Indicates a video demonstration is available for this concept.

OVERVIEW

Chapters 6 and 7 laid the theoretic basis for the structure and function of joints. Chapters 8 through 10 now examine the structure and function of the joints of the human body regionally. Chapter 8 addresses the joints of the axial body; Chapter 9 addresses the joints of the lower extremity; and Chapter 10 addresses the joints of the upper extremity. Within this chapter, Sections 8.1 and 8.2 cover the suture joints and temporomandibular joints (TMJs) of the head, respectively. Sections 8.3 through 8.10 then cover the spine. Of these, Section 8.3 begins with a study of the spinal column as an entity, and Section 8.4 covers the general structure and function of spinal joints. Sections 8.5 through 8.10 then sequentially address the various regions of the spine (e.g., cervical, thoracic, lumbar). The last section of this chapter (Section 8.11) addresses the thoracolumbar fascia and abdominal aponeurosis of the trunk.

KEY TERMS

Abdomen (AB-do-men)
Abdominal aponeurosis (ab-DOM-i-nal)
Accessory atlantoaxial ligament (at-LAN-toe-AK-see-al)
Alar ligaments of the dens (A-ar)
Annulus fibrosus (AN-you-us fi-BROS-us)
Anterior atlanto-occipital membrane (an-TEER-ee-or at-LAN-toe-ok-SIP-i-tal)
Anterior longitudinal ligament
Apical dental ligament (A-pikal)
Apical odontoid ligament (o-DONT-oid)
Apophyseal joint (a-POF-i-SEE-al)
Arcuate line (ARE-kew-it)
Atlantoaxial joint (at-LAN-oe-AK-see-al)
Atlanto-occipital joint (at-LAN-toe-ok-SIP-i-tal)
Atlanto-odontoid joint (at-LAN-toe-o-DONT-oid)
Bifid spinous processes (BI-E-fid)
Bifid transverse processes
Bucket handle movement
Cervical spine (SERV-i-kul)
Chondrosternal joints (KON-dro-STERN-al)
Costochondral joints (COS-To-KON-dral)
Costocorporeal joint (COST-o-kor-PO-ree-al)
Costospinal joints (COST-o-SPINE-al)
Costotransverse joint (COST-o-TRANS-verse)
Costotransverse ligament
Costovertebral joint (COST-o-VERT-i-bral)
Craniosacral technique (CRANE-ee-o-SAY-kral)
Cruciate ligament of the dens (KRU-shee-it, DENS)
Disc joint
Facet joint (fa-SET)
False ribs
Floating ribs
Forward-head posture
Hyperkyphotic (HI-per-ki-FOT-ik)
Hyperlordotic (HI-per-lor-DOT-ik)
Hypokyphotic (HI-po-ki-FOT-ik)
Hypolordotic (HI-po-lor-DOT-ik)
Interchondral joints (IN-ter-KON-dral)
Interchondral ligament
Interspinous ligaments (IN-ter-SPINE-us)
Intertransverse ligament (IN-ter-TRANS-verse)
Intervertebral disc joint (IN-ter-VERT-i-bral)
Joints of Von Luschka (FON LOOSH-ka)
Kyphosis, pl. kyphoses (ki-FOS-is, ki-FOS-eez)
Kyphotic (ki-FOT-ik)
Lateral collateral ligament (of the temporomandibular joint)
Lateral costotransverse ligament (COST-o-TRANS-verse)
Ligamentum flava, sing. ligamentum flavum (LIG-a-men-tum FLAY-va, FLAY-vum)
Linea alba (LIN-ee-a AL-ba)
Lordosis, pl. lordoses (lor-DOS-is, lor-DOS-eez)
Lordotic (lor-DOT-ik)
Lumbar spine (LUM-bar)
Lumbodorsal fascia (LUM-bo-DOOR-sul)
Lumbosacral joint (LUM-bo-SAY-krul)
Manubriosternal joint (ma-NOOB-ree-o-STERN-al)
Manubriosternal ligament
Medial collateral ligament (of the temporomandibular joint)
Nuchal ligament (NEW-kal)
Nucleus pulposus (NEW-klee-us pul-POS-us)
Posterior atlanto-occipital membrane (pos-TEER-ee-or at-LAN-toe-ok-SIP-i-tal)
Posterior longitudinal ligament
Primary spinal curves
Radiate ligament (of chondrosternal joint) (RAY-dee-at)
Radiate ligament (of costovertebral joint)
Rectus sheath (REK-tus)
Sacral base angle (SAY-krul)
Sacrococcygeal region (SAY-kro-kok-SI-jee-al)
Sacro-occipital technique (SAY-kro-ok-SIP-i-tal)
Scoliosis, pl. scolioses (SKO-lee-os-is, SKO-lee-os-eez)
Secondary spinal curves
Segmental level (seg-MENT-al)
Slipped disc
Sphenomandibular ligament (SFEE-no-man-DIB-you-lar)
Spinal column
Spine
Sternocostal joints (STERN-o-COST-al)
Sternoxiphoid joint (STERN-o-ZI-foid)
Sternoxiphoid ligament
Stylomandibular ligament (STY-lo-man-DIB-you-lar)
Superior costotransverse ligament (sue-PEER-ee-or COST-o-TRANS-verse)
Supraspinous ligament (SUE-pra-SPINE-us)

Tectorial membrane (tek-TOR-ee-al)
Temporomandibular joint (TEM-po-ro-man-DIB-you-lar)
Temporomandibular joint (TMJ) dysfunction (dis-FUNK-shun)
Temporomandibular ligament (TEM-po-ro-man-DIB-you-lar)
Thoracic spine (thor-AS-ik)
Thoracolumbar fascia (thor-AK-o-LUM-bar FASH-ee-a)
Thoracolumbar spine
Thorax (THOR-aks)
Transverse ligament of the atlas
True ribs
Uncinate process (UN-sin-ate)
Uncovertebral joint (UN-co-VERT-i-bral)
Vertebral arteries (VERT-i-bral)
Vertebral column
Vertebral endplate (VERT-i-bral)
Vertebral prominens (PROM-i-nens)
Z joints
Zygapophyseal joint (ZI-ga-POF-i-SEE-al)

WORD ORIGINS

- Alba—From Latin *albus*, meaning *white*
- Annulus—From Latin *anulus*, meaning *ring*
- Arcuate—From Latin *arcuatus*, meaning *bowed*
- Bifid—From Latin *bifidus*, meaning *cleft in two parts*
- Cervical—From Latin *cervicalis*, meaning *neck*
- Concavity—From Latin *con*, meaning *with*, and *cavus*, meaning *hollow, concavity*
- Convexity—From Latin *convexus*, meaning *vaulted, arched*
- Corporeal—From Latin *corpus*, meaning *body*
- Costal—From Latin *costa*, meaning *rib*
- Cruciate—From Latin *crux*, meaning *cross*
- Flavum—From Latin *flavus*, meaning *yellow*
- Kyphosis—From Greek *kyphosis*, meaning *bent, humpback*
- Linea—From Latin *linea*, meaning *line*
- Lordosis—From Greek *lordosis*, meaning *a bending backward*
- Lumbar—From Latin *lumbus*, meaning *loin*
- Mastication—From Latin *masticare*, meaning *to chew* (Note: This originates from Greek *masten*, meaning *to feed*, which in turn originates from Greek *mastos*, meaning *breast*, the first place from which a person receives sustenance.)
- Nuchal—From Latin *nucha*, meaning *back of the neck*
- Nucleus—From Latin *nucleus*, meaning *little kernel, the inside/center of a nut* (Note: Nucleus is diminutive for the Latin word *nux*, meaning *nut*.)
- Pulposus—From Latin *pulpa*, meaning *flesh*
- Radiate—From Latin *radius*, meaning *ray, to spread out in all directions*
- Scoliosis—From Greek *scoliosis*, meaning *curvature, crooked*
- Thoracic—From Greek *thorax*, meaning *breastplate, chest*
- Uncinate—From Latin *uncinatus*, meaning *shaped like a hook*
- Zygapophyseal—From Greek *zygon*, meaning *yoke* or *joining*, and *apophysis*, meaning *offshoot*

SECTION 8.1   SUTURE JOINTS OF THE SKULL

- The suture joints of the skull are located between most bones of the cranium and also between most bones of the face (Figure 8-1).

BONES:

- Suture joints are located between adjacent bones of the cranium and face.[1]
- All joints between the major bones of the cranium and face (except the temporomandibular joints [TMJs]) are suture joints. Other nonsuture joints of the skull are the joints of the teeth and the joints between middle ear ossicles.
- Joint structure classification: Fibrous joint[2]
  - Subtype: Suture joint
- Joint function classification: Synarthrotic[2]

MAJOR MOTIONS ALLOWED:

- Nonaxial

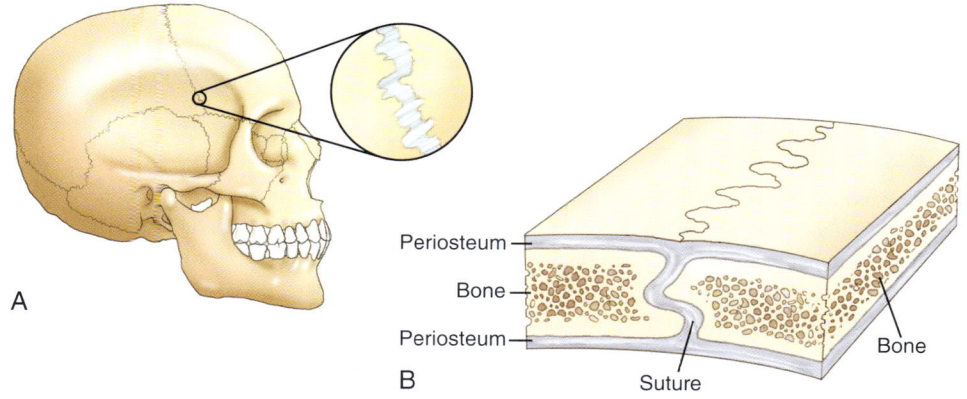

FIGURE 8-1 Suture joint of the skull. Suture joints are structurally classified as fibrous joints and allow nonaxial motion.

Miscellaneous:

- Movement at these joints is important during the birth process when the child must be delivered through the birth canal of the mother. Movement of the suture joints allows the child's head to be compressed, allowing for an easier and safer delivery.[4]
- Suture joints of the skull allow very little movement in an adult. As a person ages, many suture joints ossify and lose all ability to move[1] (Box 8-1).

 BOX 8-1

Although suture joints allow little motion, practitioners of **craniosacral technique** and **sacro-occipital technique** assert that this motion is very important. When blockage of this motion occurs, these practitioners manipulate the suture joints of the skull.

SECTION 8.2 TEMPOROMANDIBULAR JOINT (TMJ)

BONES:

- The temporomandibular joint (TMJ) is located between the temporal bone and the mandible (Figure 8-2).
  - More specifically, it is located between the mandibular fossa of the temporal bone and the condyle of the ramus of the mandible.[5]
- Joint structure classification: Synovial joint
  - Subtype: Modified hinge
- Joint function classification: Diarthrotic
  - Subtype: Uniaxial

MAJOR MOTIONS ALLOWED:

- The TMJ allows elevation and depression (axial movements) within the sagittal plane about a mediolateral axis (Figure 8-3).
- The TMJ allows protraction and retraction (nonaxial anterior and posterior glide movements) (Figure 8-4).
- The TMJ allows left and right lateral deviation (nonaxial lateral glide movements) (Figure 8-5, Box 8-2).[1]
  - Lateral deviation of the TMJ is actually a combination of spinning and glide. The condyle on the side to which the deviation is occurring spins, and the other condyle glides.

MAJOR LIGAMENTS OF THE TEMPOROMANDIBULAR JOINT (BOX 8-3):

Fibrous Joint Capsule

- The fibrous capsule (Figure 8-6) thickens medially and laterally, providing stability to the joint.[5] These thickenings are often referred to as the **medial collateral ligament** and the **lateral collateral ligament** of the TMJ. (Note: The collateral ligament thickenings are not shown in Figure 8-6.)
- However, the capsule is fairly loose anteriorly and posteriorly, allowing the condyle and disc to freely translate forward and back.

 BOX 8-2

Opening of the mouth involves both depression and protraction (i.e., anterior glide) of the mandible at the TMJs; closing the mouth involves elevation and retraction (i.e., posterior glide).

An easy way to assess the amount of depression that a TMJ should allow (i.e., how wide the mouth can be opened) is to use the proximal interphalangeal (PIP) joints of the fingers. Full depression of the TMJ should allow three PIPs to fit between the teeth.

 BOX 8-3

Ligaments of the Temporomandibular Joint (TMJ)

- Fibrous capsule (thickened medially and laterally as the medial and lateral collateral ligaments)
- Temporomandibular ligament (located laterally)
- Stylomandibular ligament (located medially)
- Sphenomandibular ligament (located medially)

- When the mandible depresses at the TMJs, it also protracts (i.e., glides anteriorly). Because the disc attaches into the anterior joint capsule, this motion pulls the disc anteriorly along with the condyle of the mandible.

Temporomandibular Ligament:
- Location: The temporomandibular ligament is located on the lateral side of the joint (see Figure 8-6, A).
- The temporomandibular ligament is primarily composed of obliquely oriented fibers.
- Function: It limits depression of the mandible and stabilizes the lateral side of the joint.[5]
- The temporomandibular ligament is also known as the **lateral ligament** of the TMJ.[5] (Not to be confused with the lateral collateral ligament thickening of the joint capsule.)
- In addition to stabilizing the lateral side of the capsule of the TMJ, the temporomandibular ligament also stabilizes the intra-articular disc. The superior head of the lateral pterygoid muscle attaches into the disc and exerts a medial pulling force on it. The temporomandibular ligament, being located laterally, opposes this pull, thereby stabilizing the medial-lateral placement of the disc within the joint.

Stylomandibular Ligament:
- Location: The stylomandibular ligament is located on the medial side of the joint (see Figure 8-6, A and B).
- More specifically, it is located from the styloid process of the temporal bone to the posterior border of the ramus of the mandible.[1]

Sphenomandibular Ligament:
- Location: The sphenomandibular ligament is located on the medial side of the joint (see Figure 8-6, B).
- More specifically, it is located from the sphenoid bone to the medial surface of the ramus of the mandible.[1]

- Function: Both the stylomandibular and sphenomandibular ligaments function to limit protraction (i.e., forward translation) of the mandible.

MAJOR MUSCLES OF THE TEMPOROMANDIBULAR JOINT:
- Lateral pterygoid, medial pterygoid, temporalis, and masseter[4] (see figures in Box 8-4).

MISCELLANEOUS:
- An intra-articular fibrocartilaginous disc is located within the TMJ (see Figure 8-6, C and D).
  - The purpose of this disc is to increase the congruence (i.e., improve the fit and stability) of the joint surfaces of the temporal bone and mandible.[1]
  - Being a soft tissue, the disc also serves to cushion the TMJ.
  - The disc divides the TMJ into two separate joint cavities: (1) an upper cavity and (2) a lower cavity.[6]
  - Technically, the lower joint of the TMJ (between the condyle of the mandible and the intra-articular disc) is a uniaxial joint. The upper joint of the TMJ (between the disc and the temporal bone) is a gliding nonaxial joint. Motions of the TMJ may occur solely at one of these joints or may occur as a combination of movements at both of these joints.
  - The intra-articular disc is attached to and moves with the condyle of the mandible.[6]
  - The intra-articular disc also has attachments into the joint capsule of the TMJ.
- The lateral pterygoid muscle has tendinous attachments directly into the fibrous joint capsule and the intra-articular disc of the TMJ.[5]
- **Temporomandibular joint (TMJ) dysfunction** is a general term that applies to any dysfunction (i.e., abnormal function) of the TMJ[7] (Box 8-5).

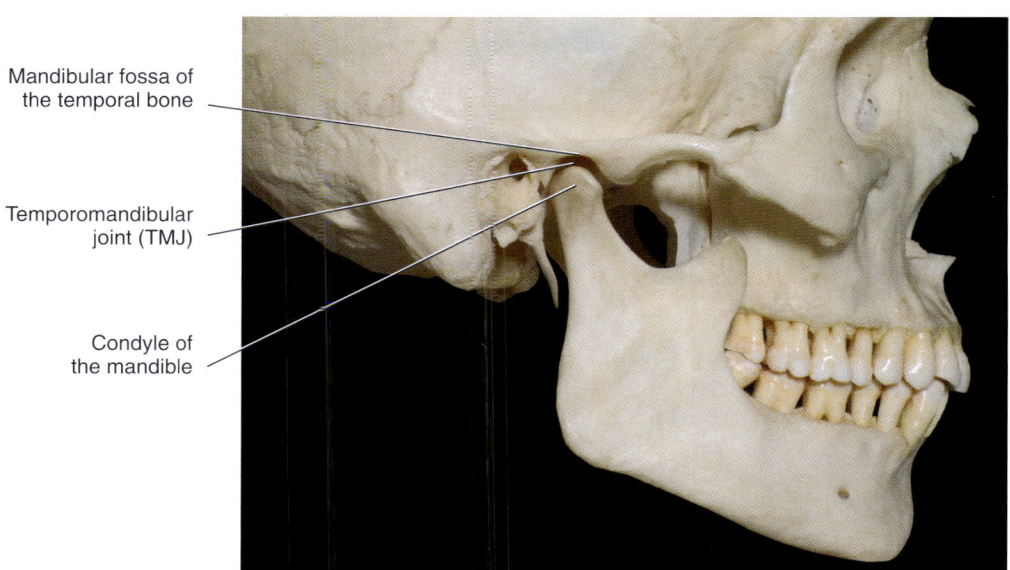

FIGURE 8-2 Lateral view of the right temporomandibular joint (TMJ). The TMJ is the **j**oint located between the **t**emporal bone and the **m**andibular bone, hence T**M**J.

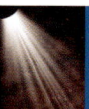

BOX 8-4 Spotlight on the Major Muscles of Mastication

- The term *mastication* means to chew, hence muscles of mastication involve moving the mandible at the temporomandibular joints (TMJs), because mandibular movement is necessary for chewing.
- Four major muscles of mastication exist: (1) temporalis, (2) masseter, (3) lateral pterygoid, and (4) medial pterygoid. The temporalis and masseter are located superficially and can be easily accessed when palpating and doing bodywork. The lateral and medial pterygoids are located deeper, and addressing these muscles with bodywork is best done from inside the mouth (see figures in this box).
- Another group of muscles that is involved with mastication is the hyoid group (see Figures 11-94 through 11-101). The hyoid muscle group is composed of eight muscles: four suprahyoids and four infrahyoids. Three of the four suprahyoids attach from the hyoid bone inferiorly to the mandible superiorly. When these suprahyoids contract, if the hyoid bone is fixed, they move the mandible, hence assisting in mastication. The infrahyoid muscles are also important with respect to mastication. Because the hyoid bone does not form an osseous joint with any other bone of the body (it is the only bone in the human body that does not articulate with another bone), it is quite mobile and needs to be stabilized for the suprahyoids to contract and move the mandible. Therefore when the suprahyoids concentrically contract and shorten to move the mandible at the TMJs, the infrahyoids simultaneously contract isometrically to fix (i.e., stabilize) the hyoid bone. With the hyoid bone fixed, all the force of the pull of the contraction of the suprahyoids will be directed toward moving the mandible.

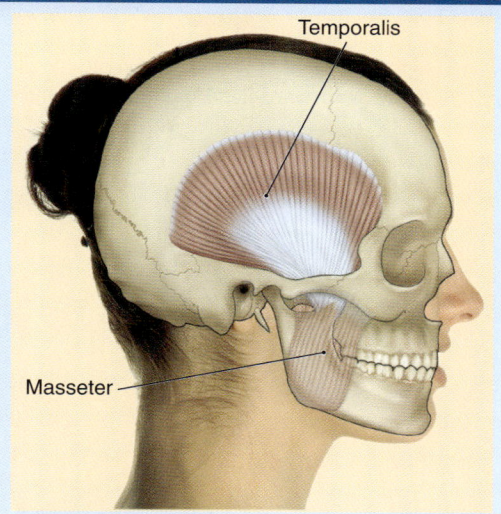

Right lateral view of the temporalis and masseter. The masseter has been ghosted in. *(From Muscolino JE: The muscular system manual: the skeletal muscles of the human body, ed 4, St Louis, 2017, Elsevier.)*

- In addition to mandibular movement at the TMJs, mastication also involves muscular action by the tongue to move food within the mouth to facilitate chewing. Therefore muscles of the tongue may also be considered to be muscles of mastication.

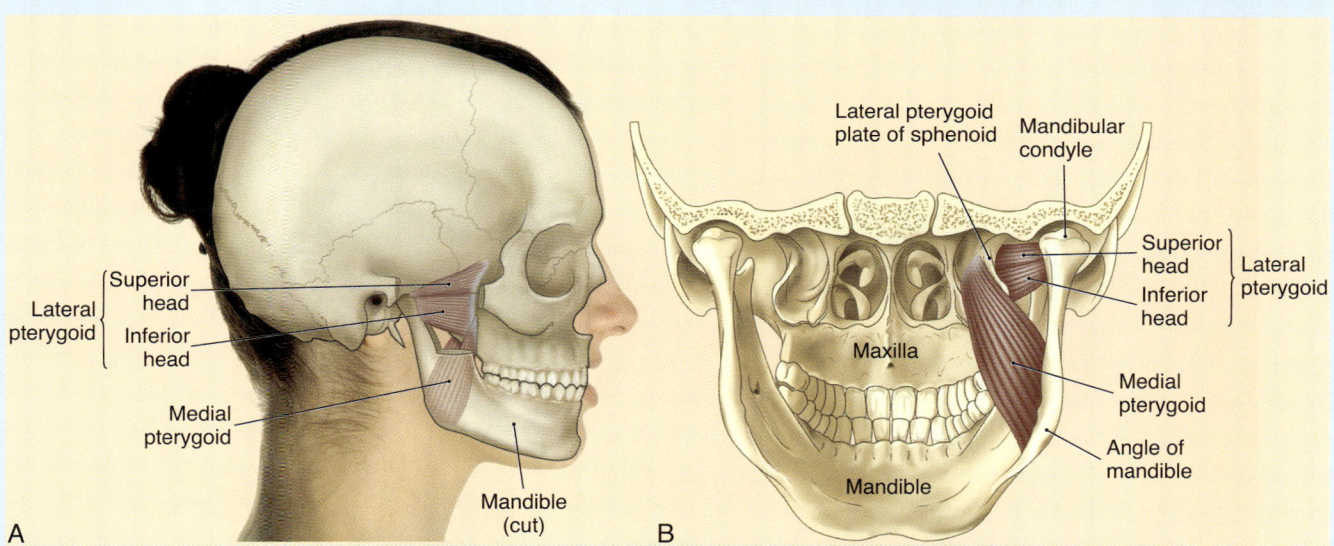

Views of the right lateral and medial pterygoids. **A,** Lateral view with the mandible partially cut away. **B,** Posterior view with the cranial bones cut away. *(From Muscolino JE: The muscular system manual: the skeletal muscles of the human body, ed 4, St Louis, 2017, Elsevier.)*

BOX 8-5

Temporomandibular joint (TMJ) dysfunction has many possible causes. Of these many causes, two may be of special interest to manual therapists. One is tightness or imbalance of the muscles that cross the TMJ (especially the lateral pterygoid because of its attachment directly into the capsule and disc). The second is **forward-head posture**, a common postural deviation in which the head and often the upper cervical vertebrae are translated anteriorly (i.e., forward). This forward-head posture is believed to create tension on the TMJs as a result of the hyoid muscles being stretched and pulled taut, resulting in a pulling force being placed on the mandible, consequently placing a tensile stress on the TMJs[5].

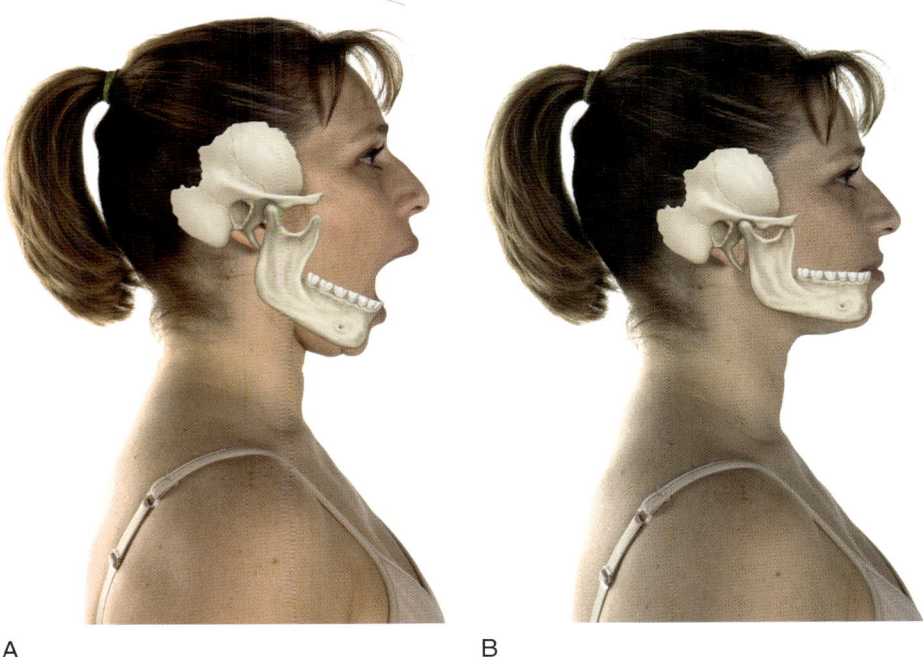

A   B

FIGURE 8-3 Lateral views that illustrate depression and elevation, respectively, of the mandible at the temporomandibular joints (TMJs). These are axial motions.

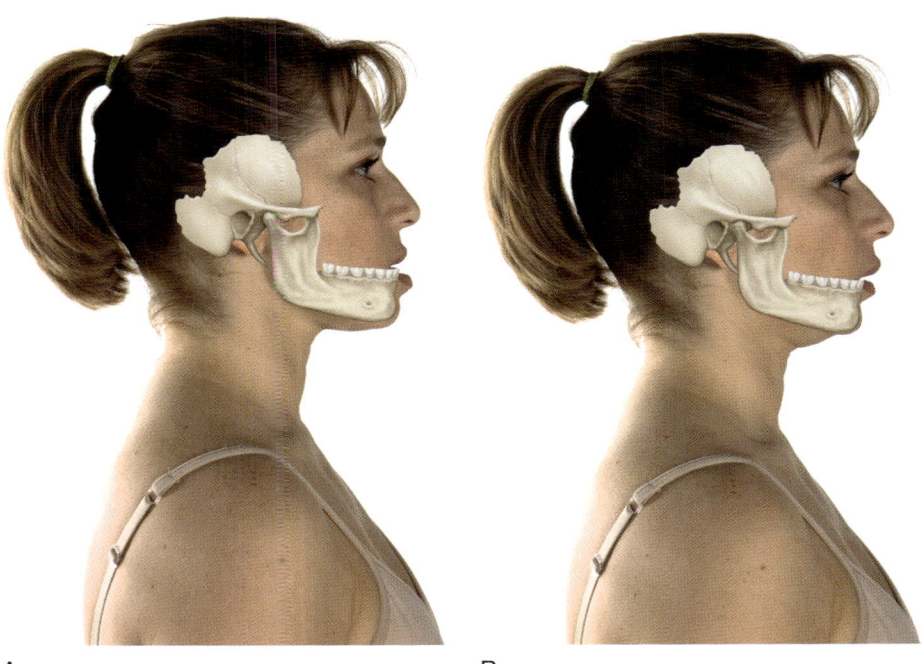

A   B

FIGURE 8-4 Lateral views that illustrate protraction and retraction, respectively, of the mandible at the temporomandibular joints (TMJs). These are nonaxial glide motions.

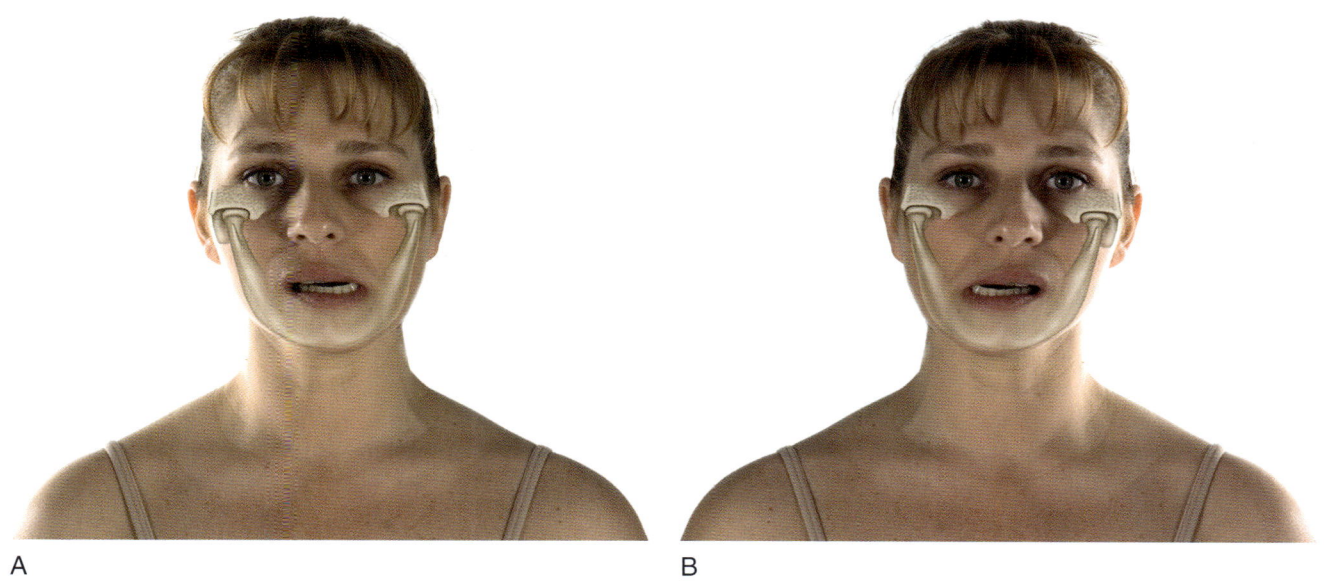

FIGURE 8-5 Anterior views that illustrate left lateral deviation and right lateral deviation, respectively, of the mandible at the temporomandibular joints (TMJs). These are nonaxial glide motions.

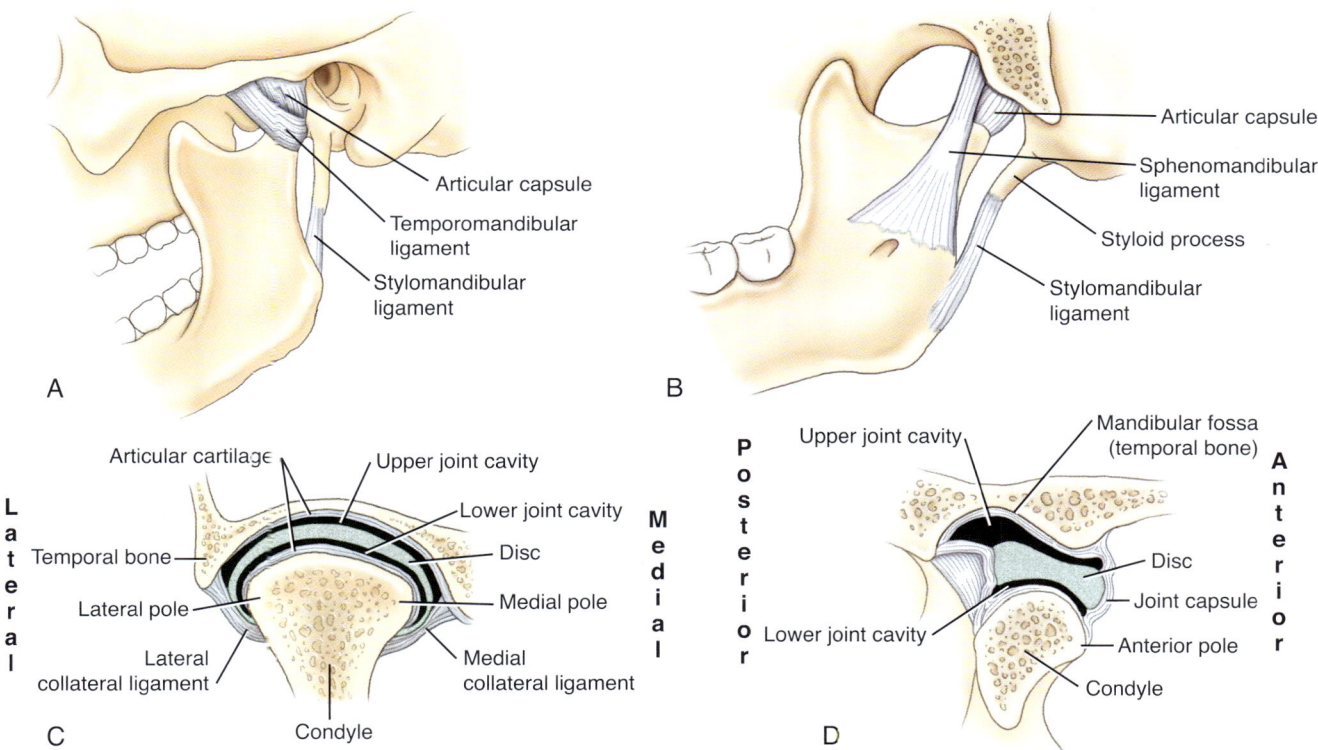

FIGURE 8-6 **A,** Left lateral view of the temporomandibular joint (TMJ). The temporomandibular ligament is located on and stabilizes the lateral side of the TMJ. **B,** Medial view illustrating the right stylomandibular and sphenomandibular ligaments. **C,** Anterior view of a coronal (i.e., frontal) section through the right TMJ. The articular disc can be seen to divide the joint into two separate joint cavities: upper and lower. **D,** Lateral view of a sagittal section of the right TMJ in the open position. The articular disc can be seen to move anteriorly along with the condyle of the mandible.

SECTION 8.3 SPINE

The **spine**, also known as the **spinal column** or **vertebral column**, is literally a column of vertebrae stacked one on top of another.[8]

ELEMENTS OF THE SPINE:

- The spine has four major regions (Figure 8-7).
- These four regions contain a total of 26 movable elements.
- The following are the four regions:
  1. **Cervical spine** (i.e., the neck), containing seven vertebrae (C1-C7)[9]
  2. **Thoracic spine** (i.e., the upper and middle back), containing 12 vertebrae (T1-T12)[9]
  3. **Lumbar spine** (i.e., the low back), containing five vertebrae (L1-L5)[9]
  4. **Sacrococcygeal spine** (within the pelvis) containing one sacrum, which is formed by the fusion of five vertebrae (S1-S5) that have never fully formed, and one coccyx, which is usually composed of four bones (Co1-Co4) that are even less developed and may partially or fully fuse as a person ages[5]

SHAPE OF THE ADULT SPINE VIEWED POSTERIORLY:

- Viewed posteriorly, the adult spine should ideally be straight (see Figure 8-7, A, Box 8-6).

SHAPE OF THE ADULT SPINE VIEWED LATERALLY:

- Viewed laterally, the adult spine should have four curves in the sagittal plane (see Figure 8-7, B).
- It has two **primary spinal curves** that are formed first (before birth) and two **secondary spinal curves** that are formed second (after birth).[9]
- The two primary curves of the spine are the thoracic and sacrococcygeal curves.
  - These curves are **kyphotic** (i.e., concave anteriorly and convex posteriorly).[9]
- The two secondary curves of the spine are the cervical and lumbar curves.
  - These curves are **lordotic** (i.e., concave posteriorly and convex anteriorly).[9]

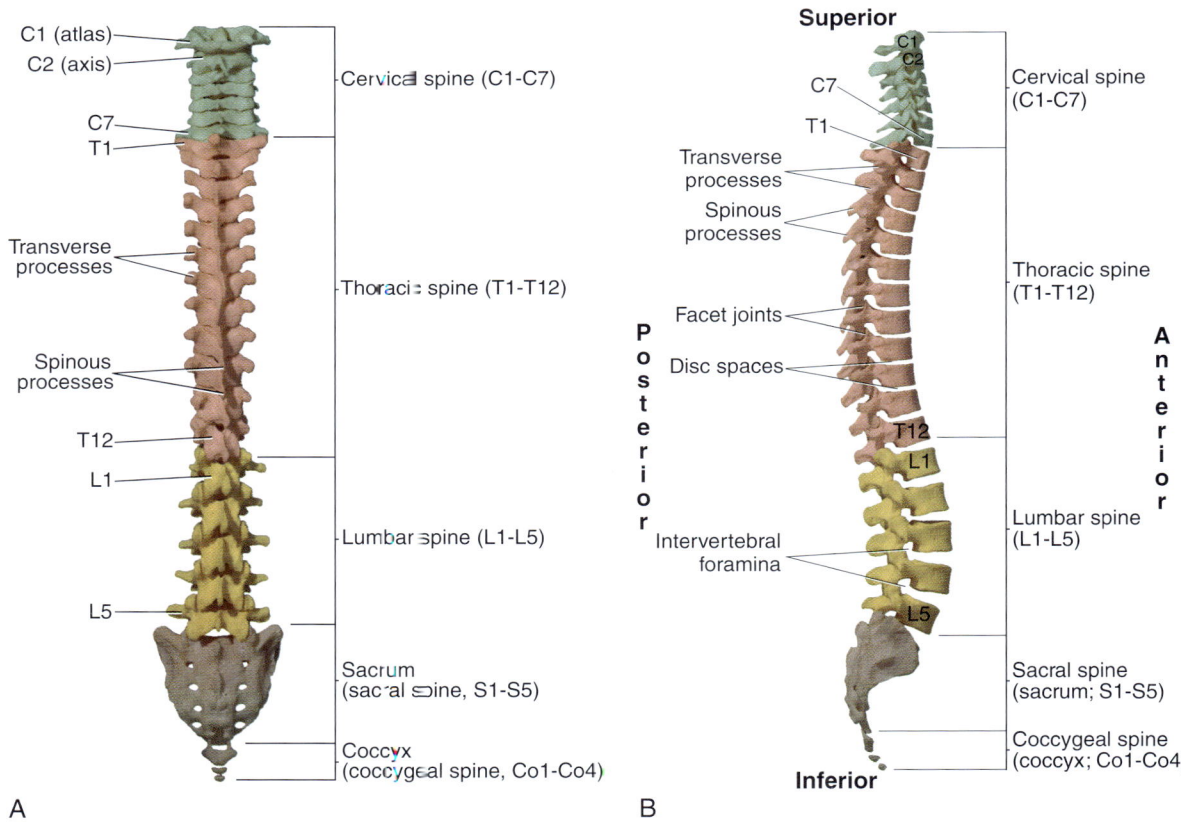

FIGURE 8-7 **A**, Posterior view of the entire spine. **B**, Right lateral view of the entire spine. The spine is composed of the cervical region containing C1-C7, the thoracic region containing T1-T12, the lumbar region containing L1-L5, and the sacrococcygeal region containing the sacrum and coccyx.

BOX 8-6

By definition, any spinal curve that exists from a posterior view is termed a **scoliosis**[7]; a scoliotic curve is a C-shaped curvature of the spine that exists within the frontal plane (and because frontal plane lateral flexion usually couples with transverse plane rotation, a scoliotic curve also involves rotation). Ideally the spine should be straight within the frontal plane; therefore a scoliosis is considered to be a postural pathology of the spine. A scoliosis is named left or right, based on the side of the curve that is convex. For example, if a curve in the lumbar spine exists that is convex to the left (therefore concave to the right), it is called a left lumbar scoliosis. A scoliosis may even have two or three curves (called an S or double-S scoliosis, respectively); again, each of the curves is named for the side of the convexity.

BOX 8-7 Spotlight on Sagittal Plane Spinal Curves

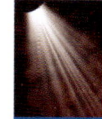

A kyphotic curve is a **kyphosis**; a lordotic curve is a **lordosis**. The terms kyphosis and lordosis are often misused in that they are used to describe an individual who has an excessive kyphotic or lordotic curve. It is normal and healthy to have a kyphosis in the thoracic and sacral spines and to have a lordosis in the cervical and lumbar spines. An excessive kyphosis should correctly be termed a hyperkyphosis or a **hyperkyphotic** curve; an excessive lordosis should correctly be termed a hyperlordosis or a **hyperlordotic** curve. Similarly, decreased curves would be termed **hypolordotic** and **hypokyphotic** curves. Many people have a hypolordotic lower cervical spine (i.e., decreased lower cervical lordotic curve)—either because the curve never fully developed or because it was lost after it developed—with a compensatory hyperlordotic upper cervical curve. This is largely because of the posture of sitting with the head forward when writing (e.g., at a desk) or working with a digital device. At a very early age we give our children crayons to draw with; then they graduate to pencils in elementary school and pens in high school and beyond. And perhaps even more of concern is that many children begin working with digital devices as early as elementary school (or even earlier). The tremendous number of hours sitting with the neck and head bent (i.e., flexed) forward over a piece of paper or a digital device causes a decrease in the extension of the lower cervical spinal joints, which is a decrease in the cervical lordotic curve. (Note: Many other postures also contribute to a loss of the lower cervical lordosis.)

DEVELOPMENT OF THE SPINAL CURVES:

- When a baby is born, only one curve to the entire spine exists, which is kyphotic. In effect, the entire spinal column is one large C-shaped kyphotic curve (Figure 8-8).
- Two activities occur during our childhood development that create the cervical and lumbar lordoses[9]:
  1. When a child first starts to lift his or her head to see the world (which is invariably higher), the spinal joints of the neck must extend, creating the cervical lordosis. This cervical lordosis is necessary to bring the position of the head posteriorly so that the head's weight is balanced over the trunk (see Figure 8-8, *B*).
  2. Next, when the child wants to sit up (and later stand up), the spinal joints of the low back must extend, creating the lumbar lordosis. This lumbar lordosis is necessary to bring the position of the trunk posteriorly so that the trunk's weight is balanced over the pelvis (see Figure 8-8, *C*). Otherwise, when the child tries to sit up, he or she would fall forward.
- In effect, the cervical and lumbar lordotic secondary curves are formed after birth, whereas the thoracic and sacrococcygeal regions retain their original primary kyphotic curves. The net result is a healthy adult spine that has four curves in the sagittal plane.
- The four kyphotic and lordotic curves of an adult spine are usually attained at approximately the age of 10 years (Box 8-7).

FUNCTIONS OF THE SPINE:

The spine has four major functions[9] (Figure 8-9):

1. To provide structural support for the body (see Figure 8-9, *A*)
   - The spine provides a base of support for the head and transmits the entire weight of the head, arms, neck, and trunk to the pelvis.
2. To allow for movement (see Figure 8-9, *B*)
   - As with all joints, the spine must find a balance between structural stability and movement. Generally, the more stable a joint is, the less mobile it is; and the more mobile a joint is, the less stable it is. The spine is a remarkable structure in that it can provide so much structural support to the body and yet also afford so much movement!

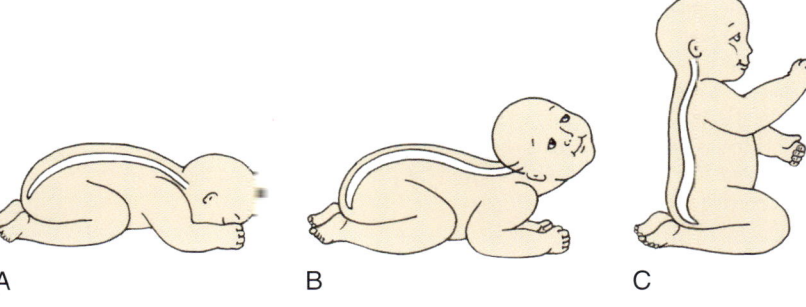

FIGURE 8-8 The developmental formation of the curves of the spine. **A,** Baby with one C-shaped kyphosis for the entire spine. **B,** Baby lifting the head, thereby creating the cervical lordosis of the neck. **C,** Baby sitting up, thereby creating the lumbar lordosis of the low back.

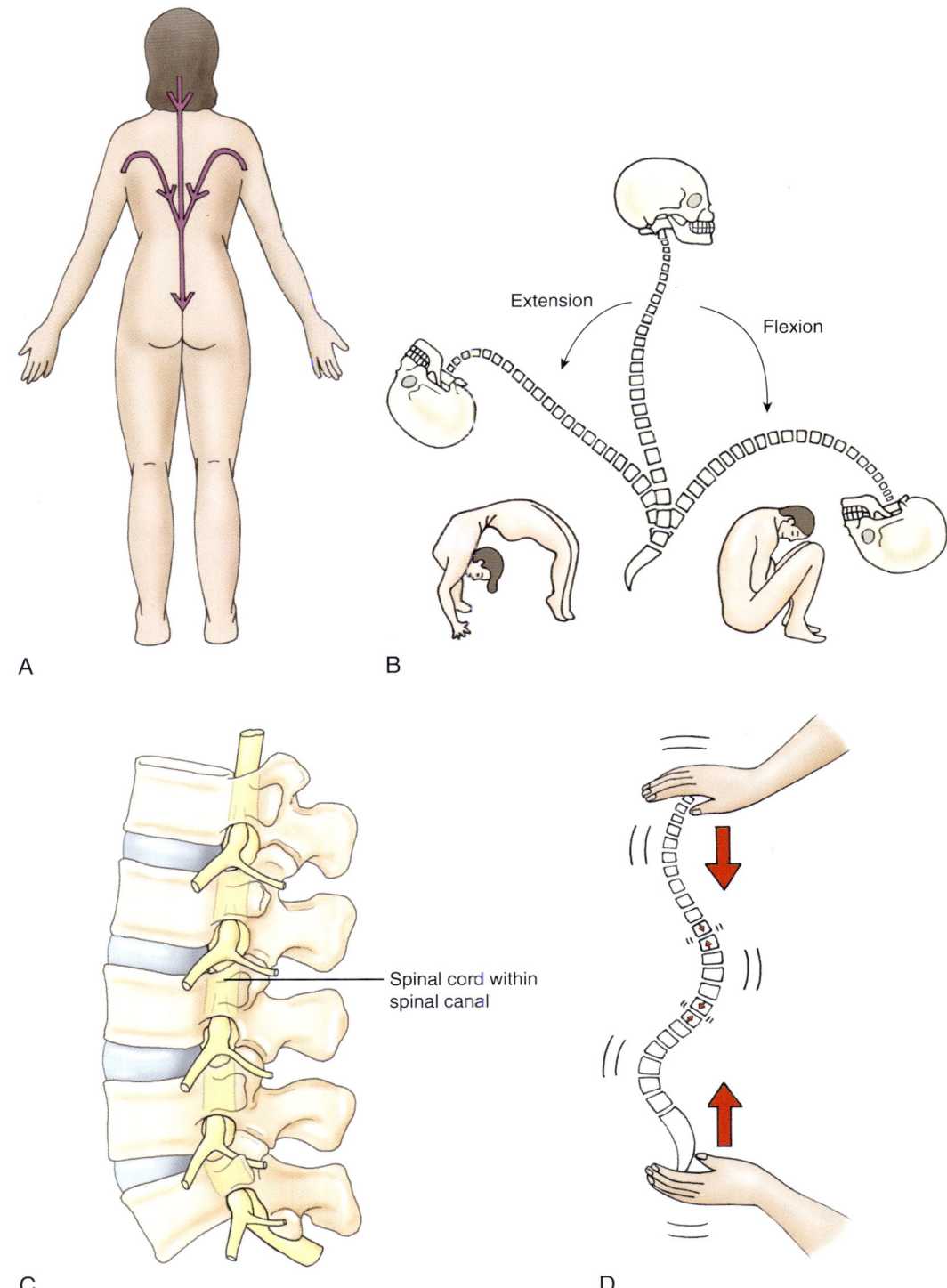

FIGURE 8-9 The four major functions of the spine. **A,** Posterior view illustrating its weight-bearing function; the lines drawn indicate the weight of the head, arms, and trunk being borne through the spine and transmitted to the pelvis. **B,** Lateral view demonstrating the tremendous movement possible of the spine (specifically, flexion and extension of the spinal joints are shown). **C,** The spine surrounds and protects the spinal cord, located within the spinal canal. **D,** Lateral view that illustrates how the spine can function to absorb shock and compressive forces; both the disc joints themselves and the spinal curves contribute to shock absorption (i.e., absorbing compression force). *(B, Modeled after Kapandji IA: Physiology of the joints: the trunk and the vertebral column, ed 2, Edinburgh, 1974, Churchill Livingstone.)*

- Although each spinal joint generally allows only a small amount of movement, when the movements of all 25 spinal segmental levels are added up, the spine allows a great deal of movement in all three planes (Table 8-1).
- The spine allows for movement of the head, neck, trunk, and pelvis. (Illustrations of these motions are shown in Sections 8.5 [head], 8.6 [neck], 8.10 [trunk], and 9.3 through 9.5 [pelvis].)
- The head can move relative to the neck at the atlanto-occipital joint (AOJ).
- The neck can move at the cervical spinal joints located within it (and/or relative to the head at the AOJ, or relative to the trunk at the C7-T1 joint).
- The trunk can move at the thoracic and lumbar spinal joints located within it (or relative to the pelvis at the lumbosacral joint).
- The pelvis can move relative to the trunk at the lumbosacral joint.

3. To protect the spinal cord (see Figure 8-9, C)
   - Neural tissue is very sensitive to damage. For this reason, the spinal cord is hidden away within the spinal canal and thereby afforded a great degree of protection from damage.
4. To provide shock absorption for the body (see Figure 8-9, D)
   - Being a weight-bearing structure, the spine provides shock absorption to the body whenever a compression force occurs, such as walking, running, or jumping. This is accomplished in two ways:
   - The nucleus pulposus in the center of the discs absorbs this compressive force.
   - The curves of the spine bend and increase slightly, absorbing some of this compressive force. They then return to their normal posture afterward.

TABLE 8-1	Average Ranges of Motion of the Entire Spine from Anatomic Position (Including the Atlanto-Occipital Joint [AOJ] between the Head and the Neck)[5]*		
Flexion	135 Degrees	Extension	120 Degrees
Right lateral flexion	90 Degrees	Left lateral flexion	90 Degrees
Right rotation	120 Degrees	Left rotation	120 Degrees

*No exact agreement exists among sources as to the average or ideal ranges of motion of joints. The ranges given in this text are approximations. Actual ranges of motion vary somewhat from one individual to another. Furthermore, ranges of motion vary enormously with age.

SECTION 8.4 SPINAL JOINTS

- Spinal joints are joints that involve two contiguous vertebrae (i.e., two adjacent vertebrae) of the spine.
- Naming a spinal joint is usually done by simply naming the levels of the two vertebrae involved. For example, the joint between the fifth cervical vertebra (C5) and the sixth cervical vertebra (C6) is called the *C5-C6 joint*.
- Again, using this example, the C5-C6 joint is one segment of the many spinal joints and is often referred to as a segmental level of the spine. The C6-C7 joint would be another, C7-T1 would be the next, and so forth.
- At any one typical segmental level of the spine, one median joint and two lateral joints exist (the median joint is located in the middle, and the lateral joints are located to the sides, hence the names).[5]
- Typically the median joint is an intervertebral disc joint and the lateral joints are the two vertebral facet joints[5] (Figure 8-10).
  - The median spinal joint at the atlanto-occipital (AOJ) and atlantoaxial joint (AAJ) are not disc joints[5] (see Section 8.5).
- When movement of one vertebra occurs relative to the contiguous vertebra, this movement is the result of movement at both the intervertebral disc joint and vertebral facet joints.

INTERVERTEBRAL DISC JOINT:

- An intervertebral disc joint is located between the bodies of two contiguous vertebrae. This joint is often referred to simply as the disc joint.[10]
- Joint structure classification: Cartilaginous joint
  - Subtype: Symphysis
- Joint function classification: Amphiarthrotic

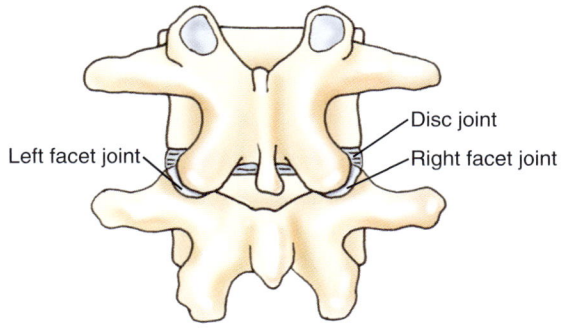

FIGURE 8-10 The median and lateral spinal joints. The median spinal joint is the disc joint; the lateral spinal joints are the facet joints.

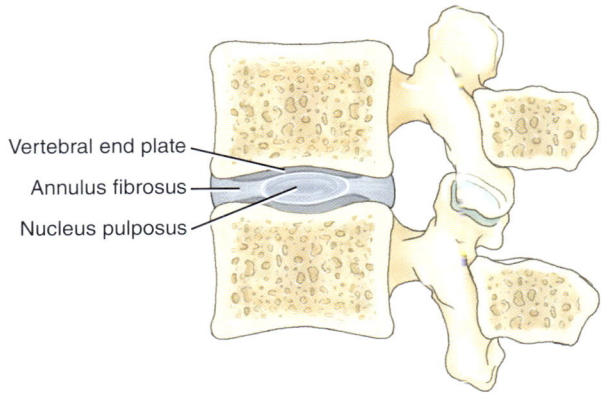

FIGURE 8-11 The three major components of the intervertebral disc joint: (1) the annulus fibrosus, (2) the nucleus pulposus and (3) the vertebral endplates of the vertebral bodies.

Miscellaneous:

- A disc joint is composed of three parts: (1) an outer annulus fibrosus, (2) an inner nucleus pulposus, and (3) the two vertebral endplates (Figure 8-11).
- Discs are actually quite thick, accounting for approximately 25% of the height of the spinal column. The thicker a disc is, the greater its shock absorption ability and the more movement it allows.
- In addition to allowing movement, two major functions of the disc joint are (1) to absorb shock and (2) to bear the weight of the body.
  - The spinal disc joint bears approximately 80% of the weight of the body above it (the other 20% is borne through the facet joints).
- The presence of a disc is also important because it maintains the opening of the intervertebral foramina (through which the spinal nerves travel) by creating a spacer between the two vertebral bodies (Box 8-8).

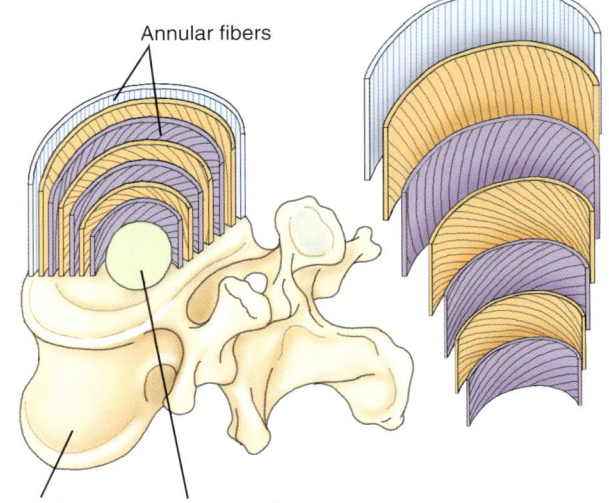

FIGURE 8-12 The basket weave configuration of the concentric layers of the annulus fibrosus of the intervertebral disc joint. The reader should note how each successive layer has a different orientation to its fibers than the previous layer. Each layer is optimal at resisting the force that runs along its direction. The sum total of having all these varying fiber directions is to resist and stabilize the disc joint along almost any line of force to which the joint may be subjected. *(Modeled after Kapandji IA: Physiology of the joints: the trunk and the vertebral column, ed 2, Edinburgh, 1974, Churchill Livingstone.)*

two vertebrae), shear forces (i.e., a horizontal sliding of one vertebra on the other), and torsion forces (i.e., a twisting of one vertebra on the other).
- The inner **nucleus pulposus** is a pulplike gel material that is located in the center of the disc and is enclosed by the annulus fibrosus.[11]
- The nucleus pulposus has a water content that is 80% or greater (Box 8-9).

BOX 8-8

If a disc thins excessively, the decreased size of an intervertebral foramen may impinge on the spinal nerve that is located within it. This is commonly known as a pinched nerve and may result in referral of pain, numbness, or weakness in the area that this nerve innervates.

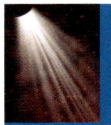

BOX 8-9 Spotlight on Pathologic Disc Conditions

When a pathologic condition of the disc occurs, it usually involves damage to the annulus fibrosus, allowing the inner nucleus pulposus to bulge or rupture (i.e., herniate) through the annular fibers. The term **slipped disc** is a nonspecific lay term that does not really mean anything. Discs do not "slip"; they either bulge or rupture. When this does occur, the most common danger is that the nearby spinal nerve may be compressed in the intervertebral foramen, resulting in a pinched nerve that refers symptoms to whatever location of the body that this nerve innervates. Another common pathologic condition of the disc is disc thinning. The reason that the nucleus pulposus has such a high water content is that it is largely composed of proteoglycans. Therefore, given the principle of thixotropy (see Section 4.6), movement of the spine is critically important toward maintaining proper disc hydration and health. Because disc hydration is responsible for the thickness of the disc, loss of disc hydration would result in thinning of the disc height (disc thinning) and approximation of the vertebral bodies, resulting in an increased likelihood of spinal nerve compression in the intervertebral foramina.

- The outer **annulus fibrosus** is a tough fibrous ring of fibrocartilaginous material that encircles and encloses the inner nucleus pulposus.[11]
  - The annulus fibrosus is composed of up to 10 to 20 concentric rings of fibrous material.
  - These rings are arranged in a basket weave configuration that allows the annulus fibrosus to resist forces from different directions (Figure 8-12).
  - More specifically, the basket weave configuration of the fibers of the annulus fibrosus gives the disc a great ability to resist distraction forces (i.e., a vertical separation of the

- The **vertebral endplate** is composed of both hyaline articular cartilage and fibrocartilage, and it lines the surface of the vertebral body.[9] Each disc joint contains two vertebral endplates: one lining the inferior surface of the superior vertebra, and the other lining the superior surface of the inferior vertebra.

VERTEBRAL FACET JOINTS:

- Technically, the correct name for a facet joint is an **apophyseal joint** or a **zygapophyseal joint**. However, these joints of the spine are usually referred to as simply the *facet joints*.[5]
- Because a facet is a smooth flat surface (think of the facets of a cut stone ring), and the facet joints are formed by the smooth flat surfaces (i.e., the facets) of the articular processes, the name *facet joint* is usually used to refer to these apophyseal (or zygapophyseal) joints of the spine. However, it must be kept in mind that in referring to these joints as *facet joints*, the context must be clear because other joints in the body involve facets. Facet joints are also often referred to as **Z joints** (Z for zygapophyseal).
- A vertebral **facet joint** is located between the articular processes of two contiguous vertebrae.[9]
  - More specifically, a facet joint of the spine is formed by the inferior articular process of the superior vertebra articulating with the superior articular process of the inferior vertebra (Figure 8-13).
- The actual articular surfaces of a facet joint are the facets of the articular processes, hence the name *facet joint*.
- There are two facet joints, paired left and right, between each two contiguous vertebrae.
- Joint structure classification: Synovial joint
  - Subtype: Plane
- Joint function classification: Diarthrotic

Miscellaneous:

- The main purpose of a facet joint is to guide movement.[9]
- The planes of the facets of the facet joint determine the movement that is best allowed at that level of the spine[9] (Figure 8-14).

- The cervical facets are generally oriented in an oblique plane that is approximately 45 degrees between the transverse and frontal planes. Therefore these facet joints freely allow transverse and frontal plane motions (i.e., right rotation and left rotation within the transverse plane, and right lateral flexion and left lateral flexion within the frontal plane).[5]
- The orientation of the cervical facets is often compared with the angle of roof shingles. However, as good as these regional rules for facet orientation are, it should be pointed out that they are generalizations. For example, the facet orientation at the upper cervical spine is nearly perfectly in the transverse plane, not a 45-degree angle like the midcervical region. Furthermore, the orientation of the facet planes is a gradual transition from one region of the spine to the next region. For example, the facet plane orientation of C6-C7 of the cervical spine is more similar to the facet plane orientation of T1-2 of the thoracic spine than it is similar to C2-3 of the cervical spine. To determine what motion is best facilitated by the facet planes at any particular segmental level, the facet joint orientation at that level should be observed.[5]
- The thoracic facets are generally oriented within the frontal plane. Therefore these facet joints freely allow right lateral flexion and left lateral flexion within the frontal plane.[5]
- The lumbar facets are generally oriented within the sagittal plane. Therefore these facet joints freely allow flexion and extension within the sagittal plane.[5]

SPINAL JOINT SEGMENTAL MOTION— COUPLING DISC AND FACET JOINTS:

Comparing and contrasting motion allowed by the disc and facet joints, the following can be stated:
- The disc joint and the two facet joints at any particular spinal joint level work together to create the movement at that segmental level.[10]
- Disc joints are primarily concerned with determining the amount of motion that occurs at a particular segmental level;

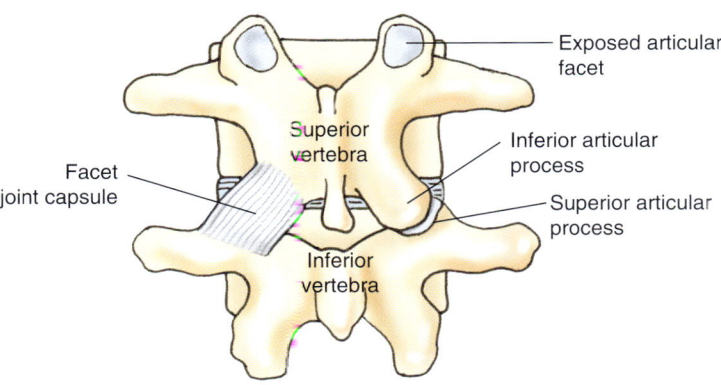
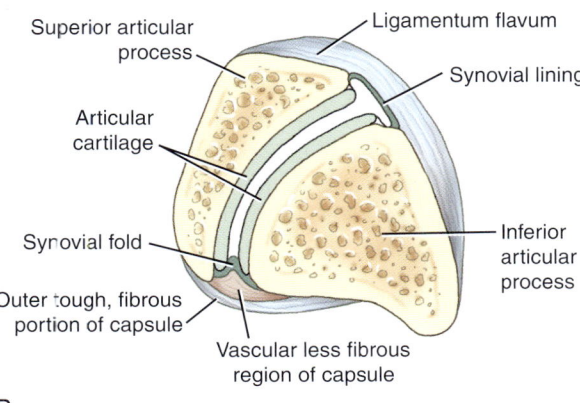

FIGURE 8-13 The vertebral facet joints. **A,** Posterior view of two contiguous vertebrae. On the left side, the facet joint capsule is seen intact. On the right side, the facet joint capsule has been removed, showing the superior and inferior articular processes; the articular facets of these processes articulate to form a facet joint. The superior articular facet surface of the right articular process of the superior vertebra is also visible. **B,** Cross-section through a facet joint showing the articular cartilage, fibrous capsule, and synovial lining.

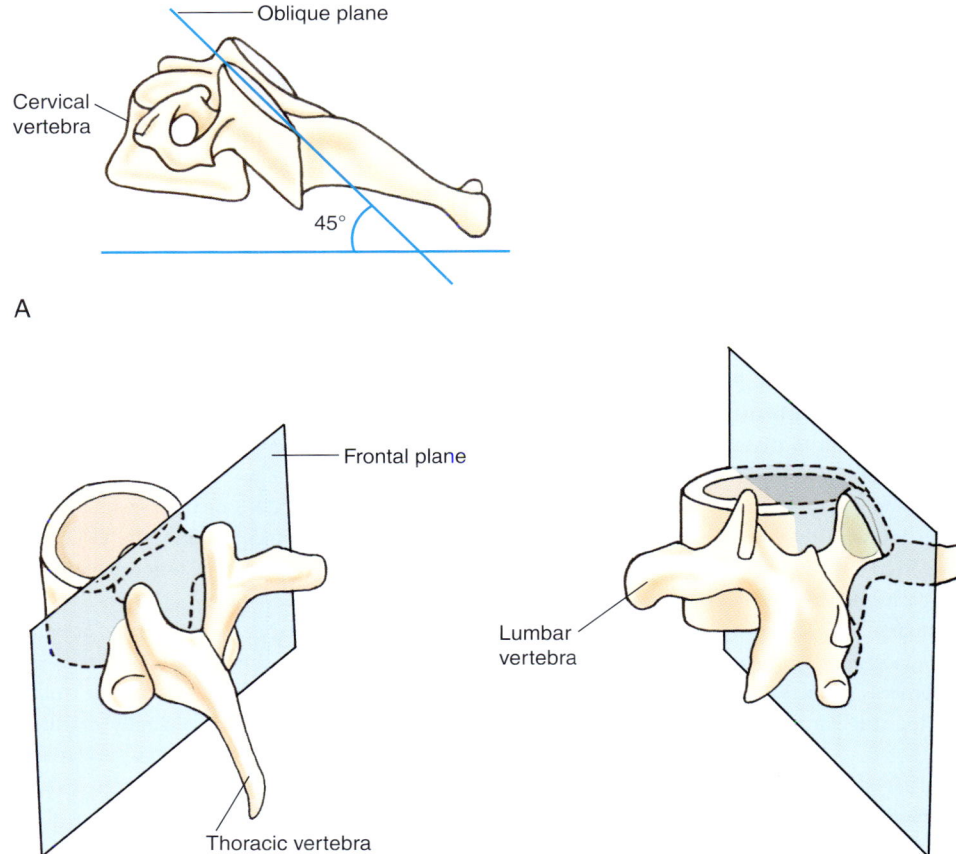

FIGURE 8-14 General orientation of the planes of the facets for the three regions of the spine. **A,** Lateral view of a cervical vertebra demonstrating the oblique plane of the cervical facet joints, which is approximately 45 degrees between the transverse and frontal planes. **B,** Posterolateral view of a thoracic vertebra demonstrating the frontal plane orientation of the thoracic facet planes. **C,** Posterolateral view of a lumbar vertebra demonstrating the sagittal plane orientation of the lumbar facet planes.

facet joints are primarily concerned with guiding the motion that occurs at that segmental level.
❍ The thicker the disc is, the more motion it allows; the orientation of the plane of the facets of that segmental level determines what type of motion is best allowed at that level.

MAJOR MOTIONS ALLOWED:

❍ Spinal joints allow flexion and extension (i.e., axial movements) within the sagittal plane around a mediolateral axis (Figure 8-15).
❍ Spinal joints allow right lateral flexion and left lateral flexion (i.e., axial movements) within the frontal plane around an anteroposterior axis (Figure 8-16).
❍ Spinal joints allow right rotation and left rotation (i.e., axial movements) within the transverse plane around a vertical axis (Figure 8-17).
❍ Spinal joints allow gliding translational movements in three directions (Figure 8-18):
  1. Right-side and left-side (lateral) translation (Perhaps the best visual example of lateral translation of the spinal joints of the neck is the typically thought of "Egyptian" dance movement wherein the head is moved from side to side.)
  2. Anterior and posterior translation
  3. Superior and inferior translation

Reverse Actions:

❍ Generally when we speak of motion at spinal joints, it is usually the more superior vertebra that is thought of as moving on the more fixed inferior vertebra; this is certainly the usual scenario for a person who is either standing or seated, because the lower part of our body is more fixed in these positions. However, it is possible, especially when we are lying down, for the more superior vertebrae to stay fixed and to move the more inferior vertebrae relative to the more fixed superior vertebrae of the spine.

MAJOR LIGAMENTS OF THE SPINAL JOINTS:

The following ligaments provide stability to the spine by limiting excessive spinal motions[5] (Figures 8-19 and 8-20; Box 8-10).
❍ Note that in all cases the ligaments of the spine limit motion that would occur in the opposite direction from where the ligament is located (this rule is true for all ligaments of the body). For example, anterior ligaments limit the posterior motion

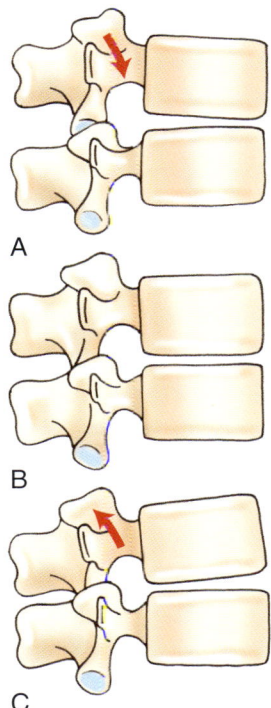

FIGURE 8-15 Flexion and extension within the sagittal plane of a vertebra on the vertebra that is below it. **A,** Flexion of the vertebra. **B,** Neutral position. **C,** Extension of the vertebra. These motions are a combination of disc and facet joint motion. (Note: All views are lateral.)

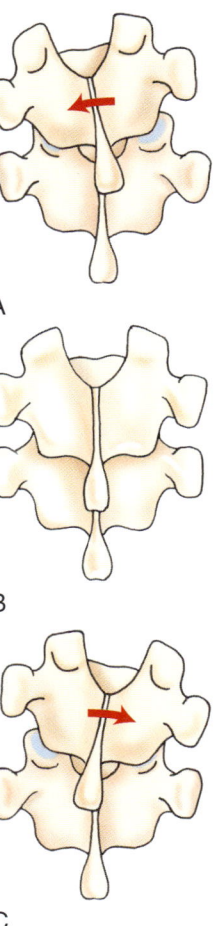

FIGURE 8-16 Left lateral flexion and right lateral flexion within the frontal plane of a vertebra on the vertebra that is below it. **A,** Left lateral flexion of the vertebra. **B,** Neutral position. **C,** Right lateral flexion of the vertebra. These motions are a combination of disc and facet joint motion. (Note: All views are posterior.)

of vertebral extension; posterior ligaments limit the anterior motion of vertebral flexion. The dividing line for anterior versus posterior is determined by where the center of motion is (i.e., where the axis of motion is located). For sagittal plane motions of the spine, the mediolateral axis of motion is located between the bodies.

Fibrous Joint Capsules of the Facet Joints:

○ Location: The fibrous joint capsules of the facet joints are located between articular processes of adjacent vertebrae of the spine (see Figure 8-13, *A*).[5]
○ Function: They stabilize the facet joints and limit the extremes of all spinal joint motions except extension (and inferior translation [i.e., compression of the two vertebrae wherein they come closer together]).

Annulus Fibrosus of the Disc Joints:

○ Location: The annulus fibrosus is located between adjacent vertebral bodies (see Figure 8-11).[5]
○ Function: It stabilizes the disc joint and limits the extremes of all spinal motions (except inferior translation).

Anterior Longitudinal Ligament:

○ Location: The **anterior longitudinal ligament** runs along the anterior margins of the bodies of the vertebrae (see Figure 8-19, *A*).[4]
○ Function: It limits extension of the spinal joints.

Posterior Longitudinal Ligament:

○ Location: The **posterior longitudinal ligament** runs along the posterior margins of the bodies of the vertebrae (within the spinal canal) (see Figure 8-19, *A*).[4]
○ Function: It limits flexion of the spinal joints.

BOX 8-10 Ligaments of the Spine

○ Fibrous capsules of the facet joints
○ Annulus fibrosus of the disc joints
○ Anterior longitudinal ligament
○ Posterior longitudinal ligament
○ Ligamenta flava
○ Interspinous ligaments
○ Supraspinous ligament
○ Intertransverse ligaments
○ Nuchal ligament

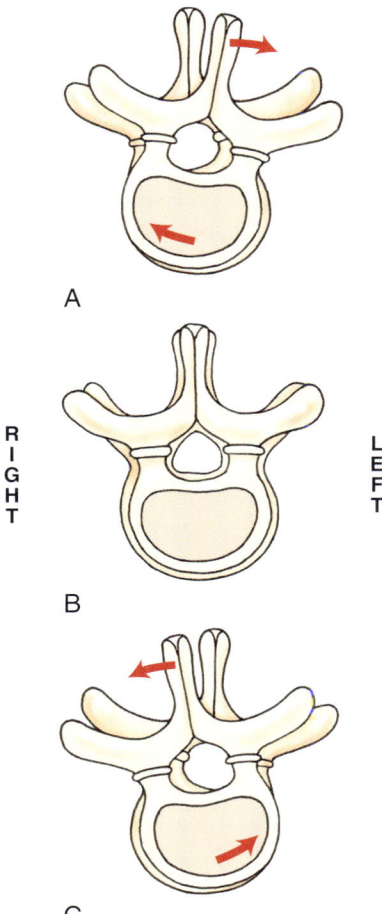

FIGURE 8-17 Left rotation and right rotation within the transverse plane of a vertebra on the vertebra that is below it. **A,** Right rotation of the vertebra. **B,** Neutral position. **C,** Left rotation of the vertebra. These motions are a combination of disc and facet joint motion. The reader should note that rotation of a vertebra is named for where the anterior aspect of the vertebra (i.e., the body) points. (Note: All views are superior.)

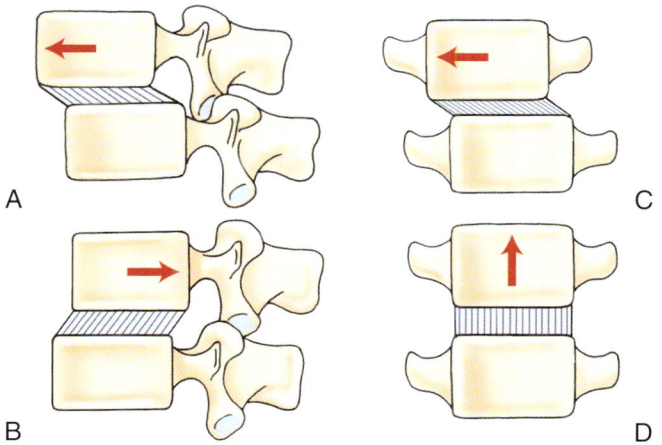

FIGURE 8-18 Translation motions of a vertebra on the vertebra that is below it. **A,** Anterior translation of the vertebra. **B,** Posterior translation. **C,** Lateral translation to the right of the vertebra (lateral translation to the left would be the opposite motion). **D,** Superior translation of the vertebra (inferior translation would be the opposite motion). All translation motions are a combination of disc and facet joint motion. A and B are lateral views; C and D are anterior views.

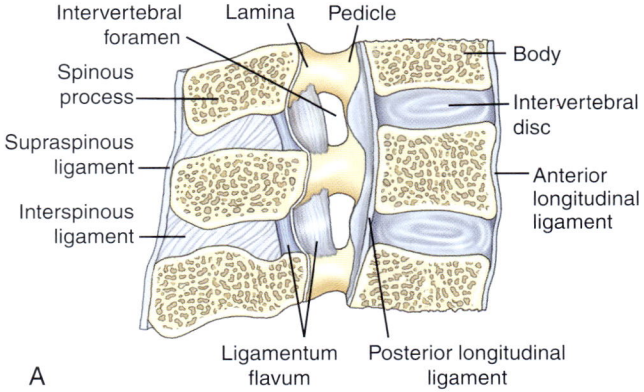

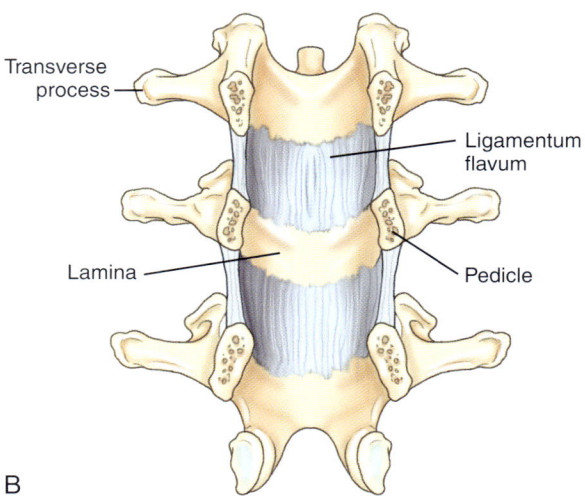

FIGURE 8-19 Ligaments of the spine. **A,** Lateral view of a sagittal cross-section. **B,** Posterior view of a coronal (frontal) plane cross-section in which all structures anterior to the pedicles have been removed. This view best illustrates the ligamenta flava running along the anterior aspect of the laminae within the spinal canal.

Ligamenta Flava:
- Two **ligamenta flava** (singular: ligamentum flavum) are located on the left and right sides of the spinal column.[5]
- Location: They run along the anterior margins of the laminae of the vertebrae within the spinal canal (see Figure 8-19).
- Function: They limit flexion of the spinal joints.

Interspinous Ligaments:
- Location: The **interspinous ligaments** are separate short ligaments that run between adjacent spinous processes of the vertebrae (see Figure 8-19, A).[5]
- Function: They limit flexion of the spinal joints.

Supraspinous Ligament:
- Location: The **supraspinous ligament** runs along the posterior margins of the spinous processes of the vertebrae (see Figure 8-19, A).[4]
- Function: It limits flexion of the spinal joints.

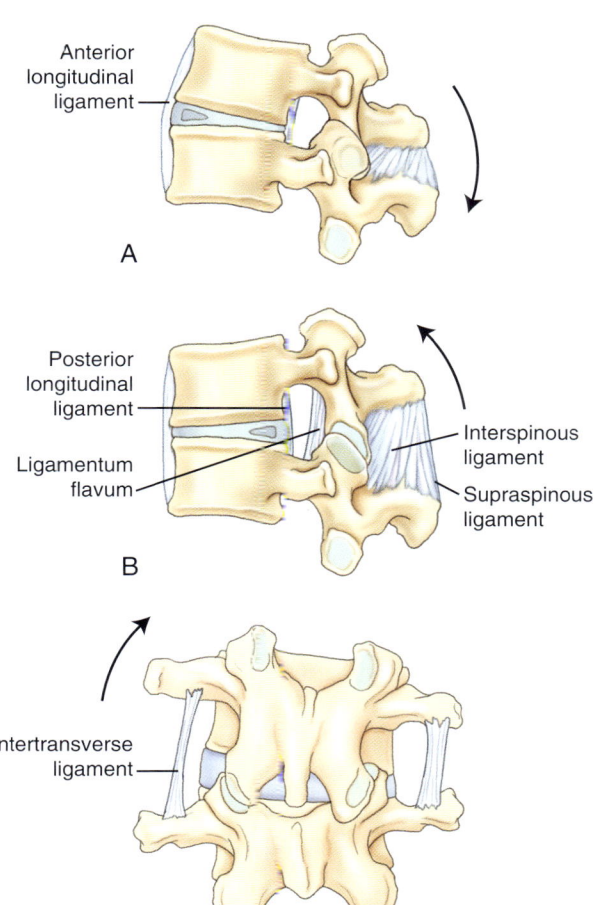

FIGURE 8-20 Demonstration of how ligaments of the spine limit motion. **A,** The superior vertebra in extension. The anterior longitudinal ligament located anteriorly becomes taut, limiting this motion. **B,** The superior vertebra in flexion. All ligaments on the posterior side (supraspinous, interspinous, ligamentum flavum, and posterior longitudinal ligaments) become taut, limiting this motion. **C,** The superior vertebra in (right) lateral flexion. The intertransverse ligament on the opposite (left) side becomes taut, limiting this motion. (Note: In this position the opposite side [left] facet joint capsule would also become taut, limiting this motion. A and B are lateral views; C is a posterior view.)

Intertransverse Ligaments:

- Location: The **intertransverse ligaments** are separate short ligaments that run between adjacent transverse processes of the vertebrae (see Figure 8-20, *C*).[4]
- Function: They limit contralateral (i.e., opposite-sided) lateral flexion of the spinal joints. They also limit rotation away from anatomic position.
- Intertransverse spinal ligaments are usually absent in the neck.

Nuchal Ligament:

- The **nuchal ligament** is a ligament that runs along and between the spinous processes from C7 to the external occipital protuberance (EOP) of the skull. The nuchal ligament is a thickening of the supraspinous ligament of the cervical region.[4]
- Function: It limits flexion of the spinal joints and provides a site of attachment for muscles of the neck (Figure 8-21).

 BOX 8-11

Some of the nuchal ligament's deepest fibers interdigitate into the dura mater. Clinically, this raises the question of whether tension on the nuchal ligament (perhaps from tight muscle attachments) may create an adverse pull on the dura mater.

- The trapezius, splenius capitis, rhomboids, serratus posterior superior, and cervical spinales (of the erector spinae group) all attach into the nuchal ligament of the neck (Box 8-11).
- The nuchal ligament is especially taut and stable in four-legged animals, such as dogs and cats. Their posture is such that their head is imbalanced in thin air (whereas our bipedal posture allows for the center of weight of our head to be centered and balanced on our trunk), allowing gravity to pull on their head and neck, making them fall into flexion. This requires a constant opposition pulling force toward extension to maintain their head in its position. The nuchal ligament gives them a strong passive force toward extension, allowing their posterior neck extensor musculature to not have to work as hard. Certainly, even with a nuchal ligament, most dogs and cats still love to have their posterior neck musculature rubbed, given its role in maintaining their neck and head posture.

MAJOR MUSCLES OF THE SPINAL JOINTS:

Many muscles cross the spinal joints. Regarding the actions of these muscles, the following general rules can be stated[12]:

- Muscles that extend the spine are located in the posterior trunk and neck and run with a vertical direction to their fibers. The erector spinae group, transversospinalis group, and other muscles in the posterior neck are examples of spinal extensors.
- Muscles that flex the spine are located in the anterior body and run with a vertical direction to their fibers. The muscles of the anterior abdominal wall and the muscles in the anterior neck are examples of spinal flexors.
- Muscles that laterally flex the spine are located on the side of the body and run with a vertical direction to their fibers. Almost all flexors and extensors are also lateral flexors, because they are usually located *anterior and lateral* or *posterior and lateral*. It should be noted that all lateral flexors are ipsilateral lateral flexors (i.e., whichever side of the body that they are located on is the side to which they laterally flex the body part [head, neck, and/or trunk]).
- Muscles that rotate the spine are more variable in their location. For example, muscles that provide right rotation of the head, neck, or trunk may be located anteriorly or posteriorly; furthermore, they may be located on the right side of the body (in which case they are ipsilateral rotators) or the left side of the body (in which case they are contralateral rotators). Prominent rotators of the trunk include the external and internal abdominal obliques and the transversospinalis group muscles. Prominent rotators of the head and/or neck include the sternocleidomastoid (SCM), upper trapezius, and splenius capitis and cervicis muscles, as well as the transversospinalis group muscles.

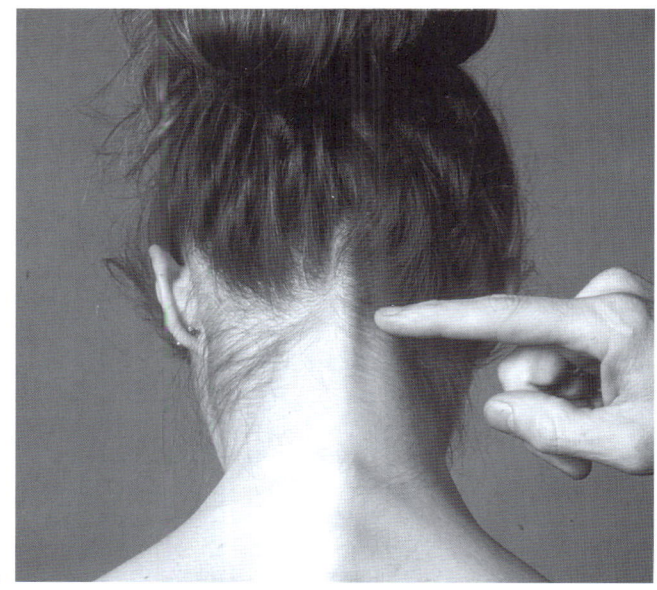

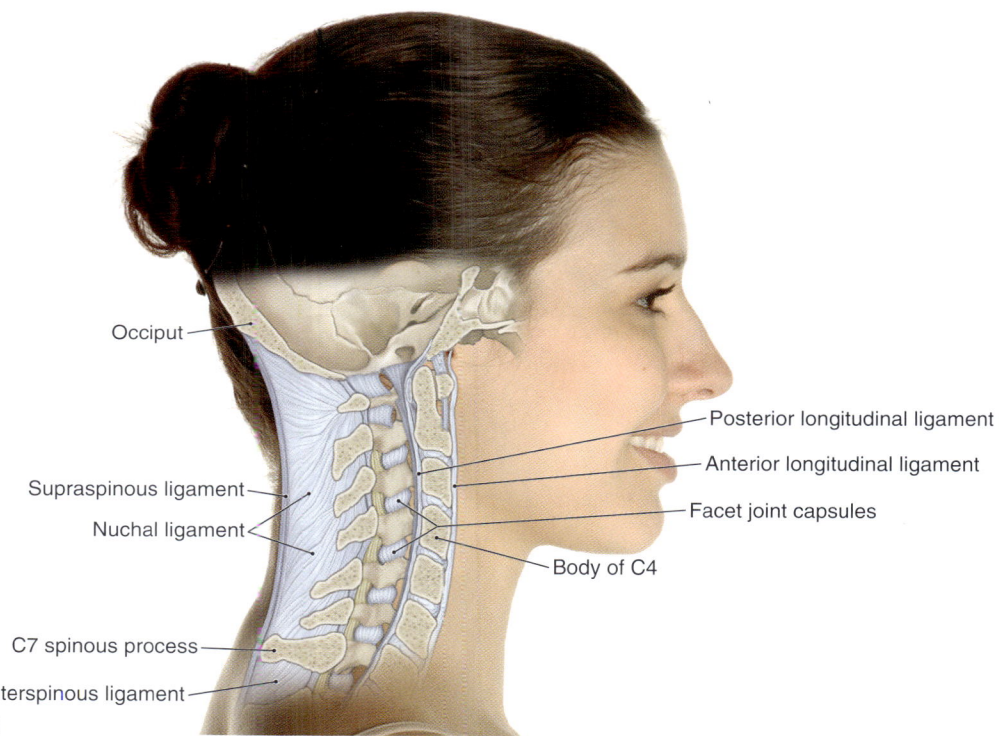

FIGURE 8-21 The nuchal ligament. **A,** Posterior view of a young woman. The nuchal ligament of the cervical region is seen to be taut as she flexes her head and neck at the spinal joints. **B,** Lateral view of the nuchal ligament. (A, From Neumann DA: *Kinesiology of the musculoskeletal system: foundations for physical rehabilitation*, ed 2 St Louis, 2010, Mosby. B, Modeled from Muscolino J: *The muscle and bone palpation manual, with trigger points, referral patterns, and stretching*, St Louis, 2009, Mosby.)

SECTION 8.5 ATLANTO-OCCIPITAL AND ATLANTOAXIAL JOINTS

Two cervical spinal joints merit special consideration:
- The **atlanto-occipital joint** (AOJ), located between the atlas (C1) and the occiput
- The **atlantoaxial joint** (AAJ or C1-C2 joint), located between the atlas (C1) and the axis (C2)

ATLANTO-OCCIPITAL JOINT:

- The AOJ (Figure 8-22) is formed by the superior articular facets of the atlas meeting the occipital condyles.
  - Therefore the AOJ has two lateral joint surfaces (i.e., two facet joints). Because the atlas has no body, no median disc joint exists as is usual for spinal joints.[5]
- The occipital condyles are convex, and the facets of the atlas are concave. This allows the occipital condyles to rock in the concave facets of the atlas.[6]
- Movement of the AOJ allows the cranium to move relative to the atlas (i.e., the head to move on the neck).
- Joint structure classification: Synovial joint
  - Subtype: Condyloid
- Joint function classification: Diarthrotic
  - Subtype: Triaxial
  - Note: The amount of rotation possible at the atlanto-occipital joint (AOJ) is considered to be negligible by many sources. Therefore these sources place the AOJ as being biaxial.

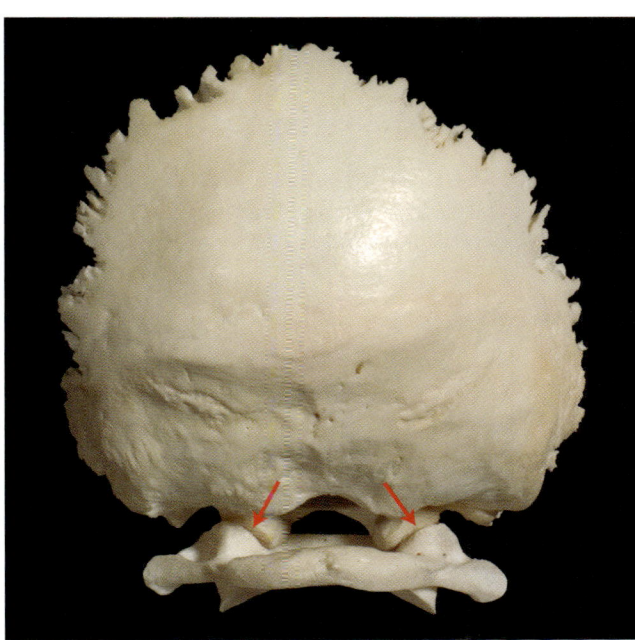

FIGURE 8-22 Posterior view of the atlanto-occipital joint (AOJ). In this photo, the occipital bone is flexed (i.e., lifted upward) to better show this joint. The AOJ is composed of two lateral joint articulations between the superior articular processes of the atlas and the condyles of the occiput.

Movement of the Head at the Atlanto-Occipital Joint:

Even though the head usually moves with the neck, the head and neck are separate body parts and can move independently of each other. The presence of the AOJ allows the head to move independently of the neck. When the head moves, it is said to move relative to the neck at the AOJ (Figures 8-23 to 8-25). Following are the movements of the head at the AOJ (the ranges of motion are given in Table 8-2):
- Flexion/extension (i.e., axial movements) in the sagittal plane around a mediolateral axis are the primary motions of the AOJ.
- The motion of nodding the head (as in indicating *yes*) is primarily created by flexing and extending the head at the AOJ.
- Right lateral flexion/left lateral flexion (i.e., axial movements) in the frontal plane around an anteroposterior axis are also allowed.
- Right rotation/left rotation (i.e., axial movements) in the transverse plane around a vertical axis are also allowed.

TABLE 8-2	Average Ranges of Motion of the Head at the Atlanto-Occipital Joint (AOJ) from Anatomic Position[5]		
Flexion	5 Degrees	Extension	10 Degrees
Right lateral flexion	5 Degrees	Left lateral flexion	5 Degrees
Right rotation	5 Degrees	Left rotation	5 Degrees

ATLANTOAXIAL (C1-C2) JOINT:

- The AAJ allows the atlas (C1) to move on the axis (C2) (Figure 8-26).
- The AAJ is composed of one median joint and two lateral joints.
- The median joint of the AAJ is the **atlanto-odontoid joint**.[5]
  - The atlanto-odontoid joint is formed by the anterior arch of the atlas meeting the odontoid process (i.e., dens) of the axis.
  - Articular facets are located on the joint surfaces of the atlas and axis (i.e., on the posterior surface of the anterior arch of the atlas and the anterior surface of the dens of the axis).
  - The atlanto-odontoid joint actually has two synovial cavities, one anterior to the dens and the other posterior to the dens.[5]
- The two lateral joints are the facet joints.
  - The facet joints of the AAJ are formed by the inferior articular facets of the atlas (C1) meeting the superior articular facets of the axis (C2).
- Joint structure classification: Synovial joints
  - Subtype
    - Atlanto-odontoid joint: Pivot joint
    - Lateral facet joints: Plane joints

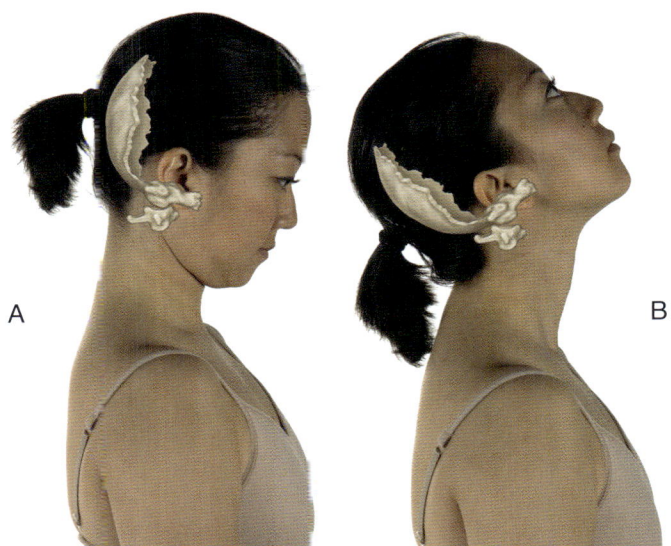

FIGURE 8-23 Lateral view illustrating sagittal plane motions of the head at the atlanto-occipital joint (AOJ). *A* illustrates flexion; *B* illustrates extension. The sagittal plane actions of flexion and extension are the primary motions of the AOJ.

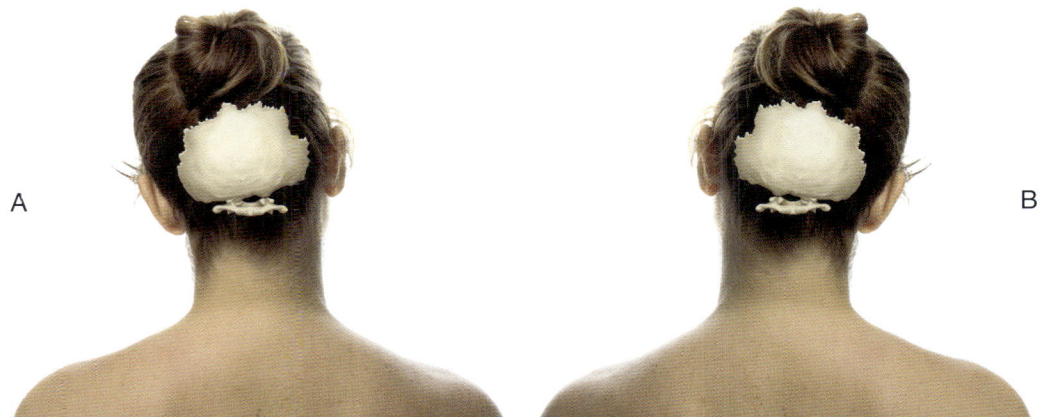

FIGURE 8-24 Posterior view illustrating lateral flexion motions of the head at the atlanto-occipital joint (AOJ). *A* Illustrates left lateral flexion; *B* illustrates right lateral flexion. These actions occur in the frontal plane.

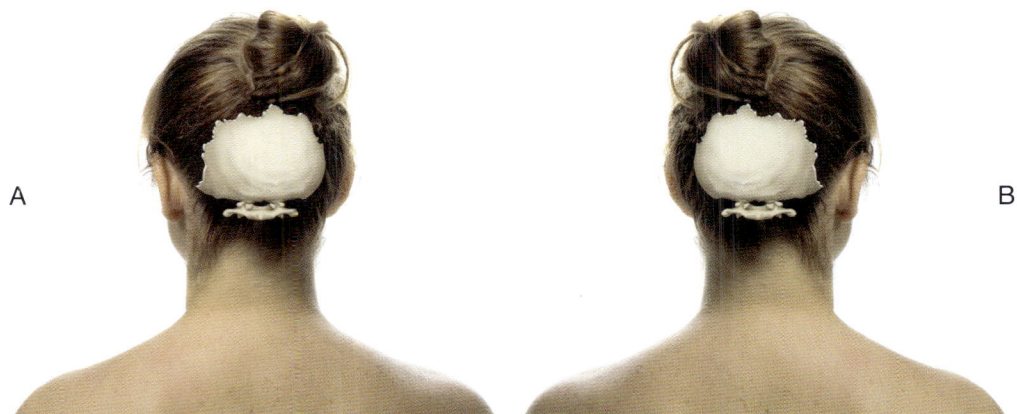

FIGURE 8-25 Posterior view that illustrates rotation motions of the head at the atlanto-occipital joint (AOJ). *A* illustrates left rotation; *B* illustrates right rotation. These actions occur in the transverse plane.

CHAPTER 8 Joints of the Axial Body

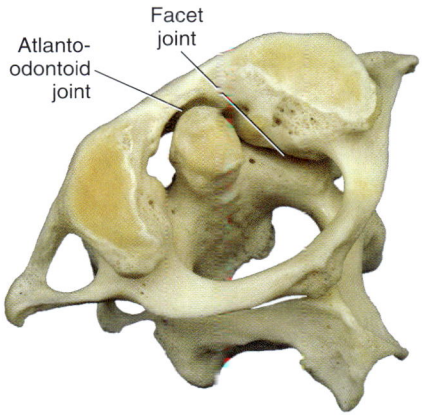

FIGURE 8-26 Oblique (superior posterolateral) view of the atlantoaxial joint (AAJ) (C1-C2). The AAJ is composed of three joints: a median atlanto-odontoid joint and two lateral facet joints.

- Joint function classification: Diarthrotic
  - Subtype: Biaxial
  - The atlanto-odontoid joint itself is often described as a *uniaxial pivot joint*. However, the AAJ complex (i.e., the median and two lateral joints) allows motion in two planes around two axes. Therefore all three AAJs together, including the atlanto-odontoid joint, technically are biaxial joints.
- Note: Intervertebral disc joints are located between bodies of adjacent vertebrae. Because the atlas has no body, there cannot be an intervertebral disc joint between the atlas and axis at the atlantoaxial (C1-C2) joint, and there cannot be an intervertebral disc joint between the atlas and occiput at the atlanto-occipital joint.

Movements of the Atlantoaxial Joint:

- Right rotation/left rotation (i.e., axial movements) in the transverse plane around a vertical axis are the primary motions of the AAJ.
  - Approximately half of all the rotation of the cervical spine occurs at the atlantoaxial joint (AAJ).[5] When you turn your head from side to side indicating *no,* the majority of that movement occurs at the AAJ.
- Flexion/extension (i.e., axial movements) in the sagittal plane around a mediolateral axis are also allowed.
- Right lateral flexion/left lateral flexion (i.e., axial movements) are negligible.
- The ranges of motion of the AAJ are given in Table 8-3.

TABLE 8-3 Average Ranges of Motion of the Atlas at the Atlantoaxial Joint (AAJ) (C1-C2 Joint) from Anatomic Position[5]

Flexion	5 Degrees	Extension	10 Degrees
Right lateral flexion	Negligible	Left lateral flexion	Negligible
Right rotation	40 Degrees	Left rotation	40 Degrees

MAJOR LIGAMENTS OF THE OCCIPITO-ATLANTOAXIAL REGION:

The following ligaments all provide stability to the AOJ and AAJ by limiting excessive motion of these joints (Box 8-12):

BOX 8-12 Ligaments of the Upper Cervical (Occipito-Atlantoaxial) Region

- Nuchal ligament
- Facet joint fibrous capsules of the atlanto-occipital joint (AOJ)
- Facet joint fibrous capsules of the atlantoaxial joint (AAJ)
- Posterior atlanto-occipital membrane
- Tectorial membrane
  - Accessory atlantoaxial ligament
- Cruciate ligament of the dens
- Alar ligaments of the dens
- Apical odontoid ligament
- Anterior longitudinal ligament
- Anterior atlanto-occipital membrane

Nuchal Ligament:

- The nuchal ligament (see Figure 8-21) of the cervical spine continues through this region to attach onto the occiput.[4]
- Functions: It limits flexion in this region and provides an attachment site for many muscles of the neck.

Facet Joint Fibrous Capsules of the Atlanto-Occipital Joint:

- Location: The facet joint fibrous capsules are located between the condyles of the occiput and the superior articular processes of the atlas (Figure 8-27).
- Function: They stabilize the atlanto-occipital facet joints.

Facet Joint Fibrous Capsules of the Atlantoaxial Joint:

- Location: The facet joint fibrous capsules are located between the inferior articular processes of the atlas and the superior articular processes of the axis (see Figure 8-27).
- Function: They stabilize the atlantoaxial facet joints.

Posterior Atlanto-Occipital Membrane:

- Location: The posterior atlanto-occipital membrane is located between the posterior arch of the atlas and the occiput.
- The posterior atlanto-occipital membrane between the atlas and occiput is the continuation of the ligamentum flavum of the spine (see Figure 8-27).
- Function: It stabilizes the AOJ.[5]

Tectorial Membrane:

- Location: The tectorial membrane is located within the spinal canal, just posterior to the cruciate ligament of the dens (Figure 8-28, *A*).

- The tectorial membrane is the continuation of the posterior longitudinal ligament in the region of C2 to the occiput.[4]
- The **accessory atlantoaxial ligament** (which runs from C2-C1) is considered to be composed of deep fibers of the tectorial membrane[13] (see Figure 8-28, *A* and *B*).
- Function: It stabilizes the AAJ and AOJ; more specifically, it limits flexion in this region.[13]

Cruciate Ligament of the Dens:

- The **cruciate ligament of the dens** attaches the dens of the axis to the atlas and occiput[13] (see Figure 8-28, *B*).
  - The cruciate ligament is given this name because it has the shape of a cross; *cruciate* means cross.
- It has three parts[13]: (1) a transverse band, (2) a superior vertical band, and (3) an inferior vertical band.
- The transverse band of the cruciate ligament is often called the **transverse ligament of the atlas**; the superior vertical band of the cruciate ligament is often called the **apical dental ligament** (located directly posterior to the apical odontoid ligament).
- Location: It is located within the spinal canal, between the tectorial membrane and the alar ligaments (anterior to the tectorial membrane and posterior to the alar ligaments).[13]
- Functions: It stabilizes the dens and limits anterior translation of the atlas at the AAJ and the head at the ACJ.[13]

Alar Ligaments of the Dens:

- Two **alar ligaments of the dens** (left and right) exist.
- Location: They run from the dens to the atlas and occiput (see Figure 8-28, *B* and *C*).
- Functions: They stabilize the dens by attaching it to the atlas and occiput, limit right and left rotation of the head at the AOJ and the atlas at the AAJ, and limit superior translation of the head at the AOJ and the atlas at the AAJ.[13]

Apical Odontoid Ligament:

- Location: The **apical odontoid ligament** runs from the dens to the occiput[4] (see Figure 8-28, *C*).
- Functions: It stabilizes the dens by attaching it to the occiput and limits superior and anterior translation of the head at the AOJ.[14]

Anterior Longitudinal Ligament:

- Location: The anterior longitudinal ligament continues through this region, attaching to the body of the axis, the anterior tubercle of the atlas, and ultimately onto the occiput[5] (Figure 8-29).
- Function: It limits extension in this region.[5]

Anterior Atlanto-Occipital Membrane:

- Location: The **anterior atlanto-occipital membrane** is located between the anterior arch of the atlas and the occiput (see Figure 8-29).
- Function: It stabilizes the AOJ.[13]

MAJOR MUSCLES OF THE OCCIPITO-ATLANTOAXIAL REGION:

Many muscles cross the AOJ and AAJ. (A complete atlas of all muscles of the body is located in Chapter 11.) Although the functional groups of spinal muscles were addressed in Section 8.4, the following muscles should be specially noted:
- Suboccipital group
  - Rectus capitis posterior major
  - Rectus capitis posterior minor
  - Obliquus capitis inferior
  - Obliquus capitis superior
- Rectus capitis anterior and rectus capitis lateralis of the prevertebral group

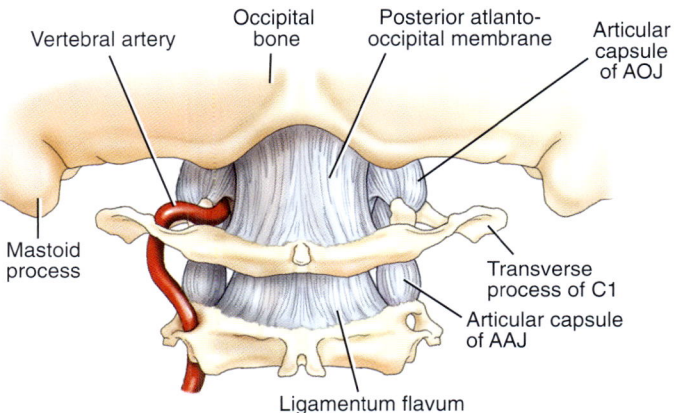

FIGURE 8-27 Posterior view of the upper cervical region demonstrating the facet joint capsules of the atlanto-occipital joint (AOJ) and atlanto-axial joint (AAJ), as well as the posterior atlanto-occipital membrane between the atlas and occiput. The posterior atlanto-occipital membrane is the continuation of the ligamentum flavum.

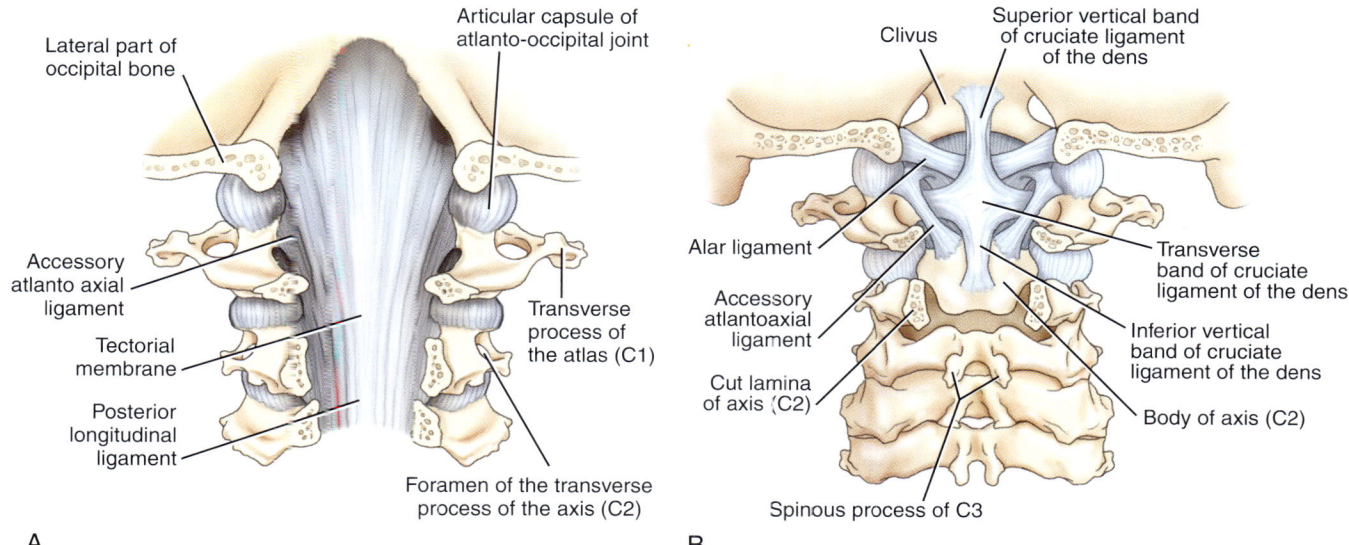

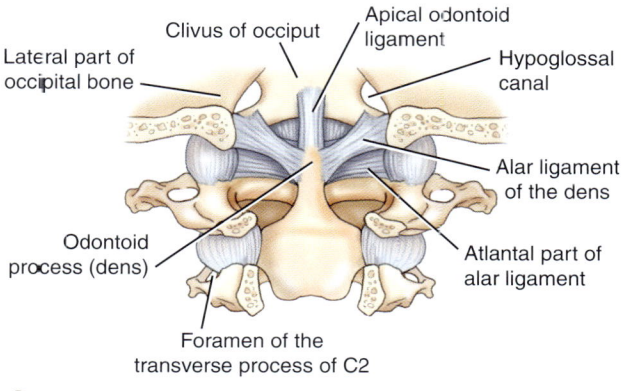

FIGURE 8-28 Posterior views of the ligaments of the upper cervical region within the spinal canal. **A,** Tectorial membrane that is the continuation of the posterior longitudinal ligament. **B,** Cruciate ligament of the dens located between the axis, atlas, and occiput. The cruciate ligament of the dens has three parts: (1) a superior vertical band, (2) an inferior vertical band, and (3) a transverse band. **C,** Apical odontoid and alar ligaments between the odontoid process of the axis and the atlas and occiput.

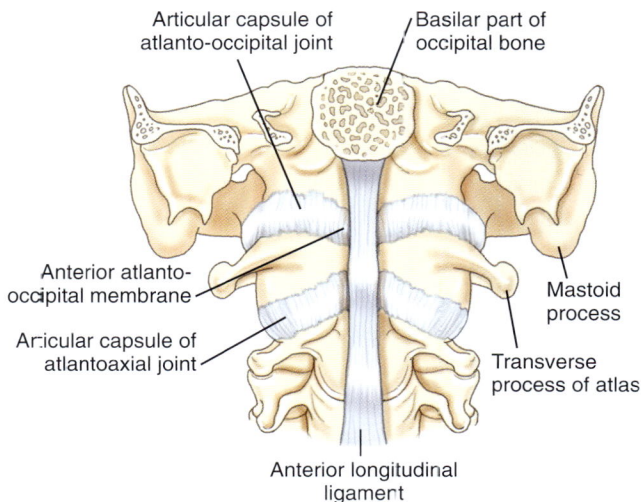

FIGURE 8-29 Anterior view of the upper cervical region demonstrating the anterior longitudinal ligament and the anterior atlanto-occipital membrane.

SECTION 8.6 CERVICAL SPINE (THE NECK)

The cervical spine defines the neck as a body part.

FEATURES OF THE CERVICAL SPINE:
Composition of the Cervical Spine:
- The cervical spine is composed of seven vertebrae (Figure 8-30).
- From superior to inferior, these vertebrae are named C1 through C7.
  - C1: The first cervical vertebra (C1) is also known as the *atlas*,[13] because it holds up the head, much as the Greek mythologic figure Atlas is depicted as holding up the world (Figure 8-31, *A*).
  - Actually, the Greek mythologic figure Atlas was forced by Zeus to hold up the sky, not the Earth. However, in artworks, Atlas is more often depicted as holding up the Earth.
  - C2: The second cervical vertebra (C2) is also known as the *axis*,[13] because the toothlike dens of C2 creates an axis of rotation around which the atlas can rotate (Figure 8-31, *B*). The spinous process of C2 is quite large and is a valuable landmark for palpation.[5]
  - C7: The seventh cervical vertebra (C7) is also known as the **vertebral prominens** because it is the most prominent cervical vertebra (and often a valuable landmark for palpation).[13]

Special Joints of the Cervical Spine:
- The joint between the atlas and the occiput is known as the *AOJ*.
- The joint between the atlas and the axis is known as the *AAJ* (or the C1-C2 joint). (See Section 8.5 for more information on the AOJ and AAJ.)

Transverse Foramina:
- Cervical vertebrae have transverse foramina in their transverse processes[2] (Figure 8-32, *A*; Box 8-13).

BOX 8-13
The cervical transverse foramina allows passage of the two **vertebral arteries** superiorly to the skull (see Figure 8-27). The vertebral arteries enter the cranial cavity to supply the posterior brain with arterial blood. If a client's head and upper neck are extended and rotated, one vertebral artery is naturally pinched off. If the other vertebral artery is blocked because of atherosclerosis or arteriosclerosis, and then the client's head is extended and rotated, the client could lose blood supply to the brain and might experience such symptoms as dizziness, lightheadedness, nausea, or ringing in the ears.

Bifid Spinous Processes:
- The cervical spine has **bifid spinous processes** (i.e., they have two points instead of one)[2] (see Figure 8-32, Box 8-14).

BOX 8-14
The presence of bifid spinous processes in the cervical spine may lead an inexperienced manual therapist to believe that a cervical vertebra has a rotational misalignment, when it does not. This is especially true of C2, because its bifid spinous process is so large and often asymmetric in shape.

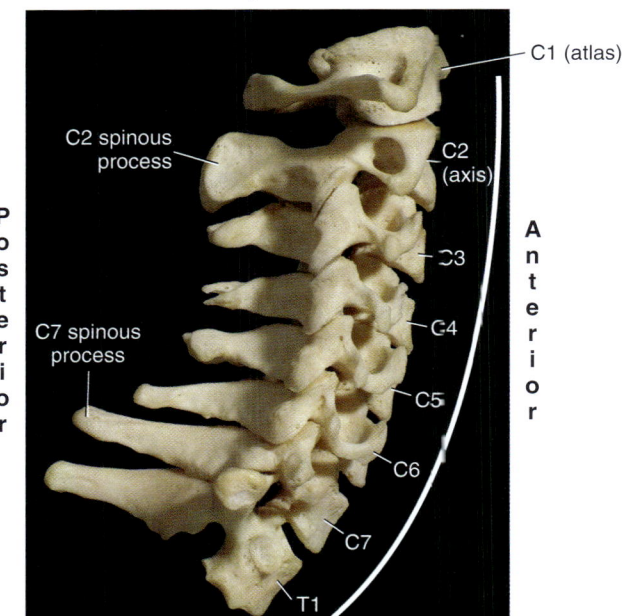

FIGURE 8-30 Right lateral view of the cervical spine. The reader should note the lordotic curve, which is concave posteriorly (and therefore convex anteriorly).

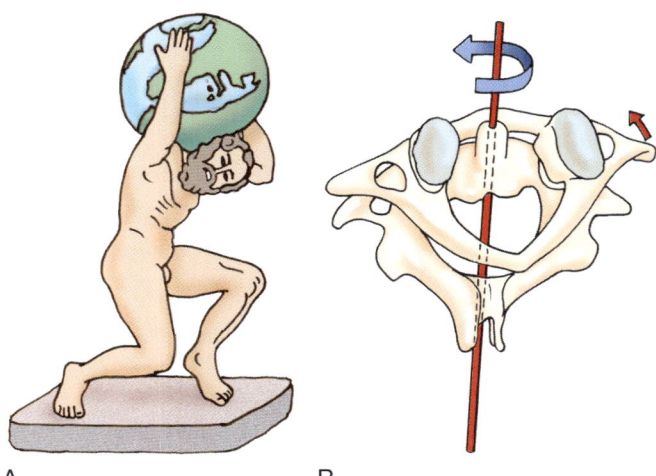

FIGURE 8-31 A, Greek mythologic figure Atlas supporting the world on his shoulders. Similarly, the first cervical vertebra (C1) supports the head. For this reason, C1 is known as the atlas. **B,** Dens of the second cervical vertebra (C2) forming an axis of rotation that the atlas can move around. For this reason, C2 is known as the axis.

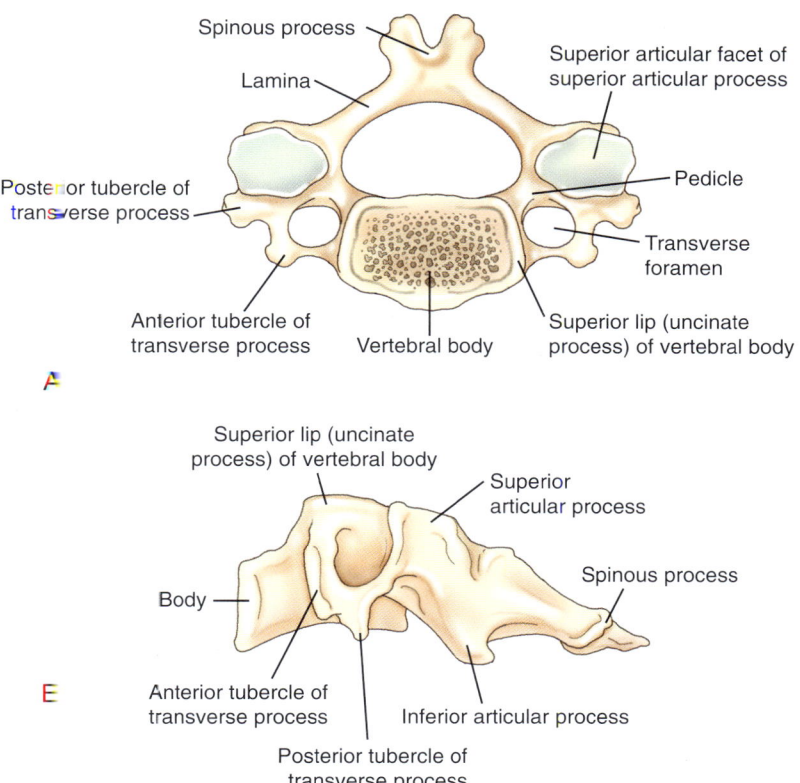

FIGURE 8-32 **A,** Superior view of a typical cervical vertebra. **B,** Lateral view. The reader should note the bifid spinous and transverse processes.

Bifid Transverse Processes:

❍ Most transverse processes of the cervical spine are **bifid transverse processes**. The two aspects are called the *anterior* and *posterior tubercles* (see Figure 8-32).

Uncinate Processes:

❍ The superior surfaces of the bodies of cervical vertebrae are not flat as in the rest of the spine; rather their lateral sides curve upward. This feature of the superior cervical body is called an **uncinate process** (see Figure 8-32).[13]
❍ Where the lateral sides of two contiguous cervical vertebrae meet each other is called an **uncovertebral joint**. (Uncovertebral joints are often called the **joints of Von Luschka**, after the person who first described them.)[13] These uncovertebral joints provide additional stability to the cervical spine because they serve to mildly limit frontal and transverse plane motions of the cervical vertebrae.

Curve of the Cervical Spine:

❍ The cervical spine has a lordotic curve[5] (i.e., it is concave posteriorly) (see Figure 8-30).

FUNCTIONS OF THE CERVICAL SPINE:

❍ Because only the head is superior to the neck, the cervical region has less of a weight-bearing function than the thoracic and lumbar regions. Having less weight-bearing function means that the cervical spine does not need to be as stable and can allow more movement.
❍ The cervical spine is the most mobile region of the spine, moving freely in all three planes [13](Tables 8-4 to 8-6).
  ❍ One reason that the cervical spine is so very mobile is the thickness of the intervertebral discs. The discs of the cervical spine account for approximately 40% of the height of the neck.

TABLE 8-4	Average Ranges of Motion of the Lower Cervical Spine (C2-C3 through C7-T1 Joints) from Anatomic Position[5]		
Flexion	40 Degrees	Extension	60 Degrees
Right lateral flexion	40 Degrees	Left lateral flexion	40 Degrees
Right rotation	40 Degrees	Left rotation	40 Degrees

TABLE 8-5 Average Ranges of Motion of the Entire Cervical Spine (i.e., the Neck; C1-C2 through C7-T1 Joints) from Anatomic Position (Numbers Include the Atlantoaxial Joint [AAJ] [C1-C2] and the Lower Cervical Spine Joints [C2-C3 through C7-T1])[5]

Flexion	45 Degrees	Extension	70 Degrees
Right lateral flexion	40 Degrees	Left lateral flexion	40 Degrees
Right rotation	80 Degrees	Left rotation	80 Degrees

TABLE 8-6 Average Ranges of Motion of the Entire Cervicocranial Region from Anatomic Position (the Neck and the Head) (Numbers Include the Entire Cervical Spine [C1-C2 through C7-T1 Joints] and the Head at the Atlanto-Occipital Joint [AOJ])[5]

Flexion	50 Degrees	Extension	80 Degrees
Right lateral flexion	45 Degrees	Left lateral flexion	45 Degrees
Right rotation	85 Degrees	Left rotation	85 Degrees

- The orientation of the cervical facet joints begins in the transverse plane at the top of the cervical spine; this accounts for the tremendous ability of the upper neck to rotate in the transverse plane.
- The cervical facet joints gradually transition from the transverse plane toward the frontal plane so that the facets of the mid to lower neck are obliquely oriented (similar to shingles on a 45-degree sloped roof) approximately halfway between the transverse and frontal planes (see Section 8.4, Figure 8-14, *A*).

MAJOR MOTIONS ALLOWED:

- The cervical spinal joints allow flexion and extension (i.e., axial movements) of the neck in the sagittal plane around a mediolateral axis (Figure 8-33, *A* and *B*).
- The cervical spinal joints allow right lateral flexion and left lateral flexion (i.e., axial movements) of the neck in the frontal plane around an anteroposterior axis (Figure 8-33, *C* and *D*).
- The cervical spinal joints allow right rotation and left rotation (i.e., axial movements) of the neck in the transverse plane around a vertical axis (Figure 8-33, *E* and *F*; Box 8-15).
- The cervical spinal joints allow gliding translational movements in all three directions[5] (see Section 8.4, Figure 8-18).

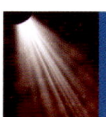

BOX 8-15 Spotlight on Coupled Cervical Motions

Because the facet joints of the cervical spine are oriented between the transverse and frontal planes, when the cervical spine laterally flexes, it ipsilaterally rotates as well. (Note: Remember that vertebral rotation is named for the direction in which the anterior bodies face; the spinous processes would therefore point in the opposite direction.) Therefore these two joint actions of lateral flexion and ipsilateral rotation are coupled together. Consequently, lateral flexion with rotation to the same side is a natural motion for the neck. **A** and **B,** Posterior views. *A* depicts the entire neck and head; *B* is a close-up of two cervical vertebrae.

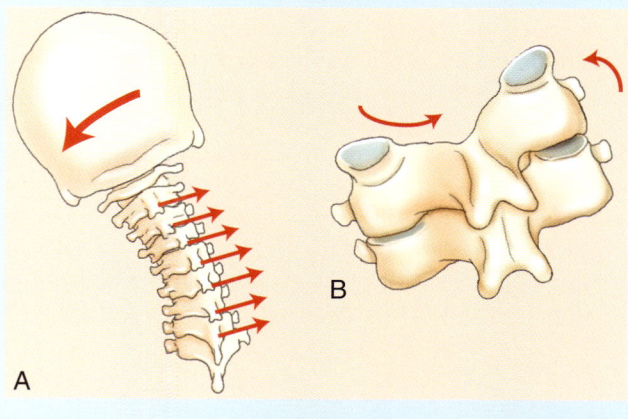

FIGURE 8-33 Motions of the neck at the spinal joints. *A* and *B* are lateral views that depict flexion and extension in the sagittal plane, respectively. *C* and *D* are posterior views that depict left lateral flexion and right lateral flexion in the frontal plane, respectively. *E* and *F* are anterior views that depict right rotation and left rotation in the transverse plane, respectively. Note: *A* through *F* depict motions of the entire craniocervical region (i.e., the head at the atlanto-occipital joint and the neck at the spinal joints).

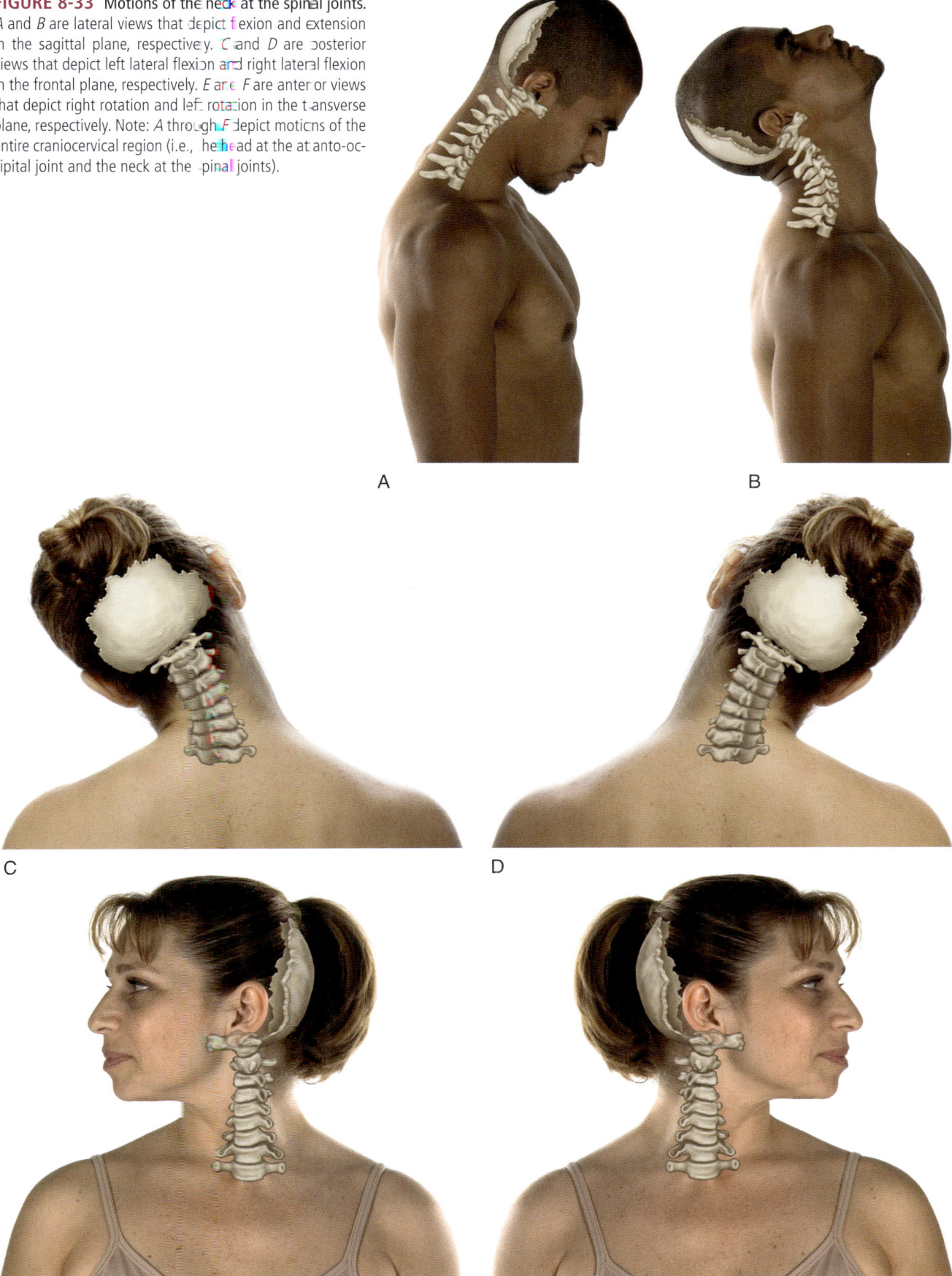

SECTION 8.7 THORACIC SPINE (THE THORAX)

- The thoracic spine defines the thorax of the body (i.e., the upper part of the trunk).
- Note: The trunk of the body is made up of the thorax and the abdomen. The **thorax** is the region of the thoracic spine, and the **abdomen** is the region of the lumbar spine.

FEATURES OF THE THORACIC SPINE:

Composition of the Thoracic Spine:
- The thoracic spine is composed of 12 vertebrae (Figure 8-34).
  - From superior to inferior, these vertebrae are named T1 through T12.
- The 12 thoracic vertebrae correspond to the 12 pairs of ribs that articulate with them.

FIGURE 8-34 Right lateral view of the thoracic spine. The reader should note the kyphotic curve, which is concave anteriorly (and therefore convex posteriorly).

Special Joints (Costospinal Joints):
- The ribs articulate with all 12 thoracic vertebrae. Generally each rib has two costospinal articulations with the spine: (1) the costovertebral joint and (2) the costotransverse joint (see Section 8.8, Figure 8-35). (For more detail on the rib joints of the thoracic spine, see Section 8.8.)
- The **costovertebral joint** is where the rib meets the bodies/disc of the spine.[5]
- The **costotransverse joint** is where the rib meets the transverse process of the spine.[5]
- Collectively, the costovertebral and costotransverse joints may be called the **costospinal joints**.

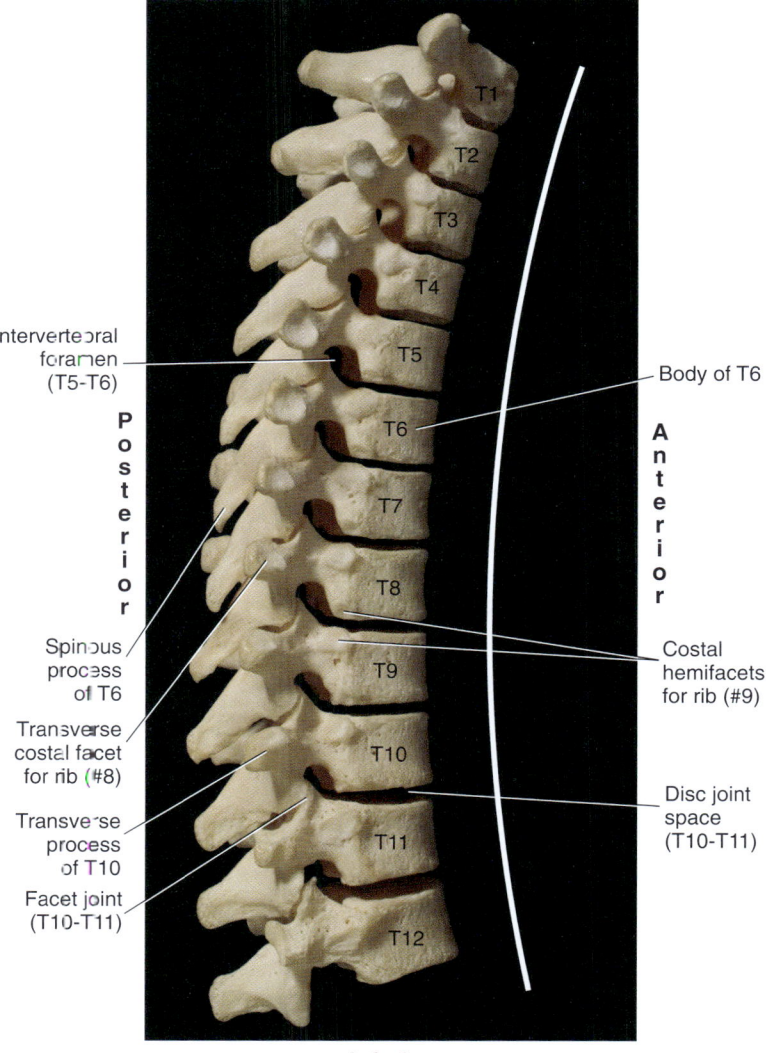

- Both the costovertebral and costotransverse joints are synovial joints.
  - These joints are nonaxial and allow gliding.
  - These joints both stabilize the ribs by giving them a posterior attachment to the spine and allow mobility of the ribs relative to the spine.
- Note: Ribs #1 through #10 also articulate with the sternum anteriorly; these joints are called *sternocostal joints*.

Curve of the Thoracic Spine:

- The thoracic spine has a kyphotic curve; in other words, it is concave anteriorly[13] (see Figure 8-34, Box 8-16).

BOX 8-16

As a person ages, it is common for a hyperkyphosis of the thoracic spine to develop. This is largely the result of activities that cause our posture to round forward, flexing the upper trunk (flexion of the upper trunk increases the thoracic kyphosis). It is also a result of the effects of gravity pulling the upper trunk down into flexion. For more on hyperkyphosis of the thoracic spine, see Section 21.3.

FUNCTIONS OF THE THORACIC SPINE:

- The thoracic region of the spine is far less mobile than the cervical and lumbar regions (Table 8-7).
- Being less mobile, the thoracic spine is more stable than the cervical and lumbar regions and therefore is injured less often.[4]
- The major reason for the lack of movement of the thoracic spine is the presence of the ribcage in this region.[4]
  - The ribcage primarily limits lateral flexion motion in the frontal plane and rotation motion in the transverse plane.
  - Lateral flexion is limited as a result of the ribs of the ribcage crowding into one another on the side to which the trunk is laterally flexed.
  - Rotation is limited as a result of the presence of the rib lateral to the vertebra.
- The spinous processes also limit range of motion of the thoracic spine. Because they are long and oriented inferiorly, they obstruct and limit extension of the thoracic spine.

TABLE 8-7 Average Ranges of Motion of the Thoracic Spine (T1-T2 through T12-L1 joints) from Anatomic Position*[5]

Flexion	35 Degrees	Extension	25 Degrees
Right lateral flexion	25 Degrees	Left lateral flexion	25 Degrees
Right rotation	30 Degrees	Left rotation	30 Degrees

*As in the cervical spine, when the thoracic spine laterally flexes, it ipsilaterally rotates to some degree as well. Therefore these two actions are coupled together.

- The orientation of the thoracic facet joints is essentially in the frontal plane (see Section 8.4, Figure 8-14, *B*), which should allow for ease of lateral flexion motion within the frontal plane; however, because of the presence of the ribcage, lateral flexion is limited.[5]
- In the lower thoracic region, the facet plane orientation gradually begins to change from the frontal plane to the sagittal plane (which is the orientation that the lumbar facets have). This sagittal orientation facilitates sagittal plane actions (i.e., flexion and extension).

MAJOR MOTIONS ALLOWED:

For motions of the thoracic spine, see Section 8.10; illustrations in Figure 8-41 demonstrate thoracolumbar motion of the trunk at the spinal joints.

- The thoracic spinal joints allow flexion and extension (i.e., axial movements) of the trunk in the sagittal plane around a mediolateral axis.
- The thoracic spinal joints allow right lateral flexion and left lateral flexion (i.e., axial movements) of the trunk in the frontal plane around an anteroposterior axis.
- The thoracic spinal joints allow right rotation and left rotation (i.e., axial movements) of the trunk in the transverse plane around a vertical axis.
- The thoracic spinal joints allow gliding translational movements in all three directions[3] (see Section 8.4, Figure 8-18).
- As in the cervical and lumbar regions, lateral flexion couples with rotation. It is generally stated that the upper thoracic spine couples lateral flexion with ipsilateral rotation (as in the cervical spine) and that the lower thoracic spine couples lateral flexion with contralateral rotation (as in the lumbar spine).

SECTION 8.8 RIB JOINTS OF THE THORAX

- As stated in Section 8.7, the ribs articulate with all 12 thoracic vertebrae posteriorly. The joints between the ribs and the spinal column are known collectively as the *costospinal joints*. Usually each rib has two articulations with the spine: (1) the costovertebral joint and (2) the costotransverse joint (Figure 8-35, *A*).
- The costovertebral joint is where the rib meets the vertebral bodies/disc.
  - The costovertebral joint where a rib articulates with the vertebral body is also known as the **costocorporeal joint**.[5] *Corpus* is Latin for body.
- The costotransverse joint is where the rib meets the transverse process of the spinal vertebra.
- Furthermore, most of the ribs articulate with the sternum anteriorly at the sternocostal joints.
- The proper movement of all rib joints is extremely important during respiration. (For more information on respiration, see Muscles of the Rib Joints later in this section and Box 8-19.)

COSTOSPINAL JOINTS IN MORE DETAIL:

Costovertebral Joint:

- The typical thoracic vertebral body has two costal hemifacets: one superiorly and one inferiorly (see Figure 8-35, B).
- The head of the rib therefore forms a joint with the inferior costal hemifacet of the vertebra above and the superior costal hemifacet of the vertebra below, as well as the intervertebral disc that is located between the two vertebral bodies[5] (see Figure 8-35, A).
- The costovertebral joint is stabilized by two ligamentous structures[5]:
  - Its fibrous joint capsule
  - The radiate ligament (see Figure 8-35, B and C, and Box 8-17)
- The typical costovertebral joint occurs between ribs #2 through #10 and the spine.
- The costovertebral joint of rib #1 meets a full costal facet at the superior end of the body of the T1 vertebra (i.e., no hemifacet on the body of C7 exists).
- The costovertebral joints of ribs #11 and #12 meet a full costal facet located at the superior body of T11 and T12, respectively.[14]

Costotransverse Joint:

- The typical thoracic vertebra has a full costal facet on its transverse processes (see Section 5.2, Figure 5-27, E and F).
- The costotransverse joint is where the tubercle of the rib meets the transverse process of the thoracic vertebra.[5]
- The costotransverse joint is stabilized by four ligamentous structures (see Box 8-17):
  - A fibrous joint capsule
  - A costotransverse ligament: This long ligament firmly attaches the neck of the rib with the entire length of the transverse process of the same level vertebra[5] (see Figure 8-35, C).
  - A lateral costotransverse ligament: This ligament attaches the costal tubercle of the rib to the lateral margin of the transverse process of the same level vertebra[13] (see Figure 8-35, C).
  - A superior costotransverse ligament: This ligament attaches the rib to the transverse process of the vertebra that is located superiorly[5] (see Figure 8-35, B).

BOX 8-17 Ligaments of the Costospinal Joints

Costovertebral joint:
- Fibrous joint capsule
- Radiate ligament

Costotransverse joint:
- Fibrous joint capsule
- Costotransverse ligament
- Lateral costotransverse ligament
- Superior costotransverse ligament

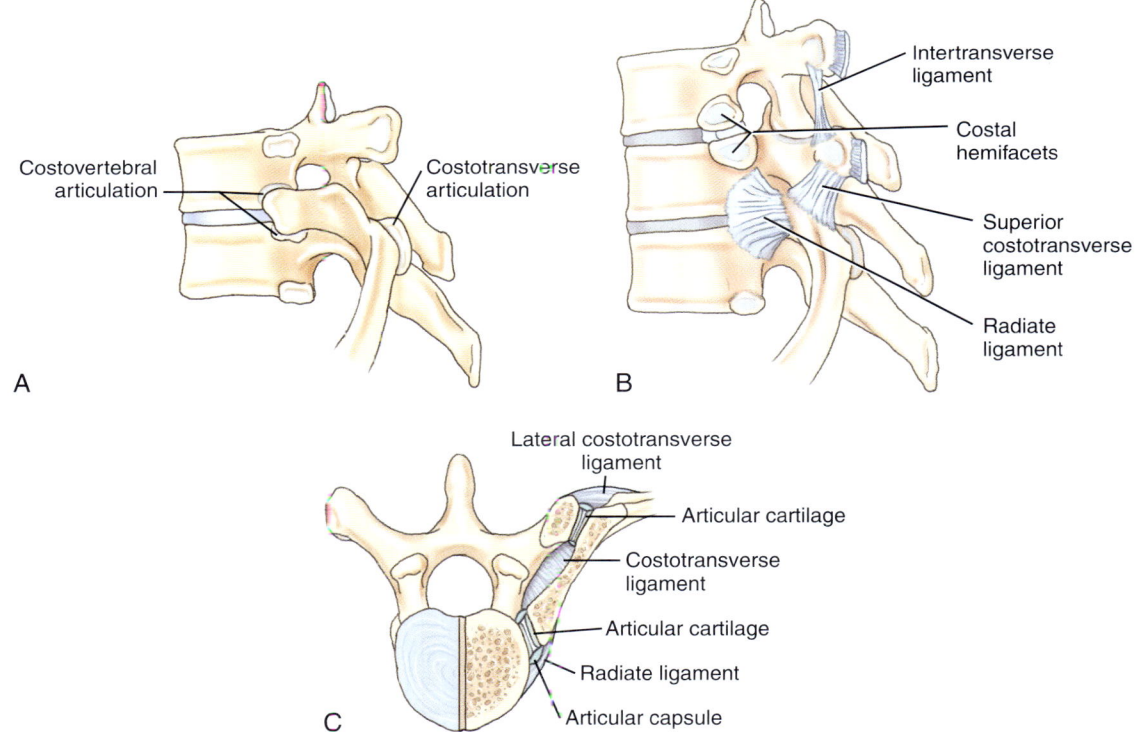

FIGURE 8-35 Joints between a rib and the spinal column (i.e., costospinal joints). **A,** Lateral view that depicts the costotransverse joint between the rib and transverse process of the vertebra and the costovertebral joint between the rib and bodies/disc of the vertebra. **B,** Lateral view depicting the radiate and superior costotransverse ligaments. **C,** Superior view in which half of the rib-vertebra complex has been horizontally sectioned to expose and illustrate the costospinal joints and the radiate, costotransverse, and lateral costotransverse ligaments.

- The typical costotransverse joints occur between ribs #1 through #10 and thoracic vertebrae #1 through #10 of the spine.[14]
- Ribs #11 and #12 do not articulate with transverse processes of the thoracic spine; hence they have no costotransverse joints.[5]

STERNOCOSTAL JOINTS:

- Seven pairs of **sternocostal joints** (Figure 8-36) attach ribs to the sternum anteriorly.[13]
- The first seven pairs of ribs attach directly to the sternum via their costal cartilages.
  - These ribs are called **true ribs**.[8]
- The ribs that do not attach directly into the sternum via their own costal cartilages are termed **false ribs**.
  - The eighth through tenth pairs of ribs join into the costal cartilage of the seventh rib pair.[13] These ribs are termed *false ribs*.[8]
  - The eleventh and twelfth rib pairs do not attach to the sternum at all; hence they are free floating anteriorly. These ribs are floating false ribs but are usually referred to simply as **floating ribs**.[14]

Sternocostal Rib Joints:

- Joint structure classification: Cartilaginous joint
  - Subtype: Synchondrosis[6]
- Joint function classification: Amphiarthrotic
  - Subtype: Gliding

Miscellaneous:

- Sternocostal joints actually involve three separate types of joints (Figure 8-37):
  1. **Costochondral joints** are located between the ribs and their cartilages.
     - A costochondral joint unites a rib directly with its costal cartilage. Neither a joint capsule nor any ligaments are present. The periosteum of the rib gradually transforms into the perichondrium of the costal cartilage. These joints permit very little motion.[5]
     - Ten pairs of costochondral joints exist (between ribs #1 through #10 and their costal cartilages).
  2. **Chondrosternal joints** are located between the costal cartilages of the ribs and the sternum.
     - A chondrosternal joint is a gliding synovial joint (except the first one, which is a synarthrosis) reinforced by its fibrous joint capsule and a **radiate ligament** (Box 8-18).[5]
     - Seven pairs of chondrosternal joints exist between costal cartilages and the sternum.[5]
  3. **Interchondral joints** are located between the costal cartilages of ribs #5 through #10.[5]
     - These joints are synovial lined[13] and reinforced by a capsule and an **interchondral ligament** (see Box 8-18)[5]

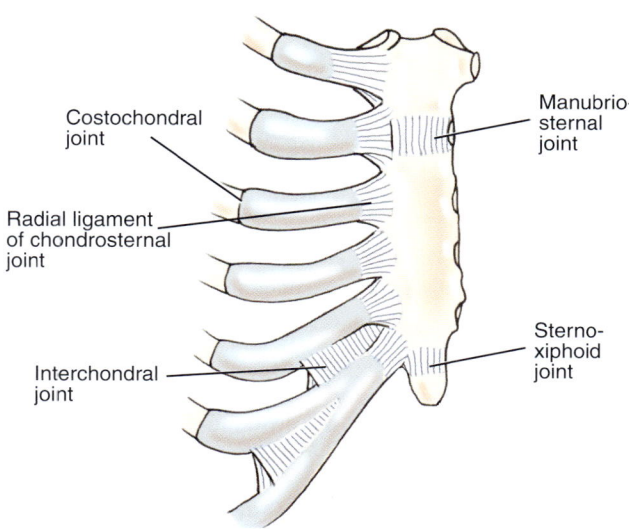

FIGURE 8-37 Anterior view of the sternum and part of the ribcage on one side of the body. Each sternocostal joint is actually composed of two articulations: (1) the costochondral joint located between a rib and its costal cartilage and (2) the chondrosternal joint located between the costal cartilage and the sternum (in addition, interchondral joints are located between adjacent costal cartilages of lower ribs). Furthermore, the manubriosternal and sternoxiphoid joints are located among the three parts of the sternum.

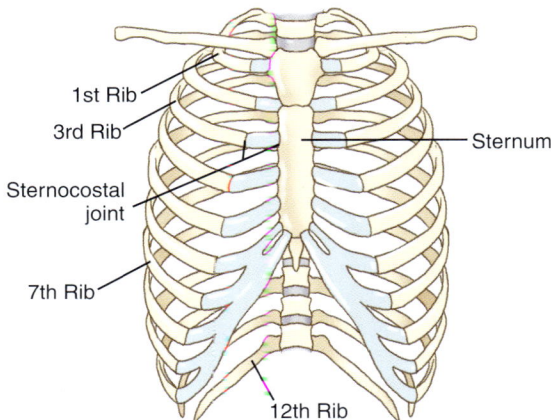

FIGURE 8-36 Anterior view of the ribcage. The sternocostal joint is located between a rib and the sternum. Seven pairs of sternocostal cartilages exist.

BOX 8-18 Ligaments of the Sternocostal and Intrasternal Joints

Chondrosternal joint:
- Fibrous joint capsule
- Radiate ligament

Interchondral joint:
- Fibrous joint capsule
- Interchondral ligament

Intrasternal joints:
- Manubriosternal and sternoxiphoid ligaments

INTRASTERNAL JOINTS:

Two intrasternal joints are located between the three parts of the sternum (see Figure 8-37).
1. The **manubriosternal joint** is located between the manubrium and body of the sternum.[13]
2. The **sternoxiphoid joint** is located between the body and xiphoid process of the sternum.[13]
   - These joints are fibrocartilaginous amphiarthrotic joints[5] that are stabilized by the manubriosternal ligament and the sternoxiphoid ligament, respectively (see Box 8-18).

MUSCLES OF THE RIB JOINTS:

- Muscles of the rib joints move the ribs at the sternocostal and costospinal joints. Moving the ribs is necessary for the process of respiration (i.e., breathing). Therefore muscles that move ribs are called *muscles of respiration*. To move the ribs, these muscles attach onto the ribs. Any muscle that attaches onto the ribcage may be considered to be a muscle of respiration (Box 8-19).

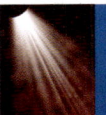

BOX 8-19 Spotlight on Muscles of Respiration

Inspiration/Expiration
Respiration is the process of taking air into and expelling air out of the lungs. Taking air into the lungs is called inspiration (i.e., inhalation); expelling air from the lungs is called expiration (i.e., exhalation). When air is taken into the lungs, the volume of the thoracic cavity expands; when air is expelled from the lungs, the volume of the thoracic cavity decreases. Therefore any muscle that has the ability to change the volume of the thoracic cavity is a muscle of respiration. Generally the volume of the thoracic cavity can be affected in two ways.

One way is to affect the ribcage by moving the ribs at the sternocostal and costospinal joints. As a general rule, elevating ribs increases thoracic cavity volume (see figure); therefore muscles that elevate ribs are generally categorized as muscles of inspiration. The primary muscle of inspiration is the diaphragm because it elevates the lower six ribs. Other inspiratory muscles include the external intercostals, scalenes, pectoralis minor, levatores costarum, and the serratus posterior superior. Conversely, muscles that depress the ribs are generally categorized as expiratory muscles and include the internal intercostals, subcostales, and serratus posterior inferior.

An exception to this concept is that musculature that depresses lower ribs can assist inspiration by stabilizing the costal (ribcage) attachment of the diaphragm so that it can more efficiently exert its force to depress its dome (see Diaphragm Function below).

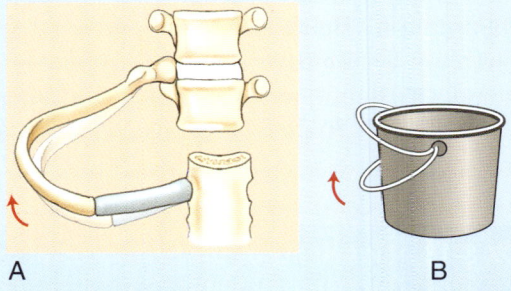

A, Anterior view illustrating the manner in which a rib lifts during inspiration. **B,** The handle of a bucket lifting. Elevation of a rib during inspiration has been described as a **bucket handle movement** because of the similarity of elevation of a rib to the elevation of a bucket handle.

The other way in which the volume of the thoracic cavity can be affected is via the abdominal region. In addition to increasing thoracic cavity volume by having the thoracic cavity expand outward when the ribcage itself expands, the thoracic cavity can also expand downward into the abdominal cavity region. Conversely, if the contents of the abdominal cavity push up into the thoracic cavity, the volume of the thoracic cavity decreases. In this regard the diaphragm is again the primary muscle of inspiration; when it contracts, in addition to raising the lower ribs, its central dome also drops down against the abdominal contents, thereby increasing the volume of the thoracic cavity. Muscles of expiration that work via the abdominal region are muscles of the abdominal wall; principal among these are the rectus abdominis, external abdominal oblique, internal abdominal oblique, and transversus abdominis.

Relaxed versus Forceful Breathing
Breathing is often divided into two types: (1) relaxed (i.e., quiet) breathing and (2) forceful breathing. During normal healthy relaxed breathing, such as when a person is calmly reading a book, the only muscle that is recruited to contract is the diaphragm. For normal healthy relaxed expiration, no muscles need to contract; instead, the diaphragm simply relaxes and the natural recoil of the tissues that were stretched during inspiration (tissues of the ribcage and abdomen) push back against the lungs, expelling the air. However, when we want to breathe forcefully, such as would occur during exercise, many other muscles of respiration are recruited. These muscles, as already mentioned, act on the thoracic cavity via the ribcage or the abdominal region. Generally speaking, whenever a pathology exists that results in labored breathing (any chronic obstructive pulmonary disorder such as asthma, emphysema, or chronic bronchitis), accessory muscles of respiration are recruited and may become hypertrophic.

Diaphragm Function
As has been stated, the diaphragm is an inspiratory muscle and increases thoracic cavity volume in two ways: (1) it expands the ribcage by lifting lower ribs, and (2) it drops down, pushing against the abdominal contents in the abdominal cavity. The manner in which the diaphragm is generally considered to function is as follows.

When the diaphragm contracts, the bony peripheral attachments are more fixed and the pull is on the central tendon, which causes the center (i.e., the top of the dome) to drop down (against the abdominal viscera). This raises the volume of the thoracic cavity to allow the lungs to inflate and expand for inspiration. This aspect of the diaphragm's contraction is usually called abdominal breathing.

As the diaphragm continues to contract, the pressure caused by the resistance of the abdominal viscera prohibits the central dome from dropping any farther and the dome now becomes less able to move (i.e., more fixed). The pull exerted by the contraction of the fibers of the diaphragm is now exerted peripherally on the ribcage, elevating the lower ribs and causing the anterior ribcage and sternum to push anteriorly. This further increases the volume of the thoracic cavity to allow the lungs to inflate and expand. This aspect of the diaphragm's contraction is usually called thoracic breathing.

SECTION 8.9 LUMBAR SPINE (THE ABDOMEN)

- The lumbar spine defines the abdomen of the body (i.e., the lower part of the trunk).
  - Most people think of the abdomen as being located only anteriorly. Actually, the abdomen is the lower (lumbar) region of the trunk that wraps 360 degrees around the body.

FEATURES OF THE LUMBAR SPINE:

Composition of the Lumbar Spine:

- The lumbar spine is composed of five vertebrae (Figure 8-38).
  - From superior to inferior, these vertebrae are named L1-L5.

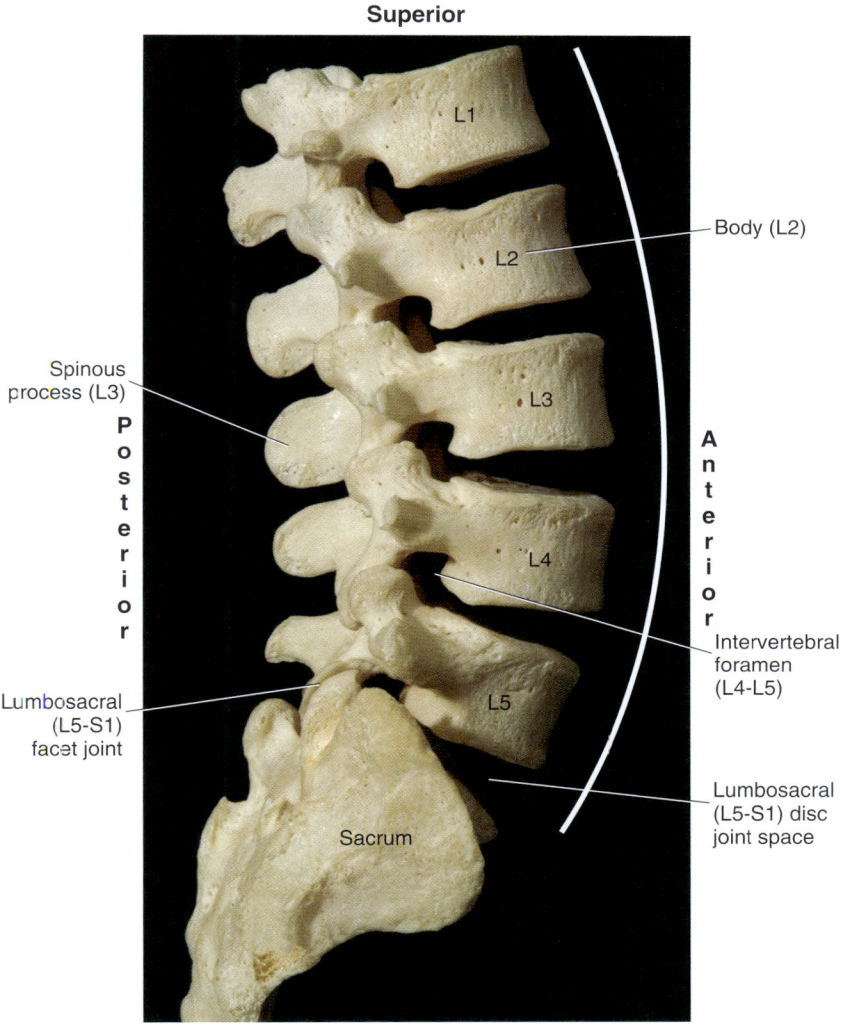

FIGURE 8-38 Right lateral view of the lumbar spine. The reader should note the lordotic curve, which is concave posteriorly (and therefore convex anteriorly).

Curve of the Lumbar Spine:

- The lumbar spine has a lordotic curve; in other words, it is concave posteriorly[5] (Box 8-20).

BOX 8-20

When the lumbar spine has a greater than normal lordotic curve, it is called a hyperlordosis. A hyperlordotic lumbar spine is involved with a postural distortion pattern known as *lower crossed syndrome*. (For more information on lower crossed syndrome, see Section 21.1.)

Functions of the Lumbar Spine:

- The lumbar spine needs to be stable because it has a greater weight-bearing role than the cervical and thoracic spinal regions.[13]
- The lumbar spine is also very mobile. Generally the lumbar spine moves freely in all ranges of motion except rotation[5] (Table 8-8).
- The orientation of the lumbar facet joints is essentially in the sagittal plane[13] (see Section 8-4, Figure 8-14, C), which allows for ease of flexion and extension motions within the sagittal plane. This is why it is so easy to bend forward and backward from our low back.
- In the lower lumbar region, the facet plane orientation changes from the sagittal plane back toward the frontal plane.[5] Clinically, this can create problems, because the upper lumbar region facilitates flexion/extension movements in the sagittal plane, but the lumbosacral joint region does not allow these sagittal plane motions as well because their facets are oriented in the frontal plane.
- Being both mobile and stable is challenging, because mobility and stability are antagonistic concepts. Usually a joint tends to be either primarily mobile or primarily stable. Having to be stable for weight bearing and yet also allowing a great amount of mobility is one of the reasons that the low back is so often injured.

MAJOR MOTIONS ALLOWED:

For motions of the lumbar spine, see Section 8.10; illustrations in Figure 8-41 demonstrate thoracolumbar motion of the trunk.

- The lumbar spinal joints allow flexion and extension (i.e., axial movements) of the trunk in the sagittal plane around a mediolateral axis.

TABLE 8-8	Average Ranges of Motion of the Lumbar Spine (L1-L2 through L5-S1 Joints) from Anatomic Position[5]		
Flexion	50 Degrees	Extension	15 Degrees
Right lateral flexion	20 Degrees	Left lateral flexion	20 Degrees
Right rotation	5 Degrees	Left rotation	5 Degrees

- The lumbar spinal joints allow right lateral flexion and left lateral flexion (i.e., axial movements) of the trunk in the frontal plane around an anteroposterior axis.
  - The lumbar spine couples lateral flexion with contralateral rotation.[5] An interesting clinical application of this is that when a client has a lumbar scoliosis (a lateral flexion deformity of the spine in the frontal plane), it can be difficult to pick this up on visual examination or palpation because the result of contralateral rotation coupling with lateral flexion is that the spinous processes rotate into the concavity, making it more difficult to see and feel the curvature of the scoliosis (Figure 8-39).
- The lumbar spinal joints allow right rotation and left rotation (i.e., axial movements) of the trunk in the transverse plane around a vertical axis.[4]
- The lumbar spinal joints allow gliding translational movements in all three directions (see Section 8.4, Figure 8-18).

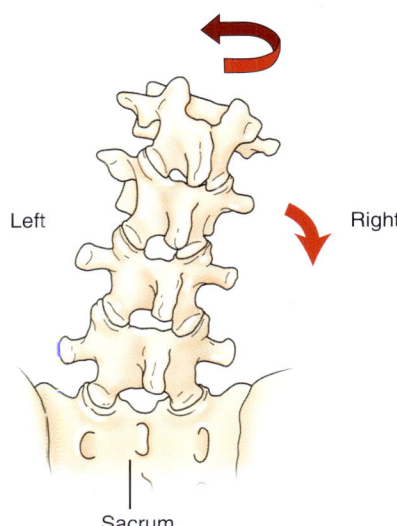

FIGURE 8-39 Posterior view illustrating the coupling pattern in the lumbar spine of lateral flexion with contralateral rotation. In this figure, the lumbar spine is right laterally flexing and rotating to the left. (Note: Remember that vertebral rotation is named for the direction in which the anterior bodies face; the spinous processes would therefore point in the opposite direction.)

SPECIAL JOINT:

- The joint between the fifth lumbar vertebra and the sacrum is known as the **lumbosacral joint** (see Figure 8-38).
- The lumbosacral joint is also known as the L5-S1 joint because it is between the fifth lumbar vertebra and the first element of the sacrum. (The sacrum is made up of five vertebrae that fused embryologically. Therefore the sacrum can be divided into its five elements, S1-S5 [from superior to inferior]).
- The lumbosacral joint is not structurally (i.e., anatomically) special. As is typical for intervertebral joints, it is made up of a median disc joint and two lateral facet joints. However, the lumbosacral joint is functionally (i.e., physiologically) special

because the lumbosacral joint is not just a joint at which the spine (specifically the fifth lumbar vertebra) can move relative to the pelvis. It is also the joint at which the pelvis can move relative to the trunk.[5]
- The pelvis can also move relative to the thighs at the hip joints.[5] (For motions of the pelvis relative to adjacent body parts, please see Sections 9.3 through 9.5.)
- Other than the usual ligaments of the spine, stabilization to the lumbosacral joint is provided by the iliolumbar ligaments (see Figure 9-4) and the thoracolumbar fascia[13] (see Section 8-11, Figure 8-42).
- The lumbosacral joint region is also important because the angle of the sacral base, termed the **sacral base angle** (Figure 8-40), determines the base that the spine sits on[5]; this determines the curvature that the spine has. Therefore the sacral base angle is an important factor toward assessing the posture of the client's spine. (See Section 9.8 for more information on the effect of the sacral base angle on the spine.)

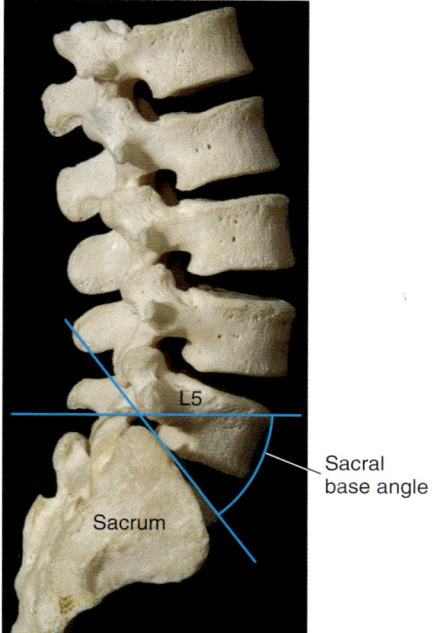

FIGURE 8-40 Right lateral view of the lumbosacral spine. The sacral base angle is formed by the intersection of a line that runs along the base of the sacrum and a horizontal line. The sacral base angle is important because it determines the degree of curvature that the lumbar spine will have.

8-6

SECTION 8.10 THORACOLUMBAR SPINE (THE TRUNK)

- Given that the thoracic spine and lumbar spine are both located in the trunk, movements of these two regions (i.e., the **thoracolumbar spine**) are often coupled and assessed together (Box 8-21). Table 8-9 provides the average ranges of motion of the thoracolumbar spine; Figure 8-41 shows the major motions of the thoracolumbar spine (i.e., the trunk).

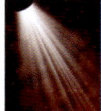

BOX 8-21 Spotlight on Reverse Actions of the Trunk

There are many reverse actions of the trunk that can occur. Reverse actions of the muscles of the thoracolumbar spine (i.e., the trunk) create actions of the pelvis at the lumbosacral joint relative to the trunk (and/or movement of the inferior vertebrae relative to the more superior vertebrae). Reverse actions of the pelvis relative to the trunk are covered in Section 8.6.

Reverse actions in which the trunk moves relative to the arm at the shoulder joint are also possible. In the accompanying illustration, the trunk is seen to move relative to the arm at the shoulder joint. A and B illustrate neutral position and right lateral deviation of the trunk at the right shoulder joint, respectively; C and D illustrate neutral position and right rotation of the trunk at the right shoulder joint, respectively; E and F illustrate neutral position and elevation of the trunk at the right shoulder joint, respectively. In all three cases, note the change in angulation between the arm and trunk at the shoulder joint (for lateral deviation B and elevation F, the elbow joint has also flexed.)

Continued

238   PART 3   Skeletal Arthrology: Study of the Joints

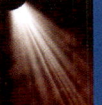 **BOX 8-21** **Spotlight on Reverse Actions of the Trunk—*Cont'd***

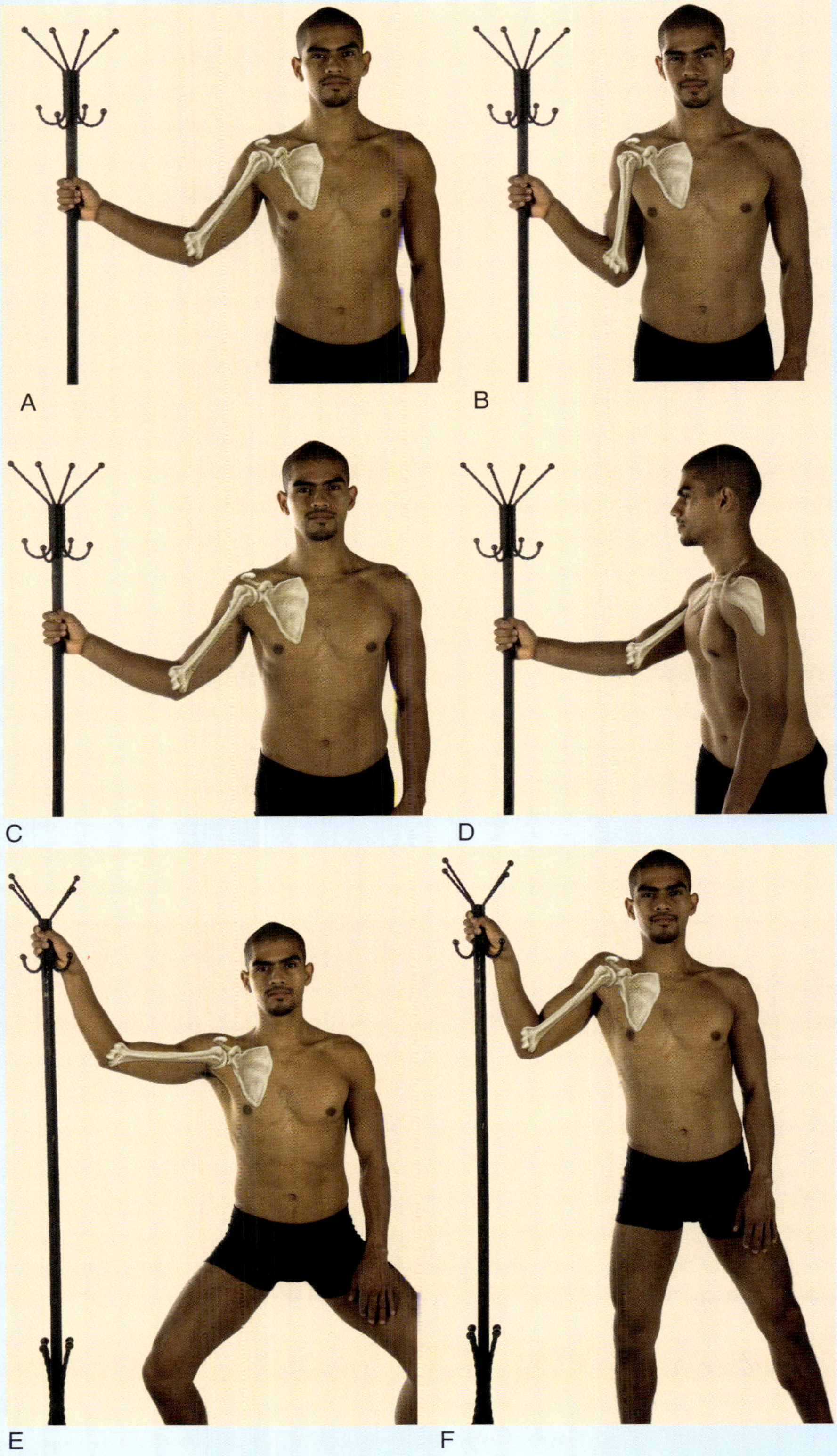

A

B

C

D

E

F

CHAPTER 8 Joints of the Axial Body   239

TABLE 8-9	Average Ranges of Motion of the Thoracolumbar Spine (i.e., the Entire Trunk from Anatomic Position) (Numbers Include the T1-T2 through L5-S1 Joints)[5]		
Flexion	85 Degrees	Extension	40 Degrees
Right lateral flexion	45 Degrees	Left lateral flexion	45 Degrees
Right rotation	35 Degrees	Left rotation	35 Degrees

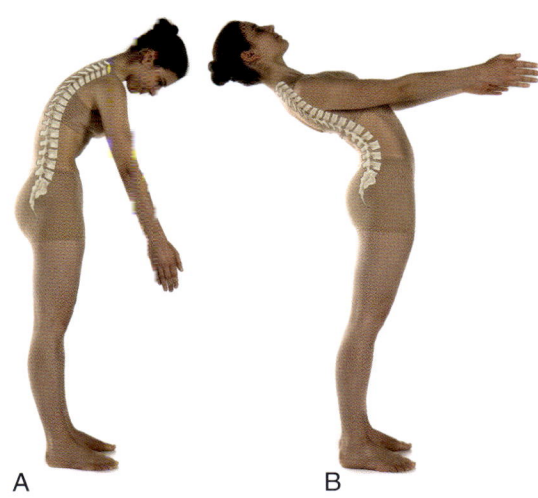
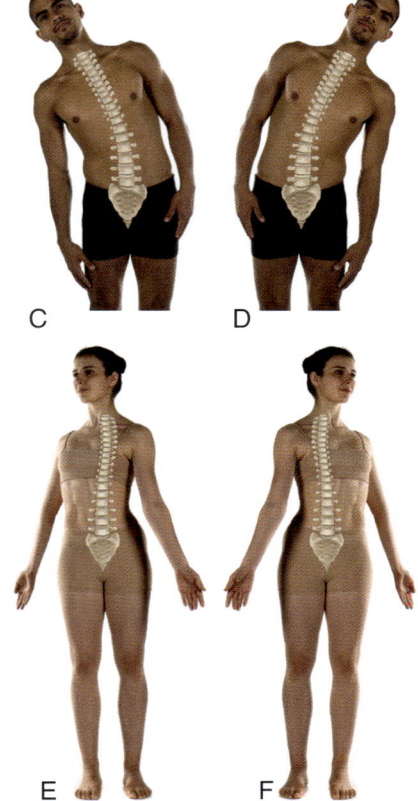

FIGURE 8-41 Motions of the thoracolumbar spine (trunk) at the spinal joints. *A* and *B* are lateral views that illustrate flexion and extension of the trunk, respectively, in the sagittal plane. *C* and *D* are anterior views that illustrate right lateral flexion and left lateral flexion of the trunk, respectively, in the frontal plane. *E* and *F* are anterior views that illustrate right rotation and left rotation of the trunk, respectively, in the transverse plane.

SECTION 8.11 THORACOLUMBAR FASCIA AND ABDOMINAL APONEUROSIS

- The thoracolumbar fascia and abdominal aponeurosis are large sheets of fibrous connective tissue located in the trunk.
- The thoracolumbar fascia is located posteriorly in the trunk.
- The abdominal aponeurosis is located anteriorly in the trunk.
- The functional importance of these structures is twofold:
    - They provide attachment sites for muscles.
    - They add to the stability of the trunk.

THORACOLUMBAR FASCIA:

- The **thoracolumbar fascia** (Figure 8-42, *A*) is located posteriorly in the trunk; as its name implies, it is a layer of fascia located in the thoracic and lumbar regions.

- The thoracolumbar fascia is also known as the **lumbodorsal fascia**.[4]
    - A sheet of thoracolumbar fascia exists on the left and right sides of the body. In other words, two sheets of thoracolumbar fascia exist.
- The thoracolumbar fascia is especially well developed in the lumbar region, where it is divided into three layers[4]: (1) anterior, (2) middle, and (3) deep (Figure 8-42, *B*).
    - The anterior layer is located between the psoas major and quadratus lumborum muscles and attaches to the anterior surface of the transverse processes (TPs).
    - The middle layer is located between the quadratus lumborum and erector spinae group musculature and attaches to the tips of the transverse processes.

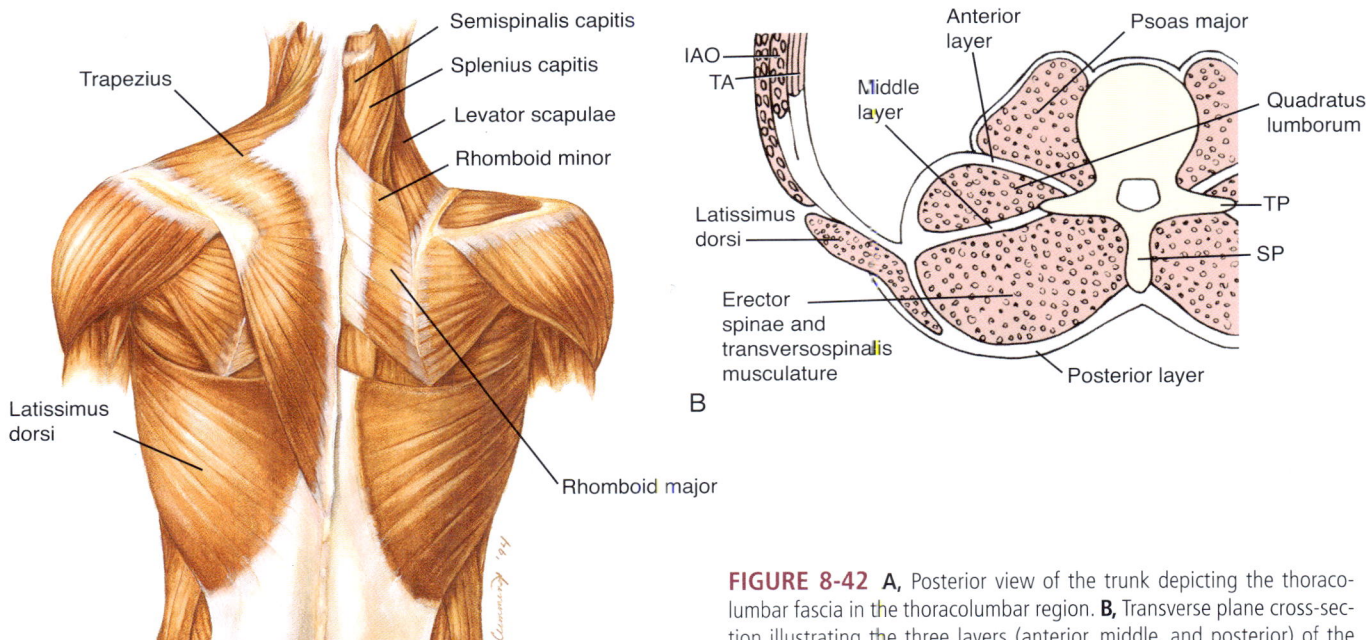

FIGURE 8-42 **A,** Posterior view of the trunk depicting the thoracolumbar fascia in the thoracolumbar region. **B,** Transverse plane cross-section illustrating the three layers (anterior, middle, and posterior) of the thoracolumbar fascia. *IAO,* Internal abdominal oblique; *TA,* transversus abdominis. *(A, From Cramer GD, Darby SA: Basic and clinical anatomy of the spine, spinal cord, and ANS, ed 2, St Louis, 2005, Mosby.)*

- The posterior layer is located posterior to the erector spinae and latissimus dorsi musculature and attaches to the spinous processes (SPs).
- The quadratus lumborum and erector spinae group muscles are encased within the thoracolumbar fascia.[4] The latissimus dorsi attaches into the spine medially via its attachment into the thoracolumbar fascia.
- All three layers of the thoracolumbar fascia meet posterolaterally where the internal abdominal oblique (IAO) and transversus abdominis (TA) muscles attach into it.[13]
- Inferiorly, the thoracolumbar fascia attaches onto the sacrum and iliac crest.[13]
- Because of its attachments onto the sacrum and ilium, the thoracolumbar fascia helps to stabilize the lumbar spinal joints and the sacroiliac joint.[13]

ABDOMINAL APONEUROSIS:

- The **abdominal aponeurosis** is located anteriorly in the abdominal region[15] (Figure 8-43).
  - An abdominal aponeurosis exists on the left and right sides of the body. In other words, two abdominal aponeuroses (left and right) exist.
  - The abdominal aponeurosis provides a site of attachment for the external abdominal oblique, the internal abdominal oblique, and the transversus abdominis muscles.
- The abdominal aponeurosis is often viewed as being an attachment site into which the abdominal wall muscles attach. Viewed another way, it can also be considered to actually be the aponeuroses of these abdominal wall muscles (namely, the external abdominal oblique, internal abdominal oblique, and transversus abdominis muscles bilaterally).
- The superior aspect of the abdominal aponeurosis has two layers (anterior and posterior), which encase the rectus abdominis.
- The inferior aspect of the abdominal aponeurosis has only one layer, which passes superficially (anteriorly) to the rectus abdominis
- The border where the abdominal aponeurosis changes its relationship to the rectus abdominis is the arcuate line. The **arcuate line** is a curved line that is located approximately halfway between the umbilicus and the symphysis pubis.[16]
- Because the abdominal aponeurosis covers and/or encases the rectus abdominis, it is also known as the **rectus sheath**.[15]
- Where the left and right abdominal aponeuroses meet in the midline is called the **linea alba**, which means *white line*.[5]
- The left and right abdominal aponeuroses, by binding the two sides of the anterior abdominal wall together, add to the stability of the trunk.

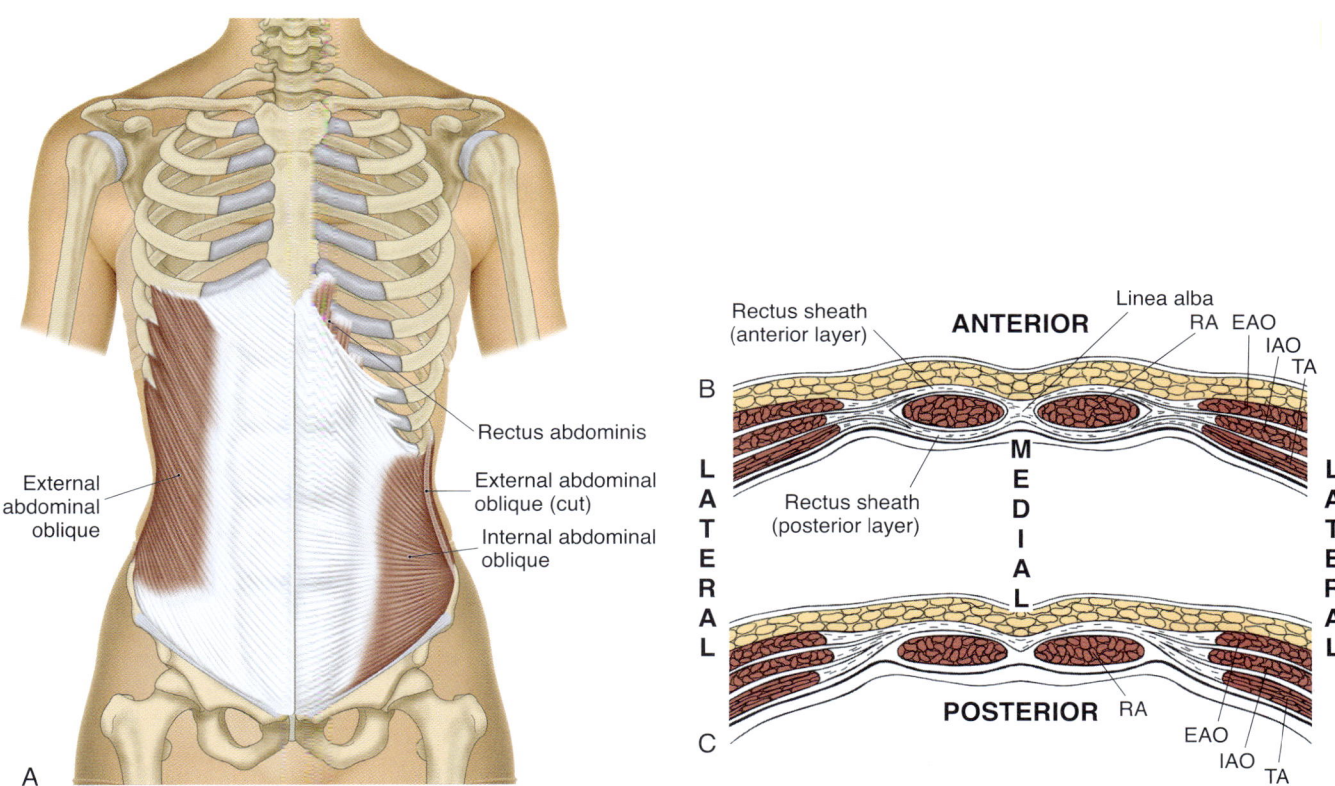

FIGURE 8-43 A, View of the anterior trunk illustrating the abdominal aponeurosis. The abdominal aponeurosis is a thick layer of fibrous tissue that is an attachment site of the transversus abdominis and external and internal abdominal oblique muscles. **B** and **C,** Transverse plane cross-section illustrating the abdominal aponeurosis superiorly and inferiorly in the trunk, respectively. *EAO,* External abdominal oblique; *IAO,* internal abdominal oblique; *RA,* rectus abdominis; *TA,* transversus abdominis. *(From Muscolino JE: The muscular system manual: the skeletal muscles of the human body, ed 4, St Louis, 2017, Mosby.)*

REVIEW QUESTIONS

evolve Answers to the following review questions appear on the Evolve website accompanying this book at: http://evolve.elsevier.com/Muscolino/kinesiology/.

1. What is the relationship between cranial suture joints and childbirth?

2. What are the four major muscles of mastication?

3. What are the four major regions of the spine, and which type of curve is found in each?

4. How many cervical vertebrae are there? How many thoracic vertebrae are there? How many lumbar vertebrae are there?

5. Developmentally, what creates the cervical lordotic curve?

6. Regarding spinal segmental motion, compare and contrast the purpose of the disc joint and the purpose of the facet joints.

7. What is the general orientation of the facet planes of the cervical, thoracic, and lumbar spinal regions?

8. Explain why the anterior longitudinal ligament limits extension of the spinal joints, and the supraspinous ligament limits flexion of the spinal joints.

9. Why is the second cervical vertebra called the *axis*?

10. Name three ligaments of the upper cervical region that stabilize the dens of the axis.

11. Which upper cervical spinous process is the most easily palpable and useful as a palpatory landmark?

12. Why are the coupled actions of extension and rotation of the upper cervical spine potentially contraindicated for clients?

13. The presence of what structure greatly decreases the range of motion of extension of the thoracic spine?

14. What are the two types of costospinal joints?

15. Why is elevation of a rib described as a *bucket handle movement*?

16. Describe the two manners in which the thoracic cavity can expand for inspiration.

17. In which plane is the lumbar spine least mobile?

18. How is the sacral base angle measured? What is its importance?

19. How many layers does the thoracolumbar fascia have in the lumbar region?

20. Why is the abdominal aponeurosis also known as the *rectus sheath*?

REFERENCES

1. Palastanga N, Field D, Soames R: Anatomy and human movement, ed 4, Oxford, 2002, Butterworth-Heinemann.
2. White TD, Folkens PA: Human osteology, ed 22, San Diego, 2000, Academic Press.
3. Behnke RS: Kinetic anatomy, ed 2, Champaign, IL, 2006, Human Kinetics.
4. Levangie PK, Norkin CC: Joint structure and function: A comprehensive analysis, ed 5, Philadelphia, 2011, FA Davis.
5. Neumann DA: Kinesiology of the musculoskeletal system: Foundations for physical rehabilitation, ed 3, St Louis, 2017, Elsevier.
6. Oatis CA: Kinesiology: The mechanics and pathomechanics of human movement, Philadelphia, 2004, Lippincott Williams & Wilkins.
7. Werner R: A massage therapist's guide to pathology, ed 4, Philadelphia, 2004, Lippincott Williams & Wilkins.
8. Watkins J: Structure and function of the musculoskeletal system, Champaign, IL, 1999, Human Kinetics.
9. Cramer GD, Darby SA: Basic and clinical anatomy of the spine, spinal cord, and ANS, St Louis, 1995, Mosby.
10. Hamill J, Knutzen KM: Biomechanical basis of human movement, ed 12, Baltimore, 2003, Lippincott Williams & Wilkins.
11. Nordin M, Frankel VH: Basic biomechanics of the musculoskeletal system, ed 3, Baltimore, 2001, Lippincott Williams & Wilkins.
12. Muscolino JE: The muscular system manual: The skeletal muscles of the human body, ed 4, St Louis, 2017, Elsevier.
13. Cramer GD, Darby SA: Basic and clinical anatomy of the spine, spinal cord, and ANS, St Louis, 1995, Mosby.
14. Smith LK, Weiss EL, Lehmkuhl LO: Brunstrom's clinical kinesiology, ed 5, Philadelphia, 1996, FA Davis.
15. Hamilton N, Weimar W, Luttgens K: Kinesiology: Scientific basis of human motion, ed 12, New York, 2012, McGraw Hill.
16. Netter FH: Atlas of human anatomy, ed 3, Teterboro, 2004, Icon Learning Systems.

CHAPTER 9
Joints of the Lower Extremity

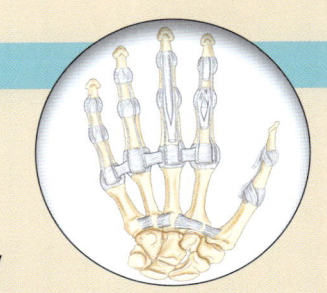

CHAPTER OUTLINE

Section 9.1	Introduction to the Pelvis and Pelvic Movement	Section 9.11	Femoropelvic Rhythm
Section 9.2	Intrapelvic Motion (Symphysis Pubis and Sacroiliac Joints)	Section 9.12	Overview of the Knee Joint Complex
		Section 9.13	Tibiofemoral (Knee) Joint
Section 9.3	Movement of the Pelvis at the Lumbosacral Joint	Section 9.14	Patellofemoral Joint
		Section 9.15	Angulations of the Knee Joint
Section 9.4	Movement of the Pelvis at the Hip Joints	Section 9.16	Tibiofibular Joints
Section 9.5	Movement of the Pelvis at the Lumbosacral and Hip Joints	Section 9.17	Overview of the Ankle/Foot Region
		Section 9.18	Talocrural (Ankle) Joint
Section 9.6	Relationship of Pelvic/Spinal Movements at the Lumbosacral Joint	Section 9.19	Subtalar Tarsal Joint
		Section 9.20	Transverse Tarsal Joint
Section 9.7	Relationship of Pelvic/Thigh Movements at the Hip Joint	Section 9.21	Tarsometatarsal (TMT) Joints
		Section 9.22	Intermetatarsal (IMT) Joints
Section 9.8	Effect of Pelvic Posture on Spinal Posture	Section 9.23	Metatarsophalangeal (MTP) Joints
Section 9.9	Hip Joint	Section 9.24	Interphalangeal (IP) Joints of the Foot
Section 9.10	Angulations of the Femur		

CHAPTER OBJECTIVES

After completing this chapter, the student should be able to perform the following:

1. Define the key terms of this chapter and state the meanings of the word origins of this chapter.
2. Do the following related to the pelvis, pelvic movement, and intrapelvic motion:
   - Describe the structure of the pelvis, and explain the difference between intrapelvic motion and motion of the pelvis relative to an adjacent body part.
   - Describe the sacral movements of nutation and counternutation.
   - List the major ligaments of the sacroiliac joint and their attachments.
3. Describe and compare movements of the pelvis at the lumbosacral and hip joints.
4. Explain the reverse action relationships between pelvic movements and movements of the trunk and thighs.
5. Explain the relationship between pelvic posture (and specifically sacral base angle) and spinal posture.
6. Discuss the hip joint, including the meaning of open-chain and closed-chain activities, and give examples of each.
7. Explain the concepts of the femoral angle of inclination and femoral torsion angle, and explain the possible consequences of these femoral angulations.
8. Describe and give an example of the concept of femoropelvic rhythm.
9. Discuss the tibiofemoral and patellofemoral joints.
10. Explain the concepts of the angulations of the knee joint, namely, genu valgum, genu varum, Q-angle, and genu recurvatum. In addition, explain the possible consequences of these knee joint angulations.

 Indicates a video demonstration is available for this concept.

11. Discuss tibiofibular joints, and describe tibial torsion.
12. Do the following related to the ankle/foot region:
    ○ List the regions of the foot and the joints of the foot.
    ○ Compare and contrast the role of stability and flexibility of the foot.
    ○ Describe the structure and function of the arches of the foot; also, relate the windlass mechanism to the arches of the foot.
    ○ Describe and give an example of the concept of bowstringing.
    ○ Define pronation and supination of the foot; list and explain the component cardinal plane actions of pronation and supination.
13. Discuss the talocrural (ankle) joint, including the bones, major motions allowed, and ligaments.
14. Discuss the subtalar tarsal joint, including the bones, major motions allowed, and ligaments.
15. Discuss the transverse tarsal joint, including the bones, major motions allowed, and ligaments.
16. Discuss the bones, major motions allowed, and ligaments of the following joints:
    ○ Tarsometatarsal (TMT) joints.
    ○ Intermetatarsal (IMT) joints.
    ○ Metatarsophalangeal (MTP) joints.
    ○ Interphalangeal (IP) joints.

OVERVIEW

9-1

Chapters 6 and 7 laid the theoretic basis for the structure and function of joints; this chapter continues our study of the regional approach of the structure and function of the joints of the body that began in Chapter 8. This chapter addresses the joints of the lower extremity. The lower extremity is primarily concerned with weight bearing and propulsion of the body through space. Toward that end, the joints of the lower extremity must work together to achieve these goals. Sections 9.1 through 9.8 concern themselves with an in-depth examination of the movements of the pelvis. Given the critical importance of the posture of the pelvis to spinal posture, a thorough understanding of the structure and function of the pelvis is crucial. Sections 9.9 through 9.11 then cover the hip joint and thigh; and Sections 9.12 through 9.16 cover the knee joint complex and leg. The last eight sections of this chapter (Sections 9.17 through 9.24) address the structure and function of the ankle joint and foot.

KEY TERMS

Acetabular labrum (AS-i-TAB-you-lar LAY-brum)
Anterior cruciate ligament (an-TEER-ree-or KRU-shee-it)
Anterior talofibular ligament (TA-low-FIB-you-lar)
Anteversion (AN-tee-ver-shun)
Arch (of the foot)
Arcuate popliteal ligament (ARE-cue-it pop-LIT-ee-al)
Arcuate pubic ligament (PYU-bik)
Bifurcate ligament (BY-fur-kate)
Bony pelvis
Bowleg
Bowstring
Bunion (BUN-yen)
Calcaneocuboid joint (kal-KANE-ee-o-CUE-boyd)
Calcaneocuboid ligament
Calcaneofibular ligament (kal-KANE-ee-o-FIB-you-lar)
Calcaneonavicular ligament (kal-KANE-ee-o-na-VIK-you-lar)
Central stable pillar (of the foot)
Cervical ligament (SERV-i-kul)
Chondromalacia patella (CON-dro-ma-LAY-she-a)
Chopart's joint (SHOW-parz)
Closed-chain activities
Coronary ligaments (CORE-o-nar-ee)
Counternutation (COUN-ter-new-TAY-shun)
Coupled action
Coxa valga (COCKS-a VAL-ga)
Coxa vara (COCKS-a VAR-a)
Coxal bone (COCKS-al)
Coxofemoral joint (COCKS-o-FEM-or-al)
Deep transverse metatarsal ligaments (MET-a-TARS-al)
Deltoid ligament (DEL-toyd)
Distal interphalangeal joints (of the foot) (IN-ter-fa-lan-GEE-al)
Distal intertarsal joints (IN-ter-TAR-sal)
Dorsal calcaneocuboid ligament (DOOR-sul kal-KANE-ee-o-CUE-boyd)
Femoral angle of inclination (FEM-or-al)
Femoral torsion angle (FEM-or-al TOR-shun)
Femoroacetabular joint (FEM-or-o-AS-i-TAB-you-lar)
Femoropelvic rhythm (FEM-or-o-PEL-vik)
Fibular collateral ligament (FIB-you-lar co-LAT-er-al)
Flat foot
Flexor retinaculum (FLEKS-or re-tin-AK-you-lum)
Forefoot (FOUR-foot)
Genu recurvatum (JEN-you REE-ker-VAT-um)
Genu valgum (VAL-gum)
Genu varum (JEN-you VAR-um)
Greater sciatic foramen (sigh-AT-ik)
Greater sciatic notch
Hallux valgus (HAL-uks VAL-gus)
Heel spur
Hindfoot (HIND-foot)
Iliofemoral ligament (IL-ee-o-FEM-or-al)
Iliolumbar ligament (IL-ee-o-LUM-bar)

Inferior extensor retinaculum (ek-STEN-sor re-tin-AK-you-lum)
Inferior fibular retinaculum (FIB-you-lar)
Infrapatellar bursa (IN-fra-pa-TELL-ar BER-sa)
Innominate bone (in-NOM-i-nate)
Intermetatarsal joints (IN-ter-MET-a-TAR-sal)
Intermetatarsal ligaments
Interosseus membrane (of the leg) (IN-ter-OS-ee-us)
Interphalangeal joints (of the foot) (IN-ter-fa-lan-GEE-al)
Ischiofemoral ligament (IS-kee-o-FEM-or-a)
Knock-knees
Lateral collateral ligament (of ankle joint)
Lateral collateral ligament (of interphalangeal joints pedis)
Lateral collateral ligament (of knee joint)
Lateral collateral ligament (of metatarsophalangeal joint)
Lateral longitudinal arch (LON-ji-TOO-di-nal)
Lateral malleolar bursa (ma-LEE-o-lar BER-sa)
Lateral meniscus (men-IS-kus)
Lesser sciatic notch (sigh-AT-ik)
Ligamentum teres (LIG-a-MEN-tum TE-reez)
Long plantar ligament (PLAN-tar)
Lower ankle joint
Lumbopelvic rhythm (LUM-bo-PEL-vik)
Lunate cartilage (LOON-ate)
Medial collateral ligament (of ankle joint)
Medial collateral ligament (of interphalangeal joints pedis)
Medial collateral ligament (of knee joint)
Medial collateral ligament (of metatarsophalangeal joint)
Medial longitudinal arch (LON-ji-TOO-di-nal)
Medial malleolar bursa (ma-LEE-o-lar BER-sa)
Medial meniscus (men-IS-kus)
Meniscal horn attachments (men-IS-kal)
Metatarsophalangeal joints (MET-a-TAR-so-FA-lan-GEE-al)
Midfoot
Mortise joint (MOR-tis)
Nutation (new-TAY-shun)
Oblique popliteal ligament (o-BLEEK pop-LIT-ee-al)
Open-chain activities
Patellar ligament (pa-TELL-ar)
Patellofemoral joint (pa-TELL-o-FEM-or-al)
Patellofemoral syndrome
Pelvic girdle (PEL-vik)
Pelvic neutral
Pes cavus (PEZ CAV-us)
Pes planus (PLANE-us)
Pigeon toes
Plantar calcaneocuboid ligament (PLAN-tar kal-KANE-ee-o-CUE-boyd)
Plantar calcaneonavicular ligament (kal-KANE-ee-o-na-VIK-you-lar)
Plantar fascia (PLAN-tar FASH-a)
Plantar fasciitis (fash-EYE-tis)
Plantar plate (of interphalangeal joints pedis) (PLAN-tar)
Plantar plate (of metatarsophalangeal joint)
Posterior cruciate ligament (pos-TEER-ree-or KRU-shee-it)
Posterior meniscofemoral ligament (men-IS-ko-FEM-or-al)
Posterior talofibular ligament (pos-TEER-ree-or TA-low-FIB-you-lar)
Prepatellar bursa (PRE-pa-TEL-ar BER-sa)
Proximal interphalangeal joints (of the foot) (IN-ter-FA-lan-GEE-al)
Pubofemoral ligament (PYU-bo-FEM-or-al)
Q-angle
Ray
Retinacular fibers (re-tin-AK-you-lar)
Retinaculum, pl retinacula (of the foot/ankle) (re-tin-AK-you-lum, re-tin-AK-you-la)
Retroversion (RET-ro-VER-shun)
Righting reflex
Rigid flat foot
Sacral base angle
Sacroiliac joint (SAY-kro-IL-ee-ak)
Sacroiliac ligaments
Sacrospinous ligament (SAY-kro-SPINE-us)
Sacrotuberous ligament (SAY-kro-TOOB-er-us)
Screw-home mechanism
Short plantar ligament (PLAN-tar)
Sinus tarsus (SIGH-nus TAR-sus)
Spring ligament
Subcutaneous calcaneal bursa (SUB-cue-TANE-ee-us KAL-ka-NEE-al BER-sa)
Subcutaneous infrapatellar bursa (IN-fra-pa-TEL-ar)
Subtendinous calcaneal bursa (sub-TEN-din-us KAL-ka-NEE-al BER-sa)
Subtalar joint (SUB-TAL-ar)
Superior extensor retinaculum (sue-PEE-ree-or eks-TEN-sor re-tin-AK-you-lum)
Superior fibular retinaculum (FIB-you-lar re-tin-AK-you-lum)
Supple flat foot
Suprapatellar bursa (SUE-pra-pa-TEL-ar BER-sa)
Symphysis pubis joint (SIM-fi-sis PYU-bis)
Talocalcaneal joint (TAL-o-kal-KANE-ee-al)
Talocalcaneal ligaments
Talocalcaneonavicular joint complex (TAL-o-kal-KANE-ee-o-na-VIK-you-lar)
Talocalcaneonaviculocuboid joint complex (TAL-o-kal-KANE-ee-o-na-VIK-you-lo-CUE-boyd)
Talocrural joint (TAL-o-KRUR-al)
Talonavicular joint (TAL-o-na-VIK-you-lar)
Tarsal joints (TAR-sal)
Tarsometatarsal joints (TAR-so-MET-a-tars-al)
Tarsometatarsal ligaments
Tibial collateral ligament (TIB-ee-al)
Tibial torsion (TOR-shun)
Tibiofemoral joint (TIB-ee-o-FEM-or-al)
Tibiofibular joints (TIB-ee-o-FIB-you-lar)
Toe-in posture
Toe-out posture
Transverse acetabular ligament (AS-i-TAB-you-lar)
Transverse arch
Transverse ligament (of knee joint)
Transverse tarsal joint (TAR-sal)
Upper ankle joint
Windlass mechanism (WIND-lus)
Y ligament
Zona orbicularis (ZONE-a or-BIK-you-la-ris)

WORD ORIGINS

- Auricle—From Latin *auris,* meaning *ear*
- Bifurcate—From Latin *bis,* meaning *two,* and *furca* meaning *fork*
- Bunion—From Old French *bugne,* meaning *bump on the head*
- Counter—From Latin *contra,* meaning *against*
- Coxa—From Latin *coxa,* meaning *hip* or *hip joint*
- Cruciate—From Latin *crux,* meaning *cross*
- Deltoid—From the Greek letter *delta,* which is triangular in shape, and *eidos,* meaning *resemblance, appearance*
- Digit—From Latin *digitus,* meaning *toe* (or *finger*)
- Hallucis—From Latin *hallucis,* meaning *of the big toe*
- Hallux—From Latin *hallex,* meaning *big toe*
- Innominate—From Latin *innominatus,* meaning *unnamed* or *nameless*
- Labrum—From Latin *labrum,* meaning *lip*
- Lunate—From Latin *luna,* meaning *moon*
- Malacia—From Greek *malakia,* meaning *softening* (related Latin *malus,* meaning *bad*)
- Meniscus—From Greek *meniskos,* meaning *crescent*
- Nutation—From Latin *annuo,* meaning *to nod*
- Pedis—From Latin *pes,* meaning *foot*
- Pelvis—From Latin *pelvis,* meaning *basin*
- Pes—From Latin *pes,* meaning *foot*
- Ray—From Latin *radius,* meaning *extending outward (radially) from a structure*
- Recurvatum—From Latin *recurvus,* meaning *bent back*
- Retinaculum—From Latin *retineo,* meaning *to hold back, restrain*
- Sacrum—From Latin *sacrum,* meaning *sacred, holy*
- Sciatic—From Latin *sciaticus* (which came from Greek *ischiadikos,* which in turn came from *ischion*), meaning *hip*
- Valga—From Latin *valgus,* meaning *twisted, bent outward, bowlegged*
- Vara—From Latin *varum,* meaning *crooked, bent inward, knock-kneed*

9-2

SECTION 9.1 INTRODUCTION TO THE PELVIS AND PELVIC MOVEMENT

- The pelvis is a body part that is located between the trunk and the thighs (see Section 1.2).
- The **bony pelvis** is the term that refers to the bones and joints of the pelvis (Figure 9-1).
- The bones located within the pelvis are the sacrum, coccyx, and the two pelvic bones.[1]
  - The sacrum is actually five vertebrae that never fully formed and that fused embryologically.
  - The coccyx is made up of four vertebrae that never fully formed. Usually the four bones of the coccyx fuse later in life.
  - Each pelvic bone is composed of an ilium, ischium, and pubis that fused embryologically.[2]
- The pelvic bone is also known as the **coxal bone, innominate bone,** or *hip bone.*
- The joints that are located within the pelvis are the symphysis pubis and two sacroiliac (SI) joints.
  - The **symphysis pubis joint** unites the two pubic bones.
  - Each **sacroiliac (SI) joint** unites the sacrum with the iliac portion of the pelvic bone on that side of the body.[2]
- The pelvis is a transitional body part that is made up of bones of both the axial skeleton and the appendicular skeleton.
  - The sacrum and coccyx of the pelvis are axial bones of the spine.
  - The two pelvic bones (each one composed of an ilium, ischium, and pubis) are appendicular pelvic girdle bones of the lower extremity.

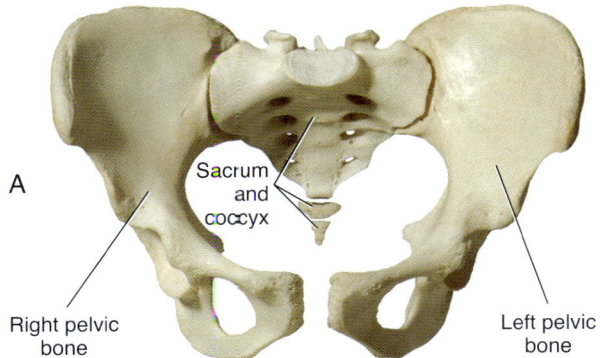
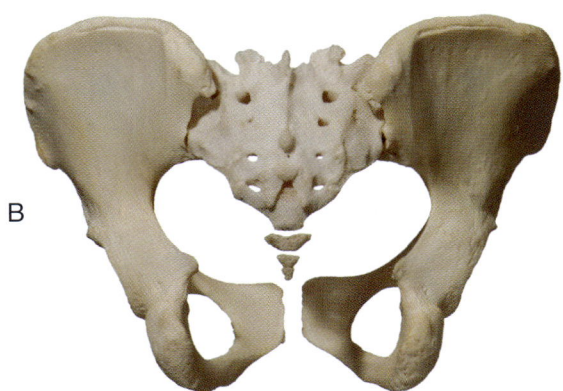

FIGURE 9-1 A, Anterior view of the bony pelvis. **B,** Posterior view. The bony pelvis is composed of the two pelvic bones and the sacrum and coccyx. The pelvic bones are part of the appendicular skeleton; the sacrum and coccyx are part of the axial skeleton. For this reason, the pelvis is considered to be a transitional body part.

- The bony pelvis is often referred to as the **pelvic girdle**.[1]
- A girdle is an article of clothing that encircles the body and provides stabilization. Similarly, the pelvic girdle encircles the body and provides a firm, stable base of attachment for the femurs.

PELVIC MOTION:

Two types of pelvic motion exist:
- Motion can occur within the pelvis (i.e., intrapelvic motion).
  - This motion can occur at the SI joints and/or at the symphysis pubis joint.
- The entire pelvis can move as one unit relative to an adjacent body part.
  - This motion can occur relative to the trunk at the lumbosacral (L5-S1) joint and/or relative to a thigh at a hip joint or to both thighs at both hip joints[3] (Box 9-1).

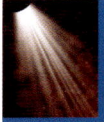

BOX 9-1 Spotlight on Pelvic Motion

Pelvic motion can be complicated and is often misunderstood. For pelvic motion to be clearly understood, it is important to be very clear about the basics of defining motion. Motion is defined as movement of one body part relative to another body part at the joint that is located between them. The pelvis is a separate body part from the trunk and can therefore move relative to the trunk at the joint that is located between them (i.e., the lumbosacral [L5-S1] joint). It is also a separate body part from the thighs and can move relative to a thigh at a hip joint (or to both thighs at both hip joints). Given that the bones within the pelvis are separated by joints, motion within the pelvis is also possible. (For more information on motion within the pelvis, see Section 9.2; for more information on motion between the pelvis and adjacent parts, see Sections 9.3 through 9.5.)

SECTION 9.2   INTRAPELVIC MOTION (SYMPHYSIS PUBIS AND SACROILIAC JOINTS)

- Because the pelvis has the symphysis pubis and sacroiliac (SI) joints located within it, the bones of the pelvis can move relative to each other at these joints; this is termed *intrapelvic motion*.
- Intrapelvic motion can occur at the symphysis pubis joint and/or the SI joints.

SYMPHYSIS PUBIS JOINT:

- The **symphysis pubis joint** is located between the two pubic bones of the pelvis.
  - More specifically, it is located between the bodies of the two pubic bones. The name *symphysis pubis* literally means joining of the bodies of the pubic bones.
- Joint structure classification: Cartilaginous joint[2]
  - Subtype: Symphysis joint
- Joint function classification: Amphiarthrotic

MAJOR MOTIONS ALLOWED:

- Nonaxial gliding

MAJOR LIGAMENTS OF THE SYMPHYSIS PUBIS JOINT:

Arcuate Pubic Ligament:

- The **arcuate pubic ligament** spans the pubic symphysis joint inferiorly, stabilizing the joint (Figure 9-2).

MISCELLANEOUS:

- The symphysis pubis joint is also stabilized (i.e., reinforced) by the fibrous aponeurotic expansions of a number of muscles of the abdominal wall and the medial thigh.[4]
  - These muscles are the rectus abdominis, external abdominal oblique, internal abdominal oblique, and transversus abdominis of the anterior abdominal wall, as well as the adductor longus, gracilis, and adductor brevis of the medial thigh.
- The end of each pubic bone of the pubic symphysis joint is lined with articular cartilage; these cartilage-covered ends are then joined by a fibrocartilaginous disc.[1]

SACROILIAC JOINTS:

- Two **sacroiliac (SI) joints** exist, paired left and right (see Figure 9-2).
- Each SI joint is located between the sacrum and the iliac portion of the pelvic bone, hence the name *SI joint*.
  - More specifically, the SI joints unite the C-shaped auricular surfaces of the sacrum with the C-shaped auricular surfaces

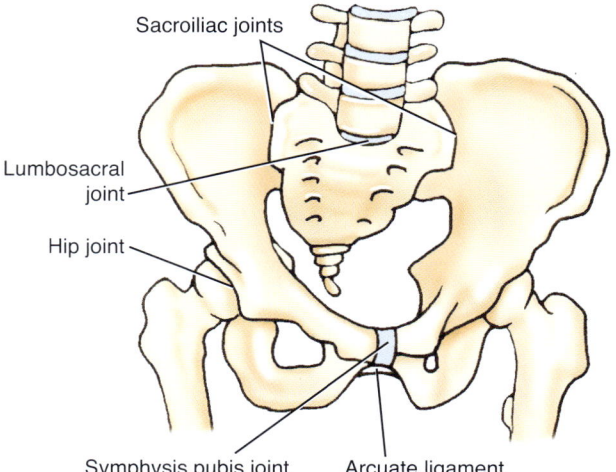

FIGURE 9-2 Anterolateral view of the pelvis. Both sacroiliac (SI) joints are shown posteriorly, and the symphysis pubis joint is shown anteriorly. The arcuate ligament of the symphysis pubis joint is also seen.

of the two pelvic bones. The term *auricular* is from the Latin *auricularis*, meaning to pertain to the ear. These articular surfaces of the sacrum and ilium are termed *auricular* because they resemble an ear in shape.
- Joint structure classification: Mixed synovial/fibrous joint[2]
  - Subtype: Plane joint
- Joint function classification: Mixed diarthrotic/amphiarthrotic
- Note: The sacroiliac (SI) joints are unusual in that they begin as diarthrotic, synovial joints; a synovial capsule and cavity are present, the bones are capped with articular cartilage, and the degree of movement allowed is appreciable. However, as a person ages, fibrous tissue is gradually placed within the joint cavity, converting this joint to a fibrous, amphiarthrotic joint.[1] The tremendous weight-bearing force from above (see Figure 9-5), wedging the sacrum into the pelvic bones, along with forces transmitted up from the lower extremities, are credited with creating the stresses that cause the changes to this joint.

MAJOR MOTIONS ALLOWED:

- Nonaxial gliding
- Nutation and counternutation[2] (axial movements in the sagittal plane) (Figure 9-3; Box 9-2)
  - **Nutation** is defined as the superior sacral base dropping anteriorly and inferiorly, while the inferior tip of the sacrum moves posteriorly and superiorly. Relatively, the pelvic bone tilts posteriorly.[5]
  - **Counternutation** is defined as the opposite of nutation; the superior sacral base moves posteriorly and superiorly, while the inferior tip of the sacrum moves anteriorly and inferiorly. Relatively, the pelvic bone tilts anteriorly.[5]

- Rotation: An individual pelvic bone can also rotate medially or laterally at the sacroiliac joint. These motions are axial motions in the transverse plane.

BOX 9-2

The amount of motion at the sacroiliac (SI) joints and the biomechanical and clinical importance of SI joint motion are extremely controversial. Many sources, especially in the traditional allopathic world, view SI motion and significance as negligible and unimportant; many sources, especially in the chiropractic and osteopathic world, view the sacrum as the keystone of the pelvis, and the SI joint, with regard to its motion and significance, as perhaps the most important joint of the "low back." It is possible to assess the degree of motion at the SI joint by performing a motion palpation assessment procedure known as the Stork Test. This involves simultaneous palpation of the posterior superior iliac spine (PSIS) and sacral tubercle as the client moves their ipsilateral (same-side) thigh into flexion.

MAJOR LIGAMENTS OF THE SACROILIAC JOINT:

All SI ligaments provide stability to the SI joint (Figure 9-4; Box 9-3).

BOX 9-3 Ligaments of the Sacroiliac Joint

- Sacroiliac (SI) ligaments (anterior, posterior, and interosseus)
- Sacrotuberous ligament
- Sacrospinous ligament
- Iliolumbar ligament

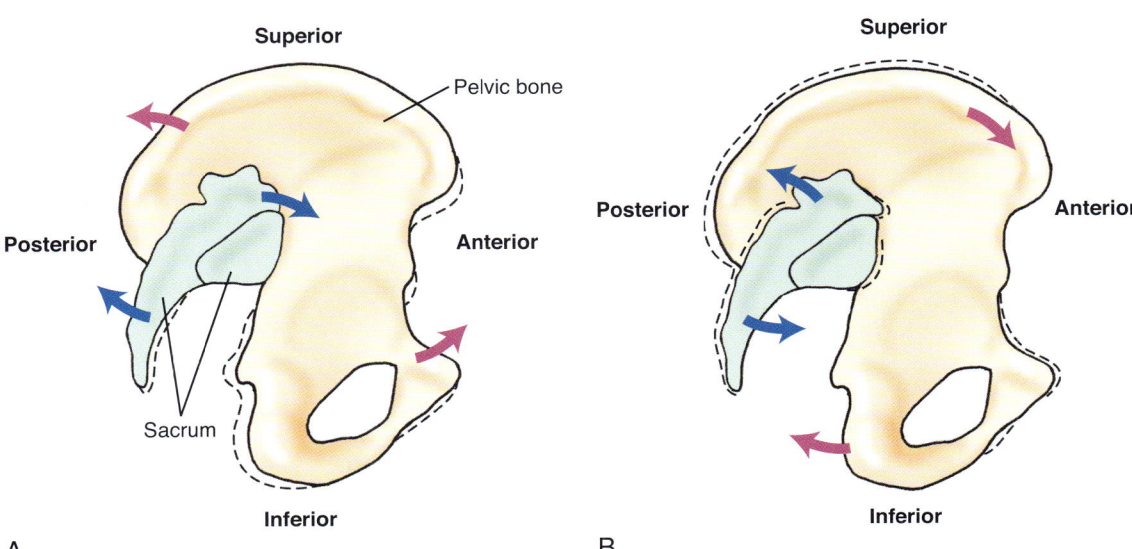

FIGURE 9-3 The sacrum can move within the pelvis relative to the two pelvic bones. **A,** Intrapelvic motion of nutation wherein the superior end of the sacrum moves anteriorly and inferiorly and the inferior end moves posteriorly and superiorly. Relatively, the pelvic bone tilts posteriorly. **B,** Intrapelvic motion of counternutation wherein the superior end of the sacrum moves posteriorly and superiorly and the inferior end moves anteriorly and inferiorly. Relatively, the pelvic bone tilts anteriorly.

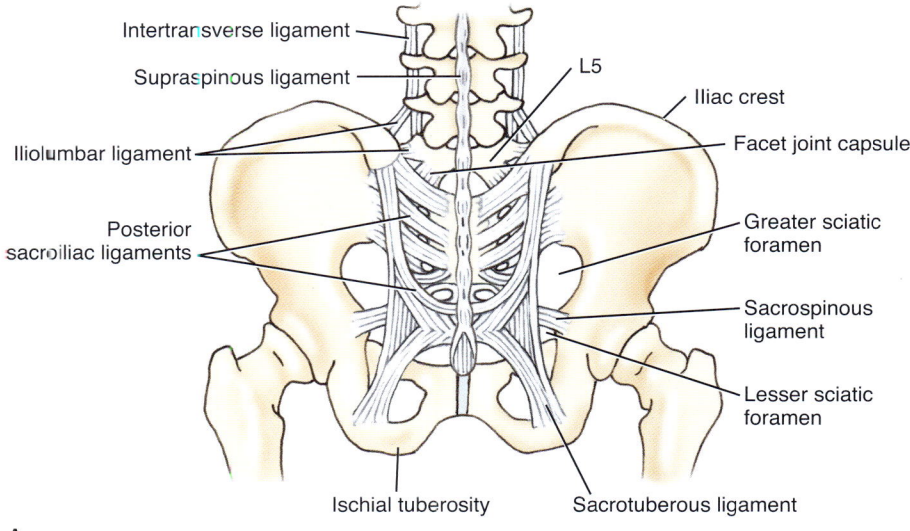

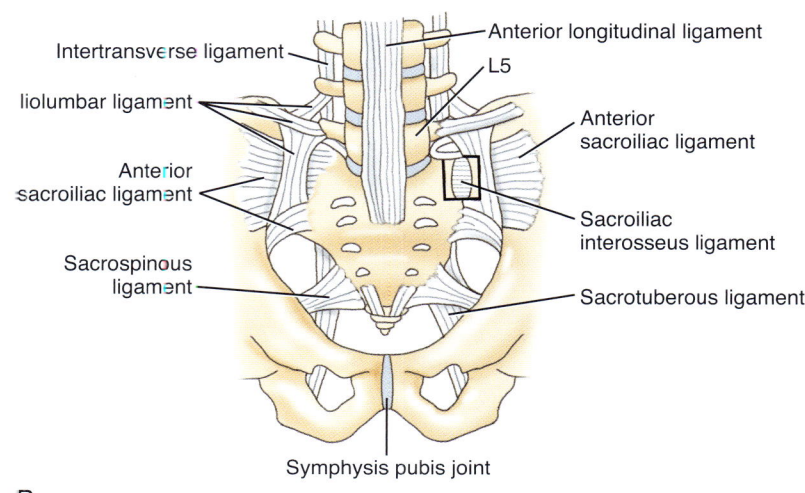

FIGURE 9-4 A, Posterior view of the ligaments of the sacroiliac (SI) joints. The major posterior ligaments of the SI joint are the posterior SI ligaments. Additional stabilization is given to this joint posteriorly by the iliolumbar, sacrotuberous, and sacrospinous ligaments. Note that the sacrospinous ligament separates the greater sciatic foramen from the lesser sciatic foramen. **B,** Anterior view of the ligaments of the SI joints. The major anterior ligaments of the SI joint are the anterior SI ligaments. On the left side (our right side), a small area of the anterior SI ligaments and the bony surfaces of the joint have been partially cut away to reveal the SI interosseus ligaments located within the joint.

Sacroiliac Ligaments:

- The **sacroiliac ligaments** span directly from the sacrum to the ilium.
- Three sets of sacroiliac (SI) ligaments exist[1]:
  - Anterior SI ligaments
  - Posterior SI ligaments (short and long)
  - SI interosseus ligaments

Sacrotuberous Ligament:

- The **sacrotuberous ligament** attaches from the sacrum to the ischial tuberosity.
- The sacrotuberous ligament does not attach directly from the sacrum to ilium; hence it provides indirect stabilization to the SI joint.

Sacrospinous Ligament:

- The **sacrospinous ligament** attaches from the sacrum to the ischial spine.
- The sacrospinous ligament does not attach directly from the sacrum to ilium; hence it provides indirect stabilization to the SI joint.
- Note: The **greater sciatic notch** and the **lesser sciatic notch** are notches in the posterior contour of the pelvic bone; the dividing point between them is created by the ischial spine. These sciatic notches become sciatic foramina with the presence of the sacrospinous and sacrotuberous ligaments (see Figure 9-4, A). (Note: The sciatic nerve exits the pelvis through the **greater sciatic foramen**.)

Iliolumbar Ligament:

- The **iliolumbar ligament** attaches from the lumbar spine to the ilium.[5]
- The iliolumbar ligament actually has a number of parts that attach the fourth and fifth lumbar vertebrae to the iliac crest.
- The iliolumbar ligaments indirectly help stabilize the SI joint. They are also important in stabilizing the lumbosacral (L5-S1) joint.

CHAPTER 9 Joints of the Lower Extremity

MISCELLANEOUS:

- The SI joint is the joint that is located at the transition of the inferior end of the axial skeleton and the proximal end of the appendicular skeleton of the lower extremity.
- The SI joints are weight-bearing joints that must transfer the weight of the axial body above to the pelvic bones of the lower extremities,[4] and transfer the ground reaction forces from below (each time our foot hits the ground, the ground hits back with equal force) through the pelvic bones and into the sacrum (Figure 9-5).
- During pregnancy, the ligaments of the SI joints loosen to allow greater movement so that the baby can be delivered through the birth canal[5] (Box 9-4).

BOX 9-4

The increased looseness of the ligaments of the sacroiliac (SI) joints that occurs during pregnancy often remains throughout the life of the woman. This increased mobility results in a decreased stability of the SI joints and an increased predisposition for low-back problems and pain.

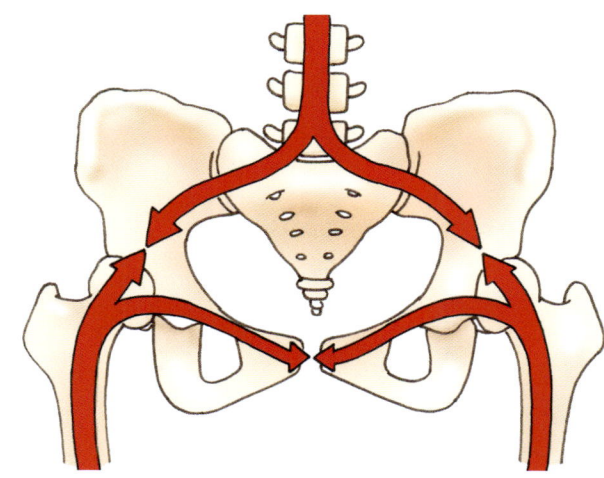

FIGURE 9-5 Illustration of the forces that are transmitted through the sacroiliac (SI) joint. These forces affect the SI joints from both above and below. Weight-bearing forces from above are represented by the *arrow* that descends the spine. Forces of impact from below that would occur when walking, running, or jumping are represented by the arrows that ascend the femurs. *(Modeled from Kapandji IA: Physiology of the joints: the trunk and the vertebral column, ed 2, Edinburgh, 1974, Churchill Livingstone.)*

SECTION 9.3 MOVEMENT OF THE PELVIS AT THE LUMBOSACRAL JOINT

MOTION OF THE PELVIS AT THE LUMBOSACRAL JOINT:

- When the pelvis moves as a unit, this motion can occur relative to the lumbar spine of the trunk at the lumbosacral joint.[4]
- Given that we usually think of the spine as moving at the spinal joints (the lumbosacral joint is a spinal joint), movement of the pelvis at the lumbosacral joint is an example of what is termed a *reverse action*. (See Section 6.29 for information on reverse actions.)
- The lumbosacral joint allows only a few degrees of motion. When the pelvis moves at the lumbosacral joint, the rest of the spine will have to begin to move once the motion of the lumbosacral joint has reached its limit. This means that the lower spine moves relative to the upper spine, which is also an example of a reverse action. This can be seen in Figure 9-6, *A* to *F* (the change in the curve of the lumbar spine should be noted).
- If no motion is occurring at the hip joints when the pelvis moves at the lumbosacral joint, then the thighs are fixed to the pelvis and will "go along for the ride," following the movement of the pelvis.

Following are motions of the pelvis at the lumbosacral joint (see Figure 9-6):

- The pelvis can anteriorly tilt and posteriorly tilt in the sagittal plane around a mediolateral axis.
- The pelvis can depress or elevate on one side in the frontal plane around an anteroposterior axis.
  - When the pelvis depresses on one side, the other side of the pelvis elevates (i.e., depression of the right pelvis creates elevation of the left pelvis). Similarly, if the pelvis elevates on one side, then the other side depresses.
  - Depression of the pelvis on one side is also called *lateral tilt* (i.e., depression of the right side of the pelvis is called *right lateral tilt of the pelvis*; depression of the left side of the pelvis is called *left lateral tilt of the pelvis*). When the side of the pelvis that elevates is described, it is often called *hiking* the hip or pelvis.
- The pelvis can rotate to the right or to the left in the transverse plane around a vertical axis.

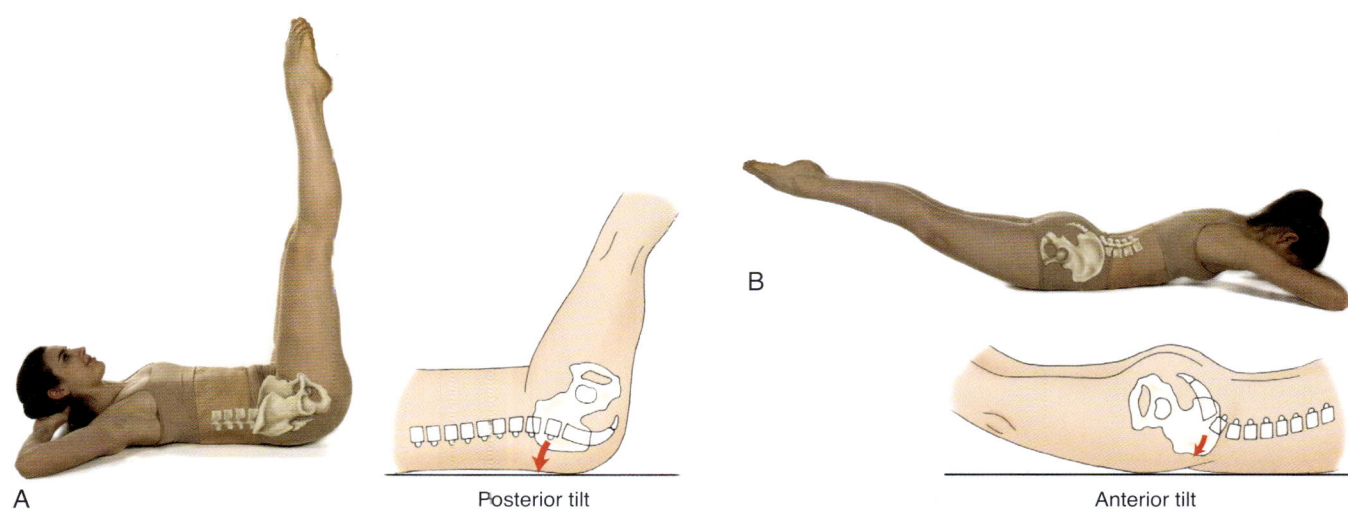

A Posterior tilt B Anterior tilt

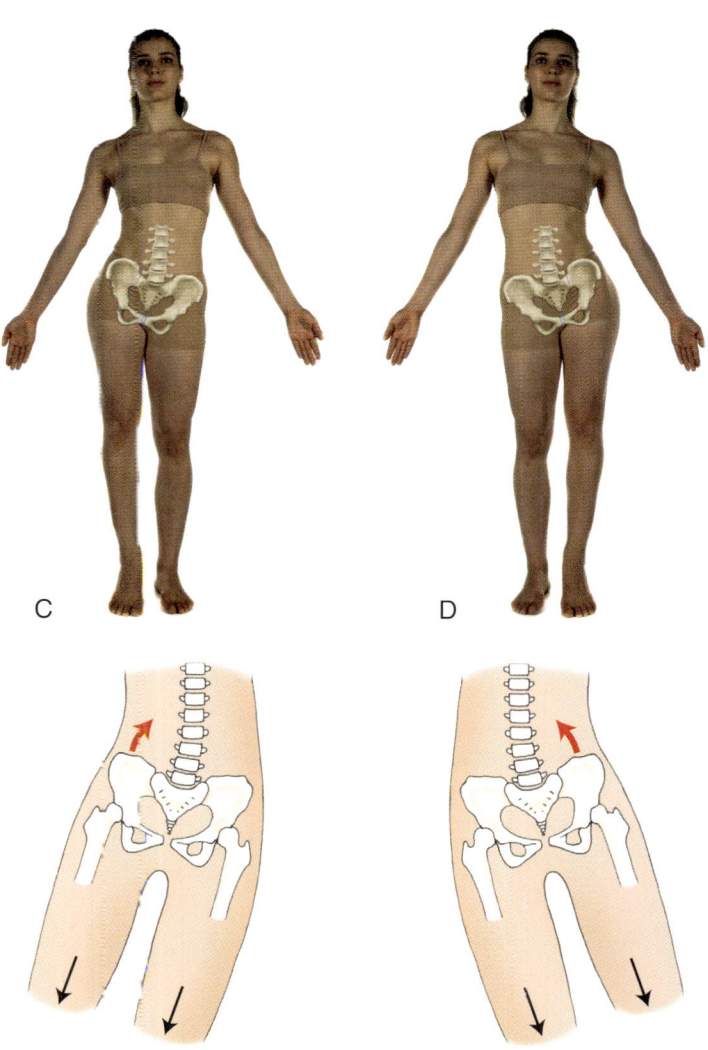

C D

Elevation of the right pelvis Elevation of the left pelvis

FIGURE 9-6 Motion of the pelvis at the lumbosacral joint. **A** and **B,** Lateral views illustrating posterior tilt and anterior tilt, respectively, of the pelvis at the lumbosacral joint. (Note: In **A** and **B,** no motion is occurring at the hip joints; therefore the thighs are shown to "go along for the ride," resulting in the lower extremities moving in space.) **C** and **D,** Anterior views illustrating elevation of the right pelvis and elevation of the left pelvis, respectively, at the lumbosacral joint. (Note: In the drawn illustration of **C** and **D,** no motion is occurring at the hip joints; therefore the thighs are shown to "go along for the ride," resulting in the lower extremities moving in space.)

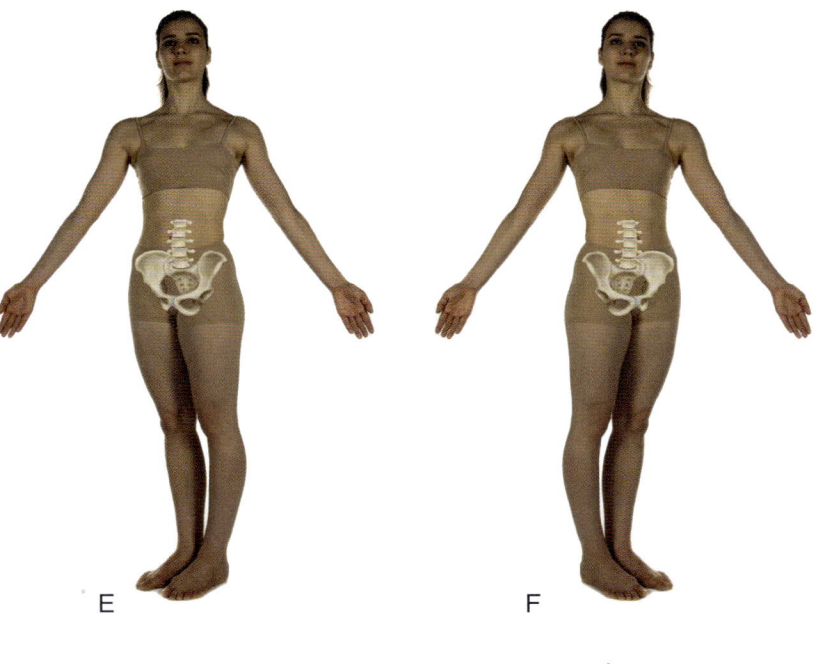

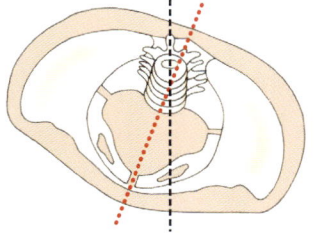

Right rotation of the pelvis

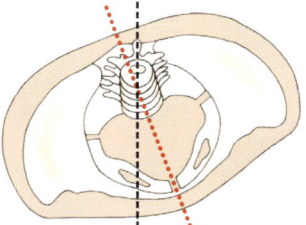

Left rotation of the pelvis

FIGURE 9-6, cont'd **E** and **F**, Anterior and superior views illustrating rotation of the pelvis to the right and rotation to the left, respectively, at the lumbosacral joint. (Note: In **E** and **F**, the dashed black line represents the orientation of the spine and the red dotted line represents the orientation of the pelvis. Given the different directions of these two lines, it is clear that the pelvis has rotated relative to the spine; this motion has occurred at the lumbosacral joint.)

SECTION 9.4 MOVEMENT OF THE PELVIS AT THE HIP JOINTS

MOTION OF THE PELVIS AS A UNIT AT THE HIP JOINTS:

- When the pelvis moves as a unit, this motion can occur relative to the thighs at the hip joints.[4]
- When the pelvis moves at the hip joints, it is possible for the pelvis to move at both hip joints at the same time; this results in the pelvis changing its position relative to both thighs. It is also possible for the pelvis to move relative to only one hip joint. In this case the pelvis moves relative only to that one thigh (at the hip joint located between the pelvis and that thigh); the other thigh stays fixed to the pelvis and "goes along for the ride."
- Given that we usually think of the thighs as moving at the hip joints, movement of the pelvis at the hip joints is an example of what is termed a *reverse action*. (See Section 6.29 for information on reverse actions.)
- If no motion is occurring at the lumbosacral joint when the pelvis moves at the hip joints, then the trunk is fixed to the pelvis and will "go along for the ride," following the movement of the pelvis (Box 9-5).

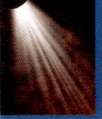 **BOX 9-5 Spotlight on Bending at the Hip Joints**

When a person is standing up and anteriorly tilts the pelvis at the hip joints (and the trunk stays fixed to the pelvis, going along for the ride) to "bend forward," this motion is often incorrectly described as flexion of the trunk or flexion of the spine. Actually, the trunk never moved in this scenario, because it did not move relative to the pelvis (it merely followed the pelvis). Furthermore, no movement ever occurred at the spinal joints. The entire movement is a result of a "flexion" of the hip joints wherein the pelvis anteriorly tilts toward the thighs.

Following are motions of the pelvis at the hip joints (Figure 9-7):
- The pelvis can anteriorly tilt and posteriorly tilt in the sagittal plane around a mediolateral axis.
- The pelvis can depress or elevate on one side in the frontal plane around an anteroposterior axis.
- The pelvis can rotate to the right or to the left in the transverse plane around a vertical axis.

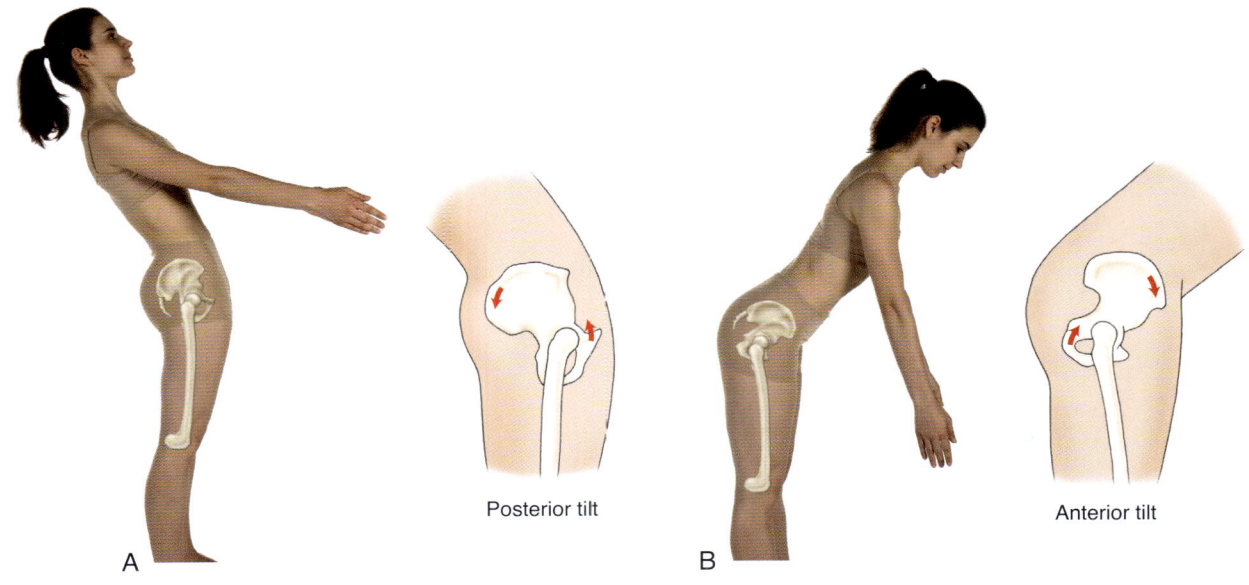
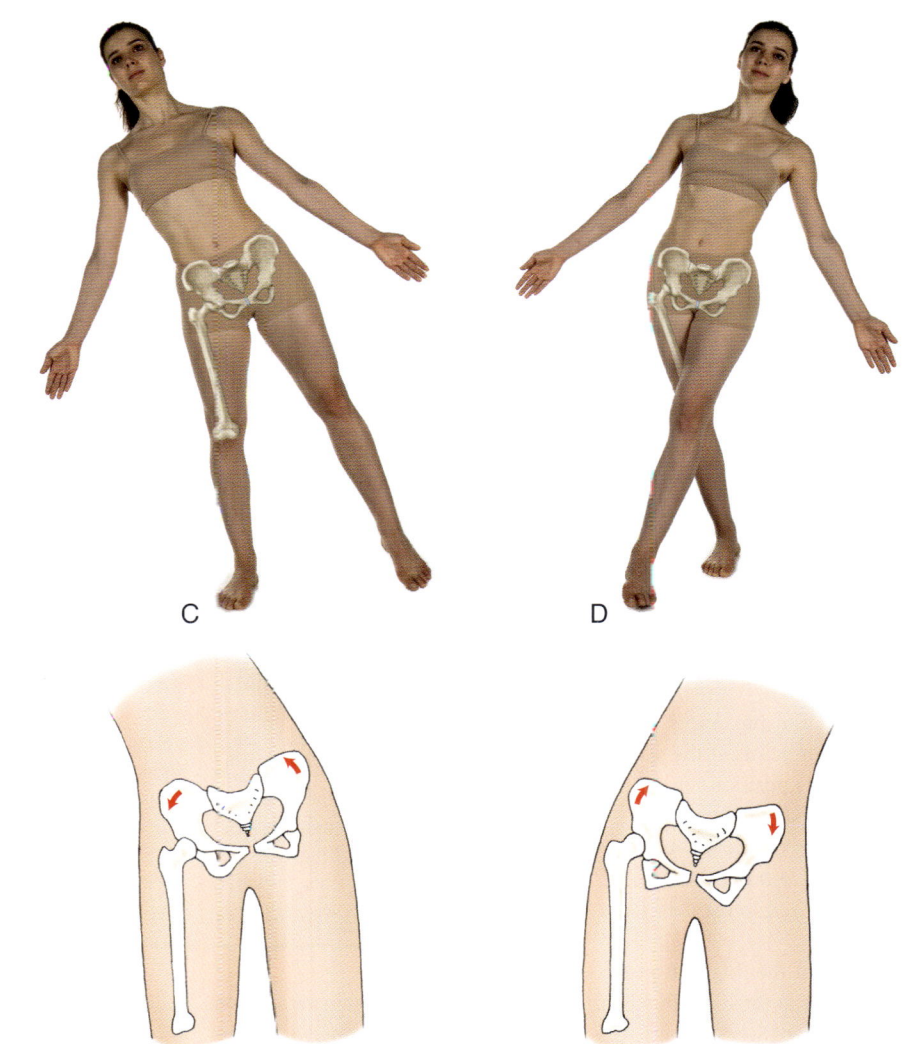

Depression of the right pelvis   Elevation of the right pelvis

FIGURE 9-7 Motion of the pelvis at the hip joint. (Note: In **A** to **D,** no motion is occurring at the lumbosacral joint; therefore the trunk is shown to "go along for the ride," resulting in the upper body changing its position in space.) **A** and **B,** Lateral views illustrating posterior tilt and anterior tilt, respectively, of the pelvis at the hip joint. **C** and **D,** Anterior views illustrating depression of the right pelvis and elevation of the right pelvis, respectively, at the right hip joint. (Note: When the pelvis elevates on one side, it depresses on the other, and vice versa.)

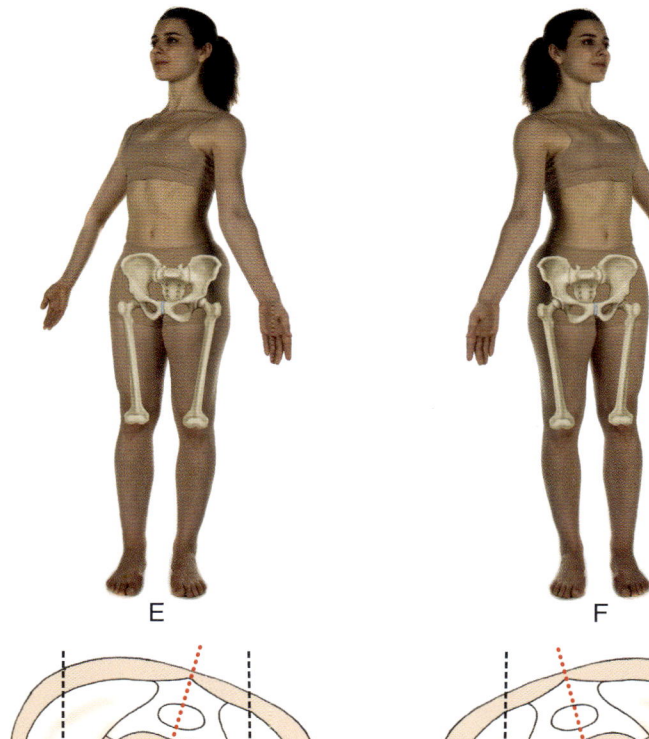

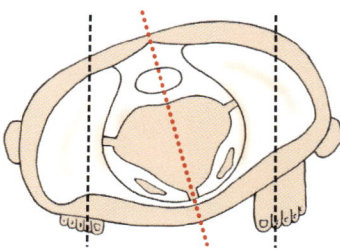

Right rotation of the pelvis   Left rotation of the pelvis

FIGURE 9-7, cont'd **E** and **F**, Anterior and superior views illustrating rotation of the pelvis to the right and rotation to the left, respectively, at the hip joints. (Note: In **E** and **F**, the black dashed line represents the orientation of the thighs and the red dotted line represents the orientation of the pelvis. Given the different directions of these lines, it is clear that the pelvis has rotated relative to the thighs; this motion has occurred at the hip joints.)

SECTION 9.5   MOVEMENT OF THE PELVIS AT THE LUMBOSACRAL AND HIP JOINTS

MOTION OF THE PELVIS AS A UNIT AT THE LUMBOSACRAL AND HIP JOINTS:

- Of course, the pelvis can move as a body part at both the lumbosacral joint and the hip joints at the same time.[4] When this occurs, two things should be noted:
  1. The pelvis moves relative to both the spine and the thigh(s).
  2. The motion has occurred at both the lumbosacral joint and the hip joint(s) (Figure 9-8). (See Table 9-1 for the average ranges of motion of the pelvis.)
- As is usual for motion of the pelvis at the lumbosacral (L5-S1) joint, when maximum motion possible at this joint is attained by the muscles that move the pelvis at the lumbosacral joint, motion will also occur successively up the spine. In other words, when the L5-S1 joint has allowed as much motion as it can, the L5 vertebra will begin to move relative to L4 at the L4-L5 joint. When this joint has moved as much as it can, then the L4 vertebra will begin to move relative to L3 at the L3-L4 joint. Motion will continue to occur successively up the spine in this manner, with the lower spine moving relative to the upper spine. Movement of the lower spine relative to the upper spine is considered to be a reverse action. Note: This spinal motion can be seen by noting the changes in the lumbar spinal curve.

TABLE 9-1	Average Ranges of Motion of the Pelvis at the Hip and Lumbosacral Joints with the Client Seated and the Thighs Flexed 90 Degrees at the Hip Joint*		
Anterior tilt	30 Degrees	Posterior tilt	15 Degrees
Right depression	30 Degrees	Left depression	30 Degrees
Right rotation	15 Degrees	Left rotation	15 Degrees

*Numbers would be different if the client were standing and would also vary based on whether the knee joint was flexed or extended.

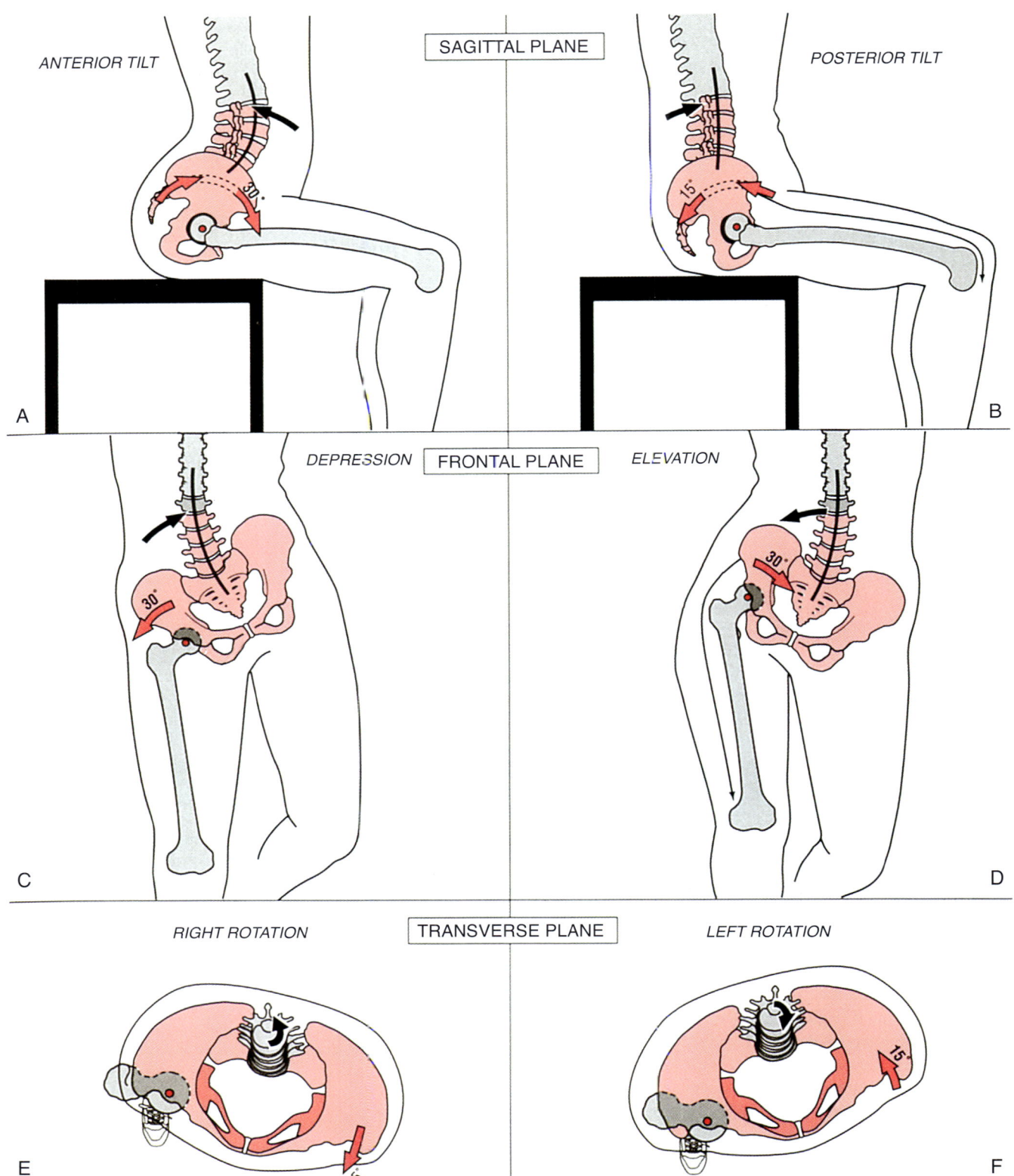

FIGURE 9-8 Motion of the pelvis at both the lumbosacral joint and the hip joints. (Note: In all illustrations the change in position of the pelvis is relative to both the spine and the femur[s].) **A** and **B**, Illustration of the sagittal plane motions of anterior tilt and posterior tilt, respectively. **C** and **D**, Frontal plane motions of depression and elevation, respectively. **E** and **F**, Transverse plane motions of right rotation and left rotation, respectively.

SECTION 9.6 RELATIONSHIP OF PELVIC/SPINAL MOVEMENTS AT THE LUMBOSACRAL JOINT

- Now that the motion of the pelvis is clearly understood, it is valuable to examine the relationship that pelvic movements have to spinal movements. If we picture the muscles that cross from the trunk to the pelvis (i.e., crossing the lumbosacral joint), then these pelvic movements would be considered the reverse actions of these muscles. The following sections describe the relationship between the pelvis and the spine for the six major movements within the three cardinal planes:

SAGITTAL PLANE MOVEMENTS:

- Posterior tilt of the pelvis at the lumbosacral joint is analogous to flexion of the trunk at the lumbosacral joint. Therefore muscles that perform flexion of the trunk also perform posterior tilt of the pelvis at the lumbosacral joint[4] (Figure 9-9).
  - Examples: The muscles of the anterior abdominal wall, such as the rectus abdominis, external abdominal oblique, and the internal abdominal oblique

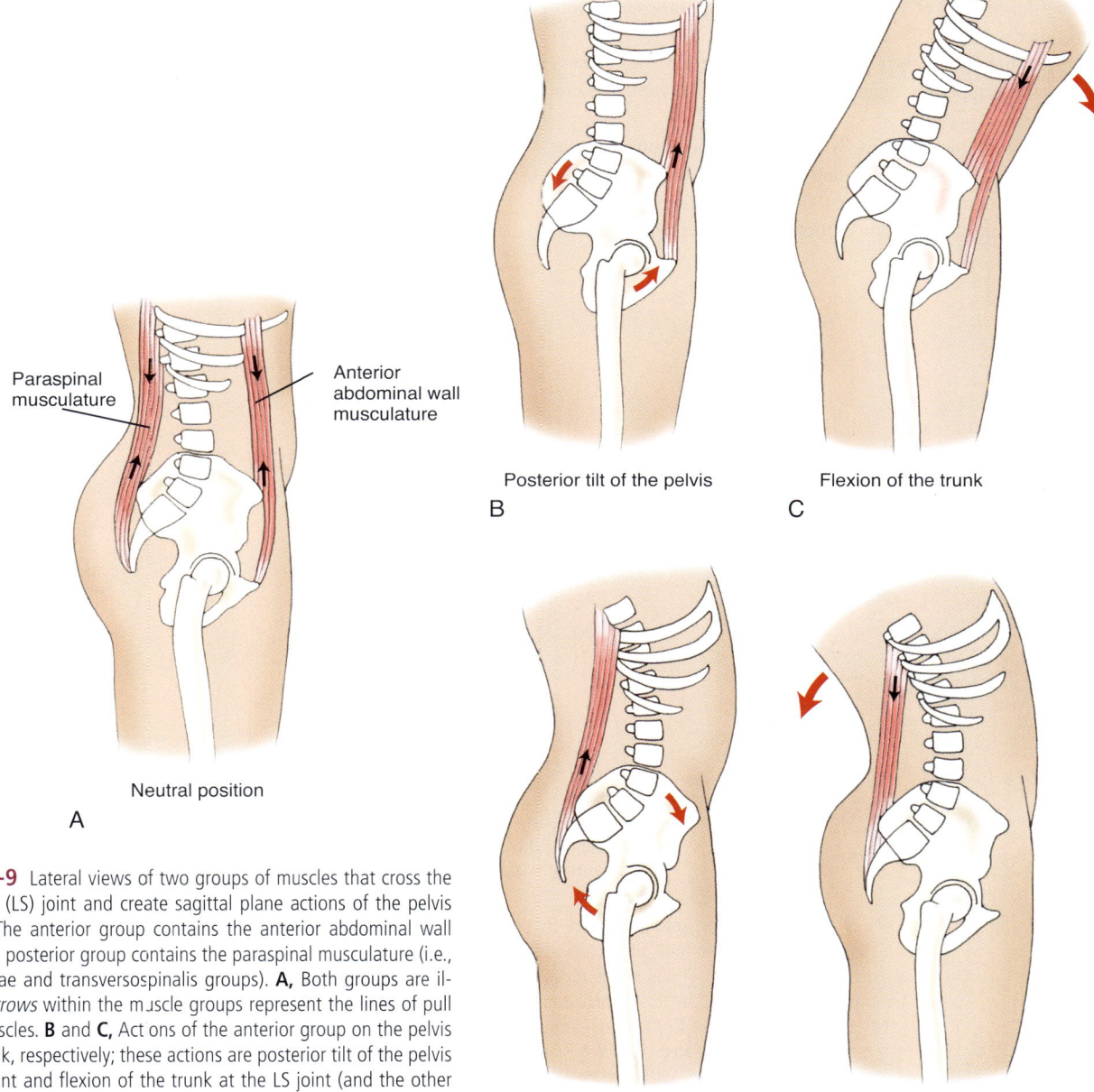

FIGURE 9-9 Lateral views of two groups of muscles that cross the lumbosacral (LS) joint and create sagittal plane actions of the pelvis and trunk. The anterior group contains the anterior abdominal wall muscles; the posterior group contains the paraspinal musculature (i.e., erector spinae and transversospinalis groups). **A,** Both groups are illustrated; *arrows* within the muscle groups represent the lines of pull of these muscles. **B** and **C,** Actions of the anterior group on the pelvis and the trunk, respectively; these actions are posterior tilt of the pelvis at the LS joint and flexion of the trunk at the LS joint (and the other spinal joints). **D** and **E,** Actions of the posterior group on the pelvis and the trunk; these actions are anterior tilt of the pelvis at the LS joint and extension of the trunk at the LS joint (and other spinal joints).

- Anterior tilt of the pelvis at the lumbosacral joint is analogous to extension of the trunk at the lumbosacral joint. Therefore muscles that perform extension of the trunk also perform anterior tilt of the pelvis at the lumbosacral joint[4] (see Figure 9-9).
  - Examples: Erector spinae group, transversospinalis group, quadratus lumborum, and latissimus dorsi

FRONTAL PLANE MOVEMENTS:

- Elevation of the right pelvis (which is also depression of the left pelvis) at the lumbosacral joint is analogous to right lateral flexion of the trunk at the lumbosacral joint. Therefore muscles that perform right lateral flexion of the trunk also perform elevation of the right pelvis (and therefore also depression of the left pelvis) at the lumbosacral joint[4] (Figure 9-10).
  - Examples: Right erector spinae group, right transversospinalis group, right quadratus lumborum, and right latissimus dorsi
- Elevation of the left pelvis (which is also depression of the right pelvis) at the lumbosacral joint is analogous to left lateral flexion of the trunk at the lumbosacral joint. Therefore muscles that perform left lateral flexion of the trunk also perform elevation of the left pelvis (and therefore also depression of the right pelvis) at the lumbosacral joint[4] (see Figure 9-10).
  - Examples: Left erector spinae group, left transversospinalis group, left quadratus lumborum, and left latissimus dorsi

TRANSVERSE PLANE MOVEMENTS:

- Right rotation of the pelvis at the lumbosacral joint is analogous to left rotation of the trunk at the lumbosacral joint. Therefore muscles that perform left rotation of the trunk also perform right rotation of the pelvis at the lumbosacral joint[4] (Figure 9-11).
  - Examples: Left-sided ipsilateral rotators of the trunk such as the left erector spinae group and left internal abdominal oblique; and right-sided contralateral rotators of the trunk such as the right transversospinalis group and right external abdominal oblique
- Left rotation of the pelvis at the lumbosacral joint is analogous to right rotation of the trunk at the lumbosacral joint. Therefore muscles that perform right rotation of the trunk also perform left rotation of the pelvis at the lumbosacral joint[4] (see Figure 9-11).
  - Examples: Right-sided ipsilateral rotators of the trunk such as the right erector spinae group and right internal abdominal oblique; and left-sided contralateral rotators of the trunk such as the left transversospinalis group and left external abdominal oblique

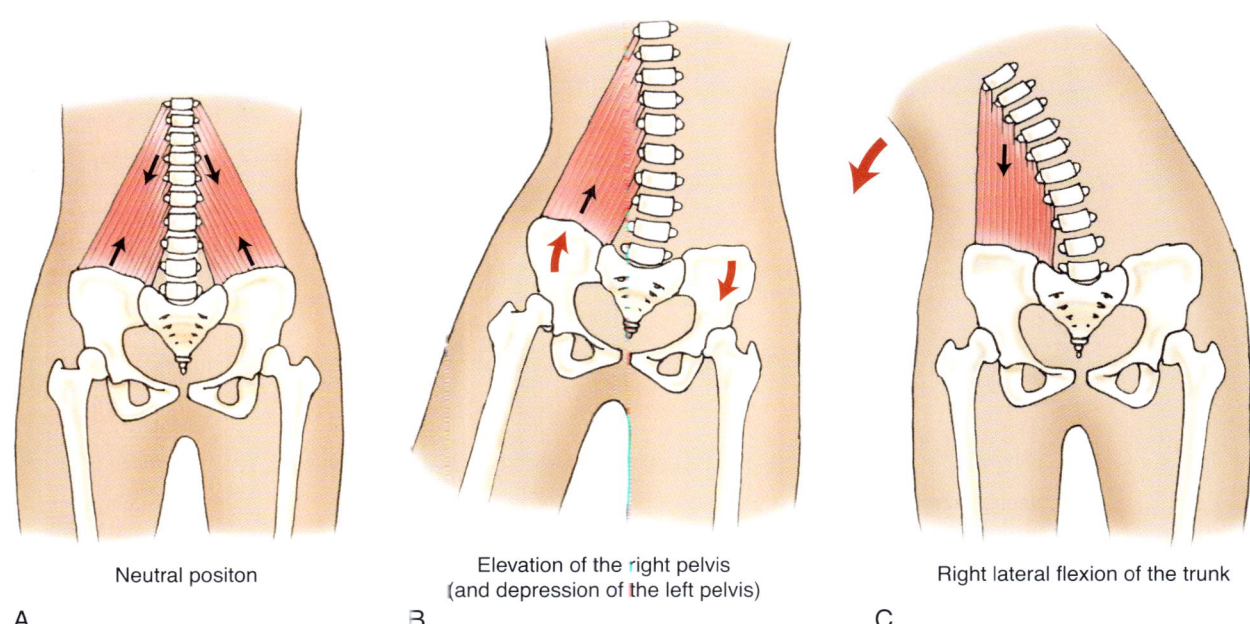

FIGURE 9-10 Anterior views of musculature that crosses the lumbosacral joint laterally and creates frontal plane actions of the pelvis and trunk at the lumbosacral joint. **A,** Illustration of this musculature bilaterally; the *arrows* demonstrate the lines of pull of the musculature. **B,** Pelvic action (i.e., elevation of the right pelvis at the lumbosacral joint) created by this musculature on the right side. (Note: When the pelvis elevates on one side, the other side depresses.) **C,** Trunk action (i.e., right lateral flexion of the trunk at the lumbosacral joint and the other spinal joints) created by this musculature on the right side. (Note: The actions for the left-sided musculature are not shown; they would be elevation of the left pelvis and left lateral flexion of the trunk.)

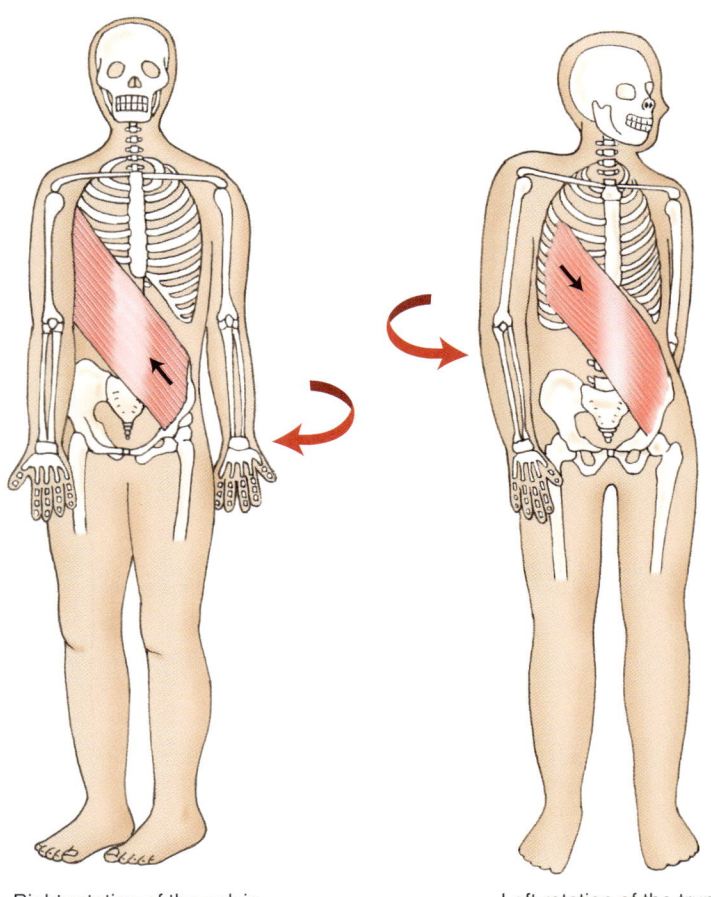

FIGURE 9-11 Anterior views of musculature that crosses the lumbosacral joint and creates transverse plane actions of the pelvis and trunk at the lumbosacral joint; this musculature is composed of the right-sided external abdominal oblique and the left-sided internal abdominal oblique. **A,** Pelvic action (i.e., right rotation of the pelvis at the lumbosacral joint) created by this musculature. **B,** Trunk action (i.e., left rotation of the trunk at the lumbosacral joint and other spinal joints) created by this musculature. (Note: The similar musculature of the left-sided external abdominal oblique and right-sided internal abdominal oblique have not been shown. Actions for this musculature would be left rotation of the pelvis and right rotation of the trunk.)

Right rotation of the pelvis
A

Left rotation of the trunk
B

SECTION 9.7   RELATIONSHIP OF PELVIC/THIGH MOVEMENTS AT THE HIP JOINT

- Just as the relationship of pelvic movements to spinal movements can be compared, the relationship between pelvic and thigh movements can also be compared. If we picture the muscles that cross from the pelvis to the thigh (i.e., crossing the hip joint), then these pelvic movements would be considered the reverse actions of these muscles. Regarding posture of the pelvis (and therefore the spine-see Section 9.8), reverse actions of the pelvis at the hip joint are more important than standard actions of the thigh at the hip joint. This is because the feet are so often rooted to the floor; hence the body is in closed chain position, requiring reverse actions at the hip joint. The following sections describe the relationship between the pelvis and the thigh for the six major movements within the three cardinal planes:

SAGITTAL PLANE MOVEMENTS:

- Anterior tilt of the pelvis at the hip joint is analogous to flexion of the thigh at the hip joint. Therefore muscles that perform anterior tilt of the pelvis at the hip joint also perform flexion of the thigh at the hip joint[6] (Figure 9-12).
  - With flexion of the thigh at the hip joint, the thigh moves up toward the pelvis anteriorly; with anterior tilt of the pelvis at the hip joint, the pelvis moves down toward the thigh anteriorly. The same muscles (i.e., flexors of the hip joint) perform both of these actions.
- Posterior tilt of the pelvis at the hip joint is analogous to extension of the thigh at the hip joint. Therefore muscles that perform posterior tilt of the pelvis at the hip joint also perform extension of the thigh at the hip joint[6] (see Figure 9-12).
  - With extension of the thigh at the hip joint, the thigh moves up toward the pelvis posteriorly; with posterior tilt of the pelvis at the hip joint, the pelvis moves down toward the thigh posteriorly. The same muscles (i.e., extensors of the hip joint) perform both of these actions.

FRONTAL PLANE MOVEMENTS:

- Depression of the right pelvis at the hip joint is analogous to abduction of the right thigh at the hip joint. Therefore muscles that perform depression of the right pelvis at the hip joint also perform abduction of the right thigh at the hip joint[6] (Figure 9-13).
  - With abduction of the right thigh at the hip joint, the right thigh moves up toward the right side of the pelvis laterally; with depression of the right side of the pelvis at the right hip joint, the right side of the pelvis moves down toward the

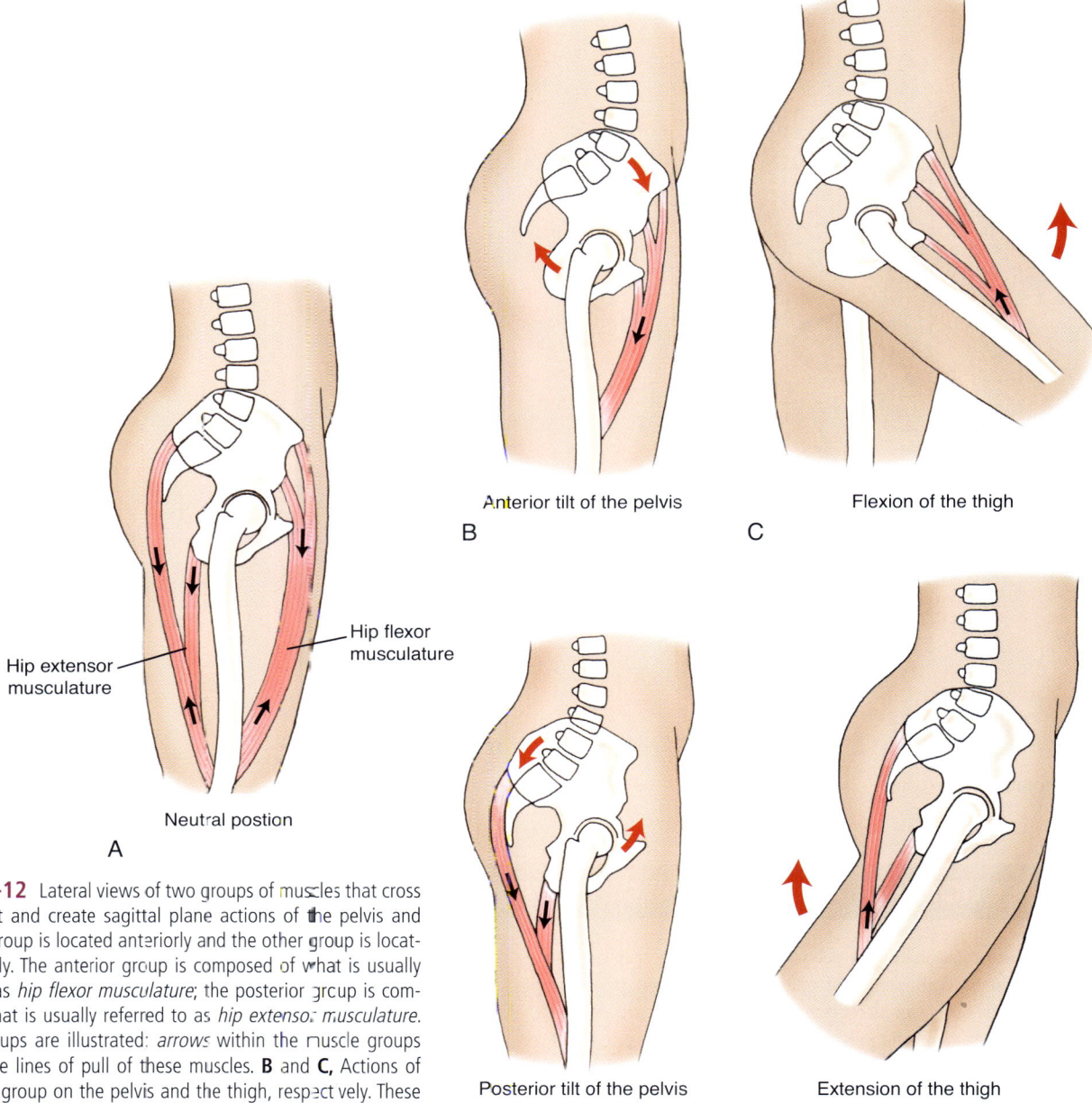

FIGURE 9-12 Lateral views of two groups of muscles that cross the hip joint and create sagittal plane actions of the pelvis and thigh; one group is located anteriorly and the other group is located posteriorly. The anterior group is composed of what is usually referred to as *hip flexor musculature*; the posterior group is composed of what is usually referred to as *hip extensor musculature*. **A,** Both groups are illustrated; *arrows* within the muscle groups represent the lines of pull of these muscles. **B** and **C,** Actions of the anterior group on the pelvis and the thigh, respectively. These actions are anterior tilt of the pelvis at the hip joint and flexion of the thigh at the hip joint. **D** and **E,** Actions of the posterior group on the pelvis and the thigh; these actions are posterior tilt of the pelvis and extension of the thigh at the hip joint.

right thigh laterally. The same muscles (i.e., abductors of the right hip joint) perform both of these actions.
- When the right side of the pelvis depresses, the left side must elevate because the pelvis largely moves as a unit. Therefore it can be said that muscles that depress the pelvis on one side of the body also elevate the pelvis on the opposite side of the body (i.e., they are opposite-side elevators, or *contralateral elevators* of the pelvis).
○ Depression of the left pelvis at the hip joint is analogous to abduction of the left thigh at the hip joint. Therefore muscles that perform depression of the left pelvis at the hip joint also perform abduction of the left thigh at the hip joint[6] (see Figure 9-13).
- The reasoning to explain this is identical to depression of the right pelvis (explained previously) except that it is on the left side of the body.
- Note: Depression of the right side of the pelvis is also known as *right lateral tilt of the pelvis*. The phrase "hiking the (left) hip" is sometimes used to refer to the other side of the pelvis, which has elevated. The same concepts would be true for depression of the left side of the pelvis.

TRANSVERSE PLANE MOVEMENTS:

○ Right rotation of the pelvis at the hip joints is analogous to medial rotation of the right thigh and lateral rotation of the left thigh at the

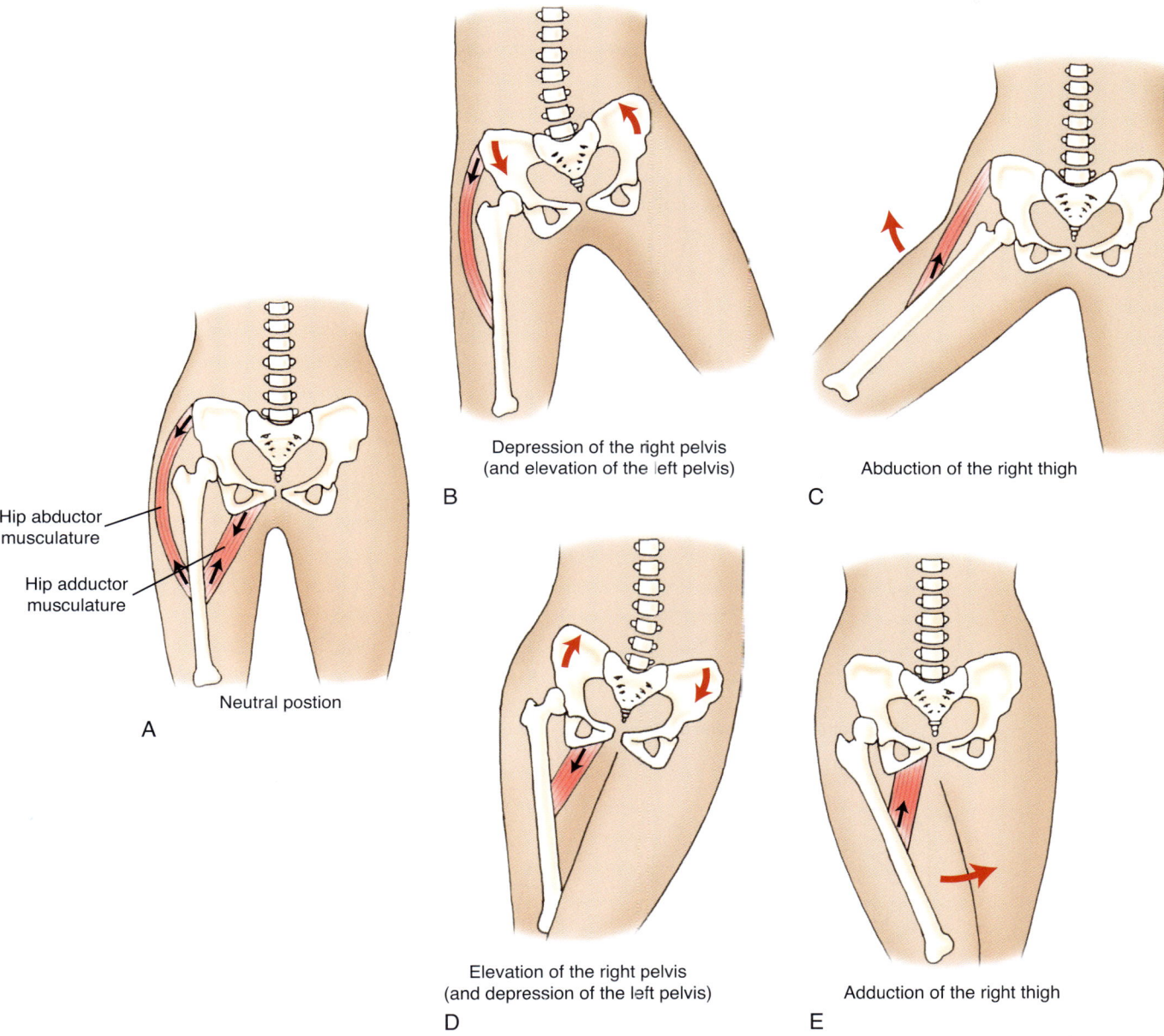

FIGURE 9-13 Anterior views of musculature that crosses the right hip joint laterally and medially and creates frontal plane actions of the pelvis and thigh at the hip joint. **A,** Both the lateral and medial groups of musculature on the right side of the body; the *arrows* demonstrate the lines of pull of the musculature. The lateral group is composed of what is usually referred to as *hip abductor musculature*; the medial group is composed of what is usually referred to as *hip adductor musculature*. **B,** Pelvic action (i.e., depression of the right pelvis) created by the lateral group of musculature. (Note: When the pelvis depresses on the right side, the left side elevates.) **C,** Thigh action (i.e., abduction of the right thigh) created by the lateral group of musculature. **D,** Pelvic action (i.e., elevation of the right pelvis) created by the medial group of musculature. (Note: When the pelvis elevates on the right side, the left side depresses.) **E,** Thigh action (i.e., adduction of the right thigh) created by the medial group of musculature. (Note: The musculature on the left side of the body is not shown.)

hip joints. Therefore muscles that perform right rotation of the pelvis at the hip joints also perform medial rotation of the right thigh and lateral rotation of the left thigh at the hip joints[6] (Figure 9-14).

❍ To best visualize this, it is helpful to picture a person who is standing up. If he or she keeps the thighs and lower extremities fixed and rotates the pelvis to the right at both hip joints, then the position that results will be identical to the position obtained if the person were to instead keep the pelvis and upper body fixed and medially rotate the right thigh at the right hip joint and laterally rotate the left thigh at the left hip joint. The result is that muscles that perform right rotation of the pelvis at the hip joints are the same

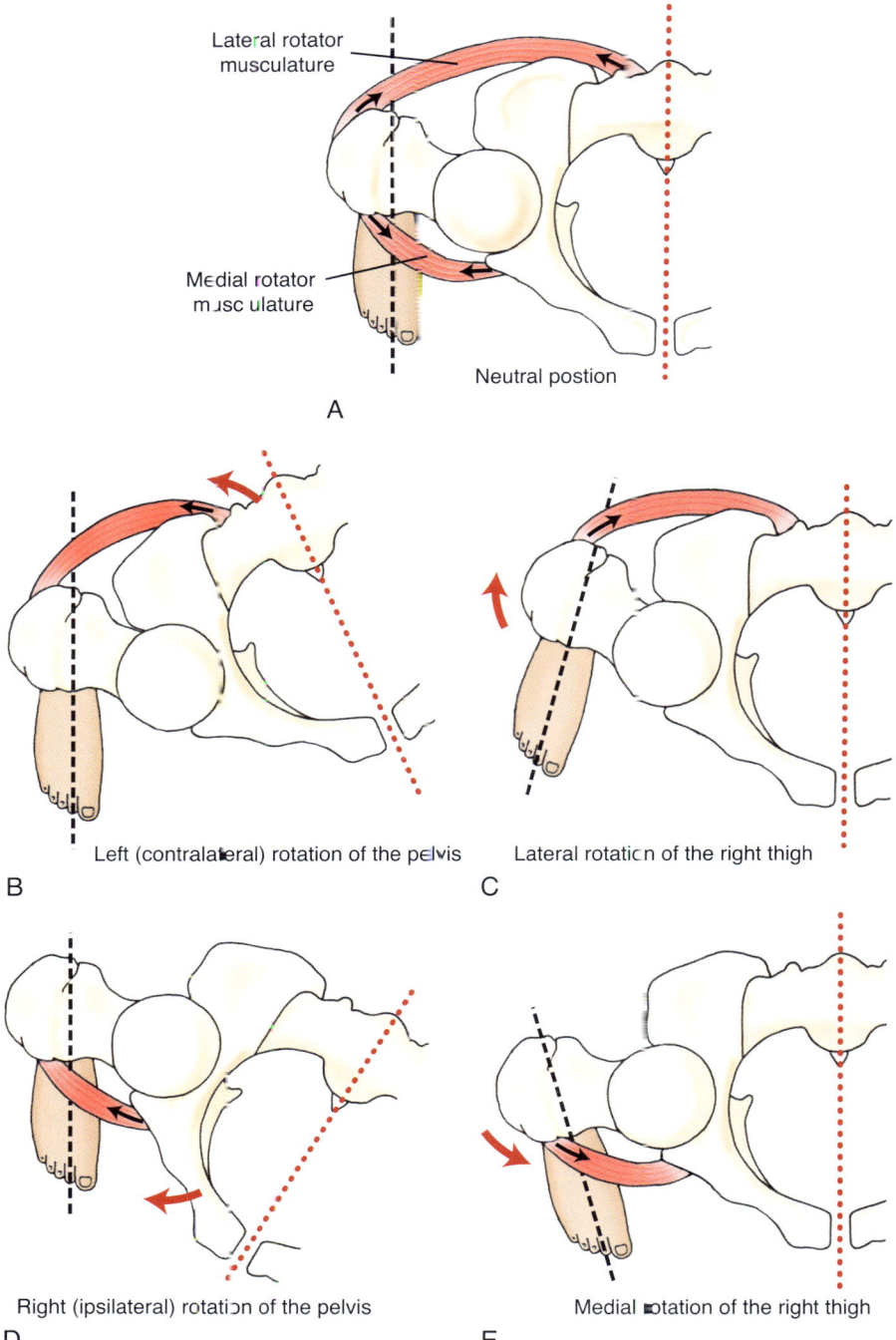

FIGURE 9-14 Superior views of musculature that crosses the right hip joint and creates transverse plane actions of the pelvis and thigh at the hip joint. **A,** The two groups of musculature: One group is posterior and is often referred to as the *lateral rotators of the hip joint;* the other group is anterior and is often referred to as the *medial rotators of the hip joint.* **B,** Pelvic action of the posterior musculature, which is left rotation of the pelvis. Given that right-sided musculature created this action, it is contralateral rotation of the pelvis. **C,** Thigh action of the posterior musculature, which is lateral rotation of the thigh created by the posterior musculature. **D,** Pelvic action of the anterior musculature, which is right rotation of the pelvis. Given that right-sided musculature created this action, it is ipsilateral rotation of the pelvis. **E,** Thigh action of the anterior musculature, which is medial rotation of the thigh created by the anterior musculature. In all figures, the black dashed line represents the orientation of the thigh; the red dotted line represents the orientation of the pelvis. (Note: The musculature on the left side of the body is not shown.)

muscles that perform medial rotation of the right thigh at the right hip joint and lateral rotation of the left thigh at the left hip joint.
- Left rotation of the pelvis at the hip joints is analogous to medial rotation of the left thigh and lateral rotation of the right thigh at the hip joints. Therefore muscles that perform left rotation of the pelvis at the hip joints also perform medial rotation of the left thigh and lateral rotation of the right thigh at the hip joints[6] (see Figure 9-14).
  - The reasoning to explain this is identical to right rotation of the pelvis at the hip joints (explained previously).
  - Therefore lateral rotator muscles of the thigh at the hip joint are contralateral rotators of the pelvis at that hip joint (see Figures 9-14, *B* and *C*); and medial rotator muscles of the thigh at the hip joint are ipsilateral rotators of the pelvis at that hip joint (see Figures 9-14, *D* and *E*; Box 9-6).

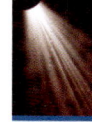

BOX 9-6 Spotlight on Pelvic Rotation Reverse Actions at the Hip Joint

Understanding the relationship of pelvic and thigh rotation movements at the hip joint in the transverse plane shows us two things:
1. The lateral rotators of the thigh at the hip joint (e.g., the posterior buttocks muscles such as the piriformis or gluteus maximus) perform rotation of the pelvis to the opposite side of the body (i.e., they are contralateral rotators of the pelvis at the hip joint). Lateral rotation of the thigh at the hip joint and contralateral rotation of the pelvis at the hip joint are reverse actions of the same muscles.
2. The medial rotators of the thigh at the hip joint (e.g., the anteriorly located tensor fasciae latae and anterior fibers of the gluteus medius) perform rotation of the pelvis to the same side of the body (i.e., they are ipsilateral rotators of the pelvis at the hip joint). Medial rotation of the thigh at the hip joint and ipsilateral rotation of the pelvis at the hip joint are reverse actions of the same muscles (see Figure 9-14).

SECTION 9.8 EFFECT OF PELVIC POSTURE ON SPINAL POSTURE

Sections 9.1 through 9.7 have spent considerable time discussing the kinesiology of the pelvis because the pelvis is probably the most important determinant of the posture and health of the spine.
- When the pelvis tilts, the sacrum tilts because it is a part of the bony pelvis. When the sacrum tilts, the base of the sacrum also tilts; this results in a sacral base that is angled relative to a horizontal line.
- This angulation of the sacral base relative to a horizontal line can be measured by the angle that is created between a line drawn along the top of the base of the sacrum and a horizontal line. This line is called the **sacral base angle**.[4]
- In effect, the sacral base angle is a measure of the degree of anterior tilt of the sacrum.
- Because the sacral base creates a base that the spinal column of vertebrae sits on, any change in the sacral base angle affects the posture of the spine.
- The relationship between the posture and movement of the pelvis and spine is often referred to as **lumbopelvic rhythm**.[6]
- One purpose of the spinal column is to bring the head to a level posture[7] (Box 9-7). If the sacral base were to be perfectly level, the spine could be totally straight and the head would be level. However, if the sacral base tilts, the spine must curve to bring the head to a level posture.

BOX 9-7

The head needs to be level so that the inner ear can function as a proprioceptive organ; having the head level also facilitates the sense of vision. The desire of the body to bring the head to a level posture is known as the **righting reflex**.

- A sacral base angle of approximately 30 degrees is considered to be normal, or what is often termed **pelvic neutral**.[7] (Note: there is controversy regarding the exact posture of pelvic neutral; however, a 30-degree sacral base angle is approximately correct.)
- A sacral base angle that is greater than 30 degrees results in increased spinal curvature; a sacral base angle that is less than 30 degrees results in decreased spinal curvature.[7] (Note: Of course, the spine does not have to compensate for a tilted sacral base [by curving] to bring the head to a level posture. The trunk can "go along for the ride" when the pelvis tilts.) (See Figure 9-7, *B*.) Figure 9-15 illustrates three different sacral base angles and the concomitant effect that these angles have on spinal posture.

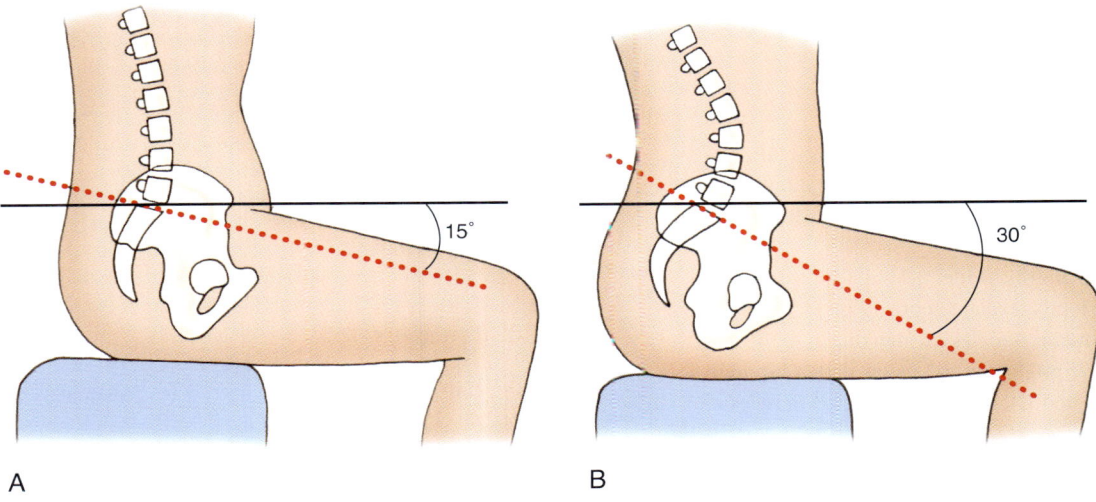
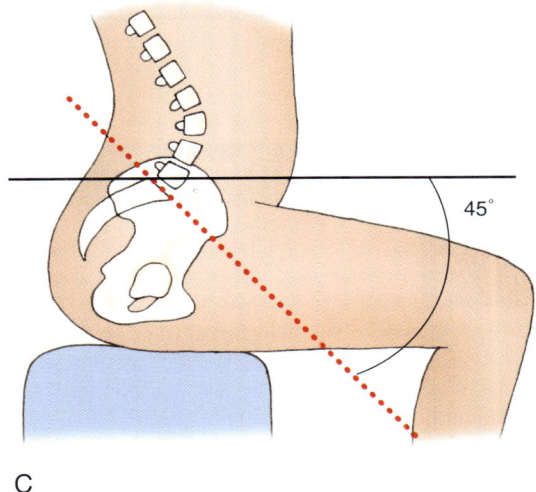

FIGURE 9-15 Effect on the spinal curve with changes in the sagittal plane tilt angle of the pelvis. When the pelvis tilts in the sagittal plane, it changes the orientation of the base of the sacrum relative to a horizontal line; a measure of this is called the sacral base angle. Because the spine sits on the sacrum, any change of the sacral base angle causes a change in the curvature of the spine if the head is to remain level. **A,** Sacral base angle of 15 degrees, which is less than normal. **B,** Normal sacral base angle of 30 degrees. **C,** Increased sacral base angle of 45 degrees. The corresponding changes in the curvature of the lumbar spine with changes in the sacral base angle should be noted.

SECTION 9.9 HIP JOINT

- The hip joint is also known as the **femoroacetabular joint**.
- Another name for the hip joint is the **coxofemoral joint** because it is between the coxal bone (the pelvic bone) and the femur.

BONES:

- The hip joint is located between the femur and the pelvic bone (Figure 9-16).
  - More specifically, it is located between the head of the femur and the acetabulum of the pelvic bone.
  - All three bones of the pelvic bone (the ilium, ischium, and pubis) contribute to the acetabulum.[4]

- The word *acetabulum* means *vinegar cup* (vinegar is *acetic* acid).
- Joint structure classification: Synovial joint
  - Subtype: Ball and socket
- Joint function classification: Diarthrotic[4]
  - Subtype: Triaxial
- Note: The socket of the hip joint (formed by the acetabulum of the pelvic bone) is very deep and provides excellent stability but relatively less mobility than a shallower socket such as the glenoid fossa of the shoulder joint.[4]

CHAPTER 9 Joints of the Lower Extremity

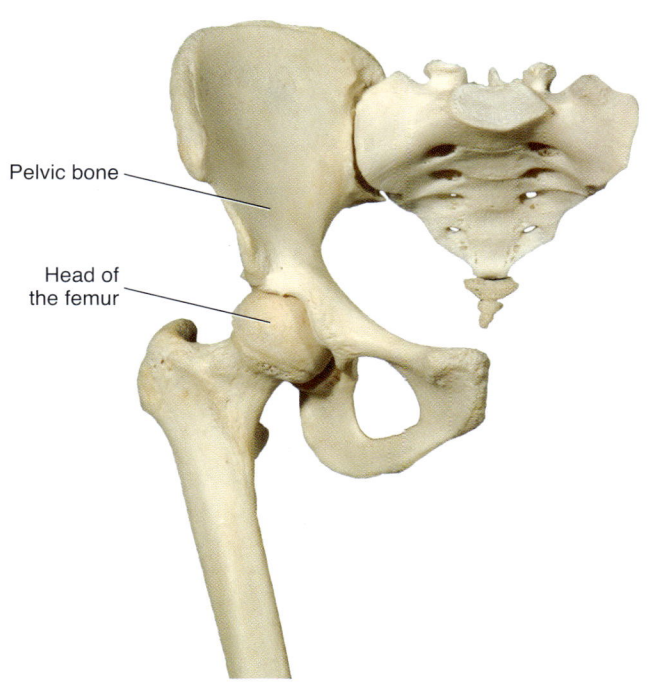

Anterior view

FIGURE 9-16 Anterior view of the right hip joint. The hip joint is a ball-and-socket joint that is formed by the head of the femur articulating with the acetabulum of the pelvic bone.

MAJOR MOTIONS ALLOWED[8]:

The average ranges of motion of the thigh at the hip joint are given in Table 9-2 (Figure 9-17). (For motions of the pelvis at the hip joint, see Section 9-4.)
- The hip joint allows flexion and extension (i.e., axial movements) within the sagittal plane around a mediolateral axis.
- The hip joint allows abduction and adduction (i.e., axial movements) within the frontal plane around an anteroposterior axis.
- The hip joint allows medial rotation and lateral rotation (i.e., axial movements) within the transverse plane around a vertical axis.

Reverse Actions:

- The muscles of the hip joint are generally considered to move the more distal thigh relative to a fixed pelvis. However, closed-chain activities are common in the lower extremity—activities in which the foot is planted on the ground; this fixes the foot/leg/thigh and requires that the pelvis moves instead. When this occurs, the pelvis can move at the hip joint instead of the thigh (Box 9-8).

- Note: Flexion and extension are measured with the knee joint extended; these ranges of motion would change with flexion of the knee joint because of the length change across the knee joint of multijoint muscles such as the hamstring group and the rectus femoris of the quadriceps femoris group.
- The reverse actions of the pelvis at the hip joint are anterior tilt and posterior tilt in the sagittal plane, depression and elevation in the frontal plane, and right rotation and left rotation in the transverse plane. These actions were covered in detail in Section 9.4, Figure 9-7.

MAJOR LIGAMENTS OF THE HIP JOINT (BOX 9-9):

Fibrous Joint Capsule:

- The capsule of the hip joint is strong and dense, providing excellent stability to the joint.
- The capsule contains strong circular deep fibers called the **zona orbicularis** that surround the neck of the femur.[8]

TABLE 9-2	Average Ranges of Motion of the Thigh at the Hip Joint[4]		
Flexion	90 Degrees	Extension	20 Degrees
Abduction	40 Degrees	Adduction	20 Degrees
Medial rotation	40 Degrees	Lateral rotation	50 Degrees

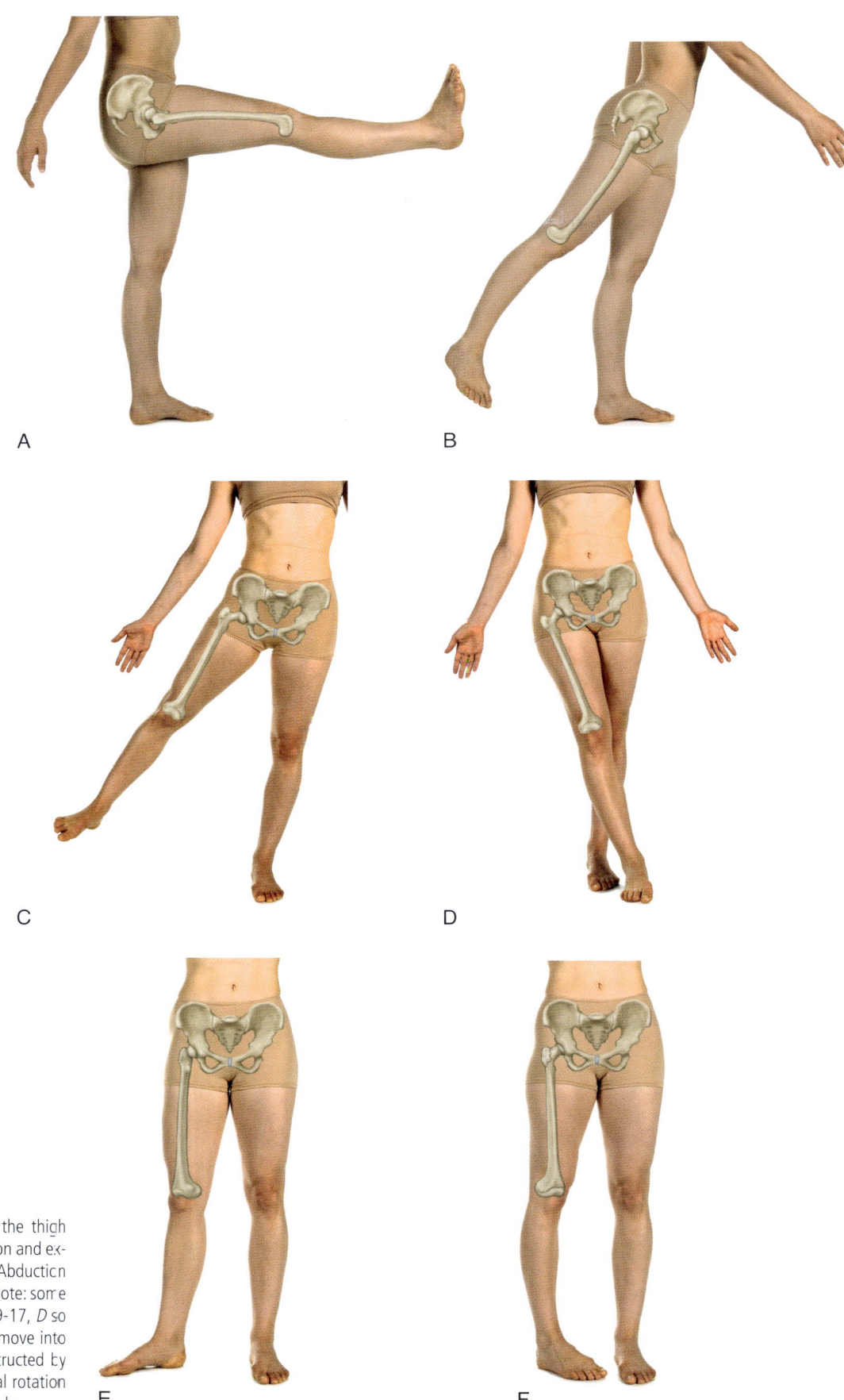

FIGURE 9-17 Motions of the thigh at the hip joint. **A** and **B,** Flexion and extension, respectively. **C** and **D,** Abduction and adduction, respectively. (Note: some flexion is also seen in Figure 9-17, *D* so that the right thigh is free to move into adduction without being obstructed by the left thigh.) **E** and **F,** Lateral rotation and medial rotation, respectively.

BOX 9-8 Spotlight on Open- and Closed-Chain Activities

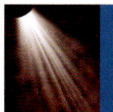

The term **open-chain activity** refers to an activity that is carried out in which the distal bone of a joint is free to move. The term **closed-chain activity** refers to an activity that is carried out in which the distal bone of a joint is fixed in some way, resulting in the proximal bone having to move when movement occurs at that joint. The most common example of a closed-chain activity is when the foot is planted on the ground and is thereby fixed; this results in the leg having to move at the ankle joint, the thigh having to move at the knee joint, and/or the pelvis having to move at the hip joint. Because muscle actions are usually thought of as moving the distal body part relative to the proximal one, these actions that occur with closed-chain activities may be termed reverse actions. Closed-chain activities are extremely common in the lower extremity. Although less common, a closed-chain activity may also occur in the upper extremity such as when the hand firmly grasps an immovable object; this results in the forearm moving at the wrist joint, the arm moving at the elbow joint, and/or the shoulder girdle moving at the glenohumeral joint. The terms *open chain* and *closed chain* refer to the idea of a chain of kinematic elements (bones/body parts, usually of the extremities) that are either open ended at their distal end (and therefore free to move distally) or not open ended (i.e., closed) at their distal end so that the distal end cannot move and the proximal end must move instead.

- The fibrous capsule of the hip joint is reinforced by three capsular ligaments, which are named based on their attachments: (1) the iliofemoral, (2) the ischiofemoral, and (3) the pubofemoral ligaments[8] (Figure 9-18).
- All three capsular ligaments of the hip joint are twisted as they pass from the pelvic bone to the femur (see Figure 9-18). This twisting reflects the medial rotation twisting that occurs to the shaft of the femur in utero.[4] The result of this femoral twisting is that the ventral (softer) surfaces of the distal thigh and leg come to face posteriorly instead of anteriorly as in the rest of the body. This also explains why flexion of the leg at the knee joint (and all movements that occur distal to the knee joint) is a posterior movement instead of an anterior movement.

BOX 9-9 Ligaments of the Hip Joint

- Fibrous joint capsule
- Iliofemoral ligament
- Ischiofemoral ligament
- Pubofemoral ligament
- Zona orbicularis
- Transverse acetabular ligament
- Ligamentum teres

Iliofemoral Ligament:
- The **iliofemoral ligament**[8] attaches from the ilium to the femur.
  - More specifically, it attaches from the anterior inferior iliac spine (AIIS) to the intertrochanteric line of the femur.
- Location: The iliofemoral ligament is a thickening of the anterosuperior capsule of the hip joint.
- Function
  - It limits extension of the thigh at the hip joint.
  - It limits posterior tilt of the pelvis at the hip joint.
- The iliofemoral ligament is also known as the **Y ligament** (because it is shaped like an upside-down letter Y) (Box 9-10).

BOX 9-10

The iliofemoral ligament is one of the thickest and strongest ligaments of the body. It is also a very important ligament posturally, because when someone stands with extension of the hip joint (whether the thigh is extended or the pelvis is posteriorly tilted), his or her body weight leans against the iliofemoral ligament.

Pubofemoral Ligament:
- The **pubofemoral ligament**[8] attaches from the pubis to the femur.
- Location: The pubofemoral ligament is a thickening of the anteroinferior capsule of the hip joint.
- Function
  - It limits abduction of the thigh at the hip joint.
  - It limits extreme extension of the thigh at the hip joint.
  - It limits depression (i.e., lateral tilt) of the pelvis at the ipsilateral hip joint.

Ischiofemoral Ligament:
- The **ischiofemoral ligament**[8] attaches from the ischium to the femur.
- Location: The ischiofemoral ligament is a thickening of the posterior capsule of the hip joint.
- Function
  - It limits medial rotation of the thigh at the hip joint.
  - It limits extension of the thigh at the hip joint.
  - It limits ipsilateral rotation of the pelvis at the hip joint.

Ligamentum Teres:
- Location: The **ligamentum teres**[8] is intra-articular, running from the internal surface of the acetabulum to the head of the femur.
- Function: The ligamentum teres does not substantially increase stability to the hip joint; its purpose is to provide a conduit for blood vessels and nerves to the femoral head.

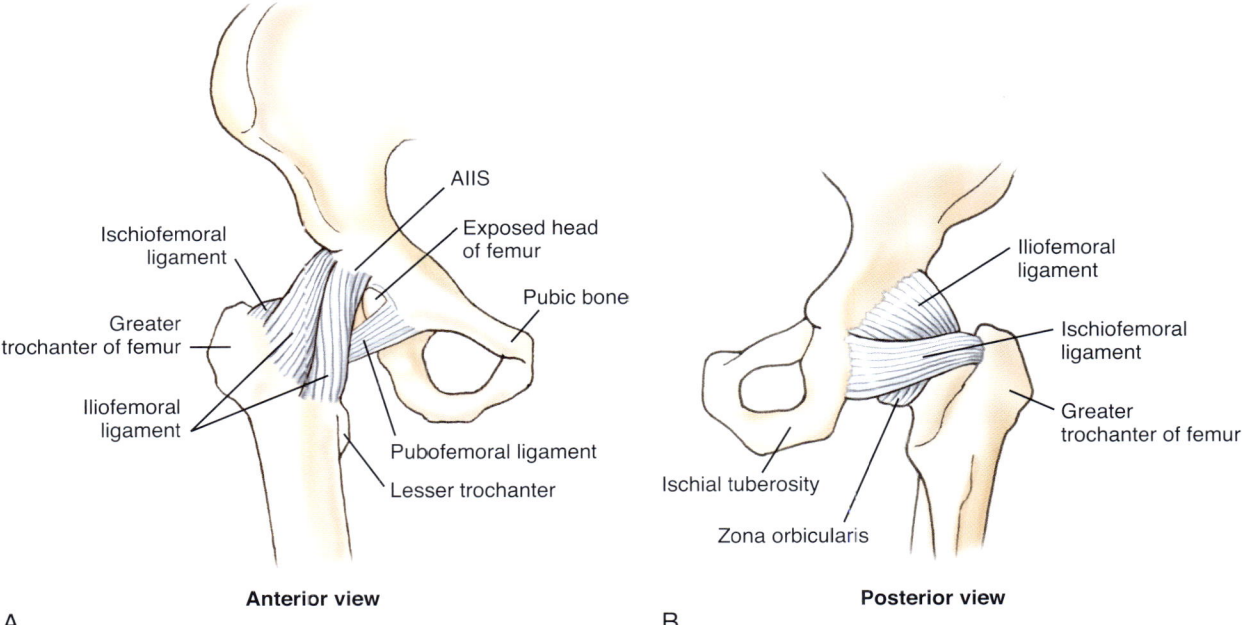
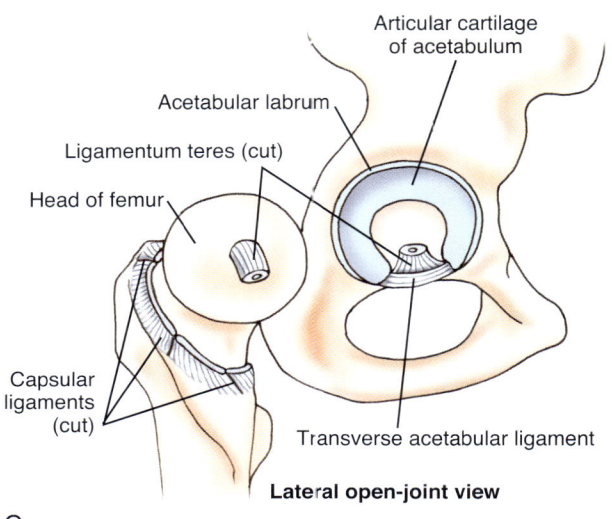

FIGURE 9-18 Ligaments of the hip joint. The major ligaments are capsular reinforcements called the iliofemoral, pubofemoral, and ischiofemoral ligaments. **A,** Anterior view of the hip joint ligaments. **B,** Posterior view. **C,** Right lateral view with the joint opened up to illustrate the ligamentum teres and transverse acetabular ligament.

CLOSED-PACKED POSITION OF THE HIP JOINT:

- Full extension[4]

MAJOR MUSCLES OF THE HIP JOINT:

- The hip joint is crossed by large muscle groups. Anteriorly, the major muscles are the iliopsoas, tensor fasciae latae, rectus femoris, sartorius, and the more anteriorly located hip joint adductors. Posteriorly are the gluteal muscles, as well as the hamstrings and the adductor magnus. Medially is the hip joint adductor group. Laterally are the gluteal muscles, tensor fasciae latae, and the sartorius. (For a detailed list of the muscles of the hip joint and their actions, see Chapter 11.) (Box 9-11)

 BOX 9-11

The relative balance of pull of musculature at the hip joint is likely the major factor in determining the posture of the pelvis, which is then the major factor in determining the posture of the spine. In the sagittal plane, it is common for the hip flexor group to become hypertonic (increase baseline tone) relative to the hip extensor group. Posturally, this plays out by anteriorly tilting the pelvis at the hip joint, thereby increasing the lumbar lordotic curve and increasing weight-bearing compression upon the lumbar facet joints. Similarly, imbalances in the frontal plane between hip joint abductors (ipsilateral pelvic depressors) and hip joint adductors (ipsilateral pelvis elevators) can affect the frontal plane posture of the pelvis, thereby possibly creating a compensatory scoliotic curve in the spine. And transverse plane imbalance of hip joint musculature can result in rotational postural distortions of the pelvis and spine. For more on postural distortions, see Chapter 21.

MISCELLANEOUS:

- The articular cartilage of the acetabulum is crescent-shaped and called the **lunate cartilage**[4] (see Figure 9-18, C).
- A fibrocartilaginous ring of tissue called the **acetabular labrum** surrounds the circumference of the acetabulum.[8]
  - The word *labrum* means *lip*; hence the acetabular labrum runs along the lip of the acetabulum.
- The acetabular labrum increases the depth of the socket of the hip joint, thereby increasing the stability of the hip joint.[4]
- The acetabular labrum does not quite form a complete ring; at the inferior margin of the acetabulum, its two ends are connected by the **transverse acetabular ligament**[8] (see Figure 9-18, C).

SECTION 9.10 ANGULATIONS OF THE FEMUR

- The femur is composed of several major components: the head, the neck, and the shaft.
- The relationship of these components is such that they are not arranged in a straight line. The angles that are measured between the head/neck and the shaft of the femur are called *femoral angulations*.
- Two femoral angulations exist[4]:
  - Femoral angle of inclination
  - Femoral torsion angle
- Note: Both the angle of inclination and the torsion angle are properties of the femur and are independent of the actual hip joint. However, abnormal angles of inclination and torsion can alter the functioning of the hip joint by creating compensations of the alignment of the bones at the hip joint and of the musculature of the hip joint.

FEMORAL ANGLE OF INCLINATION:

- The **femoral angle of inclination** is the angulation of the head/neck relative to the shaft within the frontal plane (Figure 9-19).
- The angle of inclination is normally approximately 125 degrees.[4]
- At birth the angle of inclination measures approximately 150 degrees. Because of the increased stresses of weight bearing as we age, it gradually decreases to the normal adult value of approximately 125 degrees.[4]
- An angle of inclination markedly less than 125 degrees is called a **coxa vara**.[1]
- An angle of inclination markedly greater than 125 degrees is called a **coxa valga**.[1]

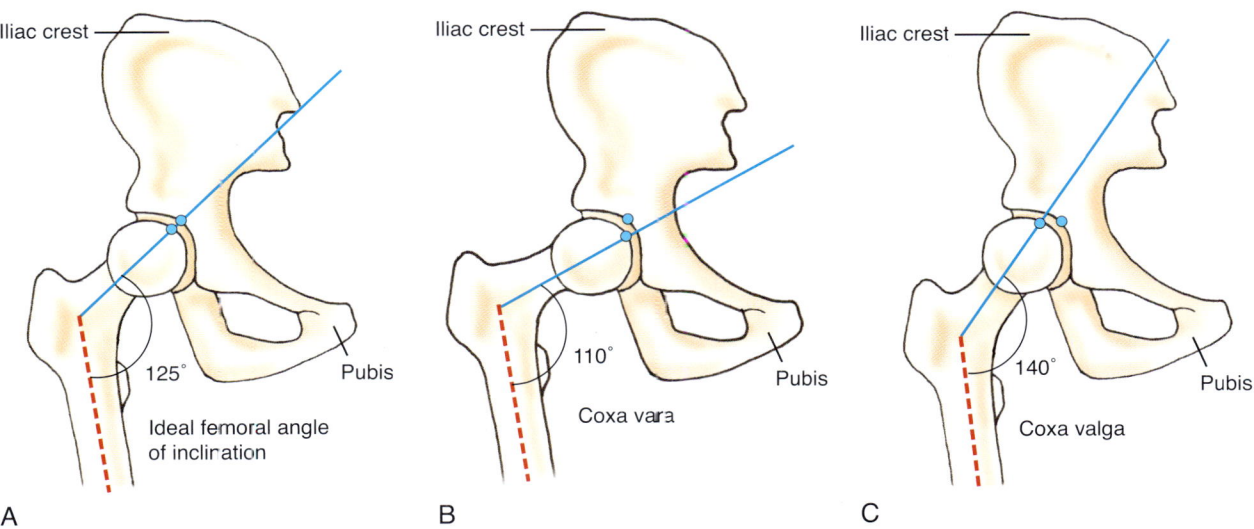

FIGURE 9-19 Various femoral angles of inclination. (Note: All views are anterior.) **A,** Angle of 125 degrees, which is considered to be normal. **B,** Decreased angle of inclination; this condition is known as coxa vara. **C,** Increased angle of inclination; this condition is known as coxa valga. The paired blue dots in each figure represent the alignment of the joint surfaces of the femoral head and acetabulum. Ideal alignment occurs at approximately 125 degrees, as seen in **A.**

- Note: The term *coxa* refers to the hip; the term *vara* means *turned inward*, and the term *valga* means *turned outward*.
  - Altered angles of inclination result in suboptimal alignment of the femoral head within the acetabulum. This can result in decreased shock absorption ability and increased degenerative (osteoarthritic) changes over time.[1]
  - A coxa valga results in a longer lower extremity; a coxa vara results in a shorter lower extremity.[1]

FEMORAL TORSION ANGLE:

- The **femoral torsion angle** is the angulation of the femoral head/neck relative to the shaft within the transverse plane[4] (Figure 9-20).
- The term **anteversion** (or *normal anteversion*) is used to refer to the femoral torsion angle.[1]
- This torsion angle represents the medial rotation of the femoral shaft that occurs embryologically[4] (Box 9-12).
- The femoral head and neck actually maintain their position while the shaft twists medially within the transverse plane. The result is a femoral shaft that is twisted medially relative to the head and neck of the femur.

BOX 9-12

An embryo begins with the limb buds (for the upper and lower extremities) pointed straight laterally. By 2 months of age, the upper and lower limb buds of the embryo adduct (i.e., point more anteriorly). However, the upper limb buds also laterally rotate, bringing the ventral surface of the upper extremities to face anteriorly; whereas the lower limb buds medially rotate, bringing the ventral surface of the lower extremities to face posteriorly. This is the reason why flexion within the lower extremity is a posterior movement from the knee joint and farther distally instead of an anterior movement as in the upper extremity.

- As noted in Section 9.9, this torsion of the femoral shaft is apparent when looking at the twisted orientation of the fibers of the ligaments of the hip joint (see Figure 9-18, *A* and *B*).
- The torsion angle is normally approximately 15 degrees.[4]
- Note: The femoral anteversion angle is a measure of the twisting of the femoral shaft that occurs within the transverse plane. Its angle is a measure of the deviation of the head and neck of the femur away from the frontal plane (see Figure 9-20).

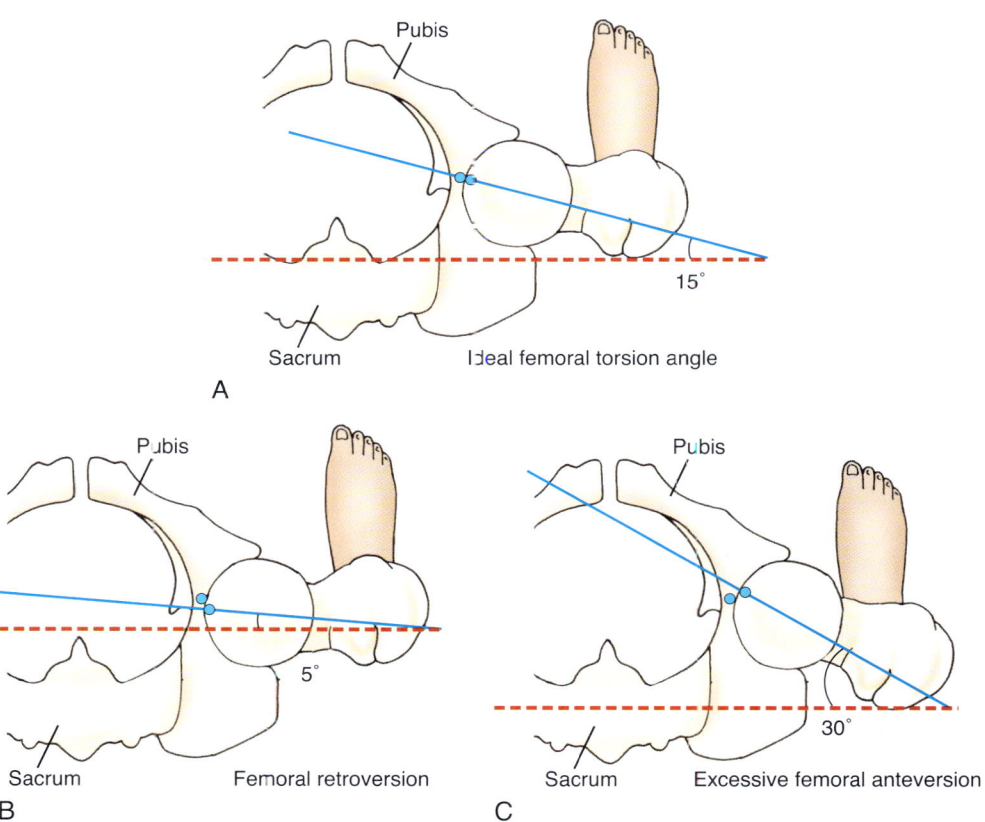

FIGURE 9-20 Various femoral torsion angles. (Note: All views are superior.) **A,** Angle of 15 degrees, which is considered to be normal. **B,** Decreased torsion angle; this condition is known as retroversion. **C,** Increased torsion angle; this condition is known as excessive anteversion. The paired blue dots in each figure represent the alignment of the joint surfaces of the femoral head and acetabulum. Ideal alignment occurs at approximately 15 degrees, as seen in **A.** To achieve optimal alignment in **B,** in which retroversion exists, a toe-out position would occur; to achieve optimal alignment in **C,** in which excessive anteversion exists, a toe-in position would occur. *(Modeled from Neumann DA: Kinesiology of the musculoskeletal system: foundations for physical rehabilitation, ed 2, St Louis, 2010, Mosby.)*

- A torsion angle markedly less than 15 degrees is called **retroversion**.[4]
- A torsion angle markedly greater than 15 degrees is called *excessive anteversion*.
  - Femoral retroversion can result in a **toe-out posture**. Toe-out posture is actually lateral rotation of the thigh at the hip joint and is a compensation to try to optimally line up the articular surfaces of the femur and acetabulum[1] (achieved by lining up the two blue dots in Figure 9-20, *B*).
  - Excessive femoral anteversion can result in a **toe-in posture**, also known as **pigeon toes**. Toe-in posture is actually medial rotation of the thigh at the hip joint and is a compensation to optimally line up the articular surfaces of the joint[1] (achieved by lining up the two blue dots in Figure 9-20, *C*).
- An altered femoral torsion angle that is uncompensated will result in suboptimal alignment of the femoral head within the acetabulum. This can result in decreased shock absorption ability and increased degenerative (osteoarthritic) changes over time.
  - Toe-in postures are very common in young children, because the femoral torsion angle is higher at birth and gradually decreases through childhood[4] (Box 9-13).

BOX 9-13

At birth the femoral torsion angle measures approximately 30 to 40 degrees. Usually by 6 years of age the torsion angle decreases to the normal adult value of 15 degrees. Because in-toeing is a common compensation for excessive femoral torsion, this postural pattern is common among children. In-toeing is usually outgrown; however, it may be retained throughout adulthood if contractures in the medial rotator muscles and adhesions in certain ligaments develop.

SECTION 9.11   FEMOROPELVIC RHYTHM

- There tends to be a rhythm to how the femur of the thigh and the pelvis move. This coordination of movement between these two body parts is often referred to as **femoropelvic rhythm**.[9]
- Femoropelvic rhythm is an example of the concept of a **coupled action** wherein two different joint actions tend to be *coupled together*[6] (i.e., if one action occurs, the other one tends to also occur).
  - Note: Coupled actions are common between the thigh and pelvis. Coupled actions also occur between the arm and the shoulder girdle (see Section 10.6). The concept of coupled actions is covered in Section 15.12.
- When the femur is moved, it is often for the purpose of raising the foot up into the air. Given the limitation of the range of motion of the thigh at the hip joint, movement of the pelvis is often created in conjunction with thigh movement to increase the ability of the foot to rise into the air.
  - For example, if a person flexes the right thigh at the hip joint for the purpose of kicking a ball, the actual range of motion of the right thigh at the hip joint is approximately 90 degrees. This is not sufficient for a strong follow-through to the kick. Therefore the pelvis is posteriorly tilted on the left thigh at the left hip joint (the *support limb* side) to increase the range of motion of the kick (Figure 9-21, *A*).

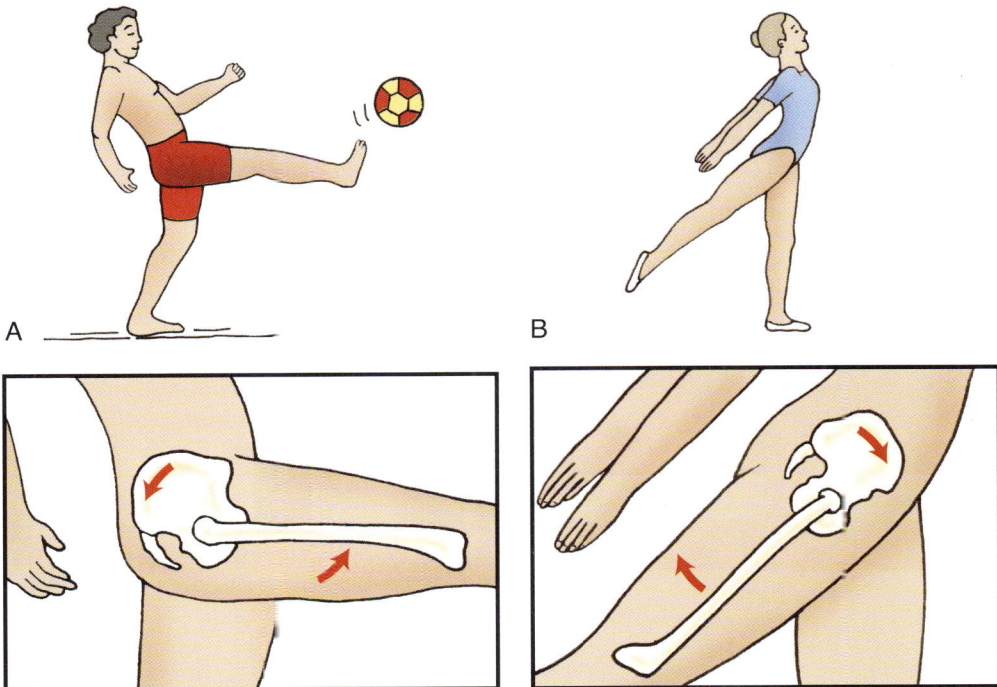

FIGURE 9-21 Concept of coupled thigh/pelvic actions, known as femoropelvic rhythm, in the sagittal plane. **A,** Soccer player who is kicking a soccer ball with his right foot. He accomplishes this by flexing his right thigh at the right hip joint and posteriorly tilting his pelvis at the left (i.e., contralateral) hip joint. These two actions couple together to enable the player to raise his right foot higher in the air. **B,** Ballet dancer who is bringing her right lower extremity up into the air behind her. She accomplishes this by extending her right thigh at her right hip joint and anteriorly tilting her pelvis at her left (i.e., contralateral) hip joint.

- Note: With femoropelvic rhythm, the nervous system is coordinating two entirely different joint actions to occur together. One joint action is of the thigh at the hip joint; the other joint action is of the pelvis at the other hip joint. These separate actions are coupled together for the larger purpose of raising the foot higher into the air.

The following are common coupled actions that occur between the thigh and the pelvis[3]:
- Thigh flexion at the hip joint is coupled with pelvic posterior tilt at the contralateral (opposite-sided [i.e., the other]) hip joint.
- Thigh extension at the hip joint is coupled with pelvic anterior tilt at the contralateral hip joint (Figure 9-21, B).
- Thigh abduction at the hip joint is coupled with pelvic depression at the contralateral hip joint.
- Thigh adduction at the hip joint is coupled with pelvic elevation at the contralateral hip joint.
- Thigh lateral rotation at the hip joint is coupled with pelvic contralateral rotation at the contralateral hip joint.
- Thigh medial rotation at the hip joint is coupled with pelvic ipsilateral rotation at the contralateral hip joint.

SECTION 9.12   OVERVIEW OF THE KNEE JOINT COMPLEX

- The knee joint is actually a joint complex, because more than one articulation exists within the joint capsule of the knee joint (Figure 9-22).
- The primary articulation at the knee joint is between the tibia and the femur.
  - This joint is known as the *tibiofemoral joint*.
- The patella also articulates with the femur within the capsule of the knee joint (see Figure 9-25 in Section 9.14).
  - This joint is known as the *patellofemoral joint*.
- The proximal tibiofibular joint between the lateral condyle of the tibia and the head of the fibula is not within the capsule of the knee joint, and the proximal tibiofibular joint is not very functionally related to the knee joint.[6]
- Generally when the context is not made otherwise clear, the knee joint is considered to be the tibiofemoral joint.

BONES:

- The **tibiofemoral joint** is located between the femur and the tibia.
  - More specifically, it is located between the medial and lateral condyles of the femur and the plateau of the tibia.
  - Because each condyle of the femur articulates separately with the tibia,[1] some sources consider the tibiofemoral joint to be two joints: (1) the medial tibiofemoral joint and (2) the lateral tibiofemoral joint.
- The **patellofemoral joint** is located between the patella and the femur.
  - More specifically, it is located between the posterior surface of the patella and the intercondylar groove of the distal femur.[4]

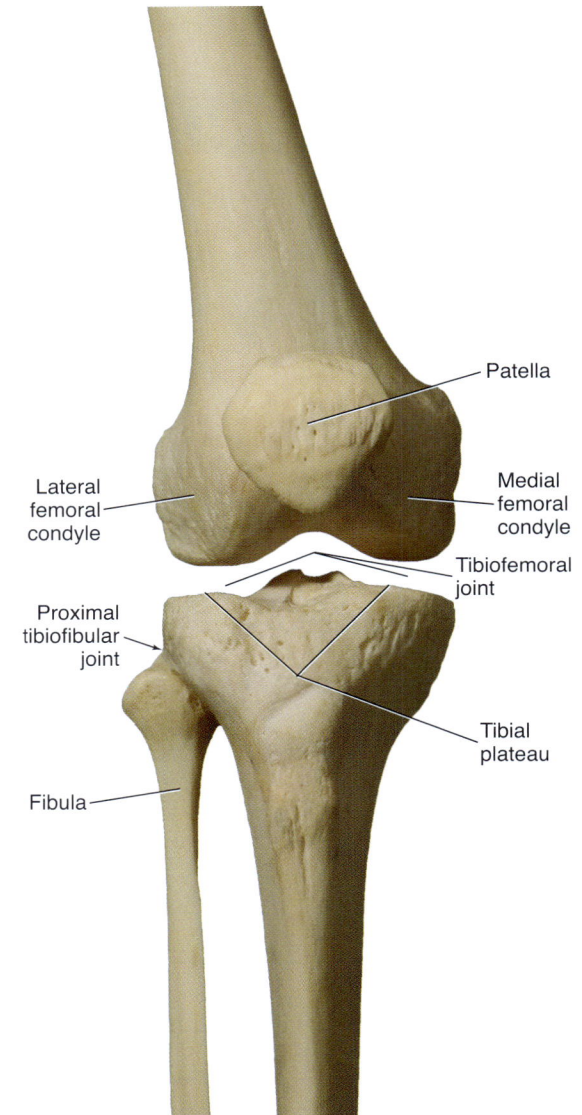

FIGURE 9-22 Anterior view of the right knee joint. The knee joint is actually a joint complex containing the tibiofemoral joint and the patellofemoral joint.

SECTION 9.13 TIBIOFEMORAL (KNEE) JOINT

BONES:

- The tibiofemoral joint is located between the femur and the tibia.
  - More specifically, it is located between the two femoral condyles and the plateau of the tibia.
- The tibiofemoral joint is located within the capsule of the knee joint along with the patellofemoral joint.
- Because each condyle of the femur articulates separately with the tibia, some sources consider the tibiofemoral joint to be two joints, the medial tibiofemoral joint and the lateral tibiofemoral joint.
- Generally when the context is not made otherwise clear, the term *knee joint* refers to the tibiofemoral joint.

TIBIOFEMORAL JOINT:

- Joint structure classification: Synovial joint
  - Subtype: Modified hinge joint
- Joint function classification: Diarthrotic
  - Subtype: Biaxial[10]
  - Note: Some sources classify the tibiofemoral joint as a double condyloid joint, with the medial condyle of the femur meeting the tibia as one condyloid joint, and the lateral condyle of the femur meeting the tibia as the other condyloid joint.

MAJOR MOTIONS ALLOWED:

Average ranges of motion of the leg at the knee joint are given in Table 9-3 (Figure 9-23).[4]

- The tibiofemoral joint allows flexion and extension (i.e., axial movements) within the sagittal plane around a mediolateral axis.
- The tibiofemoral joint allows medial rotation and lateral rotation (i.e., axial movements) within the transverse plane around a vertical axis.
  - Medial and lateral rotation of the tibiofemoral joint can occur only if the tibiofemoral joint is in a position of flexion. A fully extended tibiofemoral joint cannot rotate freely; approximately 30 degrees of knee joint flexion are needed to allow rotation (Box 9-14).

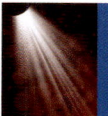

BOX 9-14 Spotlight on Tibiofemoral Joint Rotation

Rotation of the tibiofemoral (i.e., knee) joint must be carefully described. The leg can rotate when the thigh is fixed, and the thigh can rotate when the leg is fixed. Understanding and naming these reverse actions of rotation of the tibiofemoral joint is important. Medial rotation of the leg at the tibiofemoral joint is equivalent to lateral rotation of the thigh at the tibiofemoral joint. Similarly, lateral rotation of the leg at the tibiofemoral joint is equivalent to medial rotation of the thigh at the tibiofemoral joint!

Reverse Actions:

- The muscles of the tibiofemoral joint are generally considered to move the more distal leg on the more proximal thigh. However, closed-chain activities are common in the lower extremity in which the foot is planted on the ground; this fixes the leg and requires that the thigh move instead. When this occurs, the thigh moves at the tibiofemoral joint instead of the leg moving.[3]
- The thigh can flex and extend in the sagittal plane at the tibiofemoral joint.
- The thigh can medially rotate and laterally rotate in the transverse plane at the tibiofemoral joint.

LIGAMENTS OF THE TIBIOFEMORAL JOINT:

- Given the large forces that are transmitted to the tibiofemoral joint, along with the weight-bearing function and the relative lack of bony stability provided by the shape of the bones, the ligaments of the tibiofemoral joint play an important role in providing stability and consequently are often injured (Figure 9-24).

Fibrous Joint Capsule:

- The capsule of the tibiofemoral joint extends from the distal femur to the proximal tibia and includes the patella. The proximal tibiofibular joint is not included within the capsule of the knee joint.

TABLE 9-3	Average Ranges of Motion of the Leg at the Tibiofemoral (i.e., Knee) Joint[4]		
Flexion	140 Degrees	(Hyper)extension	5 Degrees
Medial rotation	15 Degrees	Lateral rotation	30 Degrees

Notes: Rotation measurements are done with the tibiofemoral joint in 90 degrees of flexion. Extension is expressed as (hyper)extension because the tibiofemoral joint is fully extended in anatomic position; any further extension is considered to be hyperextension.

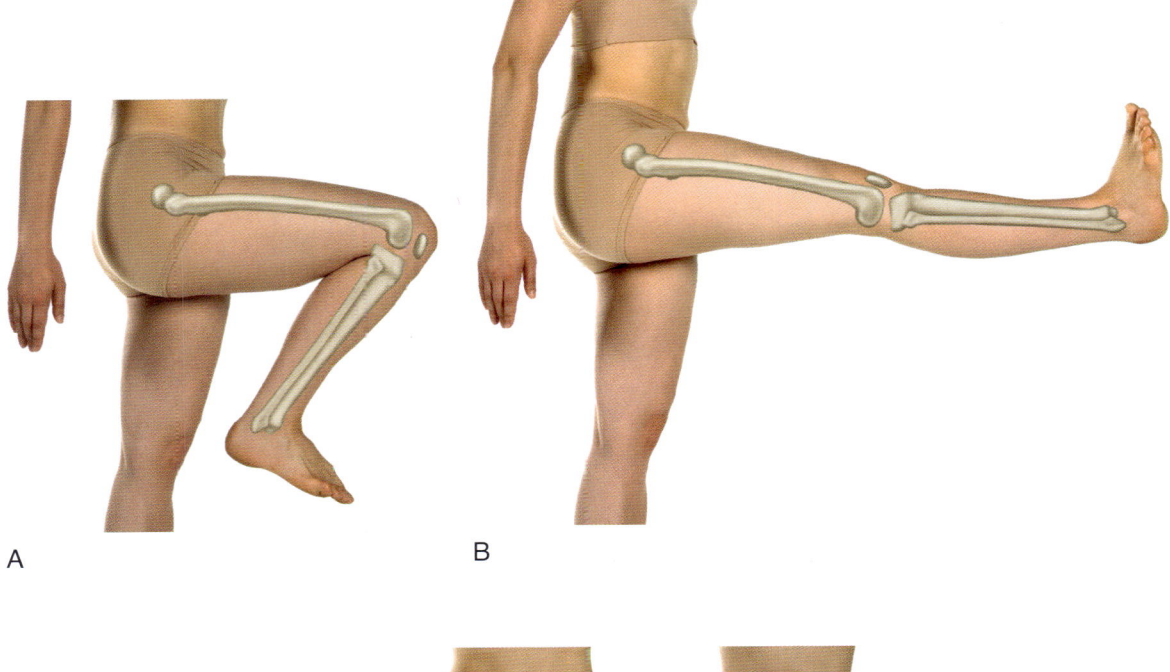
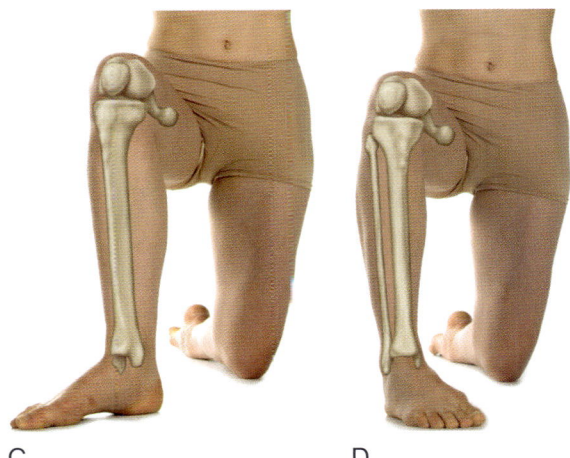

FIGURE 9-23 Motions possible at the tibiofemoral (i.e., knee) joint. **A** and **B**, Flexion and extension of the leg at the knee joint, respectively. **C** and **D**, Lateral and medial rotation of the leg at the knee joint, respectively. (Note: The knee joint can rotate only if it is first flexed.)

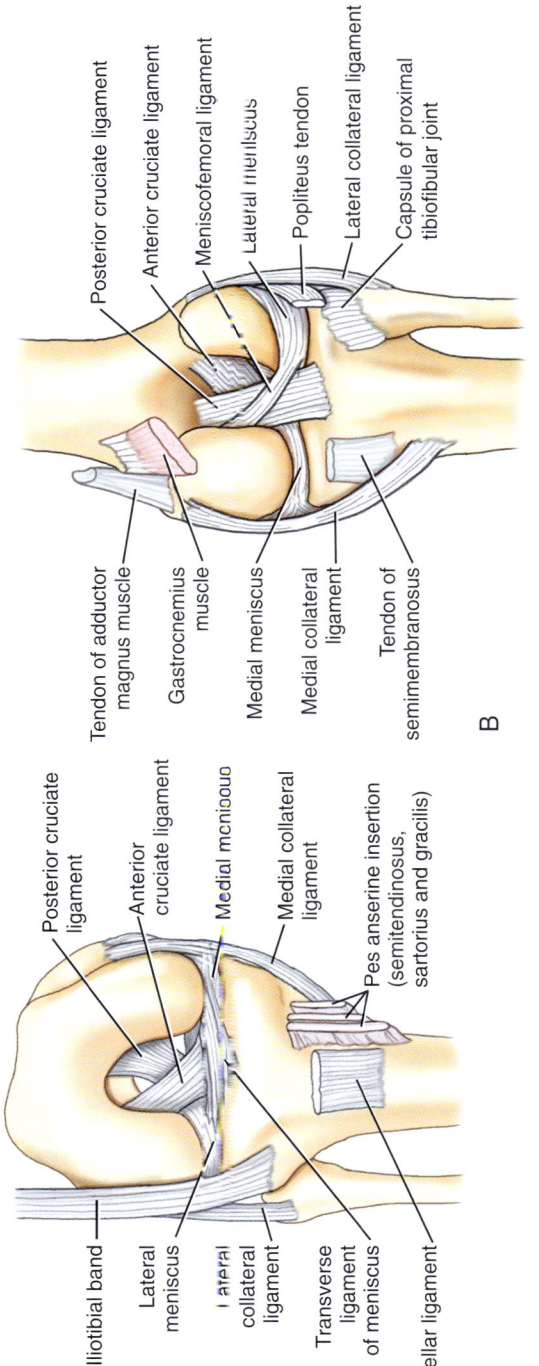
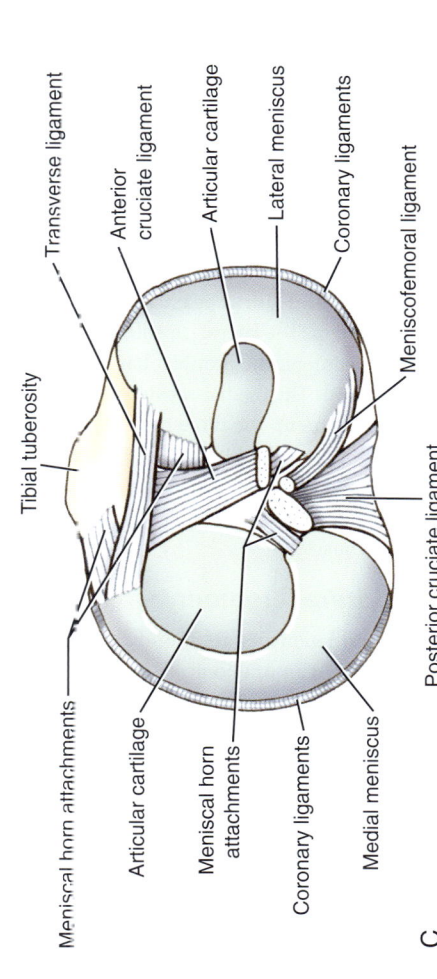

FIGURE 9-24 Ligaments of the tibiofemoral (i.e., knee) joint. **A,** Anterior view of the ligaments of the tibiofemoral joint in flexion. **B,** Posterior view of the ligaments of the tibiofemoral joint. **C,** Proximal (superior) view of the tibia, demonstrating the menisci and ligaments of the tibiofemoral joint.

BOX 9-15

The iliotibial band (ITB, also know as the iliotibial tract) is a fibrous fascial sheath, which as its name implies, runs from the ilium of the pelvic bone to the tibia. It runs from the iliac crest down the lateral side of the thigh, attaching into the proximal anterolateral tibia. In so doing, it crosses and stabilizes the hip and knee joints. Because the gluteus maximus and tensor fasciae latae attach distally into the ITB, it also functions as the distal tendon of these two muscles. Interestingly, the ITB has also been found to store elastic energy, acting like a large elastic band, to contribute to the force needed when running and walking. When the thigh moves back into extension, the ITB stretches and stores elastic energy; this elastic energy is then released when the thigh moves forward into flexion. In this manner, the ITB can be viewed as "recycling energy" to increase our efficiency and power when running. This seems to be an evolutionary adaption in humans in that the elastic rebound of the ITB is approximately 15–20 times greater than in the much-less-developed precursor structure in the chimpanzee.

- ○ The capsule of the tibiofemoral joint is somewhat lax, but it is reinforced by many ligaments, muscles, and fascia.
- ○ Specifically, the anterior capsule of the tibiofemoral joint is reinforced by the distal quadriceps femoris tendon, patella, infrapatellar ligament, and expansions of the quadriceps muscles called medial and lateral **retinacular fibers**. The lateral capsule is reinforced by the lateral collateral ligament, the iliotibial band, and lateral retinacular fibers (Box 9-15). The medial capsule is reinforced by the medial collateral ligament, the three pes anserine muscle tendons, and the medial retinacular fibers. The posterior capsule is reinforced by the oblique popliteal ligament, the arcuate popliteal ligament, and fibrous expansions of the popliteus, gastrocnemius, and hamstring muscles.[4]

Medial and Lateral Collateral Ligaments:

- ○ The medial and lateral collateral ligaments are found on both sides (*lateral* means *side*) of the tibiofemoral joint.
- ○ The two collateral ligaments are primarily important for limiting frontal plane movements of the bones of the tibiofemoral joint (Box 9-16).

BOX 9-16

- ○ Abduction of the leg at the tibiofemoral joint is defined as a lateral deviation of the leg in the frontal plane; it is not a movement that a healthy tibiofemoral joint allows. A forceful impact from the lateral side, such as "clipping" in football, could abduct the leg and rupture the medial collateral ligament; this is why clipping is not allowed. The postural condition wherein the tibiofemoral joint is abducted is called genu valgum.
- ○ Adduction of the leg at the tibiofemoral joint is defined as a medial deviation of the leg in the frontal plane; like abduction of the leg, it is not a movement that a healthy tibiofemoral joint allows. A forceful impact from the medial side of the joint would have to occur for the lateral collateral ligament to be injured. Because being hit from the medial side is less likely than being hit from the lateral side, the lateral collateral ligament is injured less often than the medial collateral ligament. The postural condition wherein the tibiofemoral joint is adducted is called genu varum. (See Section 9-15 for more information.)

Medial Collateral Ligament:
- ○ The medial collateral ligament attaches from the femur to the tibia.
  - ○ More specifically, it attaches from the medial epicondyle of the femur to the medial proximal tibia.[8]
- ○ The medial collateral ligament is also known as the **tibial collateral ligament**.
- ○ Function: It limits abduction of the leg at the tibiofemoral joint within the frontal plane.

Lateral Collateral Ligament:
- ○ The lateral collateral ligament attaches from the femur to the fibula.
  - ○ More specifically, it attaches from the lateral epicondyle of the femur to the head of the fibula.[8]
- ○ The lateral collateral ligament is also known as the **fibular collateral ligament**.
- ○ Function: It limits adduction of the leg at the tibiofemoral joint (within the frontal plane).

Anterior and Posterior Cruciate Ligaments:

- ○ The anterior and posterior cruciate ligaments cross each other (*cruciate* means *cross*). They are named for their tibial attachment.
- ○ The two cruciate ligaments are primarily important for limiting sagittal plane translation movement of the bones of the tibiofemoral joint (Box 9-17).[6]
- ○ The majority of the anterior and posterior cruciate ligaments are located between the fibrous and synovial layers of the tibiofemoral joint capsule. For this reason, they are considered to be intra-articular, yet *extrasynovial*.[8]
- ○ Together, given the various fibers of the two cruciate ligaments, they are considered able to resist the extremes of every motion at the tibiofemoral joint.

Anterior Cruciate Ligament:
- ○ The **anterior cruciate ligament** attaches from the anterior tibia to the posterior femur (see Figure 9-24).
  - ○ More specifically, it attaches from the anterior tibia to the posterolateral femur, running from the anterior intercondylar region of the tibia to the medial aspect of the lateral condyle of the femur.
- ○ Function: It limits anterior translation of the leg relative to the thigh when the thigh is fixed. It also limits the reverse action of posterior translation of the thigh relative to the leg when the leg is fixed.
- ○ The anterior cruciate ligament becomes taut at the end range of extension of the tibiofemoral joint. Therefore this ligament limits hyperextension of the tibiofemoral joint.
- ○ The anterior cruciate ligament also limits medial rotation of the leg at the tibiofemoral joint (and the reverse action of lateral rotation of the thigh at the tibiofemoral joint).
- ○ Many sources state that the anterior cruciate also limits lateral rotation of the leg at the tibiofemoral joint (and the reverse action of medial rotation of the thigh at the tibiofemoral joint) (Box 9-18).

Posterior Cruciate Ligament:
- ○ The **posterior cruciate ligament** attaches from the posterior tibia to the anterior femur (see Figure 9-24).
  - ○ More specifically, it attaches from the posterior tibia to the anteromedial femur, running from the posterior intercondylar region of the tibia to the lateral aspect of the medial condyle of the femur.
- ○ Function: It limits posterior translation of the leg relative to the thigh when the thigh is fixed. It also limits the reverse action of

BOX 9-17

Anterior and posterior translations of the tibia and femur at the tibiofemoral joint are gliding movements that occur within the sagittal plane. These movements can be assessed by anterior and posterior drawer tests.

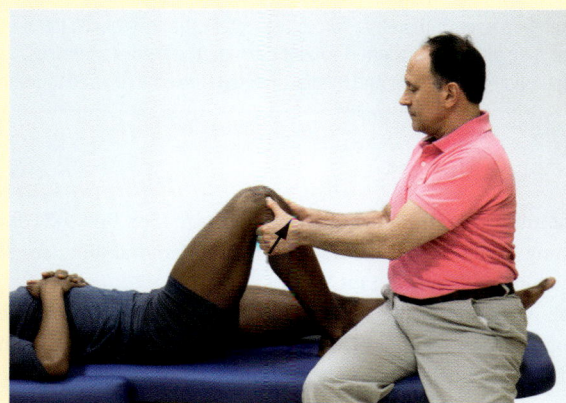

Anterior drawer test

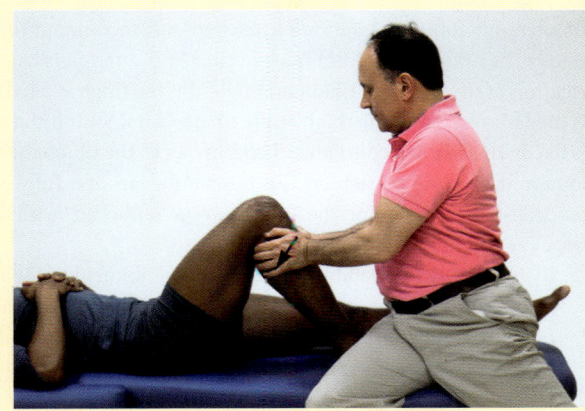

Posterior drawer test

Courtesy of Joseph E. Muscolino.

anterior translation of the thigh relative to the leg when the leg is fixed.
- The posterior cruciate ligament also becomes taut at the extreme end range of flexion of the tibiofemoral joint.

Other Ligaments of the Knee Joint:

Oblique Popliteal Ligament:
- Location: Posterior tibiofemoral joint (not seen in Figure 9-24)
  - More specifically, the **oblique popliteal ligament** attaches proximally from the lateral femoral condyle and distally into fibers of the distal tendon of the semimembranosus muscle.[4]
- Function: It reinforces the posterior capsule of the tibiofemoral joint and resists full extension of the tibiofemoral joint.

Arcuate Popliteal Ligament:
- Location: Posterior tibiofemoral joint (not seen in Figure 9-24)
  - More specifically, the **arcuate popliteal ligament** attaches distally from the fibular head and proximally into the posterior intercondylar region of the tibia and occasionally into the posterior side of the lateral femoral condyle.[6]
- Function: It reinforces the posterior capsule of the tibiofemoral joint and resists full extension of the tibiofemoral joint.

Patellar Ligament:
- Location: The **patellar ligament** is located between the patella and the tibial tuberosity[1] (see Figure 9-24).
- This ligament is actually part of the distal tendon of the quadriceps femoris group.[4]
- The patellar ligament is also known as the *infrapatellar ligament.*

Ligaments of the Menisci of the Tibiofemoral Joint:
- These ligaments stabilize the medial and lateral menisci by attaching them to adjacent structures.
- **Meniscal horn attachments**: The four horns of the two menisci are attached to the tibia via ligamentous attachments.[8]
- **Coronary ligaments**: They attach the periphery of each meniscus to the tibial condyle. These ligaments are also known as the *meniscotibial ligaments.*[4]
- **Transverse ligament**: It attaches the anterior aspects (i.e., horns) of the two menisci to each other.[8]
- **Posterior meniscofemoral ligament**: It attaches the lateral meniscus to the femur posteriorly.[4]

BOX 9-18

The anterior cruciate ligament is the most commonly injured ligament of the tibiofemoral joint. It can be injured in a number of ways. Certainly, any force that anteriorly translates the tibia relative to the femur, or posteriorly translates the femur relative to the tibia, could tear or rupture the anterior cruciate. Hyperextension of the tibiofemoral joint can also tear the anterior cruciate because tibiofemoral joint extension involves an anterior glide of the tibia and/or posterior glide of the femur at the tibiofemoral joint. Strong rotation forces to the tibiofemoral joint (especially medial rotation of the tibia or lateral rotation of the femur) can also tear the anterior cruciate ligament. "Cutting" in sports (a combination of forceful extension and rotation with the foot planted when changing direction while running) is often implicated in anterior cruciate tears because of the forceful rotation necessary.

BOX 9-19   Ligaments of the Knee Joint

- Fibrous joint capsule
- Medial (tibial) collateral ligament
- Lateral (fibular) collateral ligament
- Anterior cruciate ligament
- Posterior cruciate ligament
- Oblique popliteal ligament
- Arcuate popliteal ligament
- Patellar ligament
- Meniscal horn attachments
- Coronary ligaments
- Transverse ligament
- Posterior meniscofemoral ligament

CLOSED-PACKED POSITION OF THE TIBIOFEMORAL JOINT:

- Full extension[11]

MAJOR MUSCLES OF THE TIBIOFEMORAL JOINT:

- The tibiofemoral joint is crossed by large muscle groups. Anteriorly, the major muscles are the muscles of the quadriceps femoris group; the quadriceps femoris are extensors of the tibiofemoral joint. The gluteus maximus and tensor fasciae latae may also contribute slightly to extension of the tibiofemoral joint via their attachments into the iliotibial band. Posteriorly, the major muscle group is the hamstring group; the two heads of the gastrocnemius are also located posteriorly. These muscles are flexors of the tibiofemoral joint. No muscles move the tibiofemoral joint medially in the frontal plane; however, the three pes anserine muscles (sartorius, gracilis, semitendinosus) help to stabilize the medial side of the tibiofemoral joint. No muscles move the tibiofemoral joint laterally in the frontal plane either; however, the presence of the iliotibial band (which the gluteus maximus and tensor fasciae latae attach into) helps to stabilize the lateral side of the tibiofemoral joint.

MENISCI:

- The tibiofemoral joint has two menisci: (1) a **medial meniscus** and (2) a **lateral meniscus** (see Figure 9-24, C).
  - The menisci are located within the joint (i.e., intra-articular) on the tibia.[4]
  - They are fibrocartilaginous in structure.[4]
  - The menisci are crescent shaped.
  - The open ends of the menisci are called *horns*.
  - Note: The word *meniscus* is Greek for *crescent*.
  - The medial meniscus is shaped like a letter C; the shape of the lateral meniscus is closer to the letter O.[3]
  - The menisci are thicker peripherally and thinner centrally.[3]
  - The menisci help to increase the congruency of the tibiofemoral joint by transforming the flat tibial plateau into two shallow sockets in which the femoral condyles sit. In this manner, they increase stability of the tibiofemoral joint.[12]
  - The menisci also aid in cushioning and shock absorption of the tibiofemoral joint.[4]
  - The two menisci of the tibiofemoral joint absorb approximately half the weight-bearing force through the tibiofemoral joint.[6]
  - Meniscal attachments: The menisci are attached to the tibia at their horns; they are also attached to the tibia along their periphery via coronary ligaments. The transverse ligament attaches the anterior horns of the two menisci to each other. The posterior meniscofemoral ligament attaches the lateral meniscus to the femur.
  - The medial meniscus is more firmly attached to adjacent structures than is the lateral meniscus[3] (Box 9-20).
- Note: The menisci do not have a strong arterial blood supply; therefore they do not heal well after being injured.[6]

BOX 9-20

Because the medial meniscus is more firmly attached to adjacent structures, it has less ability to move freely. This decreased mobility is one reason why the medial meniscus is injured more frequently than the lateral meniscus. The medial meniscus is also attached into the medial collateral ligament (whereas the lateral meniscus is not attached into the lateral collateral ligament); therefore forces that stress the medial collateral ligament may also be transferred to and damage the medial meniscus. The medial collateral ligament and medial meniscus are often injured together.

MISCELLANEOUS:

- The tibiofemoral joint has many bursae.[12] (See Box 9-21 for a listing of the common bursae of the tibiofemoral joint; see also Section 7.9, Figure 7-11, C.)
- Full extension of the knee joint, unlike the elbow joint, is not stopped by a locking of the bones. Full extension of the knee joint is stopped only by the tension of soft tissues[6] (primarily those located in the posterior knee joint region).
- The term **screw-home mechanism** describes the fact that during the last 30 degrees of tibiofemoral joint extension (i.e., when the tibiofemoral joint goes into full extension), a concomitant rotation of the tibiofemoral joint must occur.[6] This rotation is lateral rotation of the leg at the tibiofemoral joint if the thigh is fixed. It is medial rotation of the thigh at the tibiofemoral joint if the leg is fixed. This associated rotation helps to "lock" the tibiofemoral joint and increase its stability. To initiate flexion of a fully extended tibiofemoral joint, the joint must be "unlocked" with the opposite rotation motion (Box 9-22).
  - By increasing the stability of the extended tibiofemoral joint, the screw-home mechanism decreases the work of the quadriceps femoris muscle group. When the knee joints are fully extended, the quadriceps femoris groups can *shut off*—in other words, they can relax. No contraction of the quadriceps femoris group is necessary to maintain a standing posture once the knee joints have fully extended.

BOX 9-21 Major Bursae of the Tibiofemoral Joint

- Suprapatellar bursa (actually part of the joint capsule)
- Prepatellar bursa
- Deep infrapatellar bursa
- Subcutaneous infrapatellar bursa
  Bursae are also present between the following:
- Biceps femoris tendon and the fibular collateral ligament (biceps femoris bursa)
- Fibular collateral ligament and the joint capsule (fibular collateral bursa)
- Iliotibial band and the joint capsule (distal iliotibial band bursa)
- Tibial collateral ligament and the pes anserine tendon (anserine bursa)
- Semimembranosus tendon and the joint capsule
- Medial head of gastrocnemius and the joint capsule (medial gastrocnemius bursa)

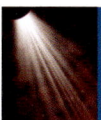

BOX 9-22 Spotlight on the Screw-Home Mechanism

The screw-home mechanism that involves tibial lateral rotation and/or femoral medial rotation as the knee joint extends does not have to be created by separate muscular action when the knee joint extends. Rather, it naturally occurs for three reasons.

One reason is the bias of the quadriceps femoris musculature pull on the tibia toward the lateral side as the quadriceps femoris pulls the tibia into extension. This occurs due to the relatively greater strength of the vastus lateralis (and vastus intermedius) compared to the vastus medialis (see Figures 11-142 through 11-144).

A second reason is the passive pull of the anterior cruciate ligament. The anterior cruciate ligament is not oriented perfectly in the sagittal plane; rather it is oriented laterally as it travels posteriorly (see Figure 9-24) so that the tibia is pulled into lateral rotation (or the femur is pulled into medial rotation) as the anterior cruciate ligament is taut as the knee joint approaches full extension.

The third reason, which is often credited as the major reason, is the asymmetry in the shape of the articular surfaces of the lateral and medial condyles of the femur. The articular surface of the medial condyle is longer and is curved approximately 30 degrees from lateral to medial as it approaches the intercondylar groove at its most anterior aspect (see Figure 5-46, B). This results in the tibia following this curved path laterally (or the femur following this curved path medially) as the knee joint approaches full extension.

This coupled rotation with extension can be observed when a person stands from a seated position. The patella is seen to orient medially—in other words, to rotate medially (the patella sits on and follows the motion of the femur). Note: The reverse action of the femur medially rotating on the fixed tibia is the tibia laterally rotating on the fixed femur.

Unlocking the fully extended tibiofemoral joint does require active muscular contraction. The popliteus is the muscle that seems to be most important in accomplishing this. If the thigh is fixed (as in open-chain movements of the lower extremity), the popliteus medially rotates the leg at the tibiofemoral joint as it begins flexion. If the leg is fixed (as in closed-chain movements of the lower extremity), the popliteus laterally rotates the thigh at the tibiofemoral joint as it begins flexion.

SECTION 9.14 PATELLOFEMORAL JOINT

BONES:

- The patellofemoral joint is formed by the articulation between the patella and the femur. (The tibia is not directly involved in the movement of the patella, therefore is not involved with the patellofemoral joint.)
  - More specifically, the patellofemoral joint is located between the posterior surface of the patella and the intercondylar groove of the femur (Figure 9-25).
- The patellofemoral joint is located within the capsule of the knee joint along with the tibiofemoral joint.

MAJOR MOTIONS ALLOWED:

- Superior and inferior gliding movements (i.e., nonaxial movements) of the patella along the femur are allowed.[11]
- As the patella moves along the femur, it is usually described as *tracking* along the femur.[11]

- Two facets exist on the posterior articular surface of the patella. The medial facet moves along the medial condyle of the femur; the lateral facet moves along the lateral condyle of the femur.[2]
- The major purpose of the patella is to act as an anatomic pulley, changing the line of pull and increasing the leverage and the force that the quadriceps femoris muscle group exerts on the tibia[11] (Figure 9-26).
  - Without a patella, the quadriceps femoris group musculature loses approximately 20% of its strength at the knee joint.[4]
- The patella also functions to reduce friction between the quadriceps femoris tendon and the femoral condyles and to protect the femoral condyles from trauma.

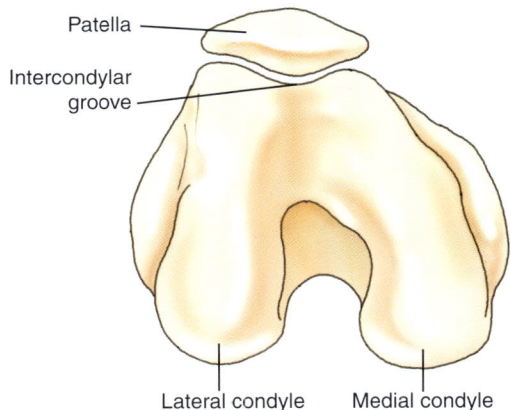

FIGURE 9-25 Distal (inferior) view of patellofemoral joint of the right lower extremity. The patella tracks along the intercondylar groove of the femur.

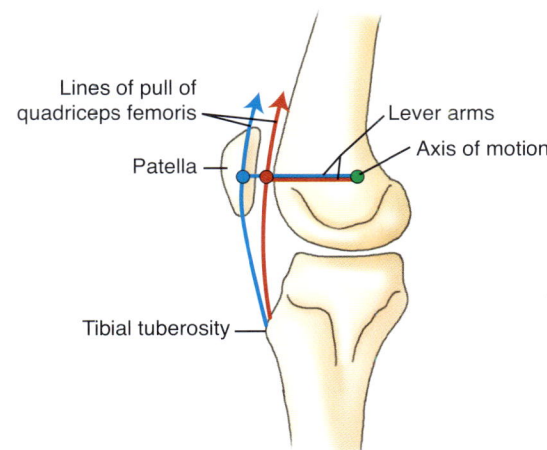

FIGURE 9-26 Lateral view of the left knee joint that illustrates the line of pull and lever arm (i.e., leverage force) of the quadriceps femoris tendon with *(blue lines)* and without *(red lines)* the presence of the patella. The increased leverage of the quadriceps femoris muscle group as a result of the presence of the patella should be noted.

- Even though the patellofemoral joint is a separate joint functionally from the tibiofemoral joint, their movements are related. When the tibiofemoral joint extends and flexes, the patella tracks up and down (i.e., moves proximally and distally) along the intercondylar groove of the femur[13] (Box 9-23).
- During forceful extension of the knee joint created by the quadriceps femoris muscle group, not all the force of the quadriceps on the tibia goes toward moving the tibia into extension. Some of the quadriceps femoris contraction force creates a compression of the patella against the femur. For this reason, the articular surface of the patella has the thickest articular cartilage of any joint in the body[4] (Box 9-24).
- When the knee joint is in full extension, the patella sits proximal to the intercondylar groove and is therefore freely movable.

BOX 9-23

Ideally, the patella should track perfectly in the middle of the intercondylar groove. However, for a variety of reasons the patella may not track perfectly. One common reason for poor tracking is an imbalance between the vastus lateralis and vastus medialis of the quadriceps femoris group; most commonly, the vastus lateralis' pull is greater than the vastus medialis' pull, resulting in an excessive force upon the patella, pulling it laterally against the lateral femoral condyle of the femur. Improper tracking can lead to damage of the articular cartilage on the underside of the patella.

- When the knee joint is flexed, the patella is located within the intercondylar groove and its mobility is greatly reduced.[13]
- Therefore, even though the closed-packed position of the knee joint (i.e., tibiofemoral joint) is full extension, the patella itself (i.e., the patellofemoral joint) is most stable when the knee joint is in flexion.[3]

BOX 9-24

The articular surface of the patella has the thickest cartilage of any joint in the body to withstand the compressive force of the patella against the femur, as well as the stress that can occur when the patella does not track perfectly along the intercondylar groove of the femur. Because of the great compressive forces to which this joint is subjected, along with the possible improper tracking of the patella, the articular cartilage of the patella often becomes damaged and breaks down. When this occurs, it is called **patellofemoral syndrome** (also known as **chondromalacia patella**).[6] There is an orthopedic assessment test that can assess this condition. With the client supine with the knee joint extended (or slightly flexed with a bolster under the knee), the therapist cups their hand along the superior pole of the patella and asks the client to gently contract the quadriceps femoris group, causing the patella to move proximally (superiorly) along the femur. With pressure placed on the superior pole, the patella pushes harder into the femur, eliciting pain and/or crepitus (joint noise) if the condition is present. It is extremely important to apply gentle pressure, and/or to slowly increase the pressure if successive repetitions are performed. Scraping or sealing the pitted and damaged articular cartilage during arthroscopic surgery is often done to repair this condition.

SECTION 9.15 ANGULATIONS OF THE KNEE JOINT

- The knee joint is composed of several components: the femur, the tibia, and the patella.
- The relationship of these components is such that they are not arranged in a straight line. The angles that are measured among the femur, tibia, and patella are called *knee joint angulations*.
- Three knee joint angulation measurements exist[2]:
  - Genu valgum/varum
  - Q-angle
  - Genu recurvatum

GENU VALGUM AND GENU VARUM:

- The genu valgum/varum angle is the angulation of the shaft of the femur relative to the shaft of the tibia within the frontal plane (Figure 9-27).[4]
- Genu valgum/varum angles are determined by the intersection of two lines: one line runs through the center of the shaft of the femur; the other line runs through the center of the shaft of the tibia.
  - **Genu valgum** is defined as an abduction of the tibia in the frontal plane relative to the femur.
  - **Genu varum** is defined as an adduction of the tibia in the frontal plane relative to the femur.
- It is normal to have a slight genu valgum at the knee joint. This normal genu valgum is the result of the femur not being vertical. Because of the angle of inclination of the femur, it slants inward as it descends. When the slanting femur meets the vertical tibia, a genu valgum is formed.
- The normal value for a genu valgum angle is approximately 5 to 10 degrees.[2]
  - A genu valgum angle greater than 10 degrees is called *excessive genu valgum* or **knock-knees**[2] (Box 9-25).
  - Note: The reported number of degrees of genu valgum can vary based on which angle is used to measure the relative positions of the shafts of the femur and tibia. The valgum angle measurement that is used to determine these figures is shown in Figure 9-27.
- If a person has a genu varum angle at the knee joint, it is called **bowleg**.[2]
- Excessive genu valgum or varum angles at the knee joint can cause increased stress and damage to the knee joint[3] (Box 9-26).

BOX 9-25

Many factors can contribute to an increased genu valgum angle at the knee joint, including overpronation of the foot (losing the arch of the foot on weight bearing), a lax medial collateral ligament of the knee, and a hip joint posture of excessive femoral medial rotation and adduction.

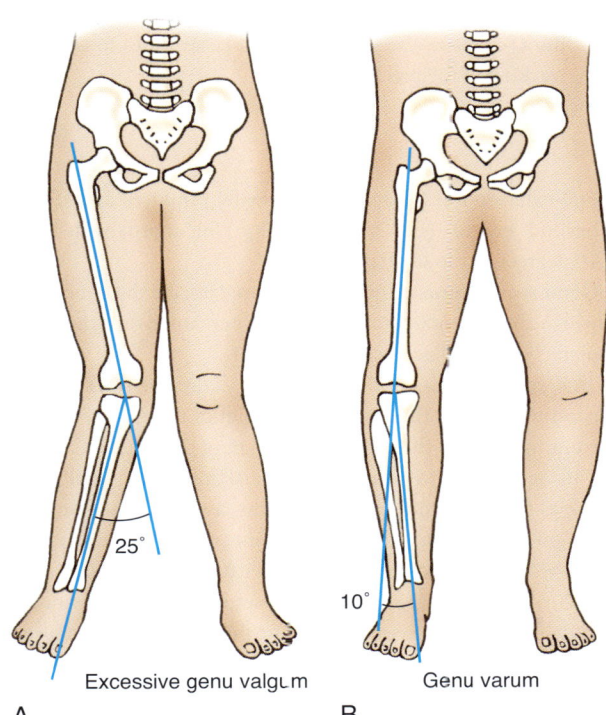

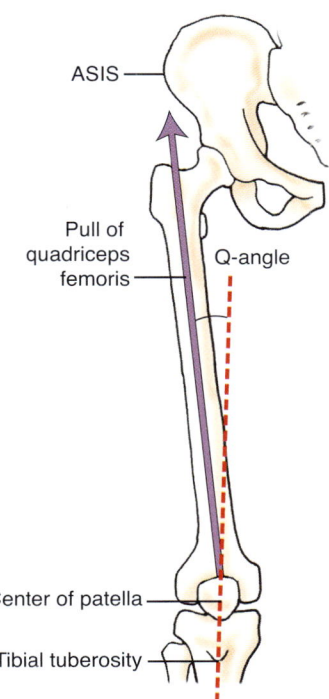

FIGURE 9-27 Anterior views of genu valgum/varum angulations of the knee joint within the frontal plane. **A,** Genu valgum angle of 25 degrees (i.e., knock-kneed). **B,** Genu varum angle of 10 degrees (i.e., bowlegged). The normal valgum/varum angle is considered to be 5 to 10 degrees of genu valgum.

FIGURE 9-28 Anterior view that illustrates the Q-angle of the knee joint. The Q-angle is formed by the intersection of two lines: one running from the tibial tuberosity to the center of the patella and the other running from the center of the patella to the anterior superior iliac spine (ASIS). The Q-angle represents the pull of the quadriceps femoris muscle group.

 BOX 9-26

An increased genu valgum angle of the knee joint results in excessive compression force at the lateral tibiofemoral joint and excessive tensile (i.e., stretching/pulling) force at the medial tibiofemoral joint. Similarly, an increased genu varum angle of the knee joint results in excessive compression force at the medial tibiofemoral joint and excessive tensile force at the lateral tibiofemoral joint.
An increased genu valgum angle also contributes to the possible development of patellofemoral syndrome (see Box 9-24)

Q-ANGLE:

- Like the angles of genu valgum and genu varum, the Q-angle is also an angulation at the knee joint that exists in the frontal plane.
- The **Q-angle** is determined by the intersection of two lines: one line runs from the tibial tuberosity to the center of the patella; the other line runs from the center of the patella to the anterior superior iliac spine (ASIS)[2] (Figure 9-28).
- The Q-angle is so named because it represents the angle of pull of the quadriceps femoris group on the patella.[6]
  - More specifically, the Q-angle measures the lateral angle of pull of the quadriceps femoris group on the patella.
- As the Q-angle increases, so does the lateral pull of the quadriceps femoris group's distal tendon on the patella. The patella is supposed to track smoothly within the center of the intercondylar groove of the femur. However, an increased Q-angle pulls the patella laterally and causes the patella to ride against the lateral side of the intercondylar groove; this may cause damage to the cartilage of the articular posterior surface of the patella[6] (Figure 9-29, Box 9-27).

 BOX 9-27

Damage to the articular posterior surface of the patella is called either patellofemoral syndrome or chondromalacia patella (see Box 9-24 in Section 9.14).

- The normal Q-angle measurement is approximately 10 to 15 degrees.[6]
- On average, the normal Q-angle for a man is approximately 10 degrees, and the normal Q-angle for a woman is approximately 15 degrees. Women usually have a greater Q-angle because the female pelvis is wider; therefore the line running up to the anterior superior iliac spine (ASIS) would be run more laterally, increasing the Q-angle.[4]
- Because the normal Q-angle is not zero degrees, it reflects the fact that the pull of the quadriceps on the patella is not even; rather it has a bias to the lateral side (Box 9-28).

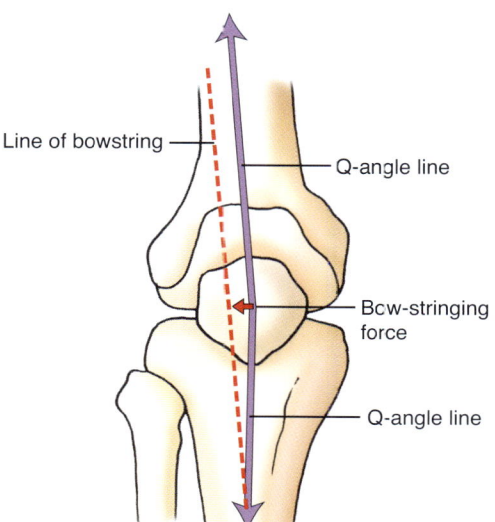

FIGURE 9-29 Anterior view that demonstrates the effect that the Q-angle has on the patella. The term *bowstringing* is used to describe the lateral pull that occurs on the patella. In this analogy the Q-angle lines represent the bow and the dashed line represents the bowstring. The bowstring force is represented by the distance between the center of the patella and the bowstring. The greater the Q-angle, the greater is the bowstringing force on the patella.

○ The lateral pull on the patella of an increased Q-angle can be explained and measured by something called the **bowstring force**.[4] Similar to how the string of a bow under tension is pulled to a position that is a straight line between the two ends of the bow where it is attached, the patella can be looked at as being located within a *string* (in this case the string is the quadriceps femoris muscle group and its distal tendon/patellar ligament) that is pulled straight between its terminal two points of attachment on the tibia and the pelvis (the anterior superior iliac spine [ASIS] is approximately correct and an easy measurement point). Thus the patella can be seen to *bowstring* laterally (see Figure 9-29). (For more on bowstringing, see *Spotlight on Bowstring Force* in Section 9.17.)
  ○ This net lateral pull of the quadriceps femoris group on the patella is caused in part by the greater relative strength of the vastus lateralis muscle compared with the vastus medialis muscle.[6]

 BOX 9-28

One recommended treatment approach for a client with an increased Q-angle is to do exercises aimed at specifically strengthening the vastus medialis muscle of the quadriceps femoris group. The idea is that a strengthened vastus medialis can counter the excessive lateral pull on the patella that occurs with an increased Q-angle. However, there is controversy over whether it is possible to specifically target the vastus medialis of the quadriceps femoris when exercising. Referral to a physical therapist, chiropractor, or trainer is recommended.

○ An increased genu valgum angle (i.e., knock-knees) increases the Q-angle at the knee joint and contributes to the lateral tracking of the patella.

GENU RECURVATUM:

○ Full extension of the knee joint usually produces an extension beyond neutral (i.e., hyperextension) of approximately 5 to 10 degrees in the sagittal plane.
○ **Genu recurvatum** is the term used to describe the condition in which the knee joint extends (i.e., hyperextends) in the sagittal plane beyond 10 degrees[4] (Figure 9-30).
○ This angle is measured by the intersection of two lines: one running through the center of the shaft of the femur; the other running through the center of the shaft of the tibia.
○ This occurs for two reasons: (1) the shape of the tibial plateau slopes slightly posteriorly, and (2) the center of a person's body weight falls anterior to the knee joint when a person is standing. Normally this tendency toward extension is resisted by the passive tension of the soft tissue structures of the posterior knee joint. When this passive tension of the soft tissue structures is unable to sufficiently resist these forces of extension and the knee joint extends (i.e., hyperextends) beyond 10 degrees, genu recurvatum results.[8]
○ The advantage to having the center of a person's body weight fall anterior to the knee joint during normal full knee joint extension is that it allows the quadriceps femoris group to relax when the person is standing.[4]

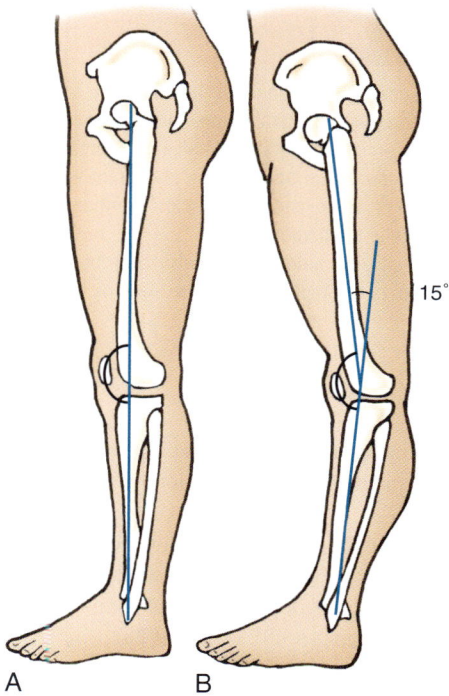

FIGURE 9-30 Genu recurvatum of the knee joint. **A,** Knee joint that is extended to zero degrees of genu recurvatum (i.e., the femur and tibia are vertically aligned). **B,** Genu recurvatum of 15 degrees.

SECTION 9.16 TIBIOFIBULAR JOINTS

BONES AND LIGAMENTS:

- The **tibiofibular joints** are located between the tibia and the fibula.
- Three tibiofibular joints exist (Figure 9-31):[8]
  - The proximal tibiofibular joint
  - The middle tibiofibular joint
  - The distal tibiofibular joint
- The proximal tibiofibular joint is located between the proximal ends of the tibia and fibula.
  - More specifically, it is located between the lateral condyle of the tibia and the head of the fibula.
  - The proximal tibiofibular joint is a plane synovial joint.
  - Its joint capsule is reinforced by anterior and posterior proximal tibiofibular ligaments.
  - Note: Even though the proximal tibiofibular joint is located close to the knee joint, it is not anatomically part of the knee joint; it has a separate joint capsule. Functionally, it is also not related to the knee joint. Structurally and functionally, all three tibiofibular joints are related to ankle joint motion.
- The middle tibiofibular joint is located between the shafts of the tibia and fibula.
  - More specifically, it is created by the **interosseous membrane** uniting the shafts of the tibia and fibula.
- The middle tibiofibular joint is a syndesmosis fibrous joint.
- By uniting the shafts of the tibia and fibula, the interosseus membrane of the leg has two purposes. One is to hold the two bones together so that they can hold the talus between them at the ankle (i.e., talocrural) joint distally. The other is to allow the force of all muscle attachments that pull on the fibula to be transferred to the tibia to move the leg at the knee joint.
- The distal tibiofibular joint is located between the distal ends of the tibia and fibula.
  - More specifically, it is created by the medial side of the lateral malleolus of the fibula articulating with the fibular notch of the distal tibia.
  - The distal tibiofibular joint is a syndesmosis fibrous joint.
  - It is reinforced by the interosseus ligament and the anterior and posterior distal tibiofibular ligaments.

MAJOR MOTIONS ALLOWED:

- The tibiofibular joints allow superior and inferior glide (i.e., nonaxial movements) of the fibula relative to the tibia.[6]
- The stability of the tibiofibular joints is dependent on the tibia and fibula being securely held to each other.
- The mobility and stability of all three tibiofibular joints are functionally related to movements of the ankle joint. (Note: For more details regarding the relationship between the ankle and tibiofibular joints, see Section 9.18.)
- The stability of the distal tibiofibular joint is particularly important to the functioning of the ankle joint, because the distal ends of the tibia and fibula at the distal tibiofibular joint must securely hold the talus between them at the ankle joint.

MISCELLANEOUS:

Tibial torsion: The term *tibial torsion* describes the fact that the shaft of the tibia twists so that the distal tibia does not face the same direction that the proximal tibia does.[6]
- The shafts of both the femur and the tibia undergo twisting or "torsion." However, the femur twists medially, but the tibia twists laterally. (For more on tibial torsion and its effects, see *Spotlight on Tibial Torsion and Talocrural Motion* in Section 9.18.)
- The result of this lateral tibial torsion is that the distal tibia faces somewhat laterally. Therefore motions at the ankle joint (i.e., dorsiflexion and plantarflexion) do not occur exactly within the sagittal plane; rather they occur in an oblique plane.

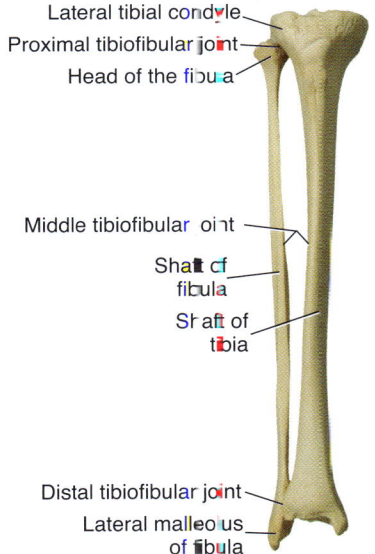

FIGURE 9-31 Anterior view that illustrates the three tibiofibular joints of the leg.

SECTION 9.17 OVERVIEW OF THE ANKLE/FOOT REGION

ORGANIZATION OF THE ANKLE/FOOT REGION:

Generally, the organization of the ankle/foot region is as follows (Figure 9-32):
- The two bones of the leg articulate with the foot at the **talocrural joint** (usually simply referred to as the *ankle joint*).
- The foot is defined as everything distal to the tibia and fibula.
  - The bones of the foot can be divided into tarsals, metatarsals, and phalanges.
  - Just as the carpal bones are the wrist bones, the tarsal bones are known as the *ankle bones*.
- The foot can be divided into three regions[6]: (1) hindfoot, (2) midfoot, and (3) forefoot.
  - The **hindfoot** consists of the talus and calcaneus, which are tarsal bones.
  - The **midfoot** consists of the navicular, the cuboid, and the three cuneiforms, which are tarsal bones.
  - The **forefoot** consists of the metatarsals and phalanges.
- The term **ray** refers (in the foot) to a metatarsal and its associated phalanges; the foot has five rays. (The first ray is composed of the first metatarsal and the two phalanges of the big toe; the second ray is composed of the second metatarsal and the three phalanges of the second toe; and so forth.)

FUNCTIONS OF THE FOOT:

- The foot is truly a marvelous structure because it must be both stable and flexible.
  - The foot must be sufficiently stable to support the tremendous weight-bearing force from the body above it, absorb the shock from landing on the ground below, and propel the body through space by pushing off the ground. Stability such as this requires the foot to be a rigid structure.[10]
  - However, the foot must also be sufficiently flexible and pliable (i.e., mobile) that it can adapt to the uneven ground surfaces that it encounters.
  - Stability and flexibility are two antagonist concepts that the foot must balance to be able to meet these divergent demands.
  - Generally, weight/shock absorption and propulsion by the foot are factors of dorsiflexion/plantarflexion of the foot at the ankle (i.e., talocrural) joint.[6]
  - Generally, adapting to uneven ground surfaces is a factor of pronation/supination (primarily composed of eversion/inversion) of the foot at the subtalar joint.[6]
  - However, it must be emphasized that the ankle joint region is a complex of joints that must function together to accomplish these tasks.[10] (Note: For more on the functions of the foot during weight bearing and the gait cycle, see Sections 20.7 and 20.8.)
  - Movements at the talocrural, subtalar, and transverse tarsal joints must occur together smoothly and seamlessly for proper functioning of the foot!

JOINTS OF THE ANKLE/FOOT REGION:

Ankle Joint:

- The ankle joint is located between the distal tibia/fibula and the talus (see Figure 9-34, A in Section 9.18).
  - This joint is usually referred to as the *talocrural joint*.[3]
  - Note: Because the ankle joint involves the distal tibia and fibula meeting the talus, the joints between the tibia and fibula (distal, middle, and proximal tibiofibular joints) are functionally related to the functioning of the ankle joint. (For more on this, see Section 9.18.)

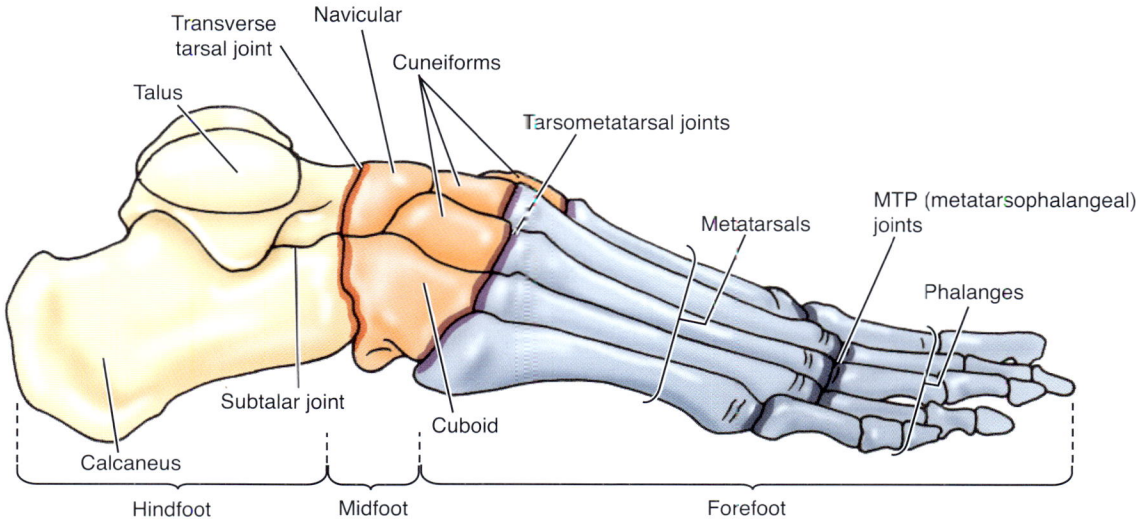

FIGURE 9-32 The three regions of the foot. The hindfoot is composed of the calcaneus and talus. The midfoot is composed of the navicular, cuboid, and the three cuneiforms. The forefoot is composed of the metatarsals and phalanges. (Note: The major joints of the foot are also labeled.)

Tarsal Joints:

- **Tarsal joints** are located between tarsal bones of the foot (see Figure 9-32).
- A number of tarsal joints are found in the foot.
- The major tarsal joint is the **subtalar joint**.
  - The subtalar joint is located between the talus and the calcaneus.
- Another important tarsal joint is the **transverse tarsal joint**.
  - The transverse tarsal joint is located between the talus/calcaneus (which are located proximally) and the navicular/cuboid (which are located distally).
- **Distal intertarsal joints** is the term used to describe all other joints formed between the tarsal bones. The individual distal intertarsal joints may also be named for the specific tarsal bones involved (e.g., the cuboidonavicular joint between the cuboid and navicular bone or the intercuneiform joints between the cuneiform bones).

Tarsometatarsal and Intermetatarsal Joints:

- The **tarsometatarsal (TMT) joints** are located between the tarsal bones located proximally and the metatarsal bones located distally (see Figure 9-32).
- **Intermetatarsal joints** are located between the metatarsal bones (see Figure 9-43 in Section 9.22).

Metatarsophalangeal Joints:

- The **metatarsophalangeal (MTP) joints** are located between the metatarsal bones located proximally and the phalanges located distally (see Figure 9-32).

Interphalangeal Joints:

- **Interphalangeal (IP) joints** are located between phalanges (see Figure 9-47 in Section 9.24)
  - **Proximal interphalangeal (PIP) joints** are located between the proximal and middle phalanges of toes #2 through #5.
  - **Distal interphalangeal (DIP) joints** are located between the middle and distal phalanges of toes #2 through #5.
  - An IP joint is located between the proximal and middle phalanges of the big toe (toe #1).

ARCHES OF THE FOOT:

- The foot is often described as having an **arch**. More accurately, it can be described as having three arches (Figure 9-33).
- Note: The arch structure of the foot is not present at birth; rather it develops as we age. Most people have their arches developed by approximately 5 years of age.
- The three arches of the foot are the medial longitudinal arch, the lateral longitudinal arch, and the transverse arch.
  - **Medial longitudinal arch**: This arch is the largest arch of the foot and runs the length of the foot on the medial side.[3] This is the arch that is normally referred to when one speaks of "the arch of the foot."
  - **Lateral longitudinal arch**: This arch runs the length of the foot on the lateral side and is not as high as the medial longitudinal arch.[3]
  - **Transverse arch**: This arch runs transversely across the foot.[3]

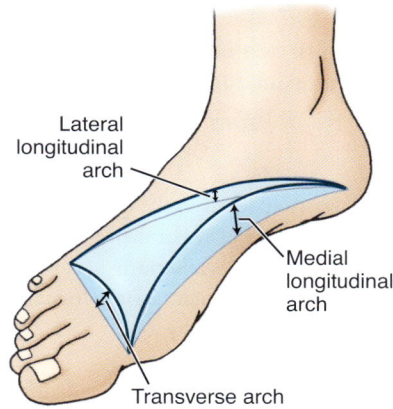

FIGURE 9-33 The three arches of the foot. Two arches run the length of the foot; they are the medial longitudinal arch, which is the largest arch of the foot, and the lateral longitudinal arch. The third arch runs across the foot; it is the transverse arch.

- Note: Because of the manner in which the bones and joints of the foot tend to function together, motion that affects one arch tends to affect all three arches. (See the discussion of subtalar pronation and supination [Section 9.19] to better understand foot motions that affect the height of the arch[es].) If one arch "drops," then all three arches drop. If one arch "raises," then all three arches raise (Box 9-29).
- An excessive arch to the foot is called **pes cavus**.[8]
- A decreased arch to the foot is called **pes planus** or is described as a **flat foot**[8] (Box 9-30).

 BOX 9-29

The client's arches can be evaluated by simply observing the feet in a weight-bearing position. This can be done from an anterior view in which the height of the arch may be directly observed. This can also be done from a posterior view in which bowing of the calcaneal (i.e., Achilles) tendon is looked at as an indication of the dropping of the arch(es) of the foot. Another very effective way that the arches of the foot can be evaluated is to spread a small amount of oil on the client's feet and then have the client step on colored construction paper. The degree of the arch can be seen by the imprint that the oil leaves on the paper.

 BOX 9-30

The clinical implications of one foot's arch that drops more than the other foot's arch are many. If one foot's arch is lower than the other foot's arch, then the height of one lower extremity will be less than the other's. This will result in a pelvis that is depressed or tilted to one side. This results in a spine that must curve in the frontal plane to bring the head to a level position (which is necessary for vision and proprioceptive balance in the inner ear). This frontal plane curve of the spine is defined as a scoliosis. Therefore evaluation of the arches of a client's feet is extremely important when the client has a scoliosis. A dropped arch will also create structural stresses on the plantar fascia of the foot, as well as the knee joint and hip joint.

PLANTAR FASCIA:

- The foot has a thick layer of dense fibrous tissue on the plantar side known as the **plantar fascia**[11] (Boxes 9-31 and 9-32).
- The plantar fascia has two layers[4]: (1) superficial and (2) deep.
  - The superficial layer is located in the dermis of the skin of the foot.
  - The deep layer is attached to the calcaneal tuberosity posteriorly and the plantar plates of the MTP joints and adjacent flexor tendons of the toes anteriorly.
- The main purpose of the plantar fascia is to maintain and stabilize the longitudinal arches of the foot.[4]

BOX 9-31

Plantar fasciitis is a condition wherein the plantar fascia of the foot becomes irritated and inflamed. Because tightening of the intrinsic muscles that attach into the plantar fascia often accompanies this condition, tension is often placed on the calcaneal attachment of the plantar fascia, which can create a **heel spur**. A common cause of plantar fasciitis is an overly pronated foot (see Section 9.19). Plantar fasciitis often responds well to soft tissue work.[14]

- Many intrinsic muscles of the foot attach into the plantar fascia. By doing so, they help to maintain the tension of the plantar fascia and therefore the arch of the foot. However, walking in shoes (compared with walking barefoot) does not require as much activity from the intrinsic muscles of the foot and may allow them to weaken. Intrinsic musculature weakness could then lead to functional weakness of the plantar fascia and a loss of the normal arch of the foot. An excessive loss of the arch of the foot when weight bearing is defined as an *overly pronating foot* (at the tarsal joints, principally the subtalar joint), which can then lead to further problems in the body.[4]

MISCELLANEOUS:

- Many retinacula are located in the ankle region. These retinacula run transversely across the ankle and act to hold down and stabilize the tendons that cross from the leg into the foot (see Box 9-33 and also Figure 9-37 in Section 9.18) (Note: In addition to the ankle region, retinacula are also located in the wrist region to hold down the tendons of the muscles of the forearm that enter the hand [see Section 10.11]).
- The word *pedis* means *foot*.
- The word *hallucis* or *hallux* means *big toe*.
- The word *digital* refers to toes #2 through #5 (or fingers #2 through #5).

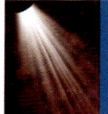

BOX 9-32 Spotlight on the Windlass Mechanism

The attachment of the plantar fascia into the flexor tendons of the toes has a functional importance. When we push ourselves off (i.e., toe-off) when walking, our metatarsals extend at the metatarsophalangeal (MTP) joints. Because of the attachment of the plantar fascia into the toe flexor tendons, the plantar fascia is pulled taut around the MTP joints. This tension of the plantar fascia then helps to stabilize the arch of the foot and make the foot more rigid, which is necessary when we push the body forward when walking or running. This mechanism is often called the **windlass mechanism**. A windlass is a pulling mechanism used for lifting the mast of a boat. It consists of a rope that can be tightened by being wound around a cylinder; the tension of the rope then pulls on and lifts the mast. In this case the MTP joint is the cylinder and the rope is the plantar fascia. When the plantar fascia is pulled taut around the MTP, it becomes taut and pulls on the two ends of the arch, increasing the height of the arch.[15]

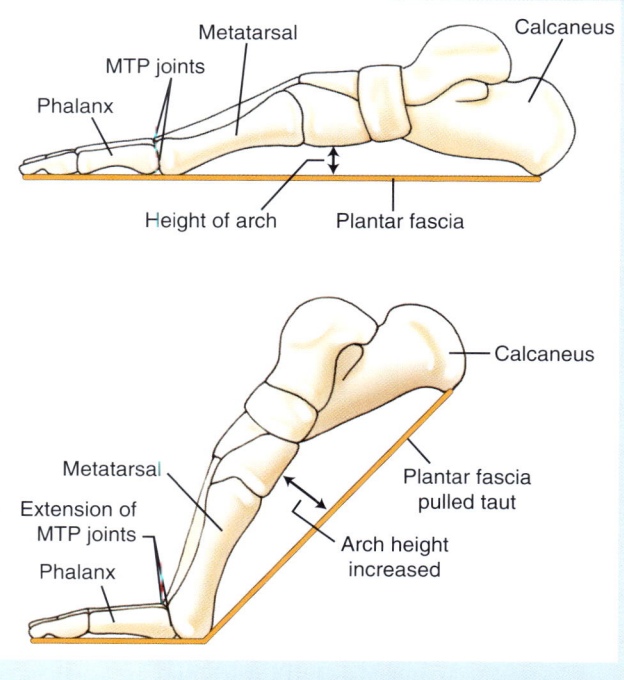

BOX 9-33 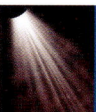 Spotlight on Bowstring Force

A **retinaculum** (plural: retinacula) acts to hold down (i.e., restrain) the tendons of the leg muscles that cross the ankle joint and enter the foot. A number of retinacula are located in the ankle region. Retinacula are needed in the ankle region, because when we contract our leg muscles to move the foot and/or toes, the pull of the muscle belly on its tendon would tend to lift the tendon away from the ankle (i.e., lift it up into the air and away from the body wall) if it were not for a retinaculum holding it down. This phenomenon is called bowstringing and weakens the strength of the muscles' ability to move the foot. Therefore the function of the retinacula of the ankle joint region is to hold these tendons down, preventing them from bowstringing away from the body.

Note: The term *bowstring* is used to describe this phenomenon because these tendons act like the string of a bow. A bow is a curved piece of wood with its string attached to both ends of the bow. When the string of a bow is placed under tension, it shortens and lifts away from the bow itself. Therefore the bowstring does not follow the curved contour of the bow; rather it lifts away to form a straight line that connects the two ends of the bow. (Note: The shortest distance between two points is a straight line.) Similarly, the leg and foot are angled relative to each other and can be likened to a curved bow. For example, when the tendons that cross the anterior ankle region are pulled taut (by the contraction of their muscle bellies), they would lift away from the ankle. Therefore we say that this lifting away is caused by the bowstring force, and it can be called bowstringing.

SECTION 9.18 TALOCRURAL (ANKLE) JOINT

9-6

○ Unless the context is made otherwise clear, when the term *ankle joint* is used, it is assumed that it refers to the talocrural joint.
○ Some sources refer to the talocrural joint as the **upper ankle joint** (the subtalar joint is then referred to as the **lower ankle joint**). The value to this description is that it emphasizes the fact that movements of the foot are primarily dependent on movements at both the talocrural and subtalar joints.

BONES:

○ The talocrural joint is located between the talus and the distal tibia and fibula (Figure 9-34, A).
  ○ More specifically, the talocrural joint is located between the trochlear surface of the dome of the talus and the rectangular cavity formed by the distal end of the tibia and the malleoli of the tibia and fibula.[8]

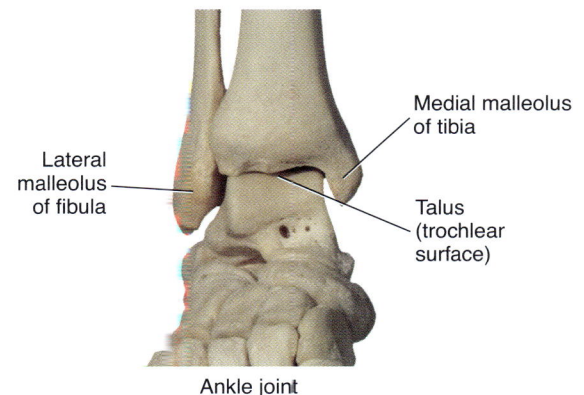

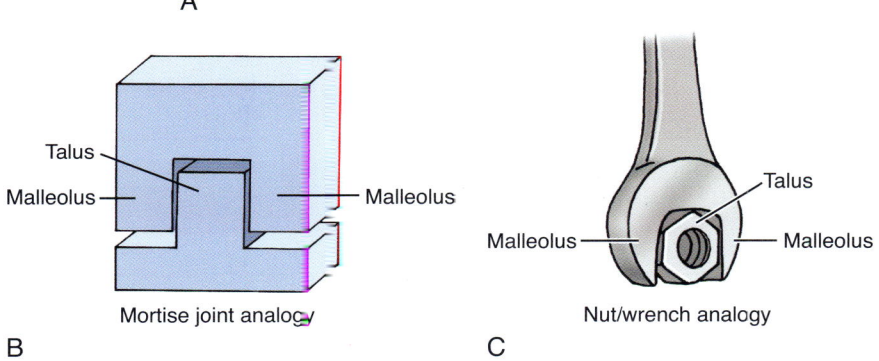

FIGURE 9-34 Talocrural (i.e., ankle) joint. **A,** Anterior view of the dorsal foot in which we see that the ankle joint is formed by the talus articulating with the distal ends of the tibia and fibula. **B,** Carpenter's mortise joint; the talocrural joint is often compared with a mortise joint. **C,** Nut held in a wrench. The talocrural joint may be compared with a nut held by a wrench. The talus is the nut, and the sides of the wrench are formed by the (malleoli of the) tibia and fibula.

- When the shape of the talocrural joint is described, it is often compared with a **mortise joint**[2] (Figure 9-34, B).
- A mortise joint was commonly used in the past by carpenters to join two pieces of wood. The mortise was formed by the end of one piece being notched out and the end of the other piece being carved to fit in this notch; a peg was then used to fasten them together. Because of its similarity in shape to a mortise joint, the talocrural (i.e., ankle) joint is often called the *mortise joint*.
- Perhaps a better analogy to visualize the shape of the talocrural joint is to compare it with a nut being held in a wrench (Figure 9-34, C).
- The bony fit of the bones of the ankle joint is so good that many sources consider it to be the most congruent joint of the human body.[3]
- Joint structure classification: Synovial joint[3]
  - Subtype: Hinge joint
- Joint function classification: Diarthrotic
  - Subtype: Uniaxial

MAJOR MOTIONS ALLOWED:

Average ranges of motion of the foot at the talocrural joint are given in Table 9-4 (Figure 9-35).[6]
- The talocrural joint allows dorsiflexion and plantarflexion (i.e., axial movements) within the sagittal plane around a mediolateral axis (Box 9-34).

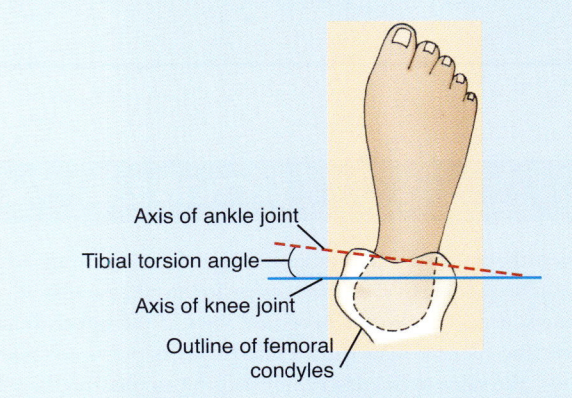

BOX 9-34 Spotlight on Tibial Torsion and Talocrural Motion

Actually, dorsiflexion and plantarflexion of the foot at the ankle joint do not occur perfectly within the sagittal plane. Because of the twisting of the tibia known as tibial torsion, talocrural motion occurs slightly in an oblique plane (tibial torsion is measured by the difference between the axis of the knee joint and the axis of the ankle joint). For this reason, talocrural joint motion is often listed as triplanar. However, use of the term *triplanar* can be misleading. Triplanar refers to the fact that its motion is across all three cardinal planes. However, the talocrural joint is uniaxial (with one degree of freedom); its motion is in one oblique plane around one oblique axis.

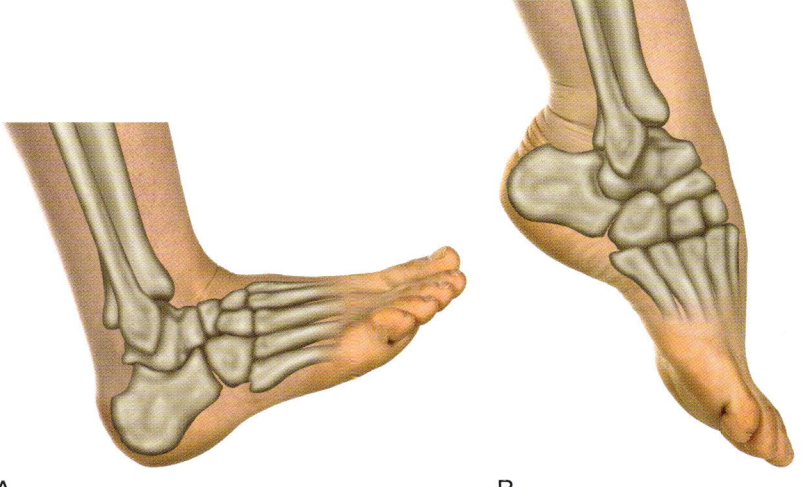

FIGURE 9-35 **A** and **B**, Dorsiflexion and plantarflexion of the foot at the talocrural (i.e., ankle) joint, respectively.

TABLE 9-4	Average Ranges of Motion of the Foot at the Talocrural Joint[5]		
Dorsiflexion	20 Degrees	Plantarflexion	50 Degrees

Note: The amount of dorsiflexion varies based on the position of the knee joint. Because the gastrocnemius (a plantarflexor of the ankle joint) crosses the knee joint posteriorly, if the knee joint is flexed, the gastrocnemius would be slackened, and more dorsiflexion would be allowed at the talocrural joint.

- ○ Functioning of the ankle and tibiofibular joints is related. The dome of the talus is not uniform in size; its anterior aspect is wider than the posterior aspect. When the foot dorsiflexes, the wider anterior aspect of the dome of the talus moves between the distal tibia and fibula; this creates a force that tends to push the tibia and fibula apart. The motion and stability of the tibiofibular joints are necessary to absorb and counter this force.

Reverse Actions:

- ○ The muscles of the talocrural joint are generally considered to move the more distal foot relative to the more proximal leg. However, closed-chain activities are common in the lower extremity in which the foot is planted on the ground; this fixes the foot and requires that the leg move relative to the foot instead. When this occurs, the leg can move at the talocrural joint instead of the foot.
- ○ The leg can dorsiflex and plantarflex in the sagittal plane at the talocrural joint.
- ○ In a closed-chain activity, when the leg moves at the talocrural joint instead of the foot, dorsiflexion of the leg at the talocrural joint is defined as the leg moving anteriorly toward the dorsum of the foot; plantarflexion of the leg at the talocrural joint is defined as the leg moving posteriorly away from the dorsum of the foot.
- ○ Dorsiflexion of the leg at the ankle joint is an extremely common motion and occurs during the gait cycle when we go from heel-strike to toe-off.

MAJOR LIGAMENTS OF THE TALOCRURAL JOINT (BOX 9-35):

Fibrous Joint Capsule

- ○ The capsule of the talocrural joint is thin and does not offer a great deal of stability.[8]

BOX 9-35   Ligaments of the Talocrural Joint

- ○ Fibrous joint capsule
- ○ Medial collateral ligament (deltoid ligament)
- ○ Lateral collateral ligament complex
  - ○ Anterior talofibular ligament
  - ○ Posterior talofibular ligament
  - ○ Calcaneofibular ligament

Medial and Lateral Collateral Ligaments:

- ○ The medial and lateral collateral ligaments are found on both sides (*lateral* means *side*) of the talocrural joint (Figure 9-36).
- ○ The collateral ligaments are primarily important for limiting frontal plane movements of the bones of the talocrural joint.[8]

Medial Collateral Ligament:
- ○ The **medial collateral ligament** is also known as the **deltoid ligament** (see Figure 9-36, *A*).
- ○ The deltoid ligament is so named because it has a delta (i.e., triangular) shape; it fans out in a triangular shape from the tibia to three tarsal bones.
- ○ It attaches from the tibia to the calcaneus, the talus, and the navicular bone.
  - ○ More specifically, it attaches from the medial malleolus of the tibia proximally, and then it fans out to attach to the medial side of the talus, the sustentaculum tali of the calcaneus, and the navicular tuberosity.
- ○ Function: It limits eversion of the foot at the talocrural joint (within the frontal plane).
  - ○ The deltoid ligament is a taut, strong ligament that does a very effective job of limiting eversion sprains of the ankle joint.
  - ○ Note: In addition to the presence of the deltoid ligament, the fact that the lateral malleolus of the fibula extends down farther distally than does the medial malleolus of the tibia also significantly helps to limit excessive eversion at the ankle joint. For this reason, eversion sprains of the ankle (i.e., talocrural) joint are very uncommon.

Lateral Collateral Ligament:
- ○ The **lateral collateral ligament** is actually a ligament complex composed of three ligaments: (1) the anterior talofibular ligament, (2) the posterior talofibular ligament, and (3) the calcaneofibular ligament (see Figure 9-36, *B*).
- ○ All three lateral collateral ligaments attach proximally to the fibula.
  - ○ More specifically, all three attach proximally to the lateral malleolus of the fibula.
- ○ Distally, the **anterior talofibular ligament** attaches to the anterior talus; the **posterior talofibular ligament** attaches to the posterior talus; and the **calcaneofibular ligament** attaches to the lateral surface of the calcaneus.
- ○ Function: The lateral collateral ligament limits inversion of the foot at the talocrural joint within the frontal plane (Box 9-36).

 BOX 9-36

Given that the medial malleolus does not extend very far distally, the lateral collateral ligaments are the only line of defense (other than musculature) against inversion sprains of the ankle joint; therefore inversion sprains are much more common than eversion sprains. Of the three lateral collateral ligaments, the anterior talofibular ligament is the most commonly sprained ligament. In fact, the anterior talofibular ligament is the most commonly sprained ligament of the human body. The reason that this particular lateral collateral ligament is more often sprained is that inversion sprains usually occur as a person is moving forward, which couples a plantarflexion motion to the foot along with the inversion. This places a particular stress on the more anteriorly placed anterior talofibular ligament.[3]

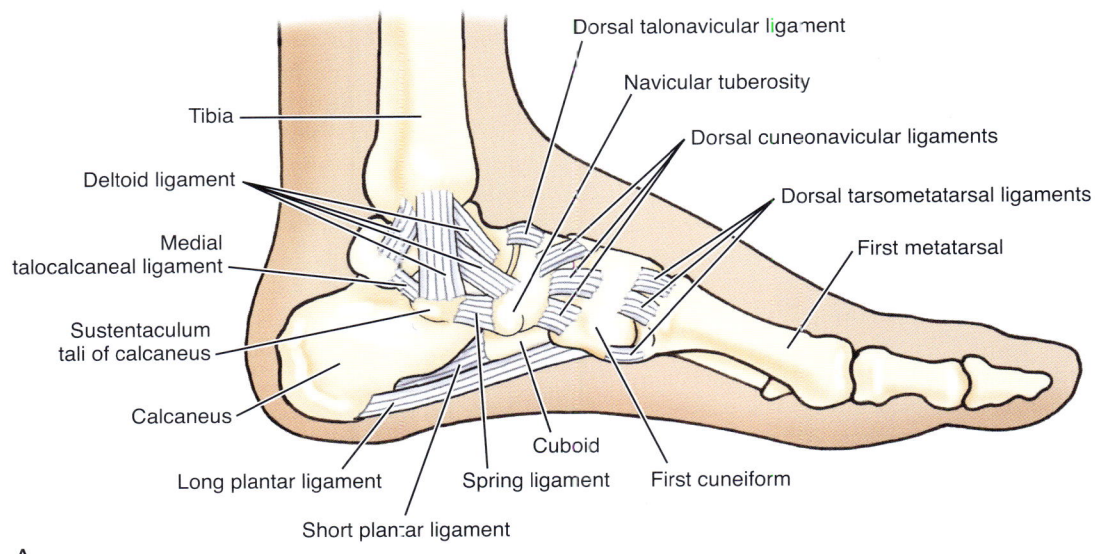

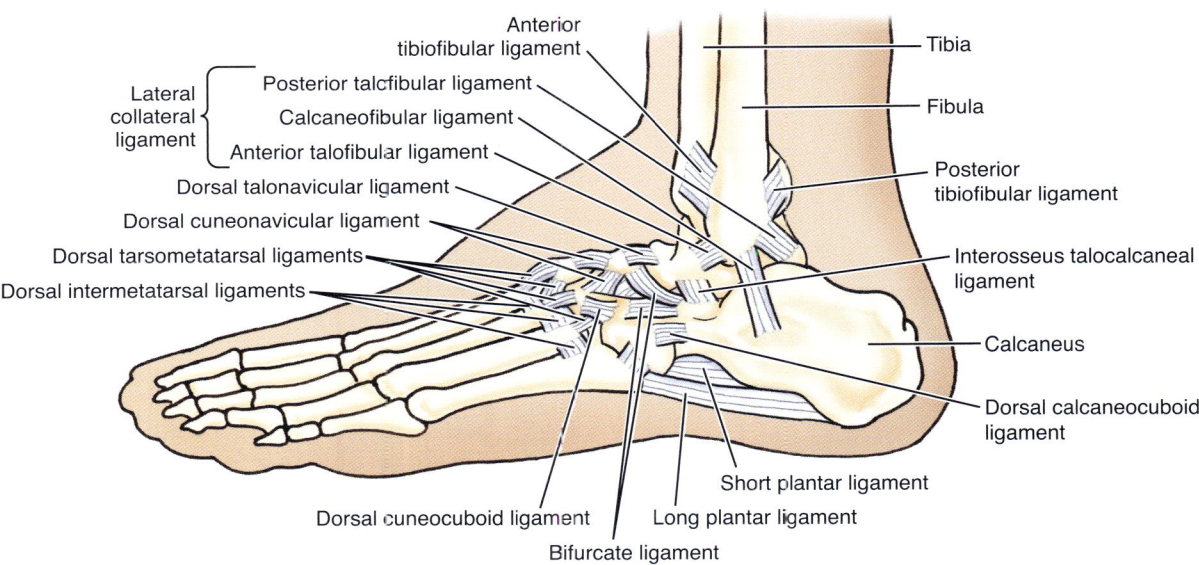

FIGURE 9-36 Ligaments of the left talocrural (i.e., ankle) and tarsal joints. **A,** Medial view. The major ligament of the medial talocrural joint is the mediolateral collateral ligament (also known as the deltoid ligament). **B,** Lateral view. The major ligament of the lateral talocrural joint is the lateral collateral ligament. The lateral collateral ligament is actually a ligament complex composed of three separate ligaments.

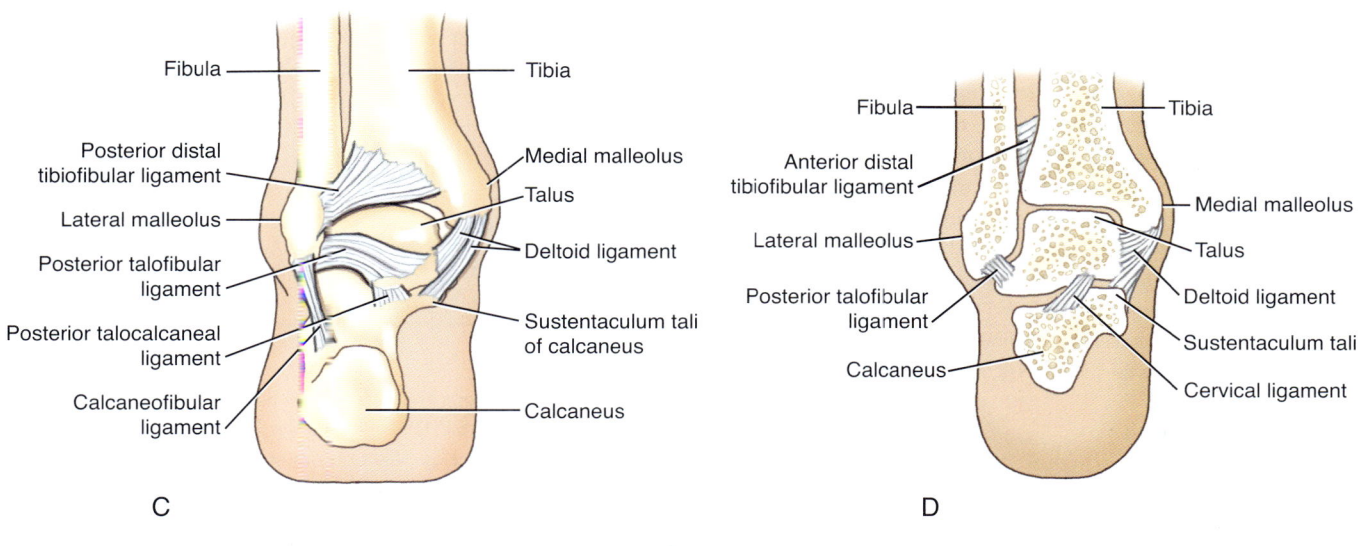
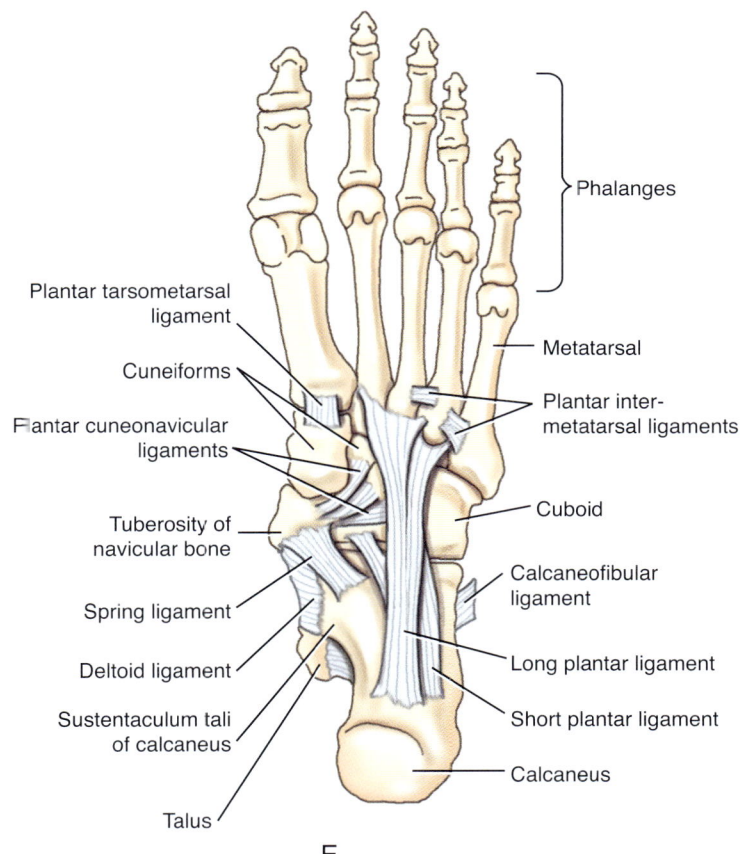

FIGURE 9-35, cont'd C and D, Posterior views. (Note: D is a frontal plane section through the bones.) E, Plantar view of the underside of the foot.

CLOSED-PACKED POSITION OF THE TALOCRURAL JOINT:

- Dorsiflexion[6]

MAJOR MUSCLES OF THE TALOCRURAL JOINT:

- The talocrural joint is crossed anteriorly by all muscles that pass anterior to the malleoli; these are the muscles of the anterior compartment of the leg (tibialis anterior, extensor digitorum longus, extensor hallucis longus, and fibularis tertius). It is crossed posteriorly by all muscles that pass posterior to the malleoli; these are the muscles located in the lateral and posterior compartments of the leg (gastrocnemius, soleus, "Tom, Dick, and Harry" muscles [i.e., tibialis posterior, flexor digitorum longus, and flexor hallucis longus], and the fibularis longus and brevis). The talocrural joint is crossed laterally by the fibularis muscles (fibularis longus, brevis, and tertius) and medially by the "Tom, Dick, and Harry" muscles.

MISCELLANEOUS:

Bursae of the Talocrural Joint:

- The talocrural joint has many bursae (Figure 9-37). (See Box 9-37 for a listing of the common bursae of the talocrural joint.)

Retinacula of the Talocrural Joint:

- Retinacula are located both anteriorly and posteriorly at the ankle joint (see Figure 9-37). These retinacula function to hold down the tendons that cross the ankle joint and prevent bowstringing of these tendons. (Note: For more information on bowstringing, see *Spotlight on Bowstring Force* in Section 9.17.) (See Box 9-37 for a listing of the retinacula of the talocrural joint.)

Tendon Sheaths:

- Tendon sheaths are found around most tendons that cross the ankle joint. They function to minimize friction between these tendons and the underlying bony structures[4] (see Figure 9-37).

> **BOX 9-37** Major Bursae and Retinacula of the Talocrural Joint (see Figure 9-37)
>
> **Bursae**
> - Medial malleolar bursa (subcutaneous)
> - Lateral malleolar bursa (subcutaneous)
> - Subcutaneous calcaneal (Achilles) bursa
> - Subtendinous calcaneal (Achilles) bursa
>
> **Retinacula**
> - Superior extensor retinaculum
> - Inferior extensor retinaculum
> - Flexor retinaculum
> - Superior fibular retinaculum
> - Inferior fibular retinaculum

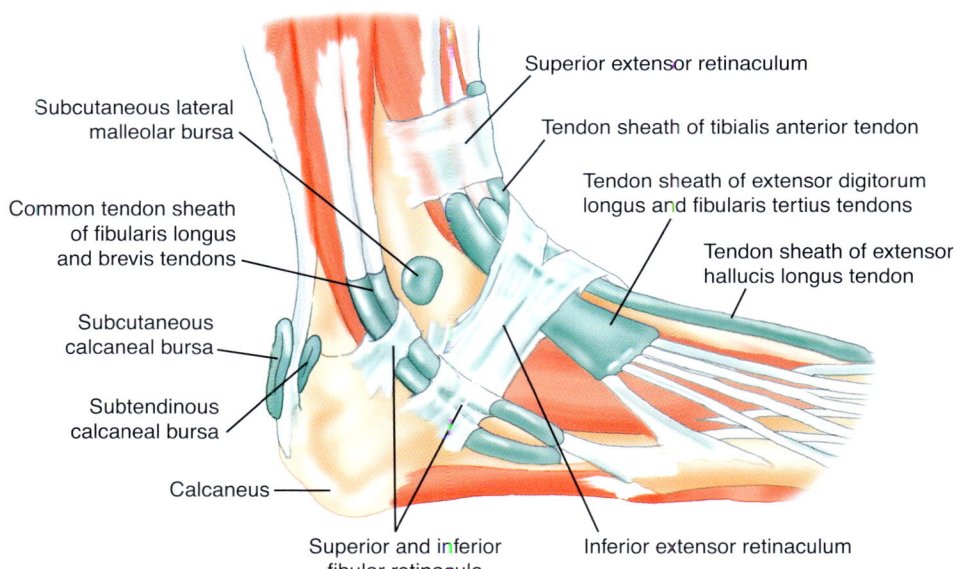

FIGURE 9-37 Lateral view that illustrates most of the bursae, tendon sheaths, and retinacula of the talocrural (i.e., ankle) joint.

CHAPTER 9 Joints of the Lower Extremity

SECTION 9.19 SUBTALAR TARSAL JOINT

BONES:

- Tarsal joints are located between tarsal bones of the foot.
- The major tarsal joint of the foot is the subtalar joint.
  - The subtalar joint is located, as its name implies, under the talus. Therefore it is located between the talus and the calcaneus (Figure 9-38, Box 9-38).

BOX 9-38

On the medial side of the foot, the talus is supported by the sustentaculum tali of the calcaneus. The sustentaculum tali is one of two easily palpable landmarks of the medial foot; the other is the tuberosity of the navicular[1] (see Figure 9-38, B).

- Therefore the subtalar joint is also known as the **talocalcaneal joint**.[6]
- The subtalar joint is sometimes referred to as the *lower ankle joint* (the talocrural joint being the upper ankle joint).

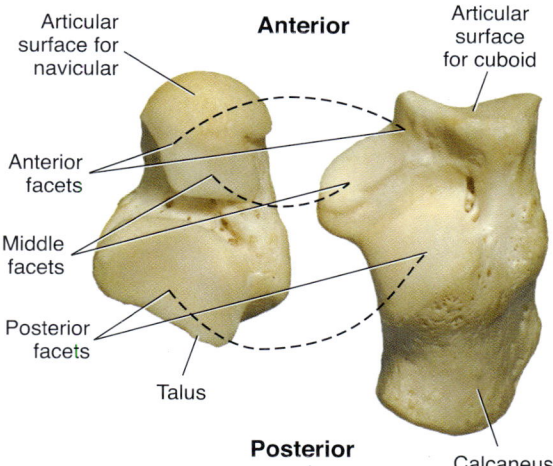

FIGURE 9-39 An "open-book" photo illustrating the facets of the subtalar joint (showing the superior surface of the calcaneus and the inferior surface of the talus). The subtalar joint is actually composed of three separate articulations. (Note: Each bone has three facets on its subtalar articular surface.) The two posterior facets are the largest of the six. Dashed lines illustrate how the facets line up with each other.

SUBTALAR JOINT ARTICULATIONS:

- The subtalar joint is actually composed of three separate talocalcaneal articulations (between the talus and calcaneus) (Figure 9-39).
  - These articulations are facet articulations that are either slightly concave/convex or flat in shape.
  - The largest articulation is between the posterior facets of the talus and calcaneus.
  - The other two articulations are between the anterior facets and middle facets of the talus and calcaneus.
- Between the talus and calcaneus, a large cavity exists called the **sinus tarsus**, which is visible from the lateral side.[14]
  - Joint structure classification: Synovial joint(s)[3]
  - Joint function classification: Diarthrotic
  - Subtype: Uniaxial
- The posterior articulation of the subtalar joint has its own distinct joint capsule, whereas the anterior and middle articulations of the subtalar joint share a joint capsule with the talonavicular joint.[1]
- Note: The subtalar joint is often referred to as being *triplanar* because it allows movement across all three cardinal planes. However, its motion is in one oblique plane around one axis (the axis for that oblique plane); hence it is uniaxial. Therefore the subtalar joint is triplanar and uniaxial.[1]

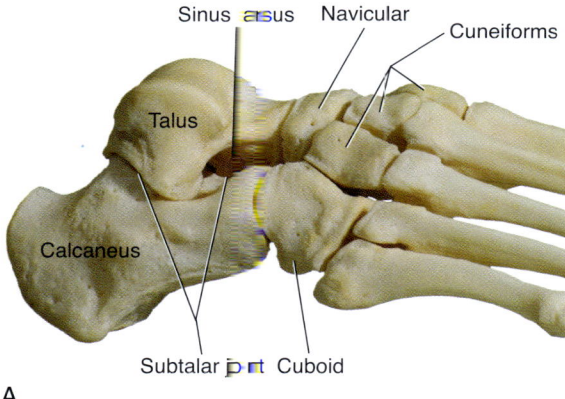

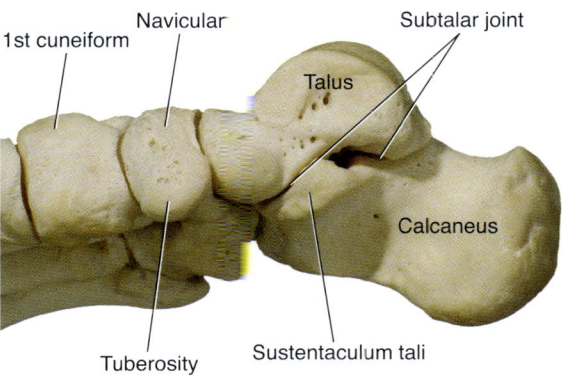

FIGURE 9-38 Subtalar joint located between the talus and the calcaneus. (Note: Subtalar means under the talus.) **A,** Lateral view. The sinus tarsus is a large cavity located between the talus and calcaneus and is visible on the lateral side. **B,** Medial view.

MAJOR MOTIONS ALLOWED:

Average ranges of motion of the foot at the subtalar joint are given in Table 9-5 (Figure 9-40).

- The subtalar joint allows pronation and supination (i.e., axial movements) in an oblique plane around an oblique axis.[4]

TABLE 9-5 Average Ranges of Motion of the (Non–Weight-Bearing) Foot at the Subtalar Joint[4]

Pronation		Supination	
Eversion	10 Degrees	Inversion	20 Degrees
Dorsiflexion	2.5 Degrees	Plantarflexion	5 Degrees
Lateral rotation (abduction)	10 Degrees	Medial rotation (adduction)	20 Degrees

Note: Determining the relative amounts of subtalar motion requires an agreed-on neutral position of the joint. Subtalar neutral position is controversial and not agreed on by all sources. The numbers here reflect the guideline that subtalar neutral is a position that allows twice as much inversion as eversion.

- The axis for subtalar motion is oblique and is located 42 degrees (anterosuperior) off the transverse plane and 16 degrees (anteromedial) off the sagittal plane.[4]
- The oblique plane movements of pronation and supination can be broken up into their component cardinal plane actions.
- Description of subtalar joint motion varies greatly from one source to another. Some sources state that eversion is pronation and inversion is supination. Technically, this is not true. Eversion and inversion are the principal cardinal plane components of the larger oblique plane pronation and supination actions (see Figure 9-40). It should be emphasized that the component cardinal plane actions of the pronation and supination cannot be isolated at the subtalar joint. All three components of pronation must occur at the subtalar joint when the foot pronates, and all three components of supination must occur at the subtalar joint when the foot supinates.

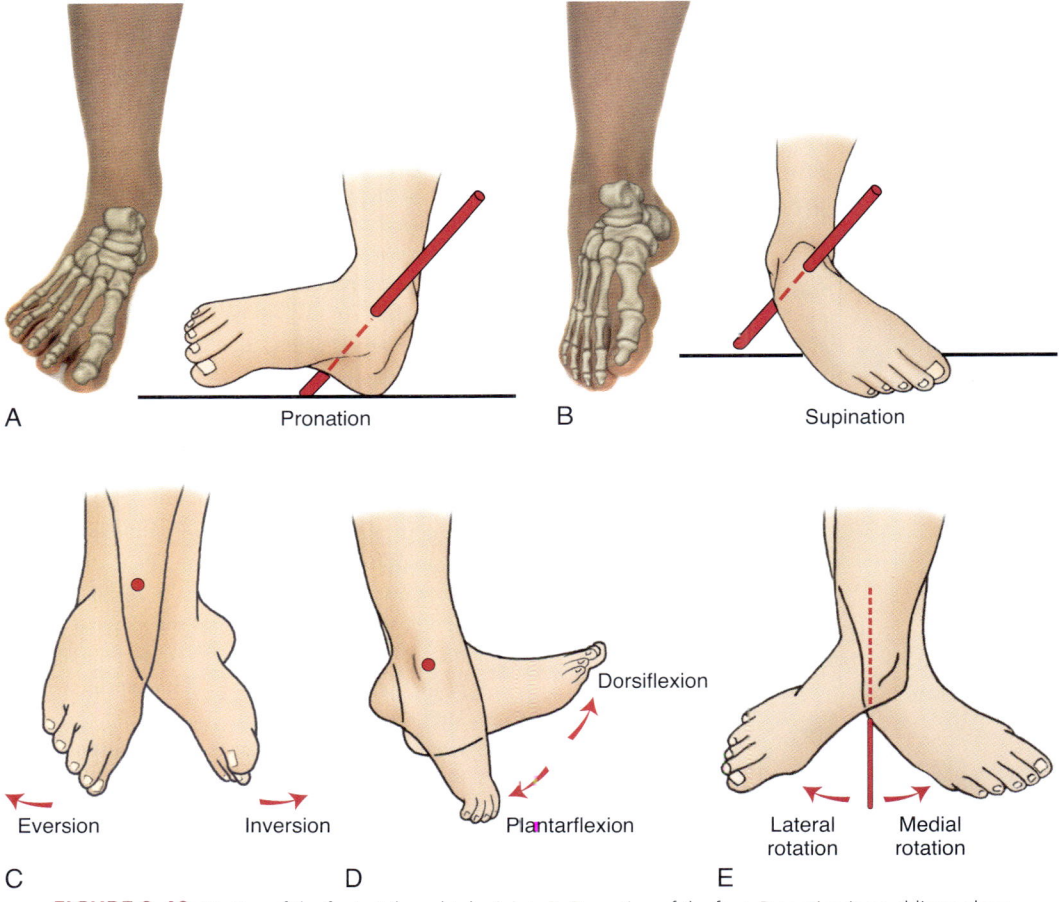

FIGURE 9-40 Motion of the foot at the subtalar joint. **A,** Pronation of the foot. Pronation is an oblique plane motion composed of three cardinal plane components: (1) eversion, (2) dorsiflexion, and (3) lateral rotation of the foot. **B,** Supination of the foot. Supination is an oblique plane motion composed of three cardinal plane components: (1) inversion, (2) plantarflexion, and (3) medial rotation of the foot. **C,** Frontal plane components of eversion/inversion. **D,** Sagittal plane components of dorsiflexion/plantarflexion. **E,** Transverse plane components of lateral rotation/medial rotation (also known as abduction/adduction, respectively). In **A, B,** and **E,** the red tube represents the axis for that motion. (Note: In **C** and **D,** the axis is represented by the red dot.)

Note: The sagittal plane subtalar joint component motions of dorsiflexion and plantarflexion are often not observed because the ankle (talocrural) joint compensates for them. In other words, subtalar joint pronation/dorsiflexion results in talocrural joint plantarflexion; and subtalar joint supination/plantarflexion results in talocrural joint dorsiflexion.

- Pronation of the foot at the subtalar joint is composed of eversion, dorsiflexion, and lateral rotation of the foot.[4]
- Supination of the foot at the subtalar joint is composed of inversion, plantarflexion, and medial rotation of the foot.[4]
  - Eversion/inversion of the foot at the subtalar joint occur within the frontal plane around an anteroposterior axis.
  - Dorsiflexion/plantarflexion of the foot at the subtalar joint occur within the sagittal plane around a mediolateral axis.
  - Lateral rotation/medial rotation of the foot at the subtalar joint occur with the transverse plane around a vertical axis.
  - Lateral rotation of the foot is also known as *abduction;* medial rotation of the foot is often described as *adduction.*

Reverse Actions:

- The previously discussed actions describe the components of pronation and supination when the more proximal talus/leg is fixed and the more distal calcaneus/foot is free to move because the foot is not weight bearing (i.e., it is an open-chain activity). However, when the foot is planted on the ground, the bones of the foot become somewhat fixed and the manner in which the components of pronation and supination of the foot at the subtalar joint are carried out changes to some degree:
  - When we stand and the foot is weight bearing, as a result of being locked between the body weight from above and the fixed bones of the foot on the ground below, the motion of the calcaneus is limited but not completely fixed. In weight bearing, the calcaneus is free to evert/invert (in the frontal plane) only. Because the calcaneus cannot freely carry out the other two components of pronation/supination (in the sagittal and transverse planes), the more proximal talus must move relative to the calcaneus at the subtalar joint for these other two aspects of pronation and supination. When the talus carries out the aspects of dorsiflexion or plantarflexion that occur in the sagittal plane, this motion is usually compensated for at the talocrural joint because the talocrural joint allows movement in the sagittal plane; therefore this motion is not transmitted up to the leg. However, because the talocrural joint does not allow any transverse plane rotation, when the talus now medially rotates or laterally rotates relative to the calcaneus in the transverse plane at the subtalar joint, the bones of the leg must move along with the talus; this results in a rotation of the leg and thigh[4] (Box 9-39).
- Summing up pronation and supination of the subtalar joint in a weight-bearing foot, we see that the calcaneus everts/inverts relative to the talus at the subtalar joint in the frontal plane, the talus dorsiflexes/plantarflexes relative to the tibia/fibula at the talocrural joint in the sagittal plane, and the talus and leg (fixed together) medially rotate/laterally rotate relative to the thigh at the knee joint or, more commonly, the talus/leg and thigh (fixed together) medially rotate/laterally rotate relative to the pelvis in the transverse plane at the hip joint (Box 9-40).

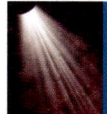

BOX 9-39 Spotlight on Reverse Action Rotations at the Subtalar Joint

When the weight-bearing foot pronates, the talus medially rotates relative to the fixed calcaneus. Because the talocrural joint does not allow rotation, the leg must medially rotate with the talus. Similarly, when the weight-bearing foot supinates, the talus laterally rotates, causing the leg to laterally rotate with it. These rotation movements of the leg will then create a rotation force/stress at the knee joint and may affect the health of the knee joint. Because more people overly pronate (which manifests as a flat foot on weight bearing) than overly supinate, the knee joint is often subjected to medial rotation stress from below.

Given that the knee joint does not allow rotation when it is extended, much of this (medial) rotation force will then be transmitted up to and affect the functioning and health of the hip joint. This can often be observed in a person by watching the orientation of the patella as the foot pronates (the patella follows the femur). In a client with excessive pronation, the patella is seen to rotate medially. For these reasons, the correction of an overly pronating foot may be extremely important toward correcting knee and hip joint problems. One solution to correct an overly pronating foot is to recommend orthotics to the client; another solution might be to recommend that the muscles of supination (i.e., inversion) of the foot at the subtalar joint be strengthened. A third is to strengthen the lateral rotation musculature of the hip joint. If these muscles are stronger, then they can help to decrease the degree of medial rotation of the thigh that occurs; this would, in turn, decrease the medial rotation of the leg and talus, thereby lessening the amount of pronation motion that occurs at the subtalar joint.

BOX 9-40

Pronation of the weight-bearing foot results in a visible drop of the arches of the foot. People who overly pronate during weight bearing are often said to be flatfooted. These people actually do have an arch when not weight bearing, but this arch is lost on weight bearing. For this reason, their condition is more accurately described as having a **supple flat foot**. A **rigid flat foot** is a foot that is flat all the time and is not a result of excessive pronation motion on weight bearing.

MAJOR LIGAMENTS OF THE SUBTALAR JOINT (BOX 9-41):

Fibrous Joint Capsule:

- The posterior aspect of the subtalar joint has its own distinct joint capsule.
- The anterior and middle aspects of the subtalar joint share a joint capsule with the talonavicular joint.[8]

Talocalcaneal Ligaments:

- Medial, lateral, posterior, and interosseus **talocalcaneal ligaments** exist (see Figures 9-36, *A* and *B*).
- They are located between the talus and calcaneus; their specific locations are indicated by their names.[8]
- The interosseous talocalcaneal ligament is located within the sinus tarsus of the subtalar joint; its function is to limit eversion (i.e., pronation) of the subtalar joint.

Cervical Ligament:

- Location: The **cervical ligament** is located within the sinus tarsus of the subtalar joint, running from the talus to the calcaneus (see Figure 9-36, *D*).
- Function: It limits inversion (i.e., supination) of the subtalar joint.[8]
- Note: The cervical ligament is named for its attachment onto the neck of the talus (*cervical* means *neck*).

Spring Ligament:

- The **spring ligament** is usually considered to be primarily important as a ligament of the transverse tarsal joint; however, it also helps to stabilize the subtalar joint (see Figure 9-36, *A* to *E*).
- Location: The spring ligament spans the subtalar joint inferiorly (on the plantar side).
- The spring ligament attaches from the calcaneus posteriorly to the navicular bone anteriorly.
  - More specifically, it attaches from the sustentaculum tali of the calcaneus to the navicular bone.[6]
- Function: It limits eversion (i.e., pronation) of the subtalar joint.
- Because of its attachment sites, the spring ligament is also known as the *plantar calcaneonavicular ligament*.

Medial Collateral Ligament of the Talocrural Joint:

- The **medial collateral ligament** is also known as the *deltoid ligament* (see Figure 9-36, *A*). (Note: For more information on the medial collateral ligament of the talocrural joint, see Section 9.18.)
- It limits eversion (i.e., pronation) of the subtalar joint.[8]

Lateral Collateral Ligament Complex of the Talocrural Joint:

- The lateral collateral ligament complex is composed of the anterior talofibular, posterior talofibular, and calcaneofibular ligaments (see Figure 9-36, *B*). (Note: For more information on the lateral collateral ligament of the talocrural joint, see Section 9.18.)
- It limits inversion (i.e., supination) of the subtalar joint.[8]

BOX 9-41 Ligaments of the Subtalar Joint

- Fibrous joint capsule(s)
- Talocalcaneal ligaments (medial, lateral, posterior, interosseus)
- Cervical ligament
- Spring ligament

Note: The medial collateral ligament and the lateral collateral ligament complex of the talocrural joint also help stabilize the subtalar joint.

CLOSED-PACKED POSITION OF THE SUBTALAR JOINT:

- Supination[3]

MISCELLANEOUS:

- It must be emphasized that in the weight-bearing foot, motion of the subtalar joint cannot occur in isolation. Its motion is intimately tied to the transverse tarsal joint and the talocrural joint, as well as every other joint of the foot, and the knee and hip joints.

SECTION 9.20 TRANSVERSE TARSAL JOINT

BONES:

- The transverse tarsal joint, as its name implies, runs transversely across the tarsal bones.
- The transverse tarsal joint is actually a compound joint, meaning that it is composed of two joints that are collectively called the *transverse tarsal joint*.
  - The two joints of the transverse tarsal joint are (1) the **talonavicular joint**, which is located between the talus and navicular bone, and (2) the **calcaneocuboid joint**, which is located between the calcaneus and cuboid[1] (Figure 9-41).
  - Of the two joints of the transverse tarsal joint, the talonavicular joint is much more mobile than the calcaneocuboid joint.[3]
  - Both of these joints are synovial joints.[8]
  - The talonavicular joint shares its joint capsule with one of the joint capsules of the subtalar joint.[3]
  - The calcaneocuboid joint has its own distinct joint capsule.
  - The transverse tarsal joint is also known as the *midtarsal* or **Chopart's joint**.[3]

MAJOR MOTIONS ALLOWED:

- Once the subtalar tarsal joint is understood, it is possible to simplify the discussion of the transverse tarsal joint.
- The motions possible at the transverse tarsal joint are pronation and supination[3] (which can be divided into their component cardinal plane actions as explained in Section 9.19).
- Any motion at the subtalar joint requires motion to occur at the transverse tarsal joint as well.
  - In fact, the named motions that occur at the subtalar joint are the same named motions that occur at the transverse tarsal joint.[8]

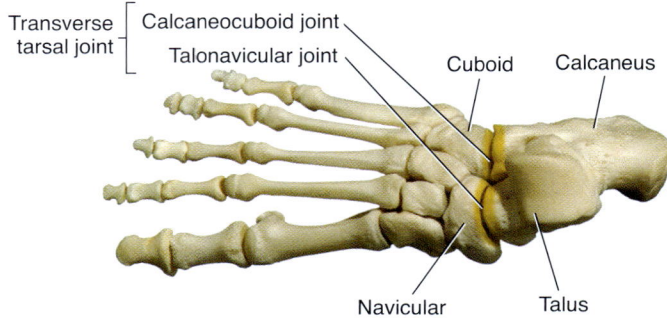

FIGURE 9-41 Dorsal view of the foot illustrating the transverse tarsal joint. The transverse tarsal joint is actually a joint complex composed of the talonavicular joint and the calcaneocuboid joint.

- The interrelationship between the subtalar and transverse tarsal joints can be understood by looking at the bones involved in each of these joints. The talus of the subtalar joint is also part of the talonavicular joint of the transverse tarsal joint; the calcaneus of the subtalar joint is also part of the calcaneocuboid joint of the transverse tarsal joint. Therefore movement of either the talus or the calcaneus requires movement at the transverse tarsal joint when these more distal navicular and cuboid bones are fixed in a weight-bearing foot.[8]
- In addition, recall that the subtalar joint has two joint capsules; of these, the anterior one is shared with the talonavicular joint of the transverse tarsal joint.
- Note: Because the talus shares a joint capsule with both the calcaneus and the navicular bone, and because motions of the subtalar and transverse tarsal joints are so intimately linked, some sources like to describe foot motion as occurring at the **talocalcaneonavicular (TCN) joint complex**.[8] Indeed, given the interrelationship of the cuboid of the transverse tarsal joint as well, one could describe foot motion as occurring at the **talocalcaneonaviculocuboid (TCNC) joint complex**!

LIGAMENTS OF THE TRANSVERSE TARSAL JOINT (BOX 9-42):

- A number of ligaments help to stabilize the transverse tarsal joint. By virtue of stabilizing the transverse tarsal joint, these ligaments also help to indirectly limit motion and thereby stabilize the subtalar joint. Ligaments of the transverse tarsal joint include the following[8]:
- The **spring ligament**: The spring ligament (covered in Section 9.19) literally forms the floor of the talonavicular joint (of the transverse tarsal joint) (see Figure 9-36, A and B).
    - The spring ligament is also known as the **plantar calcaneonavicular ligament**.
- The **long plantar ligament**: This ligament runs the length of the foot on the plantar side (see Figure 9-36, A, B, and E).

> **BOX 9-42** **Ligaments of the Transverse Tarsal Joint**
>
> - Fibrous joint capsule(s)
> - Spring ligament
> - Long plantar ligament
> - Short plantar ligament
> - Dorsal calcaneocuboid ligament
> - Bifurcate ligament
>   - Calcaneonavicular ligament
>   - Calcaneocuboid ligament

- The **short plantar ligament**: This ligament runs deep to the long plantar ligament on the plantar side of the foot between the calcaneus and the cuboid (see Figure 9-36, A, B, and E).
    - The short plantar ligament is also known as the **plantar calcaneocuboid ligament**.
- The **dorsal calcaneocuboid ligament**: This ligament is located between the calcaneus and cuboid on the dorsal side (see Figure 9-36, B).
- The **bifurcate ligament**: This Y-shaped ligament is located on the dorsal side of the foot (see Figure 9-36, B).
    - Its medial band attaches from the calcaneus to the navicular bone. Its lateral band attaches from the calcaneus to the cuboid.
    - The medial band is also known as the lateral **calcaneonavicular ligament**.
    - The lateral band is also known as the **calcaneocuboid ligament**.

CLOSED-PACKED POSITION OF THE TRANSVERSE TARSAL JOINT:

- Supination[3]

SECTION 9.21 TARSOMETATARSAL (TMT) JOINTS

BONES:

- The tarsometatarsal (TMT) joints are located between the distal row of tarsal bones and the metatarsal bones.
- Five TMT joints exist (Figure 9-42):
    1. The first TMT joint is located between the first cuneiform and the base of the first metatarsal.
    2. The second TMT joint is located between the second cuneiform and the base of the second metatarsal.
    3. The third TMT joint is located between the third cuneiform and the base of the third metatarsal.
    4. The fourth TMT joint is located between the cuboid and the base of the fourth metatarsal.
    5. The fifth TMT joint is located between the cuboid and the base of the fifth metatarsal.
- Each metatarsal and its associated phalanges make up a ray of the foot.[4]
- The TMT joints are plane synovial joints.[8]
- Only the first TMT joint has a well-developed joint capsule.
- The second and third TMT joints share a joint capsule.[8]

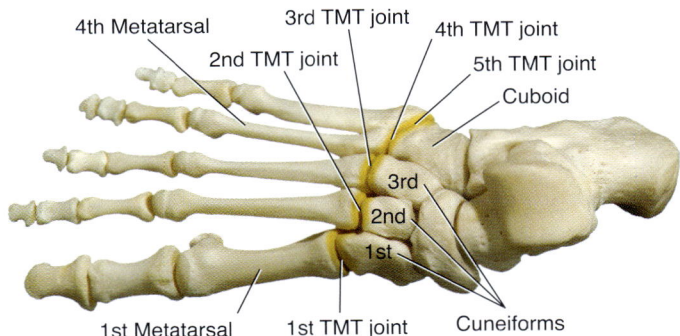

FIGURE 9-42 Dorsal view that illustrates the tarsometatarsal (TMT) joints of the foot. As the name indicates, TMT joints are located between the tarsal bones and the metatarsal bones. The TMT joints are numbered from the medial to the lateral side of the foot as MTP joints #1 through #5.

- The fourth and fifth TMT joints share a joint capsule.[8]
  - The base of the second metatarsal is set back farther posteriorly than the other metatarsal bones, causing it to be wedged between the first and third cuneiforms. This position of the second metatarsal decreases mobility of the second TMT joint. Therefore the second TMT joint is the most stable of the five TMT joints.[8] As a result, the second ray of the foot is the **central stable pillar** of the foot.
  - Because the second ray of the foot is the most stable of the five rays, an imaginary line through it (when it is in anatomic position) is the reference line for abduction and adduction of the toes. In the hand, the third ray is the most stable and is the reference line for abduction and adduction of the fingers.
- The more peripheral rays are the most mobile.
  - The first ray is the most mobile, followed by the fifth, fourth, third, and second rays (in that order).

MAJOR MOTIONS ALLOWED:

- The TMT joints allow dorsiflexion/plantarflexion and inversion/eversion.[4]
  - Dorsiflexion occurs when the distal end of the metatarsal moves dorsally; plantarflexion is the opposite motion.
  - Inversion occurs when the plantar side of the ray turns inward (i.e., medially) toward the midline of the body; eversion is the opposite action.
- These motions of the metatarsal bones at the TMT joints are important for allowing the foot to conform to the uneven surfaces of the ground on which we stand and walk.[3]
- When the metatarsals dorsiflex at the metatarsal joints, the first ray inverts and the third to fifth rays evert, and the foot flattens to meet the ground. When the metatarsals plantarflex, the first ray everts and the third to fifth rays invert, and the arch contour of the foot raises, allowing the foot to mold around a raised surface.[2]
- In addition to the fibrous joint capsules, the TMT joints are stabilized by **tarsometatarsal ligaments**[8] (see Figure 9-36, A, B, and E, and Box 9-43).
  - Dorsal, plantar, and interosseus TMT ligaments exist.

BOX 9-43 **Ligaments of the Tarsometatarsal Joint**

- Fibrous joint capsule
- Tarsometatarsal (TMT) ligaments (dorsal, plantar, and interosseus)

SECTION 9.22 INTERMETATARSAL (IMT) JOINTS

BONES AND LIGAMENTS:

- Intermetatarsal (IMT) joints are located between the metatarsal bones of the foot (Figure 9-43).
  - Proximal intermetatarsal joints and distal intermetatarsal joints exist.
- All five metatarsal bones articulate with one another, both proximally at their bases and distally at their heads.
- The proximal intermetatarsal joint between the big toe and the second toe is usually not well formed. Although ligaments are present, the joint cavity is usually not fully formed.[8]

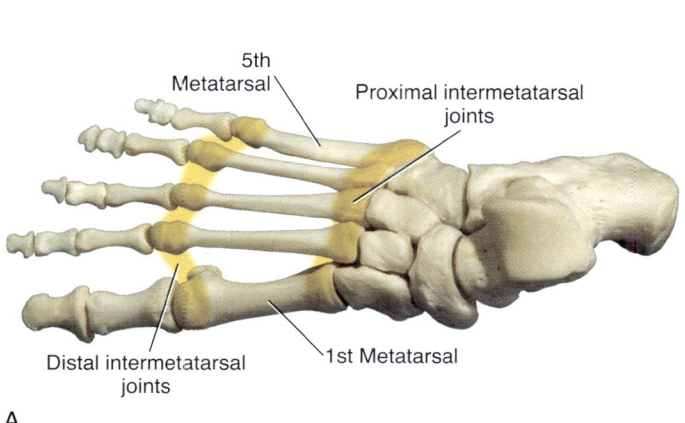
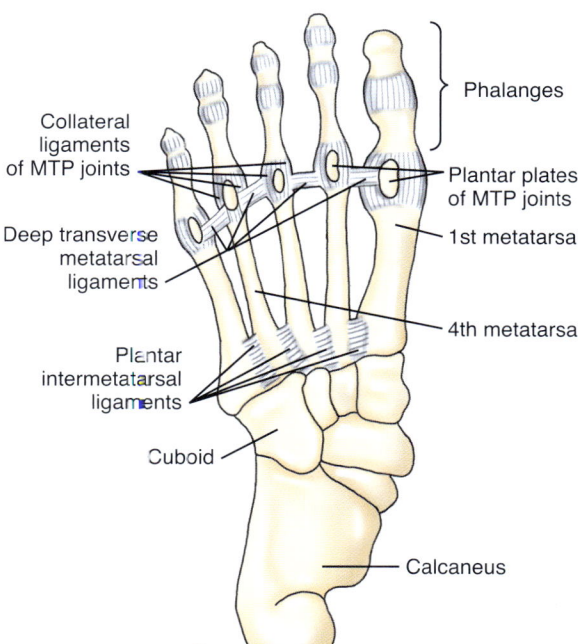

FIGURE 9-43 Intermetatarsal joints of the foot (i.e., proximal and distal intermetatarsal joints). As the name indicates, intermetatarsal joints are located between metatarsal bones. **A,** Dorsal view. **B,** Plantar view illustrates the ligaments of the plantar surface of the forefoot.

CHAPTER 9 Joints of the Lower Extremity

- The proximal intermetatarsal joints are stabilized by their fibrous joint capsules and **intermetatarsal ligaments**[16] (see Figures 9-36, B and 8-43, B).
  - Dorsal, plantar, and interosseous intermetatarsal ligaments connect the base of each metatarsal to the base of the adjacent metatarsal(s).
- The distal intermetatarsal joints are stabilized by their joint capsules and **deep transverse metatarsal ligaments**[16] (see Figure 9-43, B).
- The deep transverse metatarsal ligaments that connect the distal ends of the metatarsals to each other hold the big toe in the same plane as the other toes; therefore the big toe cannot be opposed. In the hand, the deep transverse metacarpal ligaments connect only the index through little fingers, leaving the thumb free to be opposable. Therefore the foot is designed primarily for weight bearing and propulsion, whereas the hand is designed primarily for manipulation (i.e., fine motion). In theory, the only major difference between the potential coordination of the hand and the foot is the ability to oppose digits.

BOX 9-44 Ligaments of the Intermetatarsal Joints

- Fibrous joint capsules
- Intermetatarsal ligaments (dorsal, plantar, and interosseus)
- Deep transverse metatarsal ligaments

MAJOR MOTIONS ALLOWED:

- These intermetatarsal joints are plane synovial articulations that allow nonaxial gliding motion of one metatarsal relative to the adjacent metatarsal(s).
- Because motion at a TMT joint requires the metatarsal bone to move relative to the adjacent metatarsal bone(s), intermetatarsal joints are functionally related to TMT joints.

SECTION 9.23 METATARSOPHALANGEAL (MTP) JOINTS

BONES:

- The MTP joints are located between the metatarsals and the phalanges of the toes.
  - More specifically, they are located between the heads of the metatarsals and the bases of the proximal phalanges of the toes.
- Five MTP joints exist (Figure 9-44):
  1. The first MTP joint is located between the first metatarsal and the proximal phalanx of the big (first) toe.
  2. The second MTP joint is located between the second metatarsal and the proximal phalanx of the second toe.
  3. The third MTP joint is located between the third metatarsal and the proximal phalanx of the third toe.
  4. The fourth MTP joint is located between the fourth metatarsal and the proximal phalanx of the fourth toe.
  5. The fifth MTP joint is located between the fifth metatarsal and the proximal phalanx of the little (fifth) toe.
- Joint structure classification: Synovial joint[3]
  - Subtype: Condyloid
- Joint function classification: Diarthrotic
  - Subtype: Biaxial[2]

MAJOR MOTIONS ALLOWED:

The average ranges of sagittal plane motion of the toes at the MTP joints are given in Table 9-6 (Figure 9-45).

- The MTP joint allows flexion and extension (axial movements) within the sagittal plane around a mediolateral axis[3].
- The MTP joint allows abduction and adduction (axial movements)[3].
- The sagittal plane motions of flexion and extension of the toes at the metatarsophalangeal (MTP) joints is much more important than the actions of abduction and adduction of the toes at the MTP joints. Most people have very poor motor control of abduction and adduction of their toes.[4]
- Normally, abduction and adduction movements occur within the frontal plane around an anteroposterior axis. However, because the foot is oriented perpendicular to the leg, abduction and adduction of the toes occur within the transverse plane around a vertical axis.
- The reference for abduction/adduction of the toes at the MTP joints is an imaginary line drawn through the second toe when it is in anatomic position.[4] Movement toward this imaginary line is adduction; movement away from it is abduction.
- Because transverse plane movement of the second toe in either direction is away from this imaginary line, both directions of movement are termed *abduction*. Lateral movement of the second toe is termed *fibular abduction*; medial movement of the second toe is termed *tibial abduction*.

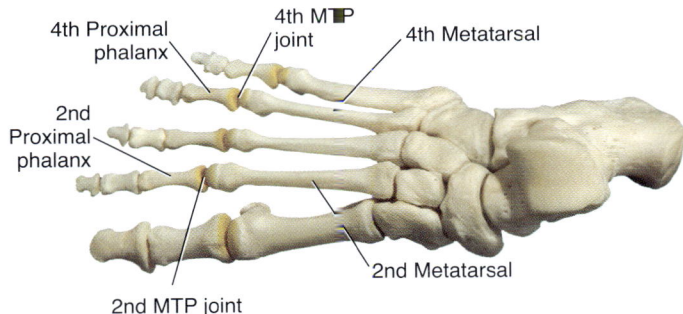

FIGURE 9-44 Dorsal view illustrating the metatarsophalangeal (MTP) joints of the foot. Five MTP joints are located between the metatarsals and the proximal phalanges of each ray of the foot. They are numbered from the medial (i.e., big toe) side to the lateral (i.e., little toe) side as MTP joints #1 through #5.

TABLE 9-6 Average Ranges of Sagittal Plane Motion of the Toes at the Metatarsophalangeal (MTP) Joints[4]

Toes #2-5			
Extension	60 Degrees	Flexion	40 Degrees
Big Toe (Toe #1)			
Extension	80 Degrees	Flexion	40 Degrees

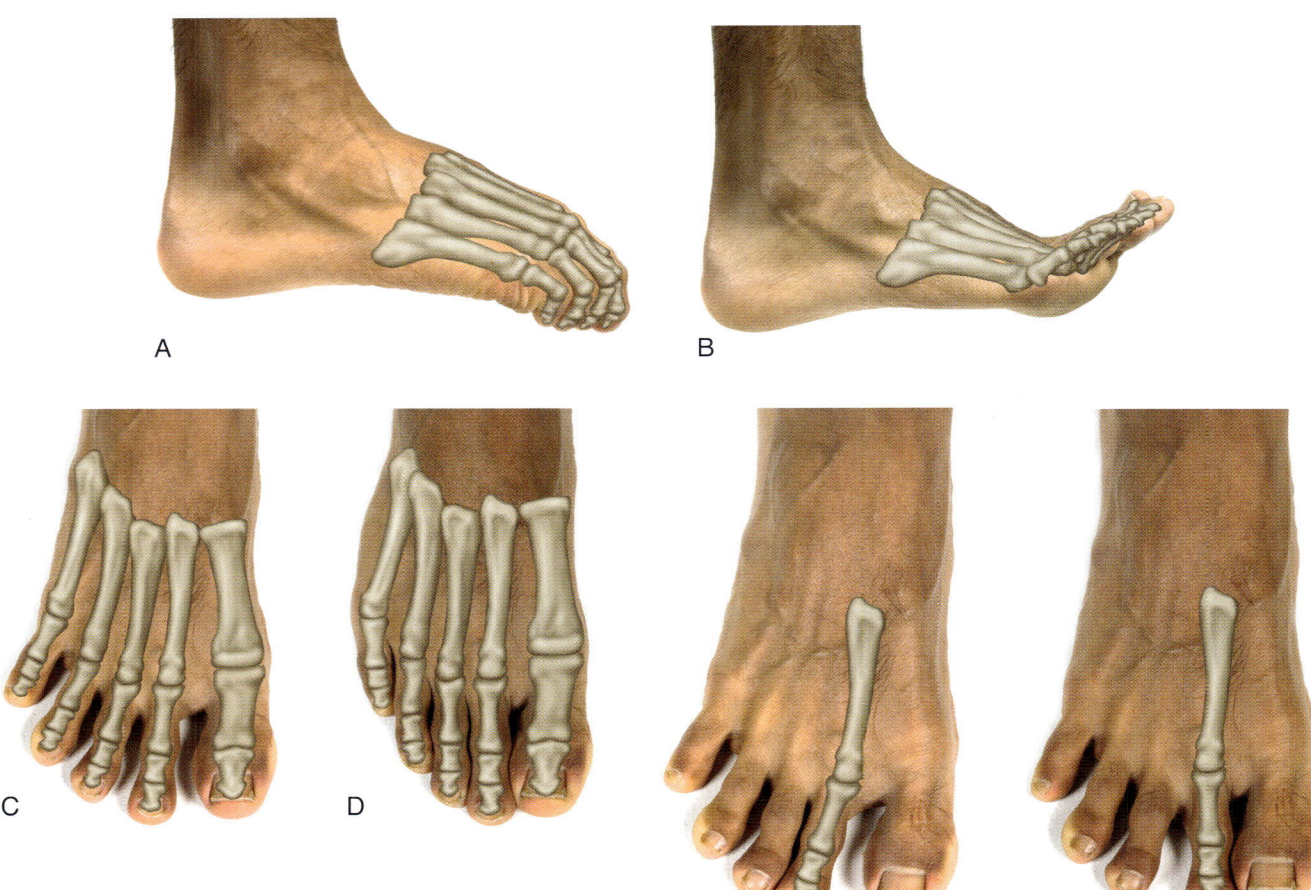

FIGURE 9-45 Motion of the toes at the metatarsophalangeal (MTP) joints **A** and **B**, flexion and extension of the toes respectively (at both the MTP and interphalangeal [IP] joints). **C** and **D**, abduction and adduction of the toes at the MTP joints. The reference line for abduction and adduction of the toes is an imaginary line through the center of the second toe when it is in anatomic position. Toes #1, #3, #4, and #5 abduct away from the second toe and adduct toward it. The second toe abducts in either direction it moves. **E,** Fibular abduction of the second toe at the MTP joint. **F,** Tibial abduction of the second toe at the MTP joint.

Reverse Actions:

- The muscles of the MTP joints are generally considered to move the more distal (proximal phalanx of the) toe relative to a fixed metatarsal bone. However, closed-chain activities are common in the lower extremity in which the foot is planted on the ground; this fixes the toes and requires that the metatarsals (and the entire foot) move relative to the toes instead. This reverse action of the MTP joints occurs every time we "toe-off" when we walk or run; our toes stay fixed on the ground and our foot hinges at the MTP joints instead, allowing the heel to rise off the ground.

LIGAMENTS OF THE METATARSOPHALANGEAL JOINTS (BOX 9-45):

Fibrous Joint Capsule:

- The capsule of the MTP joint is stabilized by collateral ligaments and the plantar plate[8] (Figure 9-46).

> **BOX 9-45** Ligaments of the Metatarsophalangeal Joint
>
> - Fibrous joint capsule
> - Medial collateral ligament
> - Lateral collateral ligament
> - Plantar plate

Collateral Ligaments:

- The **medial collateral ligament** and the **lateral collateral ligament** are thickenings of the joint capsule and are located on their respective side of the MTP joint.[8]

Plantar Plate[3]:

- The **plantar plate** is a thick, dense, fibrous tissue structure located on the plantar side of the MTP joint.
- The plantar plate's main function is to protect the head of the metatarsal during walking.

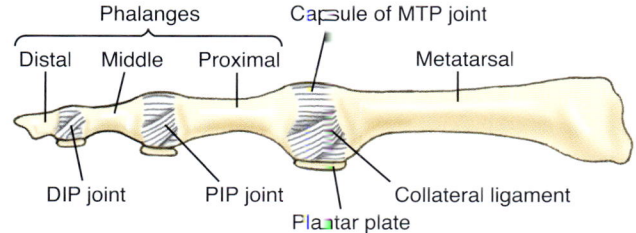

FIGURE 9-46 Fibrous capsule, collateral ligament, and plantar plate of the metatarsophalangeal (MTP) joint. (Note: These structures are also illustrated for the proximal interphalangeal [PIP] and distal interphalangeal [DIP] joints.)

❍ This is necessary because when the foot pushes off the ground, the metatarsal moves relative to the toe, exposing the articular surface of the head of the metatarsal to the ground. The plantar plate is placed between the head of the metatarsal and the ground.

CLOSED-PACKED POSITION OF THE METATARSOPHALANGEAL JOINT:

❍ Extension

MAJOR MUSCLES OF THE METATARSOPHALANGEAL JOINT:

❍ The MTP joint is crossed by both extrinsic muscles (that originate on the leg) and intrinsic muscles (wholly located within the foot).
❍ Major flexors include the flexors digitorum and hallucis longus, flexors digitorum and hallucis brevis, quadratus plantae, and flexor digiti minimi pedis, as well as the lumbricals pedis, plantar interossei, and dorsal interossei pedis.
❍ Major extensors include the extensors digitorum and hallucis longus and the extensors digitorum and hallucis brevis.
❍ Major adductors are the plantar interossei and the adductor hallucis.
❍ Major abductors are the dorsal interossei pedis, as well as the abductor hallucis and abductor digiti minimi pedis.

MISCELLANEOUS:

❍ The MTP joints are analogous to the metacarpophalangeal (MCP) joints of the hands. However, most people do not learn the same fine motor control of the toes of the foot as they have at the fingers of the hand.
❍ **Hallux valgus** is a deformity of the big toe in which the big toe (i.e., the hallux) deviates laterally (in the valgus direction) at the MTP joint[6] (Box 9-46).
  ❍ Hallux valgus also usually involves a medial deviation of the first metatarsal.[6]

 BOX 9-46

Hallux valgus, which is a lateral deviation of the big toe of the foot, may occur as a result of a genetic predisposition in certain individuals. However, overly pronated feet and incorrect footwear (high heels and/or shoes with a triangular front [i.e., toe box] that pushes the big toe laterally) seem certain to cause and/or accelerate this condition!

❍ The deformity of hallux valgus exposes the head of the first metatarsal to greater stress, resulting in inflammation of the bursa located there. In time this leads to fibrosis and excessive bone growth on the medial (and perhaps dorsal) side of the first metatarsal's head; this is called a **bunion**.[6]

SECTION 9.24 INTERPHALANGEAL (IP) JOINTS OF THE FOOT

❍ Interphalangeal (IP) joints pedis (i.e., of the foot) are located between phalanges of the toes (Figure 9-47).
  ❍ More specifically, each IP joint is located between the head of the more proximal phalanx and the base of the more distal phalanx.
  ❍ When motion occurs at an interphalangeal (IP) joint of the foot, we can say that a toe has moved at the proximal interphalangeal (PIP) or distal interphalangeal (DIP) joint. To be more specific, we could say that the distal phalanx moved at the DIP joint and/or that the middle phalanx moved at the PIP joint.[4]
  ❍ Note: IP joints are found in both the foot and the hand. To distinguish these joints from each other, the words *pedis* (denoting *foot*) and *manus* (denoting *hand*) are used.
❍ The big toe has one IP joint. It is located between the proximal and distal phalanges of the big toe.
❍ Because toes #2 to #5 each have three phalanges, two IP joints are found in each of these toes.
  ❍ The IP joint located between the proximal and middle phalanges is called the *PIP joint* (pedis).

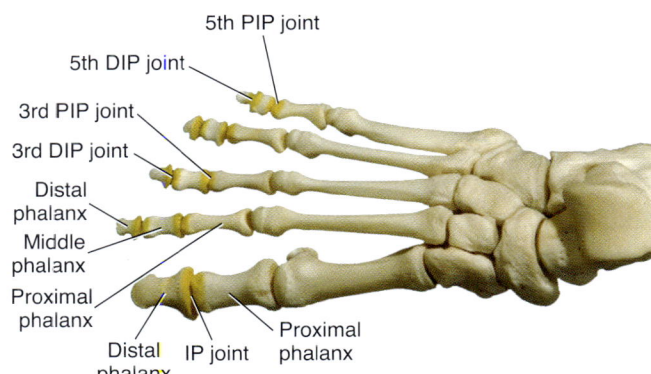

FIGURE 9-47 Dorsal view that illustrates the interphalangeal (IP) joints of the foot. Except for the big toe, which has only one IP joint, each toe has two IP joints: (1) the proximal interphalangeal (PIP) joint and (2) the distal interphalangeal (DIP) joint. Furthermore, the IP joints are numbered #1 to #5 from the medial (i.e., big toe) side to the lateral (i.e., little toe) side (Note: In this photo, the fifth DIP joint [of the little toe] has fused.)

- The IP joint located between the middle and distal phalanges is called the *DIP joint* (pedis).
- In total, nine IP joints are found in the foot (one IP, four PIPs, and four DIPs).
- Joint structure classification: Synovial joint[8]
  - Subtype: Hinge
- Joint function classification: Diarthrotic
- Subtype: Uniaxial

MAJOR MOTIONS ALLOWED:

- The average ranges of motion of the toes at the IP joints are given in Box 9-47 (see Figure 9-45 in Section 9.23).
- The IP joints allow flexion and extension (i.e., axial movements) within the sagittal plane around a mediolateral axis.[8]

BOX 9-47 Average Ranges of Motion of the Interphalangeal (IP) Joints[3]

Proximal Interphalangeal (PIP) Joints
- From a neutral position, flexion of the proximal interphalangeal (PIP) joints (and the IP joint of the big toe) is limited to approximately 90 degrees and tends to be less in the more lateral toes.
- From a neutral position, the PIP joints (and the IP joint of the big toe) do not allow any further extension.

Distal Interphalangeal (DIP) Joints
- From a neutral position, flexion of the distal interphalangeal (DIP) joints is limited to approximately 45 degrees and tends to be less in the more lateral toes.
- From a neutral position, the DIP joints do allow a small amount of further extension (i.e., hyperextension).

Reverse Actions:

- The muscles of the IP joints are generally considered to move the more distal phalanx of a toe relative to the more proximal one. However, it is possible to move the more proximal phalanx relative to the more distal one.

LIGAMENTS OF THE INTERPHALANGEAL JOINTS OF THE FOOT (BOX 9-48):

As in the MTP joints, each IP joint has a capsule that is thickened and stabilized by medial and lateral collateral ligaments; plantar plates are also present.[8] These structures are usually not as well developed as they are in the MTP joints (see Figure 9-46).

BOX 9-48 Ligaments of the Interphalangeal Joints

- Fibrous capsules
- Medial collateral ligaments
- Lateral collateral ligaments
- Plantar plates

CLOSED-PACKED POSITION OF THE INTERPHALANGEAL JOINTS OF THE FOOT:

- Extension

MAJOR MUSCLES OF THE INTERPHALANGEAL JOINTS:

- The IP joints are crossed by both extrinsic and intrinsic muscles of the foot.
- Major flexors include the flexors digitorum and hallucis longus and the flexor digitorum brevis, as well as the quadratus plantae.
- Major extensors include the extensors digitorum and hallucis longus, the extensor digitorum brevis, and the lumbricals pedis, plantar interossei, and the dorsal interossei pedis. (Some of the aforementioned muscles do not cross the DIP joint.)

MISCELLANEOUS:

- Other than the fact that toes are quite a bit shorter than fingers, the IP joints of the foot are analogous to the IP joints of the hand. However, most people do not learn the same fine motor control of the toes of the foot as they have at the fingers of the hand.[6]

REVIEW QUESTIONS

Answers to the following review questions appear on the Evolve website accompanying this book at: http://evolve.elsevier.com/Muscolino/kinesiology/.

1. When intrapelvic motion occurs, at what joint(s) does it occur?

2. When motion of the pelvis occurs relative to an adjacent body part, this motion occurs at what joint(s)?

3. What name is given to the motion of the sacrum wherein the sacral base drops anteriorly and inferiorly?

4. What are the names given to the transverse plane motions of the pelvis at the lumbosacral joint?

5. What are the names given to the sagittal plane motions of the pelvis at the hip joint?

6. A muscle that can perform lateral flexion of the trunk at the lumbosacral joint can perform what action of the pelvis at the lumbosacral joint?

7. A muscle that can perform lateral rotation of the thigh at the hip joint can perform what action of the pelvis at the hip joint?

8. What effect does an excessively anteriorly tilted pelvis usually have on the lumbar spine?

9. What are the three major ligaments that stabilize the hip joint?

10. Why are closed-chain activities more common in the lower extremities?

11. What are the two major angulations of the femur?

12. According to the usual coordination of femoropelvic rhythm, which pelvic action accompanies flexion of the thigh at the hip joint?

13. What joint actions are possible at the tibiofemoral joint?

14. What motions are limited by the medial and lateral collateral ligaments of the knee joint?

15. What is the major purpose of the patella?

16. What is abduction of the tibia (in the frontal plane) relative to the femur called?

17. What does the Q-angle of the knee joint measure?

18. Name the three tibiofibular joints.

19. What defines a ray of the foot?

20. Name the three arches of the foot.

21. What is the function of the retinacula of the ankle joint?

22. What is the name of the ankle joint ligament that limits eversion?

23. What two oblique plane motions are allowed at the subtalar joint?

24. To what two bones does the spring ligament of the foot attach?

25. The transverse tarsal joint is composed of what two joints?

26. What two bones articulate at the fourth TMT joint?

27. Which ray is the central stable pillar of the foot?

28. Name the two ligaments that stabilize the intermetatarsal joints.

29. What position of the MTP joint increases the height of the arch and the rigidity of the foot (via the windlass mechanism)?

30. Where are plantar plates of the foot located?

REFERENCES

1. Smith LK, Weiss EL, Lehmkuhl LO: Brunstrom's clinical kinesiology, ed 5, Philadelphia, 1996, FA Davis.
2. Hamill J, Knutzen KM: Biomechanical basis of human movement, ed 12, Baltimore, 2003, Lippincott Williams & Wilkins.
3. Oatis CA: Kinesiology: The mechanics & pathomechanics of human movement, Philadelphia, 2004, Lippincott Williams & Wilkins.
4. Neumann DA: Kinesiology of the musculoskeletal system: Foundations for physical rehabilitation, ed 3, St Louis, 2017, Elsevier.
5. Cramer GD, Darby SA: Basic and clinical anatomy of the spine, spinal cord, and ANS, Missouri, 1995, Mosby.
6. Levangie PK, Norkin CC: Joint structure and function: A comprehensive analysis, ed 5, Philadelphia, 2011, FA Davis.
7. Shumway-Cook A, Woollacott MH: Motor control: Translating research into clinical practice, ed 4, Baltimore, 2012, Lippincott Williams & Wilkins.
8. Palastanga N, Field D, Soames R: Anatomy and human movement, ed 4, Oxford, 2002, Butterworth-Heinemann.
9. Behnke RS: Kinetic anatomy, ed 2, Champaign, IL, 2006, Human Kinetics.
10. Hamilton N, Weimar W, Luttgens K: Kinesiology: Scientific basis of human motion, ed 12, New York, 2012, McGraw Hill.
11. Hall SJ: Basic biomechanics, ed 6, New York, 2012, McGraw Hill.
12. Thibodeau GA, Patton KT: Anatomy & physiology, ed 5, St Louis, 2003, Mosby.
13. Watkins J: Structure and function of the musculoskeletal system, Champaign, IL, 1999, Human Kinetics.
14. Werner R: A massage therapist's guide to pathology, ed 4, Philadelphia, 2004, Lippincott Williams & Wilkins.
15. Nordin M, Frankel VH: Basic biomechanics of the musculoskeletal system, ed 3, Baltimore, 2001, Lippincott Williams & Wilkins.
16. Netter FH: Atlas of human anatomy, ed 3, Teterboro, NJ, 2004, Icon Learning Systems.

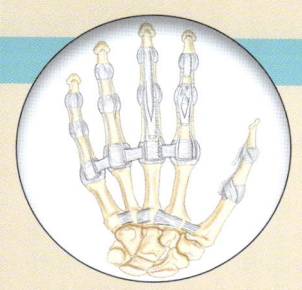

CHAPTER 10
Joints of the Upper Extremity

CHAPTER OUTLINE

Section 10.1	Shoulder Joint Complex	Section 10.10	Overview of the Wrist/Hand Region
Section 10.2	Glenohumeral Joint	Section 10.11	Wrist Joint Complex
Section 10.3	Scapulocostal Joint	Section 10.12	Carpometacarpal Joints
Section 10.4	Sternoclavicular Joint	Section 10.13	Saddle (Carpometacarpal) Joint of the Thumb
Section 10.5	Acromioclavicular Joint		
Section 10.6	Scapulohumeral Rhythm	Section 10.14	Intermetacarpal Joints
Section 10.7	Elbow Joint Complex	Section 10.15	Metacarpophalangeal Joints
Section 10.8	Elbow Joint	Section 10.16	Interphalangeal Joints of the Hand
Section 10.9	Radioulnar Joints		

CHAPTER OBJECTIVES

After completing this chapter the student should be able to perform the following:

1. Define the key terms of this chapter and state the meanings of the word origins of this chapter.
2. Do the following related to the shoulder joint complex:
   - Explain why the term shoulder joint complex is a better term than shoulder joint when describing movement of the shoulder.
   - Describe why the term shoulder corset might be a better term than shoulder girdle.
3. Describe the concepts of mobility and stability as they pertain to the glenohumeral joint, and explain why the glenohumeral joint is often called a muscular joint.
4. Explain why the scapulocostal joint is considered to be a functional joint, not an anatomic joint.
5. Do the following related to the sternoclavicular joint:
   - Explain why stabilization of the sternoclavicular joint is important toward proper functioning of the upper extremity.
   - Describe why the sternoclavicular joint can be classified as either biaxial or triaxial.
6. Describe the importance of acromioclavicular joint motion to motion of the shoulder girdle.
7. Explain the concept of scapulohumeral rhythm, and give an example for each of the six cardinal ranges of motion of the arm at the glenohumeral joint.
8. Discuss the elbow joint and the elbow joint complex, as well as describe the concept and importance of the carrying angle.
9. Describe the component motions that occur at the proximal and distal radioulnar joints that create pronation and supination of the forearm.
10. Do the following related to the wrist/hand region:
    - Describe the structure and function of the hand.
    - Describe the structure and function of the wrist, and specifically the carpal tunnel.
11. Discuss the wrist joint complex, and explain why the radiocarpal joint is the major articulation between the forearm and the hand.
12. List the five carpometacarpal joints and describe the importance of motion at the fourth and fifth carpometacarpal joints.
13. Describe the importance of motion at the first carpometacarpal joint (i.e., saddle joint of the thumb) and describe the component actions of opposition and reposition of the thumb.
14. Discuss the similarities and differences between the metacarpophalangeal joints and the interphalangeal joints.
15. Discuss the interphalangeal joints of the hand.

▶ Indicates a video demonstration is available for this concept.

OVERVIEW

Chapters 5 and 6 laid the theoretic basis for the structure and function of joints; this chapter concludes our study of the regional approach of the structure and function of the joints of the body that began in Chapters 7 and 8. This chapter addresses the joints of the upper extremity. Whereas the lower extremity is primarily concerned with weight bearing and propulsion of the body through space, the major purpose of the upper extremity is to place the hand in desired positions and to move the hand as necessary to perform whatever tasks are required. Toward that end, the many joints of the upper extremity must work together to achieve these goals. Thus there is an intimate linkage among the joints of the shoulder complex, elbow/forearm, wrist, hand, and fingers. Sections 10.1 through 10.5 concern themselves with an examination of the joints of the shoulder joint complex; Section 10.6 then completes the study of the shoulder joint complex with an in-depth exploration of the concept of scapulohumeral rhythm. Sections 10.7 through 10.9 address the joints of the elbow complex and forearm joints. Sections 10.10 through 10.16 then complete our tour of the upper extremity by examining the joints of the wrist complex and hand.

KEY TERMS

Acromioclavicular joint (a-KROM-ee-o-kla-VIK-you-lar)
Acromioclavicular ligament
Anatomic joint (an-a-TOM-ik)
Annular ligament (AN-you-lar)
Anterior oblique ligament
Anterior sternoclavicular ligament (STERN-o-kla-VIK-you-lar)
Arches (of the hand)
Basilar arthritis (BAZE-i-lar)
Bone spurs
Carpal tunnel (CAR-pal)
Carpal tunnel syndrome
Carpometacarpal joints (CAR-po-MET-a-car-pal)
Carpometacarpal ligaments
Carpus (CAR-pus)
Carrying angle
Central pillar of the hand
Check-rein ligaments (CHEK-RAIN)
Conoid ligament (CONE-oyd)
Coracoacromial arch (kor-AK-o-a-KROM-ee-al)
Coracoacromial ligament
Coracoclavicular ligament (kor-AK-o-kla-VIK-you-lar)
Coracohumeral ligament (kor-AK-o-HUME-er-al)
Costoclavicular ligament (COST-o-kla-VIK-you-lar)
Coupled movement
Cubitus valgus (CUE-bi-tus VAL-gus)
Cubitus varus (VAR-us)
De Quervain's disease (de Quervain's stenosing tenosynovitis)
Deep transverse metacarpal ligaments (MET-a-CAR-pal)
Degenerative joint disease (DJD)
Distal interphalangeal (DIP) joint (of the hand) (IN-ter-FA-lan-GEE-al)
Distal radioulnar joint (RAY-dee-o-UL-nar)
Distal transverse arch
Dorsal carpometacarpal ligaments (CAR-po-MET-a-car-pal)
Dorsal digital expansion
Dorsal hood
Dorsal intercarpal ligament (IN-ter-CAR-pal)
Dorsal intermetacarpal ligaments (IN-ter-MET-a-CAR-pal)
Dorsal radiocarpal ligament (RAY-dee-o-CAR-pal)
Dorsal radioulnar ligament (RAY-dee-o-UL-nar)
Double-jointed
Downward tilt
Extensor expansion
Extrinsic ligaments (of the wrist)
First (1st) intermetacarpal ligament (IN-ter-MET-a-CAR-pal)
Flexor retinaculum (of the wrist) (ret-i-NAK-you-lum)
Foramen of Weitbrecht (VITE-brecht)
Functional joint
Glenohumeral joint (GLEN-o-HUME-er-al)
Glenohumeral ligaments
Glenoid labrum (GLEN-oyd)
Golfer's elbow
Heberden's nodes (HE-ber-denz)
Humeroradial joint (HUME-er-o-RAY-dee-al)
Humeroulnar joint (HUME-er-o-UL-nar)
Inferior acromioclavicular ligament (a-KROM-ee-o-kla-VIK-you-lar)
Inferior glenohumeral ligament (GLEN-o-HUME-er-al)
Intercarpal joints (IN-ter-CAR-pal)
Interclavicular ligament (IN-ter-kla-VIK-you-lar)
Intermetacarpal joints (IN-ter-MET-a-CAR-pal)
Intermetacarpal ligaments
Interosseus carpometacarpal ligaments (IN-ter-OS-ee-us CAR-po-MET-a-CAR-pal)
Interosseus intermetacarpal ligaments (IN-ter-MET-a-CAR-pal)
Interosseus membrane (of the forearm) (IN-ter-OS-ee-us)
Interphalangeal joints (manus) (IN-ter-fa-lan-GEE-al)
Intertendinous connections (IN-ter-TEN-din-us)
Intrinsic ligaments (of the wrist)
Lateral collateral ligament (of the elbow joint)
Lateral epicondylitis (EP-ee-KON-di-LITE-us)
Lateral epicondylosis (EP-ee-KON-di-LOS-us)
Lateral tilt
Longitudinal arch
Medial collateral ligament (of the elbow joint)
Medial epicondylitis (EP-ee-KON-di-LITE-us)
Medial epicondylosis (EP-ee-KON-di-LOS-us)
Medial tilt
Metacarpal ligaments (MET-a-CAR-pal)
Metacarpophalangeal (MCP) joints (MET-a-CAR-po-FA-lan-GEE-al)

Metacarpus (MET-a-CAR-pus)
Midcarpal joint (MID-CAR-pal)
Middle glenohumeral ligament (GLEN-o-HUME-er-al)
Middle radioulnar joint (RAY-dee-o-UL-nar)
Muscular joint
Oblique cord
Osteoarthritis (OST-ee-o-ar-THRI-tis)
Palm
Palmar carpometacarpal ligaments (CAR-po-MET-a-CAR-pal)
Palmar fascia (FASH-a)
Palmar intercarpal ligament (IN-ter-CAR-pal)
Palmar intermetacarpal ligaments (IN-ter-MET-a-CAR-pal)
Palmar plate
Palmar radiocarpal ligaments (RAY-dee-o-CAR-pal)
Palmar radioulnar ligament (RAY-dee-o-UL-nar)
Pectoral girdle (PEK-tor-al)
Posterior oblique ligament
Posterior sternoclavicular ligament (STERN-o-kla-VIK-you-lar)
Proximal interphalangeal (PIP) joint (of the hand) (IN-ter-FA-lan-GEE-al)
Proximal radioulnar joint (RAY-dee-o-UL-nar)
Proximal transverse arch
Radial collateral ligament (of the elbow joint)
Radial collateral ligament (of the interphalangeal joints manus)
Radial collateral ligament (of the metacarpophalangeal joint)
Radial collateral ligament (of the thumb's saddle joint)
Radial collateral ligament (of the wrist joint)
Radiocapitate ligament (RAY-dee-o-KAP-i-tate)
Radiocapitular joint (RAY-dee-o-ka-PICH-you-lar)
Radiocarpal joint (RAY-dee-o-CAR-pal)
Radiolunate ligament (RAY-dee-o-LOON-ate)
Radioscapholunate ligament (RAY-dee-o-SKAF-o-LOON-ate)
Radioulnar disc (RAY-dee-o-UL-nar)
Radioulnar joints
Ray

Rheumatoid arthritis (ROOM-a-toyd ar-THRI-tis)
Saddle joint (of the thumb)
Scapuloclaviculohumeral rhythm (SKAP-you-lo-kla-VIK-you-lo-HUME-er-al)
Scapulocostal joint (SKAP-you-lo-COST-al)
Scapulohumeral rhythm (SKAP-you-lo-HUME-er-al)
Scapulothoracic joint (SKAP-you-lo-thor-AS-ik)
Shoulder corset
Shoulder girdle
Shoulder impingement syndrome
Shoulder joint complex
Sternoclavicular joint (STERN-o-kla-VIK-you-lar)
Sternoclavicular ligaments
Subacromial bursa (SUB-a-CHROME-ee-al)
Subdeltoid bursa (SUB-DELT-oyd)
Superior acromioclavicular ligament (a-KROM-ee-o-kla-VIK-you-lar)
Superior glenohumeral ligament (GLEN-o-HUME-er-al)
Tennis elbow
Tenosynovitis
Transverse carpal ligament (CAR-pal)
Trapezoid ligament (TRAP-i-zoyd)
Triangular fibrocartilage (FI-bro-KAR-ti-lij)
Ulnar collateral ligament (of the elbow joint)
Ulnar collateral ligament (of the interphalangeal joints manus)
Ulnar collateral ligament (of the metacarpophalangeal joint)
Ulnar collateral ligament (of the thumb's saddle joint)
Ulnar collateral ligament (of the wrist joint)
Ulnocarpal complex (UL-no-CAR-pal)
Ulnocarpal joint
Ulnotrochlear joint (UL-no-TRO-klee-ar)
Upward tilt
Volar plate (VO-lar)
Winging of the scapula
Wrist joint complex

WORD ORIGINS

- Annular—From Latin *anulus*, meaning *ring*
- Arthritis—From Greek *arthron*, meaning *a joint*, and *itis*, meaning *inflammation*
- Carpus—From Greek *karpos*, meaning *wrist*
- Cubitus—From Latin *cubitum*, meaning *elbow*
- Digital—From Latin *digitus*, meaning *finger* (or *toe*)
- Fore—From Old English *fore*, meaning *before, in front of*
- Manus—From Latin *manus*, meaning *hand*
- Osteoarthritis—From Greek *osteon*, meaning *bone*, and *itis*, meaning *inflammation*
- Pollicis—From Latin *pollicis*, meaning *thumb*
- Ray—From Latin *radius*, meaning *extending outward (radially) from a structure*
- Rein—From Latin *retinere*, meaning *to restrain*
- Rheumatoid—From Greek *rheuma*, meaning *discharge* or *flux*, and *eidos*, meaning *resembling, appearance*
- Thenar—From Greek *thenar*, meaning *palm*
- Trochlea—From Latin *trochlea*, meaning *pulley*

SECTION 10.1 SHOULDER JOINT COMPLEX

- When the term *shoulder joint* is used, it is usually used to describe movement of the arm relative to the scapula at the glenohumeral (GH) joint.
- However, almost every movement of the arm at the GH joint also requires a **coupled movement** of the **shoulder girdle**—in other words, the scapula and clavicle[1] (Box 10-1).

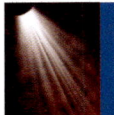

BOX 10-1 Spotlight on the Shoulder Girdle

A girdle is an article of clothing that encircles and thereby holds in and stabilizes the abdomen. Similarly, the scapulae and clavicles (along with the manubrium of the sternum) are called the shoulder girdle because they perform a similar function. They encircle the upper trunk and act as a stable base from which the upper extremity may move. However, the shoulder girdle shows a greater similarity to a corset than a girdle. Whereas a girdle completely encircles the body, a corset is open in back and requires lacing to truly encircle the body.

In this regard, the shoulder girdle is also open in back, because the two scapulae do not articulate with each other. In fact, the musculature (i.e., middle trapezius and rhomboids) that attaches the medial borders of the scapulae to the spine can be viewed as the lacing of a corset. For this reason, the term **shoulder corset** might be more appropriate! Furthermore, just as the stability of a corset is dependent on the tension of the lacing, the stability of the shoulder corset is dependent on the strength and integrity of the musculature that laces the two scapulae together.

- The shoulder girdle is also known as the **pectoral girdle**.
- The scapula and clavicle may move at the sternoclavicular (SC), acromioclavicular (AC), scapulocostal (ScC), and GH joints[1] (Figure 10-1; Table 10-1).
- Because most movement patterns of the shoulder require motion to occur at a number of these joints, the term *shoulder joint complex* is a better term to employ when describing motion of the shoulder.[2] From a "big picture" point of view, the sternoclavicular (SC) joint may be looked at as the master joint that orients the position of the scapula because motion of the clavicle at the SC joint results in motion of the scapula at the scapulocostal joint. Fine-tuning adjustments and augmentation of scapular movement also occur at the acromioclavicular (AC) joint. The net result of SC and AC joint motion is to orient the scapula to the desired position. Position of the scapula is important to facilitate humeral motion at the glenohumeral joint. Thus motion of the arm at the shoulder joint truly is dependent on a complex of joints!
- This coupling of shoulder girdle movement with arm movement is called *scapulohumeral rhythm*.[3] Given that motion of the clavicle is also required, perhaps a better term would be *scapuloclaviculohumeral rhythm*. (The concept of coupled movements [i.e., coupled actions] is addressed in Section 13.12. The coupled actions of the shoulder joint complex are described in detail in Section 10.6.)

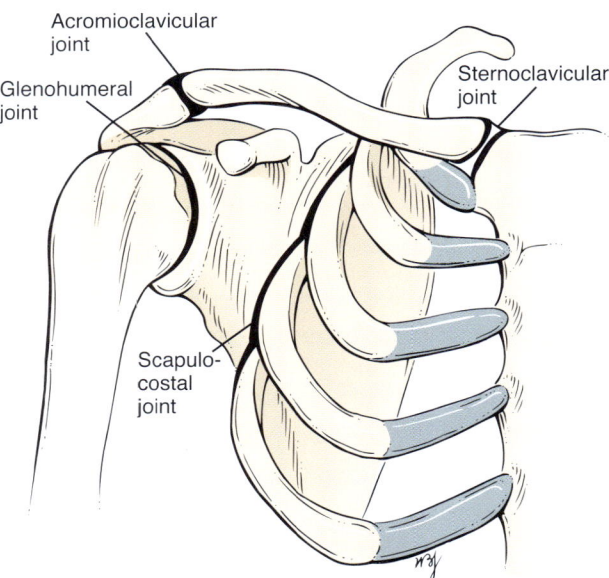

FIGURE 10-1 Anterior view illustrating the right shoulder joint complex. The shoulder joint complex is composed of many joints. The glenohumeral (GH) joint, often referred to as the shoulder joint, is located between the head of the humerus and the glenoid fossa of the scapula. The scapulocostal (ScC) joint is located between the anterior surface of the scapula and the ribcage of the trunk. The acromioclavicular (AC) joint is located between the acromion process of the scapula and the lateral end of the clavicle; the sternoclavicular (SC) joint is located between the sternum and the medial end of the clavicle. *(Modified from Swartz, M: Textbook of physical diagnosis: history and examination, ed 7, Philadelphia, 2014, Saunders.)*

- The shoulder girdle primarily moves as a unit. When this occurs, movement occurs between the clavicle of the shoulder girdle and the sternum at the SC joint, and between the scapula of the shoulder girdle and the ribcage at the ScC joint. Movement may also occur between the scapula of the shoulder girdle and the humerus at the GH joint.
- However, the scapula and clavicle of the shoulder girdle do not always move together as a fixed unit; the presence of the AC joint between these two bones allows for independent motion of the scapula and clavicle relative to each other within the shoulder girdle.[4]

TABLE 10-1	Average Ranges of Motion of the Entire Shoulder Joint Complex from Anatomic Position[7]		
Flexion	180 Degrees	Extension	150 Degrees
Abduction	180 Degrees	Adduction	0 Degrees*
Lateral rotation	90 Degrees	Medial rotation	90 Degrees

*Pure adduction from anatomic position is blocked by the presence of the trunk. However, if the arm is first flexed or extended, further adduction is possible anterior to or posterior to the trunk.

SECTION 10.2 GLENOHUMERAL JOINT

- Generally, when the context is not made otherwise clear, the term *shoulder joint* refers to the **glenohumeral (GH) joint**.

BONES:

- The GH joint is located between the scapula and the humerus.
  - More specifically, it is located between the glenoid fossa of the scapula and the head of the humerus.
- Joint structure classification: Synovial joint[1]
  - Subtype: Ball-and-socket joint
- Joint function classification: Diarthrotic
  - Subtype: Triaxial

MAJOR MOTIONS ALLOWED:

- The GH joint allows flexion and extension (i.e., axial movements) in the sagittal plane around a mediolateral axis (Figure 10-2; Table 10-2).[4]

TABLE 10-2	Average Ranges of Motion of the Arm at the Glenohumeral Joint from Anatomic Position[2,5]		
Flexion	100 Degrees	Extension	40 Degrees
Abduction	120 Degrees	Adduction	0 Degrees*
Lateral rotation	50 Degrees	Medial rotation	90 Degrees

*Pure adduction from anatomic position is blocked because of the presence of the trunk. However, if the arm is first flexed or extended, further adduction is possible anterior to or posterior to the trunk.

- The GH joint allows abduction and adduction (i.e., axial movements) in the frontal plane around an anteroposterior axis (Figure 10-3).
  - If the arm is in a neutral position or medially rotated, abduction of the arm at the glenohumeral (GH) joint will be

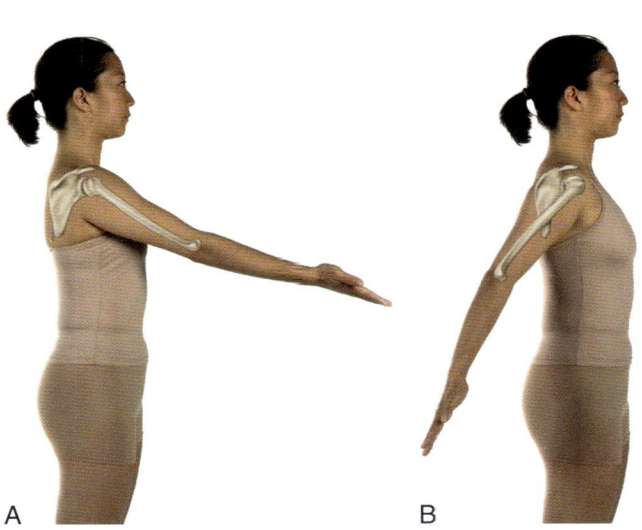

FIGURE 10-2 Sagittal plane actions of the arm at the glenohumeral joint. **A,** Flexion. **B,** Extension.

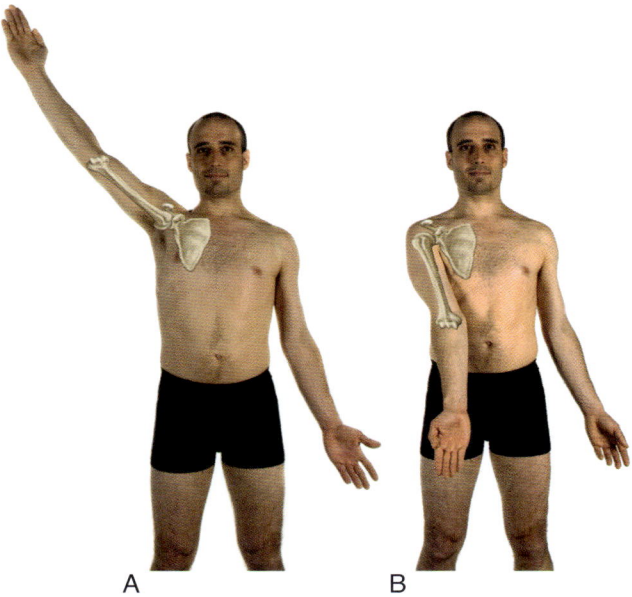

FIGURE 10-3 Frontal plane actions of the arm at the glenohumeral joint. **A,** Abduction. **B,** Adduction.

restricted because the greater tubercle of the head of the humerus will bang into the acromion process above. If the arm is laterally rotated first, then abduction of the arm at the GH joint is much greater because the greater tubercle is moved out of the way of the acromion process.[2]

○ The GH joint allows lateral rotation and medial rotation (i.e., axial movements) in the transverse plane around a vertical axis (Figure 10-4).

Reverse Actions:

○ The muscles of the GH joint are generally considered to move the more distal arm on the more proximal scapula. However, the scapula can move at the GH joint relative to the humerus; this is especially true if the arm is fixed such as when the hand is gripping an immovable object—in other words, during a closed-chain activity (Box 10-2). (For an explanation of closed-chain activities, see Section 9.9, Box 9-8.)

○ The major reverse actions of the scapula at the GH joint are upward rotation and downward rotation.

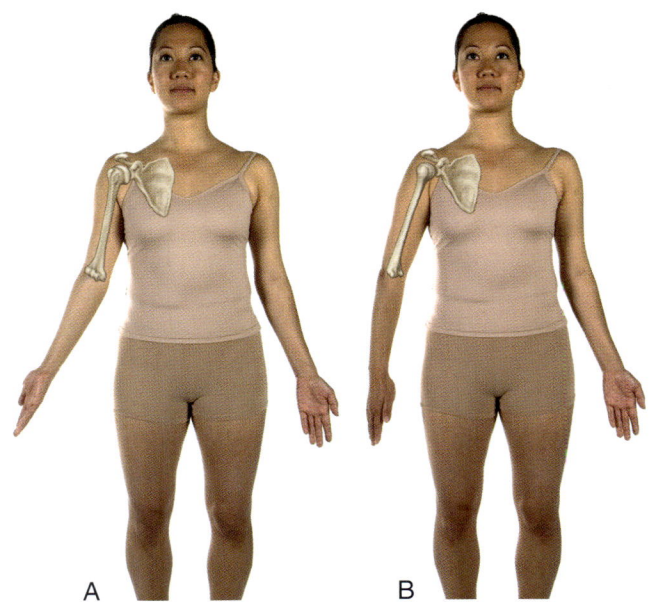

FIGURE 10-4 Transverse plane actions of the arm at the glenohumeral joint. **A,** Lateral rotation. **B,** Medial rotation.

BOX 10-2 Spotlight on Reverse Action of the Deltoid

An example of the reverse action of the scapula relative to the humerus at the glenohumeral (GH) joint can occur when the deltoid contracts to create abduction of the arm at the GH joint. Contraction of the deltoid pulls equally on the humerus and the scapula. Its pull on the scapula will cause downward rotation of the scapula if the scapula is not stabilized (fixed). This stabilization force is usually provided by the upper trapezius, which is an upward rotator of the scapula. However, if the upper trapezius is weak or inhibited, the scapula will be allowed to downwardly rotate, which can cause impingement of the rotator cuff tendon and subacromial bursa. The accompanying figure illustrates an isolated contraction of the deltoid (without stabilization of the scapula by the upper trapezius) caused by electrical muscle stimulation pads placed on the deltoid. Both abduction of the arm and downward rotation of the scapula are occurring. Note: When the reverse action of the scapula moving relative to the humerus at the GH joint occurs, the scapula moves relative to the ribcage as well. Therefore scapular actions at the GH joint can also be described as occurring at the scapulocostal (ScC) joint.

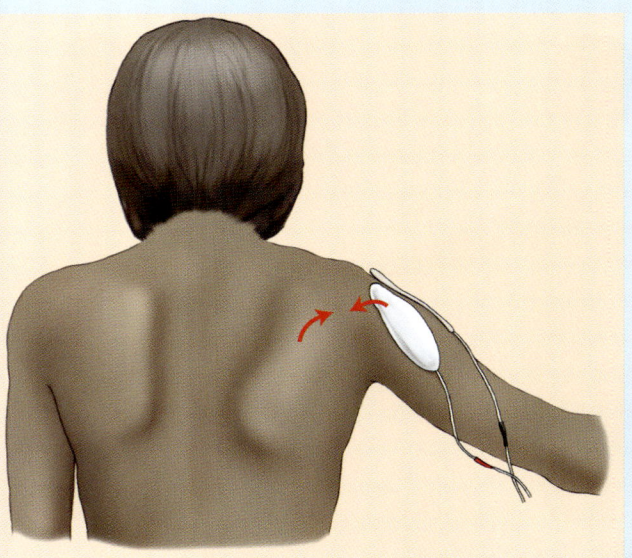

(From Muscolino JE: Back to basics: the actions and reverse actions of a muscle, Massage Ther J 46:168-170, 2007. Modeled from photographs taken by Donald A Neumann, PT, PhD, Professor, Physical Therapy Program, Marquette University.)

MAJOR LIGAMENTS OF THE GLENOHUMERAL JOINT:

- The GH joint has several major ligaments (Figures 10-5 and 10-6; Box 10-3):

Fibrous Joint Capsule:

- The capsule of the GH joint is extremely lax and permits a great deal of motion.[1]
  - The GH joint capsule is so lax that if the musculature of the shoulder joint is completely relaxed, the head of the humerus can be moved away (i.e., axially tractioned) from the glenoid fossa 1 to 2 inches (2.5 to 5.0 cm).[3]
- The GH joint capsule is thickened and strengthened by glenohumeral (GH) ligaments.
- Three GH ligaments exist: (1) the superior glenohumeral ligament, (2) the middle glenohumeral ligament, and (3) the inferior glenohumeral ligament.

Superior, Middle, and Inferior Glenohumeral Ligaments:

- These ligaments are thickenings of the anterior and inferior joint capsule.
- Function: They prevent dislocation of the humeral head anteriorly and inferiorly.[5]
- As a group, these three ligaments also limit the extremes of all GH joint motions.

BOX 10-3	Ligaments of the Glenohumeral Joint

- Fibrous joint capsule
- Superior glenohumeral (GH) ligament
- Middle GH ligament
- Inferior GH ligament
- Coracohumeral ligament*

*The coracoacromial ligament is indirectly involved with the GH joint.

- There is a small region of the anterior GH joint capsule called the **foramen of Weitbrecht** that is located between the superior and middle glenohumeral (GH) ligaments.[6] The foramen of Weitbrecht is a relatively weak region where the majority of shoulder dislocations occur.

Coracohumeral Ligament:

- Location: The coracohumeral ligament is located between the coracoid process of the scapula and the greater tubercle of the humerus.
- Function: It prevents dislocation of the humeral head anteriorly and inferiorly and limits extremes of flexion, extension, and lateral rotation.

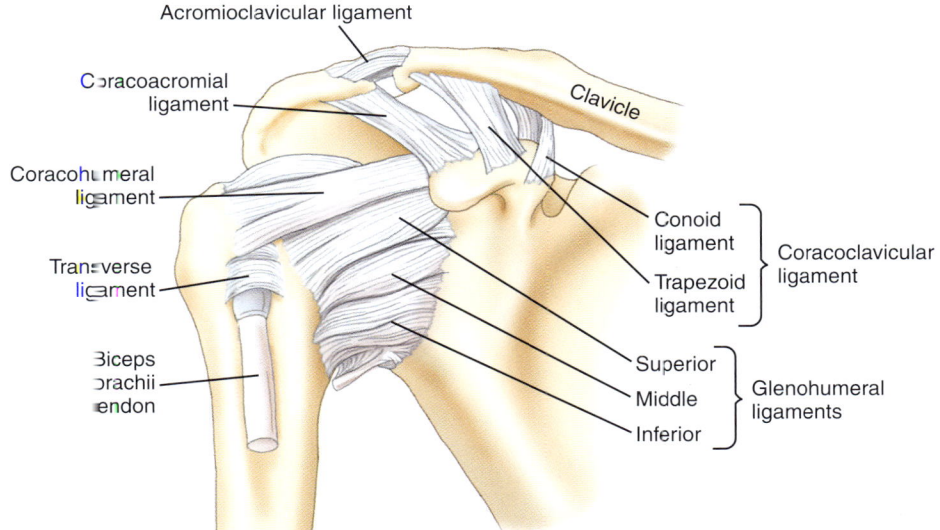

FIGURE 10-5 Anterior view of the ligaments that stabilize the right shoulder joint complex. The superior, middle, and inferior glenohumeral (GH) ligaments are thickenings of the anterior and inferior GH joint capsule. The coracohumeral ligament runs from the coracoid process of the scapula to the greater tubercle of the humerus. The coracoclavicular ligament runs from the coracoid process to the lateral clavicle; the coracoacromial ligament runs from the coracoid process to the acromion process; and the acromioclavicular (AC) ligament runs from the acromion process to the lateral clavicle. (Note: The transverse ligament that holds the long head of the biceps brachii tendon in the bicipital groove is also shown.)

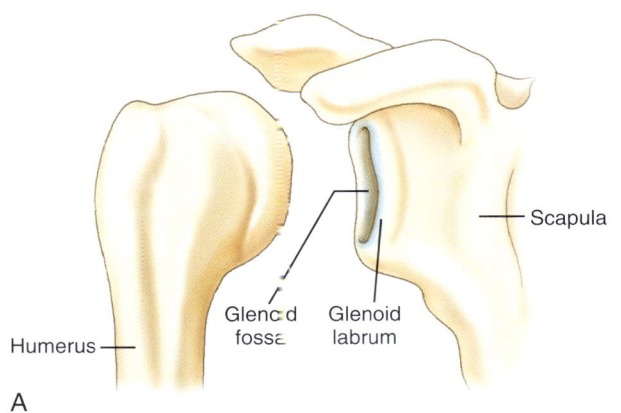
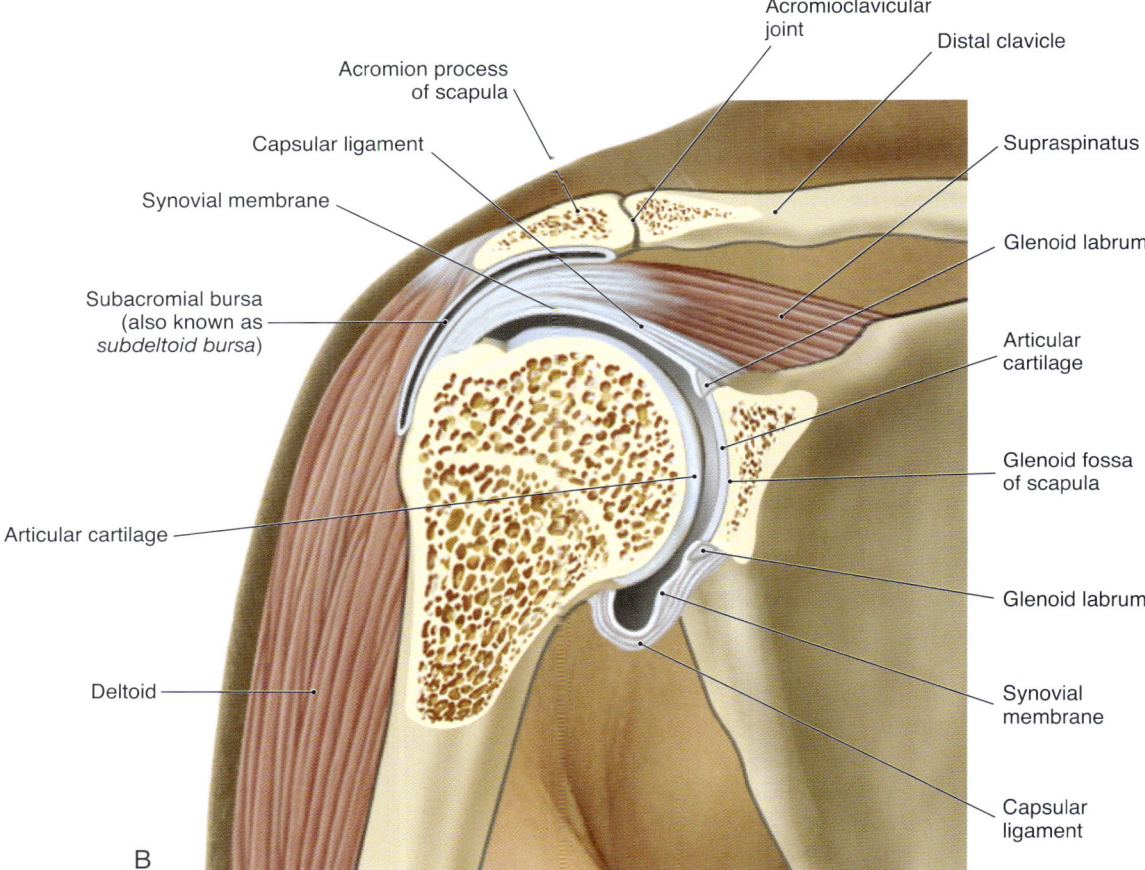

FIGURE 10-6 **A,** Anterior view of the right glenohumeral (GH) joint with the humerus separated from the scapula. The glenoid labrum, which is a rim of cartilage that surrounds the glenoid fossa of the scapula, is seen. Its functions are to deepen and cushion the GH joint. **B,** Anterior view of a frontal (i.e., coronal) plane section through the GH joint. The subacromial bursa is visualized between the acromion process of the scapula and the rotator cuff tendon of the supraspinatus muscle. (*E, From Muscolino JE: The muscular system manual, ed 4, St Louis, 2017, Elsevier.*)

CHAPTER 10 Joints of the Upper Extremity

CLOSED-PACKED POSITION OF THE GLENOHUMERAL JOINT:

- Lateral rotation and abduction.[7]

MAJOR MUSCLES OF THE GLENOHUMERAL JOINT:

- Flexors cross the GH joint anteriorly and are the anterior deltoid, pectoralis major, coracobrachialis, and biceps brachii.
- Extensors cross posteriorly and are the posterior deltoid, latissimus dorsi, teres major, and long head of the triceps brachii.
- Abductors cross superiorly (over the top of the joint) and are the deltoid and supraspinatus.
- Adductors cross below the center of the joint from the trunk to the arm and are located both anteriorly and posteriorly. Some adductors are the pectoralis major, latissimus dorsi, and teres major.
- Lateral rotators such as the posterior deltoid, infraspinatus, and teres minor cross the GH joint and wrap around the humerus, ultimately attaching to the posterior side of the humerus.
- Medial rotators such as the anterior deltoid, latissimus dorsi, teres major, and subscapularis cross the GH joint and wrap around the humerus, ultimately attaching to the anterior side of the humerus.

MISCELLANEOUS:

- A cartilaginous glenoid labrum forms a lip around the glenoid fossa[1] (see Figure 10-6).
  - The cartilaginous glenoid labrum is analogous to the acetabular labrum of the hip joint.
  - The glenoid labrum deepens the glenoid fossa and cushions the joint.
- A bursa known as the *subacromial bursa* is located between the acromion process of the scapula and the (supraspinatus) rotator cuff tendon (see Figure 10-6, 3 and Box 10-4).
  - The subacromial bursa reduces friction between the supraspinatus rotator cuff tendon inferiorly and the acromion process and deltoid muscle superiorly.

BOX 10-4

Because the subacromial bursa usually adheres to the underlying rotator cuff tendon, irritation and injury to the rotator cuff tendon will usually result in irritation and injury to the subacromial bursa as well. Hence rotator cuff tendinitis and subacromial bursa problems usually occur together.

- The subacromial bursa is also known as the **subdeltoid bursa** because it extends inferiorly/distally and is also located between the deltoid muscle and the rotator cuff tendon. This bursa is the famous shoulder joint bursa that is so often blamed for soft tissue pain of the shoulder joint.[7]
- The "roof" of the GH joint is formed by the coracoacromial arch.
- The coracoacromial arch is composed of the **coracoacromial ligament** and the acromion process of the scapula[7] (see Figure 10-5).
  - The coracoacromial ligament is a bit unusual in that it attaches to two landmarks of the same bone—the coracoid process of the scapula to the acromion process of the scapula. Most often, musculoskeletal ligaments run from one bone to a different bone.
- The coracoacromial arch functions to protect the superior structures of the GH joint (Box 10-5).
  - The long head of the biceps brachii is intra-articular (i.e., it runs through the joint cavity of the shoulder joint from the bicipital groove of the humerus to the supraglenoid tubercle of the scapula).
  - The GH joint is the most mobile (and therefore the least stable) joint of the human body. This great mobility is a result of the shallow nature of the glenoid fossa and the tremendous laxity of the joint capsule.[8]
  - The majority of stability this joint does have is provided by musculature, primarily the rotator cuff group of muscles.[2] Because the majority of the stability that the glenohumeral (GH) joint has is derived from musculature, the GH joint is often referred to as a **muscular joint**.

BOX 10-5

Activities such as carrying a bag, purse, or laptop computer on the shoulder (let alone a traumatic fall on the top of the shoulder joint) might injure the superior structures of the glenohumeral (GH) joint if it were not for the protection of the coracoacromial arch. Ironically, the presence of the coracoacromial arch can also prove to be a problem. Because it limits the space available for the superior structures of the GH joint to pass through this region (supraspinatus muscle and tendon, subacromial bursa, long head of the biceps brachii, and superior aspect of the GH joint capsule), these structures can become impinged between the head of the humerus and the coracoacromial arch, especially the acromion process. Most commonly, the supraspinatus and subacromial bursa are impinged here; indeed, this condition occurs so often that it is referred to as *shoulder impingement syndrome*. Many factors can lead to shoulder impingement syndrome, including abducting the arm above 90 degrees with the arm medially rotated, failure of the scapula to upwardly rotate when the arm abducts or flexes, and an improperly formed acromion process (or a bone spur on the underside of the acromion) that angles downward pressing into the supraspinatus tendon.

SECTION 10.3 SCAPULOCOSTAL (ScC) JOINT

- The scapulocostal (ScC) joint is also known as the scapulothoracic joint.

BONES:

- The scapula and the ribcage (Figure 10-7)
  - More specifically, the anterior surface of the scapula and the posterior surface of the ribcage
- In standing and seated positions, the scapula usually sits on the ribcage at the levels of the second through seventh ribs. However, when a client is lying prone and the arms are hanging off the table, the location of the scapula relative to the ribcage changes as the scapula protracts and upwardly rotates.
- Joint type: Functional joint[5]
  - The ScC joint is unusual in that it is not an **anatomic joint** because no actual union of the scapula and the ribcage is formed by connective tissue. (For a discussion of the anatomic structure of joints, see Section 7.1.) However, because it behaves as a joint does in that movement of the scapula relative to the ribcage occurs, it is considered to be a **functional joint**.[5]

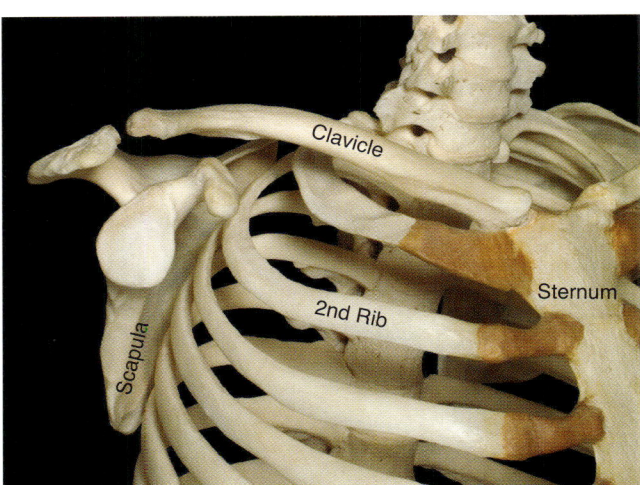

FIGURE 10-7 Anterolateral view of the upper trunk illustrating the right scapulocostal (ScC) joint located between the anterior (i.e., ventral) surface of the scapula and the posterior surface of the ribcage.

MAJOR MOTIONS ALLOWED:

Major motions allowed are as follows[5] (Figures 10-8 to 10-10, Table 10-3; Box 10-6):

- Of all the scapular actions possible, only elevation/depression and protraction/retraction can be primary movements, meaning that each one of these movements can be created separately by itself. The other scapular actions are secondary in that they must occur secondary to an action of the arm at the glenohumeral (GH) joint.[7] (See Section 10.6 for more on this topic.)
- Protraction and retraction (nonaxial movements) of the scapula
- Elevation and depression (nonaxial movements) of the scapula
- Upward rotation and downward rotation (axial movements) of the scapula
  - Note: Upward rotation and downward rotation of the scapula occur within the plane of the scapula, which is determined by the shape of the posterior rib cage wall. This plane is approximately 30–35 degrees anterior to the frontal plane (i.e., between the frontal and sagittal planes).[2]

Accessory Movements:

- Accessory movements include the following[7]:
  - **Lateral tilt** and **medial tilt** (axial movements) of the scapula
  - **Upward tilt** and **downward tilt** (axial movements) of the scapula

- Note: The accessory motions of scapular tilting are defined differently by different sources. For our purposes, a healthy scapula in anatomic position is medially and downwardly tilted, and any lateral or upward tilt of the scapula involves the medial border or the inferior angle jutting away from the body wall and is generally considered to be an unhealthy resting position of the scapulae. However, manual therapists often use positions of lateral and upward tilt to gain access to the underside (i.e., anterior side) of the scapula, enabling them to work muscles that are deep to the scapula from the posterior side of the body.
- Lateral tilt of the scapula is also known as medial rotation of the scapula because the anterior surface of the scapula comes to orient medially; medial tilt is also known as lateral rotation of the scapula because the anterior surface of the scapula comes to orient laterally.
- Lateral tilt of the scapula away from the body wall is usually referred to in lay terms as **winging of the scapula**.[7]

Reverse Actions:

- The ribcage (i.e., the trunk) can move relative to the scapula.
- One example of a reverse action at the scapulocostal (ScC) joint in which the ribcage (i.e., the trunk) moves relative to the scapula is when push-ups are done. The objective of a push-up is to exercise muscles by pushing the body up and away from

TABLE 10-3	Average Ranges of Upward Rotation and Downward Rotation Motion of the Scapula at the Scapulocostal Joint from Anatomic Position[2]		
Upward rotation	60 Degrees	Downward rotation	0 Degrees

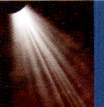

BOX 10-6 Spotlight on Scapulocostal Joint Motion

Motion of the scapula at the scapulocostal (ScC) joint cannot occur without motion also occurring at the sternoclavicular (SC) and/or acromioclavicular (AC) joint(s) as well. In other words, for the scapula to move relative to the ribcage at the ScC joint, it will also have to move relative to the clavicle at the AC joint and/or move with the clavicle when the clavicle moves relative to the sternum at the SC joint. In fact, most of scapular upward rotation at the ScC joint results from the clavicle moving (elevating) at the SC joint (see Box 10-9).

Looking at this concept from another point of view, when the scapula moves relative to the clavicle at the AC joint, it also must move relative to the ribcage at the ScC joint. Interesting to note, when the scapula moves relative to the arm at the glenohumeral (GH) joint (the reverse action of movement of the arm at the GH joint), the scapula may also move relative to the ribcage at the ScC joint, or it may stay fixed to the ribcage at the ScC joint and the entire trunk may move with the scapula relative to the arm at the GH joint.

Therefore regarding whether scapular motion can be isolated at one joint or can or must occur at more than one of its joints, we see the following: (1) Motion of the scapula at the ScC joint must always be accompanied by motion of the clavicle at the SC joint and/or by motion of the scapula at another joint (AC or GH), and (2) the only joint at which scapular motion can be isolated is the GH joint; however, this can only occur if the scapula stays fixed to the ribcage, and the trunk moves with the scapula relative to the arm.

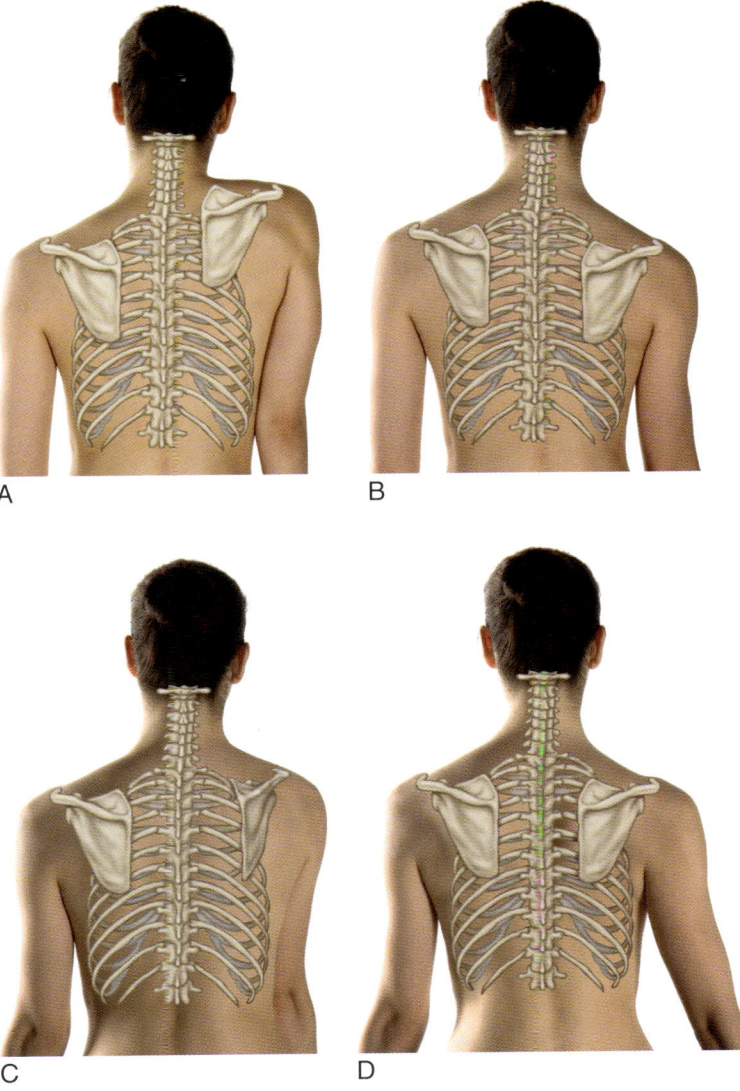

FIGURE 10-8 Nonaxial actions of elevation/depression and protraction/retraction of the scapula at the scapulocostal (ScC) joint. **A,** Elevation of the right scapula. **B,** Depression of the right scapula. **C,** Protraction of the right scapula. **D,** Retraction of the right scapula. The left scapula is in anatomic position in all figures. (Note: All views are posterior.)

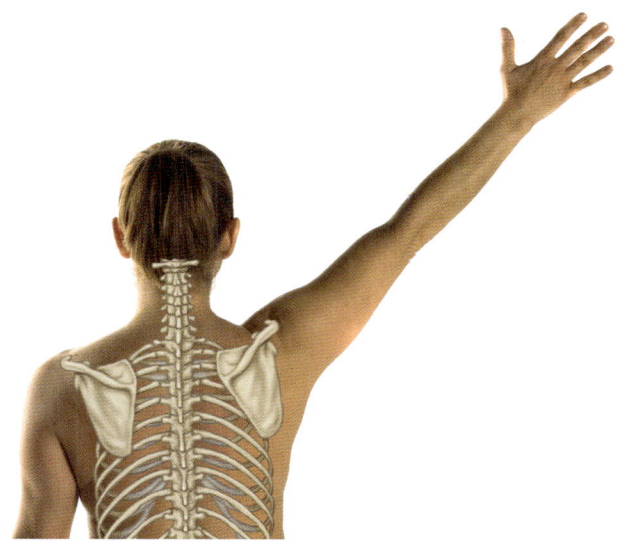

FIGURE 10-9 Upward rotation of the right scapula at the scapulocostal (ScC) joint. The left scapula is in anatomic position, which is full downward rotation. (Note: The scapular action of upward rotation cannot be isolated. It must accompany humeral motion. In this case, the humerus is abducted at the glenohumeral joint.)

scapulae (which are fixed, because the hands are planted firmly on the floor).

MAJOR MUSCLES OF THE SCAPULOCOSTAL JOINT:

- Elevators of the scapula attach from the scapula to a more superior structure; examples are the upper trapezius, levator scapulae, and rhomboids.
- Depressors attach from the scapula to a more inferior structure; examples are the lower trapezius and the pectoralis minor.
- Protractors attach from the scapula to a more anterior structure; examples are the serratus anterior and the pectoralis minor.
- Retractors attach from the scapula to a more midline structure posteriorly; examples are the middle trapezius and the rhomboids.
- Upward rotators of the scapula include the serratus anterior and the upper and lower trapezius.
- Downward rotators include the pectoralis minor, rhomboids, and levator scapulae.

MISCELLANEOUS:

- The scapula articulates with the ribcage at the ScC joint, the clavicle at the AC joint, and the humerus at the GH joint. Therefore the scapula can move relative to any of these structures, and the motion could be described as occurring at the joint located between the scapula and any one of these three bones. Keep in mind that at times the scapula moves at only one of these joints; at other times the scapula moves at more than one of these joints at the same time.

the floor. At the very end of a push-up, after the upper extremities are perfectly vertical, a little more elevation of the trunk away from the floor is possible. This motion is caused by protractors of the scapula such as the serratus anterior contracting and pulling the trunk (which is more mobile) up toward the

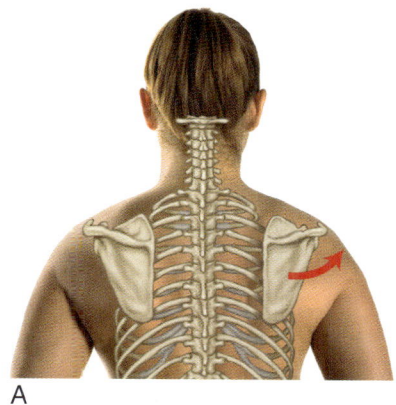
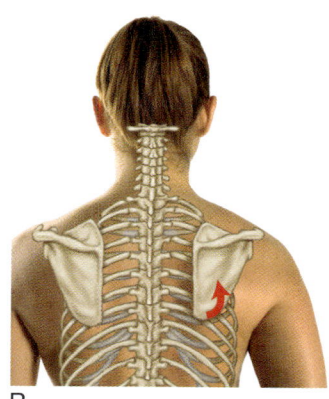

FIGURE 10-10 Tilt actions of the scapula at the scapulocostal (ScC) joint. **A,** Lateral tilt of the right scapula; the left scapula is in anatomic position of medial tilt. **B,** Upward tilt of the right scapula; the left scapula is in anatomic position of downward tilt. (Note: Both views are posterior.)

SECTION 10.4 STERNOCLAVICULAR (SC) JOINT

- The sternoclavicular joint is also known as the *SC joint*.

BONES:

- The manubrium of the sternum and the medial end of the clavicle (Figure 10-11)
- Joint structure classification: Synovial joint[1]
  - Subtype: Saddle
- Joint function classification: Diarthrotic
  - Subtype: Biaxial
  - The sternoclavicular (SC) joint actually permits motion in three planes about three axes; therefore it could also be classified as *triaxial*.[1] However, because its rotation actions cannot be isolated, this joint is most often classified as being *biaxial*. In this regard the SC joint is similar to the other more famous saddle joint of the human body, the saddle

joint of the thumb (i.e., the carpometacarpal [CMC] joint of the thumb). (For information on the saddle joint of the thumb, see Section 10.13.)

MAJOR MOTIONS ALLOWED:

Major motions allowed are as follows[5] (Figures 10-12 to 10-14; Table 10-4):
- Protraction and retraction of the clavicle (axial movements): These motions occur within the transverse plane around a vertical axis.
- Elevation and depression of the clavicle (axial movements): These motions occur within the frontal plane around an anteroposterior axis.
  - Elevation and depression motions of the clavicle at the sternoclavicular joint are not oriented perfectly in the frontal

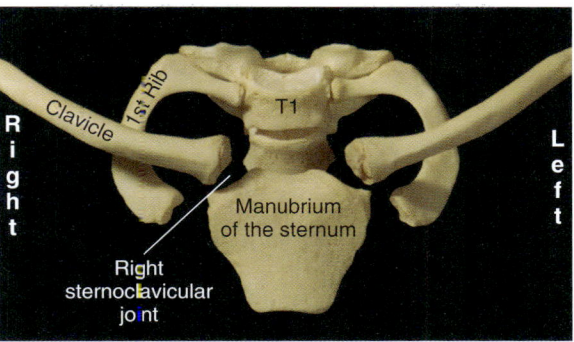

FIGURE 10-11 Anterior view of the upper trunk illustrating the sternoclavicular (SC) joints located between the manubrium of the sternum and the medial (i.e., proximal) ends of the clavicles.

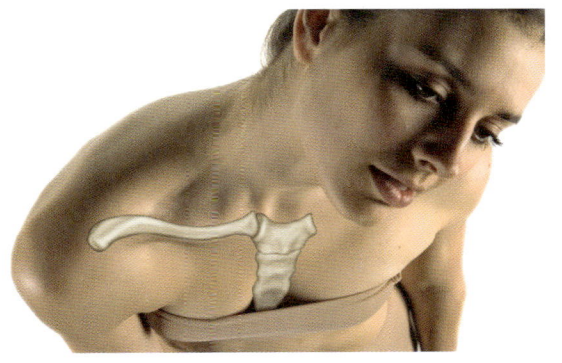 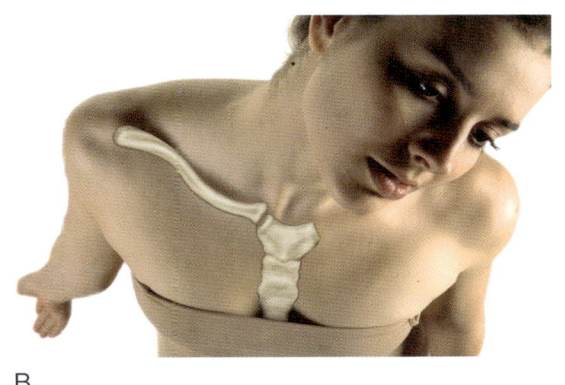

FIGURE 10-12 A, Protraction of the right clavicle at the sternoclavicular (SC) joint. **B,** Retraction of the right clavicle. (Note: Both views are anterior.)

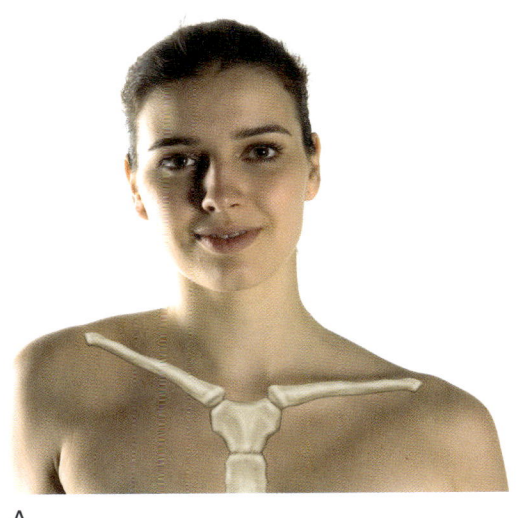 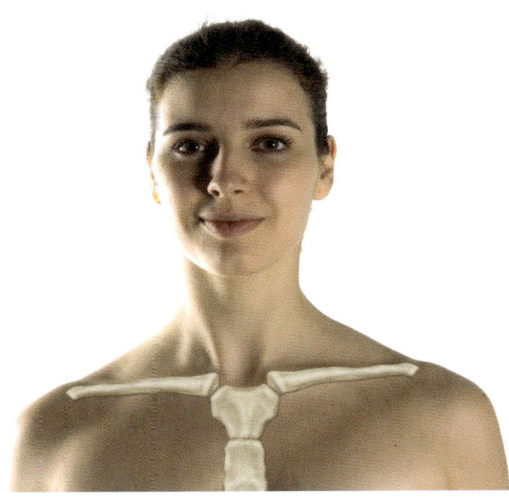

FIGURE 10-13 A, Elevation of the right clavicle at the sternoclavicular (SC) joint. **B,** Depression of the right clavicle. (Note: The left clavicle is in anatomic position. Both views are anterior.)

318   PART 3   Skeletal Arthrology: Study of the Joints

TABLE 10-4	Average Ranges of Motion of the Clavicle at the Sternoclavicular Joint from Anatomic Position[2]		
Elevation	45 Degrees	Depression	10 Degrees
Protraction	30 Degrees	Retraction	30 Degrees
Upward rotation	45 Degrees	Downward rotation	0 Degrees

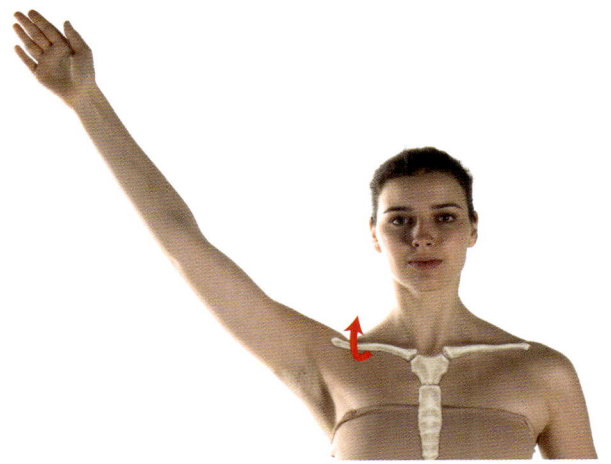

FIGURE 10-14 Anterior view that illustrates upward rotation of the right clavicle at the sternoclavicular (SC) joint; the left clavicle is in anatomic position, which is full downward rotation. (Note: Upward rotation of the clavicle cannot be isolated. In this figure the arm is abducted at the glenohumeral joint, resulting in the scapula upwardly rotating, which results in upward rotation of the clavicle.)

plane. At rest, the clavicle is actually oriented approximately 20 degrees posterior to the frontal plane.

❍ Upward rotation and downward rotation of the clavicle (axial movements): These motions occur within the sagittal plane around a mediolateral axis (this axis runs through the length of the bone).

MAJOR LIGAMENTS OF THE STERNOCLAVICULAR JOINT:

❍ The SC joint has several major ligaments (Figure 10-15; Box 10-7):
❍ The SC joint is the only osseous joint that connects the upper extremity (i.e., hand, forearm, arm, scapula, clavicle) to the axial skeleton.[2] As such, it needs to be well stabilized.
❍ The sternoclavicular (SC) joint can be considered to be the basilar joint of the entire upper extremity.[2] When the clavicle moves at the SC joint, the scapula is moved at the scapulocostal (ScC) joint. In fact, most of the motion of the scapula at the ScC joint is driven by motion of the clavicle at the SC joint.
❍ In addition to ligamentous support, the sternoclavicular joint is also stabilized by the attachments of the sternocleidomastoid, sternohyoid, and sternothyroid muscles.

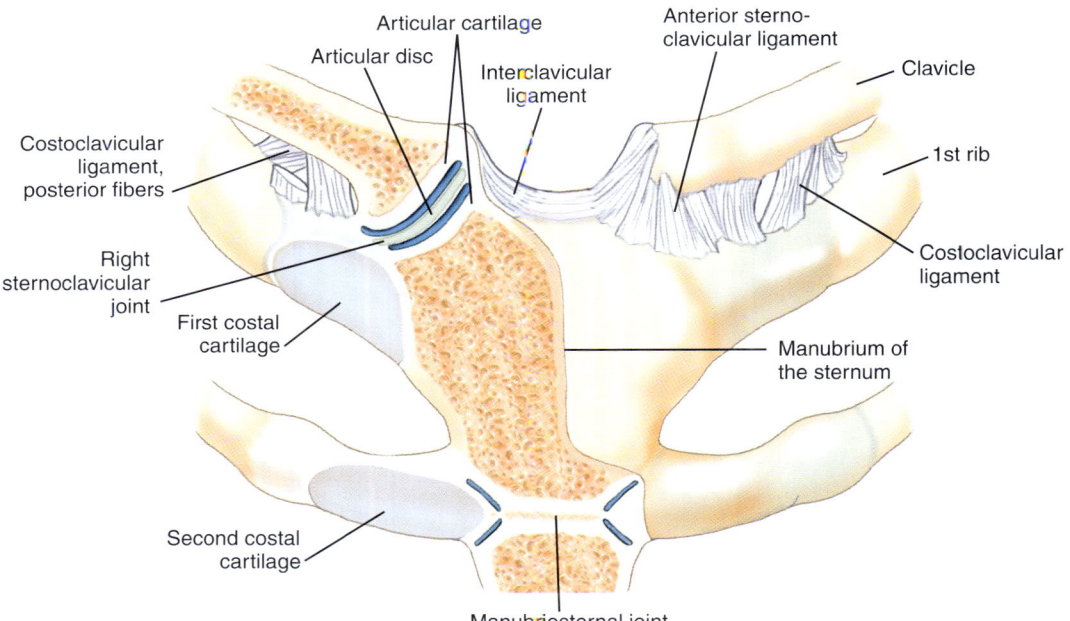

FIGURE 10-15 Anterior view of the sternoclavicular (SC) joints. The right joint is shown in a frontal (i.e., coronal) section; the left joint is left intact. The SC joint is stabilized by its fibrous capsule, anterior and posterior SC ligaments, the interclavicular ligament, and the costoclavicular ligament.

> **BOX 10-7** **Ligaments of the Sternoclavicular (SC) Joint**
>
> - Fibrous capsule
> - Anterior SC ligament
> - Posterior SC ligament
> - Interclavicular ligament
> - Costoclavicular ligament

Fibrous Joint Capsule:

- The SC joint capsule is fairly strong and is also reinforced by sternoclavicular ligaments.[8]

Anterior and Posterior Sternoclavicular Ligaments:

- Two SC ligaments exist: (1) the anterior sternoclavicular ligament and (2) the posterior sternoclavicular ligament.
- The sternoclavicular ligaments are reinforcements of the joint capsule found anteriorly and posteriorly.[8]

Interclavicular Ligament:

- The interclavicular ligament spans from one clavicle to the other clavicle.[8]

Costoclavicular Ligament:

- The costoclavicular ligament runs from the first rib to the clavicle.
  - More specifically, it runs from the costal cartilage of the first rib to the costal tuberosity on the inferior surface of the medial (i.e., proximal) end of the clavicle.
- The costoclavicular ligament has anterior and posterior fibers.
- The costoclavicular ligament limits all motions of the clavicle except depression.

CLOSED-PACKED POSITION OF THE STERNOCLAVICULAR JOINT:

- Full upward rotation of the clavicle

MISCELLANEOUS:

- A fibrocartilaginous articular disc is located within the SC joint.
- This disc helps to improve the congruence of the joint surfaces and also to absorb shock.
- It is interesting to note that the SC joint and the carpometacarpal (CMC) joint of the thumb are both saddle joints. Just as the CMC (saddle) joint of the thumb is the base joint of the thumb, the SC joint is the base joint of the entire upper extremity.

SECTION 10.5   ACROMIOCLAVICULAR (AC) JOINT

- The acromioclavicular joint is also known as the AC joint.

BONES:

- The acromion process of the scapula and the lateral (i.e., distal) end of the clavicle (Figure 10-16)
- Joint structure classification: Synovial joint[7]
  - Subtype: Plane joint
- Joint function classification: Diarthrotic
  - Subtype: Nonaxial

MOTIONS ALLOWED:

- Upward rotation and downward rotation of the scapula (axial movements) relative to the clavicle
- Without motion at the AC joint, the scapula and clavicle (i.e., the shoulder girdle) would be forced to always move as one fixed unit. The AC joint allows for independent motion between the scapula and clavicle. The major actions at the AC joint are movements of the scapula relative to the clavicle.[5] These motions of the scapula allow greater overall motion of the shoulder joint complex, which translates into the ability to move and place the hand throughout a greater range of motion (Figure 10-17; Table 10-5).

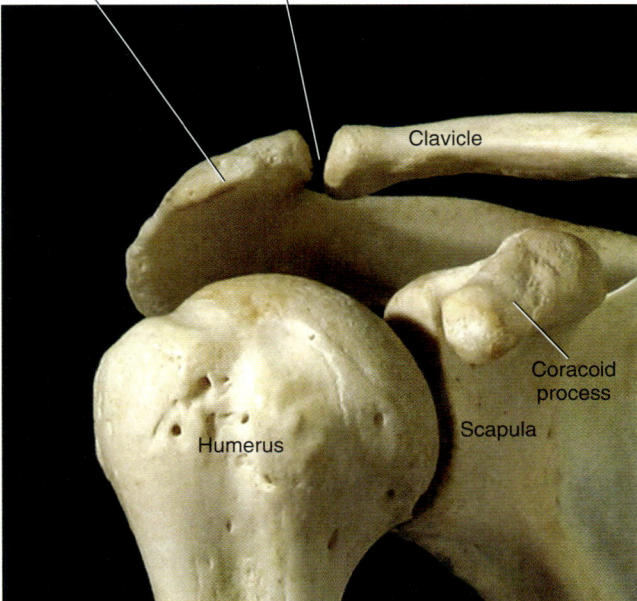

FIGURE 10-16 Anterior view of the right acromioclavicular (AC) joint formed by the union of the acromion process of the scapula and the lateral (i.e., distal) end of the clavicle.

320 PART 3 Skeletal Arthrology: Study of the Joints

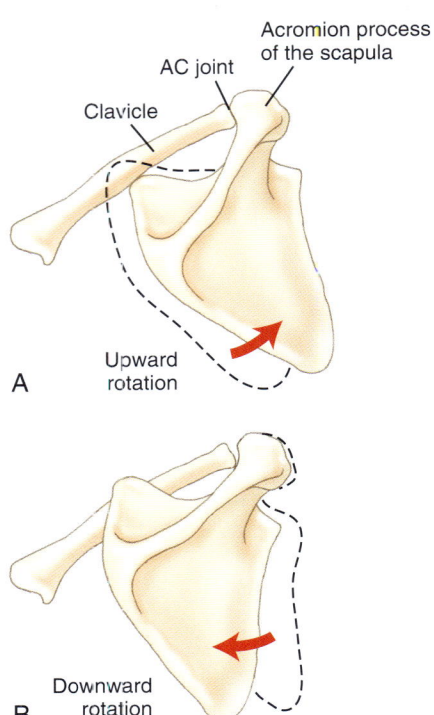

FIGURE 10-17 Motion of the scapula relative to the clavicle at the right acromioclavicular (AC) joint. **A,** Upward rotation. **B,** Downward rotation. (Note: Both views are posterior. When the scapula moves relative to the clavicle at the AC joint, it also moves relative to the ribcage at the scapulocostal [ScC] joint.)

Accessory Actions:

- Lateral tilt and medial tilt of the scapula (axial movements)
- Upward tilt and downward tilt of the scapula (axial movements)
- Note: The accessory tilt actions of the scapula are considered by many to be necessary to adjust the position of the scapula on the ribcage. Much of the motion of the scapula at the scapulocostal joint is actually driven by motion of the clavicle at the sternoclavicular joint. If there were no acromioclavicular joint, the scapula would have to follow the motion of the clavicle degree for degree. However, as the scapula moves along with the clavicle, its anterior surface may no longer remain snug against the ribcage. For this reason, fine-tuning adjustments of the scapula at the acromioclavicular joint are necessary to maintain the proper position of the scapula relative to the ribcage.[2] For illustrations of scapular tilt actions, please see Section 10.3.

TABLE 10-5	Average Ranges of Motion of the Scapula at the Acromioclavicular (AC) Joint from Anatomic Position[2]
Upward rotation	30 Degrees
Downward rotation	0 Degrees

Lateral/medial tilts and upward/downward tilts of the scapula at the AC joint have been measured at 10 to 30 degrees.

Reverse Actions:

- The clavicle can move relative to the scapula at the AC joint.

MAJOR LIGAMENTS OF THE ACROMIOCLAVICULAR JOINT:

The AC joint has several major ligaments (Figure 10-18; Box 10-8):
- In addition to the ligamentous support, the acromioclavicular (AC) joint is also stabilized by the attachments of the trapezius and deltoid muscles.

Fibrous Joint Capsule:

- The joint capsule is weak and is reinforced by the **acromioclavicular ligament**.[8]

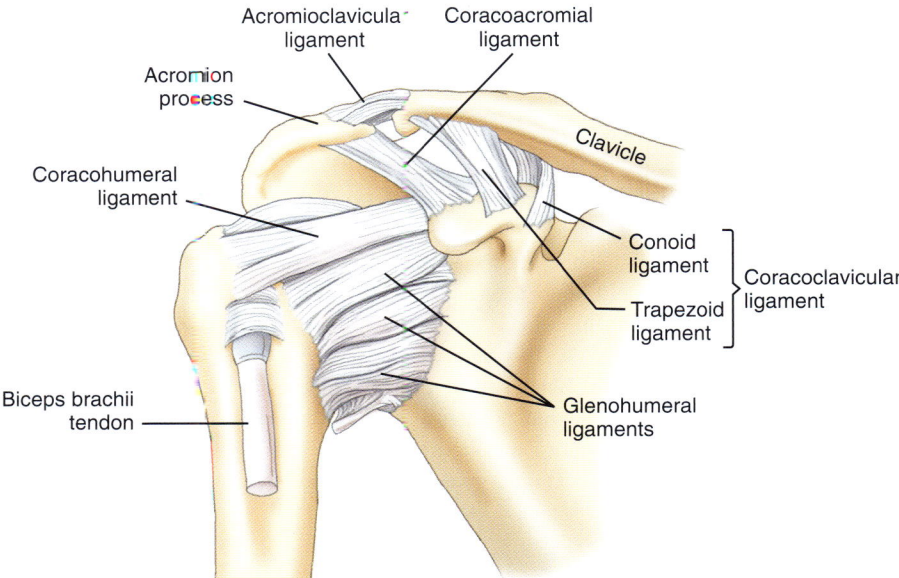

FIGURE 10-18 Anterior view of the right acromioclavicular (AC) joint. The AC joint is stabilized by its fibrous capsule, the AC ligament, and the coracoclavicular ligament. The coracoclavicular ligament has two parts: (1) the trapezoid and (2) conoid ligaments.

> **BOX 10-8** **Ligaments of the Acromioclavicular Joint**
>
> - Fibrous capsule
> - Acromioclavicular (AC) ligament
> - Coracoclavicular ligament (trapezoid and conoid)

Acromioclavicular Ligament:

- The AC ligament is a reinforcement of the AC joint capsule.
- The AC ligament is often divided into the **superior acromioclavicular ligament** and the **inferior acromioclavicular ligament**, which are reinforcements of the AC joint capsule found superiorly and inferiorly.[2]

Coracoclavicular Ligament:

- The coracoclavicular ligament has two parts: (1) the trapezoid ligament and (2) the conoid ligament.
- Location: The coracoclavicular ligament attaches from the coracoid process of the scapula to the clavicle.
  - More specifically, it attaches to the lateral (i.e., distal) end of the clavicle on the inferior surface.[8]
- The trapezoid ligament is more anterior in location and attaches from the superior surface of the coracoid process to the trapezoid line of the clavicle (on the inferior surface at the lateral end of the clavicle).
- The conoid ligament is more posterior in location and attaches from the proximal base of the coracoid process of the scapula to the conoid tubercle of the clavicle (on the inferior surface at the lateral end of the clavicle).
- Function: The coracoclavicular ligament does not directly cross the AC joint itself, but it does cross from the scapula to the clavicle and therefore adds stability to the AC joint.

CLOSED-PACKED POSITION OF THE ACROMIOCLAVICULAR JOINT:

- Full upward rotation of the scapula

MISCELLANEOUS:

- Often a fibrocartilaginous disc is located within the AC joint.[7]
- The AC joint is very susceptible to injury (e.g., a fall on an outstretched arm) and degeneration.[2]

SECTION 10.6 SCAPULOHUMERAL RHYTHM

- When a small degree of arm movement is needed, motion may occur solely at the glenohumeral (GH) joint. However, if any appreciable degree of arm motion is necessary, the entire complex of shoulder joints must become involved. The result is that arm motion requires coupled joint actions of the scapula and clavicle. (The concept of coupled actions is addressed in Section 13.12; see also Section 9.11 for coupled actions between the thigh and pelvis.) This pattern of coupled actions is called **scapulohumeral rhythm**[7]; however, given the involvement of the clavicle, it might better be termed **scapuloclaviculohumeral rhythm**.
- The reason that shoulder girdle movement must accompany arm movement is that the GH joint, albeit the most mobile joint in the human body, does not allow sufficient movement of the arm to be able to place the hand in all desired locations. For example, if one wants to reach a book that is located high up on a shelf that is located to the side of the body, it is necessary to abduct the arm at the GH joint. However, the GH joint allows only 120 degrees of abduction, which is not sufficient. Therefore for higher reaching, movement of the scapula and clavicle must occur to bring the hand up higher. When all motions of the shoulder joint complex have occurred, the arm appears to have abducted 180 degrees because the position of the arm relative to the trunk has changed 180 degrees. In reality, only 120 degrees of that motion occurred at the GH joint. The other 60 degrees (fully one third of the motion) resulted from scapular motion relative to the ribcage at the ScC joint with the arm "going along for the ride" (this scapular motion at the ScC joint is dependent on motion of the clavicle at the SC joint and motion of the scapula relative to the clavicle at the AC joint). Therefore scapulohumeral rhythm is an important concept, and a full understanding of the motions at all the joints of the shoulder joint complex is important for assessment of clients who have decreased range of motion of the arm.[5]
- The exact point at which scapular upward rotation begins to couple with arm abduction in scapulohumeral rhythm is approximately at 30 degrees of arm abduction at the GH joint. However, this number is not fixed; rather, it varies from one individual to another based on a number of factors.[7]
- Following is a list of the scapular actions at the ScC joint that couple with motions of the arm at the GH joint. In each circumstance, keep in mind that the coupled action of the scapula facilitates further movement of the arm in the direction it is moving. Furthermore, it should be noted that it is not that the arm first moves as much as it can, and then the scapula begins to move. Rather, the scapula will usually begin to move earlier on; from that point onward, motion will be a combination of arm and shoulder girdle movement.

SAGITTAL PLANE ACTIONS:

- Flexion of the arm at the GH joint couples with protraction and upward rotation of the scapula at the ScC joint.[7]
- Extension of the arm at the GH joint couples with retraction and downward rotation of the scapula at the ScC joint.[7]
- Extension of the arm at the GH joint beyond neutral (i.e., extension beyond anatomic position) couples with upward tilt of the scapula at the ScC joint.[7]

FRONTAL PLANE ACTIONS:

- Abduction of the arm at the GH joint couples with upward rotation of the scapula at the ScC joint (Figure 10-19). (For more details on scapulohumeral rhythm that occurs with abduction of the arm, see Box 10-9.)[2]
- Adduction of the arm at the GH joint couples with downward rotation of the scapula at the ScC joint.[2]

TRANSVERSE PLANE ACTIONS:

- Medial rotation of the arm at the GH joint couples with protraction of the scapula at the ScC joint.[2]
- Lateral rotation of the arm at the GH joint couples with retraction of the scapula at the ScC joint.[2]

OTHER COUPLED ACTIONS OF SCAPULOHUMERAL RHYTHM:

In addition to the usual coupled actions of scapulohumeral rhythm, two other coupled actions should be mentioned:

- When the arm abducts at the GH joint more than approximately 90 degrees, it also needs to rotate laterally at the GH joint. The reason for this is that when a medially rotated arm abducts, the greater tubercle of the head of the humerus bangs into the acromion process of the scapula. With lateral rotation of the arm, the greater tubercle is moved out of the way and the arm can fully abduct[2] (Box 10-10).
- When any motion occurs that causes the distal end of the humerus to elevate (i.e., flex, extend, abduct, or adduct) from anatomic position, the proximal end of the humerus (i.e., the head) must be held down into the glenoid fossa of the scapula. This is necessary because otherwise whatever muscle *elevates* the distal end would also *pull* and *elevate* the head of the humerus into the acromion process, resulting in impingement and damage to the tissues of the GH joint. To prevent this from occurring, other muscles must contract isometrically to fix (i.e., stabilize) the head of the humerus in place. The rotator cuff musculature is usually credited with accomplishing this. The result is that the proximal end of the humerus stays fixed in place while the distal end elevates.[4]

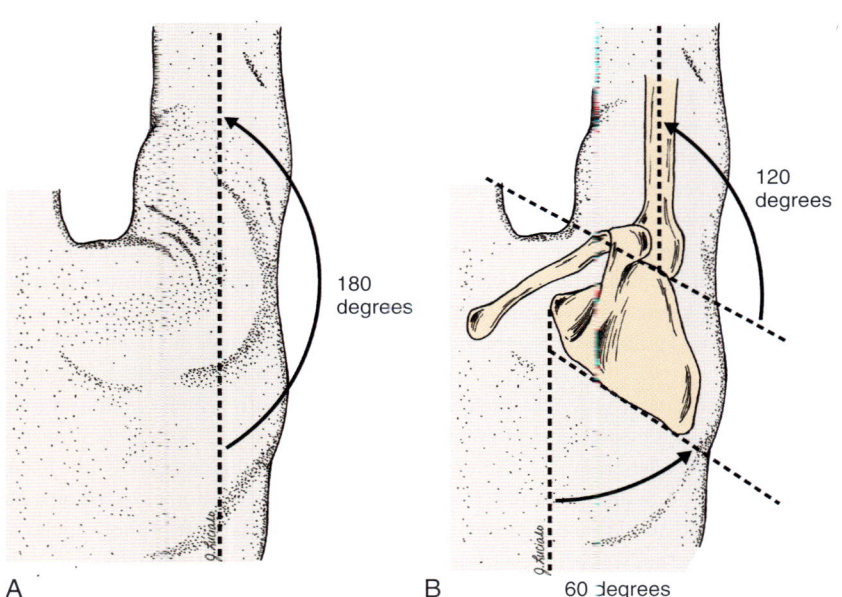

FIGURE 10-19 Concept of scapulohumeral rhythm. **A,** Right arm that has been abducted relative to the trunk 180 degrees. **B,** Of the 180 degrees of abduction of the arm relative to the trunk, only 120 degrees of that motion are the result of abduction of the arm at the glenohumeral (GH) joint; the remaining 60 degrees of motion are the result of upward rotation of the scapula at the scapulocostal (ScC) joint. Thus motion of the arm is intimately linked to motion of the scapula. (Note: Both views are posterior.)

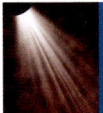

BOX 10-9 Spotlight on Scapulohumeral Rhythm of Arm Abduction

Scapulo(claviculo)humeral rhythm motion of the coupled joint actions of the shoulder joint complex that accompany frontal plane abduction of the arm at the glenohumeral (GH) joint has been extensively studied. Following is a summation of this complex of coupled actions (see Figure 10-19). (Note: The details that follow are not meant to overwhelm the reader; they are presented to manifest the beautiful complexity of scapulohumeral rhythm and illustrate the need for a larger more global assessment of shoulder joint motion in clients who have shoulder problems!)

Full frontal plane abduction of the arm is considered to be 180 degrees of arm motion relative to the trunk. Of that motion, the arm abducts 120 degrees at the GH joint, and the scapula upwardly rotates 60 degrees at the scapulocostal (ScC) joint (with the arm going along for the ride); 120 degrees + 60 degrees = 180 degrees total arm movement relative to the trunk. This total movement pattern can be divided into an early phase and a late phase, each one consisting of 90 degrees.

Early Phase (Initial 90 Degrees):
- During the early phase, the arm abducts 60 degrees at the GH joint and the scapula upwardly rotates 30 degrees at the ScC joint.
- This scapular upward rotation of 30 degrees relative to the ribcage is created by two motions:
  1. The clavicle elevates 25 degrees at the sternoclavicular (SC) joint, and the scapula goes along for the ride, thus changing its position and upwardly rotating relative to the ribcage at the ScC joint.
  2. The scapula upwardly rotates 5 degrees at the acromioclavicular (AC) joint relative to the clavicle, again changing its position and upwardly rotating relative to the ribcage at the ScC joint.

Late Phase (Final 90 Degrees):
- During the late phase, the arm abducts another 60 degrees at the GH joint and the scapula upwardly rotates another 30 degrees at the ScC joint.
- This scapular upward rotation of 30 degrees relative to the ribcage is created by two motions:
  1. The clavicle elevates another 5 degrees at the SC joint and the scapula goes along for the ride, again changing its position and upwardly rotating relative to the ribcage at the ScC joint.
  2. The scapula upwardly rotates another 25 degrees at the AC joint relative to the clavicle, again changing its position and upwardly rotating relative to the ribcage at the ScC joint.

Summation of Early and Late Phases:
- The arm has abducted at the GH joint relative to the scapula 120 degrees.
- The scapula has upwardly rotated at the ScC joint relative to the ribcage 60 degrees.
- This scapular upward rotation relative to the ribcage is composed of 30 degrees of elevation of the clavicle at the SC joint and 30 degrees of upward rotation of the scapula at the AC joint.

A Detailed Explanation of How and Why These Motions of the Scapula Occur
The scapula and clavicle are linked together at the AC joint as the shoulder girdle. Hence muscular contraction that pulls and moves one bone of the shoulder girdle tends to result in movement of the entire shoulder girdle. Therefore muscles that pull and cause upward rotation of the scapula tend to also pull the clavicle into elevation; conversely, muscles that pull the clavicle into elevation also result in the scapula upwardly rotating.

Early Phase
- The force of muscular contraction (by scapular upward rotators and clavicular elevators) results in elevation of the clavicle at the SC joint relative to the sternum (25 degrees); by simply going along for the ride, the scapula succeeds in upwardly rotating relative to the ribcage (i.e., at the ScC joint). The clavicle elevates until it encounters resistance to this motion by the costoclavicular ligament (see Figure 10-15) becoming taut, which limits further motion.
- Once the costoclavicular ligament becomes taut, because the clavicle cannot elevate further, the force of the scapular upward rotation musculature continues to pull on the scapula and results in upward rotation of the scapula relative to the clavicle at the AC joint (5 degrees). The scapula upwardly rotates at the AC joint until the coracoclavicular ligament (see Figure 10-18) becomes taut, which limits further motion.
- The muscles of upward rotation of the scapula continue to pull on the scapula. However, the clavicle cannot elevate any further at the SC joint, and the scapula cannot upwardly rotate any further at the AC joint.

Late Phase
- This continued pull of the scapular upward rotation musculature creates a pull on the scapula that creates tension on the coracoclavicular ligaments. This tension of the coracoclavicular ligaments then pulls on the clavicle in such a way that the clavicle is pulled into upward rotation at the SC joint (the clavicle upwardly rotates approximately 35 degrees).
- Once the clavicle is upwardly rotated at the SC joint, the clavicle can now elevate an additional 5 degrees at the SC joint (because the costoclavicular ligament was slackened) and, more important, the scapula can now upwardly rotate at the AC joint another 25 degrees.

Conclusion
It can be seen that abduction of the arm in the frontal plane is strongly dependent on scapular movement; thus the importance of the term scapulohumeral rhythm. However, it is just as clear that the scapular motion of upward rotation is strongly dependent on clavicular motion; thus the importance of amending the term to scapuloclaviculohumeral rhythm! Therefore in assessment of a client with limited frontal plane motion of the arm, it is crucially important to assess not just GH joint motion but also ScC joint motion; assessing ScC joint motion then necessitates assessment of SC and AC joint motion as well. Thus a case study of frontal plane arm abduction truly manifests the need for healthy coordinated functioning of all components of the shoulder joint complex!

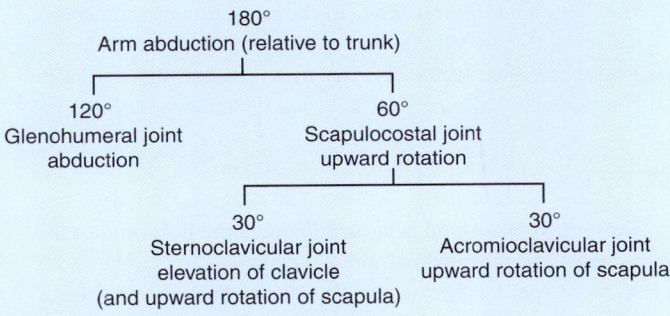

BOX 10-10

If the head of the humerus bangs into the acromion process of the scapula, the tissues located between these two bones will be pinched. The supraspinatus rotator cuff tendon and subacromial bursa are located in this precarious position. Understanding this, imagine the possible health consequences to a client who has a chronic posture of rounded shoulders (i.e., protracted scapulae and medially rotated humeri). As this client perpetually raises the medially rotated arm into abduction, damage to these soft tissues will occur. This condition is known as *shoulder impingement syndrome*. Note also the importance of avoiding abduction motion of the arm above 90 degrees with the arm medially rotated.

SECTION 10.7 ELBOW JOINT COMPLEX

- The elbow joint is unusual in that three articulations are enclosed within one joint capsule.
- These three articulations are (1) the **humeroulnar joint**, (2) the **humeroradial joint**, and (3) the **proximal radioulnar joint**[7] (Figure 10-20).
- Because all three of these articulations are enclosed within one joint capsule and share one joint cavity, anatomically (i.e., structurally) they can be considered to be one joint, or one joint complex. However, because three separate articulations are involved, physiologically (i.e., functionally) they can be considered to be three separate joints.
- Classically, when one speaks of the "elbow joint," it is the humeroulnar and humeroradial joints to which one refers.
- Of these two joints, it is the humeroulnar joint that is functionally more important. Movement at the humeroradial joint is of less significance.[2]
- The proximal radioulnar joint is functionally separate from the elbow joint and will be considered as a part of the radioulnar joints (see Section 10.9).

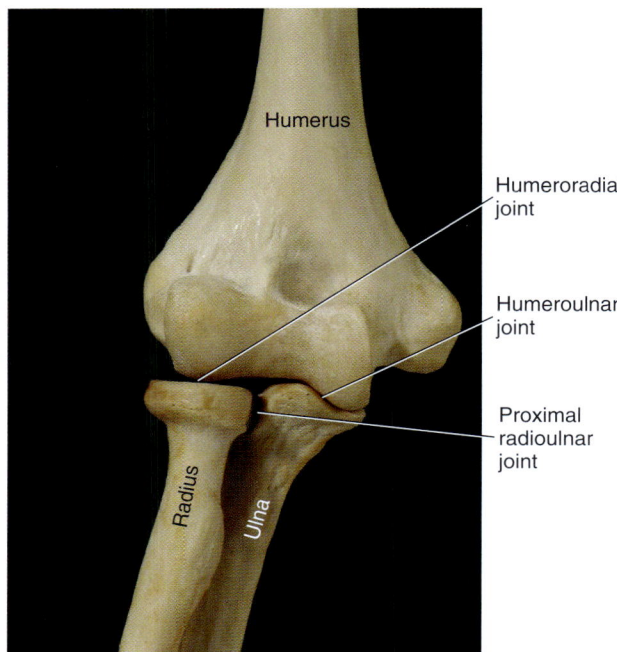

FIGURE 10-20 Anterior view of the right elbow joint complex. Three joints share the same joint capsule; these joints are the humeroulnar and humeroradial joints between the distal humerus and the ulna and radius, respectively, and the proximal radioulnar joint between the head of the radius and the proximal ulna.

SECTION 10.8 ELBOW JOINT

- The elbow joint is composed of the humeroulnar and humeroradial joints (Figure 10-21).
- The humeroulnar joint is also known as the **ulnotrochlear joint**.
- The humeroradial joint is also known as the **radiocapitular joint**.

BONES:

- The humeroulnar joint is located between the distal end of the humerus and the proximal end of the ulna.
  - More specifically, the trochlea of the humerus articulates with the trochlear notch of the ulna.

- The humeroradial joint is located between the distal end of the humerus and the proximal end of the radius.
  - More specifically, the humeroradial joint is located between the capitulum of the humerus and the head of the radius.

HUMEROULNAR JOINT:

- Joint structure classification: Synovial joint[2]
  - Subtype: Hinge
- Joint function classification: Diarthrotic
  - Subtype: Uniaxial

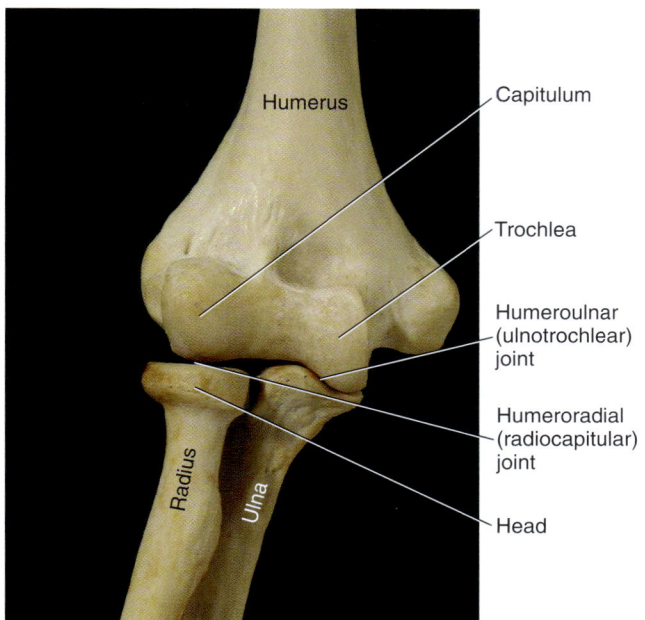

FIGURE 10-21 Anterior view of the right humeroulnar and humeroradial joints. When motion occurs at the elbow joint, it occurs at these two joints; the humeroulnar joint is functionally more important. The humeroulnar joint is also known as the ulnotrochlear joint because the ulna articulates with the trochlea of the distal humerus. The humeroradial joint is also known as the radiocapitular joint because the radius articulates with the capitulum of the distal humerus.

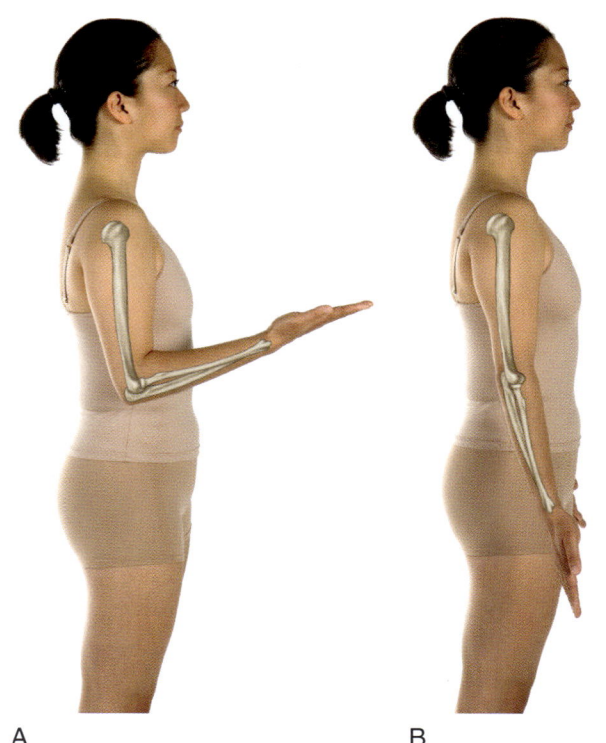

FIGURE 10-22 Motion at the elbow joint. The elbow joint is uniaxial and allows only flexion and extension in the sagittal plane. **A,** Flexion of the forearm at the elbow joint. **B,** Extension of the forearm at the elbow joint. (Note: Both views are lateral.)

HUMERORADIAL JOINT:

- Joint structure classification: Synovial joint[2]
  - Subtype: Atypical ball-and-socket joint
- Joint function classification: Diarthrotic
  - Subtype: Biaxial
  - In addition to the movement that occurs at the humeroradial joint in the sagittal plane as the elbow joint flexes and extends, the head of the radius can also spin relative to the distal end of the humerus (in the transverse plane) as the radius pronates and supinates at the radioulnar joints.

MAJOR ACTIONS OF THE ELBOW JOINT:

- Flexion and extension of the forearm in the sagittal plane around a mediolateral axis (Figure 10-22; Table 10-6).[2]

TABLE 10-6 Average Ranges of Motion of the Forearm at the Elbow Joint from Anatomic Position[2]

Flexion	145 Degrees	Extension	0 Degrees

From anatomic position, usually 5 degrees of hyperextension of the forearm are possible at the elbow joint.

Reverse Actions:

- The arm can move relative to the forearm at the elbow joint.
- Flexion of the arm at the elbow joint is one of the classic reverse actions that is typically used to explain the concept of reverse actions. For example, a pull-up involves flexion of the arm at the elbow joint. (For more on the concept of reverse actions, see Section 6.29.)

MAJOR LIGAMENTS OF THE ELBOW JOINT (HUMEROULNAR AND HUMERORADIAL JOINTS):

The elbow joint has several major ligaments (Figure 10-23; Box 10-11):

BOX 10-11 Ligaments of the Elbow Joint

- Fibrous capsule
- Medial (i.e., ulnar) collateral ligament
- Lateral (i.e., radial) collateral ligament

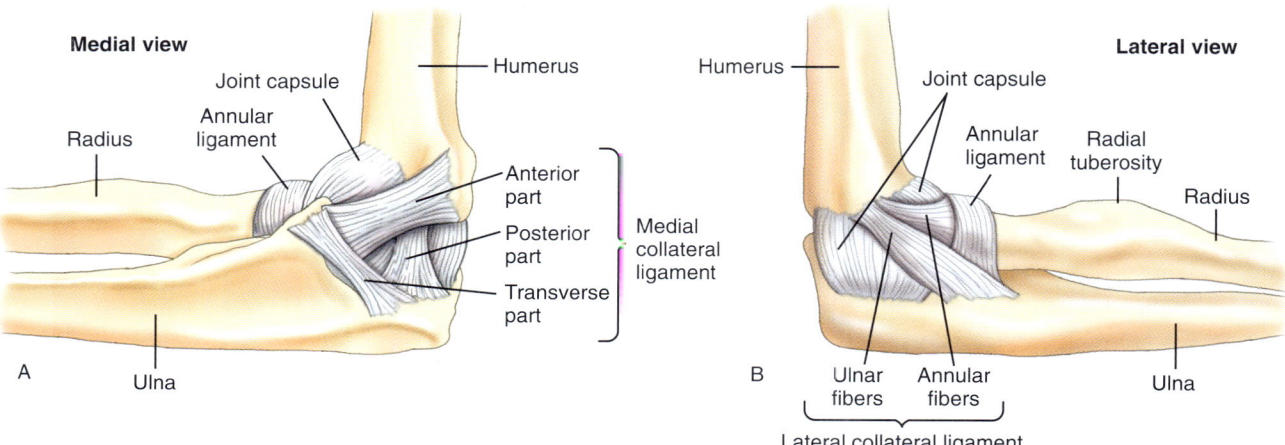

FIGURE 10-23 Ligaments of the right elbow joint. **A,** Medial view demonstrating the joint capsule and the medial collateral ligament. The medial collateral ligament has three parts: (1) anterior, (2) posterior, and (3) transverse. **B,** Lateral view demonstrating the joint capsule, lateral collateral ligament, and annular ligament of the proximal radioulnar (RU) joint. The lateral collateral ligament has two parts: (1) annular fibers that blend into the annular ligament and (2) ulnar fibers that attach onto the ulna.

Medial Collateral Ligament:

- The **medial collateral ligament** consists of three parts: (1) anterior, (2) posterior, and (3) transverse fibers.
- The majority of the fibers of the medial collateral ligament attach from the medial epicondyle of the humerus to the ulna.
- The functions are to stabilize the medial side of the elbow joint and to prevent abduction of the forearm at the elbow joint.[1]
- The medial collateral ligament is also known as the **ulnar collateral ligament**.

Lateral Collateral Ligament:

- The **lateral collateral ligament** consists of two parts: (1) annular fibers and (2) ulnar fibers.
- The lateral collateral ligament attaches from the lateral epicondyle of the humerus to the annular ligament that lies over the radial head, and to the ulna.
- The functions are to stabilize the lateral side of the elbow joint and to prevent adduction of the forearm at the elbow joint.[1]
- The lateral collateral ligament is also known as the **radial collateral ligament**.

CLOSED-PACKED POSITION OF THE ELBOW JOINT:

- Extension

MAJOR MUSCLES OF THE ELBOW JOINT:

- Because the elbow joint is a hinge joint, its actions are restricted to flexion and extension. All muscles that cross the elbow joint anteriorly can perform flexion, and all muscles that cross posteriorly can perform extension.
  - The major flexors at the elbow joint are the brachialis, biceps brachii, brachioradialis, and pronator teres.
  - The major extensor of the elbow joint is the triceps brachii. The anconeus and extensor carpi ulnaris can also extend the elbow joint.

- Note: Two other groups of muscles (the wrist flexor group and wrist extensor group) have bellies that are located near the elbow joint and proximal tendons that originate and attach onto the humerus. The wrist flexor group attaches to the medial epicondyle of the humerus via the common flexor belly/tendon; the wrist extensor group primarily attaches to the lateral epicondyle of the humerus via the common extensor belly/tendon. Even though these muscles do cross the elbow joint and therefore can move the elbow joint, their primary actions (as their names imply) are at the wrist joint (Box 10-12).

 BOX 10-12

Tennis elbow and golfer's elbow are the names given to irritation and/or inflammation of the common extensor belly/tendon and common flexor belly/tendon, respectively (and/or their attachments onto the humerus). Technically, tennis elbow is called **lateral epicondylitis** or **lateral epicondylosis**, and golfer's elbow is called **medial epicondylitis** or **medial epicondylosis**. These conditions are considered to be tendinitis or tendinosis problems; they usually also involve hypertonicity of the involved muscles. (Note: Tendinosis is distinguished from tendinitis by an absence of inflammation; *itis* means "inflammation," and *osis* simply means "condition of" and implies degeneration of the fascial tissue). Even though these conditions are named as elbow problems, they are not elbow joint problems; rather, they are functionally related to use of the hand at the wrist joint.

MISCELLANEOUS:

- From the anterior perspective, it can be seen that the humerus and ulna are not aligned in a perfectly straight line within the frontal plane; rather, the ulna deviates laterally.[2] This lateral deviation of the ulna relative to the humerus is known as the **carrying angle** (Figure 10-24).
  - The usual carrying angle is approximately 5 to 15 degrees. It is usually between 5 and 10 degrees in men and 10 and 15 degrees in women.

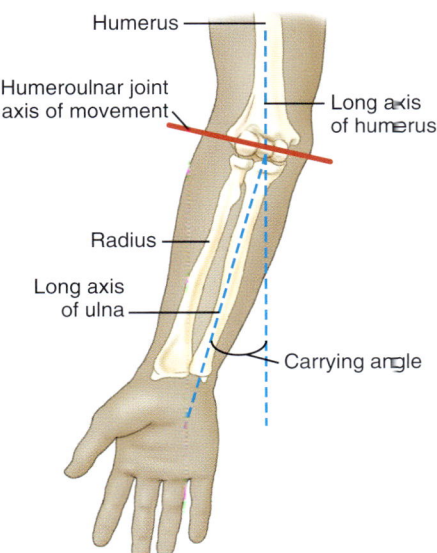

FIGURE 10-24 Carrying angle of the upper extremity. The carrying angle is formed by the intersection of two lines: one through the long axis of the humerus and the other through the long axis of the ulna. The usual carrying angle is 5 to 15 degrees. The carrying angle is formed because the axis of movement of the humeroulnar joint is not horizontal.

- This carrying angle is also known as **cubitus valgus**.
- The term *valgus* refers to a lateral deviation of a body part—in this case the ulna. A carrying angle that is appreciably greater than 15 degrees is referred to as an *excessive cubitus valgus*, and a carrying angle appreciably less than 15 degrees is referred to as **cubitus varus**.
- The reason that the carrying angle exists is that the axis of movement at the elbow (i.e., humeroulnar) joint is not purely horizontal (see Figure 10-24). Rather, from medial to lateral, it is directed slightly superiorly, because the medial lip of the trochlea protrudes farther than does the lateral lip of the trochlea (see Figure 5-64).
- The advantage of a carrying angle is that objects carried in the hand are naturally held away from the body.
- For this reason, the carrying angle is larger for women because the female pelvis is wider than the male pelvis.

SECTION 10.9 RADIOULNAR JOINTS

- When the radius moves relative to the ulna during pronation and supination, these actions occur at the **radioulnar (RU) joints**.[8]
- Three radioulnar joints exist: (1) the **proximal radioulnar joint**, (2) the **middle radioulnar joint**, and (3) the **distal radioulnar joint**[3] (Figure 10-25).
- Although all three RU joints are functionally related in that their combined movements allow pronation and supination of the forearm, they are anatomically distinct from one another.
  - In fact, the proximal RU joint shares its joint capsule with the elbow joint, whereas the distal RU joint shares its joint capsule with the radiocarpal joint of the wrist joint complex.

BONES:

- The RU joints are located between the radius and ulna.
- The proximal RU joint is located between the proximal radius and the proximal ulna.
  - More specifically, the proximal RU joint is located between the head of the radius and the radial notch of the ulna.
- The middle RU joint is formed by the interosseus membrane that connects the shafts of the radius and ulna.
- The distal RU joint is located between the distal radius and the distal ulna.
  - More specifically, the distal RU joint is located between the ulnar notch of the radius and the head of the ulna.

PROXIMAL RADIOULNAR JOINT:

- Joint structure classification: Synovial joint
  - Subtype: Pivot
- Joint function classification: Diarthrotic
  - Subtype: Uniaxial[5]

MIDDLE RADIOULNAR JOINT:

- Joint structure classification: Fibrous joint
  - Subtype: Syndesmosis
- Joint function classification: Amphiarthrotic
  - Subtype: Uniaxial[2]

DISTAL RADIOULNAR JOINT:

- Joint structure classification: Synovial joint
  - Subtype: Pivot
- Joint function classification: Diarthrotic
  - Subtype: Uniaxial (Box 10-13)[7]

328　PART 3　Skeletal Arthrology: Study of the Joints

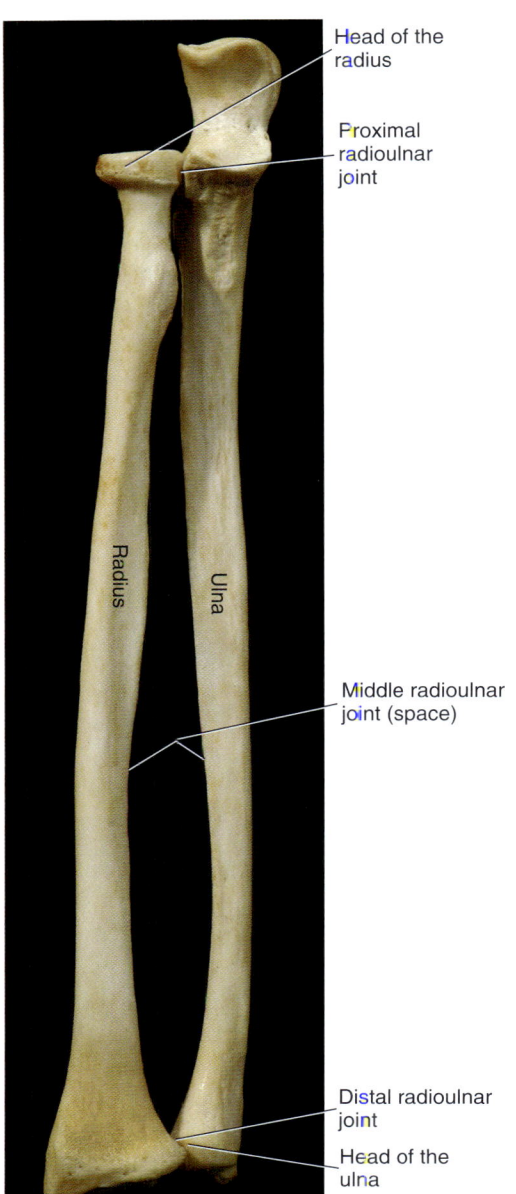

FIGURE 10-25 Anterior view that illustrates the three radioulnar (RU) joints of the right forearm.

MAJOR ACTIONS OF THE RADIOULNAR JOINTS:

- The combined movements at the RU joints allow for pronation and supination of the forearm (Figure 10-26; Table 10-7; and see Figures 5-68 and 5-72.)
- During pronation and supination of the forearm, it is usually the radius that accomplishes the majority of the motion around a relatively fixed ulna.[6] However, when the hand is fixed (i.e., closed-chain activity), the radius becomes fixed during pronation and supination motions, and it is the ulna that performs the majority of the motion (see Section 13.9, Figure 13-15).

 | BOX 10-13 | Spotlight on Motion at the Distal Radioulnar Joint |

The terms pronation and supination are used to describe motions of the radius, because the radius does not move in a typical manner for a long bone. During pronation of the radius, the head of the radius clearly medially rotates relative to the proximal ulna. This medial rotation involves the proximal radius spinning medially and remaining "in place." However, the distal radioulnar (RU) joint does not allow the distal radius to perform pure medial rotation and stay in its same location in space (medial rotation and lateral rotation of a long bone usually occur around an axis that runs through the shaft of the bone; consequently the bone spins in place). When the proximal radius medially rotates, the distal radius is forced to rotate and "swing around" the distal ulna.

This *rotating-and-swinging* motion can be described in terms of roll, spin, and glide (see Sections 6.7 and 6.8). In this case the distal radius rolls and glides in the same direction, as is usual for a concave bone moving relative to a convex bone. However, what is unusual about the roll/glide dynamics here is that the roll and glide occur in a line that is perpendicular to the long axis of the radius; roll and glide usually occur in the same line as the long axis of the bone.

Describing distal RU motion in the terminology system of flexion/extension, abduction/adduction, and medial rotation/lateral rotation is even more awkward because it does not fit well into any one of these categories. If one were to try to place this motion into one of these categories of motion, the closest fit would be to say that the distal radius medially rotates, but that this rotation occurs around an axis that lies outside of the shaft of the radius. Because this axis runs through the distal ulna (see Section 6.18, Figure 6-18), pronation and supination of the radius at the distal RU joint involve the distal end of the radius actually rotating and "swinging" around the distal ulna.

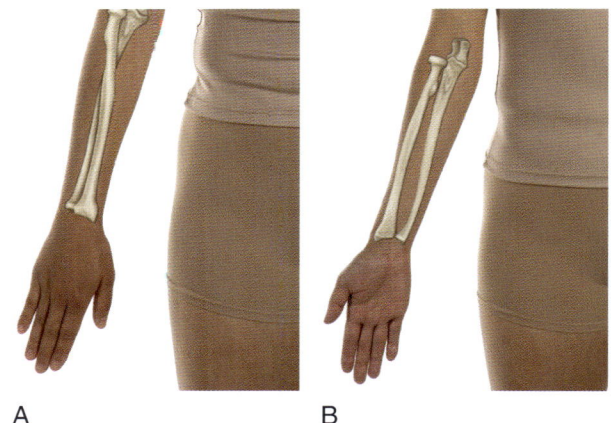

A　　　　　　　　　　B

FIGURE 10-26 Pronation and supination of the right forearm at the radioulnar (RU) joints. **A,** Pronation. **B,** Supination, which is anatomic position for the forearm (Note: Both figures are anterior views of the forearm.)

- This action of the radius occurs around an axis that runs from the head of the radius to the head of the ulna; this axis is not purely vertical (see Section 6.18, Figure 6-18).
  - Movement at the proximal RU joint: The head of the radius medially rotates during pronation of the forearm; the

TABLE 10-7	Average Ranges of Motion of the Forearm at the Radioulnar Joints from Anatomic Position		
Pronation	160 Degrees	Supination	0 Degrees

Forearm pronation and supination motions are often measured from a neutral "thumbs-up" position. From this neutral position, 85 degrees of forearm supination and 75 degrees of forearm pronation are possible.[2]

> **BOX 10-14**   **Ligaments of the Radioulnar Joints**
>
> **Proximal Radioulnar (RU) Joint**
> - Fibrous joint capsule
> - Annular ligament
>
> **Middle RU Joint**
> - Interosseus membrane
> - Oblique cord
>
> **Distal RU Joint**
> - Fibrous joint capsule
> - RU disc (triangular fibrocartilage)

- head of the radius laterally rotates during supination of the forearm.
- Movement at the distal RU joint: The distal radius swings around the distal ulna.

MAJOR LIGAMENTS OF THE RADIOULNAR JOINTS:

- The proximal, middle, and distal RU joints have several major ligaments (Figure 10-27; Box 10-14):

Proximal Radioulnar Joint:

- Fibrous capsule
- Annular ligament
  - The **annular ligament** attaches to the anterior ulna, wraps around the head of the radius, and then attaches to the posterior ulna.
  - Function: It stabilizes the proximal RU joint and creates a cavity within which the head of the radius can rotate.[8]

Middle Radioulnar Joint:

- Interosseus membrane of the forearm
  - The **interosseus membrane** is a fibrous sheet of tissue that unites the radius and ulna of the forearm, forming the middle RU joint.
  - Function: It stabilizes the middle RU joint by binding the radius and ulna together.[8]
  - The interosseus membrane, by binding the radius and ulna together, helps to stabilize the two bones of the forearm (i.e., the middle radioulnar [RU] joint). However, it also serves another important function. When compression forces travel up from the hand into the radius of the forearm (e.g., during an activity such as a push-up), these forces need to be transferred into the arm and from there into the trunk. However, the radius is not the principal bone of the elbow joint to be able to transfer this force

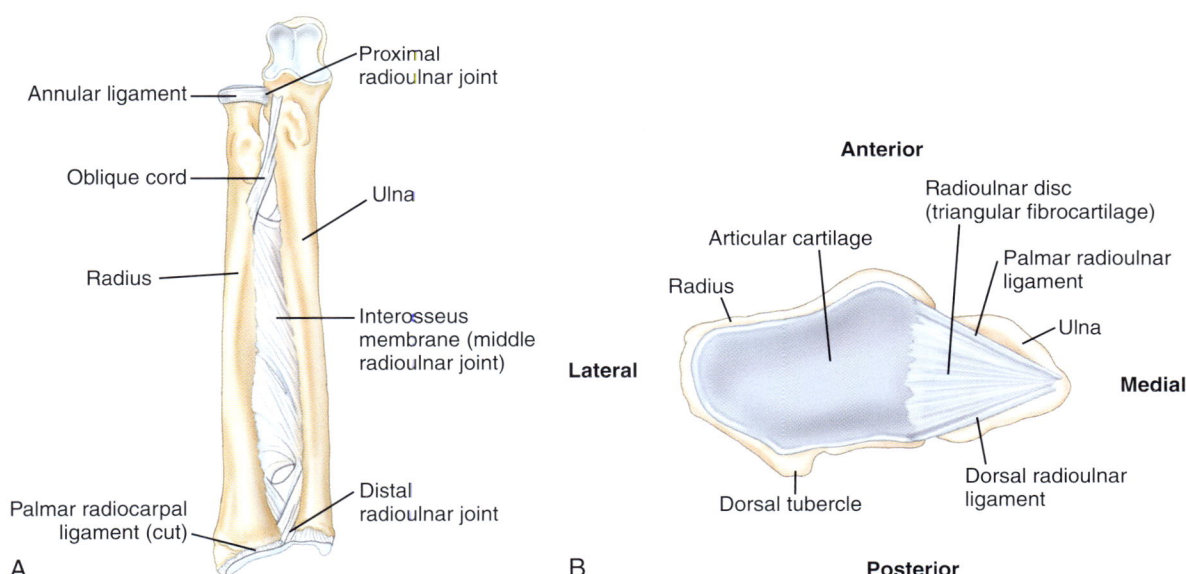

FIGURE 10-27 Ligamentous structures of the right radioulnar (RU) joints. **A,** Anterior view demonstrating the interosseus membrane and oblique cord, which form the middle RU joint, and the annular ligament of the proximal RU joint. Part of the joint capsule of the distal RU joint (which it shares with the wrist joint) is also shown. **B,** View of the distal ends of the radius and ulna, depicting the radioulnar disc of the distal RU joint. (Reader should note its triangular shape; hence its other name, the triangular fibrocartilage.)

330   PART 3   Skeletal Arthrology: Study of the Joints

to the humerus; it is the ulna that forms the major articulation at the elbow joint with the humerus. Therefore to efficiently transfer this force up to the arm, the radius must first transfer it to the ulna. This is accomplished by the interosseus membrane. Because of the direction of the fibers of the interosseus membrane (see Figure 10-27), if an upward force travels through the radius, the interosseus membrane will transfer this force to the ulna by pulling upward on the ulna. This force can then be transferred across the humeroulnar (i.e., elbow) joint to the humerus. Similarly, a downward force that travels from the trunk and through the arm will cross the elbow joint into the ulna. The interosseus membrane will then transfer that force into the radius (given its fiber direction, a downward force on the ulna will create a downward pulling force on the radius), which can then be transferred across the radiocarpal (i.e., wrist) joint into the hand.

- Oblique cord
  - The oblique cord runs from the proximal ulna to the proximal radius. Its fibers are oriented perpendicular to the fibers of the interosseus membrane.
  - Function: It assists the interosseus membrane in stabilizing the middle RU joint.

Distal Radioulnar Joint:

- Fibrous capsule
  - The fibrous capsule is thickened on the dorsal and palmar sides.
  - The dorsal and palmar thickenings of the fibrous capsule of the distal radioulnar (RU) joint are called the **dorsal radioulnar ligament** and the **palmar radioulnar ligament** (see Figure 10-27, B).[7]

Radioulnar Disc:

- The RU disc runs from the distal radius to the distal ulna.
- It also blends into the capsular/ligamentous structure of the distal RU joint.
- Function: It stabilizes the distal RU joint.[7]
- The RU disc is also known as the **triangular fibrocartilage**.
- Because the distal radioulnar (RU) joint and the radiocarpal joint share the same joint capsule, the radioulnar (RU) disc, also known as the *triangular fibrocartilage,* is involved with both joints. It blends into the capsular/ligamentous structure of both the distal RU joint and the radiocarpal joint and adds to the stability of both these joints. (For more information on the RU disc, see Section 10.11; for information on the radiocarpal joint, see Sections 10.10 and 10.11.)

MISCELLANEOUS:

- The proximal RU joint shares its joint capsule with the elbow joint.
- The distal RU joint shares its joint capsule with the radiocarpal joint of the wrist joint complex.

SECTION 10.10   OVERVIEW OF THE WRIST/HAND REGION

- The wrist/hand region involves a number of bones and a number of joints. Generally the organization of the wrist/hand region is as follows (Figure 10-28):
- The two bones of the forearm—the radius and ulna—articulate with the hand at the wrist joint.
- The hand is defined as everything distal to the radius and ulna.
  - The bones of the hand can be divided into carpals, metacarpals, and phalanges.
  - Just as the tarsal bones are the ankle bones, the carpal bones are known as the *wrist bones.*
- The hand can be divided into three regions[2]:
  1. The **carpus** is composed of the eight carpal bones.
  2. The **metacarpus**, also known as the *body of the hand,* contains the five metacarpal bones. The **palm** is the anterior region of the metacarpus of the hand.
  3. The fingers contain the phalanges.
- The term **ray** refers to a metacarpal and its associated phalanges; the hand has five rays:
  - The first ray is composed of the first metacarpal and the two phalanges of the thumb.
  - The second ray is composed of the second metacarpal and the three phalanges of the index finger (i.e., second finger).
  - The third ray is composed of the third metacarpal and the three phalanges of the middle finger (i.e., third finger).
  - The fourth ray is composed of the fourth metacarpal and the three phalanges of the ring finger (i.e., fourth finger).
  - The fifth ray is composed of the fifth metacarpal and the three phalanges of the little finger (i.e., fifth finger).

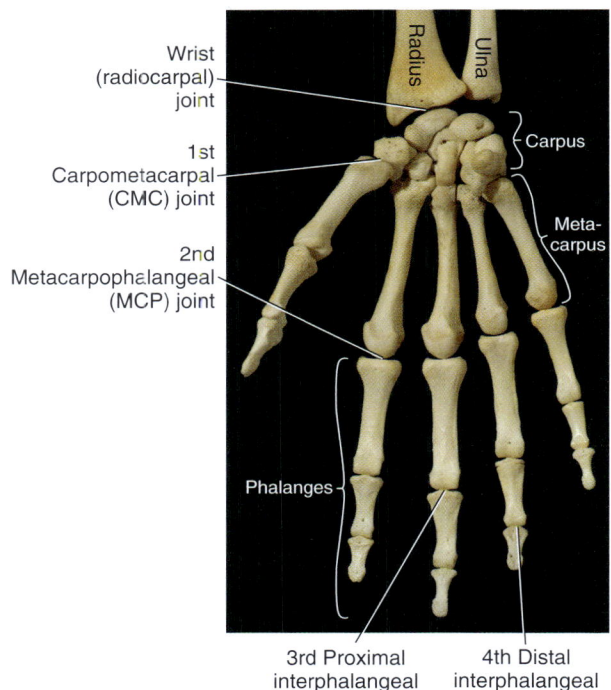

FIGURE 10-28 Anterior view of the skeletal structure of the right distal forearm and hand. The hand is located distal to the radius and ulna of the forearm. The hand can be divided into three parts: (1) the carpus, (2) the metacarpus, and (3) the phalanges.

CHAPTER 10 Joints of the Upper Extremity

FUNCTIONS OF THE HAND:

- The human hand is an amazing structure. With the presence of an opposable thumb, the hand allows us to create, grasp, and use tools. The brain is usually credited as the distinguishing structure that has allowed human beings to advance and create civilization; however, some give equal credit to the hand. Although the brain conceptually designs civilization, the hand actually creates it. In this regard the hand may be viewed as the tool of expression of our brain!
- To free our hands for use, a bipedal stance on two legs instead of four is necessary. It is then up to the joints of the upper extremity to move our hand through space and place it in whatever location is necessary for the desired task. Because the upper extremity joints are freed from their weight-bearing responsibility, they have been able to trade off stability for the increased mobility necessary to place the hand in almost any position in all three cardinal planes.

GENERAL ORGANIZATION OF THE JOINTS OF THE WRIST/HAND REGION:

Wrist Joint:

- The wrist joint is actually a complex of two major joints: (1) the **radiocarpal joint** and (2) the **midcarpal joint**.[9]
  - The radiocarpal joint is located between the distal end of the radius and the proximal row of carpal bones.
  - The midcarpal joint is located between the proximal row of carpal bones and the distal row of carpal bones.

Carpometacarpal Joints:

- The carpometacarpal (CMC) joints are located between the distal row of carpals and the metacarpal bones.[5]
  - The first CMC joint (of the thumb) is a saddle joint that is specialized to allow a great degree of movement.

Intermetacarpal Joints:

- The intermetacarpal (IMC) joints are located between adjacent metacarpal bones.[8]

Metacarpophalangeal Joints:

- The metacarpophalangeal (MCP) joints are located between the metacarpal bones and the phalanges.[8]

Interphalangeal Joints (of the Hand):

- The interphalangeal (IP) joints are located between phalanges of a finger (see Figure 10-28).[2]
  - Proximal interphalangeal (PIP) joints are located between the proximal and middle phalanges of fingers #2 through #5.
  - Distal interphalangeal (DIP) joints are located between the middle and distal phalanges of fingers #2 through #5.
  - The IP joint of the thumb is located between the proximal and middle phalanges of the thumb (i.e., finger #1).

ARCHES OF THE HAND:

- Although the foot is usually thought of when arches are discussed, the hand also has arches. The arches of the hand create a concavity of the palm and a concavity of the fingers that helps the hand fit more securely around objects that are held, increasing the security of one's grasp (Figure 10-29).
- The hand has three arches:[10]
  - **Proximal transverse arch**: The proximal transverse arch of the hand runs transversely (i.e., across the hand) and is formed by the two rows (proximal and distal) of carpal bones.
  - **Distal transverse arch**: The distal transverse arch runs transversely (i.e., across the hand) and is located at the MCP joints.
    - Unlike the proximal transverse arch, which is fairly rigid, the distal transverse arch is quite mobile. When an object is held in the hand, the mobile first, fourth, and fifth

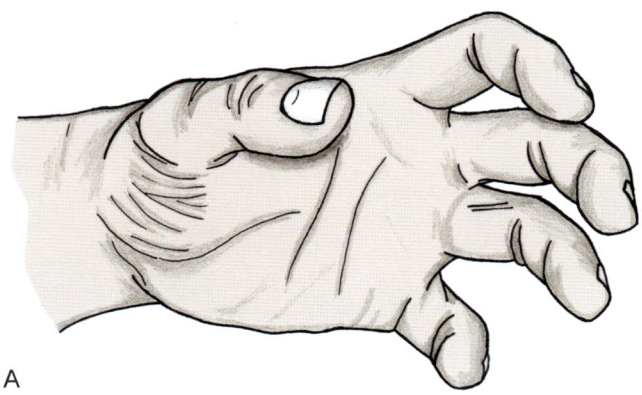

A

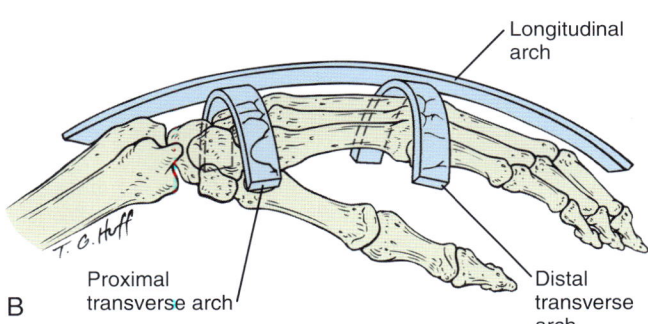

B

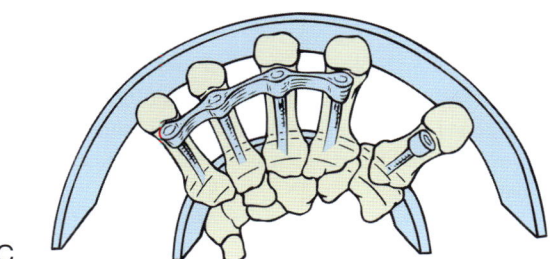

C

FIGURE 10-29 Arches of the hand. The hand has three arches: (1) a proximal transverse arch formed by the carpals, (2) a distal transverse arch formed at the metacarpophalangeal (MCP) joints, and (3) the longitudinal arch formed by the length of the metacarpals and phalanges. (**A**, *Courtesy Joseph E. Muscolino;* **B** *and* **C**: Browner BD, Jupiter JB, Levine AM, et al. *Skeletal trauma: basic science, management, and reconstruction,* ed 4, Philadelphia, 2008, Saunders).

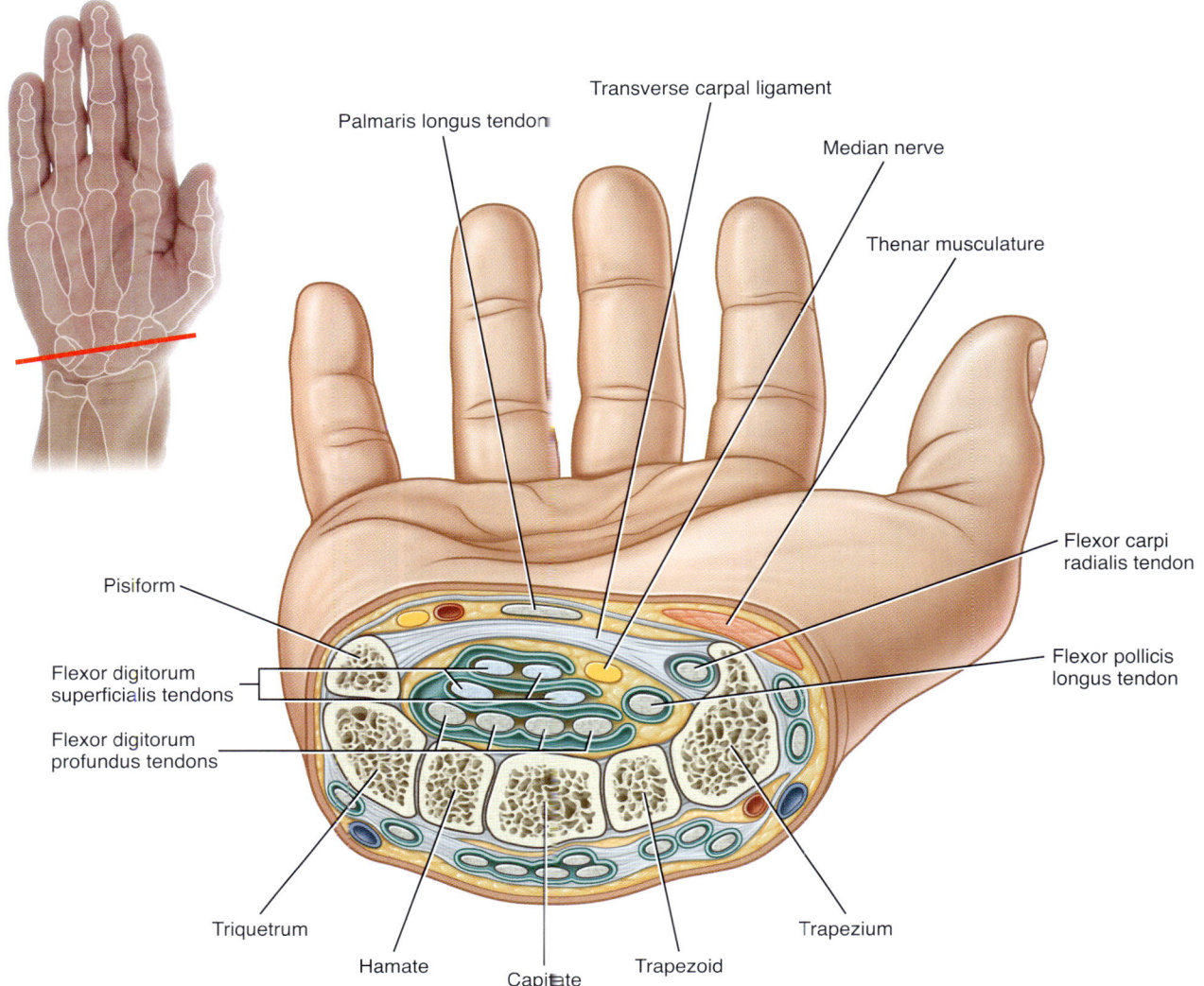

FIGURE 10-30 Illustration looking distally into the right hand. The tunnel formed by the carpal bones (i.e., the carpal tunnel) can be seen. The floor of the carpal tunnel is formed by the carpal bones; the roof is formed by the transverse carpal ligament. The carpal tunnel contains the median nerve and nine extrinsic flexor tendons of the fingers. Note: Cross section cuts through the distal row of carpal bones and the triquetrum and pisiform of the proximal row. *(Modified from Drake, R: Gray's atlas of anatomy, ed 2, Philadelphia, 2015, Churchill Livingstone.)*

metacarpals wrap around the stable second and third metacarpals.
- **Longitudinal arch**: The longitudinal arch runs the length of the hand and is formed by the shape of the metacarpals and fingers. The shape of the metacarpals is somewhat fixed, but flexion of the fingers increases the longitudinal arch of the hand.

CARPAL TUNNEL:

- The carpal tunnel is located anteriorly at the wrist and is a tunnel formed by the arrangement of the carpal bones (Figure 10-30).
  - It is located between the archlike transverse concavity of the carpal bones and the **transverse carpal ligament** that spans across the top of the carpal bones.[2]
- The transverse carpal ligament is also known as the **flexor retinaculum** (of the wrist) because it functions as a retinaculum to hold down the extrinsic finger flexor muscles that enter the hand from the forearm. It attaches to the pisiform and hook of the hamate on the ulnar side and to the tubercles of the trapezium and scaphoid on the radial side (see Figure 10-30).
- The carpal tunnel provides a safe passageway for the median nerve and the distal tendons of the extrinsic finger flexor muscles of the forearm to enter the hand (Box 10-15).
- The distal tendons of the extrinsic finger flexor muscles located within the carpal tunnel are the four tendons of the flexor digitorum superficialis (FDS), four tendons of the flexor digitorum profundus (FDP), and the tendon of the flexor pollicis longus.
- The radial (lateral) part of the transverse carpal ligament has a superficial part and a deep part. Running between these

BOX 10-15

If the carpal tunnel is injured, the median nerve may be impinged, causing sensory and/or motor symptoms within the region of the hand that is innervated by the median nerve. This condition is known as **carpal tunnel syndrome**. Sensory symptoms may occur on the anterior side of the thumb, index, middle, and radial half of the ring finger, as well as the posterior side of the fingertips of the same fingers; motor symptoms may result in weakness of the intrinsic thenar muscles of the thumb that are innervated by the median nerve. Individuals who work with their hands, especially manual therapists and trainers, are particularly susceptible to this condition. Placing excessive pressure through the wrist when doing massage, bodywork, and training should be avoided. Prolonged postures of wrist joint extension with finger flexion, falls on outstretched hands, and swelling within the wrist can also cause carpal tunnel syndrome.

two parts is the distal tendon of the flexor carpi radialis. Technically, the distal tendon of the flexor carpi radialis is not located within the carpal tunnel.

PALMAR FASCIA:

- The hand has a thick layer of dense fibrous tissue on the palmar side known as the **palmar fascia**. Although not as significant as the plantar fascia of the foot, the palmar fascia does increase the structural stability of the hand.

DORSAL DIGITAL EXPANSION:

- The **dorsal digital expansion** is a fibrous aponeurotic expansion of the distal attachment of the extensor digitorum muscle on the fingers (index, middle, ring, and little) (Figure 10-31).[2]
  - The dorsal digital expansion serves as a movable hood of tissue when the fingers flex and extend.
  - The dorsal digital expansion begins on the dorsal, medial, and lateral sides of the proximal phalanx of each finger and ultimately attaches onto the dorsal side of the middle and distal phalanges.
  - The dorsal digital expansion serves as an attachment site for a number of muscles.
  - These muscles are the lumbricals manus, palmar interossei, dorsal interossei manus, and abductor digiti minimi manus.
  - Because the dorsal digital expansion eventually attaches onto the dorsal side of the middle and distal phalanges, it crosses the proximal interphalangeal (PIP) joint and the distal interphalangeal (DIP) joint on the dorsal side. Consequently, when any muscle that attaches into the dorsal digital expansion contracts, the pull of its contraction is transferred across these interphalangeal (IP) joints. Therefore all muscles that attach into the dorsal digital expansion can perform extension of the fingers at the PIP and DIP joints.
  - The dorsal digital expansion is also known as the **extensor expansion** or the **dorsal hood**.
  - A dorsal digital expansion of the thumb is formed by the distal tendon of the extensor pollicis longus.

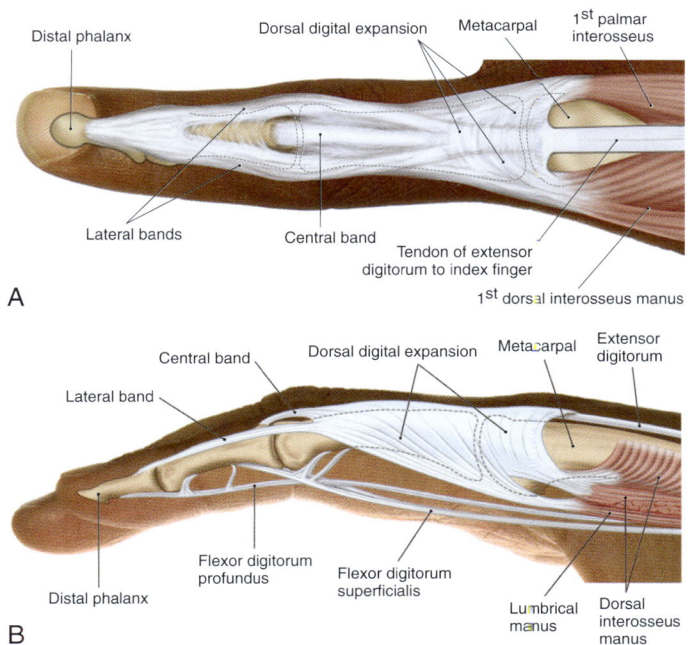

FIGURE 10-31 Dorsal digital expansion of the right hand. **A,** Dorsal view. **B,** Lateral view. The dorsal digital expansion is a fibrous expansion on fingers #2 through #5 of the distal tendons of the extensor digitorum muscle. Dotted lines represent borders of underlying bones. *(From Muscolino JE. The muscular system manual: the skeletal muscles of the human body, ed 4, St Louis, 2017, Elsevier.)*

SECTION 10.11 WRIST JOINT COMPLEX

- Movement at the wrist joint actually occurs at two joints: (1) the radiocarpal joint and (2) the midcarpal joint. For this reason, the wrist joint is better termed the **wrist joint complex** (Figure 10-32).
- In addition to the radiocarpal and midcarpal joints, a great number of smaller **intercarpal joints** are located between the individual carpal bones of the wrist (e.g., the scapholunate joint is an intercarpal joint located between the scaphoid and lunate bones). However, these individual intercarpal joints do not contribute to movement of the hand relative to the forearm at the wrist joint.

RADIOCARPAL JOINT:

Bones:

- The radiocarpal joint is located between the radius and the carpals.
  - More specifically, the distal end of the radius articulates with the proximal row of carpal bones.
- The proximal row of carpals is made up of the scaphoid, lunate, and triquetrum. (Note: Even though the pisiform is in the proximal row of carpals, it does not participate in either the radiocarpal joint or the midcarpal joint. The pisiform is considered to be a sesamoid bone and functions to increase the contraction force of the flexor carpi ulnaris and also serve as an attachment site for the transverse carpal ligament that covers the carpal tunnel[2].)

- Because more than two bones are involved, the radiocarpal joint is a compound joint.
- The entire radiocarpal joint is enclosed within one joint cavity.[1]
  - Note: The joint between the forearm and the carpal bones is called the *radiocarpal joint* because it is the radius that primarily articulates with the carpals. The ulna itself does not directly articulate with the carpal bones, because many soft tissue structures (of the ulnocarpal complex) are located between them. However, when we look at the wrist joint complex functionally, the **ulnocarpal joint** does transmit 20% of the load from the hand to the forearm when compression forces occur through the wrist (e.g., when doing a push-up). Therefore even though the radiocarpal joint is by far the more significant joint between the forearm and carpus, the ulnocarpal joint does have some functional significance.
- In addition, an intra-articular disc is located within the radiocarpal joint.[2]
  - This intra-articular disc is known as the *radioulnar disc* or the *triangular fibrocartilage*.
- The radiocarpal joint shares its joint cavity with the distal radioulnar (RU) joint. (For information on the distal RU joint, see Section 10.9.) Because the radiocarpal joint and the distal RU joint share the same joint capsule, the radioulnar disc (i.e., triangular fibrocartilage) located within this joint capsule is involved with both of these joints.

MIDCARPAL JOINT:

Bones:

- The midcarpal joint is located between the proximal row of carpal bones and the distal row of carpal bones.[5]
  - More specifically, the midcarpal joint is located between the scaphoid, lunate, and triquetrum proximally and the trapezium, trapezoid, capitate, and hamate distally.
- Because more than two bones are involved, the midcarpal joint is a compound joint.
- The joint capsule of the midcarpal joint is anatomically separate from the joint capsule of the radiocarpal joint.
- The joint surfaces and capsule of the midcarpal joint are fairly irregular in shape and are continuous with the individual intercarpal joints of all the bones involved.
- Because the midcarpal joint is so irregular in shape and the joint capsule is continuous with the joint spaces between the separate intercarpal joints involved, the midcarpal joint is often described as being more of a functional joint than an anatomic joint.
- The midcarpal joint is usually divided into a medial compartment and a lateral compartment.[1]
  - The medial compartment is larger, and its orientation is similar to the radiocarpal joint; its proximal surface is concave and its distal surface is convex. It is a compound joint formed between the proximal pole of the scaphoid and the

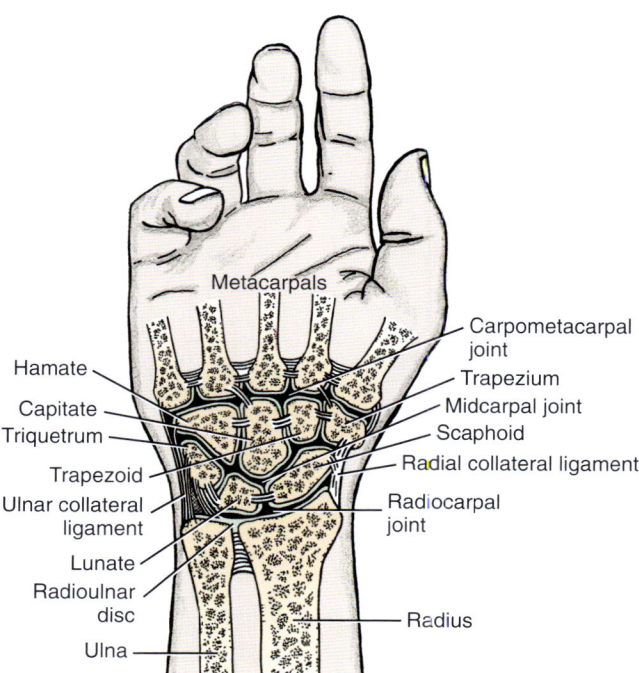

FIGURE 10-32 Anterior view of the wrist/hand region that illustrates the two major joints of the wrist joint complex. The more proximal joint is the radiocarpal joint; the more distal joint is the midcarpal joint. *(Courtesy Joseph E. Muscolino.)*

lunate and triquetrum proximally, and the capitate and hamate distally.
- The lateral compartment is smaller, and its orientation is opposite that of the medial compartment; its proximal surface is convex and its distal surface is concave. It is a compound joint formed between the distal pole of the scaphoid proximally and the trapezium and trapezoid distally.

BOTH RADIOCARPAL AND MIDCARPAL JOINTS:

- Joint structure classification: Synovial joint[2]
  - Subtype: Condyloid
- Joint function classification: Diarthrotic
  - Subtype: Biaxial

MAJOR MOTIONS ALLOWED:

- Flexion and extension of the hand (i.e., axial actions) in the sagittal plane around a mediolateral axis (Figure 10-33, A and B; Table 10-8)
  - Flexion is greater at the radiocarpal joint, and extension is greater at the midcarpal joint

TABLE 10-8	Average Ranges of Motion of the Hand at the Wrist Joint from Anatomic Position[2]
Flexion	80 Degrees
Extension	70 Degrees
Radial deviation	15 Degrees
Ulnar deviation	30 Degrees

- Radial deviation and ulnar deviation (i.e., axial actions) of the hand in the frontal plane around an anteroposterior axis (Figure 10-33, C and D)
  - From anatomic position, radial deviation of the hand at the wrist joint is minimal as a result of the impingement of the carpus against the styloid process of the radius, which is located at the radial side of the radius. Ulnar deviation is not as limited because the styloid process of the ulna is located posteriorly, not on the ulnar side of the ulna.[8]
  - Radial deviation is greater at the midcarpal joint, and ulnar deviation occurs equally at the radiocarpal and midcarpal joints.
  - Note: Radial deviation is also known as *abduction;* ulnar deviation is also known as *adduction.*

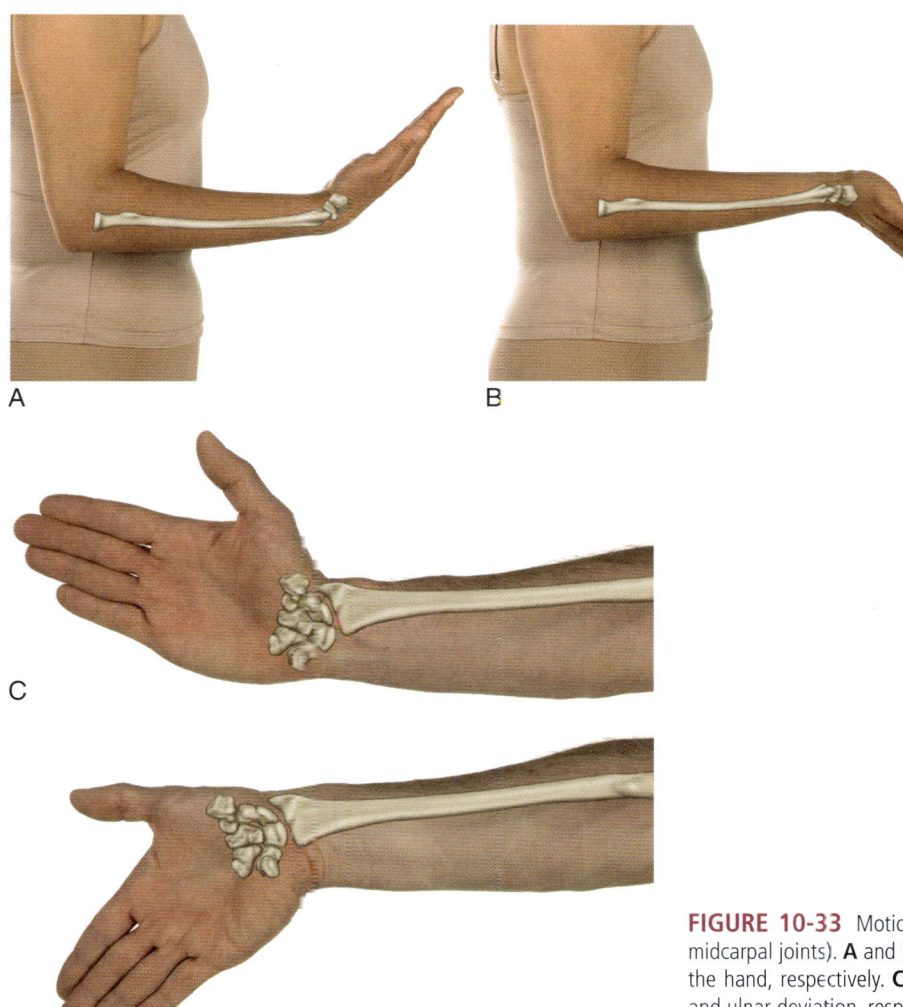

FIGURE 10-33 Motions of the hand at the wrist joint (radiocarpal and midcarpal joints). **A** and **B,** Lateral views illustrating flexion and extension of the hand, respectively. **C** and **D,** Anterior views illustrating radial deviation and ulnar deviation, respectively. Radial deviation of the hand is also known as abduction; ulnar deviation is also known as adduction.

Accessory Motions:
- The carpal bones permit a great deal of gliding motion.[8]

Reverse Actions:
- The forearm can move relative to the hand at the wrist joint. This would occur when the hand is fixed (closed-chain activity), perhaps grasping an immovable object.

MAJOR LIGAMENTS OF THE WRIST JOINT COMPLEX:

The wrist joint complex has many ligaments (Figure 10-34; Box 10-16). These ligaments include the joint capsules of the radiocarpal and midcarpal joints, the radioulnar disc, the transverse carpal ligament, and extrinsic and intrinsic ligaments of the wrist.

BOX 10-16 Ligaments of the Wrist Joint Complex

- Joint capsule of the radiocarpal joint
- Radioulnar (RU) disc (i.e., triangular fibrocartilage)
- Joint capsule of the midcarpal joint
- Transverse carpal ligament

Extrinsic Ligaments
- Dorsal radiocarpal ligament
- Palmar radiocarpal ligaments
- Radial collateral ligament
- Ulnar collateral ligament

Intrinsic Ligaments
- Short
- Intermediate
- Long

Joint Capsule of the Radiocarpal Joint:
- The radiocarpal joint capsule is thickened and strengthened by the dorsal radiocarpal, palmar radiocarpal, radial collateral, and ulnar collateral ligaments.[8]

Joint Capsule of the Midcarpal Joint:
- The midcarpal joint capsule is less a single joint capsule than a series of interconnected joint capsules of the many bones of the midcarpal joint.

Radioulnar Disc (Triangular Fibrocartilage):
- As its name indicates, the **radioulnar disc** is attached to the radius and ulna.[2]
- It adds to the stability of the radiocarpal joint because it blends into the capsular/ligamentous structure of the radiocarpal joint.
- The radioulnar disc is also known as the triangular fibrocartilage (TFC) because of its shape.

Transverse Carpal Ligament:
- The transverse carpal ligament forms the roof of the carpal tunnel.
- It attaches to the tubercles of the scaphoid and trapezium radially and to the pisiform and hook of hamate on the ulnar side.
- Its function is to enclose and stabilize the carpal tunnel.[5]
- It also functions as a retinaculum for the extrinsic finger flexor muscles of the forearm that enter the hand.
- The transverse carpal ligament is also known as the *flexor retinaculum of the wrist*.

Extrinsic Ligaments:
- **Extrinsic ligaments** attach onto one or both of the forearm bones and then attach distally onto carpal bones. Their primary function is to stabilize the radiocarpal joint. If they cross the midcarpal joint, they add to the stability of that joint as well. There are radiocarpal (dorsal and palmar) and collateral (radial and ulnar) extrinsic ligaments. All radiocarpal ligaments attach the radius to carpal bones, as their names imply.

Dorsal Radiocarpal Ligament:
- Location: The **dorsal radiocarpal ligament** is located on the dorsal (i.e., posterior) side from the radius to the carpal bones.
  - The dorsal radiocarpal ligament attaches the radius to the capitate, lunate, and scaphoid bones.
- Function: It limits full flexion.[8]

Palmar Radiocarpal Ligaments:
- Location: The **palmar radiocarpal ligaments** are located on the palmar (i.e., anterior) side from the radius to the carpal bones.
- Function: They limit full extension.[8]
- There are three palmar radiocarpal ligaments. They are (1) the **radiocapitate ligament**, (2) the **radiolunate ligament**, and (3) the **radioscapholunate ligament**. These ligaments attach the radius to the bones stated within their names.[5]

Radial Collateral Ligament:
- Location: The **radial collateral ligament** is located on the radial side, from the radius to the carpal bones.
  - More specifically, it is located from the styloid process of the radius to the scaphoid and trapezium.
- Function: It limits ulnar deviation (i.e., adduction).[8]

Ulnar Collateral Ligament:
- Location: The **ulnar collateral ligament** is located on the ulnar side, from the ulna to the carpal bones.
- Note: Many sources describe the ligaments between the distal end of the ulna and the carpus on the ulnar side of the wrist as being the **ulnocarpal complex**; included in this complex are the ulnar collateral ligament, the palmar ulnocarpal ligament, and the radioulnar disc (triangular fibrocartilage).[5]
  - More specifically, it is located from the styloid process of the ulna to the triquetrum.
- Function: It limits radial deviation (i.e., abduction).

Intrinsic Ligaments:
- **Intrinsic ligaments** attach proximally and distally onto carpal bones, crossing and stabilizing motion between carpal bones, primarily at the midcarpal joint.
- The intrinsic ligaments of the wrist are divided into short, intermediate, and long ligaments.[5]
  - Short: Short intrinsic ligaments connect the distal row of carpal bones to each other.

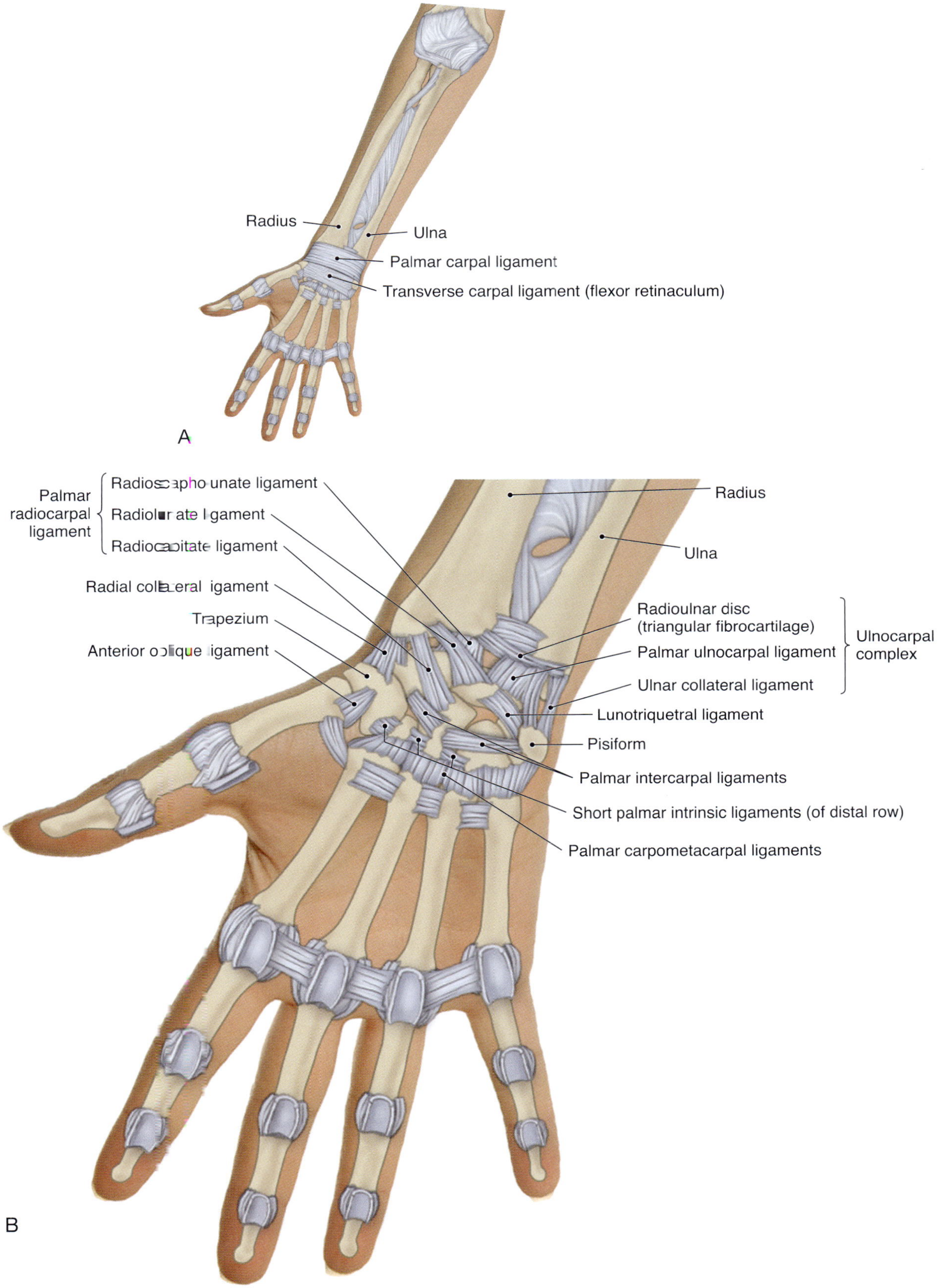

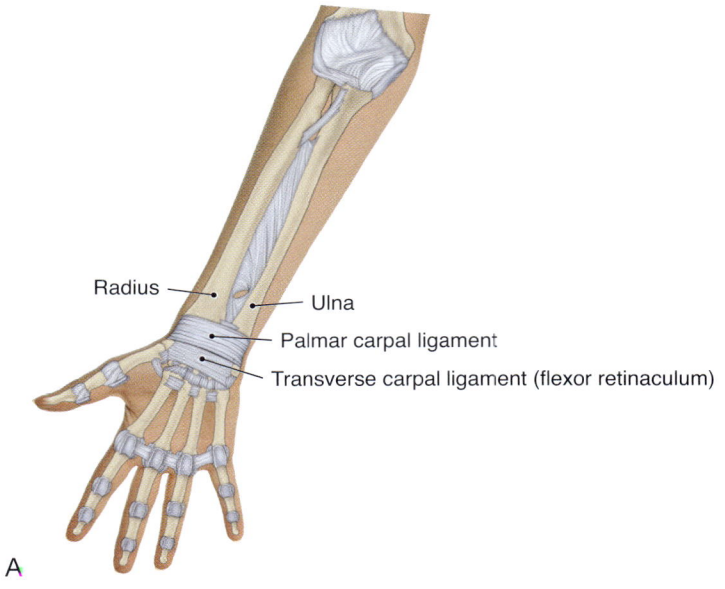

FIGURE 10-34 Ligaments of the right wrist joint complex region. **A** and **B,** Superficial and deep palmar (i.e., anterior) views respectively. **C** and **D,** Superficial and deep dorsal (i.e., posterior) views respectively. Most of the wrist joint complex ligaments are divided into two broad categories: (1) extrinsic ligaments that originate in the forearm and then attach onto the carpus, and (2) intrinsic ligaments that originate and insert (i.e., are wholly located within) onto the carpus.

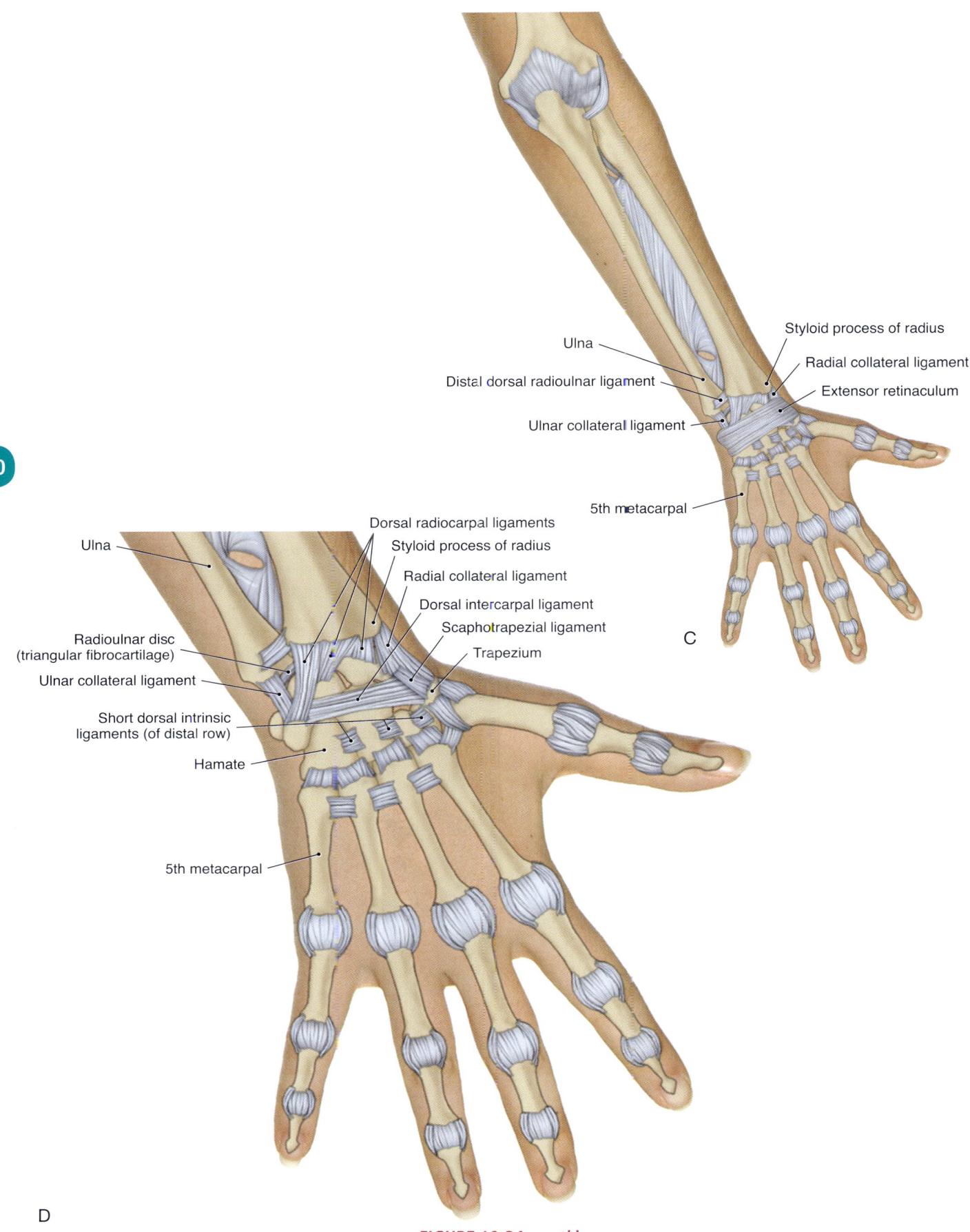

FIGURE 10-34, cont'd

- ○ Intermediate: The intermediate ligaments primarily function to connect the bones of the proximal row together.
- ○ Long: The long intrinsic ligaments connect the scaphoid, triquetrum, and capitate to each other.
- ○ Note: Two long ligaments exist: (1) the **dorsal intercarpal ligament** and (2) the **palmar intercarpal ligament**.

CLOSED-PACKED POSITION OF THE WRIST JOINT:

- ○ Extension and slight ulnar deviation[5]
  - ○ Having extension as the closed-packed position of the wrist joint complex allows for greater stability during such activities as crawling on hands and knees and performing push-ups.

MAJOR MUSCLES OF THE WRIST JOINT:

- ○ The muscles that cross the wrist joint may be divided into four major groups: those that cross on the anterior, posterior, radial, and/or on the ulnar side.
- ○ The anterior muscles can all perform flexion.
  - ○ The major flexors are the flexor carpi radialis, palmaris longus, and flexor carpi ulnaris (collectively known as the *wrist flexor group*), as well as the finger flexors (flexors digitorum superficialis and profundus).
- ○ The posterior muscles can all perform extension.
  - ○ The major extensors are the extensor carpi radialis longus, extensor carpi radialis brevis, and extensor carpi ulnaris (collectively known as the *wrist extensor group*), as well as the finger extensors (extensors digitorum and digiti minimi).
- ○ The radial muscles all can perform radial deviation (i.e., abduction).
  - ○ The major radial deviators are the flexor carpi radialis and extensors carpi radialis longus and brevis.
- ○ The ulnar muscles can all perform ulnar deviation (i.e., adduction).
  - ○ The major ulnar deviators are the flexor carpi ulnaris and extensor carpi ulnaris.
- ○ Of course all other muscles that cross the wrist can also create motion at the wrist joint; the specific action would be determined by which side(s) of the wrist joint the muscle crosses.
- ○ Many retinacula are located in the wrist region. These retinacula run transversely across the distal forearm and act to hold down and stabilize the tendons of muscles that cross from the forearm into the hand. (Note: In addition to the wrist region, retinacula are also located in the ankle region to hold down the tendons of the muscles of the leg that enter the foot (see Box 9-31 in Section 9.17.)

SECTION 10.12   CARPOMETACARPAL JOINTS

- ○ The carpometacarpal (CMC) joints are located between the distal row of carpal bones and the metacarpal bones (Figure 10-35).
- ○ Five CMC joints exist[8]:
  1. The first CMC joint is located between the trapezium and the base of the first metacarpal.
  2. The second CMC joint is located between the trapezoid and the base of the second metacarpal.
  3. The third CMC joint is located between the capitate and the base of the third metacarpal.
  4. The fourth CMC joint is located between the hamate and the base of the fourth metacarpal.
  5. The fifth CMC joint is located between the hamate and the base of the fifth metacarpal.
- ○ Note: Each metacarpal and its associated phalanges make up a ray of the hand.

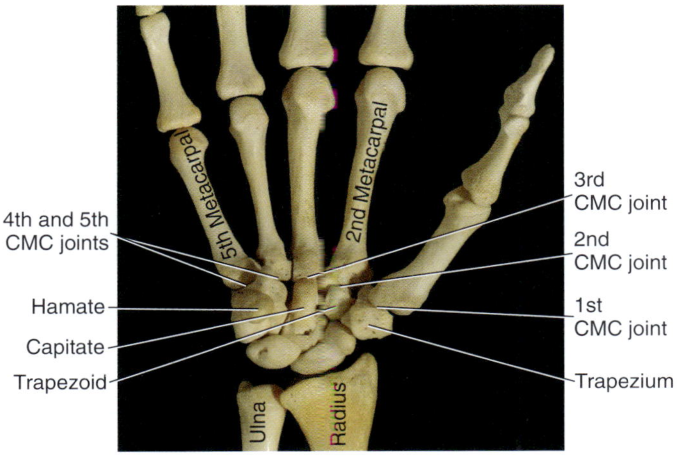

SECOND AND THIRD CMC JOINTS:

- ○ Joint structure classification: Synovial joint
  - ○ Subtype: Plane[2]
- ○ Joint function classification: Synarthrotic
  - ○ Subtype: Nonaxial[2]

FIRST, FIFTH, AND FOURTH CMC JOINTS:

- ○ Joint structure classification: Synovial joint
  - ○ Subtype: Saddle[2]
- ○ Joint function classification: Diarthrotic
  - ○ Subtype: Biaxial[2]

CMC JOINT MOTION:

- ○ The peripheral CMC joints are more mobile, creating more mobile rays (Figure 10-36).[7]
- ○ The (first) CMC saddle joint of the thumb is the most mobile, allowing the thumb to oppose the other fingers (i.e., move toward the center of the palm) (see Section 10.13, Figure 10-39, or

FIGURE 10-35 Anterior view of the carpometacarpal (CMC) joints. Five CMC joints are formed between the distal row of carpals and the metacarpal bones.

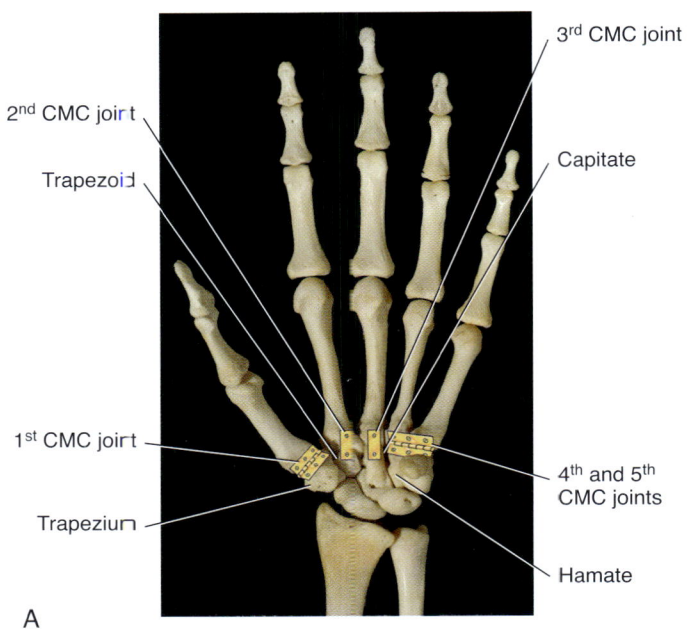
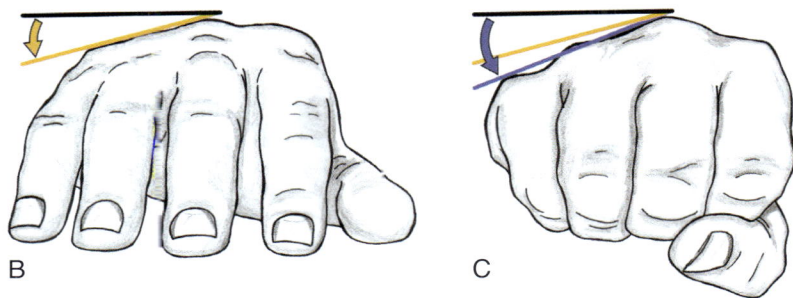

FIGURE 10-36 Motion of the carpometacarpal (CMC) joints of the hand. **A,** Anterior view of the right hand that depicts the concept of the relative mobility of the first, fifth, and fourth CMC joints and the relative rigidity/stability of the second and third CMC joints. The second and third rays form the stable central pillar of the hand. **B** and **C,** Two views of the hand that show the motion of the fourth and fifth CMC joints that is evident when the fingers flex. (**B** and **C,** Courtesy Joseph E. Muscolino.)

Section 6.23, Figure 6.24). (For more details on the CMC joint of the thumb, see Section 10.13.)[7]

- The fifth and fourth CMC joints are also fairly mobile, allowing the ulnar side of the hand (the fifth and fourth metacarpals) to fold toward the center of the palm.[2]
- Therefore the first ray is the most mobile, followed by the fifth and then the fourth rays.
- The ability of the fourth, fifth, and first metacarpals to fold toward the center of the palm increases the distal transverse arch of the hand, creating a better grip on objects held.
- The second and third CMC joints are relatively rigid, forming a stable **central pillar of the hand.** When the hand grasps and closes in around an object, the central pillar of the hand stays fixed and the other rays close in around it.

MAJOR MOTIONS ALLOWED:

- The CMC joints primarily allow flexion/extension (see Figure 10-36; Table 10-9).[2]

- Some abduction/adduction occurs at the fourth and fifth CMC joints. Some lateral rotation/medial rotation occurs at the fifth CMC joints. The abduction/adduction and lateral/medial rotation motions of the fifth metacarpal at the fifth CMC joint allow for opposition/reposition of the little finger.[7]

TABLE 10-9	Average Ranges of Motion from Anatomic Position of the Metacarpals at the Second through Fifth Carpometacarpal (CMC) Joints*[5]	
	Flexion	Extension
Fifth CMC Joint	20 Degrees	0 Degrees
Fourth CMC Joint	10 Degrees	0 Degrees
Third CMC Joint	0 Degrees	0 Degrees
Second CMC Joint	0-2 Degrees	0 Degrees

*Ranges of motion of the metacarpal of the thumb at the first CMC joint are covered in Section 10.13, Table 10-10.

MAJOR LIGAMENTS OF THE CMC JOINTS:

- The CMC joints are stabilized by their joint capsules, as well as **carpometacarpal (CMC) ligaments**.[8]
  - The CMC ligaments are the dorsal carpometacarpal ligaments, the palmar carpometacarpal ligaments, and the interosseus carpometacarpal ligaments (Figure 10-37, Box 10-17).

BOX 10-17 Ligaments of the Carpometacarpal (CMC) Joints

- Fibrous capsules

CMC Ligaments
- Dorsal CMC ligaments
- Palmar CMC ligaments
- Interosseus CMC ligaments

MISCELLANEOUS:

- As stated, a metacarpal and its associated phalanges make up a ray. Therefore motion of a metacarpal at its CMC joint is functionally related to motion of the phalanges of that ray at the MCP and IP joints. In other words, metacarpal movement is related to finger movement.
- The word *pollicis* means *thumb*.
- The word *digital* refers to fingers #2 through #5 (or toes #2 through #5).

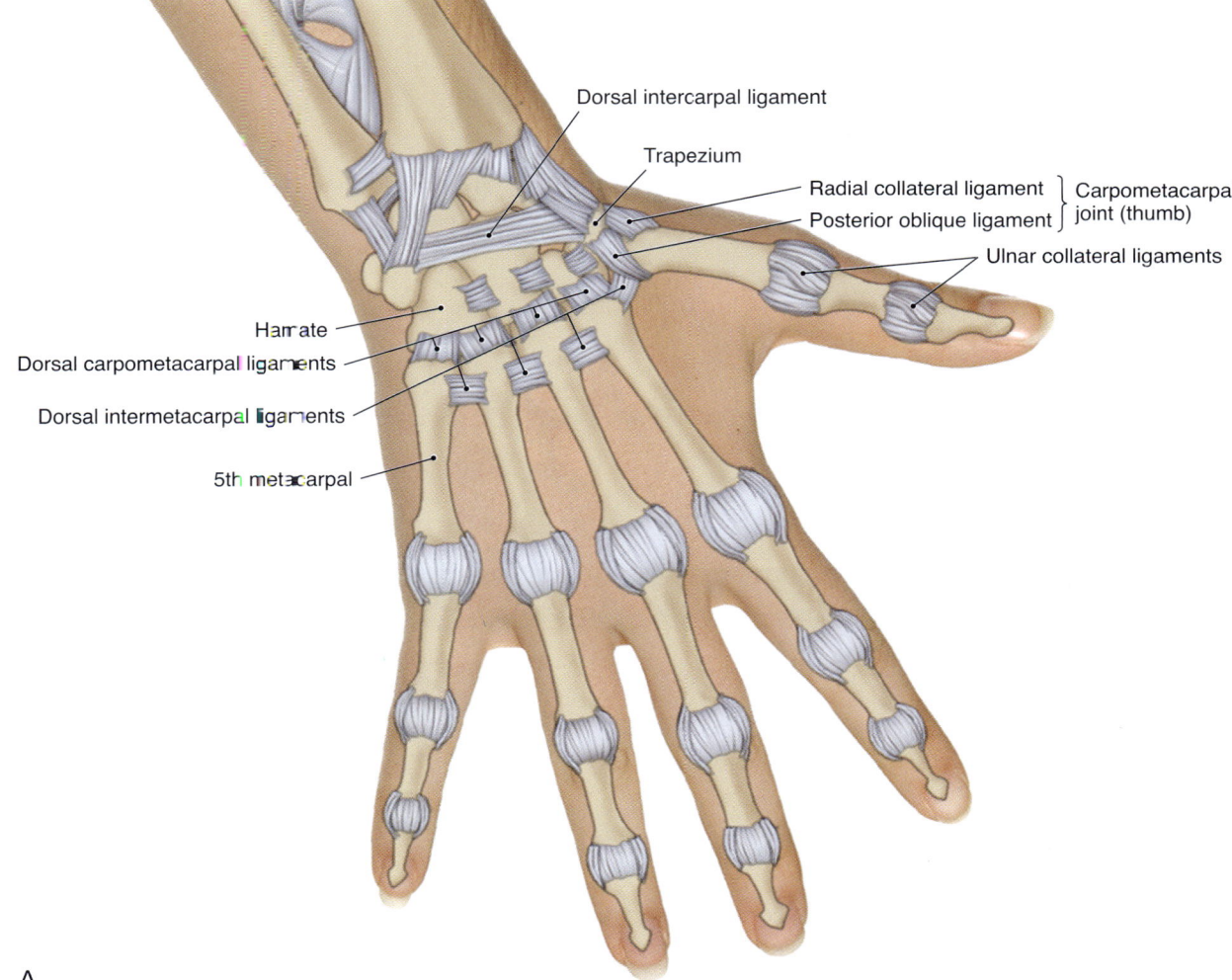

FIGURE 10-37 Dorsal and palmar carpometacarpal (CMC) ligaments of the CMC joints of fingers #2 through #5 of the right hand. **A,** Dorsal (i.e., posterior) view.

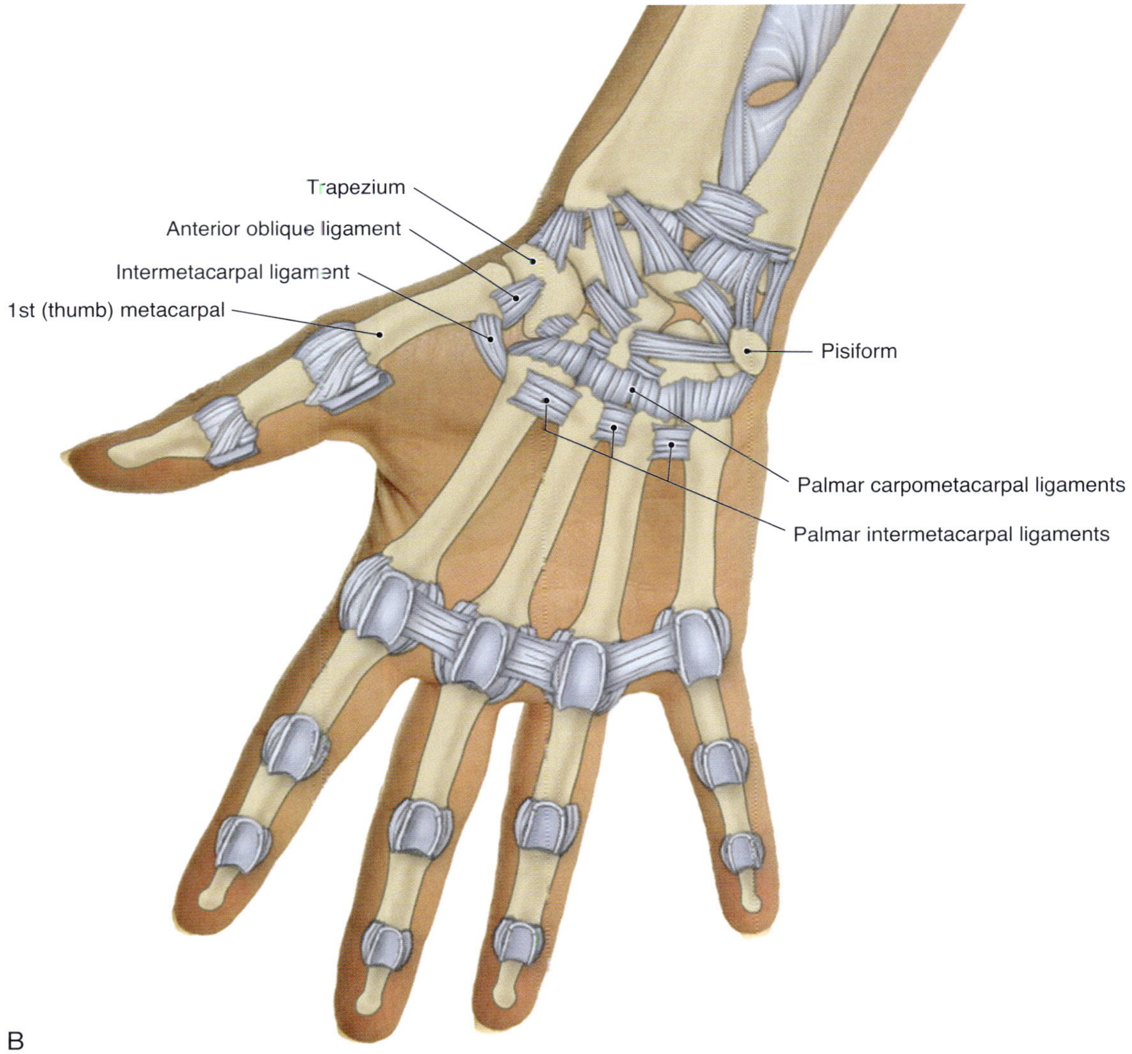

FIGURE 10-37, cont'd B, Palmar (i.e., anterior) view. (Note: The carpometacarpal ligaments of the saddle joint of the thumb are also shown.)

SECTION 10.13   SADDLE (CARPOMETACARPAL) JOINT OF THE THUMB

- The saddle joint of the thumb is the first CMC joint (Figure 10-38).
- The **saddle joint of the thumb** is the classic example of a saddle joint in the human body. (See Section 7.11 for more information on saddle joints.)

BONES:

- The saddle joint of the thumb is located between the trapezium and the first metacarpal—in other words, the metacarpal of the thumb (Box 10-18).
  - More specifically, the distal end of the trapezium articulates with the base of the first metacarpal.
- Joint structure classification: Synovial[1]
  - Subtype: Saddle

> **BOX 10-18**
>
> Because of the thumb's tremendous use, degenerative arthritic changes are commonly found at the saddle joint of the thumb. This condition is called **basilar arthritis** because the saddle joint of the thumb is the base joint of the entire thumb.

- Joint function classification: Diarthrotic
  - Subtype: Biaxial
  - The saddle joint of the thumb is classified as a *biaxial joint*. It actually permits motion in all three cardinal planes; therefore some might be tempted to classify it as *triaxial*. However, its rotation actions in the transverse plane cannot

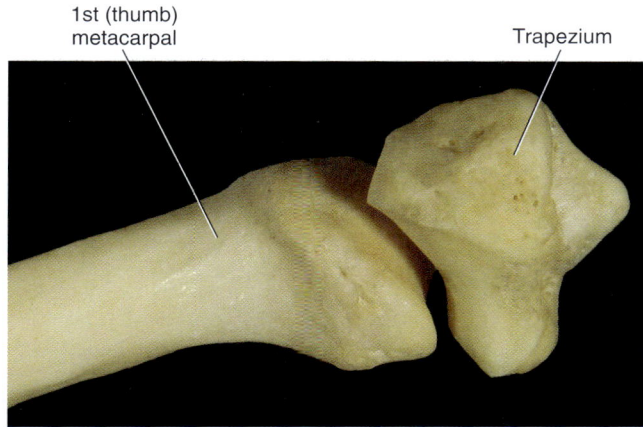

FIGURE 10-38 Palmar (i.e., anterior) view of the first carpometacarpal (CMC) (i.e., saddle) joint of the thumb of the right hand. The reason that this joint is called a saddle joint is evident—that is, each articular surface is concave in one direction and convex in the other. Furthermore, the convexity of one bone fits into the concavity of the other bone.

be actively isolated, and its flexion/extension actions in the frontal plane cannot be isolated. Because of the shape of the bones of the joint, medial rotation of the first metacarpal must accompany flexion of the first metacarpal, and lateral rotation must accompany extension. Therefore the saddle joint of the thumb can move in the sagittal plane around a mediolateral axis and it can move in the oblique plane that is a combination of the frontal and transverse planes around the axis for this plane. For this reason, it is classified as being *biaxial*.[1]

MAJOR MOTIONS ALLOWED:

- Note: It is usually stated that the thumb moves at the saddle (i.e., carpometacarpal [CMC]) joint. To be more specific, it can be stated that the first metacarpal (of the thumb) moves at the thumb's saddle joint. The thumb can also move at its metacarpophalangeal (MCP) and interphalangeal (IP) joints. The proximal phalanx moves at the MCP joint, and the distal phalanx moves at the IP joint.[4]
- The saddle joint of the thumb allows several major motions (Figure 10-39; Table 10-10):

TABLE 10-10	Average Ranges of Motion of the Metacarpal of the Thumb at the Thumb's Saddle Joint from Anatomic Position[2]		
Abduction	60 Degrees	Adduction	10 Degrees
Flexion	40 Degrees	Extension	10 Degrees
Medial rotation	45 Degrees	Lateral rotation	0 Degrees

Anatomic position has the thumb in full lateral rotation and near full extension and adduction.

- Opposition and reposition of the thumb
  - Opposition and reposition of the thumb are not specific actions, they are combinations of actions (Box 10-19).
  - Opposition is a combination of abduction, flexion, and medial rotation of the thumb's metacarpal; reposition is a combination of adduction, extension, and lateral rotation of the thumb's metacarpal. (For more on opposition/reposition, see Section 6.23.)
- Flexion and extension of the thumb in the frontal plane around an anteroposterior axis
- Abduction and adduction of the thumb in the sagittal plane around a mediolateral axis
- Medial rotation and lateral rotation of the thumb in the transverse plane around a vertical axis
  - Note: Because of the rotation of the thumb that occurs embryologically, flexion and extension occur within the frontal plane instead of the sagittal plane, and abduction and adduction occur within the sagittal plane instead of the frontal plane. (For more on opposition/reposition of the thumb, see Section 6.23.)

Reverse Actions:

- The trapezium of the wrist (along with the remainder of the hand) could move relative to the metacarpal of the thumb.

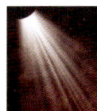 **BOX 10-19 Spotlight on Opposition of the Thumb**

Opposition is usually defined simply as the pad of the thumb meeting the pad of another finger. Most textbooks will then state that opposition is a combination of three component actions: (1) abduction, (2) flexion, and (3) medial rotation of the thumb (more specifically, the metacarpal of the thumb at the carpometacarpal [CMC] joint [i.e., the saddle joint] of the thumb) because these are the motions that must occur for the thumb to meet the pad of another finger when starting opposition from anatomic position. However, the exact component motions and the degrees of these component motions that are necessary to create opposition against the pad of another finger can vary based on three factors:
1. The starting position of the thumb: If the thumb begins opposition from anatomic position, more abduction is needed than if the thumb begins opposition from the relaxed position of the thumb, wherein it is already in some degree of abduction.
2. The finger to which the thumb is being opposed: For example, it takes relatively more flexion to oppose the thumb to the little finger than it does to oppose the thumb to the index finger.
3. The position of the finger to which the thumb is being opposed: If the finger to which the thumb is being opposed is held fixed in or close to anatomic position (it does not move toward the thumb), then the thumb may have to adduct, depending on the position from which it began opposition. If instead the finger to which the thumb is being opposed is flexed toward the thumb, then the thumb would most likely not need to adduct.

Given this discussion, it should be clear that the opponens pollicis is not the only muscle that can help create opposition of the thumb. The degree to which each muscle contributes to opposition will vary based on the exact component motions of opposition in a particular situation.

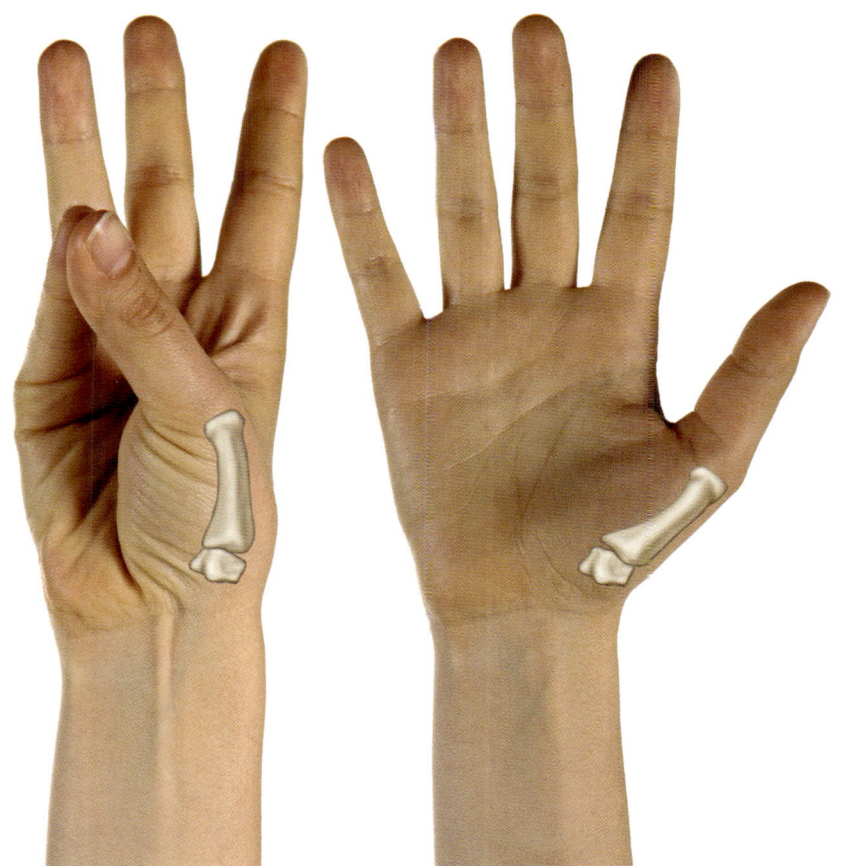

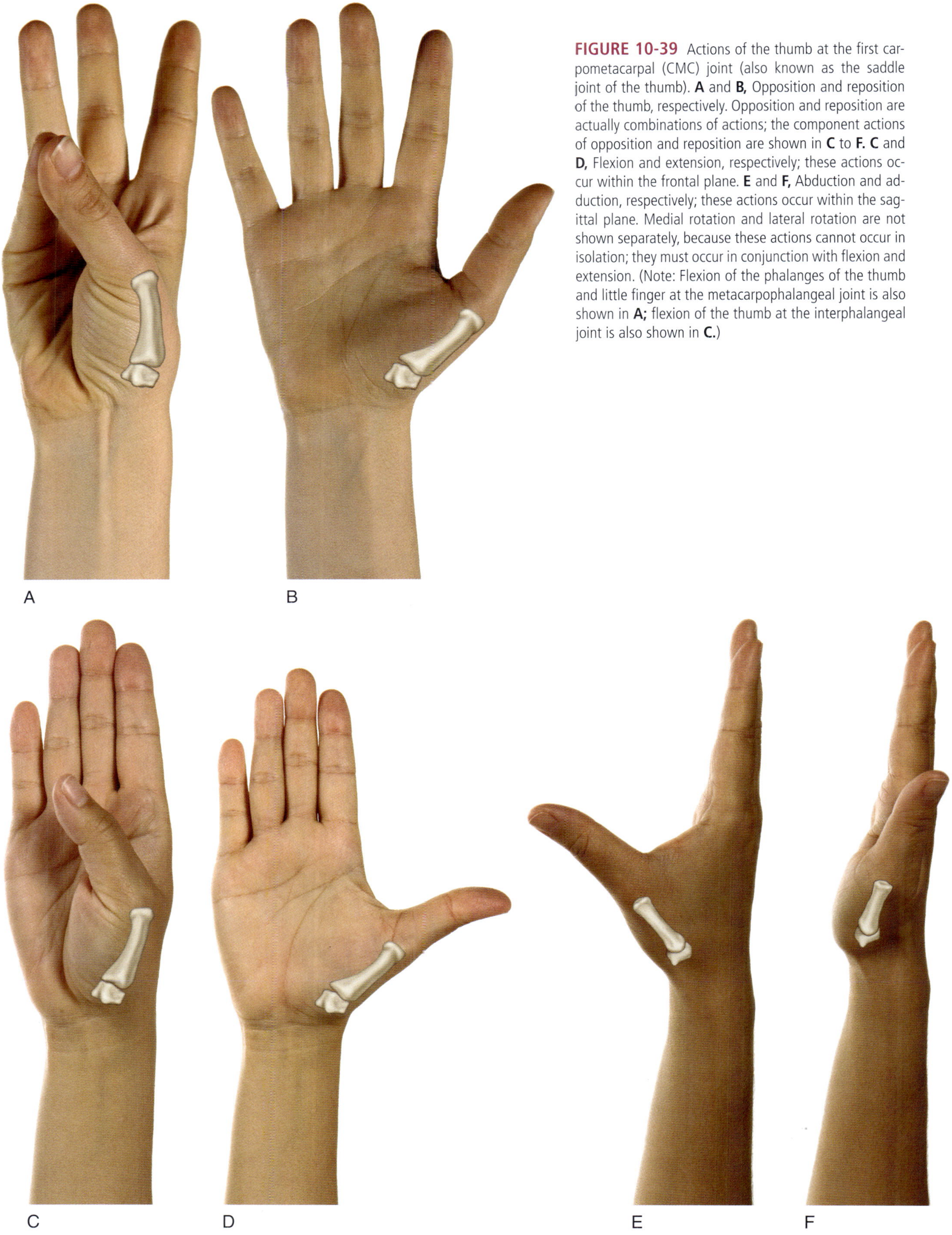

FIGURE 10-39 Actions of the thumb at the first carpometacarpal (CMC) joint (also known as the saddle joint of the thumb). **A** and **B,** Opposition and reposition of the thumb, respectively. Opposition and reposition are actually combinations of actions; the component actions of opposition and reposition are shown in **C** to **F. C** and **D,** Flexion and extension, respectively; these actions occur within the frontal plane. **E** and **F,** Abduction and adduction, respectively; these actions occur within the sagittal plane. Medial rotation and lateral rotation are not shown separately, because these actions cannot occur in isolation; they must occur in conjunction with flexion and extension. (Note: Flexion of the phalanges of the thumb and little finger at the metacarpophalangeal joint is also shown in **A;** flexion of the thumb at the interphalangeal joint is also shown in **C.**)

CHAPTER 10 Joints of the Upper Extremity

MAJOR LIGAMENTS OF THE SADDLE JOINT OF THE THUMB:

The saddle joint of the thumb has several major ligaments (Figure 10-40; Box 10-20):
- The CMC joint of the thumb is stabilized by its fibrous joint capsule and five major ligaments.
- The fibrous joint capsule of the thumb is loose, allowing large ranges of motion.
- Generally the ligaments of the thumb become taut in full opposition and/or full abduction or full extension.

Radial Collateral Ligament:
- Location: The **radial collateral ligament** is located on the radial side of the joint.
  - More specifically, it is located from the radial surface of the trapezium to the base of the metacarpal of the thumb.[8]

Ulnar Collateral Ligament:
- Location: The **ulnar collateral ligament** is located on the ulnar side of the joint.
  - More specifically, it is located from the transverse carpal ligament to the base of the metacarpal of the thumb.[2]

Anterior Oblique Ligament:
- Location: The **anterior oblique ligament** is located on the anterior side of the joint.
  - More specifically, it is located from the tubercle of the trapezium to the base of the metacarpal of the thumb.[8]

> **BOX 10-20** Ligaments of the Saddle Joint (Carpometacarpal [CMC] Joint) of the Thumb
>
> - Fibrous capsule
> - Radial collateral ligament
> - Ulnar collateral ligament
> - Anterior oblique ligament
> - Posterior oblique ligament
> - First intermetacarpal (IMC) ligament

Posterior Oblique Ligament:
- Location: The **posterior oblique ligament** is located on the posterior side of the joint.
  - More specifically, it is located from the posterior surface of the trapezium to the palmar-ulnar surface of the base of the metacarpal of the thumb.[8]

First Intermetacarpal Ligament:
- Location: The **first intermetacarpal ligament** is located between metacarpals of the thumb and index finger (i.e., the first and second metacarpals).
  - More specifically, it is located from the base of the metacarpal of the index finger to the base of the metacarpal of the thumb.[1]

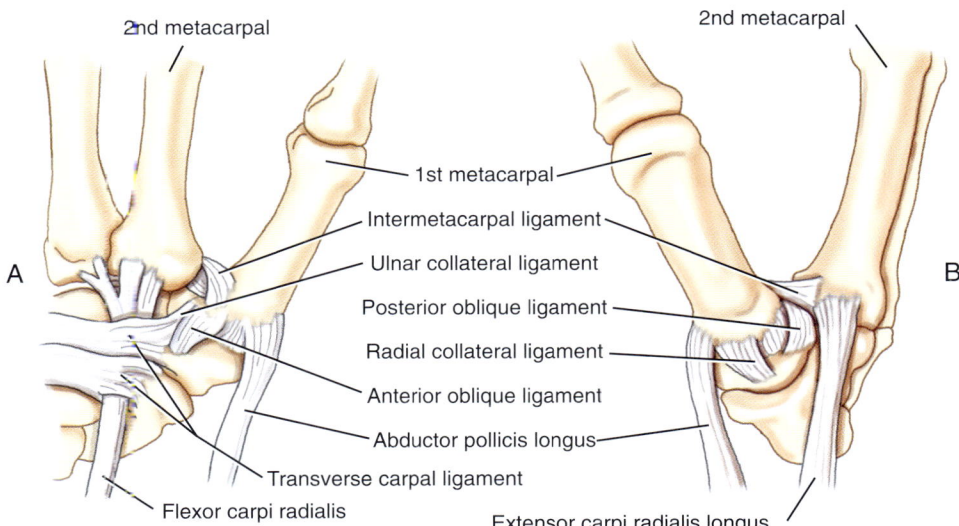

FIGURE 10-40 Ligaments of the first carpometacarpal (CMC) (i.e., saddle) joint of the right thumb. **A,** Palmar (i.e., anterior) view in which the ulnar collateral and anterior oblique ligaments are shown. **B,** Radial (i.e., lateral) view in which the radial collateral and posterior oblique ligaments are shown. (Note: The intermetacarpal [IMC] ligament between the thumb and index finger is also shown.) *(Modeled from Neumann DA: Kinesiology of the musculoskeletal system: foundations for physical rehabilitation, ed 2, St Louis, 2010, Mosby.)*

CLOSED-PACKED POSITION OF THE SADDLE JOINT OF THE THUMB:

- Full opposition[2]

MAJOR MUSCLES OF THE SADDLE JOINT OF THE THUMB:

- The muscles of the saddle joint of the thumb can be divided into extrinsic muscles (that originate on the arm and/or forearm) and intrinsic muscles (wholly located within the hand).
  - The extrinsic muscles are the flexor pollicis longus, extensors pollicis longus and brevis, and abductor pollicis longus (Box 10-21).
  - The intrinsic muscles of the thumb are the three muscles of the thenar eminence (i.e., the abductor and flexor pollicis brevis and the opponens pollicis) and the adductor pollicis.

BOX 10-21

Muscles that cross the wrist to enter the hand (and that cross the ankle to enter the foot) encounter friction as they slide along the underlying bony structures. For this reason, they are encased in synovial tendon sheaths. However, these sheaths are not always capable of withstanding this friction and may become inflamed themselves. When this occurs, the condition is called **tenosynovitis** (in effect, inflammation of the synovial sheath of a tendon). The most common form of wrist tenosynovitis is known as **de Quervain's disease** (or **de Quervain's stenosing tenosynovitis**) and occurs at the common synovial sheath of the abductor pollicis longus and extensor pollicis brevis tendons as the sheath rubs against the styloid process of the radius with use (usually overuse) of the thumb.

SECTION 10.14 INTERMETACARPAL JOINTS

BONES:

- **Intermetacarpal (IMC) joints** are located between the metacarpal bones of the hand (Figure 10-41, *A*).
- Proximal IMC joints and distal IMC joints exist.
- All five metacarpals (#1-#5) articulate with one another proximally at their bases; hence four proximal IMC joints exist.
- Only metacarpals #2 through #5 articulate with one another distally at their heads; hence three distal IMC joints exist.[3]

IMC MOTION:

- These IMC joints allow nonaxial gliding motion of one metacarpal relative to the adjacent metacarpal(s).[1]
- Apart from the motion between the first and second metacarpals, the joint between the fifth and fourth metacarpals allows the most motion.
- Motion between the metacarpals at the IMC joints increases the ability of the hand to close in around an object and grasp it securely.[1] For this reason, the first and fifth metacarpals (i.e., the metacarpals on either side of the hand) are the most mobile.
- Joint structure classification: Synovial joint[8]
  - Subtype: Plane
- Joint function classification: Amphiarthrotic
  - Subtype: Nonaxial

INTERMETACARPAL LIGAMENTS:

- IMC joints are stabilized by their fibrous capsules and ligaments[3] (see Figure 10-41, *B* and Box 10-22).
- The proximal IMC joints are stabilized by the **intermetacarpal (IMC) ligaments** that connect the base of each of the five metacarpals to the base of the adjacent metacarpal(s).[8]
  - Three sets of intermetacarpal (IMC) ligaments stabilize the proximal IMC joints: (1) **dorsal intermetacarpal ligaments**, (2) **palmar intermetacarpal ligaments**, and (3) **interosseus intermetacarpal ligaments**. (Note: IMC ligaments of the proximal IMC joints are also known simply as **metacarpal ligaments**.) Stability of the proximal intermetacarpal joints indirectly helps to stabilize the associated carpometacarpal (CMC) joints of the hand.[8]
- The distal IMC joints (between metacarpals #2-#5) are stabilized by **deep transverse metacarpal ligaments** that connect the heads of metacarpals #2 through #5.[3]
  - Although all five distal ends of the metatarsals in the foot are connected by deep intermetatarsal ligaments, the hand does not have a deep transverse metacarpal ligament connecting the distal ends of the metacarpals of the thumb and index finger. The absence of this ligament between the thumb and index finger is one aspect that allows the thumb much greater range of motion than the big toe of the foot. Therefore the hand is designed primarily for manipulation (i.e., fine motion), whereas the foot is designed primarily for weight bearing and propulsion. In theory, the only major difference between the potential coordination of the hand and the foot is the ability to oppose digits.

BOX 10-22 Ligaments of the Intermetacarpal Joints

Proximal Intermetacarpal (IMC) Joints[7]
- Fibrous capsules
- IMC ligaments

Distal IMC Joints[7]
- Fibrous capsules
- Deep transverse metacarpal ligaments

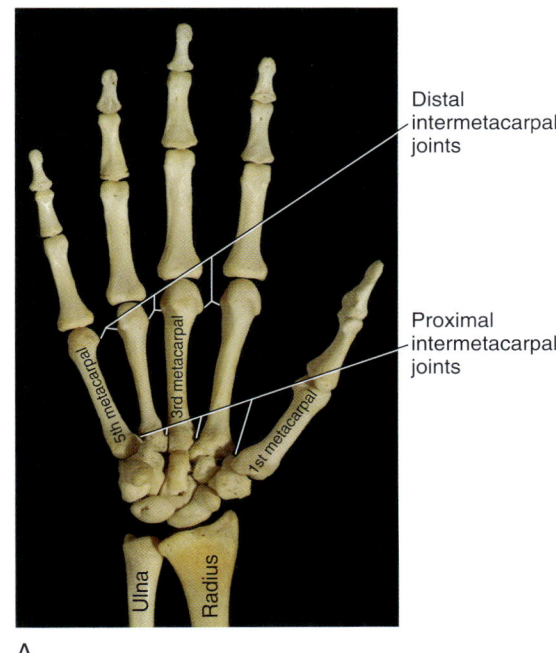

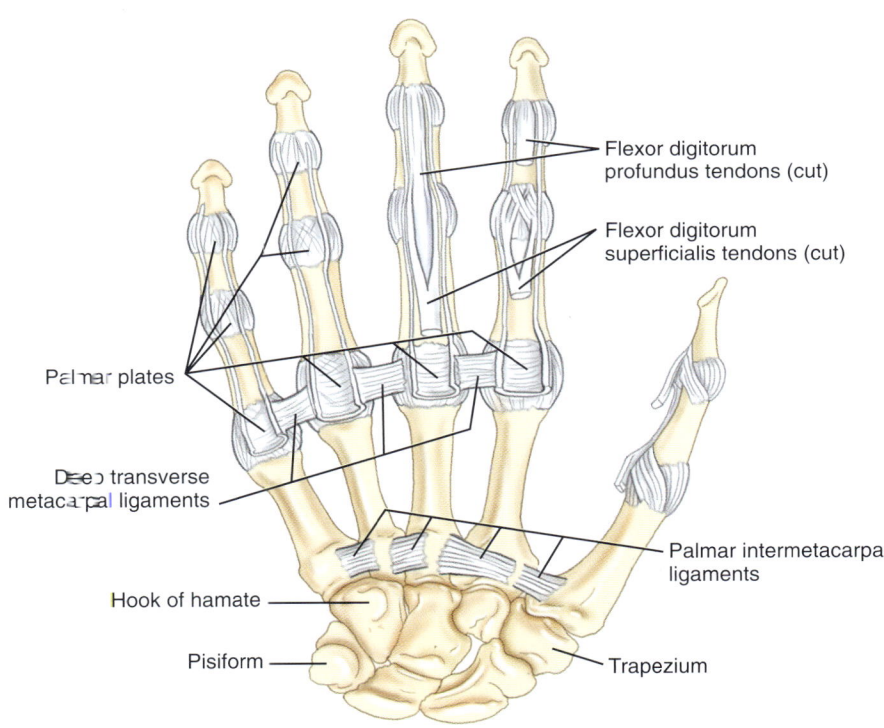

Palmar (anterior) view

FIGURE 10-1 Intermetacarpal (IMC) joints of the hand. **A,** Anterior view shows the osseous joints. (Note: Four proximal IMC joints and three distal IMC joints exist.) **B,** Anterior view illustrates the ligaments of the proximal and distal IMC joints. Proximal IMC joints are stabilized by intermetacarpal ligaments. Distal IMC joints are stabilized by deep transverse metacarpal ligaments. (Note: Palmar plates of the metacarpophalangeal and interphalangeal joints are also shown.)

348   PART 3   Skeletal Arthrology: Study of the Joints

SECTION 10.15   METACARPOPHALANGEAL (MCP) JOINTS

BONES:

- The **metacarpophalangeal (MCP) joints** are located between the metacarpals of the palm and the phalanges of the fingers (Figure 10-42; Box 10-23).
  - More specifically, they are located between the heads of the metacarpals and the bases of the proximal phalanges of the fingers.
- Five MCP joints exist[2]:
  - The first MCP joint is located between the first metacarpal and the proximal phalanx of the thumb (i.e., finger #1).
  - The second MCP joint is located between the second metacarpal and the proximal phalanx of the index finger (i.e., finger #2).
  - The third MCP joint is located between the third metacarpal and the proximal phalanx of the middle finger (i.e., finger #3).
  - The fourth MCP joint is located between the fourth metacarpal and the proximal phalanx of the ring finger (i.e., finger #4).
  - The fifth MCP joint is located between the fifth metacarpal and the proximal phalanx of the little finger (i.e., finger #5).
- Joint structure classification: Synovial[2]
  - Subtype: Condyloid
- Joint function classification: Diarthrotic
  - Subtype: Biaxial

 BOX 10-23

Rheumatoid arthritis (RA) is a progressive degenerative arthritic condition that weakens and destroys the capsular connective tissue of joints. Although this condition attacks many joints, the metacarpophalangeal joints (MCP) of the hand are particularly hard hit. Clients with RA will usually develop a characteristic ulnar deviation deformity of the proximal phalanges at the MCP joints. This occurs because the capsules of the MCP joints are no longer sufficiently stable to be able to resist the forces that push against the fingers in an ulnar direction when objects are held between the thumb and the other fingers (opposition of the thumb to another finger to grasp an object creates an ulnar force against that finger).

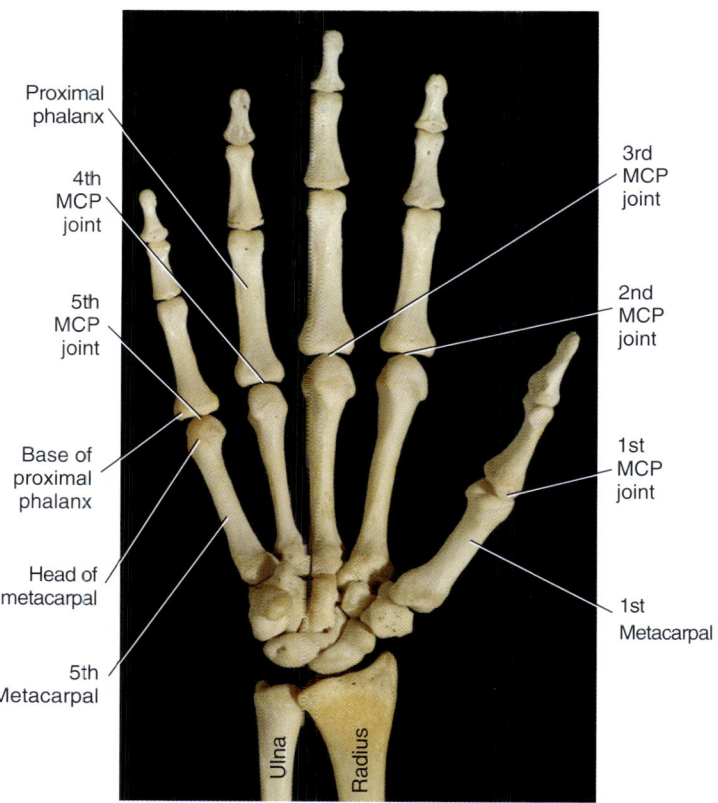

FIGURE 10-42 Metacarpophalangeal (MCP) joints of the hand. MCP joints are located between the heads of the metacarpals and the bases of the proximal phalanges of the fingers. They are numbered #1 through #5, starting on the radial (i.e., lateral) side with the thumb.

CHAPTER 10 Joints of the Upper Extremity

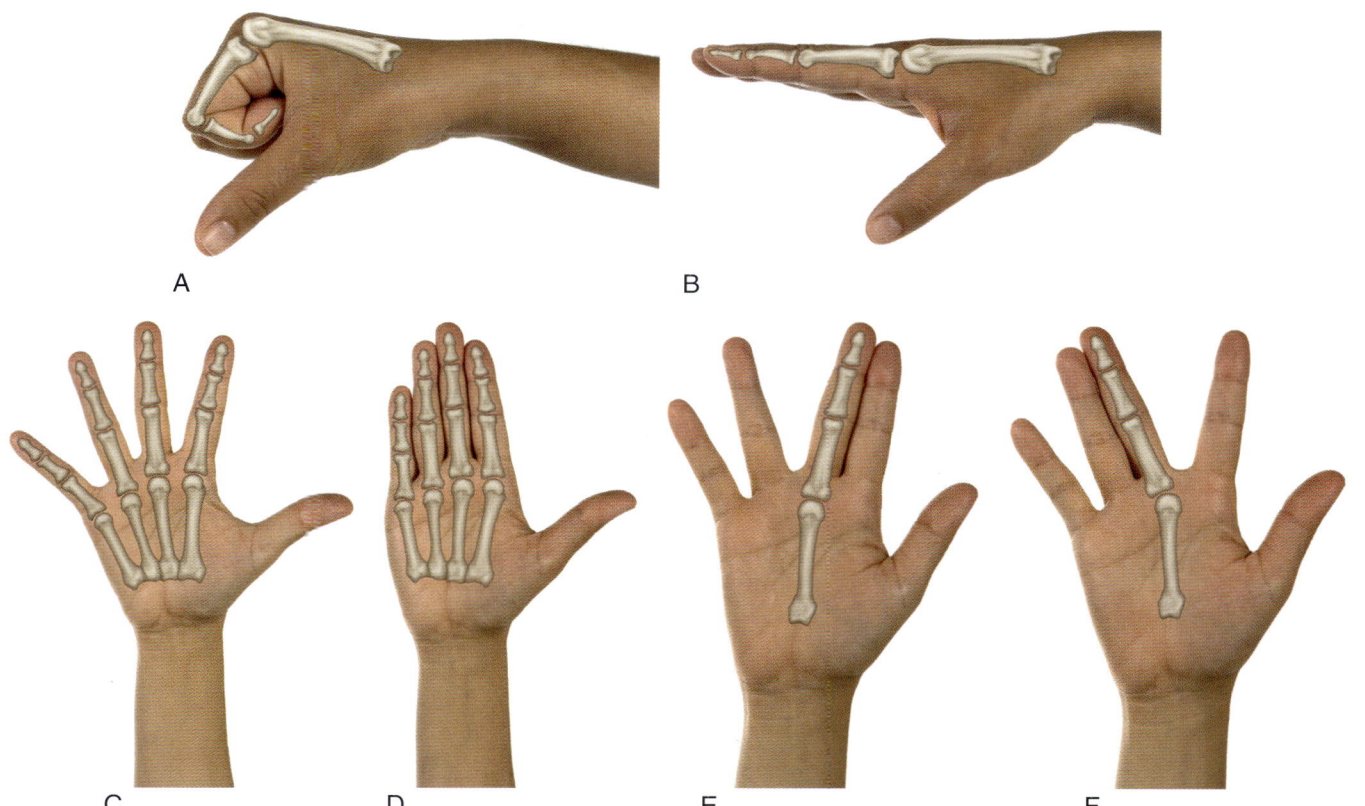

FIGURE 10-43 Actions of the fingers at the metacarpophalangeal (MCP) joints of the hand. **A** and **B,** Radial (i.e., lateral) views illustrating flexion and extension, respectively, of fingers #2 through #5 at the MCP joints. (Note: Flexion of the fingers at the interphalangeal joints is also shown.) **C** and **D,** Abduction and adduction of fingers #2 through #5 at the MCP joints, respectively. (Note: The reference line for abduction/adduction of the fingers is an imaginary line through the center of the middle finger when in anatomic position.) **E** and **F,** Radial abduction and ulnar abduction of the middle finger at the third MCP joint, respectively.

MAJOR MOTIONS ALLOWED:

The MCP joint allows several major motions (Figure 10-43; Tables 10-11 and 10-12):
- The MCP joint allows flexion and extension (i.e., axial movements) within the sagittal plane around a mediolateral axis[3] (Box 10-24).
- The MCP joint allows abduction and adduction (i.e., axial movements) within the frontal plane around an anteroposterior axis.[3]
- The reference for abduction/adduction of the fingers at the MCP joints is an imaginary line drawn through the middle finger when it is in anatomic position. Movement toward this imaginary line is adduction; movement away from this imaginary line is abduction.[3] Because frontal plane movement of the middle finger in either direction (starting from anatomic position) is away from this imaginary line, both directions of movement are termed *abduction*. Lateral movement of the middle finger is termed *radial abduction;* medial movement of the middle finger is termed *ulnar abduction* (see Figure 10-43, *E* and *F*).

TABLE 10-11	Average Ranges of Motion of the Proximal Phalanx of Fingers #2 through #5 at a Metacarpophalangeal (MCP) Joint from Anatomic Position[2]		
Flexion	90–110 Degrees*	Extension	0-20 Degrees†
Abduction	20 Degrees	Adduction	20 Degrees

*Flexion is greatest at the little finger and least at the index finger.
†From anatomic position, sources differ on how much active extension (hyperextension) is possible at the MCP joints. However, most sources agree that passive extension (hyperextension) of 30 to 40 degrees is possible.

TABLE 10-12	Average Ranges of Motion of the Proximal Phalanx of the Thumb at the First Metacarpophalangeal Joint from Anatomic Position[2]		
Flexion	60 Degrees	Extension	0 Degrees

Abduction/adduction are negligible and considered to be accessory motions. Passive hyperextension of the thumb at the metacarpophalangeal (MCP) joint is minimal as compared with the MCP joints of fingers #2 through #5.

350   PART 3   Skeletal Arthrology: Study of the Joints

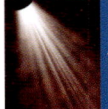

| BOX 10-24 | Spotlight on the Extensor Digitorum's Tendons |

The extensor digitorum is an extrinsic finger extensor muscle. Its belly, which is located in the posterior forearm, gradually transitions into four tendons. These four tendons attach onto the dorsal side of the middle and distal phalanges of fingers #2 through #5 (one tendon into each finger). However, these tendons do not remain fully separated from one another; they have what are called **intertendinous connections** (see Figure 11-35). As a result, extension of one finger can be influenced by the position of other fingers. If the hand is placed in the position shown in the accompanying photograph, the person will find that it is difficult if not impossible to raise the ring finger (i.e., extend the fourth finger at the metacarpophalangeal [MCP] joint). The reason is that maximally flexing the middle finger as shown pulls the tendon of the middle finger of the extensor digitorum distally, making it very taut. Because of the orientation of the intertendinous connection between the middle and ring fingers, when the distal tendon of the middle finger is pulled distally, the distal tendon of the ring finger is also pulled distally, resulting in its proximal aspect becoming taut and its distal aspect becoming slackened. Now, when the fibers of the extensor digitorum that would normally extend the ring finger contract, they cannot generate sufficient tension to pull on the tendon to the ring finger to move it proximally because they cannot overcome the distal pull on the proximal aspect of the ring finger's tendon and there is slack in the distal aspect of the ring finger's tendon. As a result, in this position it is difficult or impossible to extend the ring finger at the MCP joint. (Photo courtesy Joseph E. Muscolino.)

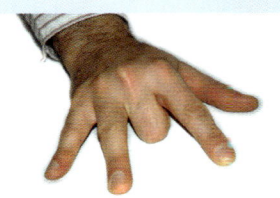

○ When people are described in lay terms as being **double-jointed**, they do not have double joints; rather, they have ligaments that are so lax that they permit a greater than normal passive range of motion. Passive extension beyond normal (i.e., hyperextension) of the fingers at the metacarpophalangeal (MCP) joints is a very common location for this type of ligament laxity that is described as double-jointed.

Reverse Actions:

○ The muscles of the MCP joints are generally considered to move the proximal phalanx of the finger (i.e., the more distal bone) toward a fixed metacarpal bone (i.e., the more proximal bone). However, a metacarpal of the palm of the hand can move toward the proximal phalanx of a finger instead.

Accessory Motions:

○ The MCP joints allow a great deal of passive glide in all directions (i.e., anterior to posterior, medial to lateral, and axial distraction), as well as passive rotation. These accessory motions help the hand to better fit around objects that are being held, resulting in a firmer and more secure grasp.

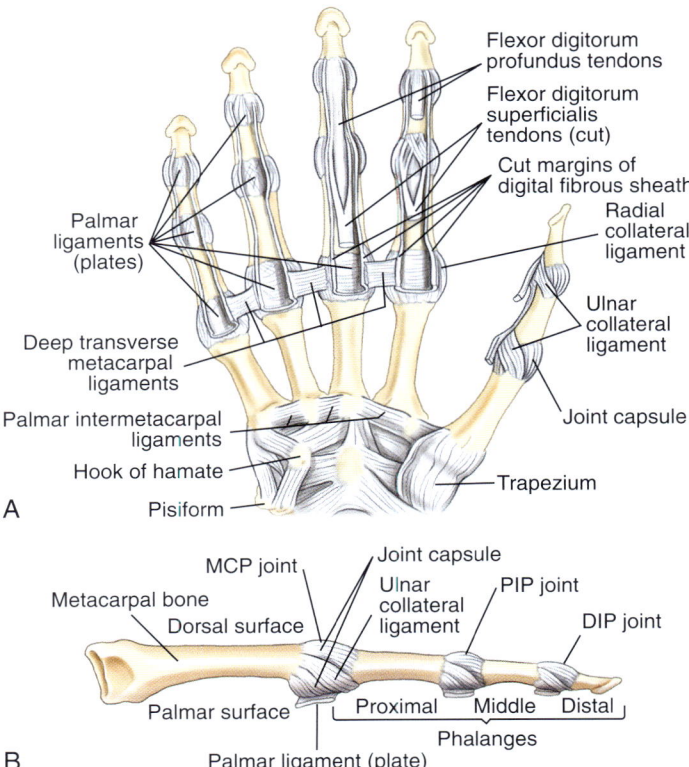

FIGURE 10-44 Ligaments of the metacarpophalangeal (MCP) joints of the hand. **A,** Anterior (palmar) view. **B,** Ulnar (i.e., medial) view. Note: Ligaments of the interphalangeal (IP) joints are also seen. *DIP,* Distal interphalangeal; *PIP,* Proximal interphalangeal.

MAJOR LIGAMENTS OF THE METACARPOPHALANGEAL JOINTS:

○ Each MCP joint is stabilized by a fibrous capsule and ligaments[8] (Figure 10-44; Box 10-25).
○ The fibrous capsule of the MCP joint is lax when the joint is in extension and becomes somewhat taut when the joint is in flexion.[7]
○ Three ligaments of the MCP joint exist[8]:
  ○ The **radial collateral ligament** is located on the radial side of the MCP joint.
  ○ The **ulnar collateral ligament** is located on the ulnar side of the MCP joint.
    ○ More specifically, both the radial and ulnar collateral ligaments attach proximally onto the head of the metacarpal and attach distally onto the base of the proximal phalanx.

| BOX 10-25 | Ligaments of the Metacarpophalangeal Joints |

○ Fibrous capsules
○ Radial collateral ligaments
○ Ulnar collateral ligaments
○ Palmar plates

- ○ The radial and ulnar collateral ligaments of the MCP joint are considered to have two parts: (1) the part that attaches onto the proximal phalanx is called the *cord,* and (2) the part that attaches into the palmar plate is called the *accessory part.*
- ○ The **palmar plate** is a ligamentous-like thick disc of fibrocartilage.[7]
  - ○ Location: It is located on the palmar side of the joint, superficial to the fibrous capsule.
    - ○ More specifically, it is located from just proximal to the head of the metacarpal to the base of each proximal phalanx.
  - ○ The purpose of the palmar plate is to stabilize the MCP joint and resist extension beyond anatomic position (i.e., resist hyperextension).
  - ○ The palmar plate is also known as the **volar plate**.
  - ○ Attaching between the palmar plates of the MCP joints are the deep transverse metacarpal ligaments of the distal intermetacarpal joints[5] (see Section 10.14).
  - ○ Attaching superficially to the anterior side of the palmar plates are fibrous sheaths that create tunnels for the extrinsic finger flexors (i.e., flexors digitorum superficialis and profundus) to travel to their attachment sites on the fingers[7] (see Figure 10-44, *A*).

CLOSED-PACKED POSITION:

- ○ 70 degrees of flexion[2]

MAJOR MUSCLES OF THE MCP JOINTS:

- ○ The muscles of the MCP joints move fingers and can be divided into extrinsic muscles (that originate on the arm and/or forearm) and intrinsic muscles (wholly located within the hand).
- ○ The extrinsic muscles of the MCP joints of fingers #2 through #5 are the flexors digitorum superficialis and profundus, extensor digitorum, extensor digiti minimi, and extensor indicis.
- ○ The extrinsic muscles of the MCP joint of the thumb are the flexor pollicis longus and extensors pollicis longus and brevis.
- ○ The intrinsic muscles of the MCP joints of fingers #2 through #5 are the abductor digiti minimi manus, flexor digiti minimi manus, opponens digiti minimi, lumbricales manus, palmar interossei, and dorsal interossei manus.
- ○ The intrinsic muscles of the MCP joint of the thumb are the abductor pollicis brevis, flexor pollicis brevis, opponens pollicis, and adductor pollicis.

MISCELLANEOUS:

- ○ When the fingers are flexed at the MCP joints, the frontal plane movements of abduction and adduction are either greatly diminished or absent entirely.[11]
  - ○ This reduced frontal plane movement when in flexion is a result of both the tension in the ligaments and the shape of the bones of the joint.
- ○ Usually a pair of sesamoid bones is located on the palmar side of the MCP joint of the thumb.[1]
- ○ Note: The frontal plane movements of abduction and adduction of the thumb at the metacarpophalangeal (MCP) joint are negligible and considered to be accessory motions. Abductor and adductor muscles that do cross the MCP joint of the thumb also cross the carpometacarpal (CMC) joint of the thumb and create abduction/adduction at that joint.

SECTION 10.16 INTERPHALANGEAL (IP) JOINTS OF THE HAND

- ○ **Interphalangeal (IP) joints** of the hand are located between phalanges of the fingers (Figure 10-45; Box 10-26).
  - ○ More specifically, each IP joint is located between the head of a phalanx and the base of the phalanx distal to it.
  - ○ Interphalangeal (IP) joints are located in both the hand and the foot. To distinguish these joints from each other, the words *manus* (denoting hand) and *pedis* (denoting foot) are often used.

BOX 10-26

Osteoarthritis (OA) is a progressive degenerative arthritic condition caused by increased physical stress to a joint. It weakens and destroys the articular cartilage of the joint and results in calcium deposition at the bony joint margins. Although this condition attacks many joints, the distal interphalangeal (DIP) joints of the hand are particularly hard hit. Clients with OA will usually develop characteristic increased bony formations, known as **bone spurs**, at the affected joints. Bone spurs at the DIP joints are called **Heberden's nodes**. OA is also known as **degenerative joint disease (DJD)**.

- ○ One IP joint in the thumb exists. It is located between the proximal and distal phalanges of the thumb.[5]
- ○ Because each of fingers #2 through #5 has three phalanges, two IP joints exist in each of these fingers[5]: (A) a **proximal interphalangeal (PIP) joint** and (B) a **distal interphalangeal (DIP) joint**.
  - ○ The IP joint located between the proximal and middle phalanges is called the *PIP joint (manus).*
  - ○ The IP joint located between the middle and distal phalanges is called the *DIP joint (manus).*
- ○ In total, nine IP joints are found in the hand (one IP, four PIPs, and four DIPs).
- ○ Joint structure classification: Synovial joint
  - ○ Subtype: Hinge
- ○ Joint function classification: Diarthrotic
  - ○ Subtype: Uniaxial

MAJOR MOTIONS ALLOWED:

The IP joints allow two major motions (Figure 10-46; Table 10-13):
- ○ The IP joints allow flexion and extension (i.e., axial movements) within the sagittal plane about a mediolateral axis.[11]

352 PART 3 Skeletal Arthrology: Study of the Joints

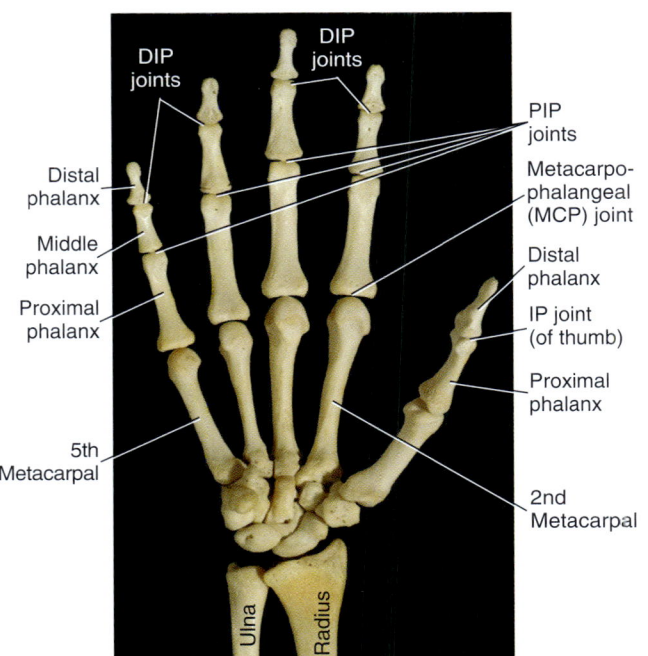

FIGURE 10-45 Anterior view that illustrates the interphalangeal (IP) joints of the hand. The thumb has one IP joint; each of the other four fingers has two IP joints: (1) a proximal interphalangeal (PIP) joint and (2) a distal interphalangeal (DIP) joint. IP joints are uniaxial hinge joints allowing only flexion and extension in the sagittal plane.

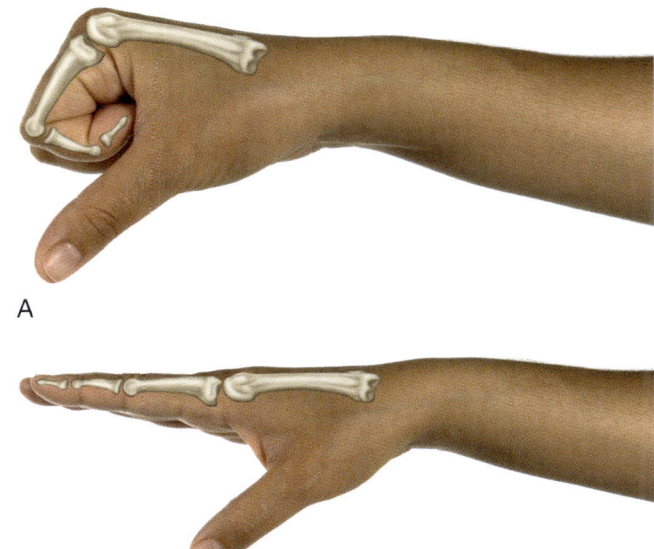

FIGURE 10-46 Flexion and extension of the fingers at the interphalangeal (IP) joints of fingers #2–5. (Note: All views are radial [i.e., lateral].) **A,** Flexion of the fingers at the proximal interphalangeal (PIP) and distal interphalangeal (DIP) joints. (Note: Flexion is also shown at the metacarpophalangeal [MCP] joints. **B,** Extension of the fingers at the PIP and DIP joints. (Note: Extension is also shown at the MCP joints.)

- When motion occurs at an IP joint of the hand, we can say that a finger moves at the proximal or distal IP joint. To be more specific, we could say that the middle phalanx moves at the proximal interphalangeal (PIP) joint, and/or that the distal phalanx moves at the distal interphalangeal (DIP) joint.
- The amount of passive extension beyond anatomic position (i.e., hyperextension) of the IP joint of the thumb is normally approximately 20 degrees.[2] However, this amount often increases with use because of a loosening of the ligamentous structure of the joint. Massage therapists and other manual therapists are prone to having this problem[8] (i.e., thumbs that bend backward) and must be careful not to overuse their thumbs, especially when doing deep work. When using the thumb for deep tissue work, it can be helpful to use a double contact (i.e., support your thumb that is in contact with the client with the thumb or fingers of the other hand). This will increase the stability of the IP joint of the thumb and lessen the deleterious effects of hyperextension forces.

Reverse Actions:

- The muscles of the IP joints are generally considered to move the more distal phalanx of a finger relative to the more proximal phalanx. However, it is possible to move the more proximal phalanx relative to the more distal one.

TABLE 10-13 Average Ranges of Motion of the Fingers at the Interphalangeal Joints from Anatomic Position[2]

Proximal Interphalangeal (PIP) Joints			
Flexion	100-120 Degrees*	Extension	0 Degrees
Distal Interphalangeal (DIP) Joints			
Flexion	80-90 Degrees*	Extension	0 Degrees[†]
Interphalangeal (IP) Joint of the Thumb			
Flexion	80 Degrees	Extension	0 Degrees[‡]

*The amount of flexion at the PIP and DIP joints gradually increases from the radial side to the ulnar side fingers.
[†]From anatomic position, no further active extension is possible at the PIP and DIP joints; however, further passive extension (i.e., hyperextension) of approximately 30 degrees is possible at the DIP joints.
[‡]From anatomic position, no further active extension is possible at the IP joint of the thumb; however, further passive extension (i.e., hyperextension) of 20 degrees is possible.

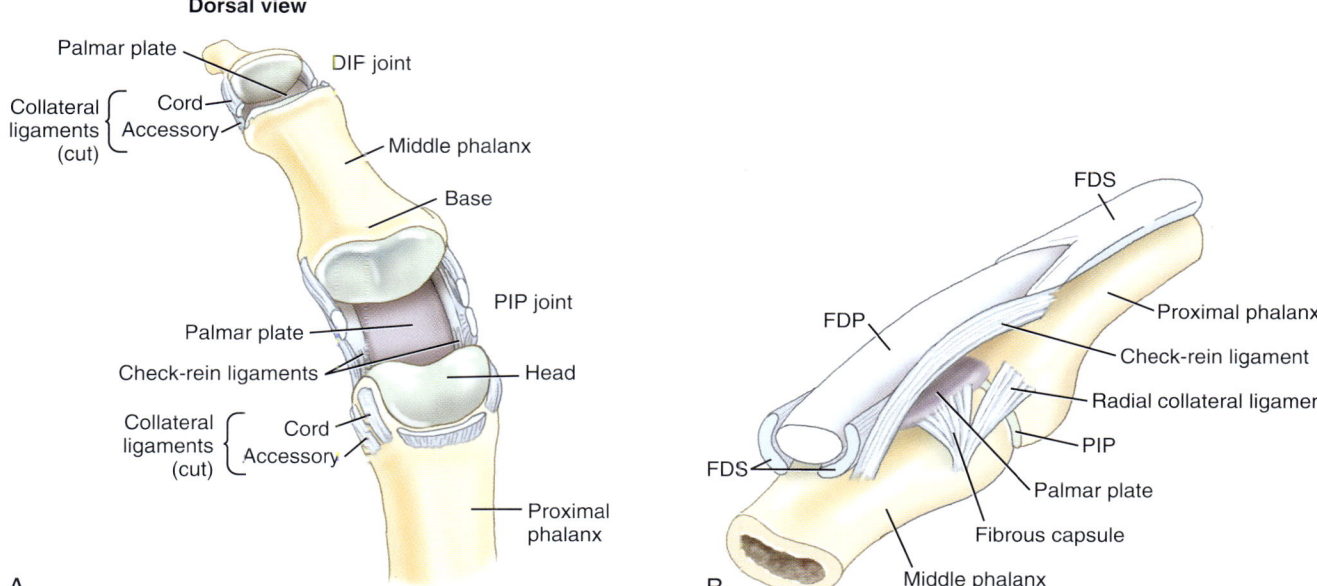

FIGURE 10-47 Ligaments of the interphalangeal (IP) joints (both the proximal interphalangeal [PIP] joints and the distal interphalangeal [DIP] joints). **A,** Dorsal (i.e., posterior) view with the IP joints opened up. Note: The fibrous capsule is not shown. **B,** A view of the palmar (i.e. anterior) surface of the PIP joint. In this view the relationship of the check-rein ligaments can be seen relative to the palmar plate and the tendons of the flexor digitorum superficialis (FDS) and the flexor digitorum profundus (FDP). *(Modeled from Neumann DA: Kinesiology of the musculoskeletal system: foundations for physical rehabilitation, ed 2, St Louis, 2010, Mosby.)*

MAJOR LIGAMENTS OF THE INTERPHALANGEAL (IP) JOINTS:

- The ligament complex of the IP joints is very similar to that of the MCP joints (Figure 10-47; Box 10-27).
- The PIP joint is stabilized by a fibrous capsule, two collateral ligaments (radial and ulnar), a palmar plate, and an additional structure called the *check-rein ligament*.[5]
- The DIP joint is stabilized by a fibrous capsule, two collateral ligaments (radial and ulnar), and a palmar plate.[5]
- The ligamentous structure of the IP joint of the thumb is similar to the DIP joint of fingers #2 through #5.

Radial and Ulnar Collateral Ligaments:

- The **radial collateral ligament** is on the radial side of the joint.
- The **ulnar collateral ligament** is on the ulnar side of the joint.
  - More specifically, both the radial and ulnar collateral ligaments attach proximally onto the head of the more proximal phalanx and distally onto the base of the phalanx that is located more distally.[8]
- The collateral ligaments of the interphalangeal (IP) joints are essentially identical to the collateral ligaments of the metacarpophalangeal (MCP) joint. The IP joint's collateral ligaments also have two parts: (1) a cord that attaches into the more distal bone of the joint and (2) an accessory part that attaches into the palmar plate.
- Function: The radial collateral ligament limits motion of the phalanx to the ulnar side; the ulnar collateral ligament limits motion of the phalanx to the radial side. Ulnar and radial motions are frontal plane motions that should not occur at the IP joints (aside from some passive joint play). These collateral ligaments help to restrict these frontal plane motions.

Palmar Plate:

- Each **palmar plate** is a ligamentous-like thick disc of fibrocartilage.
- Location: It is located on the palmar side of the joint, superficial to the fibrous capsule.[7]
  - More specifically, it is located from just proximal to the head of the more proximal phalanx to the base of the more distal phalanx.
- The purpose of the palmar plate is to stabilize the IP joint and resist extension beyond anatomic position (i.e., hyperextension).
- The palmar plate is also known as the **volar plate**.

Check-Rein Ligaments:

- The **check-rein ligaments** are located only at the PIP joint (not the DIP joint or the MCP joint).

BOX 10-27 **Ligaments of the Interphalangeal (Proximal Interphalangeal [PIP] and Distal Interphalangeal [DIP]) Joints**

- Fibrous capsules
- Radial collateral ligaments
- Ulnar collateral ligaments
- Palmar plates
- Check-rein ligaments (PIP joint only)

- They are located immediately anterior to the palmar plate (and on either side of the long finger flexor muscles' tendons) (i.e., flexors digitorum superficialis and profundus).[8]
- The check-rein ligaments strengthen the connection between the palmar plate and the bones of the joint. As with the palmar plate, the check-rein ligaments restrict hyperextension.
- Note: Passive hyperextension, which is possible at the metacarpophalangeal (MCP) and distal interphalangeal (DIP) joints, is not possible at the proximal interphalangeal (PIP) joint because of the presence of the check-rein ligaments.

CLOSED-PACKED POSITION OF THE INTERPHALANGEAL JOINTS:

- Approximately full extension[12]

MAJOR MUSCLES OF THE INTERPHALANGEAL JOINTS:

- The IP joints are crossed by both extrinsic muscles (that originate on the arm and/or forearm) and intrinsic muscles (wholly located within the hand).
- Extrinsic flexors of fingers #2 through #5 are the flexor digitorum superficialis (FDS) (which crosses only the PIP joint) and the flexor digitorum profundus (FDP). The flexor pollicis longus is an extrinsic flexor of the thumb.
- No intrinsic flexors of the IP joints of the hand exist.
- Extrinsic extensors of fingers #2 through #5 are the extensor digitorum, extensor digiti minimi manus, and extensor indicis. The extensor pollicis longus is an extrinsic extensor of the thumb.
- Intrinsic extensors of the IP joints of the hand include all intrinsics that attach into the dorsal digital expansion; they are the lumbricales manus, palmar interossei, dorsal interossei manus, and abductor digiti minimi manus.

MISCELLANEOUS:

- Other than the fact that fingers are quite a bit longer than toes, the IP joints of fingers #2 through #5 of the hand are essentially identical to the IP joints of toes #2 through #5 of the foot. However, most people do not learn the same fine-motor neural control of the toes of the foot as they have of the fingers of the hand.
- It is usually difficult to isolate finger flexion at the DIP joint.

REVIEW QUESTIONS

evolve *Answers to the following review questions appear on the Evolve website accompanying this book at: http://evolve.elsevier.com/Muscolino/kinesiology/.*

1. Name the four joints of the shoulder joint complex.

2. What is the term that describes the concept that scapular (and clavicular) movements accompany arm movements at the GH joint?

3. What are the names of the three ligaments that are thickenings of the anterior and inferior capsule of the GH joint?

4. Where do all extensors of the arm at the shoulder joint cross the shoulder joint?

5. Why is the scapulocostal joint considered to be a functional joint and not an anatomic joint?

6. How many degrees of upward rotation of the scapula at the scapulocostal joint are possible?

7. What is the only osseous articulation between the upper extremity and the axial skeleton?

8. What bones can move at the acromioclavicular joint?

9. What are the two parts of the coracoclavicular ligament?

10. What scapular joint action couples with abduction of the arm at the shoulder joint?

11. What three articulations of the elbow joint complex share the same joint capsule?

12. What is the principal articulation at the elbow joint complex?

13. Where do all muscles that flex the forearm cross the elbow joint?

14. What is the reverse action of flexion of the forearm at the elbow joint?

15. Name the three radioulnar joints.

16. What is the major ligament of the proximal radioulnar joint?

17. What defines a ray of the hand?

18. Name the arches of the hand.

19. What structures are contained within the carpal tunnel?

20. What bones are involved in the radiocarpal joint?

21. Name the joint actions possible at the wrist joint.

22. Which wrist joint ligament limits radial deviation (i.e., abduction) of the hand at the wrist joint?

23. Other than the first carpometacarpal (CMC) joint, which CMC joint is the most mobile?

24. What is the significance of the central pillar of the hand?

25. Around how many axes does the saddle joint of the thumb allow motion?

26. What are the component cardinal plane actions of opposition of the thumb at the first CMC joint?

27. What is the name of the ligament that stabilizes the distal intermetacarpal joint?

28. What is the functional classification of the metacarpophalangeal joint?

29. What are the names of the structures that stop passive extension beyond neutral (i.e., hyperextension) at the proximal interphalangeal joint?

30. What is the reference line for abduction/adduction of the fingers?

REFERENCES

1. Oatis CA: Kinesiology: The mechanics and pathomechanics of human movement, Philadelphia, 2004, Lippincott Williams & Wilkins.
2. Neumann DA: Kinesiology of the musculoskeletal system: Foundations for physical rehabilitation, ed 3, St Louis, 2017, Elsevier.
3. Hamilton N, Weimar W, Luttgens K: Kinesiology: Scientific basis of human motion, ed 12, New York, 2012, McGraw Hill.
4. Jenkins DB: Hollinshead's functional anatomy of the limbs and back, ed 8, Philadelphia, 2002, WB Saunders.
5. Smith LK, Weiss EL, Lehmkuhl LO: Brunstrom's clinical kinesiology, ed 5, Philadelphia, 1996, FA Davis.
6. Stedman's medical dictionary, ed 27, Baltimore, 2000, Lippincott Williams & Wilkins.
7. Levangie PK, Norkin CC: Joint structure and function: A comprehensive analysis, ed 5, Philadelphia, 2001, FA Davis.
8. Palastanga N, Field D, Soames R: Anatomy and human movement, ed 4, Oxford, 2002, Butterworth-Heinemann.
9. Behnke RS: Kinetic anatomy, ed 2, Champaign, IL, 2006, Human Kinetics.
10. Nordin M, Frankel VH: Basic biomechanics of the musculoskeletal system, ed 3, Baltimore, 2001, Lippincott Williams & Wilkins.
11. Hamill J, Knutzen KM: Biomechanical basis of human movement, ed 12, Baltimore, 2003, Lippincott Williams & Wilkins.
12. Hall SJ: Basic biomechanics, ed 6, New York, 2012, McGraw Hill.

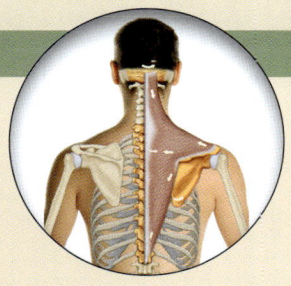

PART IV

Myology: Study of the Muscular System

CHAPTER 11
Attachments and Actions of Muscles

CHAPTER OUTLINE

Section 11.1	Overview of the Skeletal Muscles of the Body	Section 11.8	Muscles of the Spinal Joints
		Section 11.9	Muscles of the Ribcage Joints
Section 11.2	Muscles of the Shoulder Girdle	Section 11.10	Muscles of the Temporomandibular Joints
Section 11.3	Muscles of the Glenohumeral Joint	Section 11.11	Muscles of Facial Expression
Section 11.4	Muscles of the Elbow and Radioulnar Joints	Section 11.12	Muscles of the Hip Joint
		Section 11.13	Muscles of the Knee Joint
Section 11.5	Muscles of the Wrist Joint	Section 11.14	Muscles of the Ankle and Subtalar Joints
Section 11.6	Extrinsic Muscles of the Finger Joints	Section 11.15	Extrinsic Muscles of the Toe Joints
Section 11.7	Intrinsic Muscles of the Finger Joints	Section 11.16	Intrinsic Muscles of the Toe Joints

CHAPTER OBJECTIVES

After completing this chapter, the student should be able to perform the following:

1. Define the key terms of this chapter and state the meanings of the word origins of this chapter.
2. Discuss the attachments and functions of the muscles of the shoulder girdle, glenohumeral, elbow, radioulnar, wrist, and finger joints.
3. Discuss the attachments and functions of the muscles of the spinal, ribcage, and temporomandibular joints, as well as the muscles of facial expression.
4. Discuss the attachments and functions of the muscles of the hip, knee, ankle, subtalar, and toe joints.

OVERVIEW

The skeletal muscles of the human body are organs of the musculoskeletal system (more accurately, the neuro-myo-fascio-skeletal system) that are specialized to contract and create pulling forces. These pulling forces may cause movement, modify movement, or stop movement. This chapter is an atlas of the skeletal muscles and presents an illustration of each muscle along with its attachments and its major concentric/shortening (standard open-chain and/or reverse closed-chain) mover actions (for a more thorough atlas of muscle actions, see *The Muscular System Manual: The Skeletal Muscles of the Human Body, 4th Edition*. Elsevier, 2017). Note: The bones to which each featured muscle attaches have been colored orange.

357

KEY TERMS

Abductor digiti minimi manus (of hypothenar eminence group) (ab-DUK-tor DIJ-i-tee MIN-i-mee MAN-us)
Abductor digiti minimi pedis (ab-DUK-tor DIJ-i-tee MIN-i-mee PEED-us)
Abductor hallucis (ab-DUK-tor hal-OO-sis)
Abductor pollicis brevis (of thenar eminence group) (ab-DUK-tor POL-i-sis LONG-us)
Abductor pollicis longus (of deep distal four group) (ab-DUK-tor POL-i-sis LONG-us)
Adductor brevis (of adductor group) (ad-DUK-tor BRE-vis)
Adductor hallucis (ad-DUK-tor hal-OO-sis)
Adductor longus (of adductor group) (ad-DUK-tor LONG-us)
Adductor magnus (of adductor group) (ad-DUK-tor MAG-nus)
Adductor pollicis (of central compartment group) (ad-DUK-tor POL-i-sis)
Anconeus (an-KO-nee-us)
Anterior scalene (of scalene group) (an-TEE-ri-or SKAY-leen)
Articularis genus (ar-TIK-you-LA-ris JEH-new)
Auricularis group (aw-RIK-u-la-ris)
Biceps brachii (BY-seps BRAY-key-eye)
Biceps femoris (of hamstring group) (BY-seps FEM-o-ris)
Brachialis (BRAY-key-AL-is)
Brachioradialis (of radial group) (BRAY-key-o-RAY-dee-AL-is)
Buccinator (BUK-sin-A-tor)
Coracobrachialis (KOR-a-ko-BRA-key-AL-is)
Corrugator supercilii (KOR-uh-GAY-tor SOOP-er-SIL-lee-eye)
Deltoid (DEL-toid)
Depressor anguli oris (dee-PRES-or ANG-you-lie OR-is)
Depressor labii inferioris (dee-PRES-or LAY-be-eye in-FEE-ri-OR-is)
Depressor septi nasi (dee-PRES-or SEP-ti NAY-zi)
Diaphragm (DI-a-fram)
Digastric (of hyoid group) (di-GAS-trik)
Dorsal interossei manus (of central compartment group) (DOR-sul IN-ter-OSS-ee-I MAN-us)
Dorsal interossei pedis (DOR-sul in-ter-OSS-ee-eye PEED-us)
Erector spinae group (ee-REK-tor SPEE-nee)
Extensor carpi radialis brevis (of wrist extensor and radial groups) (eks-TEN-sor KAR-pie RAY-de-A-lis BRE-vis)
Extensor carpi radialis longus (of wrist extensor and radial groups) (eks-TEN-sor KAR-pie RAY-dee-A-lis LONG-us)
Extensor carpi ulnaris (of wrist extensor group) (eks-TEN-sor KAR-pie ul-NA-ris)
Extensor digiti minimi (eks-TEN-sor DIJ-i-tee MIN-i-mee)
Extensor digitorum (eks-TEN-sor dij-i-TOE-rum)
Extensor digitorum brevis (eks-TEN-sor dij-i-TOE-rum BRE-vis)
Extensor digitorum longus (eks-TEN-sor dij-i-TOE-rum LONG-us)
Extensor hallucis brevis (eks-TEN-sor hal-OO-sis BRE-vis)
Extensor hallucis longus (eks-TEN-sor hal-OO-sis LONG-us)
Extensor indicis (of deep distal four group) (eks-TEN-sor IN-di-sis)
Extensor pollicis brevis (of deep distal four group) (eks-TEN-sor POL-i-sis BRE-vis)
Extensor pollicis longus (of deep distal four group) (eks-TEN-sor POL-i-sis LONG-us)
External abdominal oblique (of anterior abdominal wall) (EKS-turn-al ab-DOM-in-al o-BLEEK)
External intercostals (EKS-turn-al in-ter-KOS-tals)
Fibularis brevis (fib-you-LA-ris BRE-vis)
Fibularis longus (fib-you-LA-ris LONG-us)
Fibularis tertius (fib-you-LA-ris TER-she-us)
Flexor carpi radialis (of wrist flexor group) (FLEKS-or KAR-pie RAY-dee-A-lis)
Flexor carpi ulnaris (of wrist flexor group) (FLEKS-or KAR-pie ul-NA-ris)
Flexor digiti minimi manus (of hypothenar eminence group) (FLEKS-or DIJ-i-tee MIN-i-mee MAN-us)
Flexor digiti minimi pedis (FLEKS-or DIJ-i-tee MIN-i-mee PEED-us)
Flexor digitorum brevis (FLEKS-or dij-i-TOE-rum BRE-vis)
Flexor digitorum longus (*Dick* of *Tom*, *Dick* and *Harry* group) (FLEKS-or dij-i-TOE-rum LONG-us)
Flexor digitorum profundus (FLEKS-or dij-i-TOE-rum pro-FUN-dus)
Flexor digitorum superficialis (FLEKS-or dij-i-TOE-rum SOO-per-fish-ee-A-lis)
Flexor hallucis brevis (FLEKS-or hal-OO-sis BRE-vis)
Flexor hallucis longus (*Harry* of *Tom*, *Dick*, and *Harry* group) (FLEKS-or hal-OO-sis LONG-us)
Flexor pollicis brevis (of thenar eminence group) (FLEKS-or POL-i-sis BRE-vis)
Flexor pollicis longus (FLEKS-or POL-i-sis LONG-us)
Gastrocnemius ("*gastrocs*") (of triceps surae group) (GAS-trok-NEE-me-us)
Geniohyoid (of hyoid group) (JEE-nee-o-HI-oyd)
Gluteus maximus (of gluteal group) (GLOO-tee-us MAX-i-mus)
Gluteus medius (of gluteal group) (GLOO-tee-us MEED-ee-us)
Gluteus minimus (of gluteal group) (GLOO-tee-us MIN-i-mus)
Gracilis (of adductor group) (gra-SIL-is)
Iliacus (of iliopsoas) (i-lee-AK-us)
Iliocostalis (of erector spinae group) (IL-ee-o-kos-TA-lis)
Inferior gemellus (of deep lateral rotator group) (in-FEE-ree-or jee-MEL-us)
Infraspinatus (of rotator cuff group) (IN-fra-spy-NAY-tus)
Internal abdominal oblique (of anterior abdominal wall) (in-TURN-al ab-DOM-in-al o-BLEEK)
Internal intercostals (IN-turn-al in-ter-KOS-tals)
Interspinales (IN-ter-spy-NA-leez)
Intertransversarii (IN-ter-trans-ver-SA-ri-eye)
Lateral pterygoid (LAT-er-al TER-i-goyd)
Latissimus dorsi ("lat") (la-TIS-i-mus DOOR-si)
Levator anguli oris (le-VAY-tor ANG-you-lie O-ris)
Levator labii superioris (le-VAY-tor LAY-be-eye soo-PEE-ri-O-ris)
Levator labii superioris alaeque nasi (le-VAY-tor LAY-be-eye soo-PEE-ri-o-ris a-LEE-kwe NAY-si)
Levator palpebrae superioris (LE-vay-tor pal-PEE-bree su-PEE-ri-OR-is)
Levator scapulae (le-VAY-tor, SKAP-you-lee)
Levatores costarum (le-va-TO-rez [singular: le-VAY-tor] kos-TAR-um)

Longissimus (of erector spinae group) (lon-JIS-i-mus)
Longus capitis (of prevertebral group) (LONG-us KAP-i-tis)
Longus colli (of prevertebral group) (LONG-us KOL-eye)
Lumbricals manus (of central compartment group) (LUM-bri-kuls MAN-us)
Lumbricals pedis (LUM-bri-kuls PEED-us)
Masseter (MA-sa-ter)
Medial pterygoid (MEE-dee-al TER-i-goyd)
Mentalis (men-TA-lis)
Middle scalene (of scalene group) (MI-dil SKAY-leen)
Multifidus (of transversospinalis group) (mul-TIF-id-us MY-nor)
Mylohyoid (of hyoid group) (MY-lo-HI-oyd)
Nasalis (nay-SA-lis)
Obliquus capitis inferior (of suboccipital group) (ob-LEE-kwus KAP-i-tis in-FEE-ri-or)
Obliquus capitis superior (of suboccipital group) (ob-LEE-kwus KAP-i-tis sue-PEE-ri-or)
Obturator externus (of deep lateral rotator group) (ob-too-RAY-tor ex-TER-nus)
Obturator internus (of deep lateral rotator group) (ob-too-RAY-tor in-TER-nus)
Occipitofrontalis (of epicranius) (ok-SIP-i-to-fron-TA-lis)
Omohyoid (of hyoid group) (O-mo-HI-oyd)
Opponens digiti minimi (of hypothenar eminence group) (op-PO-nens DIJ-i-tee MIN-i-mee)
Opponens pollicis (of thenar eminence group) (op-PO-nens POL-i-sis)
Orbicularis oculi (or-BIK-you-la-ris OK-you-lie)
Orbicularis oris (or-BIK-you-LA-ris OR-is)
Palmar interossei (of central compartment group) (PAL-mar IN-ter-OSS-ee-I)
Palmaris brevis (pall-MA-ris BRE-vis)
Palmaris longus (of wrist flexor group) (pall-MA-ris LONG-us)
Pectineus (of adductor group) (pek-TIN-ee-us)
Pectoralis major (PEK-to-ra-lis MAY-jor)
Pectoralis minor (PEK-to-ra-lis MY-nor)
Piriformis (of deep lateral rotator group) (pi-ri-FOR-mis)
Plantar interossei (PLAN-tar in-ter-OSS-ee-eye)
Plantaris (plan-TA-ris)
Platysma (pla-TIZ-ma)
Popliteus (pop-LIT-ee-us)
Posterior scalene (of scalene group) (pos-TEE-ri-or SKAY-leen)
Procerus (pro-SAIR-rus)
Pronator quadratus (pro-NAY-tor kwod-RAY-tus)
Pronator teres (pro-NAY-tor TE-reez)
Psoas major (of iliopsoas) (SO-as MAY-jor)
Psoas minor (SO-as MY-nor)
Quadratus femoris (of deep lateral rotator group) (kwod-RATE-us FEM-o-ris)
Quadratus lumborum (QL) (kwod-RAY-tus lum-BOR-um)
Quadratus plantae (kwod-RAY-tus PLAN-tee)
Rectus abdominis (of anterior abdominal wall) (REK-tus ab-DOM-i-nis)
Rectus capitis anterior (of prevertebral group) (REK-tus KAP-i-tis an-TEE-ri-or)
Rectus capitis lateralis (of prevertebral group) (REK-tus KAP-i-tis la-ter-A-lis)
Rectus capitis posterior major (of suboccipital group) (REK-tus KAP-i-tis pos-TEE-ri-or MAY-jor)
Rectus capitis posterior minor (of suboccipital group) (REK-tus KAP-i-tis pos-TEE-ri-or)
Rectus femoris (of quadriceps femoris group) (REK-tus FEM-o-ris)
Rhomboids major and minor (ROM-boyd, MAY-jor, MY-nor)
Risorius (ri-ZOR-ee-us)
Rotatores (of transversospinalis group) (ro-ta-TO-reez)
Sartorius (sar-TOR-ee-us)
Semimembranosus (of hamstring group) (SEM-i-MEM-bra-NO-sus)
Semispinalis (of transversospinalis group) (SEM-ee-spy-NA-lis)
Semitendinosus (of hamstring group) (SEM-i-TEN-di-NO-sus)
Serratus anterior (ser-A-tus, an-TEE-ri-or)
Serratus posterior inferior (ser-A-tus pos-TEE-ri-or in-FEE-ri-or)
Serratus posterior superior (ser-A-tus pos-TEE-ri-or sue-PEE-ri-or)
Soleus (of triceps surae group) (SO-lee-us)
Spinalis (of erector spinae group) (spy-NA-lis)
Splenius capitis (SPLEE-nee-us KAP-i-tis)
Splenius cervicis (SPLEE-nee-us SER-vi-sis)
Sternocleidomastoid (SCM) (STER-no-KLI-do-MAS-toyd)
Sternohyoid (of hyoid group) (STER-no-HI-oyd)
Sternothyroid (of hyoid group) (STER-no-THI-royd)
Stylohyoid (of hyoid group) (STI-lo-HI-oyd)
Subclavius (sub-KLAY-vee-us)
Subcostales (sub-kos-TAL-eez)
Subscapularis (of rotator cuff group) (sub-skap-u-LA-ris)
Superior gemellus (of deep lateral rotator group) (su-PEE-ree-or jee-MEL-us)
Supinator (SUE-pin-AY-tor)
Supraspinatus (of rotator cuff group) (SOO-pra-spy-NAY-tus)
Temporalis (tem-po-RA-lis)
Temporoparietalis (of epicranius) (TEM-po-ro-pa-RI-i-TAL-is)
Tensor fasciae latae (TFL) (TEN-sor FASH-ee-a LA-tee)
Teres major (TE-reez MAY-jor)
Teres minor (of rotator cuff group) (TE-reez MY-nor)
Thyrohyoid (of hyoid group) (THI-ro-HI-oyd)
Tibialis anterior (tib-ee-A-lis an-TEE-ri-or)
Tibialis posterior (Tom of Tom, Dick, and Harry group) (tib-ee-A-lis pos-TEE-ri-or)
Transversospinalis group (trans-VER-so-spy-NA-lis)
Transversus abdominis (of anterior abdominal wall) (trans-VER-sus ab-DOM-i-nis)
Transversus thoracis (trans-VER-sus thor-AS-is)
Trapezius ("trap") (tra-PEE-zee-us)
Triceps brachii (TRY-seps BRAY-key-eye)
Vastus intermedius (of quadriceps femoris group) (VAS-tus in-ter-MEE-dee-us)
Vastus lateralis (of quadriceps femoris group) (VAS-tus lat-er-A-lis)
Vastus medialis (of quadriceps femoris group) (VAS-tus mee-dee-A-lis)
Zygomaticus major (ZI-go-MAT-ik-us MAY-jor)
Zygomaticus minor (ZI-go-MAT-ik-us MY-nor)

WORD ORIGINS

- Abdominal/Abdominis—From Latin, *refers to the abdomen*
- Abductor—From Latin, *a muscle that abducts a body part*
- Adductor—From Latin, *a muscle that adducts a body part*
- Anconeus—From Greek, *elbow*
- Alaeque—From Latin, *refers to the ala* (alar cartilage)
- Anguli—From Latin, *refers to the angle*
- Anterior—From Latin, *before, in front of*
- Articularis—From Latin, *refers to a joint*
- Auricularis—From Latin, *ear*
- Biceps—From Latin, *two heads*
- Brachialis/Brachii/Brachio—From Latin, *refers to the arm*
- Brevis—From Latin, *shorter*
- Buccinator—From Latin, *trumpeter, refers to the cheek*
- Capitis—From Latin, *refers to the head*
- Carpi—From Latin, *of the wrist*
- Cervicis—From Latin, *refers to the cervical spine*
- Clavius—From Latin, *key*
- Cleido—From Greek, *refers to the clavicle*
- Colli—From Latin, *refers to the neck*
- Coraco—From Greek, *refers to the coracoid process of the scapula*
- Corrugator—From Latin, *to wrinkle together*
- Costalis/Costals/Costarum—From Latin, *refers to the rib*
- Delta—From Greek, *the letter delta (Δ) (triangle shape)*
- Depressor—From Latin, *depressor*
- Di—From Greek, *two*
- Diaphragm—From Greek, *partition*
- Digiti/Digitorum—From Latin, *refers to a digit* (finger/toe)
- Dorsal/Dorsi—From Latin, *back*
- Erector—From Latin, *to make erect*
- Extensor—From Latin, *a muscle that extends a body part*
- External—From Latin, *outside*
- Fasciae—From Latin, *band/bandage*
- Femoris—From Latin, *refers to the femur*
- Fibularis—From Latin, *refers to the fibula*
- Fidus—From Latin, *to split*
- Flexor—From Latin, *a muscle that flexes a body part*
- Gastroc—From Greek, *belly*
- Gemellus—From Latin, *twin*
- Genio—From Greek, *chin*
- Genu—From Latin, *refers to the knee*
- Gluteus—From Greek, *buttock*
- Gracilis—From Latin, *slender, graceful*
- Hallucis—From Latin, *refers to the big toe*
- Hyoid—From Greek, *refers to the hyoid bone*
- Iliacus/Ilio—From Latin, *refers to the ilium*
- Indicis—From Latin, *index finger* (finger two)
- Inferior/Inferioris—From Latin, *below/lower*
- Infraspinatus—From Latin, *below the spine* (of the scapula)
- Inter—From Latin, *between*
- Internal/Internus—From Latin, *inside/inner*
- Interossei—From Latin, *between bones*
- Labii—From Latin, *refers to the lip*
- Latae—From Latin, *broad, refers to the side*
- Lateral/Lateralis—From Latin, *side*
- Latissimus—From Latin, *wide*
- Levator—From Latin, *lifter*
- Longissimus—From Latin, *very long*
- Longus—From Latin, *longer*
- Lumborum—From Latin, *loin* (low back)
- Lumbricals—From Latin, *earthworms*
- Magnus—From Latin, *great, larger*
- Major—From Latin, *larger*
- Manus—From Latin, *refers to the hand*
- Masseter—From Greek, *chewer*
- Mastoid—From Greek, *refers to the mastoid process*
- Maximus—From Latin, *greatest*
- Medial/Medius—From Latin, *toward the middle*
- Membranosus—From Latin, *refers to its flattened, membranous tendon*
- Mentalis—From Latin, *the chin*
- Middle—From Latin, *middle* (between)
- Minimi/Minimus—From Latin, *least*
- Minor—From Latin, *smaller*
- Multi—From Latin, *many*
- Mylo—From Greek, *mill* (refers to the molar teeth)
- Nasalis/Nasi—From Latin, *nose*
- Nemius—From Greek, *leg*
- Oblique/Obliquus—From Latin, *oblique, slanting, diagonal*
- Obturator—From Latin, *to stop up, obstruct* (refers to the obturator foramen)
- Occipitofrontalis—From Latin, *refers to the occipital and frontal bones*
- Oculi—From Latin, *refers to the eyes*
- Oid—From Greek, *shape, resemblance*
- Omo—From Greek, *shoulder*
- Opponens—From Latin, *opposing*
- Orbicularis—From Latin, *a small circle*
- Oris—From Latin, *mouth*
- Palmar/Palmaris—From Latin, *refers to the palm*
- Parietals—From Latin, *refers to the parietal bone*
- Pectineus—From Latin, *comb*
- Pectoralis—From Latin, *refers to the chest*
- Pedis—From Latin, *refers to the foot*
- Piriformis—From Latin, *pear shaped*
- Plantae/Plantaris—From Latin, *refers to the plantar surface of the foot*
- Platysma—From Greek, *broad, plate*
- Pollicis—From Latin, *thumb*
- Popliteus—From Latin, *ham of the knee* (refers to the poster or knee)
- Posterior—From Latin, *behind, toward the back*
- Procerus—From Latin, *a chief noble, prince*
- Profundus—From Latin, *deep*
- Pronator—From Latin, *a muscle that pronates a body part*
- Psoas—From Greek, *loin* (low back)
- Pterygoid—From Greek, *wing shaped*
- Quadratus—From Latin, *squared*

- Radialis—From Latin, *refers to the radius*
- Rectus—From Latin, *straight*
- Rhomb—From Greek, *rhombos* (the geometric shape)
- Risorius—From Latin, *laughing*
- Rotatores—From Latin, *to turn, a muscle revolving a body part on its axis*
- Sartorius—From Latin, *tailor*
- Scalene—From Latin, *uneven, ladder*
- Scapulae—From Latin, *of the scapula*
- Semi—From Latin, *half*
- Septi—From Latin, *refers to the nasal septum*
- Serratus—From Latin, *a notching*
- Soleus—From Latin, *sole of the foot*
- Spinae—From Latin, *thorn* (refers to the spine)
- Spinalis—From Latin, *refers to the spinous processes*
- Splenius—From Greek, *bandage*
- Sterno—From Greek, *refers to the sternum*
- Stylo—From Greek, *refers to the styloid process*
- Sub—From Latin, *under*
- Subscapularis—From Latin, *refers to the subscapular fossa*
- Supercilii—From Latin, *refers to the eyebrow*
- Superficialis—From Latin, *superficial* (near the surface)
- Superior—From Latin, *above*
- Supinator—From Latin, *a muscle that supinates a body part*
- Supraspinatus—From Latin, *above the spine* (of the scapula)
- Temporalis/Temporo—From Latin, *refers to the temple/temporal bone*
- Tendinosus—From Latin, *refers to its long tendon*
- Tensor—From Latin, *stretcher*
- Teres—From Latin, *round*
- Thoracis—From Greek, *refers to the thorax* (chest)
- Thyroid—From Greek, *refers to the thyroid cartilage*
- Tibialis—From Latin, *refers to the tibia*
- Transversarii/Transverso—From Latin, *refers to the transverse process*
- Transversus—From Latin, *running transversely*
- Trapezius—From Greek, *a little table* (or trapezoid shape)
- Triceps—From Latin, *three heads*
- Ulnaris—From Latin, *refers to the ulnar side* (of the forearm)
- Vastus—From Latin, *vast, large*
- Zygomaticus—From Greek, *refers to the zygomatic bone*

362 PART 4 Myology: Study of the Muscular System

SECTION 11.1 OVERVIEW OF THE SKELETAL MUSCLES OF THE BODY

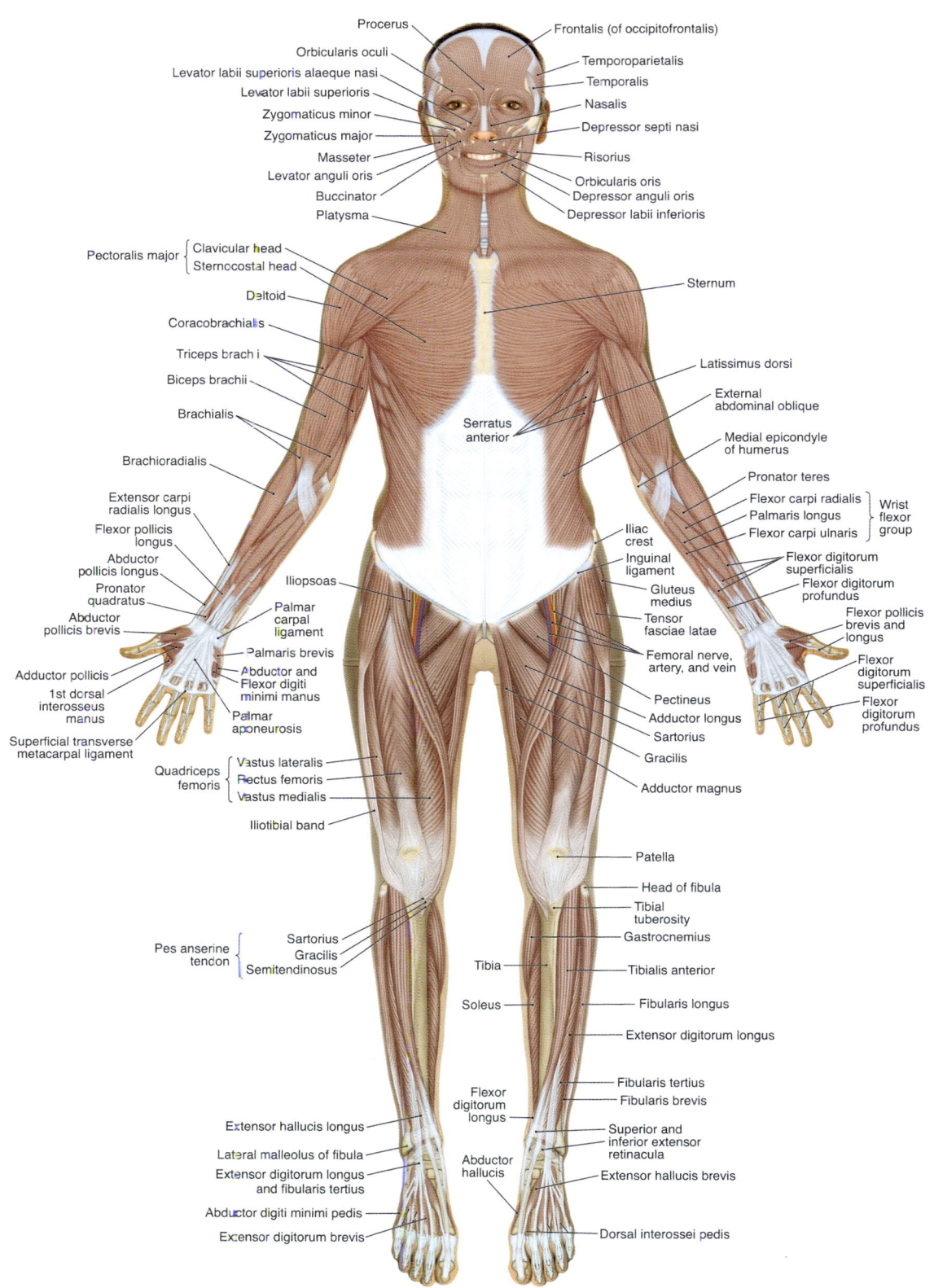

FIGURE 11-1 Anterior view of the body.

CHAPTER 11 Attachments and Actions of Muscles

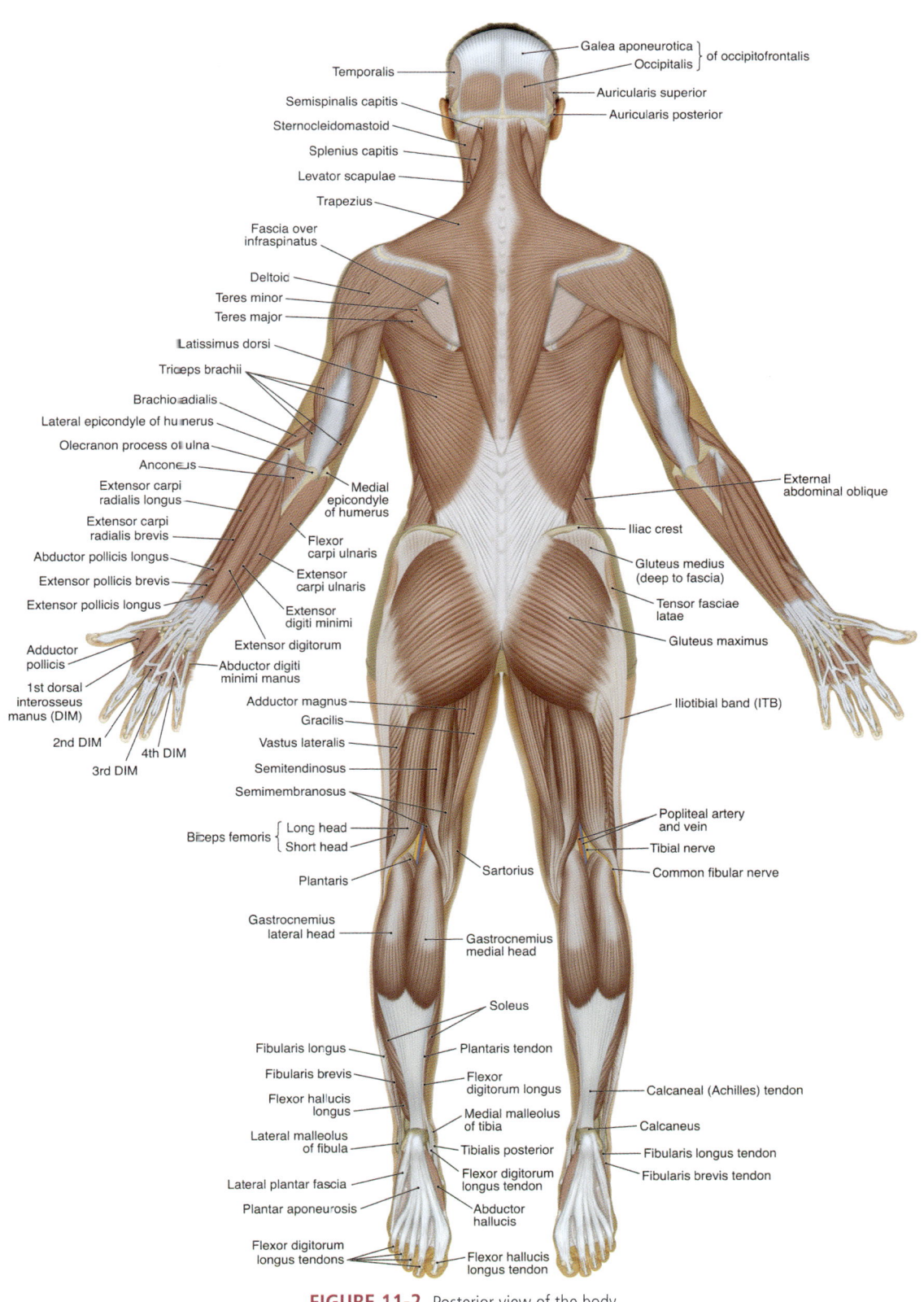

FIGURE 11-2 Posterior view of the body.

SECTION 11.2 MUSCLES OF THE SHOULDER GIRDLE

TRAPEZIUS ("TRAP"):

Attachments:

- **Entire Muscle: External Occipital Protuberance, Medial ⅓ of the Superior Nuchal Line of the Occiput, Nuchal Ligament, and Spinous Processes of C7-T12**
  - UPPER: the external occipital protuberance, the medial ⅓ of the superior nuchal line of the occiput, the nuchal ligament, and the spinous process of C7
  - MIDDLE: the spinous processes of T1-T5
  - LOWER: the spinous processes of T6-T12

to the

- **Entire Muscle: Lateral ⅓ of the Clavicle, Acromion Process, and the Spine of the Scapula**
  - UPPER: lateral ⅓ of the clavicle and the acromion process of the scapula
  - MIDDLE: acromion process and spine of the scapula
  - LOWER: the tubercle at the root of the spine of the scapula

Functions:

Major Standard Mover Actions	Major Reverse Mover Actions
UPPER	
1. Elevates the scapula at the ScC joint[1-6]	1. Extends the head and neck at the spinal joints[1-7]
2. Retracts the scapula at the ScC joint[1,3-6]	2. Contralaterally rotates the head and neck at the spinal joints[3-7]
3. Upwardly rotates the scapula at the ScC joint[1-7]	3. Laterally flexes the head and neck at the spinal joints[1-7]
MIDDLE	
4. Retracts the scapula at the ScC joint[1-6]	
LOWER	
5. Depresses the scapula at the ScC joint[2-6]	

ScC joint = scapulocostal joint

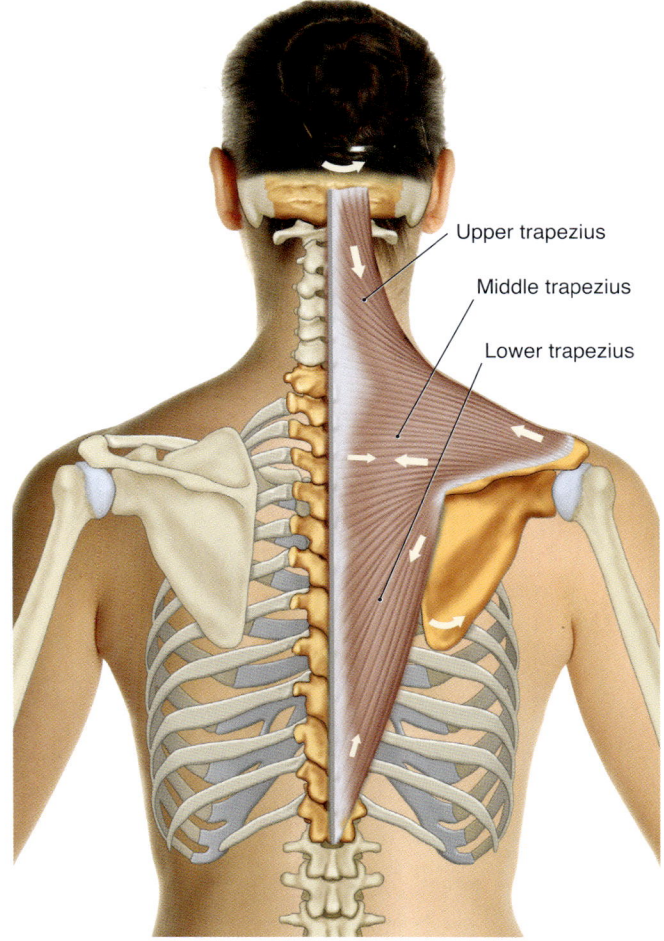

FIGURE 11-3 Posterior view of the right trapezius.

RHOMBOIDS MAJOR AND MINOR:

Attachments:

- **THE RHOMBOIDS: Spinous Processes of C7-T5**
  - MINOR: spinous processes of C7-T1 and the inferior nuchal ligament
  - MAJOR: spinous processes of T2-T5

to the

- **THE RHOMBOIDS: Medial Border of the Scapula from the Root of the Spine to the Inferior Angle of the Scapula**
  - MINOR: at the root of the spine of the scapula
  - MAJOR: between the root of the spine and the inferior angle of the scapula

Functions:

Major Standard Mover Actions
1. Retracts the scapula at the ScC joint[1–7]
2. Elevates the scapula at the ScC joint[1–7]
3. Downwardly rotates the scapula at the ScC joint[2–7]

ScC joint = scapulocostal joint

LEVATOR SCAPULAE:

Attachments:

- **Transverse Processes of C1-C4**
  - the posterior tubercles of the transverse processes of C3 and C4

to the

- **Medial Border of the Scapula, from the Superior Angle to the Root of the Spine of the Scapula**

Functions:

Major Standard Mover Action	Major Reverse Mover Actions
1. Elevates the scapula at the ScC joint[1–7]	1. Extends the neck at the spinal joints[2–7]
	2. Laterally flexes the neck at the spinal joints[1,3–6]

ScC joint = scapulocostal joint

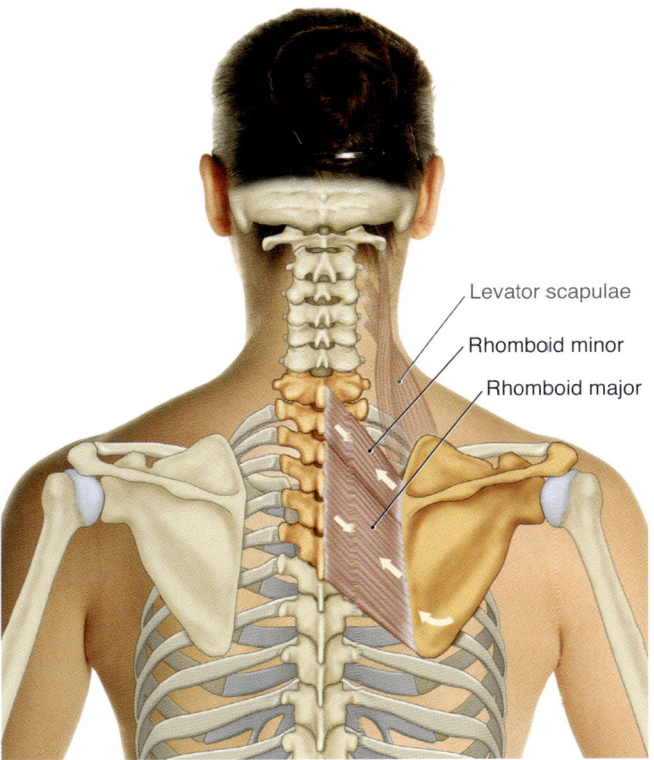

FIGURE 11-4 Posterior view of the right rhomboids major and minor. The levator scapulae has been ghosted in.

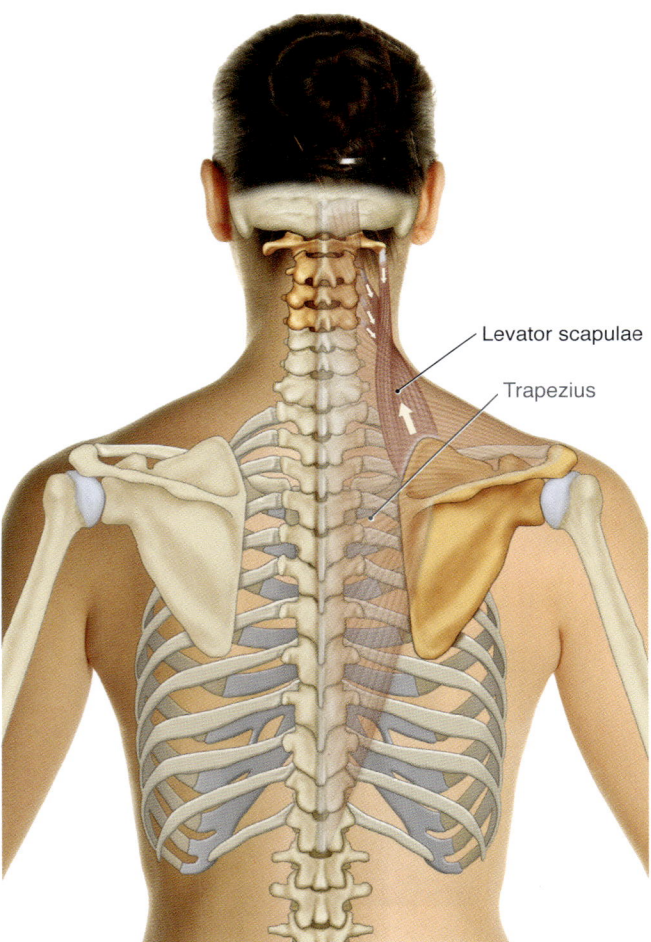

FIGURE 11-5 Posterior view of the right levator scapulae. The trapezius has been ghosted in.

SERRATUS ANTERIOR:

Attachments:

- **Ribs One through Nine**
  - anterolaterally

to the

- **Anterior Surface of the Entire Medial Border of the Scapula**

Functions:

Major Standard Mover Actions
1. Protracts the scapula at the ScC joint[1-6]
2. Upwardly rotates the scapula at the ScC joint[1-7]

ScC joint = scapulocostal joint

PECTORALIS MINOR:

Attachments:

- **Ribs Three through Five**

to the

- **Coracoid Process of the Scapula**
  - the medial aspect

Functions:

Major Standard Mover Actions	Major Reverse Mover Action
1. Protracts the scapula at the ScC joint[1,3-7]	1. Elevates ribs three through five at the sternocostal and costospinal joints[1-7]
2. Depresses the scapula at the ScC joint[1-7]	
3. Downwardly rotates the scapula at the ScC joint[1-7]	

ScC joint = scapulocostal joint

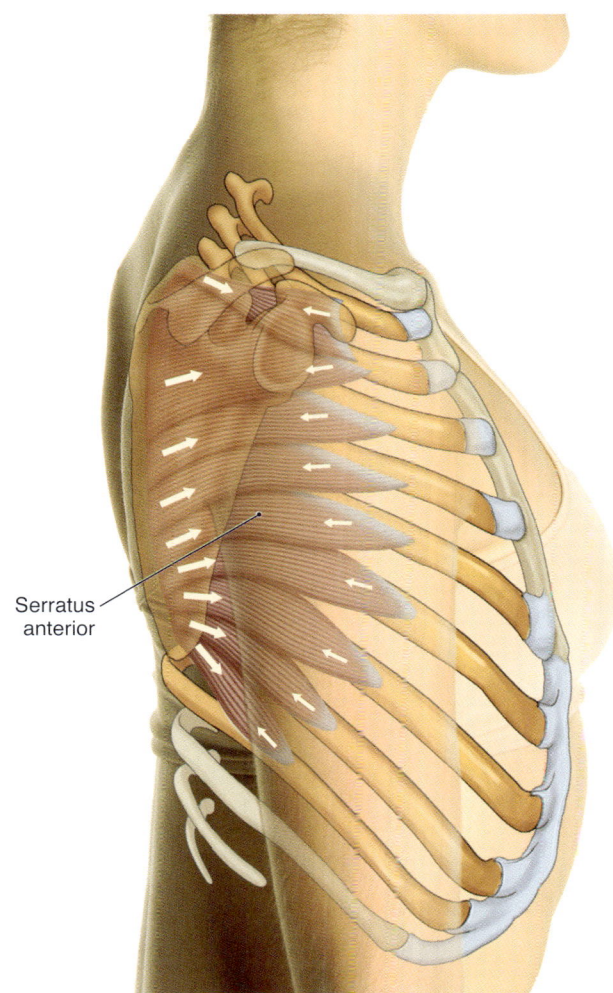

FIGURE 11-6 Lateral view of the right serratus anterior.

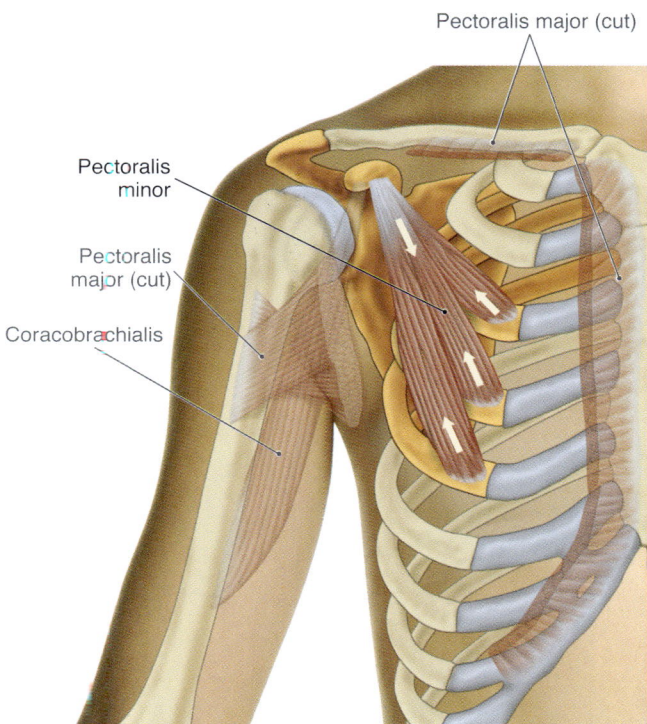

FIGURE 11-7 Anterior view of the right pectoralis minor. The coracobrachialis and cut pectoralis major have been ghosted in.

SUBCLAVIUS:

Attachments:

- **First Rib**
  - at the junction with its costal cartilage
- *to the*
- **Clavicle**
  - the middle of the inferior surface

Functions:

Major Standard Mover Action	Major Reverse Mover Action
1. Depresses the clavicle at the SC joint[2,4–6]	1. Elevates the first rib at the sternocostal and costospinal joints[2,5–7]

SC joint = sternoclavicular joint

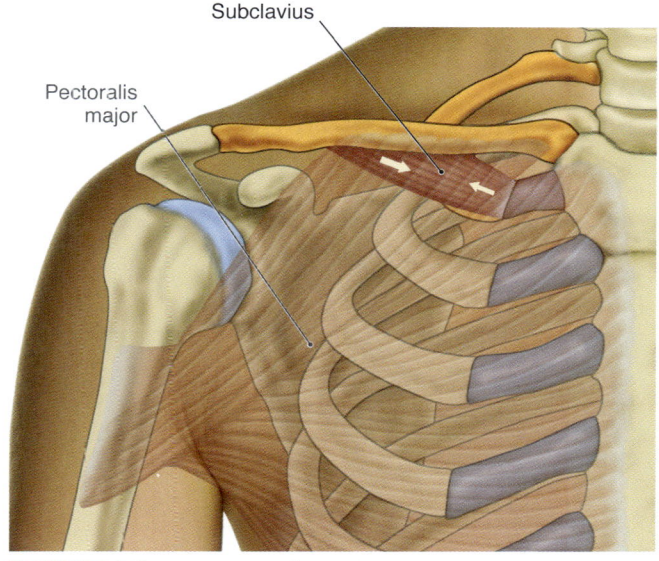

FIGURE 11-8 Anterior view of the right subclavius. The pectoralis major has been ghosted in.

SECTION 11.3 MUSCLES OF THE GLENOHUMERAL JOINT

DELTOID:

Attachments:

- **Lateral Clavicle, Acromion Process, and the Spine of the Scapula**
  - the lateral ⅓ of the clavicle
- *to the*
- **Deltoid Tuberosity of the Humerus**

Functions:

Major Standard Mover Actions	Major Reverse Mover Action
1. Abducts the arm at the GH joint (entire muscle)[1–7]	1. Downwardly rotates the scapula at the GH and scapulocostal joints[2,3,5–7]
2. Flexes the arm at the GH joint (anterior deltoid)[1–7]	
3. Medially rotates the arm at the GH joint (anterior deltoid)[1,3–6]	
4. Horizontally flexes the arm at the GH joint (anterior deltoid)[3–5]	
5. Extends the arm at the GH joint (posterior deltoid)[1,3–7]	
6. Laterally rotates the arm at the GH joint (posterior deltoid)[1–6]	
7. Horizontally extends the arm at the GH joint (posterior deltoid)[3–5,7]	

GH joint = glenohumeral joint

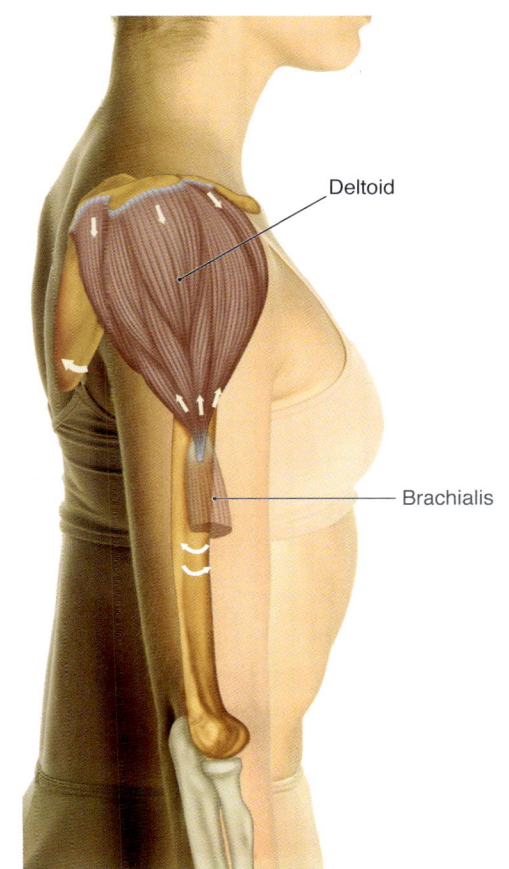

FIGURE 11-9 Lateral view of the right deltoid. The proximal end of the brachialis has been ghosted in.

CORACOBRACHIALIS:

Attachments:
- **Coracoid Process of the Scapula**
  - the apex

to the

- **Medial Shaft of the Humerus**
  - the middle ⅓

Functions:

Major Standard Mover Actions
1. Flexes the arm at the GH joint[1-6]
2. Adducts the arm at the GH joint[1,4-6]

GH joint = glenohumeral joint

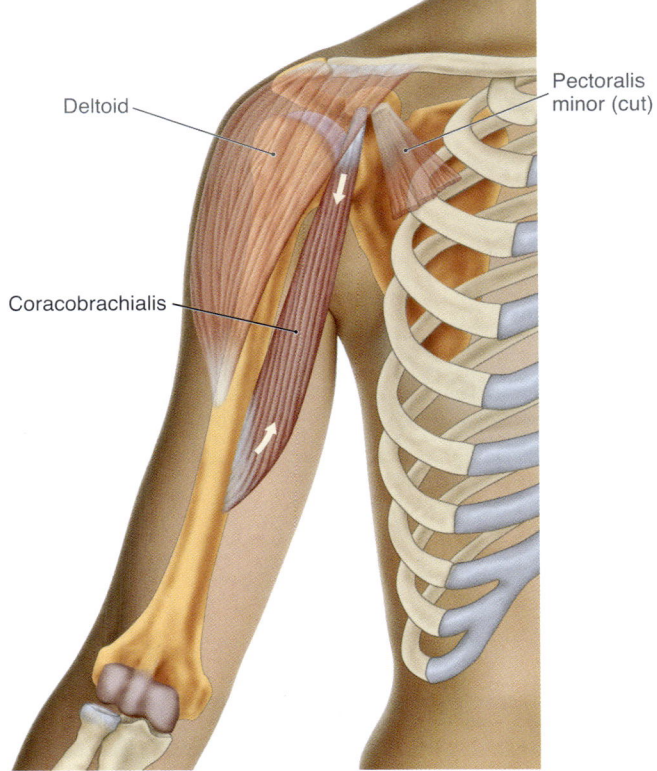

FIGURE 11-10 Anterior view of the right coracobrachialis. The deltoid and proximal end of the pectoralis minor have been ghosted in.

PECTORALIS MAJOR:

Attachments:
- **Medial Clavicle, Sternum, and the Costal Cartilages of Ribs One through Seven**
  - the medial ½ of the clavicle, and the aponeurosis of the external abdominal oblique

to the

- **Lateral Lip of the Bicipital Groove of the Humerus**

Functions:

Major Standard Mover Actions
1. Adducts the arm at the GH joint[1-7]
2. Medially rotates the arm at the GH joint[1,3-7]
3. Flexes the arm at the GH joint (clavicular head)[1,3-6]
4. Extends the arm at the GH joint (sternocostal head)[2-5,7]

GH joint = glenohumeral joint

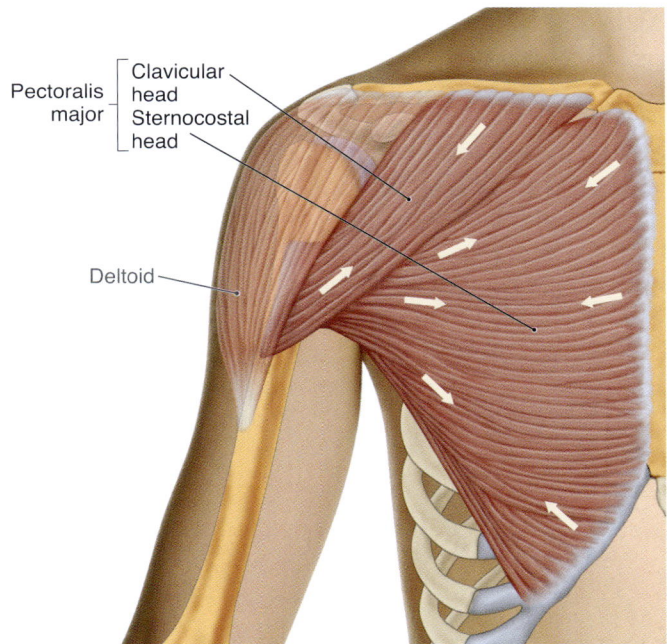

FIGURE 11-11 Anterior view of the right pectoralis major. The deltoid has been ghosted in.

LATISSIMUS DORSI ("LAT"):

Attachments:

- **Spinous Processes of T7-L5, Posterior Sacrum, and the Posterior Iliac Crest**
  - all via the thoracolumbar fascia
  - and the lowest three to four ribs and the inferior angle of the scapula

to the

- **Medial Lip of the Bicipital Groove of the Humerus**

Functions:

Major Standard Mover Actions
1. Medially rotates the arm at the GH joint[1,3–7]
2. Adducts the arm at the GH joint[1–7]
3. Extends the arm at the GH joint[1–7]

GH joint = glenohumeral joint

TERES MAJOR:

Attachments:

- **Inferior Angle and Inferior Lateral Border of the Scapula**
  - the inferior on the dorsal surface

to the

- **Medial Lip of the Bicipital Groove of the Humerus**

Functions:

Major Standard Mover Actions
1. Medially rotates the arm at the GH joint[1,3–7]
2. Adducts the arm at the GH joint[2–7]
3. Extends the arm at the GH joint[1,3–7]

GH joint = glenohumeral joint

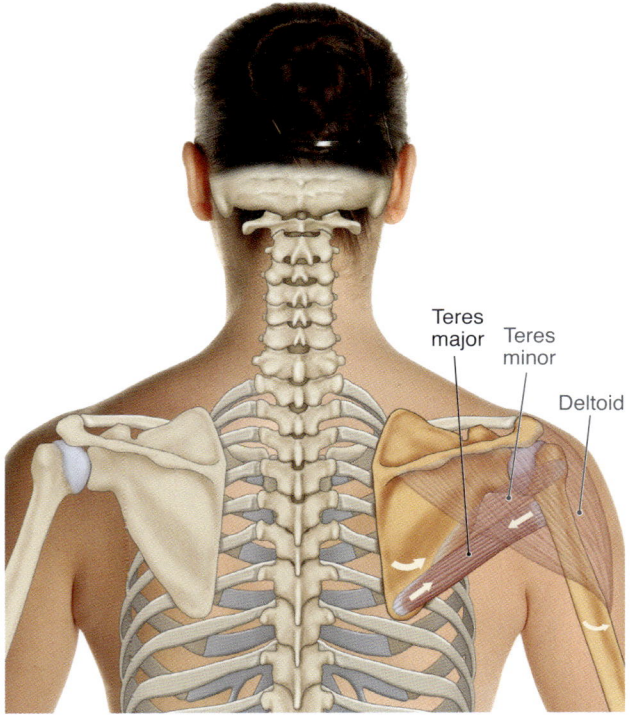

FIGURE 11-13 Posterior view of the right teres major. The deltoid and teres minor have been ghosted in.

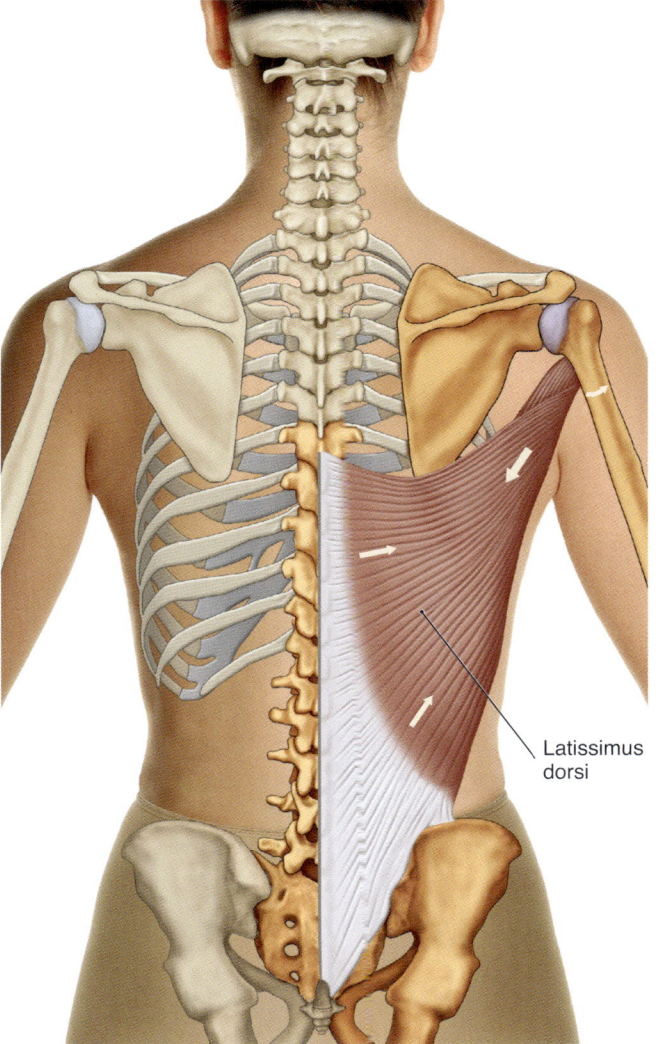

FIGURE 11-12 Posterior view of the right latissimus dorsi.

SUPRASPINATUS (OF ROTATOR CUFF GROUP):

Attachments:

- **Supraspinous Fossa of the Scapula**
  - the medial ⅔

to the

- **Greater Tubercle of the Humerus**
  - the superior facet

Functions:

Major Standard Mover Actions
1. Abducts the arm at the GH joint[1-7]
2. Flexes the arm at the GH joint[3,5]

GH joint = glenohumeral joint

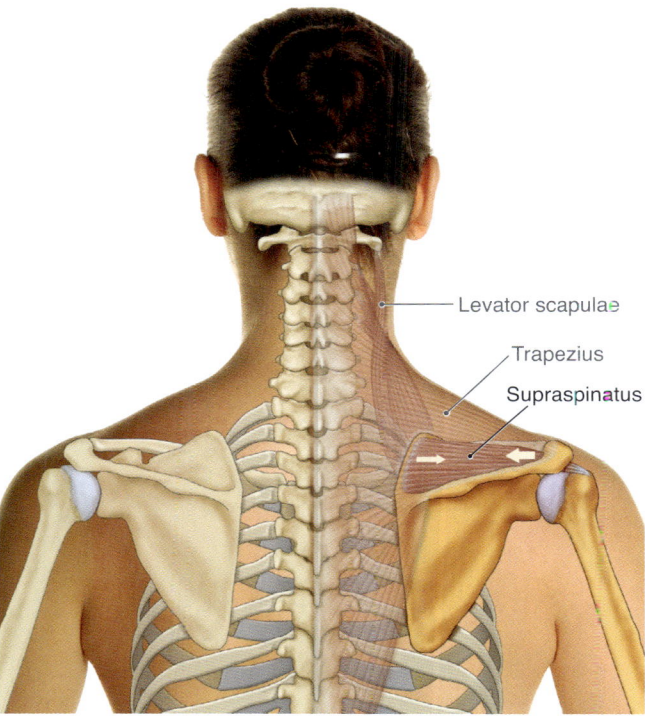

FIGURE 11-14 Posterior view of the right supraspinatus. The trapezius and levator scapulae have been ghosted in.

INFRASPINATUS (OF ROTATOR CUFF GROUP):

Attachments:

- **Infraspinous Fossa of the Scapula**
  - the medial ⅔

to the

- **Greater Tubercle of the Humerus**
  - the middle facet

Functions:

Major Standard Mover Action
1. Laterally rotates the arm at the GH joint[1-5,7]

GH joint = glenohumeral joint

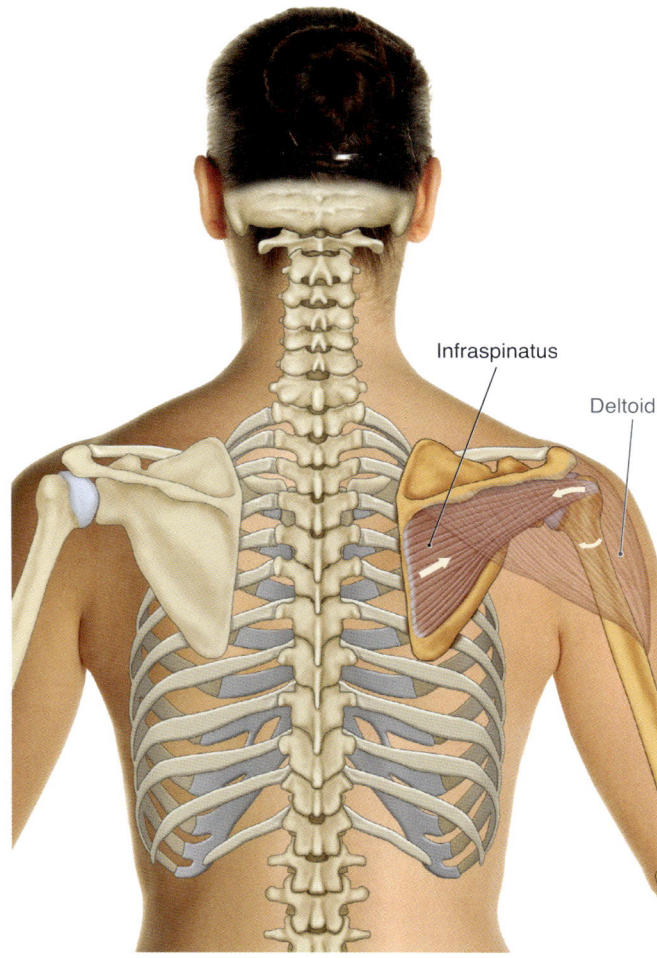

FIGURE 11-15 Posterior view of the right infraspinatus. The deltoid has been ghosted in.

TERES MINOR (OF ROTATOR CUFF GROUP):

Attachments:

- **Superior Lateral Border of the Scapula**
  - the superior ⅔ of the dorsal surface
- *to the*
- **Greater Tubercle of the Humerus**
  - the inferior facet

Functions:

Major Standard Mover Action
1. Laterally rotates the arm at the GH joint[1–4,6,7]

GH joint = glenohumeral joint

SUBSCAPULARIS (OF ROTATOR CUFF GROUP):

Attachments:

- **Subscapular Fossa of the Scapula**

to the

- **Lesser Tubercle of the Humerus**

Functions:

Major Standard Mover Action
1. Medially rotates the arm at the GH joint[1,3–7]

GH joint = glenohumeral joint

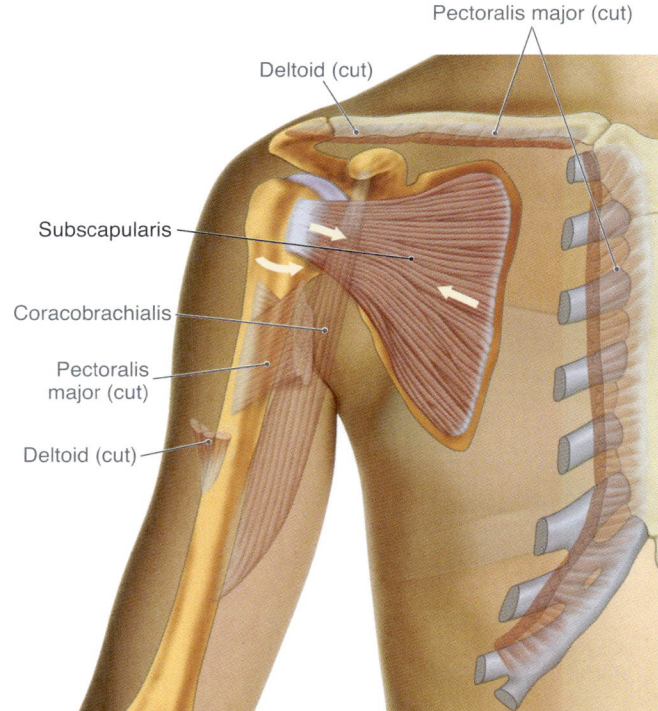

FIGURE 11-17 Anterior view of the right subscapularis. Most of the rib cage has been removed. The coracobrachialis has been ghosted in. The pectoralis major and deltoid have been cut and ghosted in.

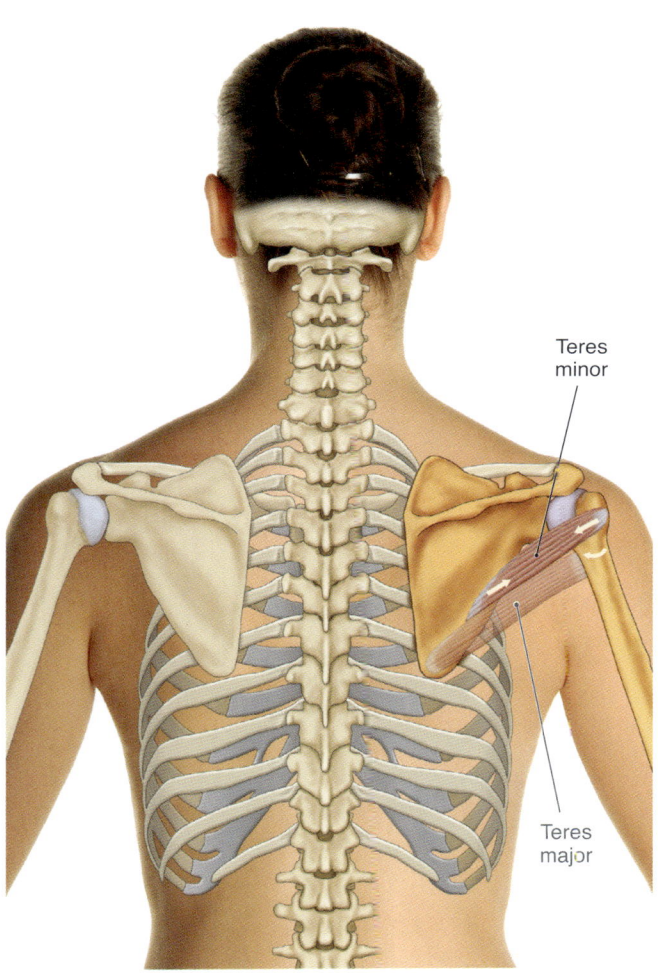

FIGURE 11-16 Posterior view of the right teres minor. The teres major has been ghosted in.

SECTION 11.4 MUSCLES OF THE ELBOW AND RADIOULNAR JOINTS

BICEPS BRACHII:

Attachments:
- **LONG HEAD:** Supraglenoid Tubercle of the Scapula
- **SHORT HEAD:** Coracoid Process of the Scapula
  - the apex

to the
- **Radial Tuberosity**
  - and the bicipital aponeurosis into deep fascia overlying the common flexor belly/tendon

Functions:

Major Standard Mover Actions
1. Flexes the forearm at the elbow joint[1-6]
2. Supinates the forearm at the RU joints[1-5,7]
3. Flexes the arm at the GH joint[1-7]

GH joint = glenohumeral joint; RU joints = radioulnar joints

BRACHIALIS:

Attachments:
- Distal ½ of the Anterior Shaft of the Humerus

to the
- **Ulnar Tuberosity**
  - and the coronoid process of the ulna

Functions:

Major Standard Mover Action
1. Flexes the forearm at the elbow joint[1-7]

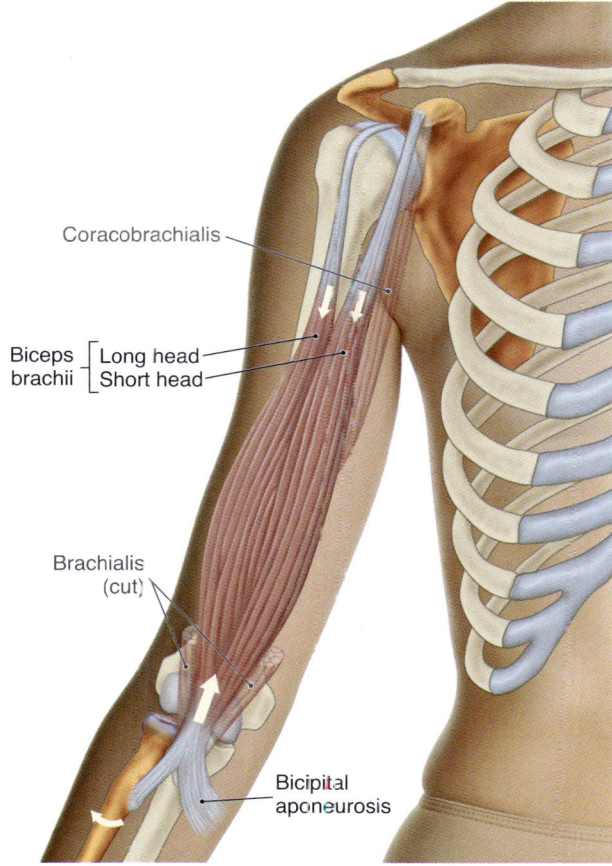

FIGURE 11-18 Anterior view of the right biceps brachii. The coracobrachialis and distal end of the brachialis have been ghosted in.

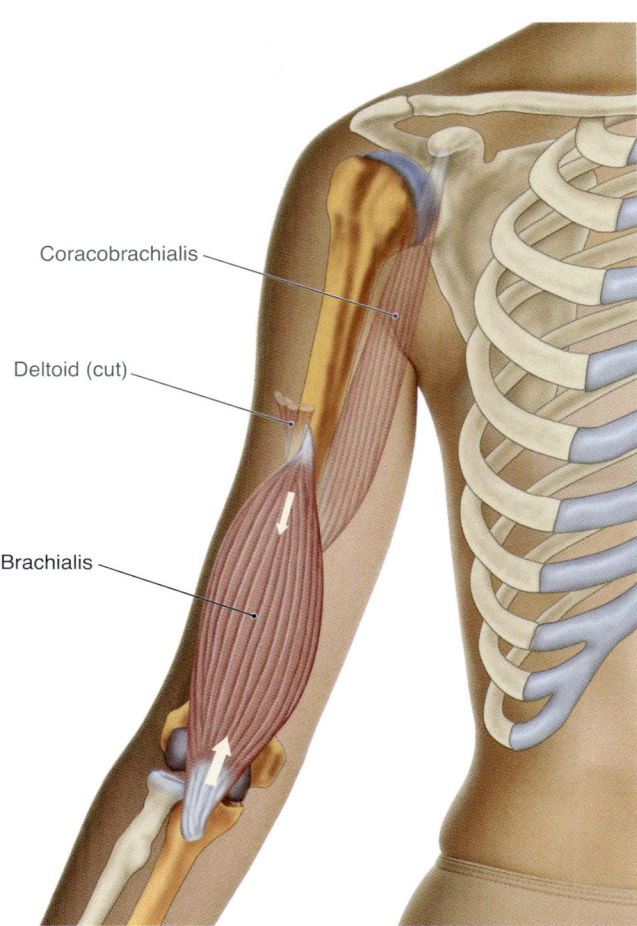

FIGURE 11-19 Anterior view of the right brachialis; the coracobrachialis and distal end of the deltoid have been ghosted in.

BRACHIORADIALIS (OF RADIAL GROUP):

Attachments:

- **Lateral Supracondylar Ridge of the Humerus**
  - the proximal ⅔

to the

- **Styloid Process of the Radius**
  - the lateral side

Functions:

Major Standard Mover Actions
1. Flexes the forearm at the elbow joint[1-7]
2. Supinates the forearm at the RU joints[2-7]
3. Pronates the forearm at the RU joints[2-7]

RU joints = radioulnar joints

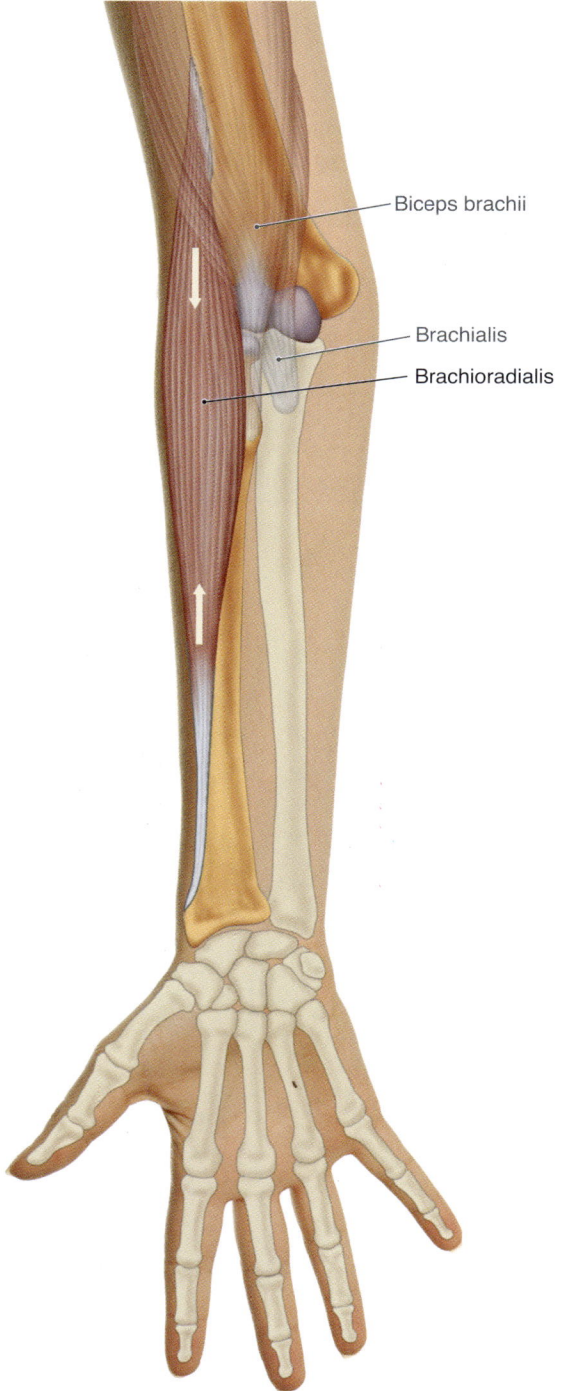

FIGURE 11-20 Anterior view of the right brachioradialis. The biceps brachii and brachialis have been ghosted in.

TRICEPS BRACHII:

Attachments:

- **LONG HEAD:** Infraglenoid Tubercle of the Scapula
- **LATERAL HEAD:** Posterior Shaft of the Humerus
  - the proximal ⅓
- **MEDIAL HEAD:** Posterior Shaft of the Humerus
  - the distal ⅔

to the

- **Olecranon Process of the Ulna**

Functions:

Major Standard Mover Actions
1. Extends the forearm at the elbow joint[1-7]
2. Extends the arm at the GH joint (long head)[1-7]

GH joint = glenohumeral joint

ANCONEUS:

Attachments:

- **Lateral Epicondyle of the Humerus**

to the

- **Posterior Proximal Ulna**
  - the lateral side of the olecranon process of the ulna and the proximal ¼ of the posterior ulna

Functions:

Major Standard Mover Action
1. Extends the forearm at the elbow joint[1-7]

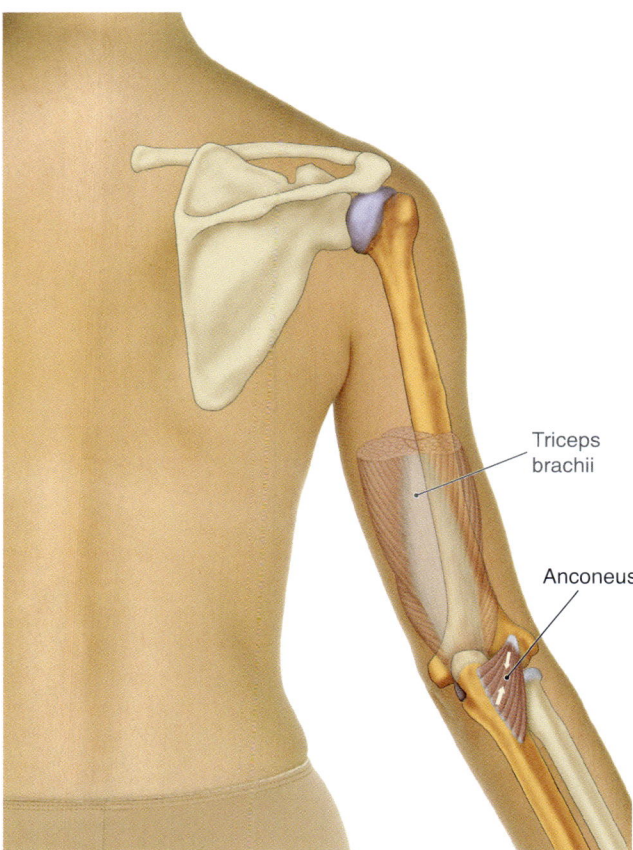

FIGURE 11-22 Posterior view of the right anconeus. The triceps brachii has been cut and ghosted in.

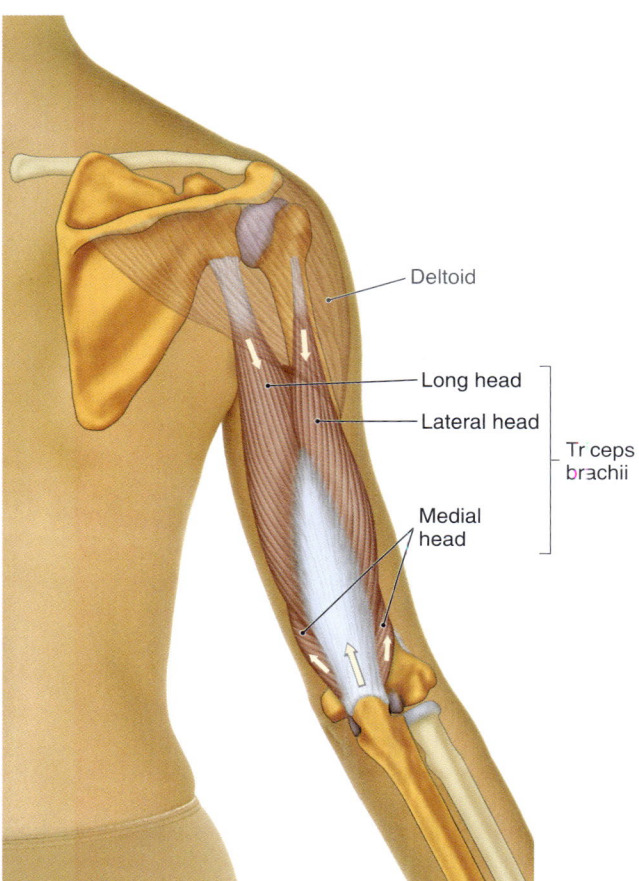

FIGURE 11-21 Superficial view of the right triceps brachii. The deltoid has been ghosted in.

PRONATOR TERES:

Attachments:

- **HUMERAL HEAD: Medial Epicondyle of the Humerus (via the Common Flexor Tendon)**
  - and the medial supracondylar ridge of the humerus
- **ULNAR HEAD: Coronoid Process of the Ulna**
  - the medial surface

to the

- **Lateral Radius**
  - the middle ⅓

Functions:

Major Standard Mover Actions
1. Pronates the forearm at the RU joints[1-7]
2. Flexes the forearm at the elbow joint[1-7]

RU joints = radioulnar joints

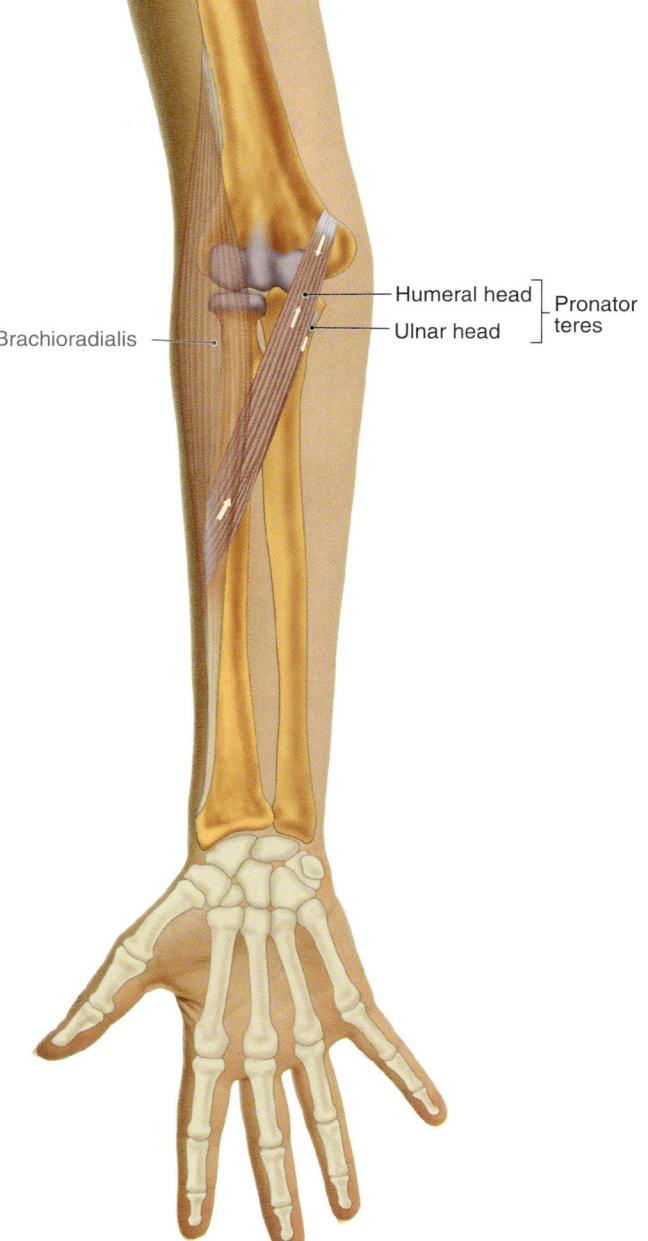

FIGURE 11-23 Anterior view of the right pronator teres. The brachioradialis has been ghosted in.

PRONATOR QUADRATUS:

Attachments:

- **Anterior Distal Ulna**
  - the distal ¼

to the

- **Anterior Distal Radius**
  - the distal ¼

Functions:

Major Standard Mover Action
1. Pronates the forearm at the RU joints[1–4,6,7]

RU joints = radioulnar joints

SUPINATOR:

Attachments:

- **Lateral Epicondyle of the Humerus and the Proximal Ulna**
  - the supinator crest of the ulna

to the

- **Proximal Radius**
  - the proximal ⅓ of the posterior, lateral, and anterior sides

Functions:

Major Standard Mover Action
1. Supinates the forearm at the RU joints[1–7]

RU joints = radioulnar joints

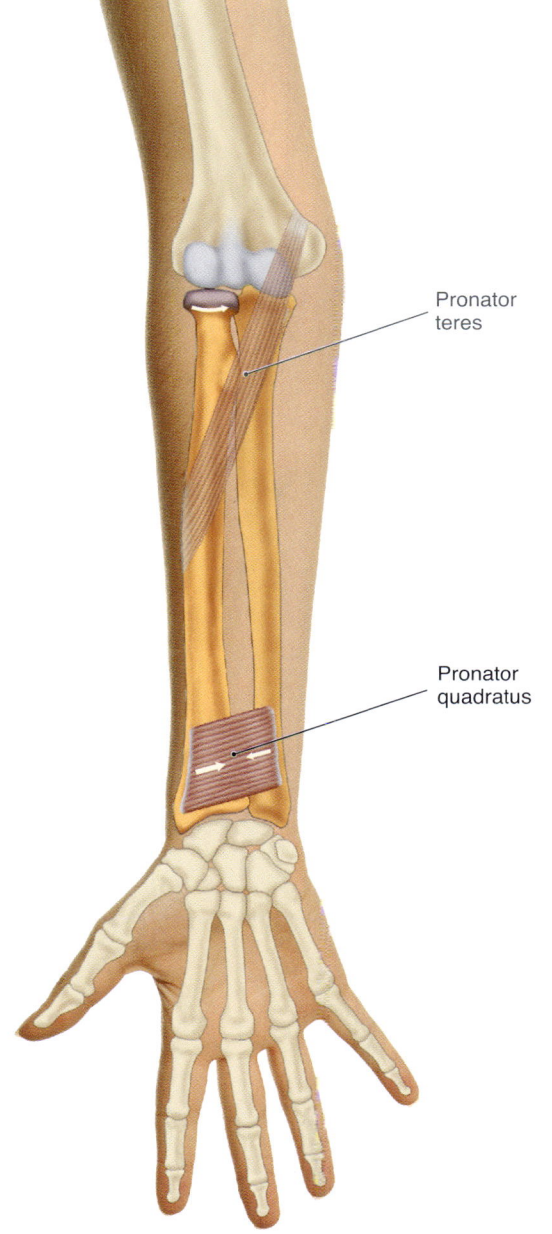

FIGURE 11-24 Anterior view of the right pronator quadratus. The pronator teres has been ghosted in.

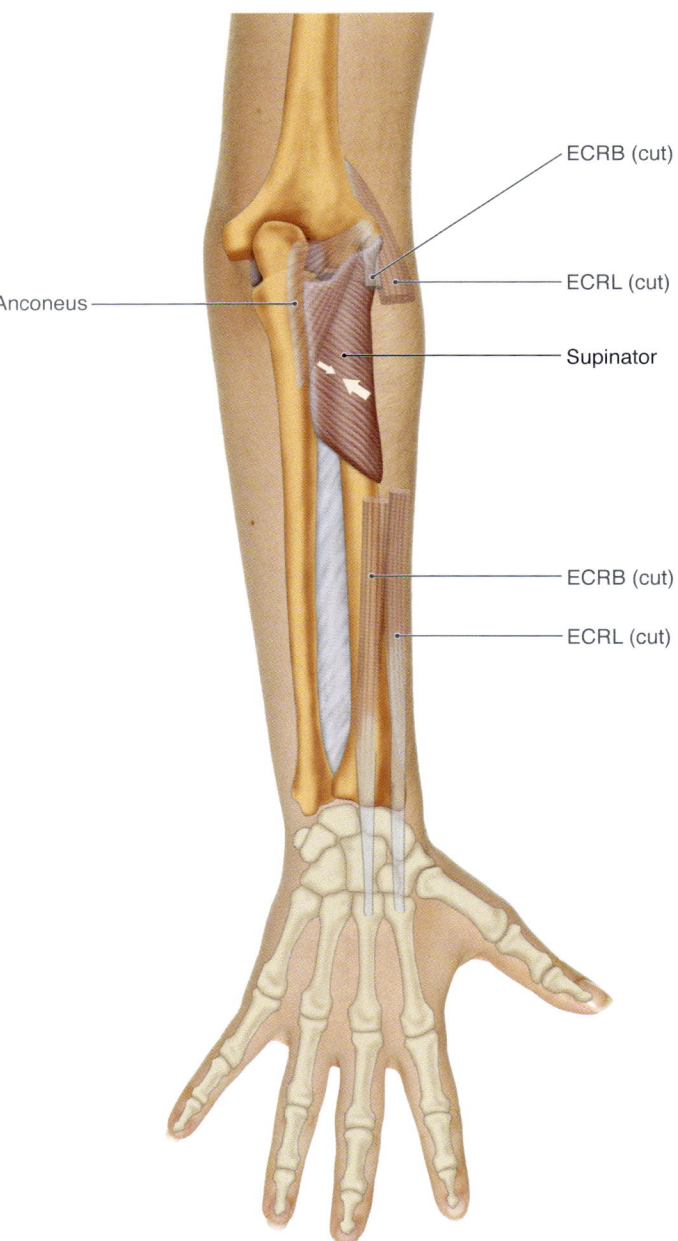

FIGURE 11-25 Posterior view of the right supinator. The anconeus has been ghosted in. The extensor carpi radialis longus (ECRL) and extensor carpi radialis brevis (ECRB) have been cut and ghosted in.

SECTION 11.5 MUSCLES OF THE WRIST JOINT

FLEXOR CARPI RADIALIS (OF WRIST FLEXOR GROUP):

Attachments:

- **Medial Epicondyle of the Humerus via the Common Flexor Belly/Tendon**

to the

- **Anterior Hand on the Radial Side**
  - the anterior side of the bases of the second and third metacarpals

Functions:

Major Standard Mover Actions
1. Flexes the hand at the wrist joint[1-7]
2. Radially deviates the hand at the wrist joint[1-7]

PALMARIS LONGUS (OF WRIST FLEXOR GROUP):

Attachments:

- **Medial Epicondyle of the Humerus via the Common Flexor Belly/Tendon**

to the

- **Palm of the Hand**
  - the palmar aponeurosis and the flexor retinaculum

Functions:

Major Standard Mover Action
1. Flexes the hand at the wrist joint[1-7]

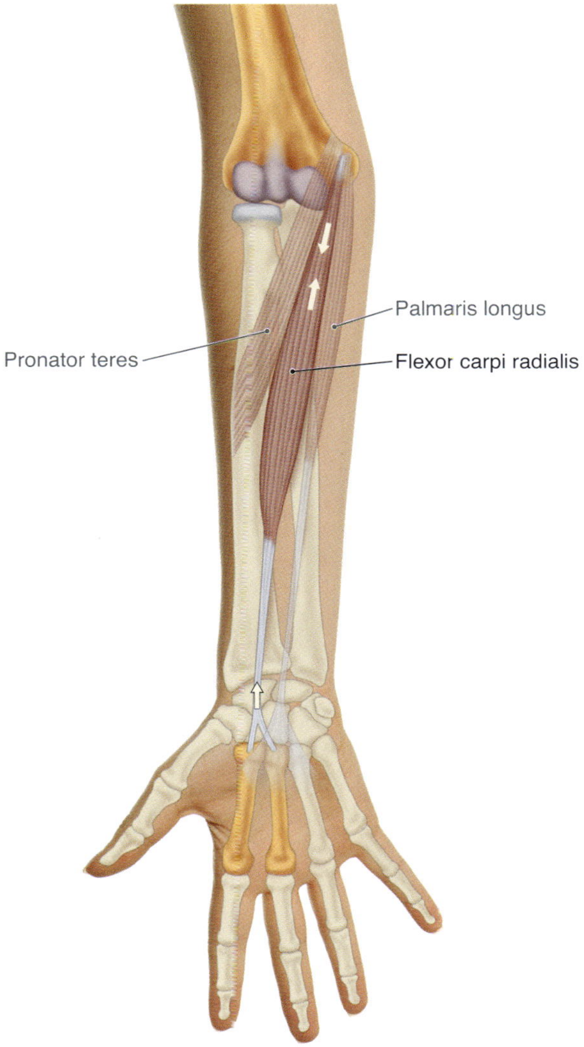

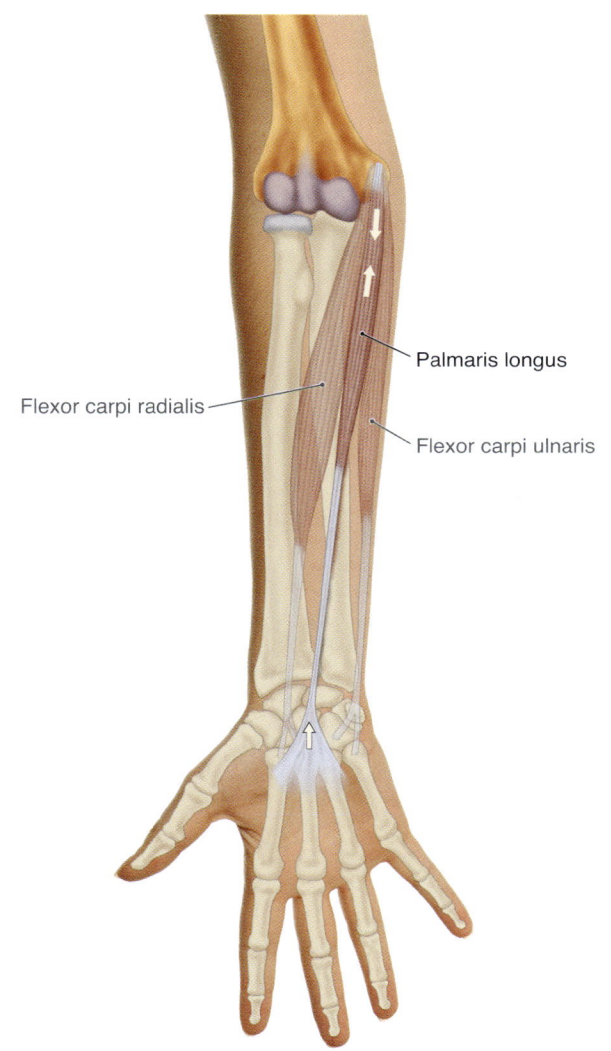

FIGURE 11-26 Anterior view of the right flexor carpi radialis. The pronator teres and palmaris longus have been ghosted in.

FIGURE 11-27 Anterior view of the right palmaris longus. The flexor carpi radialis and flexor carpi ulnaris have been ghosted in.

FLEXOR CARPI ULNARIS (OF WRIST FLEXOR GROUP):

Attachments:
- **Medial Epicondyle of the Humerus via the Common Flexor Belly/Tendon, and the Ulna**
  - the medial margin of the olecranon and the posterior proximal ⅔ of the ulna

to the

- **Anterior Hand on the Ulnar Side**
  - the pisiform, the hook of the hamate, and the base of the fifth metacarpal

Functions:

Major Standard Mover Actions
1. Flexes the hand at the wrist joint[1-7]
2. Ulnar deviates the hand at the wrist joint[1-7]

EXTENSOR CARPI RADIALIS LONGUS (OF WRIST EXTENSOR AND RADIAL GROUPS):

Attachments:
- **Lateral Supracondylar Ridge of the Humerus**
  - the distal ⅓

to the

- **Posterior Hand on the Radial Side**
  - the posterior side of the base of the second metacarpal

Functions:

Major Standard Mover Actions
1. Extends the hand at the wrist joint[1-7]
2. Radially deviates the hand at the wrist joint[1-7]

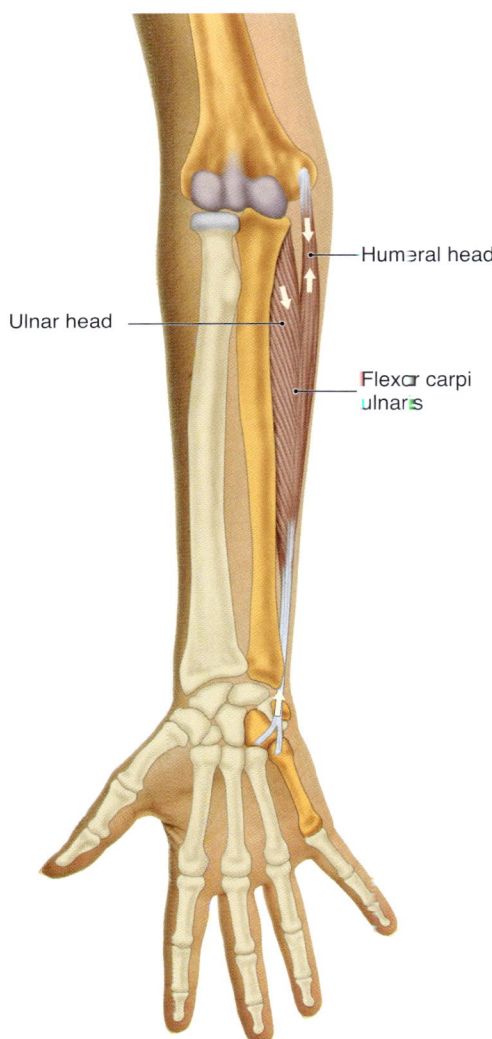

FIGURE 11-28 Anterior view of the right flexor carpi ulnaris.

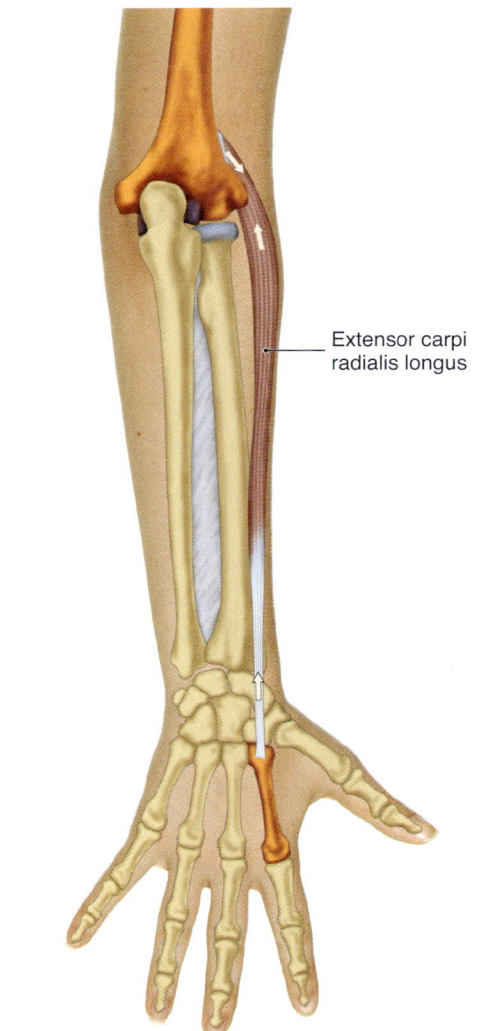

FIGURE 11-29 Posterior view of the right extensor carpi radialis longus.

EXTENSOR CARPI RADIALIS BREVIS (OF WRIST EXTENSOR AND RADIAL GROUPS):

Attachments:

- **Lateral Epicondyle of the Humerus via the Common Extensor Belly/Tendon**

to the

- **Posterior Hand on the Radial Side**
  - the posterior side of the base of the third metacarpal

Functions:

Major Standard Mover Actions
1. Extends the hand at the wrist joint[1-7]
2. Radially deviates the hand at the wrist joint[1-6]

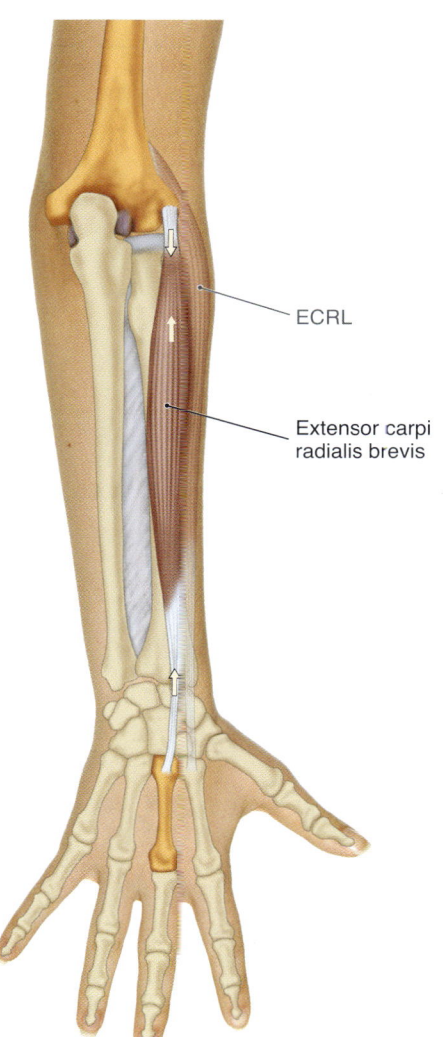

FIGURE 11-30 Posterior view of the right extensor carpi radialis brevis. The extensor carpi radialis longus (ECRL) has been ghosted in.

EXTENSOR CARPI ULNARIS (OF WRIST EXTENSOR GROUP):

Attachments:

- **Lateral Epicondyle of the Humerus via the Common Extensor Belly/Tendon, and the Ulna**
  - the posterior middle ⅓ of the ulna

to the

- **Posterior Hand on the Ulnar Side**
  - the posterior side of the base of the fifth metacarpal

Functions:

Major Standard Mover Actions
1. Extends the hand at the wrist joint[1-7]
2. Ulnar deviates the hand at the wrist joint[1-7]

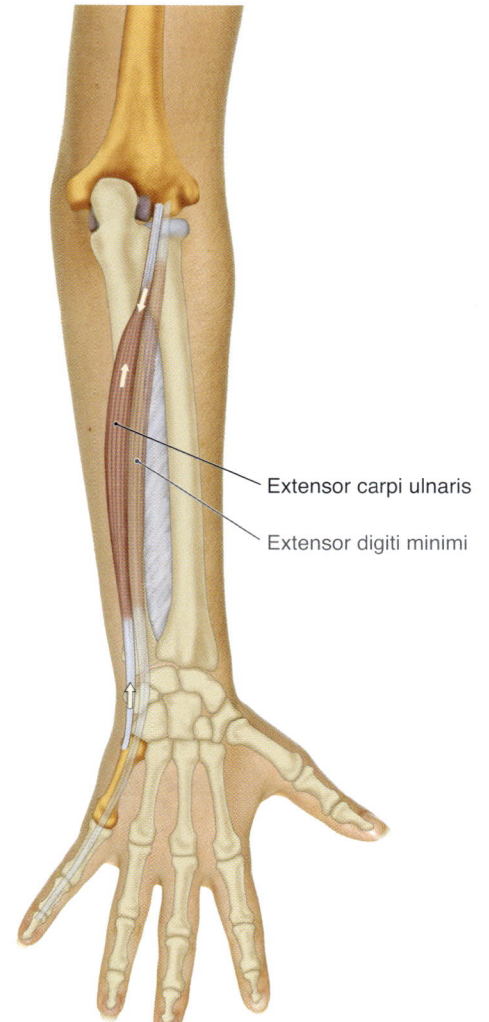

FIGURE 11-31 Posterior view of the right extensor carpi ulnaris. The extensor digiti minimi has been ghosted in.

SECTION 11.6 EXTRINSIC MUSCLES OF THE FINGER JOINTS

FLEXOR DIGITORUM SUPERFICIALIS:

Attachments:

- **Medial Epicondyle of the Humerus via the Common Flexor Belly/Tendon, and the Anterior Ulna and Radius**
  - HUMEROULNAR HEAD: medial epicondyle of the humerus (via the common flexor belly/tendon) and the coronoid process of the ulna
  - RADIAL HEAD: proximal ½ of the anterior shaft of the radius (starting just distal to the radial tuberosity)

to the

- **Anterior Surfaces of Fingers Two through Five**
  - each of the four tendons divides into two slips that attach onto the sides of the anterior surface of the middle phalanx

Functions:

Major Standard Mover Actions
1. Flexes fingers two through five at the MCP and PIP joints[1–7]
2. Flexes the hand at the wrist joint[1–7]

MCP joints = metacarpophalangeal joints; PIP joints = proximal interphalangeal joints

FLEXOR DIGITORUM PROFUNDUS:

Attachments:

- **Medial and Anterior Ulna**
  - the proximal ½ (starting just distal to the ulnar tuberosity) and the interosseus membrane

to the

- **Anterior Surfaces of Fingers Two through Five**
  - the distal phalanges

Functions:

Major Standard Mover Actions
1. Flexes fingers two through five at the MCP, PIP, and DIP joints[1–7]
2. Flexes the hand at the wrist joint[1,2,4–7]

DIP joints = distal interphalangeal joints; MCP joints = metacarpophalangeal joints; PIP joints = proximal interphalangeal joints

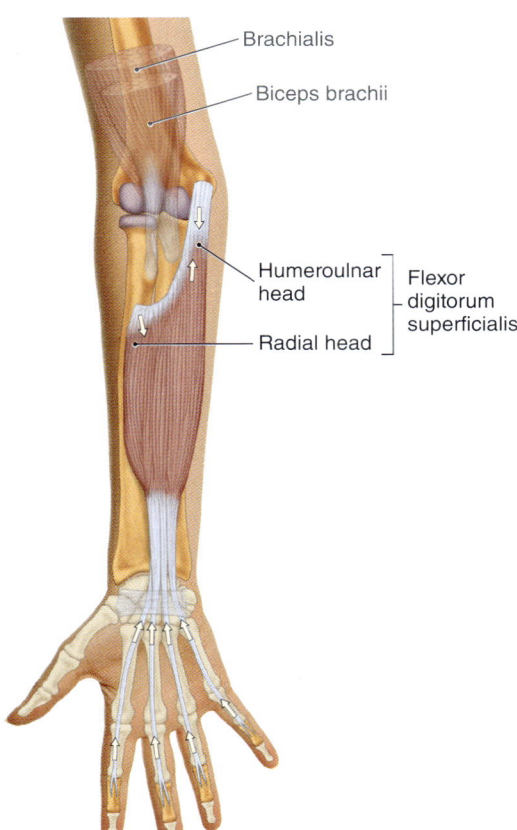

FIGURE 11-32 Anterior view of the right flexor digitorum superficialis. The distal ends of the biceps brachii and brachialis have been ghosted in.

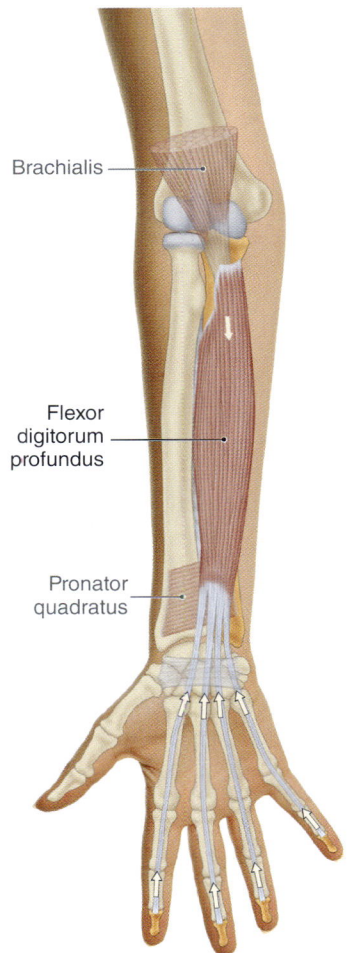

FIGURE 11-33 Anterior view of the right flexor digitorum profundus. The pronator quadratus and distal end of the brachialis have been ghosted in.

FLEXOR POLLICIS LONGUS:

Attachments:

- **Anterior Surface of the Radius**
  - and the interosseus membrane, the medial epicondyle of the humerus, and the coronoid process of the ulna

to the

- **Thumb**
  - the anterior aspect of the base of the distal phalanx

Functions:

Major Standard Mover Actions
1. Flexes the thumb at the CMC, MCP, and IP joints[1–7]
2. Flexes the hand at the wrist joint[2,4–7]

CMC joint = carpometacarpal joint; IP joint = interphalangeal joint; MCP joint = metacarpophalangeal joint

EXTENSOR DIGITORUM:

Attachments:

- **Lateral Epicondyle of the Humerus via the Common Extensor Belly/Tendon**

to the

- **Phalanges of Fingers Two through Five**
  - via its dorsal digital expansion onto the posterior surfaces of the middle and distal phalanges

Functions:

Major Standard Mover Actions
1. Extends fingers two through five at the MCP, PIP, and DIP joints[1–7]
2. Extends the hand at the wrist joint[1–7]

DIP joints = distal interphalangeal joints; MCP joints = metacarpophalangeal joints; PIP joints = proximal interphalangeal joints

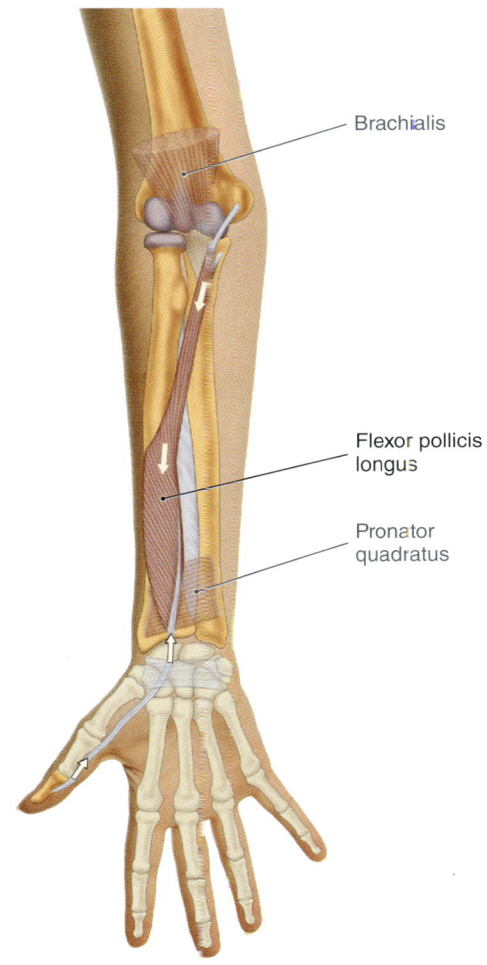

FIGURE 11-34 Anterior view of the right flexor pollicis longus. The pronator quadratus and distal end of the brachialis have been ghosted in.

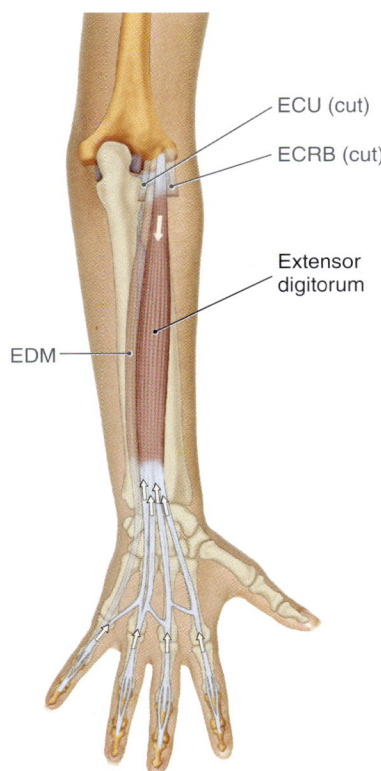

FIGURE 11-35 Posterior view of the right extensor digitorum. The extensor digiti minimi (EDM) and the cut extensor carpi ulnaris (ECU) and cut extensor carpi radialis brevis (ECRB) have been ghosted in.

EXTENSOR DIGITI MINIMI:

Attachments:
- **Lateral Epicondyle of the Humerus via the Common Extensor Belly/Tendon**

to the

- **Phalanges of the Little Finger (Finger Five)**
  - attaches into the ulnar side of the tendon of the extensor digitorum muscle (to attach onto the posterior surface of the middle and distal phalanges of the little finger via the dorsal digital expansion)

Functions:

Major Standard Mover Actions
1. Extends the little finger (finger five) at the MCP, PIP, and DIP joints[1,2,4,6,7]
2. Extends the hand at the wrist joint[1,2,4,7]

DIP joint = distal interphalangeal joint; MCP joint = metacarpophalangeal joint; PIP joint = proximal interphalangeal joint

ABDUCTOR POLLICIS LONGUS (OF DEEP DISTAL FOUR GROUP):

Attachments:
- **Posterior Radius and Ulna**
  - approximately the middle ⅓ of the radius, ulna, and interosseus membrane

to the

- **Thumb**
  - the lateral side of the base of the first metacarpal

Functions:

Major Standard Mover Actions
1. Abducts the thumb at the CMC joint[1–4,6,7]
2. Extends the thumb at the CMC joint[1–4,6]

CMC joint = carpometacarpal joint (of the thumb; saddle joint of the thumb)

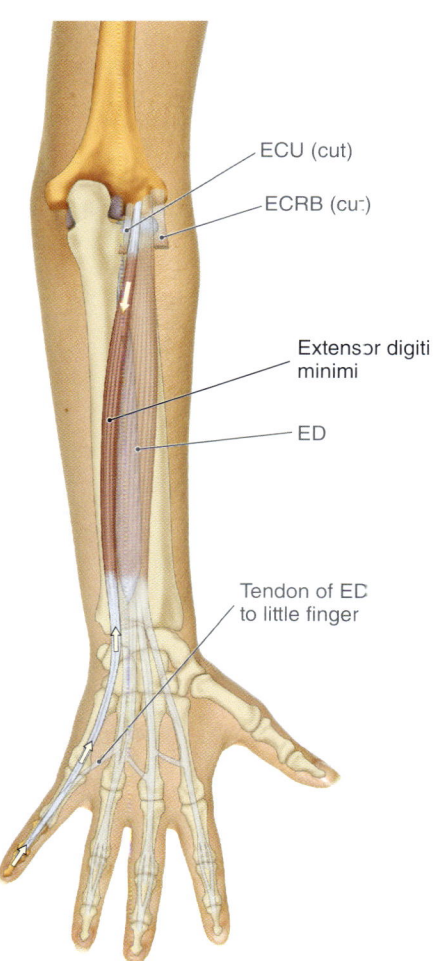

FIGURE 11-36 Posterior view of the right extensor digiti minimi. The extensor digitorum (ED) and the cut extensor carpi ulnaris (ECU) and cut extensor carpi radialis brevis (ECRB) have been ghosted in.

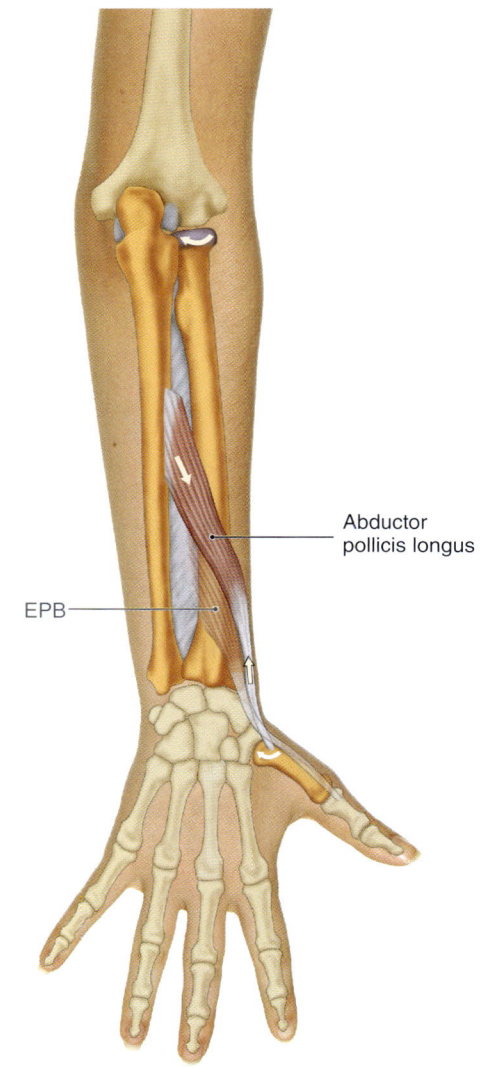

FIGURE 11-37 Posterior view of the right abductor pollicis longus. The extensor pollicis brevis (EPB) has been ghosted in.

EXTENSOR POLLICIS BREVIS (OF DEEP DISTAL FOUR GROUP):

Attachments:
- **Posterior Radius**
  - the distal ⅓ and the adjacent interosseus membrane

to the

- **Thumb**
  - the posterolateral base of the proximal phalanx

Functions:

Major Standard Mover Actions
1. Extends the thumb at the CMC and MCP joints[1–4,6,7]
2. Abducts the thumb at the CMC joint[3,4,6,7]

CMC joint = carpometacarpal joint (of the thumb; saddle joint of the thumb); MCP joint = metacarpophalangeal joint

EXTENSOR POLLICIS LONGUS (OF DEEP DISTAL FOUR GROUP):

Attachments:
- **Posterior Ulna**
  - the middle ⅓ and the adjacent interosseus membrane

to the

- **Thumb**
  - via its dorsal digital expansion onto the posterior surface of the distal phalanx of the thumb

Functions:

Major Standard Mover Action
1. Extends the thumb at the CMC, MCP, and IP joints[1–4,6,7]

CMC joint = carpometacarpal joint (of the thumb; saddle joint of the thumb); IP joint = interphalangeal joint; MCP joint = metacarpophalangeal joint

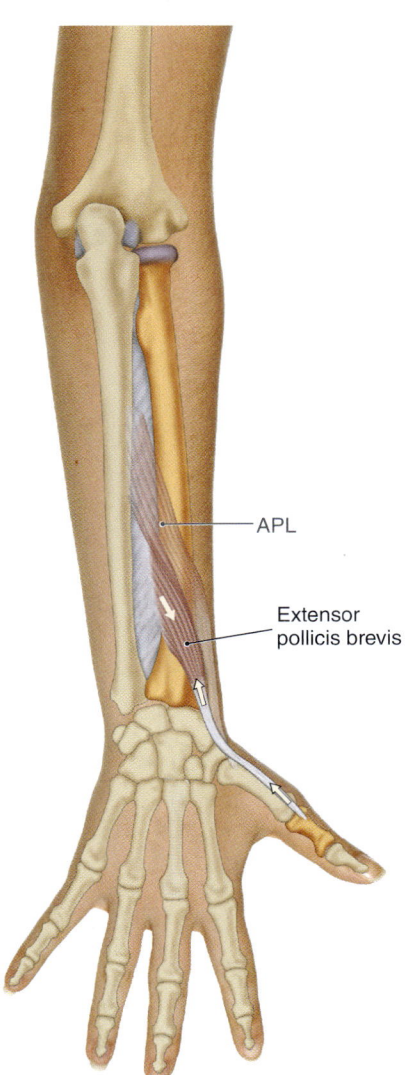

FIGURE 11-38 Posterior view of the right extensor pollicis brevis. The abductor pollicis longus (APL) has been ghosted in.

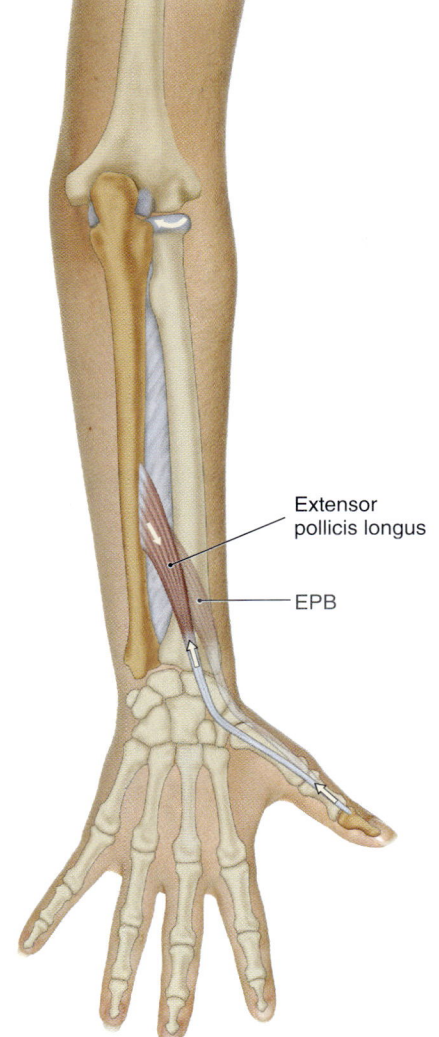

FIGURE 11-39 Posterior view of the extensor pollicis longus. The extensor pollicis brevis (EPB) has been ghosted in.

EXTENSOR INDICIS (OF DEEP DISTAL FOUR GROUP):

Attachments:
- **Posterior Ulna**
  - the distal ⅓ and the interosseus membrane

to the

- **Index Finger (Finger Two)**
  - attaches into the ulnar side of the tendon of the extensor digitorum muscle (to attach onto the posterior surface of the middle and distal phalanges of the index finger via the dorsal digital expansion)

Functions:

Major Standard Mover Actions

1. Extends the index finger at the MCP, PIP, and DIP joints[1,2,4–7]
2. Extends the hand at the wrist joint[1,2,4,7]

DIP joint = distal interphalangeal joint; MCP joint = metacarpophalangeal joint; PIP joint = proximal interphalangeal joint

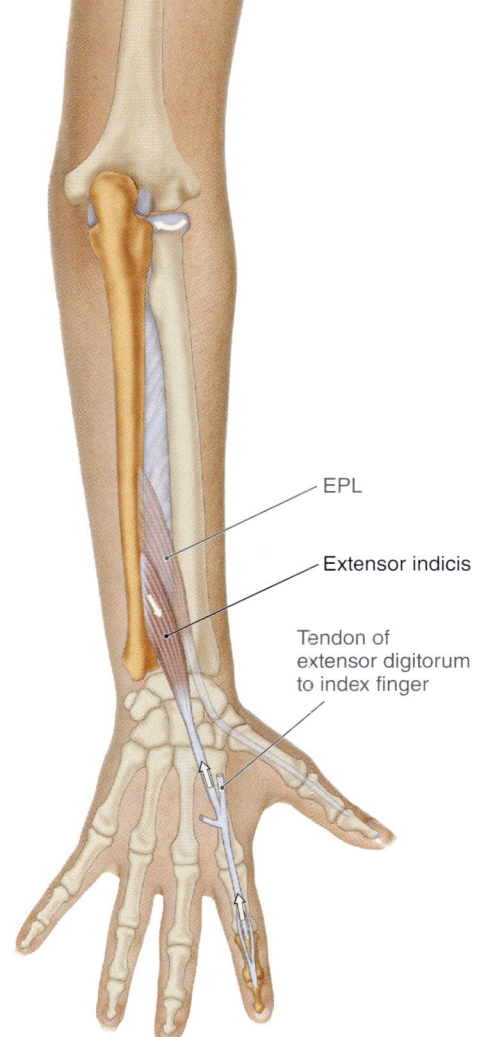

FIGURE 11-40 Posterior view of the extensor indicis. The extensor pollicis longus (EPL) has been ghosted in.

SECTION 11.7 INTRINSIC MUSCLES OF THE FINGER JOINTS

ABDUCTOR POLLICIS BREVIS (OF THENAR EMINENCE GROUP):

Attachments:

- **The Flexor Retinaculum and the Scaphoid and the Trapezium**
  - the tubercle of the scaphoid and the tubercle of the trapezium

to the

- **Proximal Phalanx of the Thumb**
  - the radial (lateral) side of the base of the proximal phalanx and the dorsal digital expansion

Functions:

Major Standard Mover Action

1. Abducts the thumb at the CMC joint[1–4,6]

CMC joint = carpometacarpal joint (of the thumb; saddle joint of the thumb)

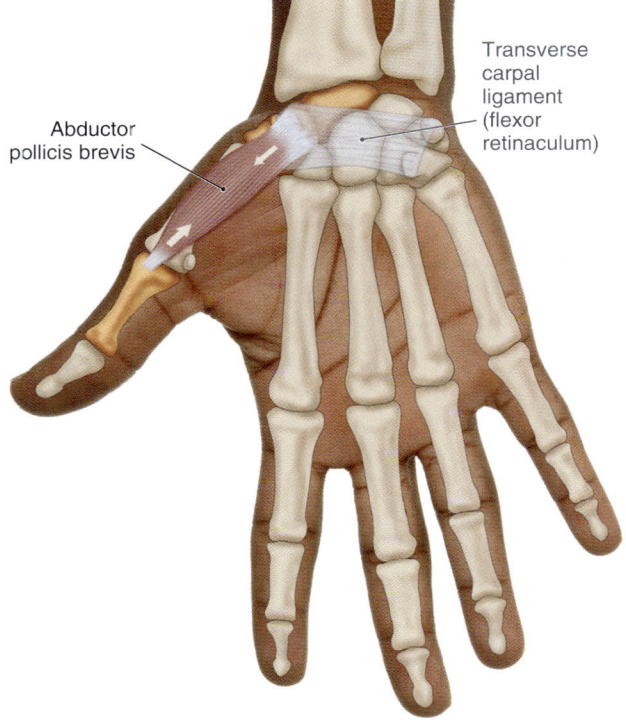

FIGURE 11-41 Anterior view of the right abductor pollicis brevis.

FLEXOR POLLICIS BREVIS (OF THENAR EMINENCE GROUP):

Attachments:

- **The Flexor Retinaculum and the Trapezium**

to the

- **Proximal Phalanx of the Thumb**
  - the radial (lateral) side of the base of the proximal phalanx

Functions:

Major Standard Mover Action

1. Flexes the thumb at the CMC and MCP joints[1–4,6]

CMC joint = carpometacarpal joint (of the thumb; saddle joint of the thumb); MCP joint = metacarpophalangeal joint

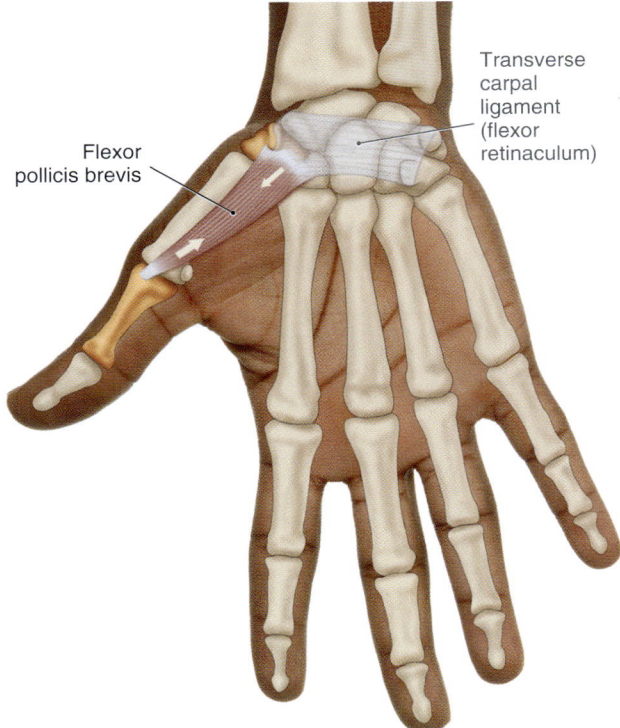

FIGURE 11-42 Anterior view of the right flexor pollicis brevis.

OPPONENS POLLICIS (OF THENAR EMINENCE GROUP):

Attachments:

- **The Flexor Retinaculum and the Trapezium**
  - the tubercle of the trapezium

to the

- **First Metacarpal (of the Thumb)**
  - the anterior surface and radial (lateral) border

Functions:

Major Standard Mover Action
1. Opposes the thumb at the CMC joint[2-6]

CMC joint = carpometacarpal joint (of the thumb; saddle joint of the thumb)

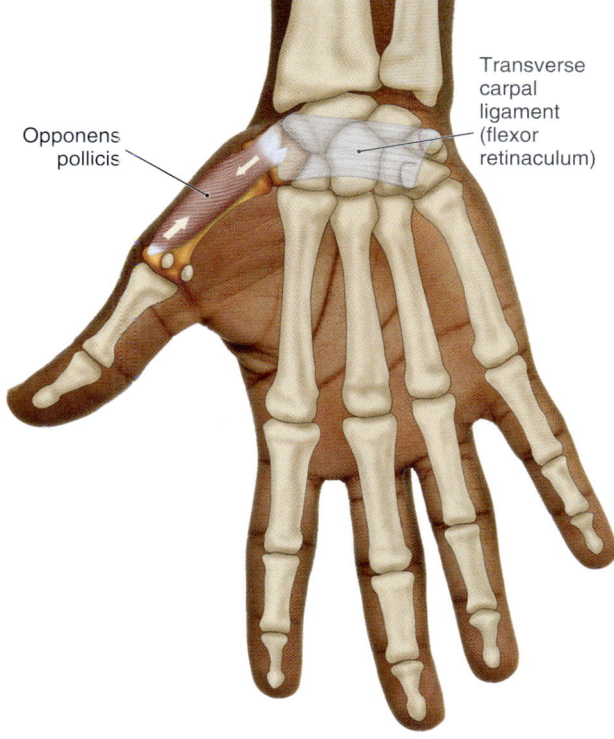

FIGURE 11-43 Anterior view of the right opponens pollicis.

ABDUCTOR DIGITI MINIMI MANUS (OF HYPOTHENAR EMINENCE GROUP):

Attachments:

- **The Pisiform**
  - and the tendon of the flexor carpi ulnaris

to the

- **Proximal Phalanx of the Little Finger (Finger Five)**
  - the ulnar (medial) side of the base of the proximal phalanx and the dorsal digital expansion

Functions:

Major Standard Mover Action
1. Abducts the little finger at the MCP joint[1-4,6,7]

MCP joint = metacarpophalangeal joint

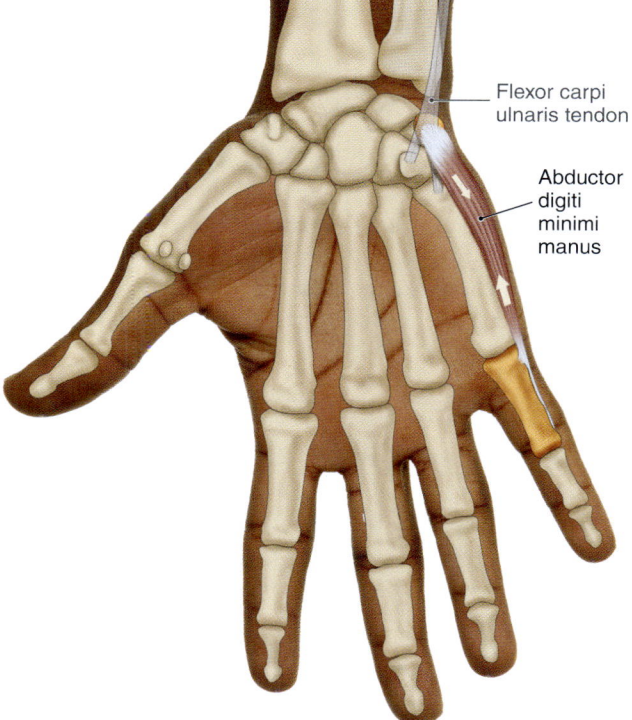

FIGURE 11-44 Anterior view of the right abductor digiti minimi manus. The flexor carpi ulnaris tendon has been ghosted in.

FLEXOR DIGITI MINIMI MANUS (OF HYPOTHENAR EMINENCE GROUP):

Attachments:
- **The Flexor Retinaculum and the Hamate**
  - the hook of the hamate
- to the
- **Proximal Phalanx of the Little Finger (Finger Five)**
  - the ulnar (medial) side of the base of the proximal phalanx

Functions:

Major Standard Mover Action
1. Flexes the little finger at the MCP joint[1-4,6]

MCP joint = metacarpophalangeal joint

OPPONENS DIGITI MINIMI (OF HYPOTHENAR EMINENCE GROUP):

Attachments:
- **The Flexor Retinaculum and the Hamate**
  - the hook of the hamate
- to the
- **Fifth Metacarpal (of the Little Finger)**
  - the anterior surface and the medial (ulnar) border of the fifth metacarpal

Functions:

Major Standard Mover Action
1. Opposes the little finger at the CMC joint[1-4,6]

CMC joint = carpometacarpal joint

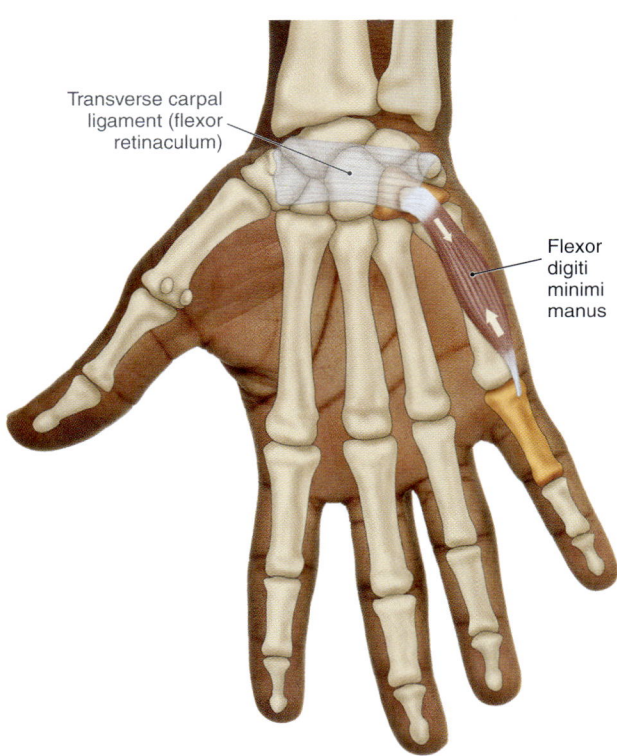

FIGURE 11-45 Anterior view of the right flexor digiti minimi manus.

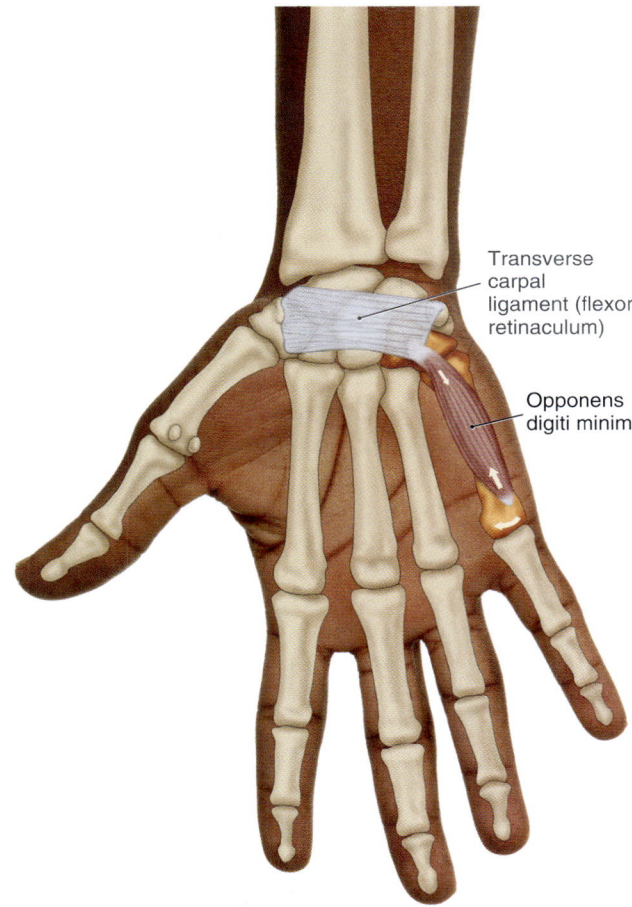

FIGURE 11-46 Anterior view of the right opponens digiti minimi.

ADDUCTOR POLLICIS (OF CENTRAL COMPARTMENT GROUP):

Attachments:

- **Third Metacarpal**
  - OBLIQUE HEAD: the anterior bases of the second and third metacarpals and the capitate
  - TRANSVERSE HEAD: the distal ⅔ of the anterior surface of the third metacarpal

to the

- **Proximal Phalanx of the Thumb**
  - OBLIQUE HEAD: the medial side of the base of the proximal phalanx and the dorsal digital expansion
  - TRANSVERSE HEAD: the medial side of the base of the proximal phalanx

Functions:

Major Standard Mover Action
1. Adducts the thumb at the CMC joint[1-6]

CMC joint = carpometacarpal joint (of the thumb; saddle joint of the thumb)

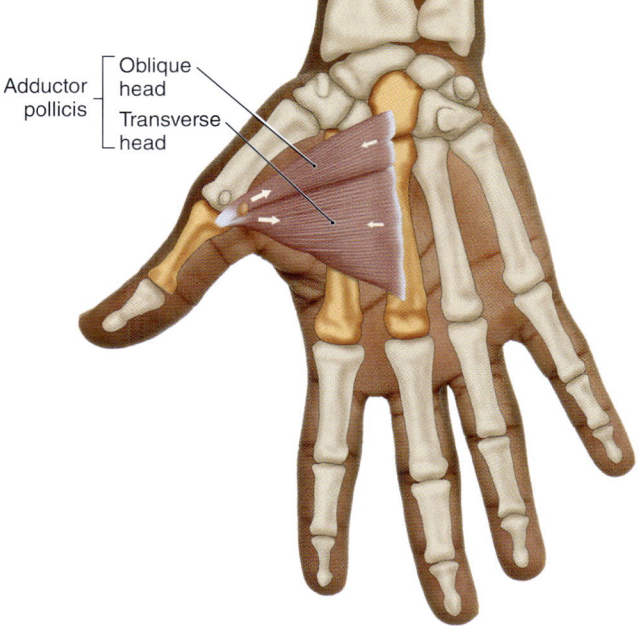

FIGURE 11-47 Anterior view of the right adductor pollicis.

LUMBRICALS MANUS (OF CENTRAL COMPARTMENT GROUP):

Attachments:

- **The Distal Tendons of the Flexor Digitorum Profundus**
  - **One**: the radial (lateral) side of the tendon of the index finger (finger two)
  - **Two**: the radial side of the tendon of the middle finger (finger three)
  - **Three**: the ulnar (medial) side of the tendon of the middle finger (finger three) and the radial side of the tendon of the ring finger (finger four)
  - **Four**: the ulnar side of the tendon of the ring finger (finger four) and the radial side of the tendon of the little finger (finger five)

to the

- **Distal Tendons of the Extensor Digitorum (the Dorsal Digital Expansion)**
  - the radial side of the tendons merging into the dorsal digital expansion
    - **One**: into the tendon of the index finger (finger two)
    - **Two**: into the tendon of the middle finger (finger three)
    - **Three**: into the tendon of the ring finger (finger four)
    - **Four**: into the tendon of the little finger (finger five)

Functions:

Major Standard Mover Actions
1. Extend fingers two through five at the PIP and DIP joints[1-7]
2. Flex fingers two through five at the MCP joints[1-7]

DIP joints = distal interphalangeal joints; MCP joints = metacarpophalangeal joints; PIP joints = proximal interphalangeal joints

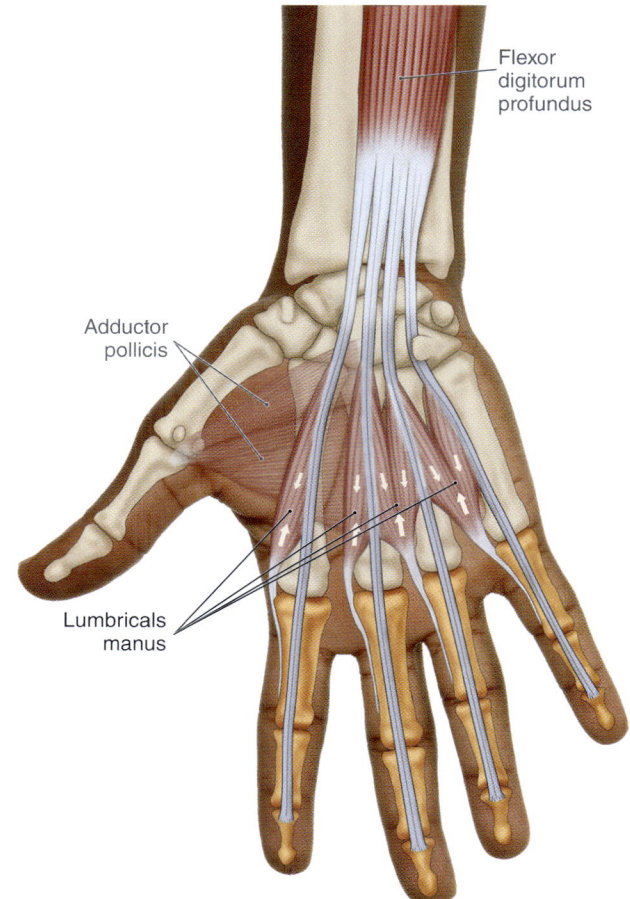

FIGURE 11-48 Anterior view of the right lumbricals manus. The adductor pollicis has been ghosted in.

PALMAR INTEROSSEI (OF CENTRAL COMPARTMENT GROUP):

Attachments:

- The Metacarpals of Fingers Two, Four, and Five
  - The anterior side and on the "middle finger side" of the metacarpals:
    - **One**: attaches to the metacarpal of the index finger (finger two)
    - **Two**: attaches to the metacarpal of the ring finger (finger four)
    - **Three**: attaches to the metacarpal of the little finger (finger five)

to the

- Proximal Phalanges of Fingers Two, Four, and Five on the "Middle Finger Side"
  - The base of the proximal phalanx and the dorsal digital expansion:
    - **One**: attaches to the index finger (finger two)
    - **Two**: attaches to the ring finger (finger four)
    - **Three**: attaches to the little finger (finger five)

Functions:

Major Standard Mover Action
1. Adduct fingers two, four, and five at the MCP joints[1-7]

MCP joints = metacarpophalangeal joints

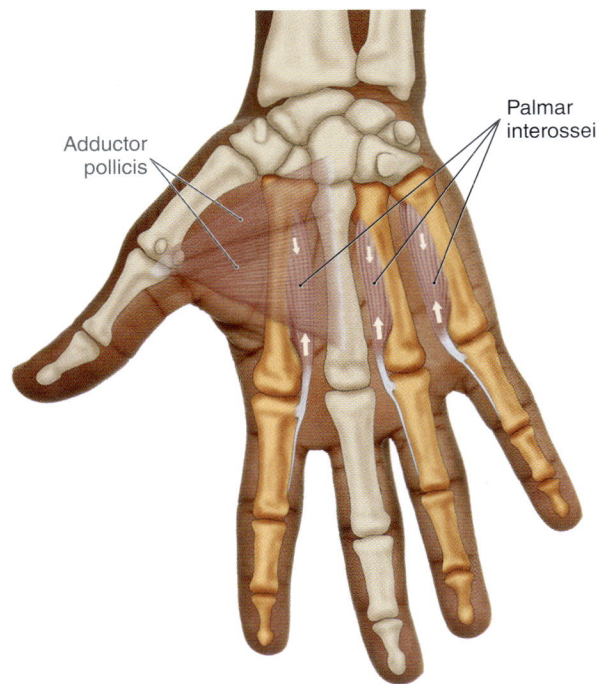

FIGURE 11-49 Anterior view of the right palmar interossei. The adductor pollicis has been ghosted in.

DORSAL INTEROSSEI MANUS (OF CENTRAL COMPARTMENT GROUP):

Attachments:

- The Metacarpals of Fingers One through Five
  - Each one arises from the adjacent sides of two metacarpals:
    - **One**: attaches onto the metacarpals of the thumb and index finger (fingers one and two)
    - **Two**: attaches onto the metacarpals of the index and middle fingers (fingers two and three)
    - **Three**: attaches onto the metacarpals of the middle and ring fingers (fingers three and four)
    - **Four**: attaches onto the metacarpals of the ring and little fingers (fingers four and five)

to the

- Proximal Phalanges of Fingers Two, Three, and Four on the Side That Faces Away from the Center of the Middle Finger
  - The base of the proximal phalanx and the dorsal digital expansion:
    - **One**: attaches to the lateral side of the index finger (finger two)
    - **Two**: attaches to the lateral side of the middle finger (finger three)
    - **Three**: attaches to the medial side of the middle finger (finger three)
    - **Four**: attaches to the medial side of the ring finger (finger four)

Functions:

Major Standard Mover Action
1. Abduct fingers two through four at the MCP joints[1-7]

MCP joints = metacarpophalangeal joints

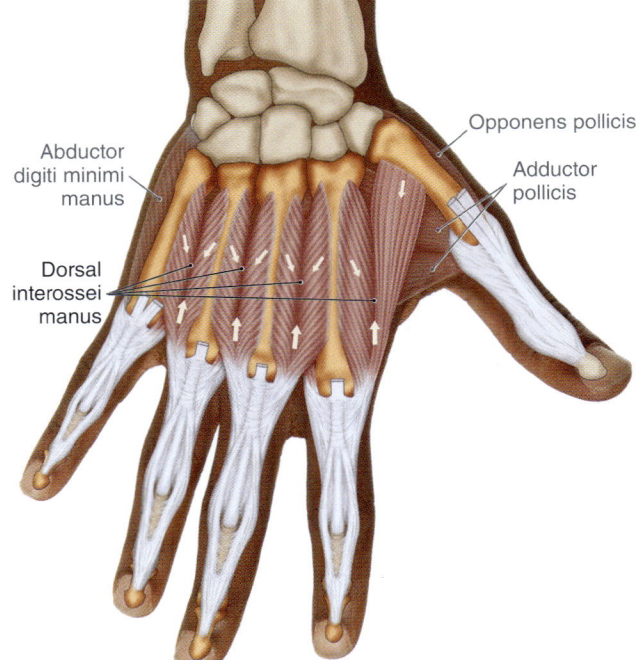

FIGURE 11-50 Posterior view of the right dorsal interossei manus. The adductor pollicis, opponens pollicis, and abductor digiti minimi manus have been ghosted in.

PALMARIS BREVIS:

Attachments:
- The Flexor Retinaculum and the Palmar Aponeurosis

to the
- Dermis of the Ulnar (Medial) Border of the Hand

Functions:

Major Standard Mover Action
1. Wrinkles the skin of the palm[1,2,6]

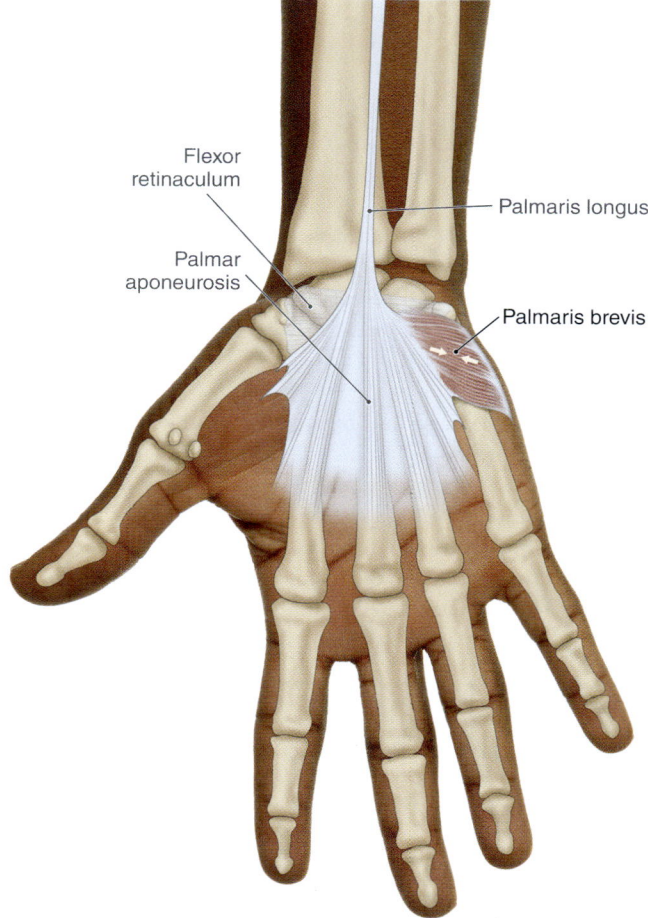

FIGURE 11-51 Anterior view of the right palmaris brevis.

SECTION 11.8 MUSCLES OF THE SPINAL JOINTS

Full Spine:
ERECTOR SPINAE GROUP:

Attachments:
- Pelvis

to the
- Spine, Rib Cage, and Head

Functions:

Major Standard Mover Actions	Major Reverse Mover Action
1. Extends the trunk, neck, and head at the spinal joints[1–5,7]	1. Anteriorly tilts the pelvis at the LS joint and extends the lower spine relative to the upper spine[2–5,7]
2. Laterally flexes the trunk, neck, and head at the spinal joints[1–5,7]	

LS joint = lumbosacral joint

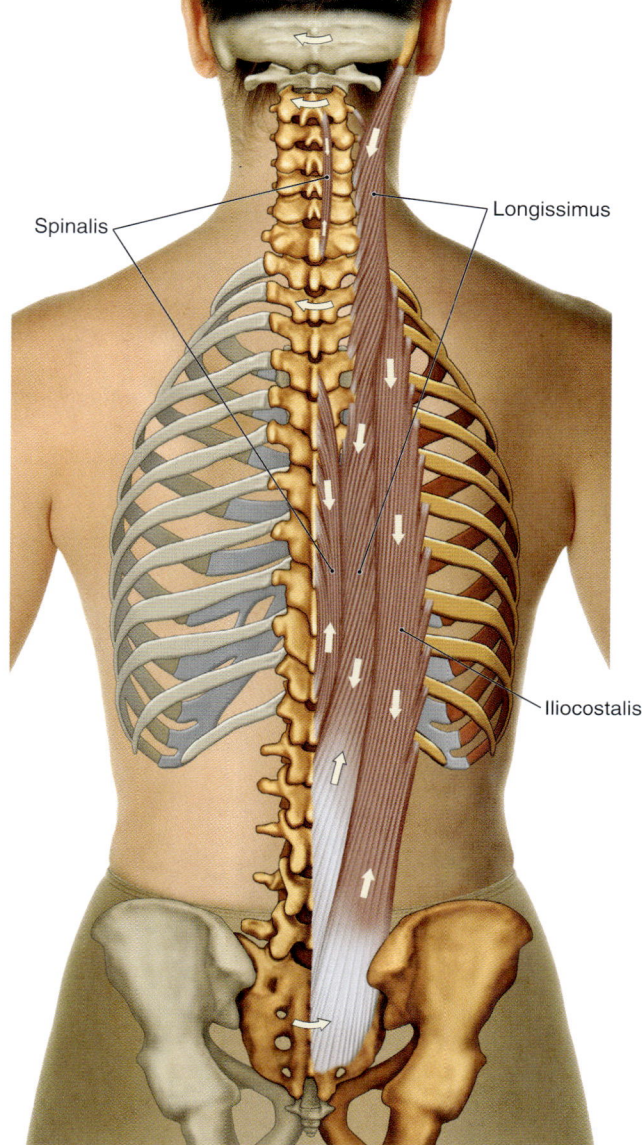

FIGURE 11-52 Posterior view of the right erector spinae group.

ILIOCOSTALIS (OF ERECTOR SPINAE GROUP):

Attachments:

- **ENTIRE ILIOCOSTALIS: Sacrum, Iliac Crest, and Ribs Three through Twelve**
  - ILIOCOSTALIS LUMBORUM: Medial iliac crest and the medial and lateral sacral crests
  - ILIOCOSTALIS THORACIS: Angles of ribs seven through twelve
  - ILIOCOSTALIS CERVICIS: Angles of ribs three through six

to the

- **ENTIRE ILIOCOSTALIS: Ribs One through Twelve and Transverse Processes of C4-C7**
  - ILIOCOSTALIS LUMBORUM: Angles of ribs seven through twelve
  - ILIOCOSTALIS THORACIS: Angles of ribs one through six and the transverse process of C7
  - ILIOCOSTALIS CERVICIS: Transverse processes of C4-C6

Functions:

Major Standard Mover Actions	Major Reverse Mover Action
1. Extends the trunk and neck at the spinal joints[2-6]	1. Anteriorly tilts the pelvis at the LS joint and extends the lower spine relative to the upper spine[2-6]
2. Laterally flexes the trunk and neck at the spinal joints[2-6]	

LS joint = lumbosacral joint

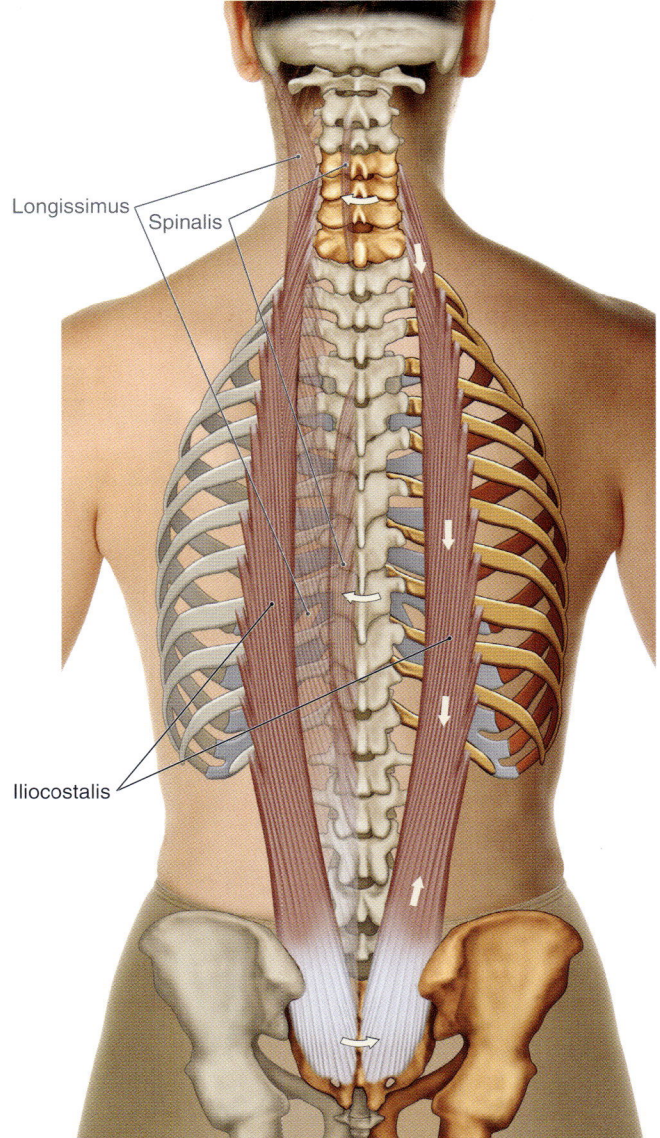

FIGURE 11-53 Posterior view of the iliocostalis bilaterally. The other two erector spinae muscles have been ghosted in on the left side.

LONGISSIMUS (OF ERECTOR SPINAE GROUP):

Attachments:

- **ENTIRE LONGISSIMUS: Sacrum, Iliac Crest, Transverse Processes of L1-L5 and T1-T5, and the Articular Processes of C5-C7**
  - LONGISSIMUS THORACIS: Medial iliac crest, posterior sacrum, and the transverse processes of L1-L5
  - LONGISSIMUS CERVICIS: Transverse processes of the upper five thoracic vertebrae
  - LONGISSIMUS CAPITIS: Transverse processes of the upper five thoracic vertebrae and the articular processes of the lower three cervical vertebrae

to the

- **ENTIRE LONGISSIMUS: Ribs Four through Twelve, Transverse Processes of T1-T12 and C2-C6, and the Mastoid Process of the Temporal Bone**
  - LONGISSIMUS THORACIS: Transverse processes of all the thoracic vertebrae and the lower nine ribs (between the tubercles and the angles)
  - LONGISSIMUS CERVICIS: Transverse processes of C2-C6 (posterior tubercles)
  - LONGISSIMUS CAPITIS: Mastoid process of the temporal bone

Functions:

Major Standard Mover Actions	Major Reverse Mover Action
1. Extends the trunk, neck, and head at the spinal joints[2-6]	1. Anteriorly tilts the pelvis at the LS joint and extends the lower spine relative to the upper spine[2-6]
2. Laterally flexes the trunk, neck, and head at the spinal joints[2-7]	

LS joint = lumbosacral joint

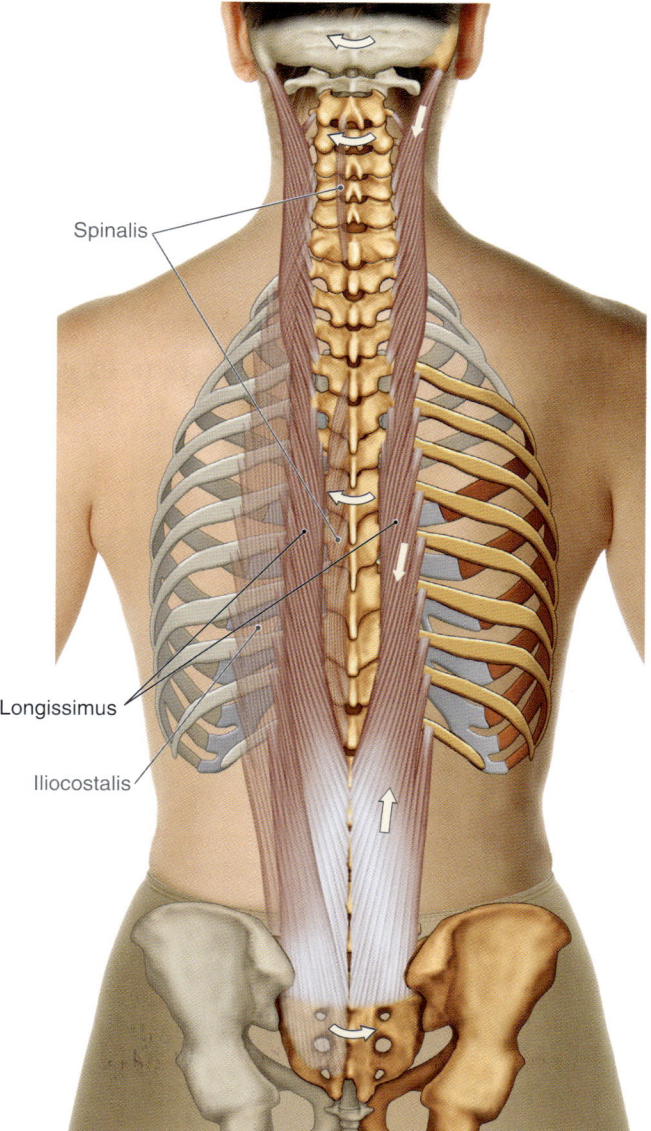

FIGURE 11-54 Posterior view of the longissimus bilaterally. The other two erector spinae muscles have been ghosted in on the left side.

SPINALIS (OF ERECTOR SPINAE GROUP):

Attachments:

- **ENTIRE SPINALIS: Spinous Processes of T11-L2; and the Spinous Process of C7 and the Nuchal Ligament**
  - SPINALIS THORACIS: Spinous processes of T11-L2
  - SPINALIS CERVICIS: Inferior nuchal ligament and the spinous process of C7
  - SPINALIS CAPITIS: Usually considered to be the medial part of the semispinalis capitis

to the

- **ENTIRE SPINALIS: Spinous Processes of T4-T8; and the Spinous Process of C2**
  - SPINALIS THORACIS: Spinous processes of T4-T8
  - SPINALIS CERVICIS: Spinous process of C2
  - SPINALIS CAPITIS: Usually considered to be the medial part of the semispinalis capitis

Functions:

Major Standard Mover Actions
1. Extends the trunk and neck at the spinal joints[2-6]
2. Laterally flexes the trunk and neck at the spinal joints[2-5]

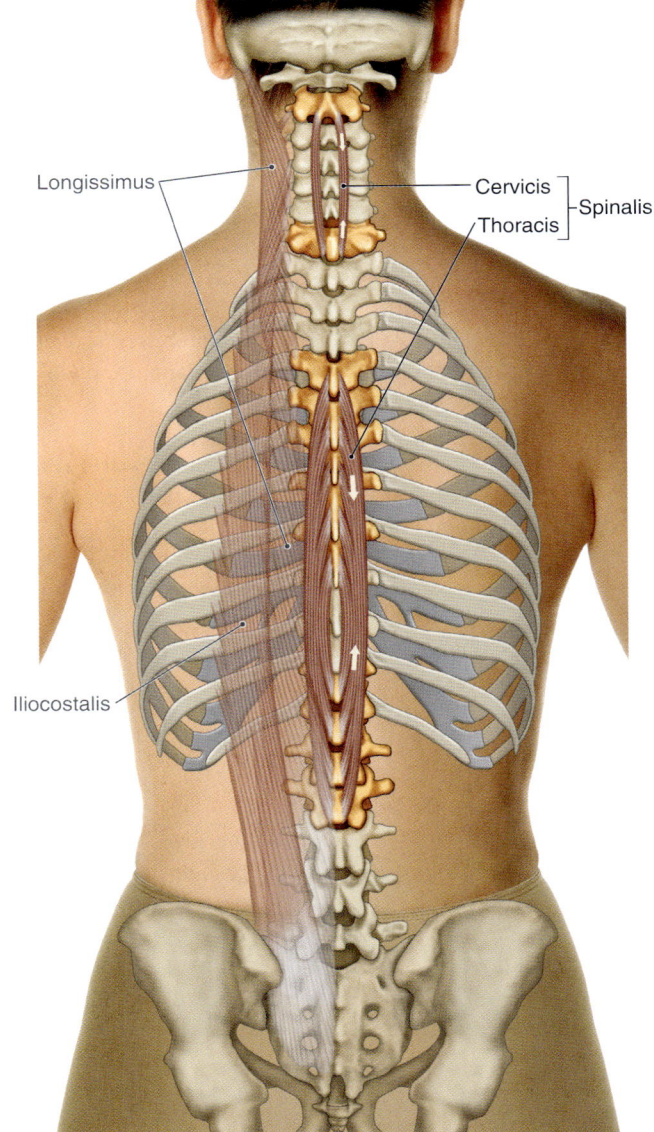

FIGURE 11-55 Posterior view of the spinalis bilaterally. The other two erector spinae muscles have been ghosted in on the left side.

TRANSVERSOSPINALIS GROUP:

Attachments:

- **Pelvis**

to the

- **Spine and the Head**
  - Generally running from transverse process below to spinous process above

Functions:

Major Standard Mover Actions	Major Reverse Mover Action
1. Extends the trunk, neck, and head at the spinal joints[1–4,7]	1. Anteriorly tilts the pelvis at the LS joint and extends the lower spine relative to the upper spine[2–4]
2. Laterally flexes the trunk, neck, and head at the spinal joints[2–4]	
3. Contralaterally rotates the trunk and neck at the spinal joints[2–4]	

LS joint = lumbosacral joint

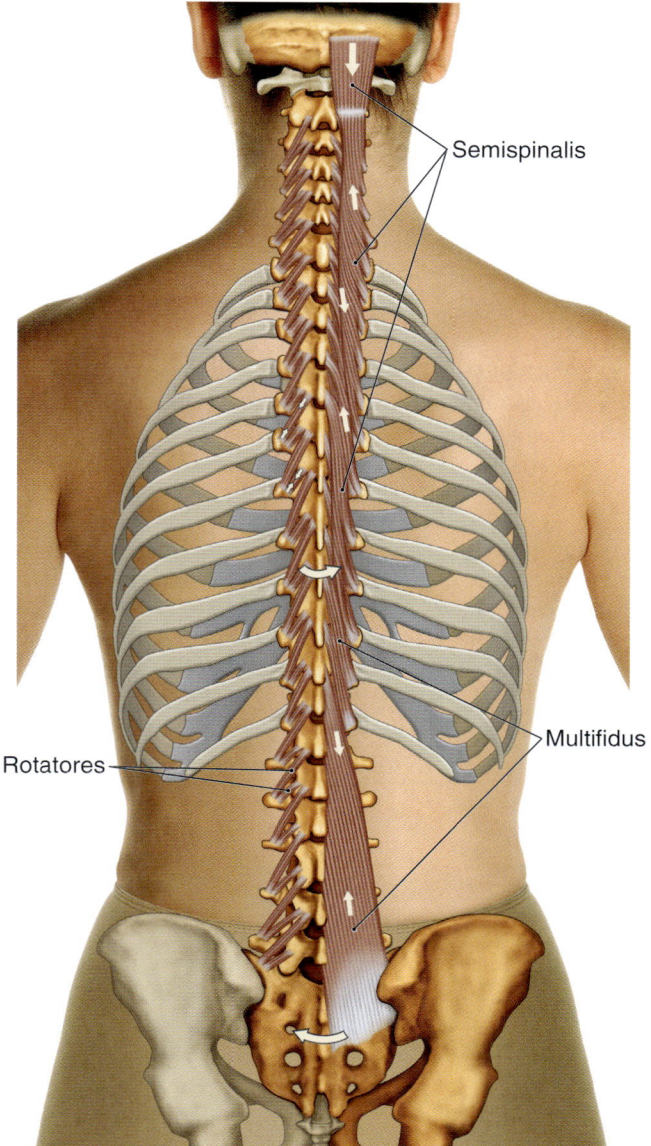

FIGURE 11-56 Posterior view of the transversospinalis group. The semispinalis and multifidus are seen on the right; the rotatores are seen on the left.

SEMISPINALIS (OF TRANSVERSOSPINALIS GROUP):

Attachments:

- **ENTIRE SEMISPINALIS:** Transverse Processes of C7-T10 and the Articular Processes of C4-C6
  - SEMISPINALIS THORACIS: Transverse processes of T6-T10
  - SEMISPINALIS CERVICIS: Transverse processes of T1-T5
  - SEMISPINALIS CAPITIS: Transverse processes of C7-T6 and articular processes of C4-C6

to the

- **ENTIRE SEMISPINALIS:** Spinous Processes of C2-T4 and the Occipital Bone (Five-Six Segmental Levels Superior to the Inferior Attachment)
  - SEMISPINALIS THORACIS: Spinous processes of C6-T4
  - SEMISPINALIS CERVICIS: Spinous processes of C2-C5
  - SEMISPINALIS CAPITIS: Occipital bone between the superior and inferior nuchal lines

Functions:

Major Standard Mover Actions
1. Extends the trunk, neck, and head at the spinal joints[1-7]
2. Laterally flexes the trunk, neck, and head at the spinal joints[2-4]
3. Contralaterally rotates the trunk and neck at the spinal joints[2-6]

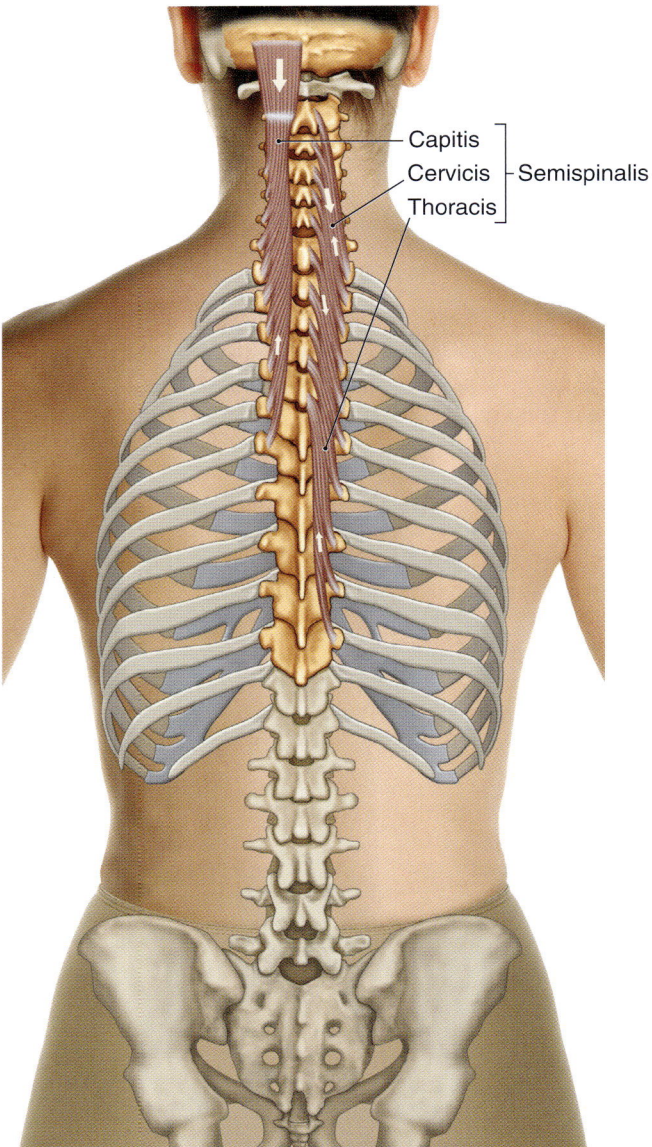

FIGURE 11-57 Posterior view of the semispinalis. The semispinalis thoracis and cervicis are seen on the right; the semispinalis capitis is seen on the left.

MULTIFIDUS (OF TRANSVERSOSPINALIS GROUP):

Attachments:

- **Posterior Sacrum, Posterior Superior Iliac Spine (PSIS), Posterior Sacroiliac Ligament, and L5-C4 Vertebrae**
  - LUMBAR REGION: All mammillary processes (not transverse processes)
  - THORACIC REGION: All transverse processes
  - CERVICAL REGION: The articular processes of C4-C7 (not transverse processes)

to the

- **Spinous Processes of Vertebrae Three-Four Segmental Levels Superior to the Inferior Attachment**

Functions:

Major Standard Mover Actions	Major Reverse Mover Action
1. Extends the trunk and neck at the spinal joints[1-7]	1. Anteriorly tilts the pelvis at the LS joint and extends the lower spine relative to the upper spine[2-7]
2. Laterally flexes the trunk and neck at the spinal joints[2-5]	
3. Contralaterally rotates the trunk and neck at the spinal joints[2-6]	

LS joint = lumbosacral joint

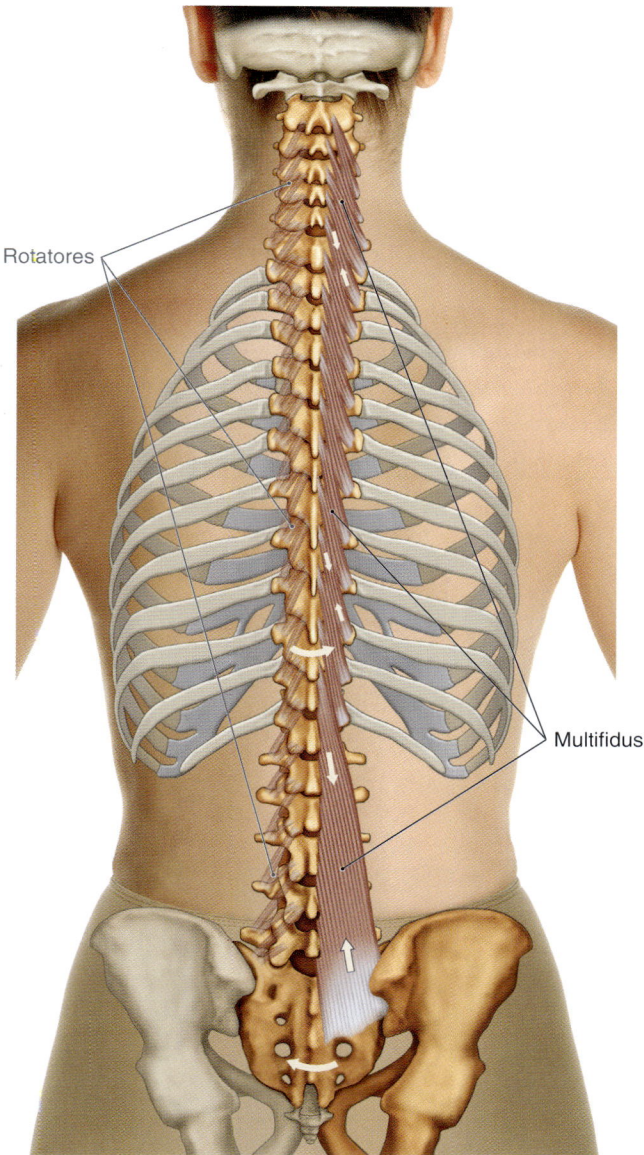

FIGURE 11-58 Posterior view of the right multifidus. The rotatores have been ghosted in on the left.

ROTATORES (OF TRANSVERSOSPINALIS GROUP):

Attachments:
- **Transverse Process (inferiorly)**

to the
- **Lamina (superiorly)**
  - One-two segmental levels superior to the inferior attachment

Functions:

Major Standard Mover Actions
1. Contralaterally rotate the trunk and neck at the spinal joints[2-6]
2. Extend the trunk and neck at the spinal joints[1-6]
3. Laterally flex the trunk and neck at the spinal joints[2-4]

INTERSPINALES:

Attachments:
- **From a Spinous Process**

to the
- **Spinous Process Directly Superior**
  - CERVICAL REGION: There are six pairs of interspinales located between T1-C2.
  - THORACIC REGION: There are two pairs of interspinales located between T2-T1 and T12-T11.
  - LUMBAR REGION: There are four pairs of interspinales located between L5-L1.

Functions:

Major Standard Mover Action
1. Extend the neck and trunk at the spinal joints[2,3,6]

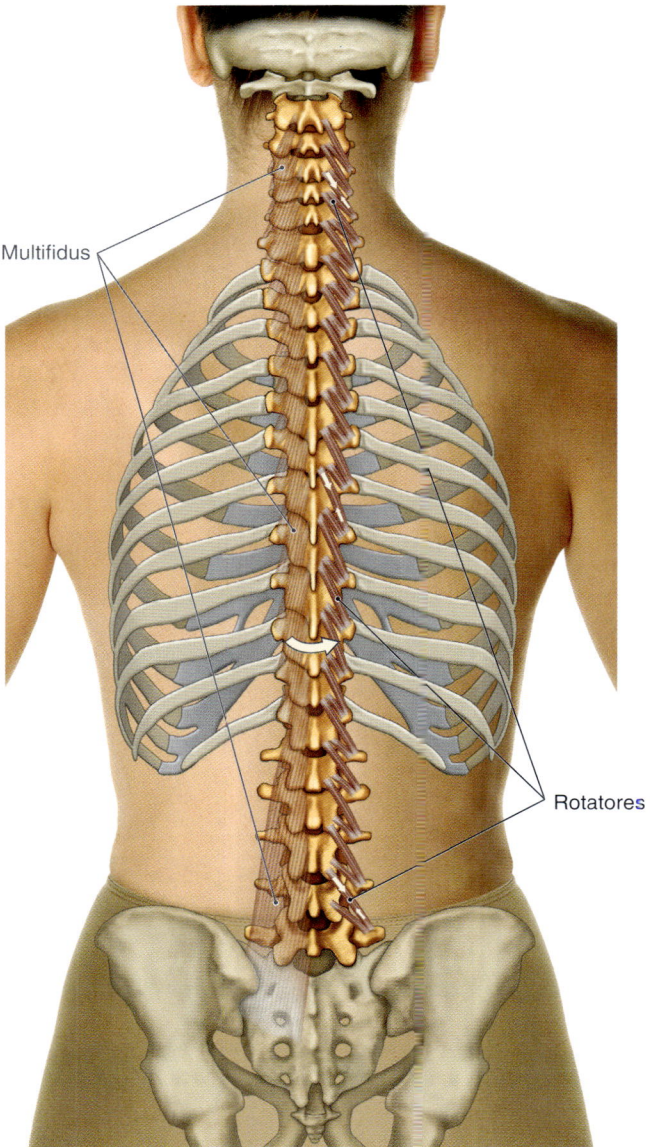

FIGURE 11-59 Posterior view of the right rotatores. The multifidus has been ghosted in on the left.

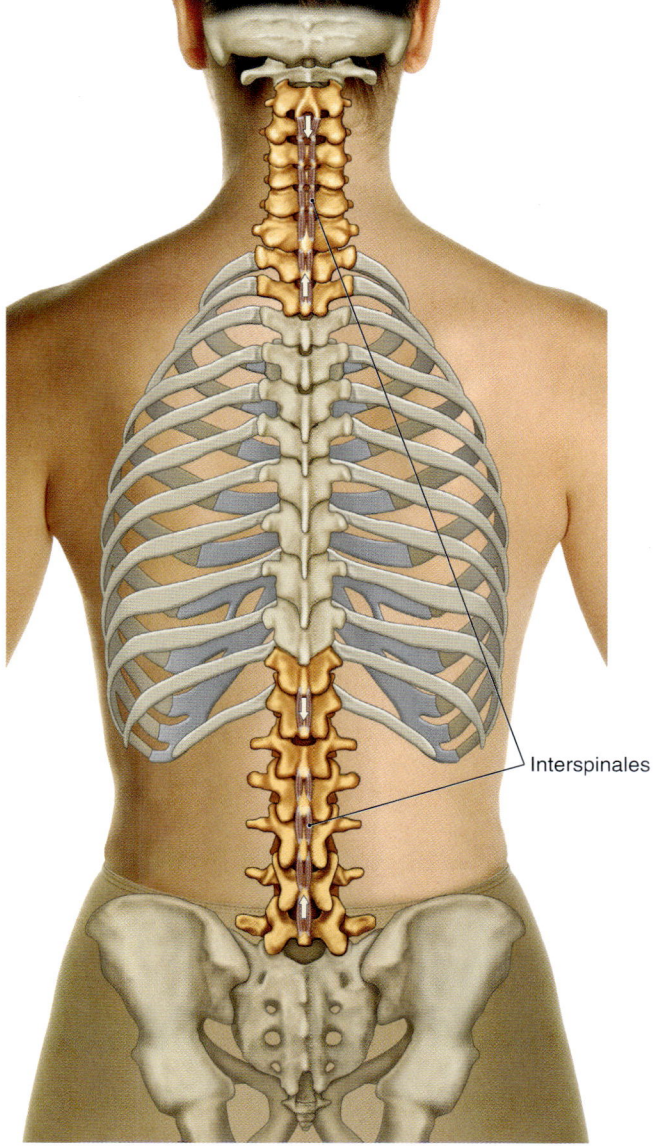

FIGURE 11-60 Posterior view of the right and left interspinales.

INTERTRANSVERSARII:

Attachments:
- **From a Transverse Process**

to the

- **Transverse Process Directly Superior**
  - CERVICAL REGION: There are seven pairs of intertransversarii muscles (anterior and posterior sets) located between C1 and T1 on each side of the body.
  - THORACIC REGION: There are three intertransversarii muscles between T10 and L1 on each side of the body.
  - LUMBAR REGION: There are four pairs of intertransversarii muscles (medial and lateral sets) located between L1 and L5 on each side of the body.

Functions:

Major Standard Mover Action

1. Laterally flex the neck and trunk at the spinal joints[2–4,6,7]

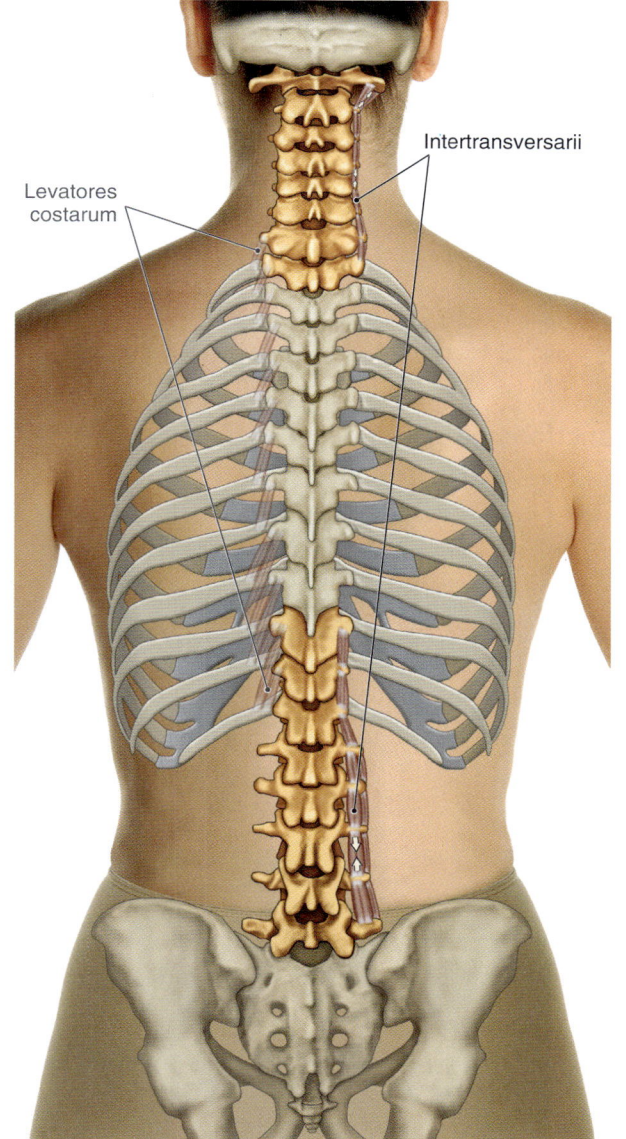

FIGURE 11-61 Posterior view of the right intertransversarii. The levatores costarum have been ghosted in on the left.

Neck:
STERNOCLEIDOMASTOID (SCM):

Attachments:
- **STERNAL HEAD: Manubrium of the Sternum**
  - the anterior superior surface
- **Clavicular Head: Medial Clavicle**
  - the medial ⅓

to the
- **Mastoid Process of the Temporal Bone**
  - and the lateral ½ of the superior nuchal line of the occipital bone

Functions:

Major Standard Mover Actions
1. Flexes the lower neck at the spinal joints[1-7]
2. Extends the upper neck and head at the spinal joints[1,2,4-7]
3. Laterally flexes the neck and head at the spinal joints[1-7]
4. Contralaterally rotates the neck and head at the spinal joints[1-7]

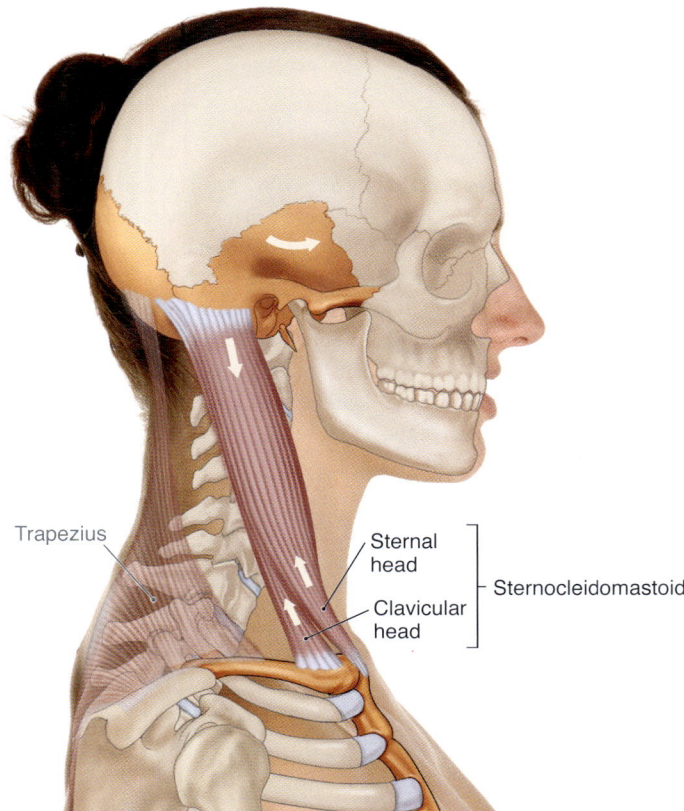

FIGURE 11-62 Lateral view of the right sternocleidomastoid. The trapezius has been ghosted in.

ANTERIOR SCALENE (OF SCALENE GROUP):

Attachments:
- **Transverse Processes of the Cervical Spine**
  - the anterior tubercles of C3-C6

to the
- **First Rib**
  - the scalene tubercle on the inner border

Functions:

Major Standard Mover Actions	Major Reverse Mover Action
1. Flexes the neck at the spinal joints[1-7]	1. Elevates the first rib at the sternocostal and costospinal joints[1-7]
2. Laterally flexes the neck at the spinal joints[1-7]	

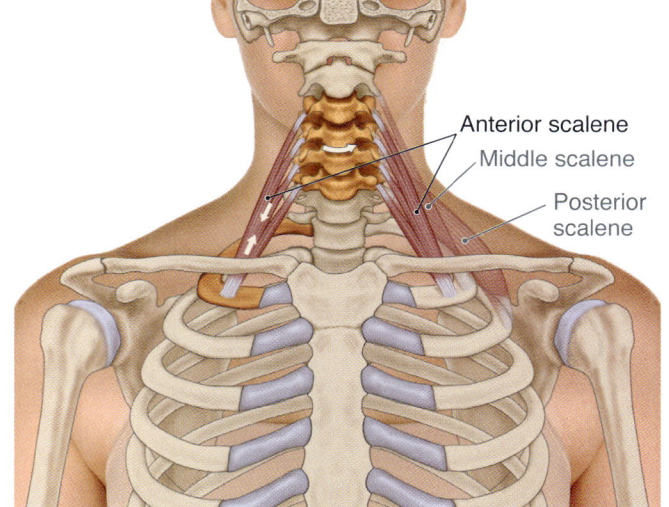

FIGURE 11-63 Anterior view of the anterior scalene bilaterally. The other two scalenes have been ghosted in on the left side.

MIDDLE SCALENE (OF SCALENE GROUP):

Attachments:

- **Transverse Processes of the Cervical Spine**
  - the posterior tubercles of C2-C7

to the

- **First Rib**
  - the superior surface

Functions:

Major Standard Mover Actions	Major Reverse Mover Action
1. Flexes the neck at the spinal joints[2-5]	1. Elevates the first rib at the sternocostal and costospinal joints[1-7]
2. Laterally flexes the neck at the spinal joints[1,2,4-6]	

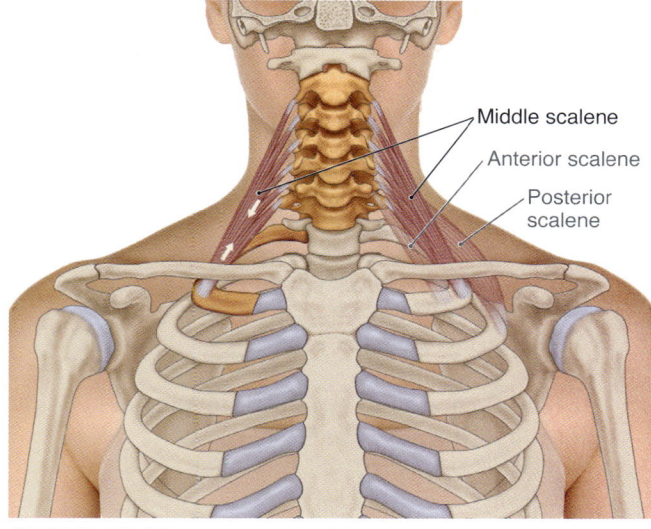

FIGURE 11-64 Anterior view of the middle scalene bilaterally. The other two scalenes have been ghosted in on the left side.

POSTERIOR SCALENE (OF SCALENE GROUP):

Attachments:

- **Transverse Processes of the Cervical Spine**
  - the posterior tubercles of C5-C7

to the

- **Second Rib**
  - the external surface

Functions:

Major Standard Mover Action	Major Reverse Mover Action
1. Laterally flexes the neck at the spinal joints[1-7]	1. Elevates the second rib at the sternocostal and costospinal joints[1-7]

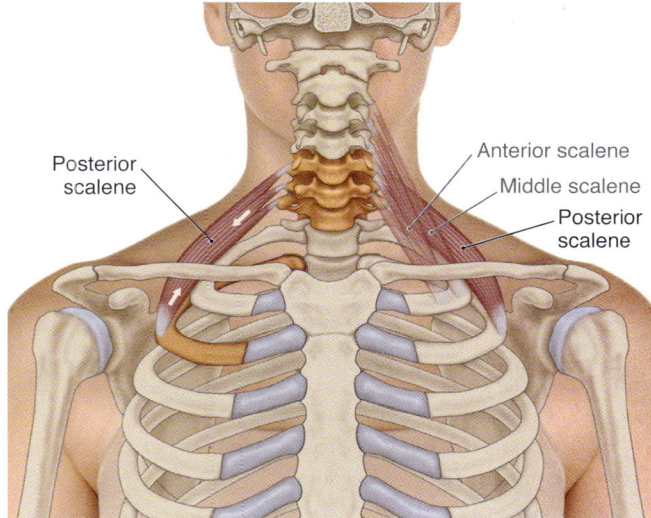

FIGURE 11-65 Anterior view of the posterior scalene bilaterally. The other two scalenes have been ghosted in on the left side.

LONGUS COLLI (OF PREVERTEBRAL GROUP):

Attachments:

- **Entire Muscle: Transverse Processes and Anterior Bodies of C3-T3 Vertebrae**
  - SUPERIOR OBLIQUE PART:
    - the transverse processes of C3-C5
  - INFERIOR OBLIQUE PART:
    - the anterior bodies of T1-T3
  - VERTICAL PART:
    - the anterior bodies of C5-T3

to the

- **Entire Muscle: Transverse Processes and Anterior Bodies of C2-C6 and the Anterior Arch of C1**
  - SUPERIOR OBLIQUE PART:
    - the anterior arch of C1
  - INFERIOR OBLIQUE PART:
    - the transverse processes of C5-C6
  - VERTICAL PART:
    - the anterior bodies of C2-C4

Functions:

Major Standard Mover Action

1. Flexes the neck at the spinal joints[1-7]

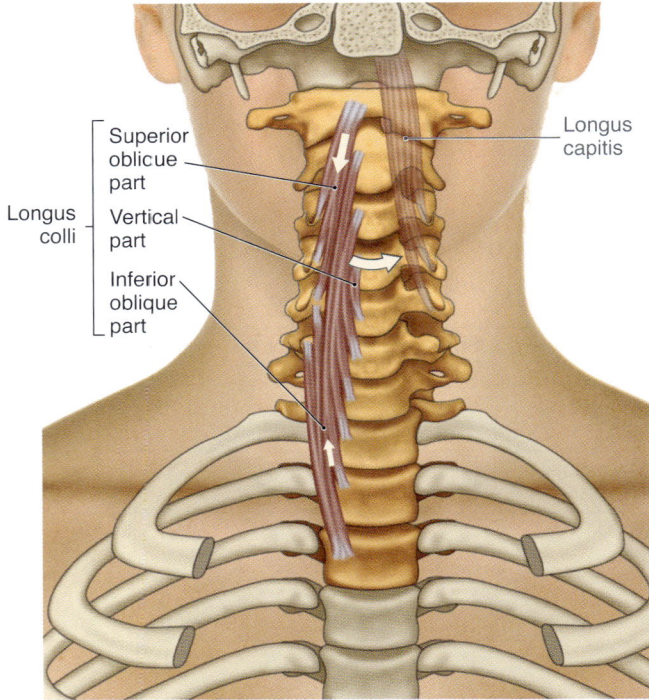

FIGURE 11-66 Anterior view of the right longus colli. The longus capitis has been ghosted in on the left.

LONGUS CAPITIS (OF PREVERTEBRAL GROUP):

Attachments:

- **Transverse Processes of the Cervical Spine**
  - the anterior tubercles of C3-C5

to the

- **Occiput**
  - the inferior surface of the basilar part of the occiput (just anterior to the foramen magnum)

Functions:

Major Standard Mover Action

1. Flexes the neck and head at the spinal joints[1-7]

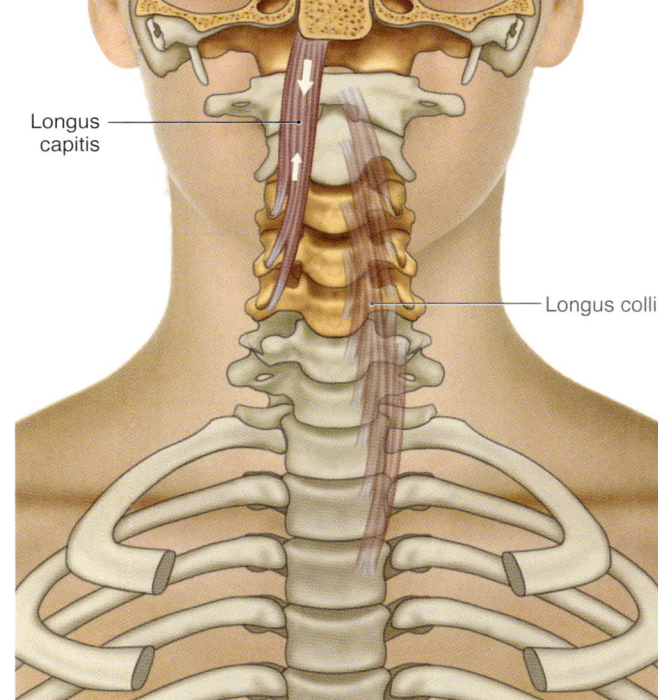

FIGURE 11-67 Anterior view of the right longus capitis. The longus colli has been ghosted in on the left.

RECTUS CAPITIS ANTERIOR (OF PREVERTEBRAL GROUP):

Attachments:

- **Atlas (C1)**
  - the anterior surface of the base of the transverse process

to the

- **Occiput**
  - the inferior surface of the basilar part of the occiput (just anterior to the foramen magnum)

Functions:

Major Standard Mover Action
1. Flexes the head at the AOJ[1-7]

AOJ = atlanto-occipital joint

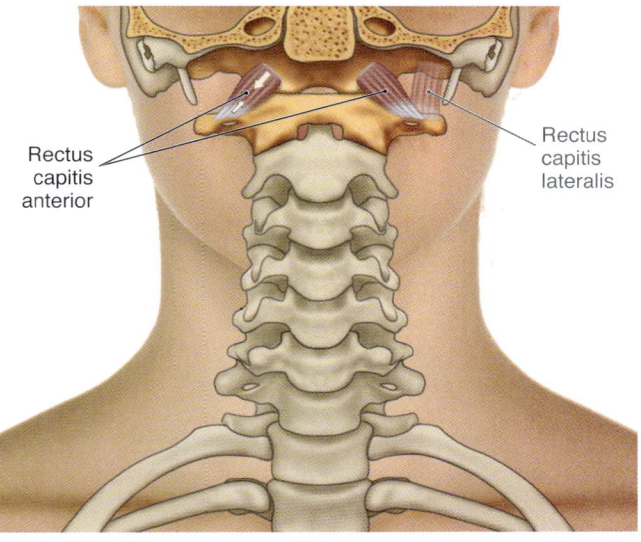

FIGURE 11-68 Anterior view of the rectus capitis anterior bilaterally. The rectus capitis lateralis has been ghosted in on the left.

RECTUS CAPITIS LATERALIS (OF PREVERTEBRAL GROUP):

Attachments:

- **The Atlas (C1)**
  - the superior surface of the transverse process

to the

- **Occiput**
  - the inferior surface of the jugular process of the occiput

Functions:

Major Standard Mover Action
1. Laterally flexes the head at the AOJ[1-7]

AOJ = atlanto-occipital joint

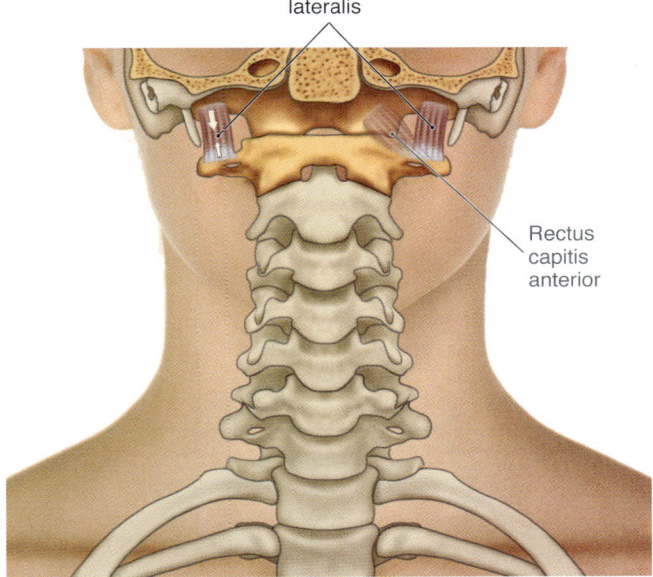

FIGURE 11-69 Anterior view of the rectus capitis lateralis bilaterally. The rectus capitis anterior has been ghosted in on the left.

SPLENIUS CAPITIS:

Attachments:

- **Nuchal Ligament from C3-C6 and the Spinous Processes of C7-T4**

to the

- **Mastoid Process of the Temporal Bone and the Occipital Bone**
  - the lateral ⅓ of the superior nuchal line of the occiput

Functions:

Major Standard Mover Actions
1. Extends the head and neck at the spinal joints[1-7]
2. Laterally flexes the head and neck at the spinal joints[2-4,6]
3. Ipsilaterally rotates the head and neck at the spinal joints[1-7]

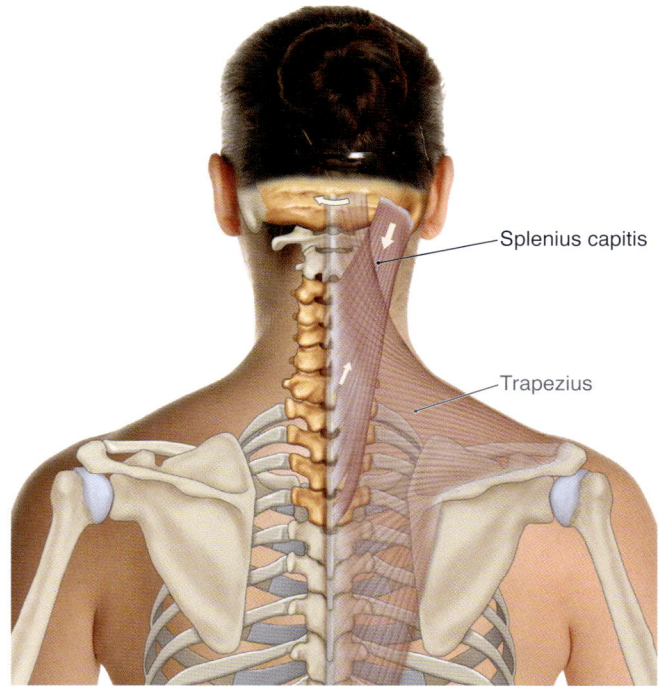

FIGURE 11-70 Posterior view of the right splenius capitis. The trapezius has been ghosted in.

SPLENIUS CERVICIS:

Attachments:

- **Spinous Processes of T3-T6**

to the

- **Transverse Processes of C1-C3**
  - the posterior tubercles of the transverse processes

Functions:

Major Standard Mover Actions
1. Extends the neck at the spinal joints[1-7]
2. Laterally flexes the neck at the spinal joints[2-6]
3. Ipsilaterally rotates the neck at the spinal joints[1-7]

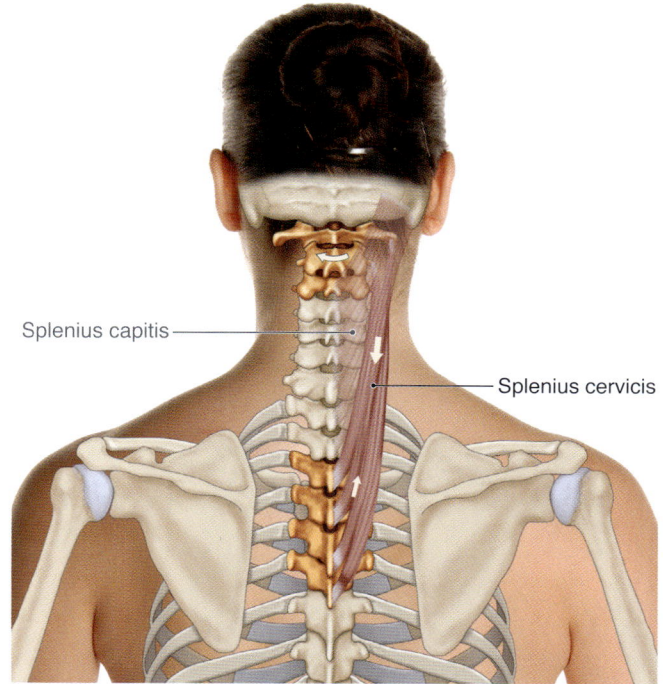

FIGURE 11-71 Posterior view of the right splenius cervicis. The splenius capitis has been ghosted in.

RECTUS CAPITIS POSTERIOR MAJOR (OF SUBOCCIPITAL GROUP):

Attachments:
- The Spinous Process of the Axis (C2)

to the
- Occiput
  - the lateral ½ of the inferior nuchal line

Functions:

Major Standard Mover Action
1. Extends the head at the AOJ[1-7]

AOJ = atlanto-occipital joint

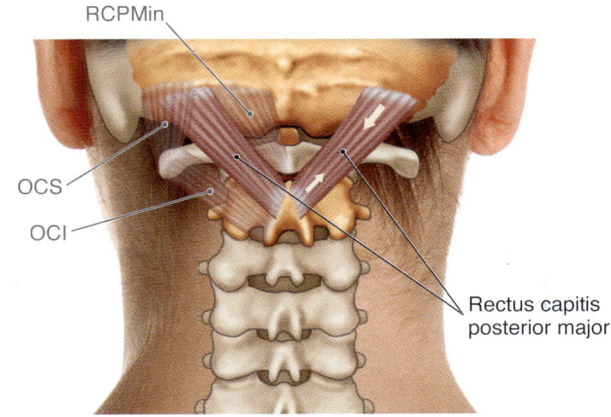

FIGURE 11-72 Posterior view (bilaterally) of the rectus capitis posterior major. The other three suboccipital muscles have been ghosted in on the left. OCI, Obliquus capitis inferior; OCS, Obliquus capitis superior; RCPMin, Rectus capitis posterior minor.

RECTUS CAPITIS POSTERIOR MINOR (OF SUBOCCIPITAL GROUP):

Attachments:
- The Posterior Tubercle of the Atlas (C1)

to the
- Occiput
  - the medial ½ of the inferior nuchal line

Functions:

Major Standard Mover Action
1. Protracts the head at the AOJ[2,8]

AOJ = atlanto-occipital joint

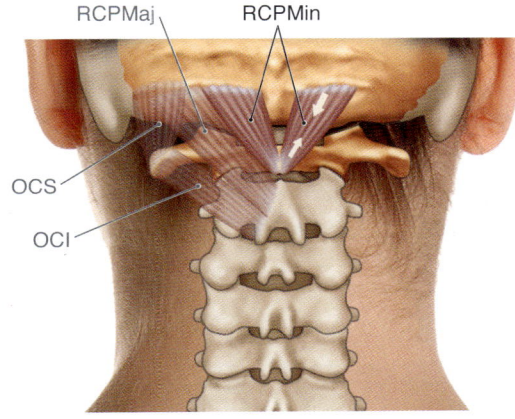

FIGURE 11-73 Posterior view (bilaterally) of the rectus capitis posterior minor (RCPMin). The other three suboccipital muscles have been ghosted in on the left. OCI, Obliquus capitis inferior; OCS, Obliquus capitis superior; RCPMaj, Rectus capitis posterior major.

OBLIQUUS CAPITIS INFERIOR (OF SUBOCCIPITAL GROUP):

Attachments:
- The Spinous Process of the Axis (C2)

to the
- Transverse Process of the Atlas (C1)

Functions:

Major Standard Mover Action
1. Ipsilaterally rotates the atlas at the AAJ[1-7]

AAJ = atlantoaxial joint

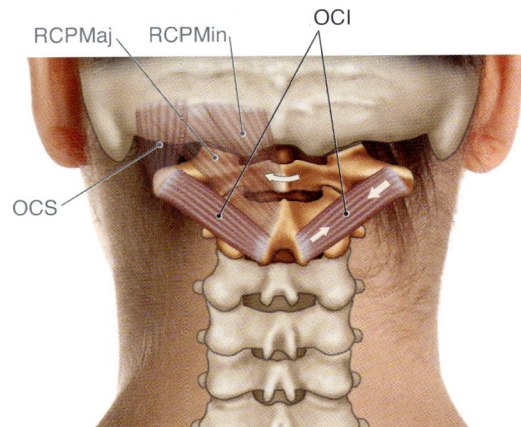

FIGURE 11-74 Posterior view (bilaterally) of the obliquus capitis inferior (OCI). The other three suboccipital muscles have been ghosted in on the left. OCS, Obliquus capitis superior; RCPMaj, Rectus capitis posterior major; RCPMin, Rectus capitis posterior minor.

OBLIQUUS CAPITIS SUPERIOR (OF SUBOCCIPITAL GROUP):

Attachments:

- **The Transverse Process of the Atlas (C1)**

to the

- **Occiput**
  - between the superior and inferior nuchal lines

Functions:

Major Standard Mover Action
1. Protracts the head at the AOJ[2,9]

AOJ = atlanto-occipital joint

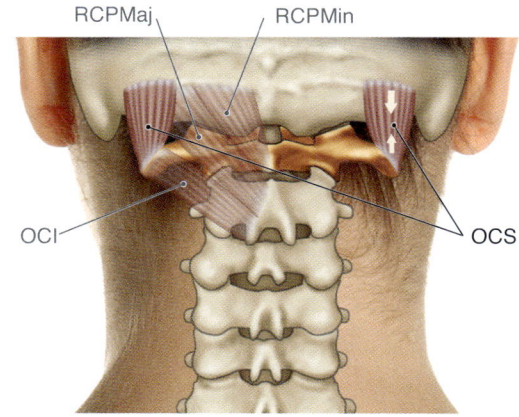

FIGURE 11-75 Posterior view (bilaterally) of the obliquus capitis superior OCS. The other three suboccipital muscles have been ghosted in on the left. OCI, Obliquus capitis inferior; RCPMaj, Rectus capitis posterior major; RCPMin, Rectus capitis posterior minor.

Low Back:
QUADRATUS LUMBORUM (QL):

Attachments:

- **Twelfth Rib and the Transverse Processes of L1-L4**
  - the medial of the inferior border of the twelfth rib

to the

- **Posterior Iliac Crest**
  - the posteromedial iliac crest and the iliolumbar ligament

Functions:

Major Standard Mover Actions	Major Reverse Mover Actions
1. Elevates the same-side pelvis at the LS joint and laterally flexes the lower lumbar spine relative to the upper lumbar spine[2,3,6,7,10]	1. Laterally flexes the trunk at the spinal joints[1–3,6,7,10]
2. Anteriorly tilts the pelvis at the LS joint and extends the lower lumbar spine relative to the upper lumbar spine[2,6]	2. Depresses the twelfth rib at the costospinal joints[1,2,6,7,10]
	3. Extends the trunk at the spinal joints[1,2,6,10]

LS joint = lumbosacral joint

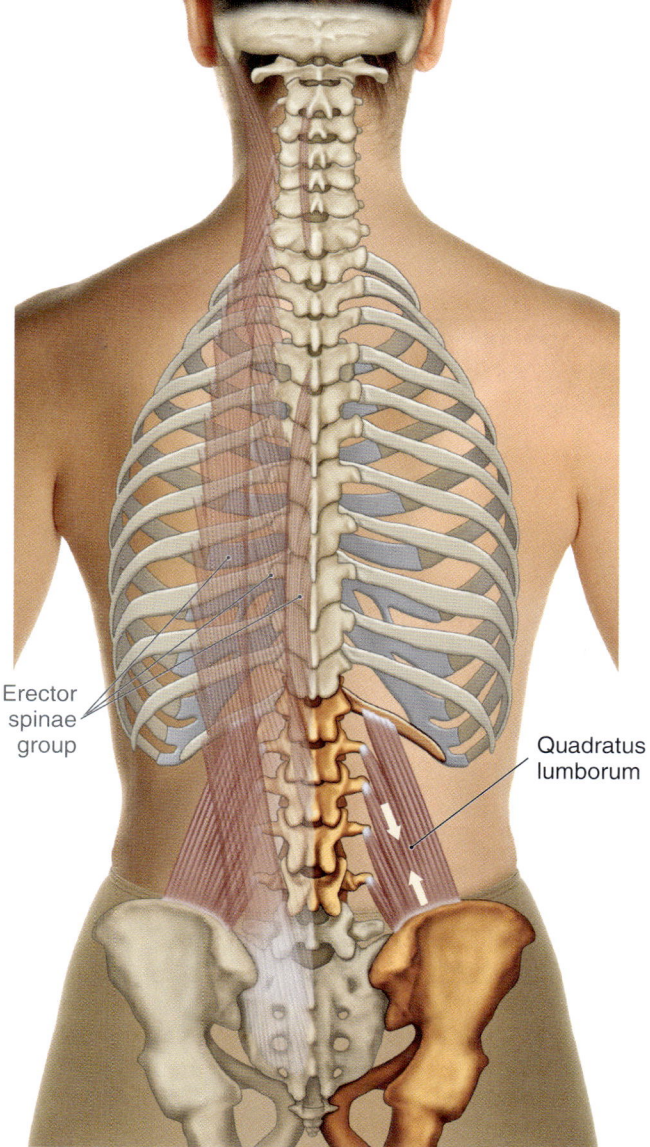

FIGURE 11-76 Posterior view of the quadratus lumborum (QL). The erector spinae group has been ghosted in on the left side.

RECTUS ABDOMINIS (OF ANTERIOR ABDOMINAL WALL):

Attachments:

- Pubis
  - the crest and symphysis of the pubis

to the

- Xiphoid Process and the Cartilage of Ribs Five through Seven

Functions:

Major Standard Mover Actions	Major Reverse Mover Action
1. Flexes the trunk at the spinal joints[1-7]	1. Posteriorly tilts the pelvis at the LS joint and flexes the lower trunk relative to the upper trunk[2-7]
2. Laterally flexes the trunk at the spinal joints[2,3]	

LS joint = lumbosacral joint

EXTERNAL ABDOMINAL OBLIQUE (OF ANTERIOR ABDOMINAL WALL):

Attachments:

- Anterior Iliac Crest, Pubic Bone, and the Abdominal Aponeurosis
  - the pubic crest and tubercle

to the

- Lower Eight Ribs (Ribs Five through Twelve)
  - the inferior border of the ribs

Functions:

Major Standard Mover Actions	Major Reverse Mover Action
1. Flexes the trunk at the spinal joints[2-6]	1. Posteriorly tilts the pelvis at the LS joint and flexes the lower trunk relative to the upper trunk[2-6]
2. Laterally flexes the trunk at the spinal joints[1-6]	
3. Contralaterally rotates the trunk at the spinal joints[2-6]	

LS joint = lumbosacral joint

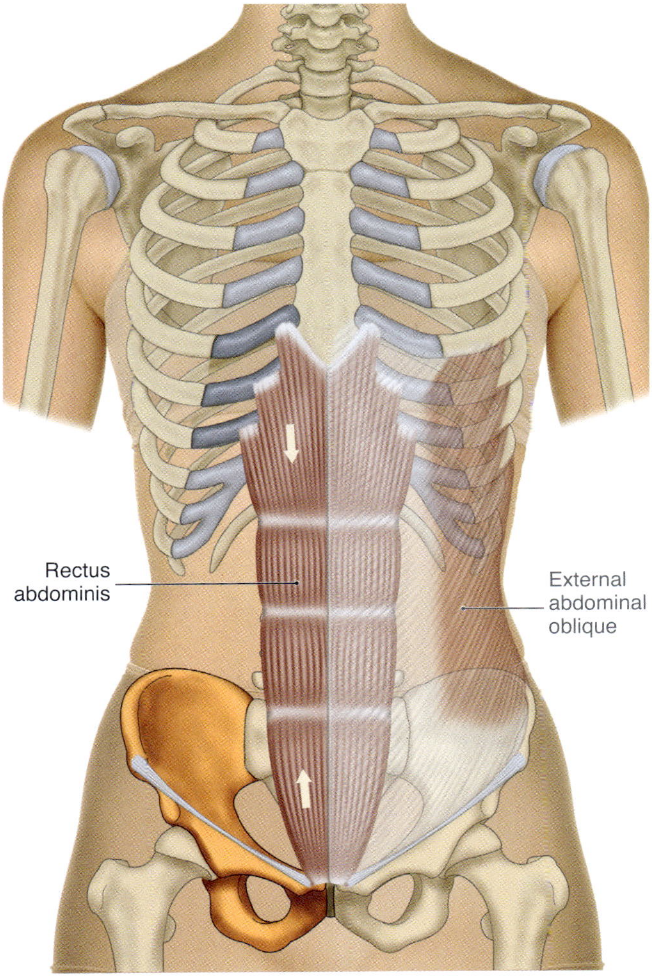

FIGURE 11-77 Anterior view of the rectus abdominis bilaterally. The external abdominal oblique has been ghosted in on the left.

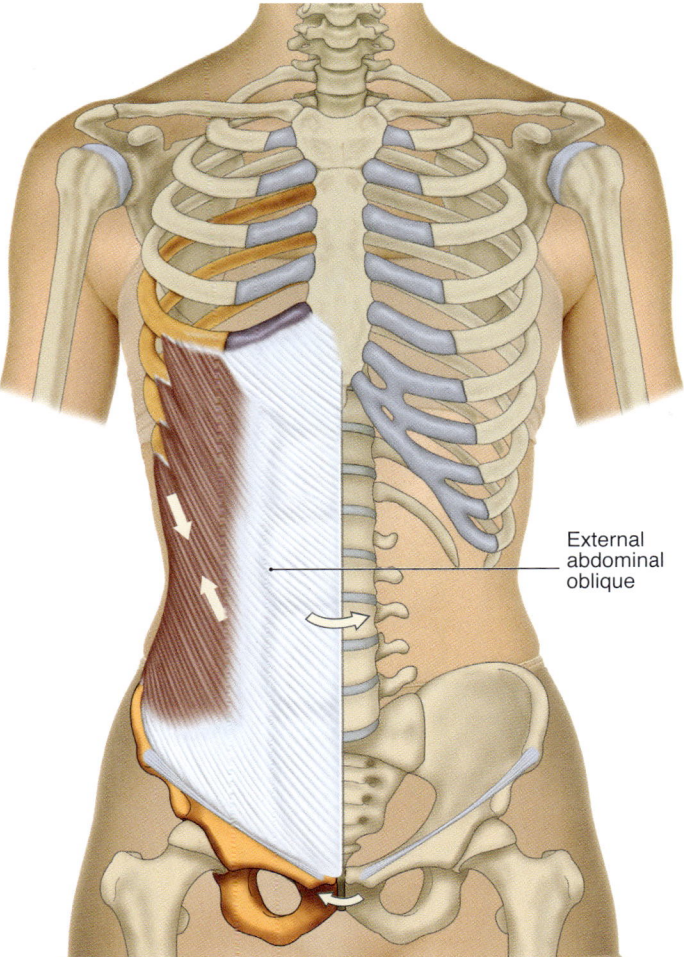

FIGURE 11-78 Anterior view of the right external abdominal oblique.

INTERNAL ABDOMINAL OBLIQUE (OF ANTERIOR ABDOMINAL WALL):

Attachments:

- **Inguinal Ligament, Iliac Crest, and Thoracolumbar Fascia**
  - the lateral ⅔ of the inguinal ligament

to the

- **Lower Three Ribs (Ten through Twelve) and the Abdominal Aponeurosis**

Functions:

Major Standard Mover Actions	Major Reverse Mover Action
1. Flexes the trunk at the spinal joints[2-6]	1. Posteriorly tilts the pelvis at the LS joint and flexes the lower trunk relative to the upper trunk[2-6]
2. Laterally flexes the trunk at the spinal joints[1-6]	
3. Ipsilaterally rotates the trunk at the spinal joints[2-6]	

LS joint = lumbosacral joint

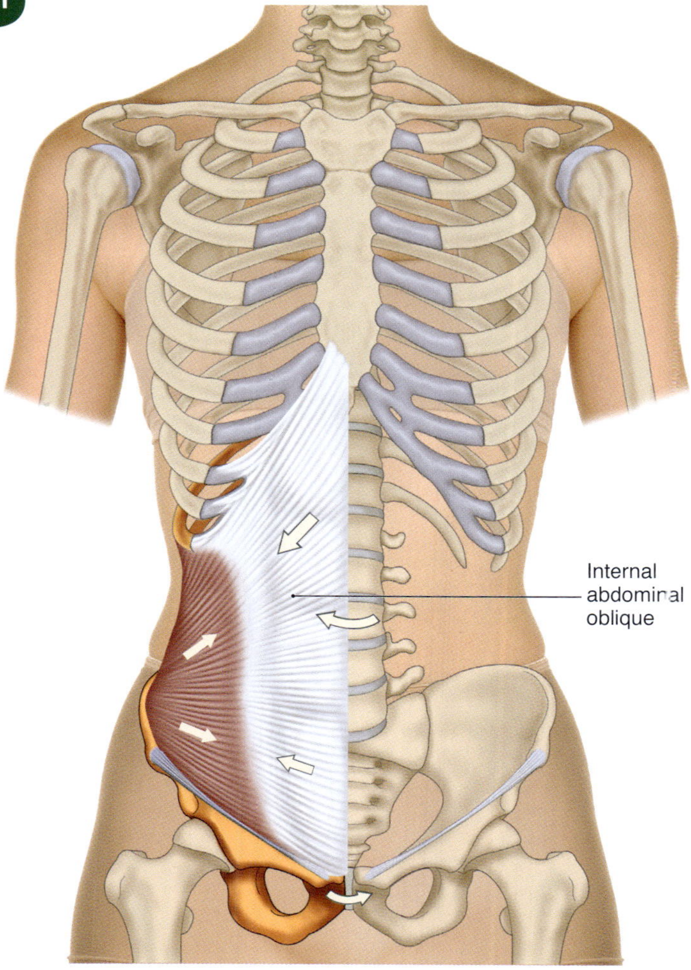

TRANSVERSUS ABDOMINIS (OF ANTERIOR ABDOMINAL WALL):

Attachments:

- **Inguinal Ligament, Iliac Crest, Thoracolumbar Fascia, and the Lower Costal Cartilages**
  - the lateral ⅔ of the inguinal ligament; the lower six costal cartilages (of ribs seven through twelve)

to the

- **Abdominal Aponeurosis**

Functions:

Major Standard Mover Action
1. Compresses abdominopelvic cavity[1-3,5,7]

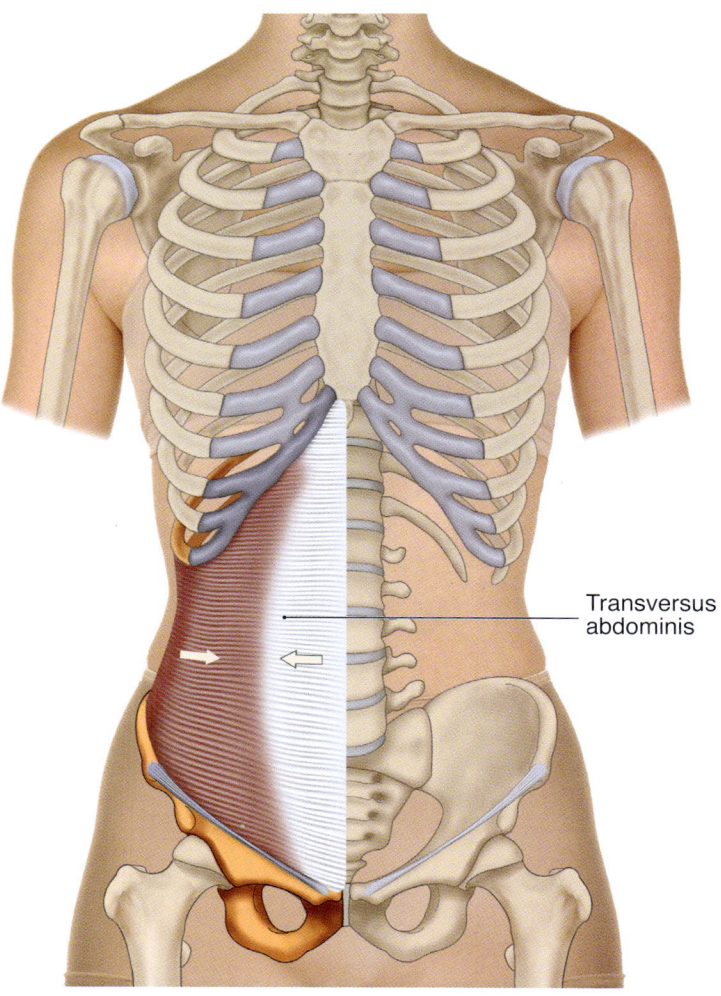

FIGURE 11-80 Anterior view of the right transversus abdominis.

FIGURE 11-79 Anterior view of the right internal abdominal oblique.

PSOAS MINOR:

Attachments:
- **Anterolateral Bodies of T12 and L1**
  - and the disc between T12 and L1

to the

- **Pubis**
  - the pectineal line of the pubis and the iliopectineal eminence (of the ilium and the pubis)

Functions:

Major Standard Mover Action	Major Reverse Mover Action
1. Flexes the trunk at the spinal joints[1,2,4,6]	1. Posteriorly tilts the pelvis at the LS joint and flexes the lower trunk relative to the upper trunk[2,4,6,10]

LS joint = lumbosacral joint

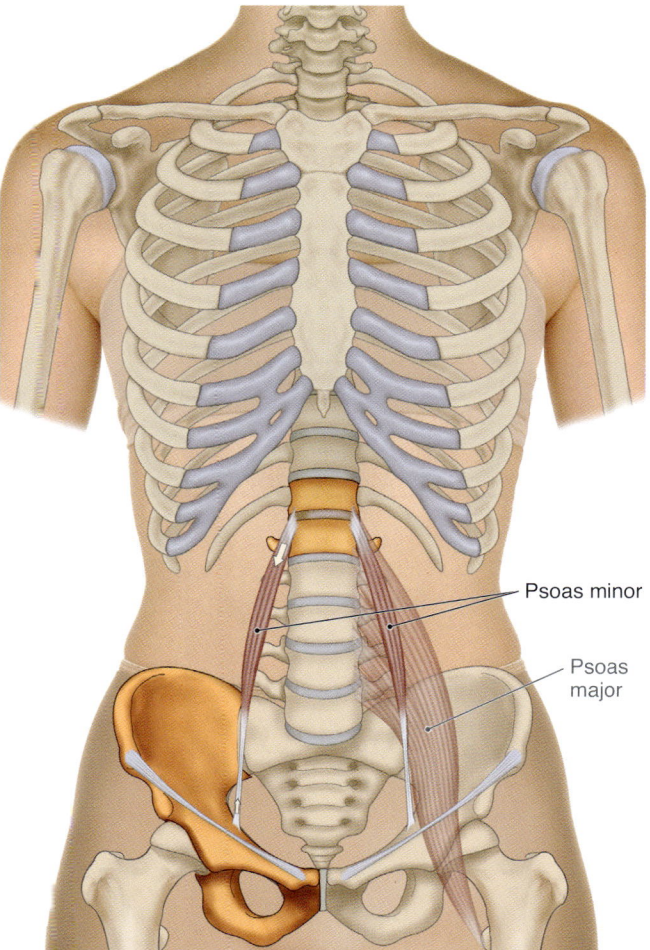

FIGURE 11-81 Anterior view of the psoas minor bilaterally. The psoas major has been ghosted in on the left.

SECTION 11.9 MUSCLES OF THE RIBCAGE JOINTS

EXTERNAL INTERCOSTALS:

Attachments:
- In the Intercostal Spaces of Ribs One through Twelve
  - Each external intercostal attaches from the inferior border of one rib to the superior border of the rib directly inferior.

Functions:

Major Standard Mover Actions
1. Elevate ribs two through twelve at the sternocostal and costospinal joints[2,4,6]
2. Rotate contralaterally the trunk at the spinal joints[2,4,5,7]

INTERNAL INTERCOSTALS:

Attachments:
- In the Intercostal Spaces of Ribs One through Twelve
  - Each internal intercostal attaches from the superior border of one rib and its costal cartilage to the inferior border of the rib and its costal cartilage that is directly superior.

Functions:

Major Standard Mover Actions
1. Depress ribs one through eleven at the sternocostal and costospinal joints[2,4,6,7]
2. Rotate ipsilaterally the trunk at the spinal joints[2,4,5,7]

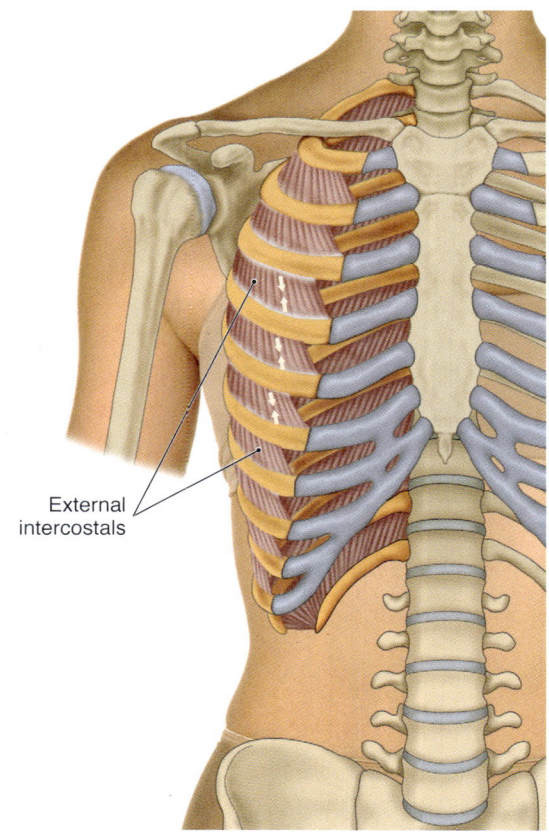

FIGURE 11-82 Anterior view of the right external intercostals.

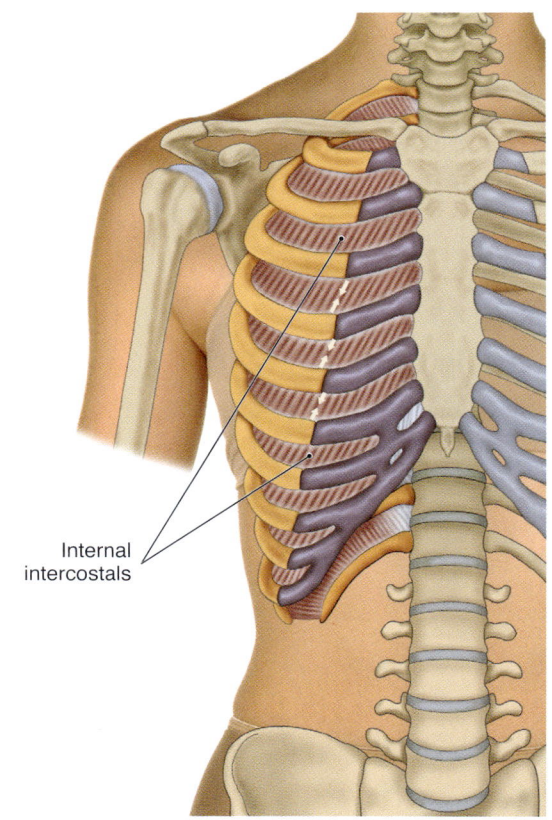

FIGURE 11-83 Anterior view of the right internal intercostals.

TRANSVERSUS THORACIS:

Attachments:

- **Internal Surfaces of the Sternum, the Xiphoid Process, and the Adjacent Costal Cartilages**
  - the inferior ⅔ of the sternum, and the costal cartilages of ribs four through seven

to the

- **Internal Surface of Costal Cartilages Two through Six**

Functions

Major Standard Mover Action
1. Depresses ribs two through six at the sternocostal and costospinal joints[1–4,6,7]

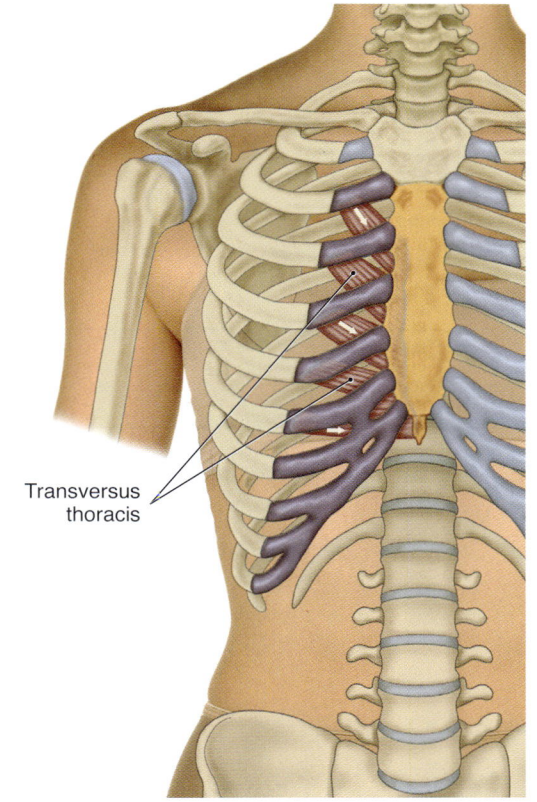

FIGURE 11-84 Anterior view of the right transversus thoracis.

DIAPHRAGM:

Attachments:

- **ENTIRE MUSCLE: Internal Surfaces of the Rib Cage and Sternum, and the Spine**
  - COSTAL PART: Internal surface of the lower six ribs (ribs seven through twelve) and their costal cartilages
  - STERNAL PART: Internal surface of the xiphoid process of the sternum
  - LUMBAR PART: L1-L3
    - The lumbar attachments consist of two aponeuroses, called the medial and lateral arcuate ligaments, and two tendons, called the right and left crura (singular: crus).

to the

- **Central Tendon (Dome) of the Diaphragm**

Functions:

Major Standard Mover Action	Major Reverse Mover Action
1. Increases the volume of (expands) the thoracic cavity via abdominal breathing[1–7]	1. Increases the volume of (expands) the thoracic cavity via thoracic breathing[2–6]

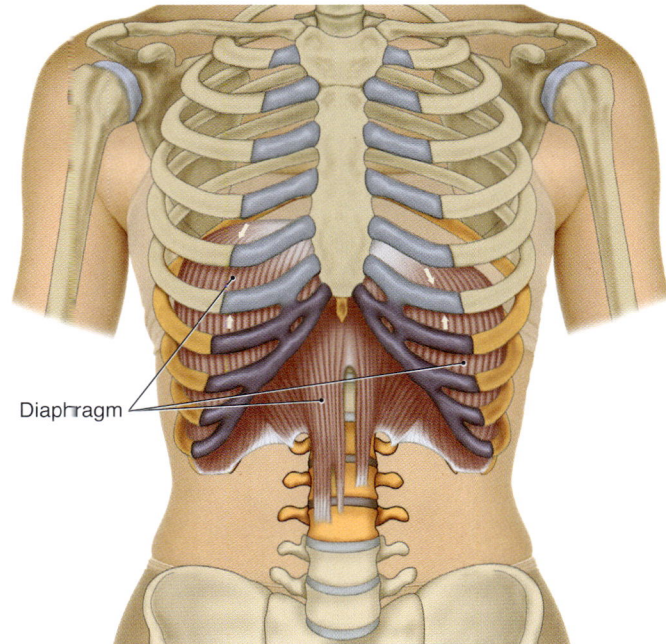

FIGURE 11-85 Anterior view of the diaphragm.

SERRATUS POSTERIOR SUPERIOR:

Attachments:
- **Spinous Processes of C7-T3**
  - and the lower nuchal ligament

to
- **Ribs Two through Five**
  - the superior borders and the external surfaces

Functions:

Major Standard Mover Action

1. Elevates ribs two through five at the sternocostal and costospinal joints[1-6]

SERRATUS POSTERIOR INFERIOR:

Attachments:
- **Spinous Processes of T11-L2**

to
- **Ribs Nine through Twelve**
  - the inferior borders and the external surfaces

Functions:

Major Standard Mover Action

1. Depresses ribs nine through twelve at the sternocostal and costospinal joints[1-6]

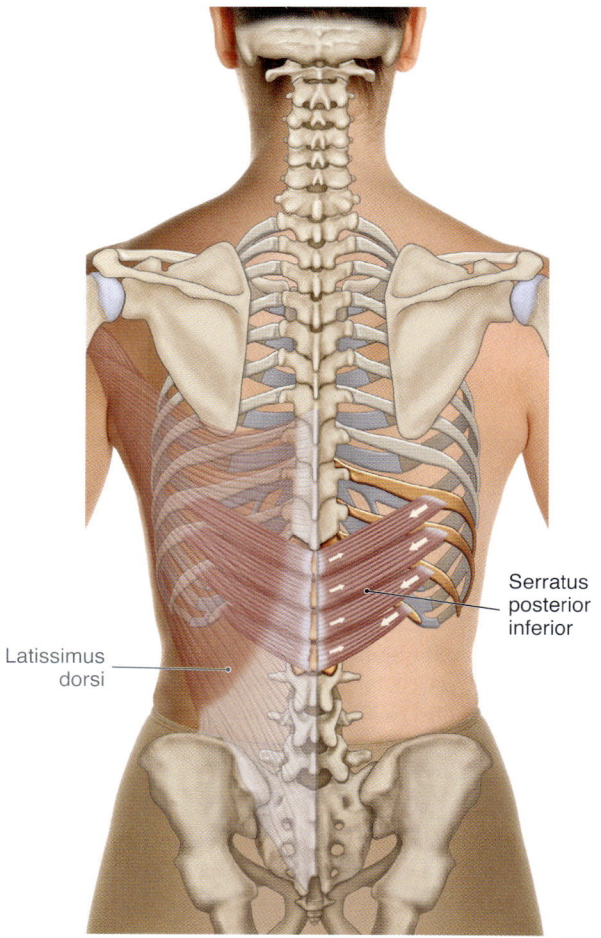

FIGURE 11-87 Posterior view of the serratus posterior inferior bilaterally. The latissimus dorsi has been ghosted in on the left side.

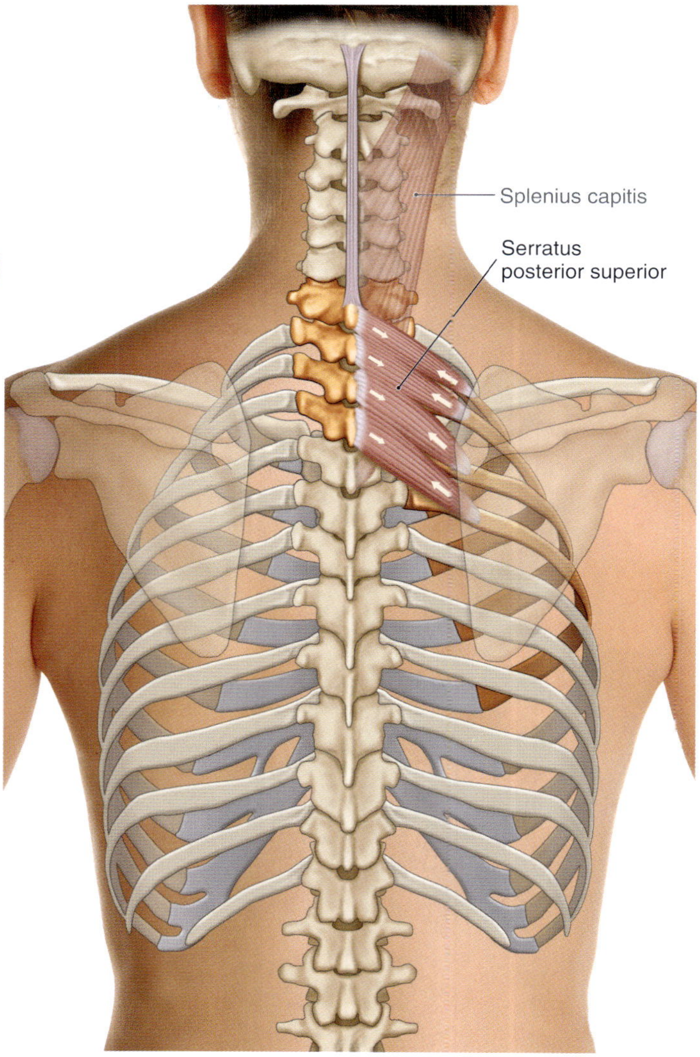

FIGURE 11-86 Posterior view of the right serratus posterior superior. The splenius capitis has been ghosted in.

LEVATORES COSTARUM:

Attachments:

- **Transverse Processes of C7-T11**
  - the tips of the transverse processes

to

- **Ribs One through Twelve (inferiorly)**
  - the external surfaces of the ribs, between the tubercle and the angle

Functions:

Major Standard Mover Action

1. Elevate the ribs at the sternocostal and costospinal joints[1,2,4–7]

SUBCOSTALES:

Attachments:

- **Ribs Ten through Twelve**
  - the internal surface of the ribs, near the angle

to

- **Ribs Eight through Ten**
  - the internal surfaces of the ribs, near the angle

Functions:

Major Standard Mover Action

1. Depress ribs eight through ten at the sternocostal and costospinal joints[1,4]

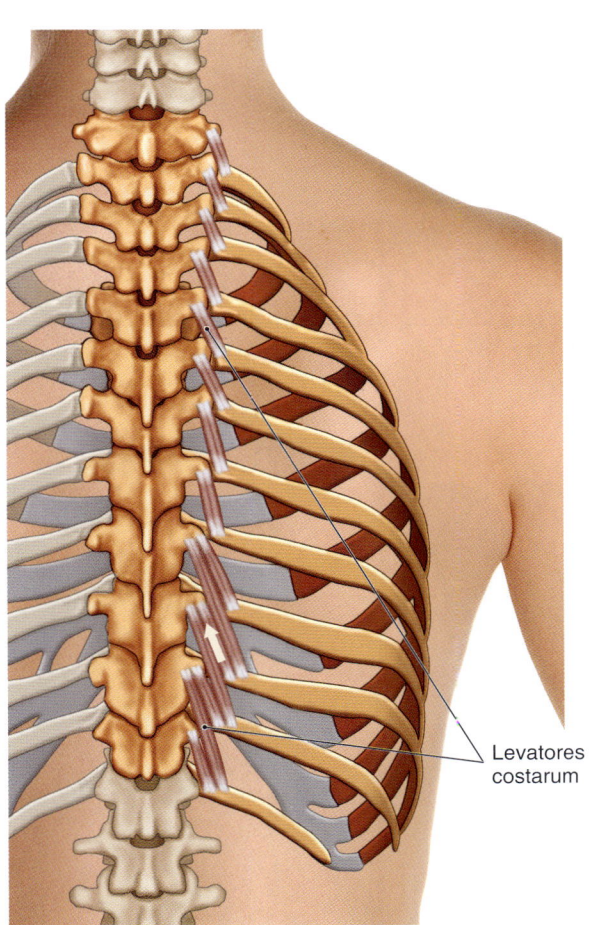

FIGURE 11-88 Posterior view of the right levatores costarum.

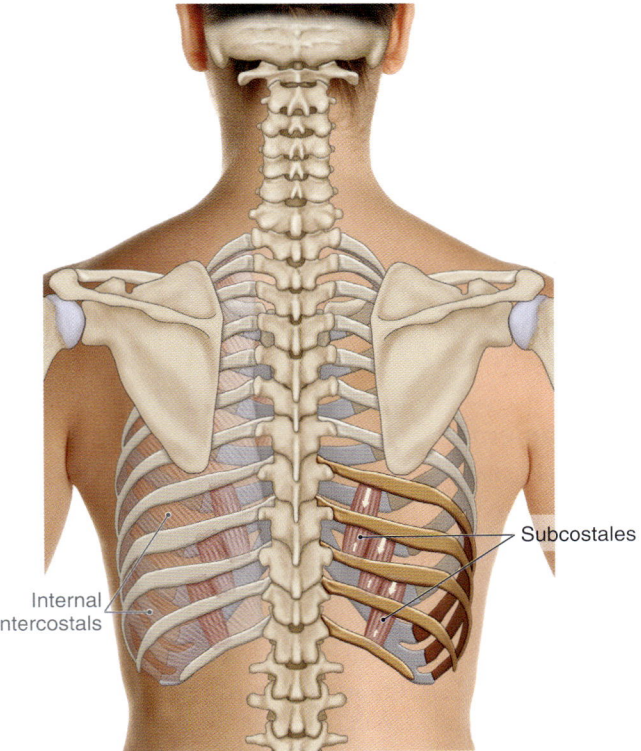

FIGURE 11-89 Posterior view of the subcostales bilaterally. The internal intercostals have been ghosted in on the left side.

SECTION 11.10 MUSCLES OF THE TEMPOROMANDIBULAR JOINTS

TEMPORALIS:

Attachments:

- **Temporal Fossa**
  - the entire temporal fossa except the portion on the zygomatic bone

to the

- **Coronoid Process and the Ramus of the Mandible**
  - the anterior border, apex, posterior border, and internal surface of the coronoid process of the mandible, as well as the anterior border of the ramus of the mandible

Functions:

Major Standard Mover Action
1. Elevates the mandible at the TMJs[1,2,4–7]

TMJs = temporomandibular joints

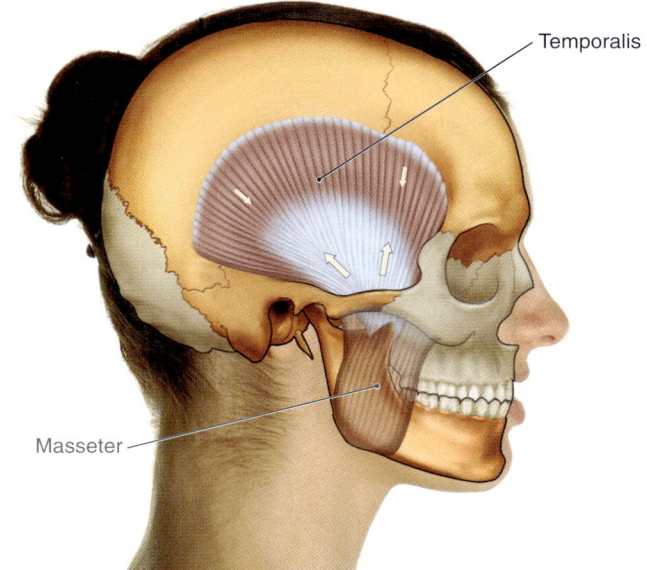

FIGURE 11-90 Lateral view of the right temporalis. The masseter has been ghosted in.

MASSETER:

Attachments:

- **Inferior Margins of Both the Zygomatic Bone and the Zygomatic Arch of the Temporal Bone**
  - SUPERFICIAL LAYER: the inferior margins of the zygomatic bone and the zygomatic arch
  - DEEP LAYER: the inferior margin and the deep surface of the zygomatic arch

to the

- **Angle, Ramus, and Coronoid Process of the Mandible**
  - SUPERFICIAL LAYER: the angle and the inferior of the external surface of the ramus of the mandible
  - DEEP LAYER: the external surface of the coronoid process, and the superior ½ of the external surface of the ramus of the mandible

Functions:

Major Standard Mover Action
1. Elevates the mandible at the TMJs[1,2,4–7]

TMJs = temporomandibular joints

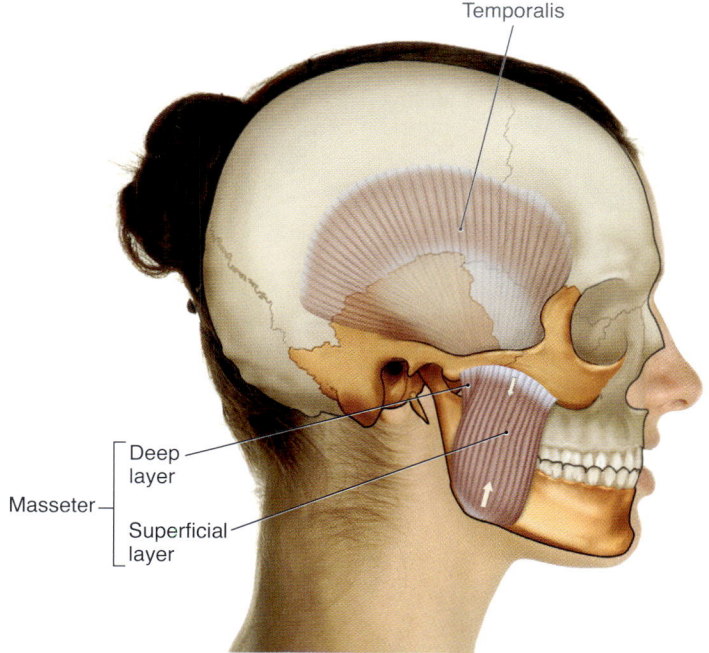

FIGURE 11-91 Lateral view of the right masseter. The temporalis has been ghosted in.

LATERAL PTERYGOID:

Attachments:

- **Entire Muscle: Sphenoid Bone**
  - SUPERIOR HEAD: the greater wing of the sphenoid
  - INFERIOR HEAD: the lateral surface of the lateral pterygoid plate of the pterygoid process of the sphenoid

to the

- **Mandible and the Temporomandibular Joint (TMJ)**
  - SUPERIOR HEAD: the capsule and articular disc of the TMJ
  - INFERIOR HEAD: the neck of the mandible

Functions:

Major Standard Mover Actions
1. Protracts the mandible at the TMJs[1,2,4-7]
2. Contralaterally deviates the mandible at the TMJs[1,2,4-7]

TMJs = temporomandibular joints

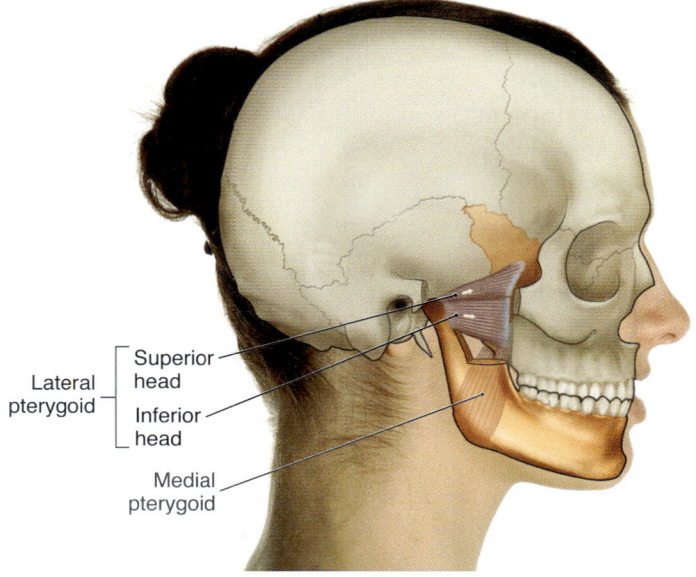

FIGURE 11-92 Lateral view of the right lateral pterygoid with the medial pterygoid ghosted in and with the mandible partially cut away.

MEDIAL PTERYGOID:

Attachments:

- **Entire Muscle: Sphenoid Bone**
  - DEEP HEAD: the medial surface of the lateral pterygoid plate of the pterygoid process of the sphenoid, the palatine bone, and the tuberosity of the maxilla
  - SUPERFICIAL HEAD: the palatine bone and the maxilla

to the

- **Internal Surface of the Mandible**
  - at the angle and the inferior border of the ramus of the mandible

Functions:

Major Standard Mover Actions
1. Elevates the mandible at the TMJs[1,2,4-7]
2. Protracts the mandible at the TMJs[1,2,4,5,7]
3. Contralaterally deviates the mandible at the TMJs[1,2,4,5,7]

TMJs = temporomandibular joints

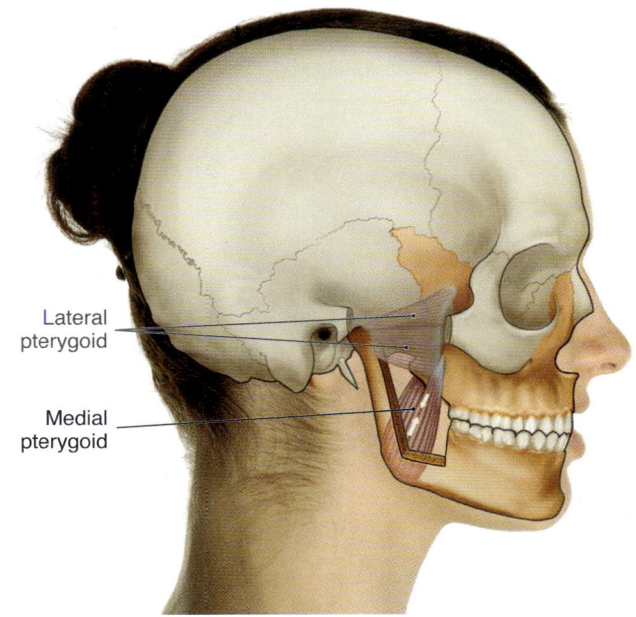

FIGURE 11-93 Lateral view of the right medial pterygoid with the lateral pterygoid ghosted in and with the mandible partially cut away.

DIGASTRIC (OF HYOID GROUP):

Attachments:
- **POSTERIOR BELLY:**
  - **Temporal Bone**
    - the mastoid notch of the temporal bone

  to the
  - **Hyoid**
    - the central tendon is bound to the hyoid bone at the body and the greater cornu

- **ANTERIOR BELLY:**
  - **Mandible**
    - the inner surface of the inferior border (the digastric fossa)

  to the
  - **Hyoid**
    - the central tendon is bound to the hyoid bone at the body and the greater cornu

Functions:

Major Standard Mover Actions	Major Reverse Mover Action
1. Depresses the mandible at the TMJs[1,2,4,5,7]	1. Elevates the hyoid bone[1,2,4,5,7]
2. Flexes the head and neck at the spinal joints[3,8,11]	

TMJs = temporomandibular joints

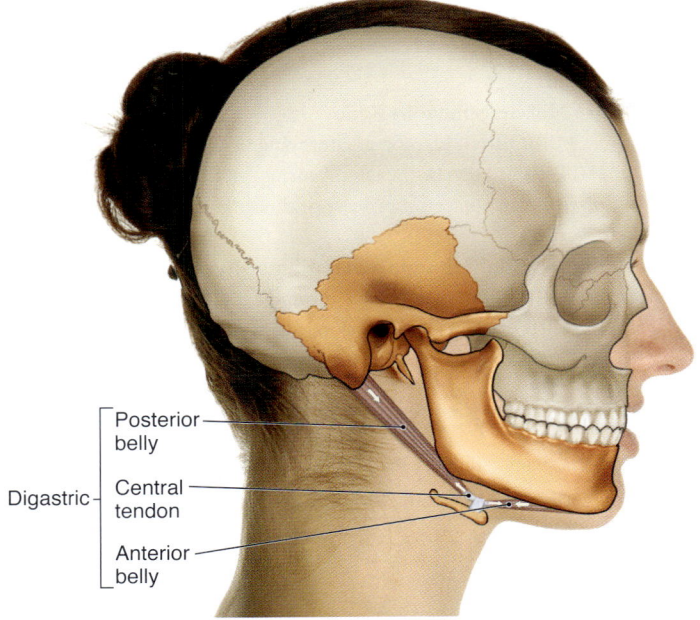

FIGURE 11-94 Lateral view of the right digastric.

MYLOHYOID (OF HYOID GROUP):

Attachments:
- **Inner Surface of the Mandible**
  - the mylohyoid line of the mandible (from the symphysis menti to the molars)

to the
- **Hyoid**
  - the anterior surface of the body of the hyoid

Functions:

Major Standard Mover Actions	Major Reverse Mover Action
1. Depresses the mandible at the TMJs[1,2,4,7]	1. Elevates the hyoid bone[1,2,4,5,7]
2. Flexes the head and neck at the spinal joints[3,8,11]	

TMJs = temporomandibular joints

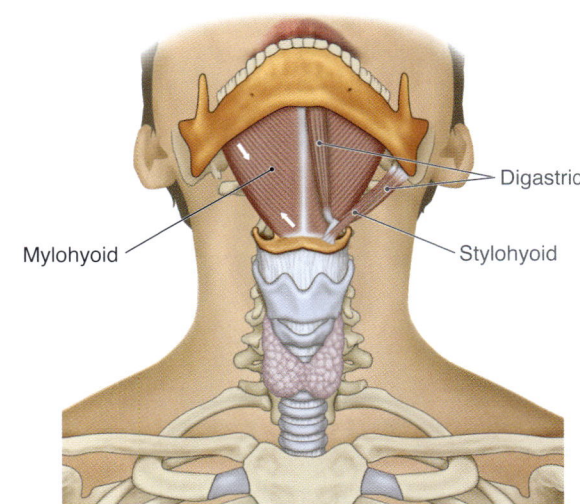

FIGURE 11-95 Anterior view of the mylohyoid bilaterally with the digastric and stylohyoid shown on the client's left side.

GENIOHYOID (OF HYOID GROUP):

Attachments:
- **Inner Surface of the Mandible**
  - the inferior mental spine of the mandible

to the

- **Hyoid**
  - the anterior surface of the body of the hyoid

Functions:

Major Standard Mover Actions	Major Reverse Mover Action
1. Depresses the mandible at the TMJs[1,2,4,5,7]	1. Elevates the hyoid bone[1,2,4,5,7]
2. Flexes the head and neck at the spinal joints[3,8]	

TMJs = temporomandibular joints

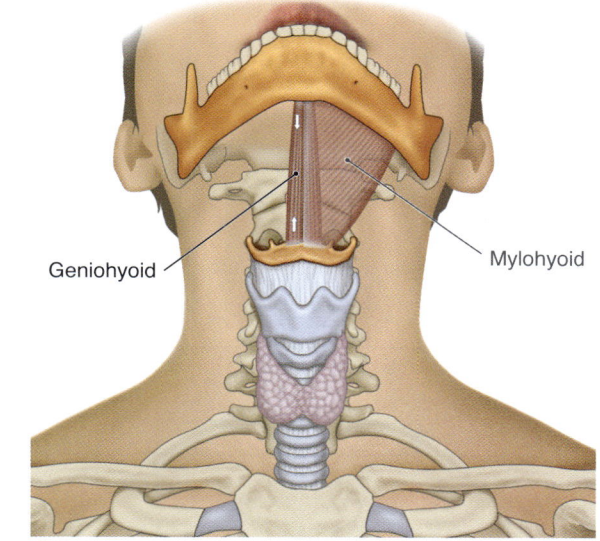

FIGURE 11-96 Anterior view of the geniohyoid bilaterally with the mylohyoid ghosted in on the client's left side.

STYLOHYOID (OF HYOID GROUP):

Attachments:
- **Styloid Process of the Temporal Bone**
  - the posterior surface

to the

- **Hyoid**
  - at the junction of the body and the greater cornu of the hyoid bone

Functions:

Major Standard Mover Action
1. Elevates the hyoid bone[1,2,4,5,7]

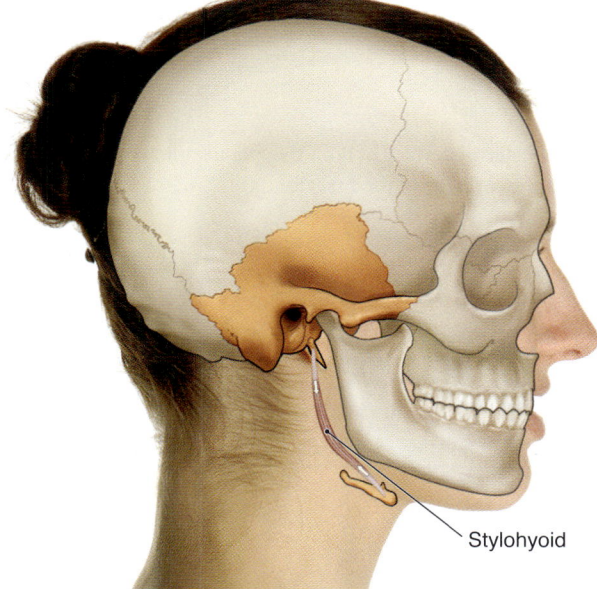

FIGURE 11-97 Lateral view of the right stylohyoid.

STERNOHYOID (OF HYOID GROUP):

Attachments:
- **Sternum**
  - the posterior surface of both the manubrium of the sternum and the medial clavicle
- *to the*
- **Hyoid**
  - the inferior surface of the body of the hyoid

Functions:

Major Standard Mover Actions
1. Depresses the hyoid bone[1,4,5,7]
2. Flexes the neck and head at the spinal joints[3,1]

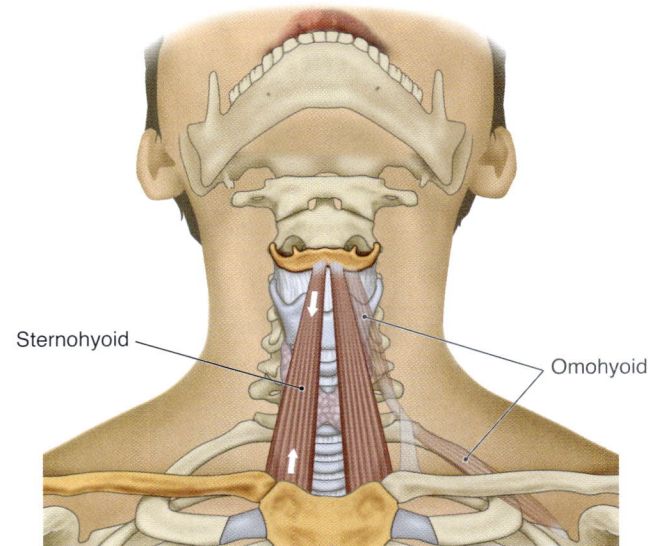

FIGURE 11-98 Anterior view of the sternohyoid bilaterally. The omohyoid has been ghosted in on the client's left side.

STERNOTHYROID (OF HYOID GROUP):

Attachments:
- **Sternum**
  - the posterior surface of both the manubrium of the sternum and the cartilage of the first rib
- *to the*
- **Thyroid Cartilage**
  - the lamina of the thyroid cartilage

Functions:

Major Standard Mover Actions
1. Depresses the thyroid cartilage[4,5,7]
2. Flexes the neck and head at the spinal joints[3,6]

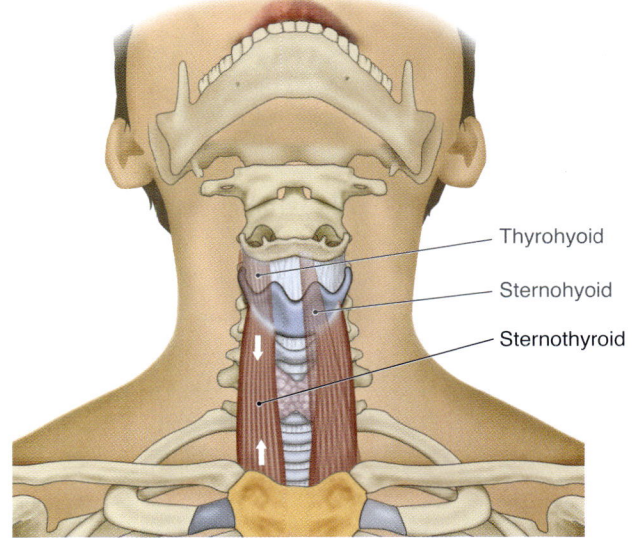

FIGURE 11-99 Anterior view of the sternothyroid bilaterally. The left sternohyoid and right thyrohyoid have been ghosted in.

THYROHYOID (OF HYOID GROUP):

Attachments:

- **Thyroid Cartilage**
  - the lamina of the thyroid cartilage

to the

- **Hyoid**
  - the inferior surface of the greater cornu of the hyoid

Functions:

Major Standard Mover Actions
1. Depresses the hyoid bone[1,4,5,7]
2. Flexes the neck and head at the spinal joints[3,4]

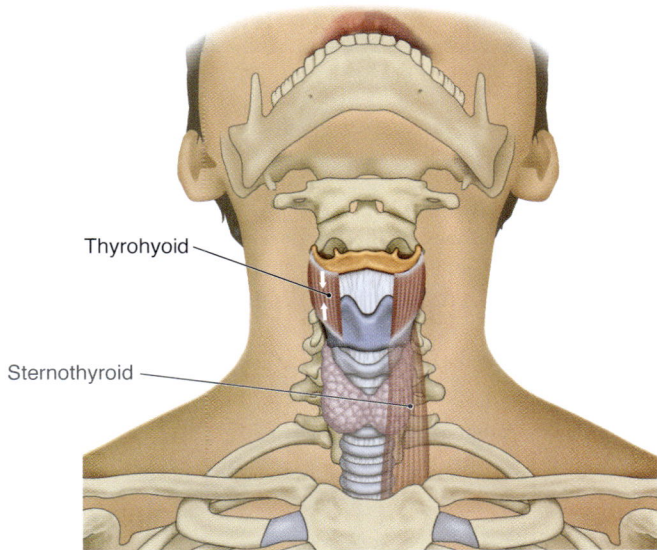

FIGURE 11-100 Anterior view of the thyrohyoid bilaterally. The sternothyroid has been ghosted in on the client's left side.

OMOHYOID (OF HYOID GROUP):

Attachments:

- **INFERIOR BELLY:**
  - **Scapula**
    - the superior border

to the

  - **Clavicle**
    - the central tendon is bound to the clavicle

- **SUPERIOR BELLY:**
  - **Clavicle**
    - the central tendon is bound to the clavicle

to the

  - **Hyoid**
    - the inferior surface of the body of the hyoid

Functions:

Major Standard Mover Actions
1. Depresses the hyoid bone[1,4,5,7]
2. Flexes the neck and head at the spinal joints[3,4]

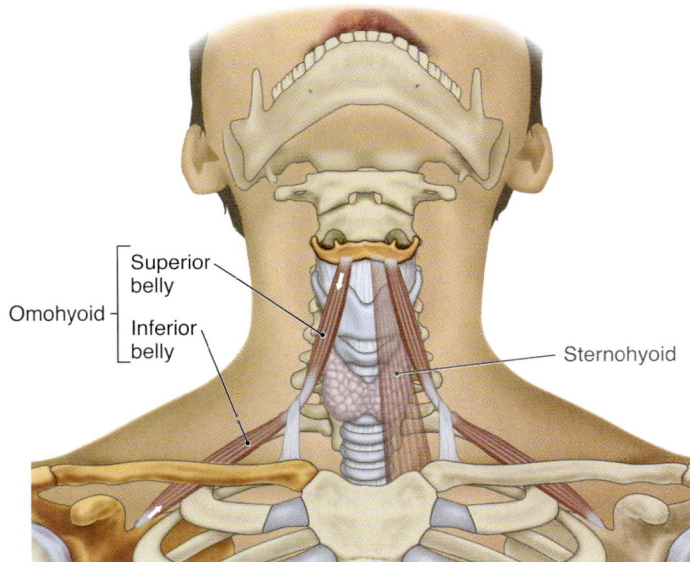

FIGURE 11-101 Anterior view of the omohyoid bilaterally. The sternohyoid has been ghosted in on the client's left side.

SECTION 11.11 MUSCLES OF FACIAL EXPRESSION

OCCIPITOFRONTALIS (OF EPICRANIUS):

Attachments:
- **OCCIPITALIS:**
  - Occipital Bone and the Temporal Bone
    - The lateral ⅔ of the highest nuchal line of the occipital bone and the mastoid area of the temporal bone

  to the
  - Galea Aponeurotica

- **FRONTALIS:**
  - Galea Aponeurotica

  to the
  - Fascia and Skin overlying the Frontal Bone

Functions:

Major Mover Action
1. Draws the scalp posteriorly (elevation of the eyebrow)[1,4–6]

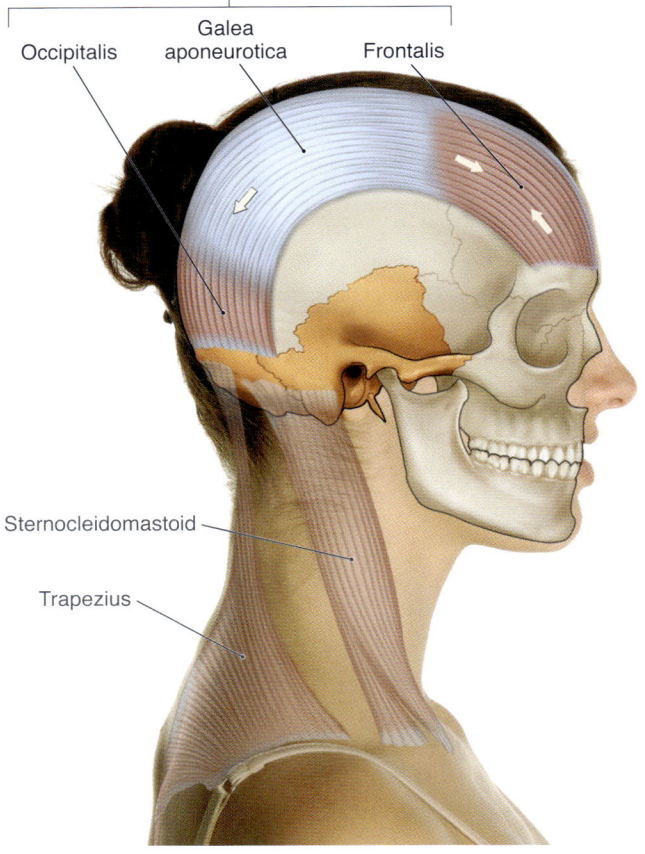

FIGURE 11-102 Lateral view of the right occipitofrontalis. The trapezius and sternocleidomastoid have been ghosted in.

TEMPOROPARIETALIS (OF EPICRANIUS):

Attachments:
- Fascia Superior to the Ear

to the
- Lateral Border of the Galea Aponeurotica

Functions:

Major Mover Action
1. Elevates the ear[8,12]

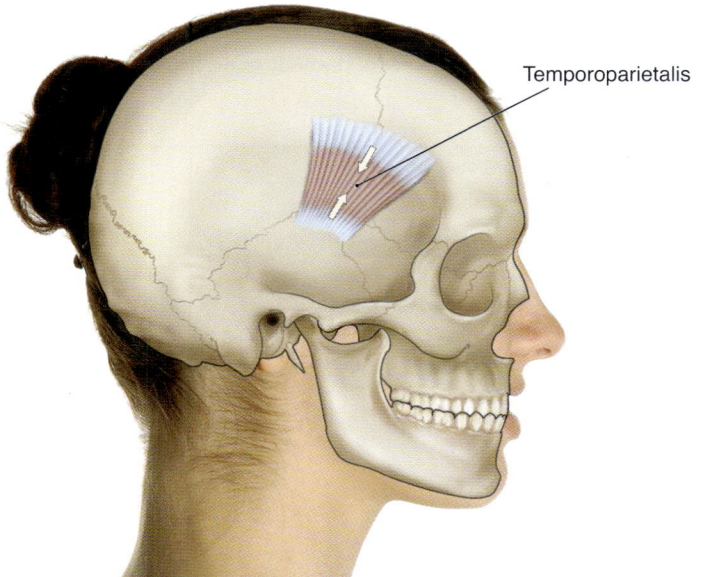

FIGURE 11-103 Lateral view of the right temporoparietalis.

AURICULARIS GROUP:

Attachments:

- **AURICULARIS ANTERIOR:**
Galea Aponeurotica
  - the lateral margin

to the

Anterior Ear
  - the spine of the helix

- **AURICULARIS SUPERIOR:**
Galea Aponeurotica
  - the lateral margin

to the

Superior Ear
  - the superior aspect of the cranial surface

- **AURICULARIS POSTERIOR:**
Temporal Bone
  - the mastoid area of the temporal bone

to the

Posterior Ear
  - the ponticulus of the eminentia conchae

Functions:

Major Mover Actions
1. Draws the ear anteriorly (auricularis anterior)[8,13,14]
2. Elevates the ear (auricularis superior)[8,13,14]
3. Draws the ear posteriorly (auricularis posterior)[8,13,14]

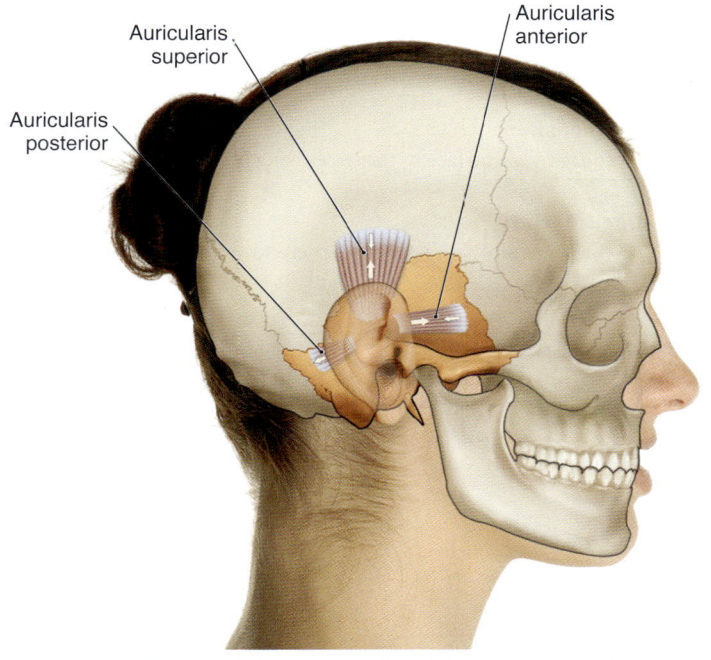

FIGURE 11-104 Lateral view of the right auricularis muscles.

ORBICULARIS OCULI:

Attachments:

- **Medial Side of the Eye**
  - ORBITAL PART: the nasal part of the frontal bone, the frontal process of the maxilla, and the medial palpebral ligament
  - PALPEBRAL PART: the medial palpebral ligament
  - LACRIMAL PART: the lacrimal bone

to the

- **Medial Side of the Eye (returns to the same attachment, encircling the eye)**
  - ORBITAL PART: returns to the same attachment (these fibers encircle the eye)
  - PALPEBRAL PART: the lateral palpebral ligament (these fibers run through the connective tissue of the eyelids)
  - LACRIMAL PART: the medial palpebral raphe (these fibers are deeper in the eye socket)

Functions:

Major Mover Action
1. Closes and squints the eye (orbital part)[1,4–6]

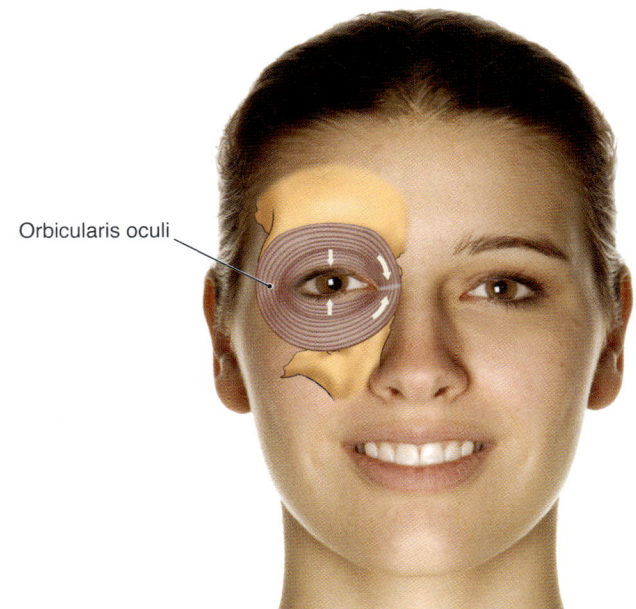

FIGURE 11-105 Anterior view of the right orbicularis oculi.

LEVATOR PALPEBRAE SUPERIORIS:

Attachments:
- **Sphenoid Bone**
  - the anterior surface of the lesser wing of the sphenoid
- *to the*
- **Upper Eyelid**
  - the fascia and skin of the upper eyelid

Functions:

Major Mover Action
1. Elevates the upper eyelid[1,4–6]

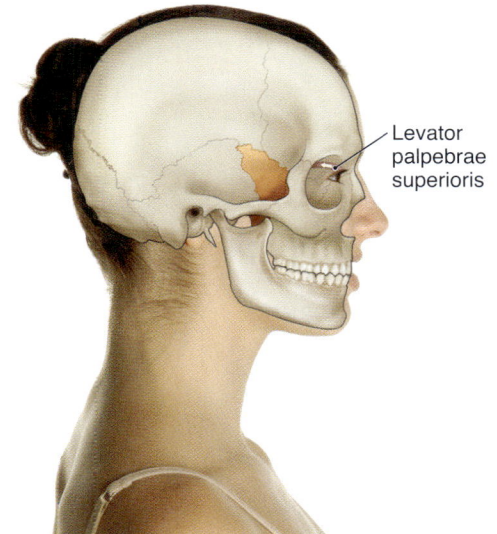

FIGURE 11-106 Lateral view of the right levator palpebrae superioris.

CORRUGATOR SUPERCILII:

Attachments:
- **Inferior Frontal Bone**
  - the medial end of the superciliary arch of the frontal bone
- *to the*
- **Fascia and Skin Deep to the Eyebrow**

Functions:

Major Mover Action
1. Draws the eyebrow inferomedially[1,4,6]

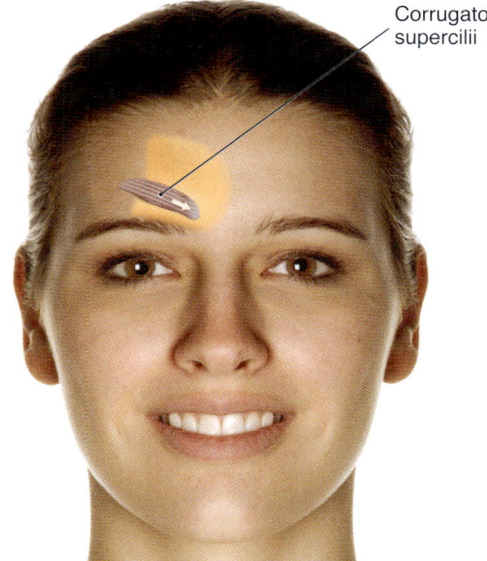

FIGURE 11-107 Anterior view of the right corrugator supercilii.

PROCERUS:

Attachments:
- Fascia and Skin over the Nasal Bone

to the
- Fascia and Skin Medial to the Eyebrow

Functions:

Major Mover Action
1. Wrinkles the skin of the nose upward[1,4,6]
2. Draws down the medial eyebrow[1,4,6]

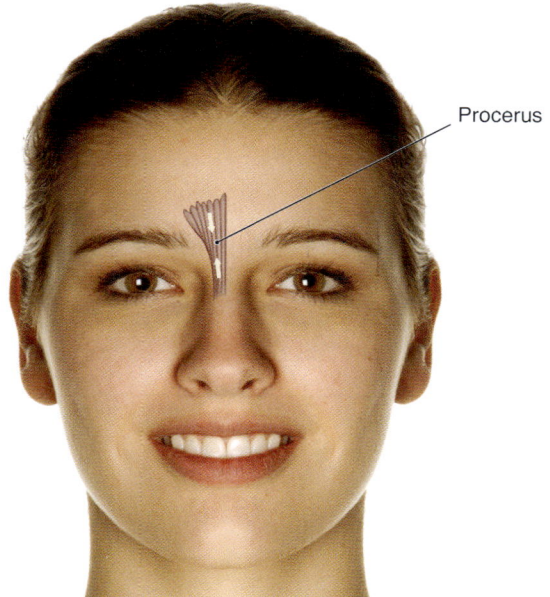

FIGURE 11-108 Anterior view of the right procerus.

NASALIS:

Attachments:
- **Maxilla**
  - ALAR PART: the maxilla, lateral to the lower part of the nose
  - TRANSVERSE PART: the maxilla, lateral to the upper part of the nose

to the
- **Cartilage of the Nose and the Opposite-Side Nasalis Muscle**
  - ALAR PART: the alar cartilage of the nose
  - TRANSVERSE PART: the opposite-side nasalis over the upper cartilage of the nose

Functions:

Major Mover Actions
1. Flares the nostril[1,4,6]
2. Constricts the nostril[1,4,6]

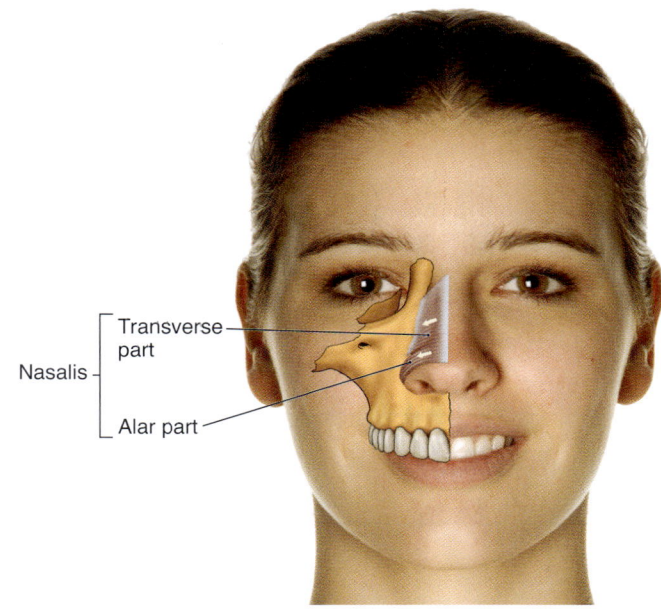

FIGURE 11-109 Anterior view of the right nasalis.

DEPRESSOR SEPTI NASI:

Attachments:

- **Maxilla**
  - the incisive fossa of the maxilla

to the

- **Cartilage of the Nose**
  - the septum and the alar cartilage of the nose

Functions:

Major Mover Action
1. Constricts the nostril[6,14]

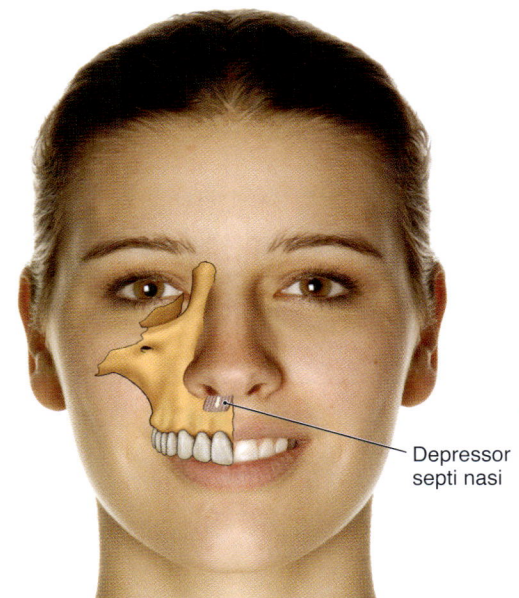

FIGURE 11-110 Anterior view of the right depressor septi nasi.

LEVATOR LABII SUPERIORIS ALAEQUE NASI:

Attachments:

- **Maxilla**
  - the frontal process of the maxilla near the nasal bone

to the

- **Upper Lip and the Nose**
  - LATERAL SLIP: the muscular substance of the lateral part of the upper lip
  - MEDIAL SLIP: the alar cartilage and the fascia and skin of the nose

Functions:

Major Mover Actions
1. Elevates the upper lip[1,4,6]
2. Flares the nostril[1,4]

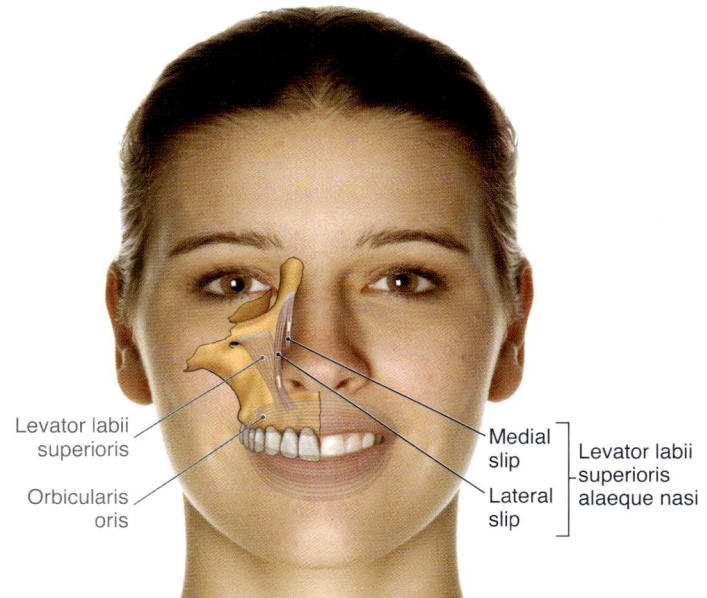

FIGURE 11-111 Anterior view of the right levator labii superioris alaeque nasi. The levator labii superioris and the orbicularis oris have been ghosted in.

LEVATOR LABII SUPERIORIS:

Attachments:

- **Maxilla**
  - at the inferior orbital margin of the maxilla

to the

- **Upper Lip**
  - the muscular substance of the upper lip

Functions:

Major Mover Action
1. Elevates the upper lip[1,4,6]

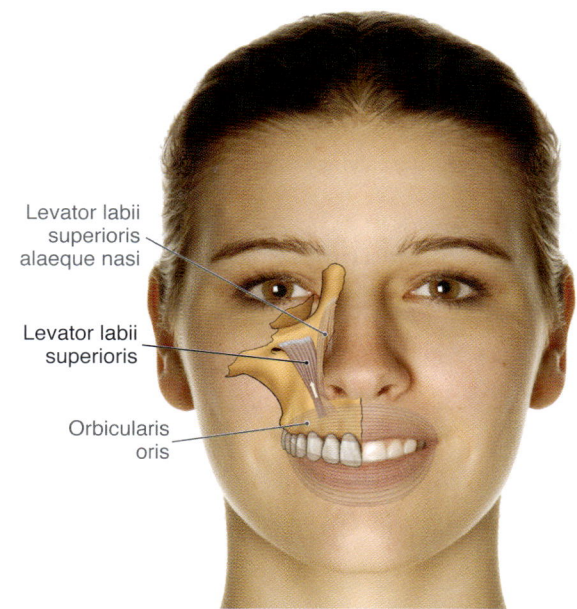

FIGURE 11-112 Anterior view of the right levator labii superioris. The levator labii superioris alaeque nasi and the orbicularis oris have been ghosted in.

ZYGOMATICUS MINOR:

Attachments:

- **Zygomatic Bone**
  - near the zygomaticomaxillary suture

to the

- **Upper Lip**
  - the muscular substance of the upper lip

Functions:

Major Mover Action
1. Elevates the upper lip[1,4-6]

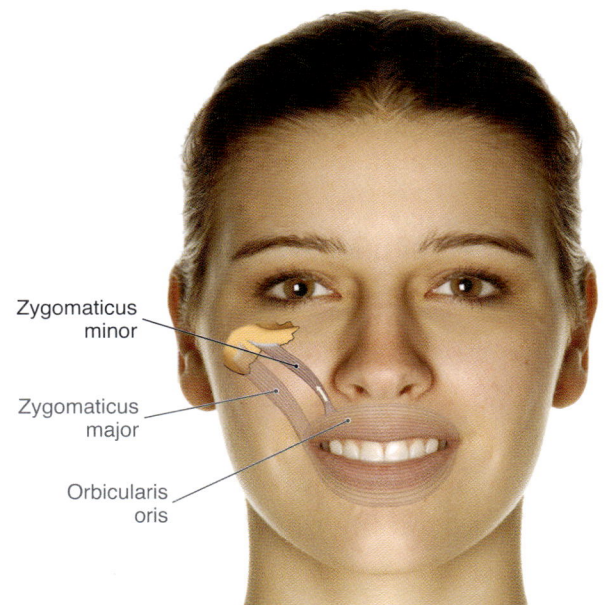

FIGURE 11-113 Anterior view of the right zygomaticus minor. The zygomaticus major and the orbicularis oris have been ghosted in.

ZYGOMATICUS MAJOR:

Attachments:

- **Zygomatic Bone**
  - near the zygomaticotemporal suture

to the

- **Angle of the Mouth**
  - the modiolus, just lateral to the angle of the mouth

Functions:

Major Mover Action
1. Elevates the angle of the mouth[1,4–6]

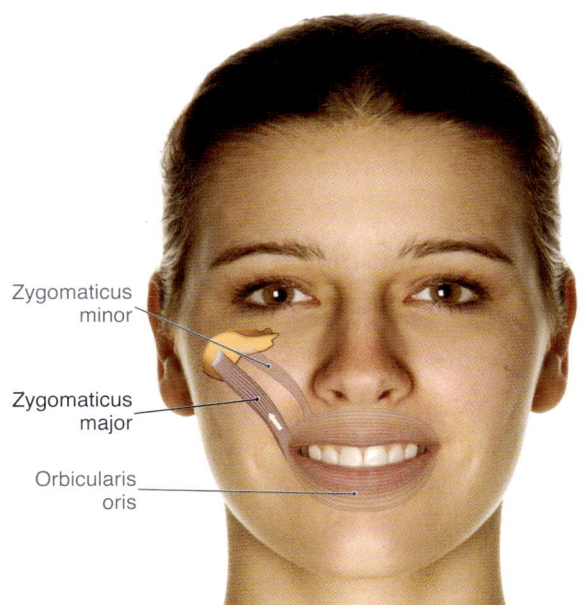

FIGURE 11-114 Anterior view of the right zygomaticus major. The zygomaticus minor and the orbicularis oris have been ghosted in.

LEVATOR ANGULI ORIS:

Attachments:

- **Maxilla**
  - the canine fossa of the maxilla (just inferior to the infraorbital foramen)

to the

- **Angle of the Mouth**
  - the modiolus, just lateral to the angle of the mouth

Functions:

Major Mover Action
1. Elevates the angle of the mouth[1,4,6]

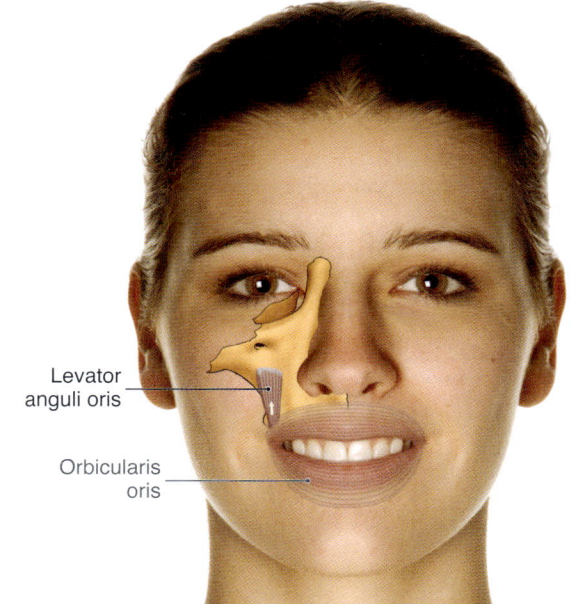

FIGURE 11-115 Anterior view of the right levator anguli oris. The orbicularis oris has been ghosted in.

RISORIUS:

Attachments:

- **Fascia and Skin Superficial to the Masseter**
to the
- **Angle of the Mouth**
  - the modiolus, just lateral to the angle of the mouth

Functions:

Major Mover Action
1. Draws laterally the angle of the mouth[1,4,6]

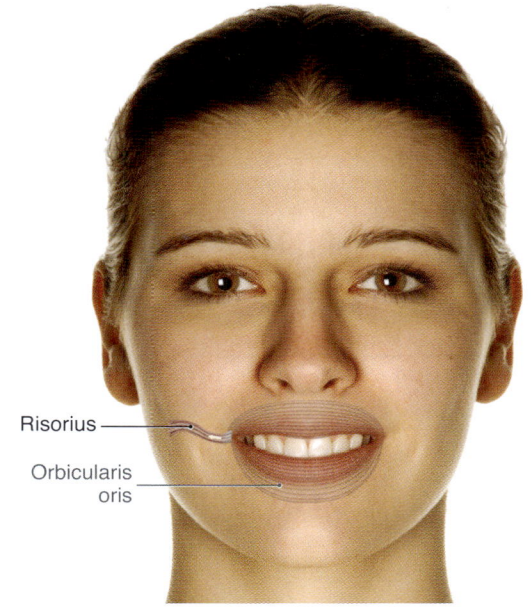

FIGURE 11-116 Anterior view of the right risorius. The orbicularis oris has been ghosted in.

DEPRESSOR ANGULI ORIS:

Attachments:

- **Mandible**
  - the oblique line of the mandible, inferior to the mental foramen
to the
- **Angle of the Mouth**
  - the modiolus, just lateral to the angle of the mouth

Functions:

Major Mover Action
1. Depresses the angle of the mouth[1,4,6]

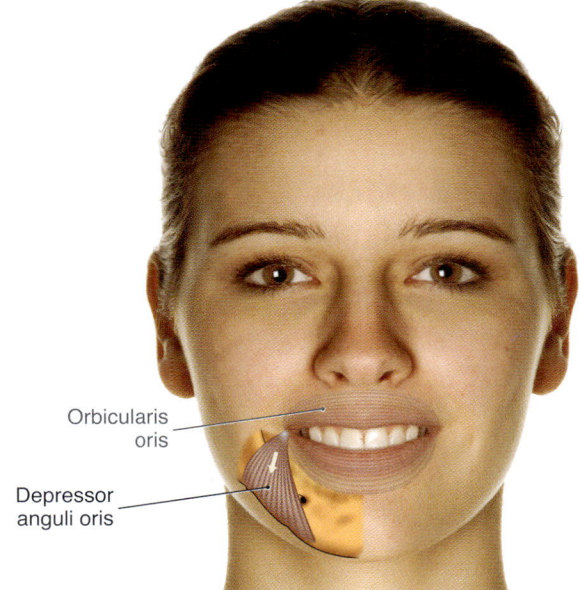

FIGURE 11-117 Anterior view of the right depressor anguli oris. The orbicularis oris has been ghosted in.

DEPRESSOR LABII INFERIORIS:

Attachments:

- **Mandible**
  - the oblique line of the mandible, between the symphysis menti and the mental foramen

to the

- **Lower Lip**
  - the midline of the lower lip

Functions:

Major Mover Action
1. Depresses the lower lip[1,4,6]

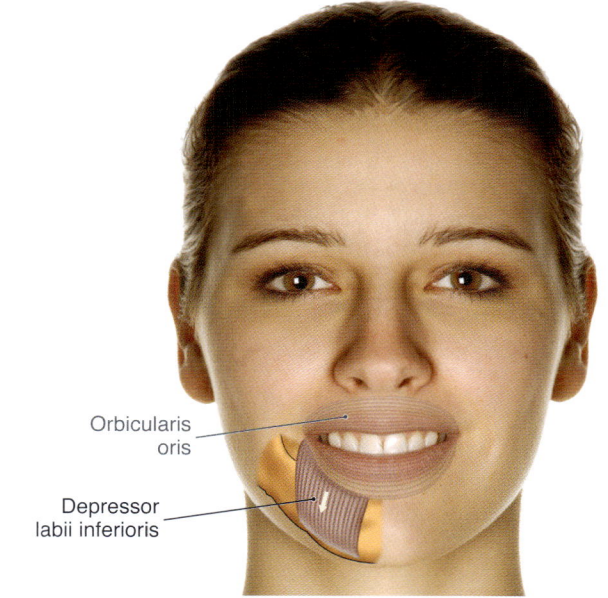

FIGURE 11-118 Anterior view of the right depressor labii inferioris. The orbicularis oris has been ghosted in.

MENTALIS:

Attachments:

- **Mandible**
  - the incisive fossa of the mandible

to the

- **Fascia and Skin of the Chin**

Functions:

Major Mover Action
1. Elevates the lower lip[1,4,6]
2. Everts and protracts the lower lip[1,4,6]

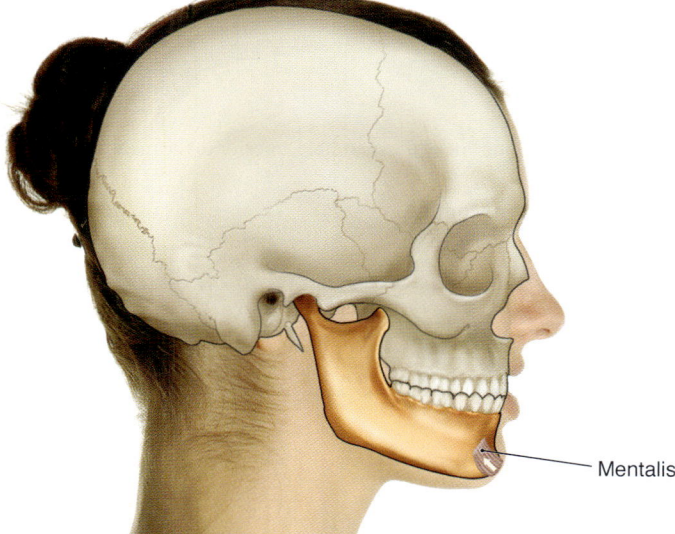

FIGURE 11-119 Right lateral view of the mentalis.

BUCCINATOR:

Attachments:

- **Maxilla and the Mandible**
  - the external surfaces of the alveolar processes of the mandible and the maxilla (opposite the molars), and the pterygomandibular raphe

to the

- **Lips**
  - deeper into the musculature of the lips and the modiolus, just lateral to the angle of the mouth

Functions:

Major Mover Action
1. Compresses the cheek against the teeth[1,4–6]

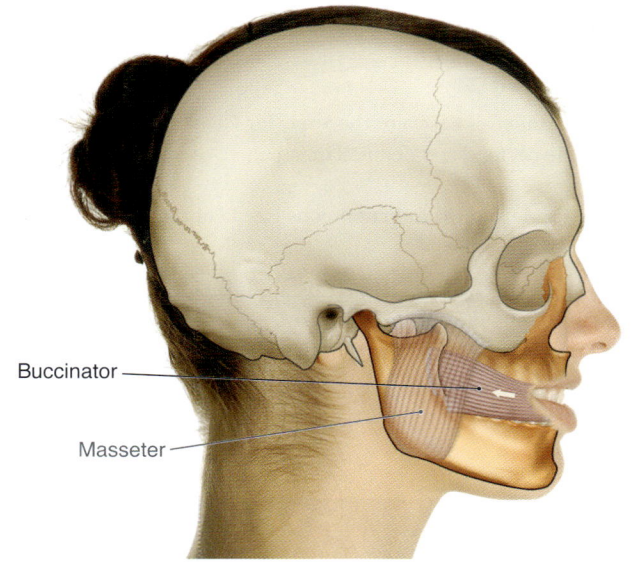

FIGURE 11-120 Right lateral view of the buccinator. The masseter has been ghosted in.

ORBICULARIS ORIS:

Attachments:

- **Orbicularis oris is a muscle that, in its entirety, surrounds the mouth.**
  - In more detail, there are four parts to the orbicularis oris: two on the left (upper and lower) and two on the right (upper and lower). Therefore there is one part in each of the four quadrants. Each of these four parts of the orbicularis oris anchors to the modiolus on that side. From there, the fibers traverse through the tissue of the upper or the lower lips. At the midline, the fibers on each side interlace with each other, thereby attaching into each other.

Functions:

Major Mover Actions
1. Closes the mouth[4,6]
2. Protracts the lips[6,13–15]

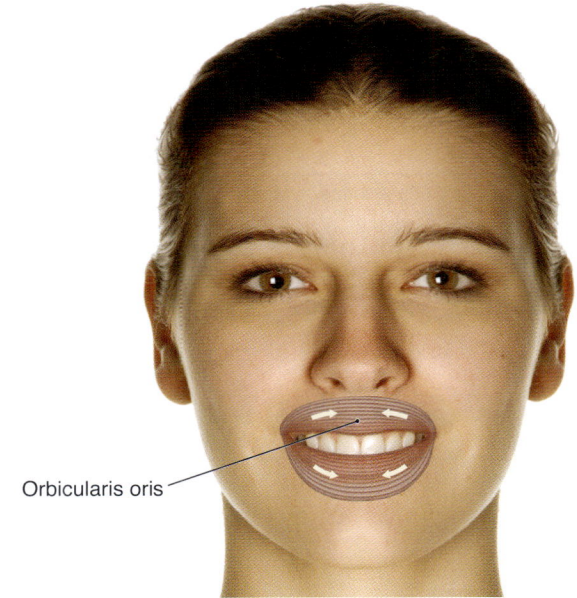

FIGURE 11-121 Anterior view of the orbicularis oris.

430 PART 4 Myology: Study of the Muscular System

PLATYSMA:

Attachments:

- **Subcutaneous Fascia of the Superior Chest**
  - the pectoral and deltoid fascia

to the

- **Mandible and the Subcutaneous Fascia of the Lower Face**

Functions:

Major Mover Action
1. Draws up the skin of the superior chest and neck, creating ridges of skin of the neck[1,5]

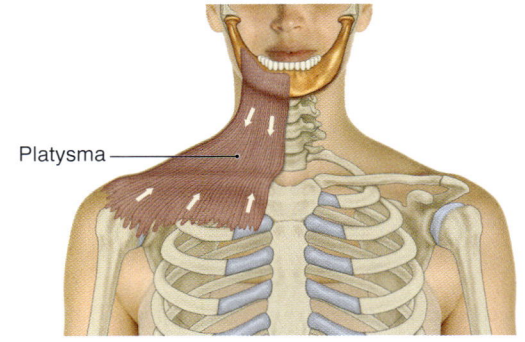

FIGURE 11-122 Anterior view of the right platysma.

SECTION 11.12 MUSCLES OF THE HIP JOINT

PSOAS MAJOR (OF ILIOPSOAS)

Attachments:

- **Anterolateral Lumbar Spine**
  - anterolaterally on the bodies of T12-L5 and the intervertebral discs between, and anteriorly on the TPs of L1-L5

to the

- **Lesser Trochanter of the Femur**

Functions:

Major Standard Mover Actions	Major Reverse Mover Actions
1. Flexes the thigh at the hip joint[1-4,6,7,10]	1. Flexes the trunk at the spinal joints[1-4,5,7,10]
2. Posteriorly tilts the pelvis at the LS joint[2,16,17]	2. Anteriorly tilts the pelvis at the hip joint[1-3,6,7,10]
3. Abducts the thigh at the hip joint[5,6,20,21]	
4. Laterally rotates the thigh at the hip joint[1,2,4,6,10]	3. Laterally flexes the trunk at the spinal joints[2-4,6,20]

LS joint = lumbosacral joint

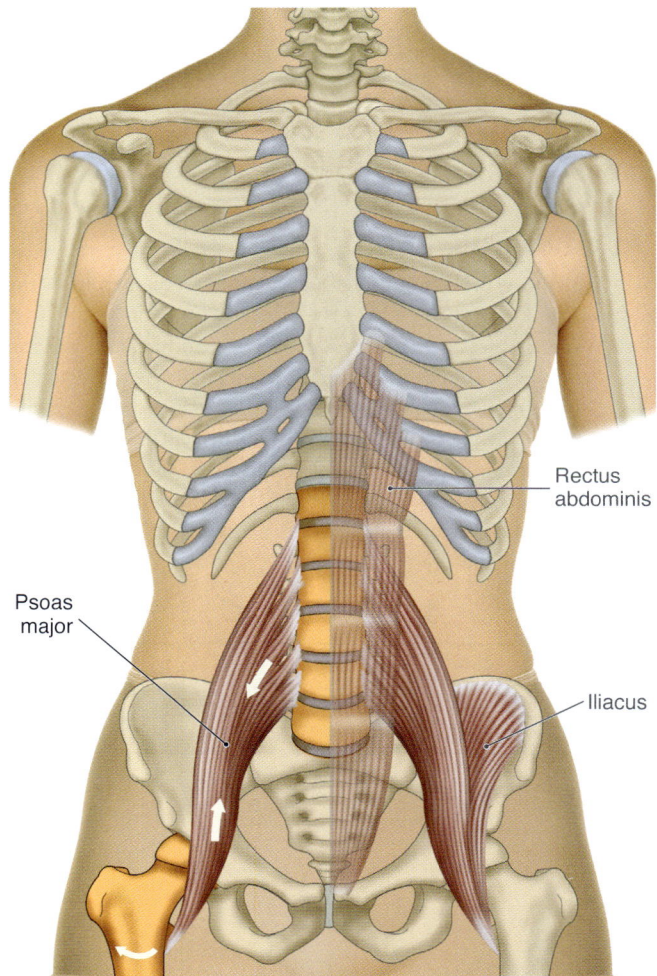

FIGURE 11-123 Anterior view of the psoas major bilaterally. The left iliacus has been drawn in, and the left rectus abdominis has been ghosted in.

ILIACUS (OF ILIOPSOAS):

Attachments:

- **Internal Ilium**
  - the upper of the iliac fossa, and the anterior inferior iliac spine (AIIS) and the sacral ala

to the

- **Lesser Trochanter of the Femur**

Functions:

Major Standard Mover Actions	Major Reverse Mover Action
1. Flexes the thigh at the hip joint[1–4,6,7,10]	1. Anteriorly tilts the pelvis at the hip joint[1–4,6,7]
2. Laterally rotates the thigh at the hip joint[1,2,4,6,10]	

TENSOR FASCIAE LATAE (TFL):

Attachments:

- **Anterior Superior Iliac Spine (ASIS)**
  - and the anterior iliac crest

to the

- **Iliotibial Band (ITB)**
  - ⅓ of the way down the thigh

Functions:

Major Standard Mover Actions	Major Reverse Mover Actions
1. Flexes the thigh at the hip joint[2–4,6,7,10]	1. Anteriorly tilts the pelvis at the hip joint[2–4,6,7,10]
2. Abducts the thigh at the hip joint[1–4,6,7,10]	2. Depresses the same-side pelvis at the hip joint[2–4,6,7,10]
3. Medially rotates the thigh at the hip joint[1,2,4,6,7,10]	

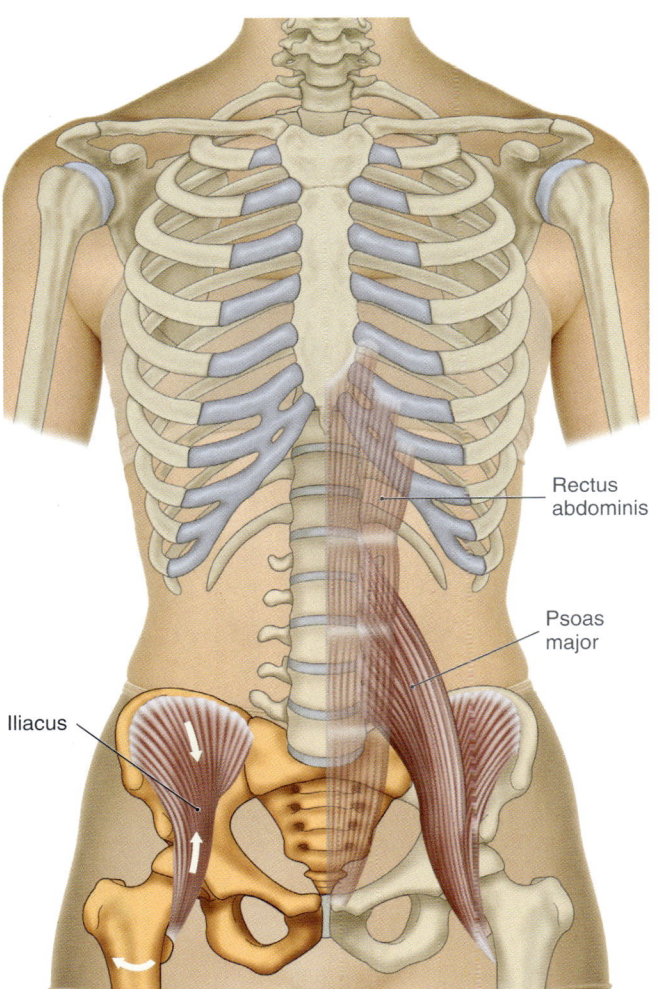

FIGURE 11-124 Anterior view of the iliacus bilaterally. The left psoas major has been drawn in, and the left rectus abdominis has been ghosted in.

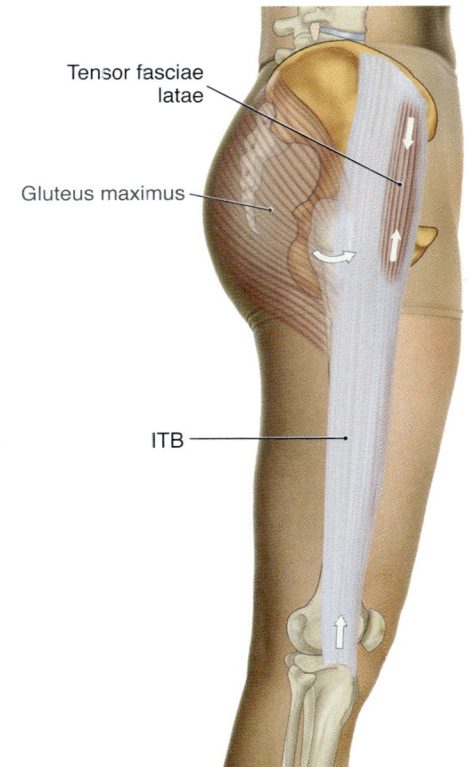

FIGURE 11-125 Lateral view of the right tensor fasciae latae (TFL). The gluteus maximus has been ghosted in. ITB, Iliotibial band.

SARTORIUS:

Attachments:

- Anterior Superior Iliac Spine (ASIS)

to the

- Pes Anserine Tendon (at the Proximal Anteromedial Tibia)

Functions:

Major Standard Mover Actions	Major Reverse Mover Action
1. Flexes the thigh at the hip joint[1–4,6,7,10]	1. Anteriorly tilts the pelvis at the hip joint[2–4,6,7,10]
2. Abducts the thigh at the hip joint[1–4,7,10]	
3. Laterally rotates the thigh at the hip joint[1–4,6,7]	
4. Flexes the leg at the knee joint[1–4,6,7,10]	

PECTINEUS (OF ADDUCTOR GROUP):

Attachments:

- Pubis
  - the pectineal line on the superior pubic ramus

to the

  - the pectineal line of the femur

Functions:

Major Standard Mover Actions	Major Reverse Mover Action
1. Flexes the thigh at the hip joint[1–7,6,7,10]	1. Anteriorly tilts the pelvis at the hip joint[2–4,6,7,10]
2. Adducts the thigh at the hip joint[1–4,6,7,10]	

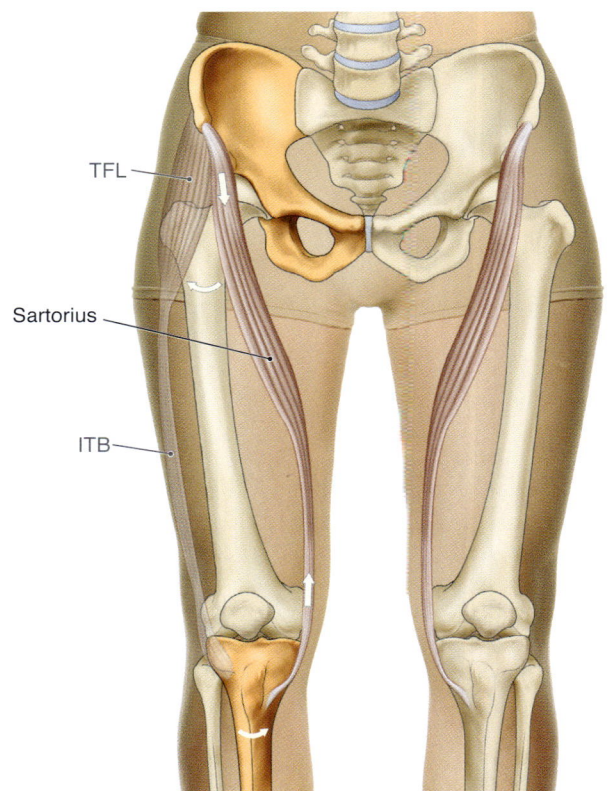

FIGURE 11-126 Anterior view of the sartorius bilaterally. The tensor fasciae latae (TFL) and iliotibial band (ITB) have been ghosted in on the right.

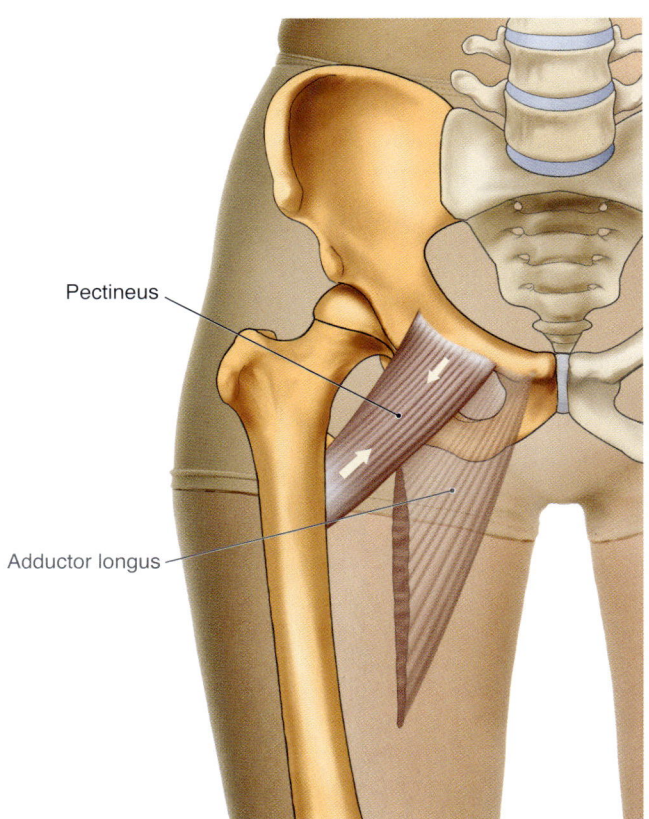

FIGURE 11-127 Anterior view of the right pectineus. The adductor longus has been cut and ghosted in.

ADDUCTOR LONGUS (OF ADDUCTOR GROUP):

Attachments:

- **Pubis**
  - the anterior body

to the

- **Linea Aspera of the Femur**
  - the middle ⅓ at the medial lip

Functions:

Major Standard Mover Actions	Major Reverse Mover Action
1. Adducts the thigh at the hip joint[1-4,6,7,10]	1. Anteriorly tilts the pelvis at the hip joint[2-4,6,7,10]
2. Flexes the thigh at the hip joint[2-4,6,7,10]	

GRACILIS (OF ADDUCTOR GROUP):

Attachments:

- **Pubis**
  - the anterior body and the inferior ramus

to the

- **Pes Anserine Tendon (at the Proximal Anteromedial Tibia)**

Functions:

Major Standard Mover Actions	Major Reverse Mover Action
1. Adducts the thigh at the hip joint[1-4,6,7,10]	1. Anteriorly tilts the pelvis at the hip joint[2,3,7,10]
2. Flexes the thigh at the hip joint[2,3,7,10]	
3. Flexes the leg at the knee joint[1-4,6,7,10]	

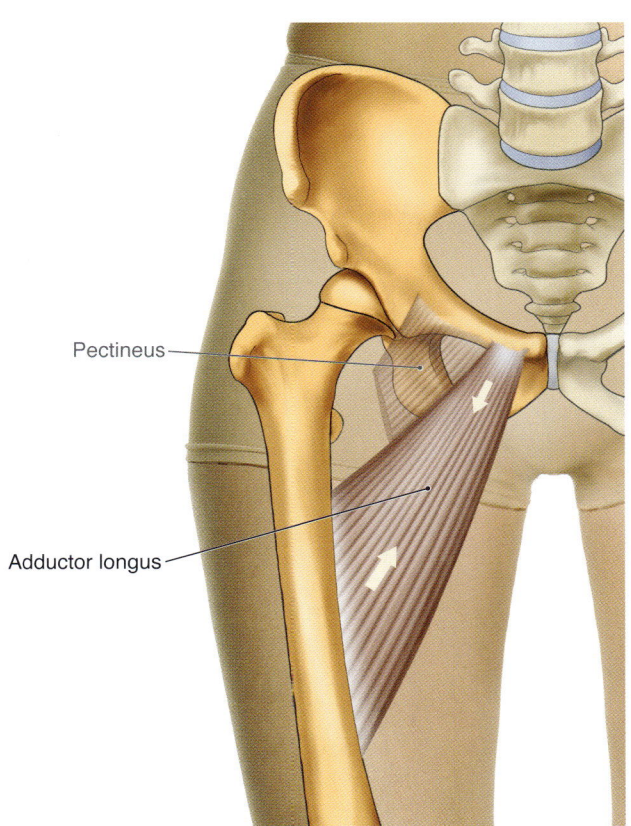

FIGURE 11-128 Anterior view of the right adductor longus. The pectineus has been cut and ghosted in.

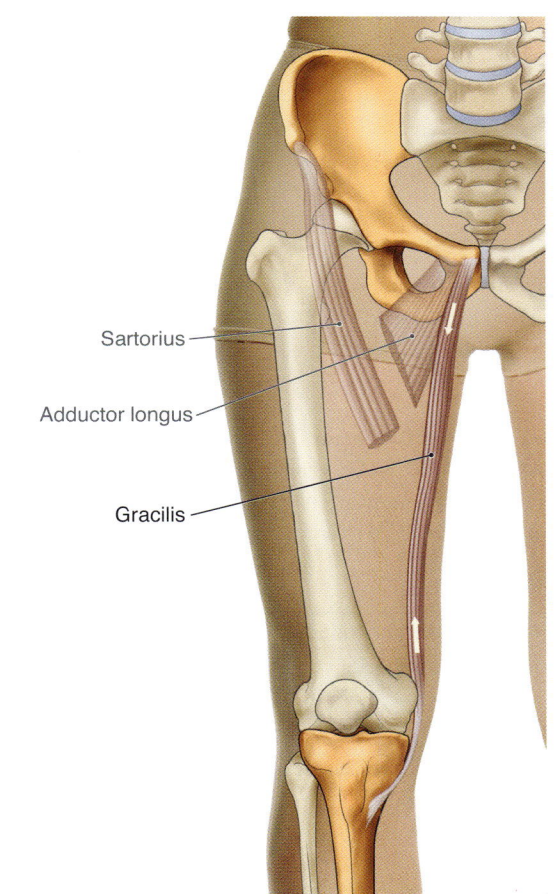

FIGURE 11-129 Anterior view of the right gracilis. The adductor longus and sartorius have been cut and ghosted in.

ADDUCTOR BREVIS (OF ADDUCTOR GROUP):

Attachments:

- **Pubis**
  - the inferior ramus

to the

- **Linea Aspera of the Femur**
  - the proximal ⅓

Functions:

Major Standard Mover Actions	Major Reverse Mover Action
1. Adducts the thigh at the hip joint[1-4,6,7,10]	1. Anteriorly tilts the pelvis at the hip joint[2-4,6,10]
2. Flexes the thigh at the hip joint[2-4,6,10]	

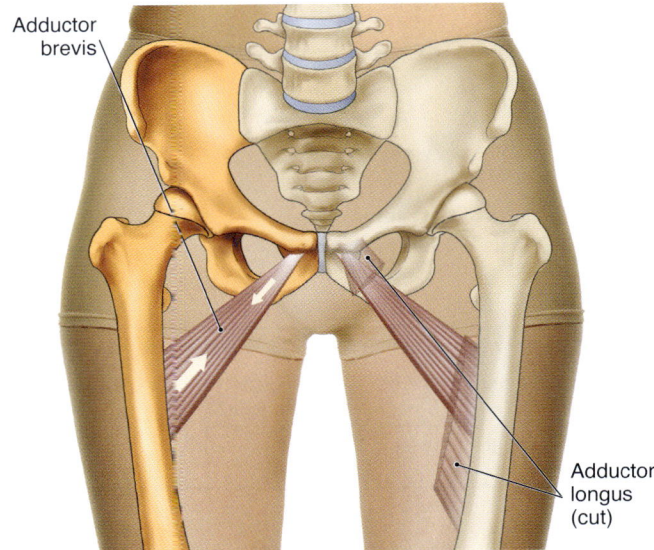

FIGURE 11-130 Anterior view of the adductor brevis bilaterally. The adductor longus has been cut and ghosted in on the left.

ADDUCTOR MAGNUS (OF ADDUCTOR GROUP):

Attachments:

- **Pubis and Ischium**
  - ANTERIOR HEAD: inferior pubic ramus and the ramus of the ischium
  - POSTERIOR HEAD: ischial tuberosity

to the

- **Linea Aspera of the Femur**
  - ANTERIOR HEAD: gluteal tuberosity, linea aspera, and medial supracondylar line of the femur
  - POSTERIOR HEAD: adductor tubercle of the femur

Functions:

Major Standard Mover Actions	Major Reverse Mover Action
1. Adducts the thigh at the hip joint[1-4,6,7,10]	1. Posteriorly tilts the pelvis at the hip joint[2-4,6,7,10]
2. Extends the thigh at the hip joint[1-4,6,7,10]	

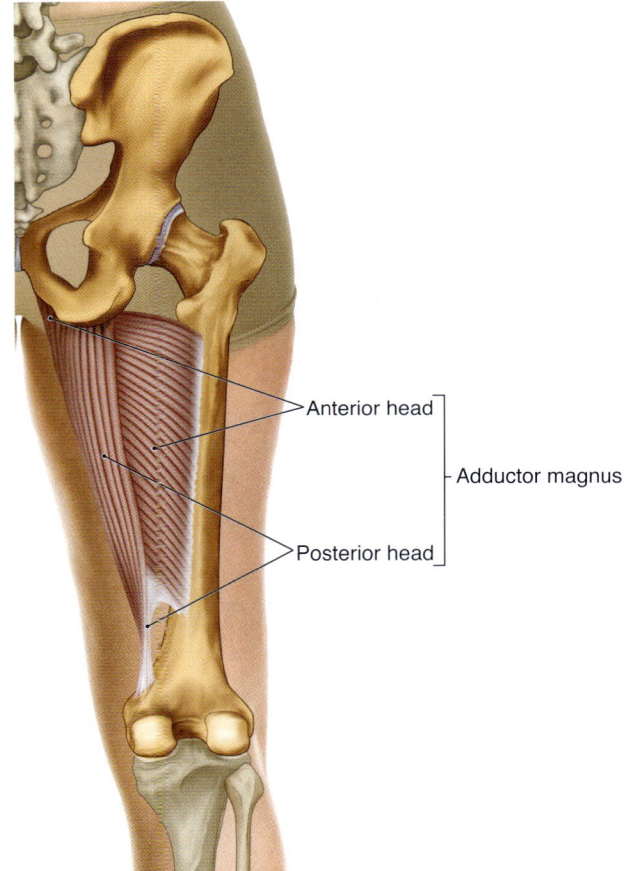

FIGURE 11-131 Posterior view of the right adductor magnus.

CHAPTER 11 Attachments and Actions of Muscles

GLUTEUS MAXIMUS (OF GLUTEAL GROUP):

Attachments:

- **Posterior Iliac Crest, the Posterolateral Sacrum, and the Coccyx**
  - and the sacrotuberous ligament, the thoracolumbar fascia, and the fascia over the gluteus medius

to the

- **Iliotibial Band (ITB) and the Gluteal Tuberosity of the Femur**

Functions:

Major Standard Mover Actions	Major Reverse Mover Actions
1. Extends the thigh at the hip joint[1–4,6,7,10]	1. Posteriorly tilts the pelvis at the hip joint[1–4,6,7,10]
2. Laterally rotates the thigh at the hip joint[1–4,6,7,10]	2. Contralaterally rotates the pelvis at the hip joint[2–4,6,7,10]
3. Abducts the thigh at the hip joint (upper ⅓)[1,3,4,6,7,10]	
4. Adducts the thigh at the hip joint (lower ⅔)[2–4,6,10]	

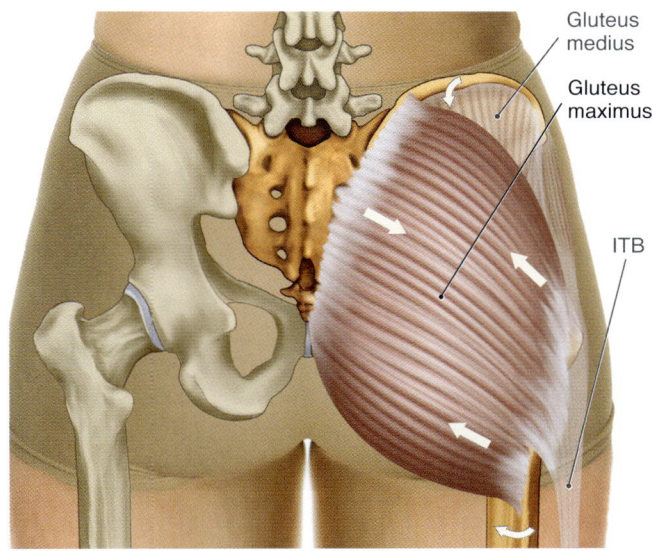

FIGURE 11-132 Posterior view of the right gluteus maximus. The gluteus medius and iliotibial band (ITB) have been ghosted in.

GLUTEUS MEDIUS (OF GLUTEAL GROUP):

Attachments:

- **External Ilium**
  - inferior to the iliac crest and between the anterior and posterior gluteal lines

to the

- **Greater Trochanter of the Femur**
  - the lateral surface

Functions:

Major Standard Mover Actions	Major Reverse Mover Actions
1. Abducts the thigh at the hip joint (entire muscle)[1–4,6,7,10]	1. Depresses the same-side pelvis at the hip joint[1–4,6,7,10]
2. Extends the thigh at the hip joint (posterior fibers)[2,6,7]	2. Posteriorly tilts the pelvis at the hip joint[2,6,7]
3. Flexes the thigh at the hip joint (anterior fibers)[6,7,10]	3. Anteriorly tilts the pelvis at the hip joint[6,7,10]
4. Laterally rotates the thigh at the hip joint (posterior fibers)[2,4,6,7,10]	4. Contralaterally rotates the pelvis at the hip joint[2,4,6,7,10]
5. Medially rotates the thigh at the hip joint (anterior fibers)[1–4,6,7,10]	

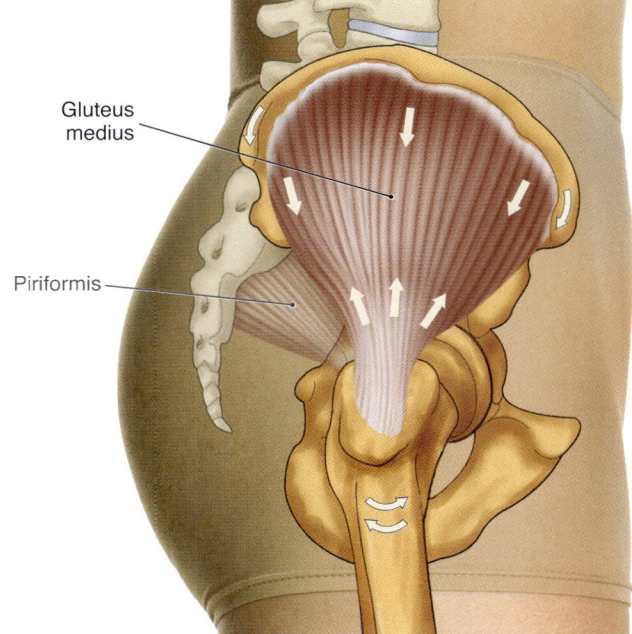

FIGURE 11-133 Lateral view of the right gluteus medius. The piriformis has been ghosted in.

GLUTEUS MINIMUS (OF GLUTEAL GROUP):

Attachments:

- **External Ilium**
  - between the anterior and inferior gluteal lines

to the

- **Greater Trochanter of the Femur**
  - the anterior surface

Functions:

Major Standard Mover Actions	Major Reverse Mover Actions
1. Abducts the thigh at the hip joint (entire muscle)[1-4,6,7,10]	1. Depresses the same-side pelvis at the hip joint[2-4,6,7,10]
2. Flexes the thigh at the hip joint (anterior fibers)[2,6,7,18]	2. Anteriorly tilts the pelvis at the hip joint[2,6,7,18]
3. Extends the thigh at the hip joint (posterior fibers)[12,13,19]	3. Posteriorly tilts the pelvis at the hip joint[1,2,13,19]
4. Medially rotates the thigh at the hip joint (anterior fibers)[1-4,6,7,10]	
5. Laterally rotates the thigh at the hip joint (posterior fibers)[2,4,7,10]	4. Contralaterally rotates the pelvis at the hip joint[2,4,7,10]

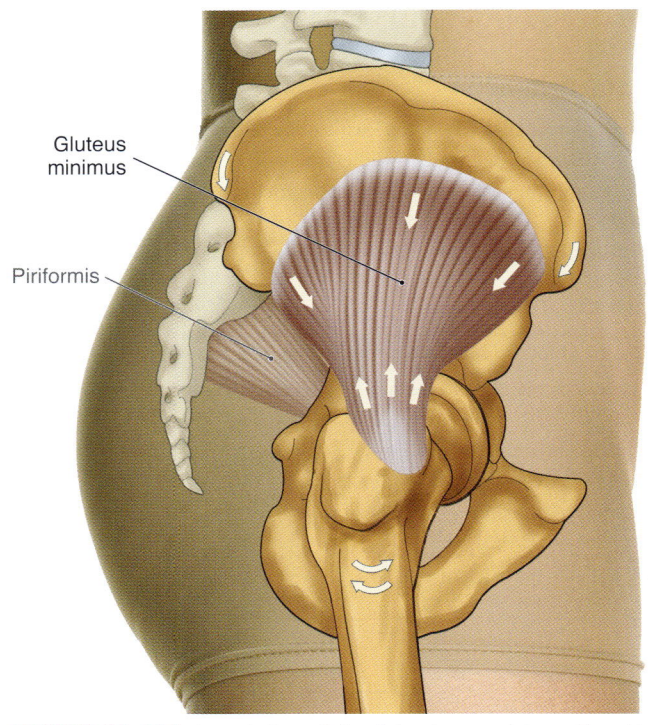

FIGURE 11-134 Lateral view of the right gluteus minimus. The piriformis has been ghosted in.

PIRIFORMIS (OF DEEP LATERAL ROTATOR GROUP):

Attachments:

- **Anterior Sacrum**
  - and the anterior surface of the sacrotuberous ligament

to the

- **Greater Trochanter of the Femur**
  - the superomedial surface

Functions:

Major Standard Mover Actions	Major Reverse Mover Action
1. Laterally rotates the thigh at the hip joint[1-4,6,7,10]	1. Contralaterally rotates the pelvis at the hip joint[2-4,7]
2. Horizontally extends the thigh at the hip joint[1,10]	
3. Medially rotates the thigh at the hip joint[2,4,7,10]	

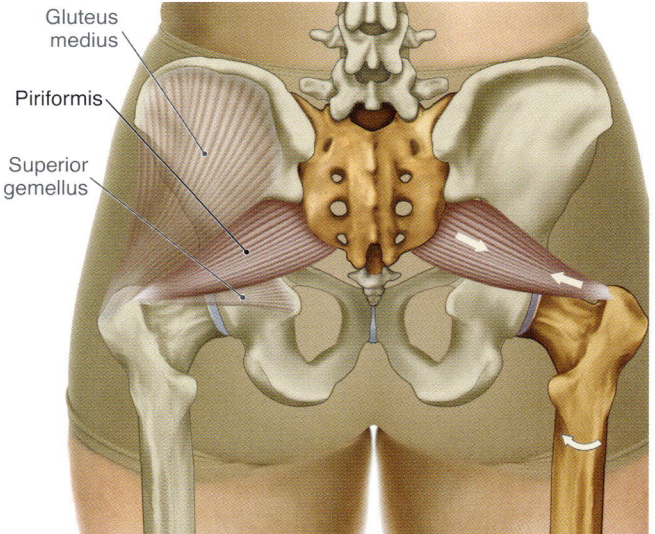

FIGURE 11-135 Posterior view of the piriformis bilaterally. The gluteus medius and superior gemellus have been ghosted in on the left.

SUPERIOR GEMELLUS (OF DEEP LATERAL ROTATOR GROUP):

Attachments:
- **Ischial Spine**

to the
- **Greater Trochanter of the Femur**
  - the medial surface

Functions:

Major Standard Mover Action	Major Reverse Mover Action
1. Laterally rotates the thigh at the hip joint[2-4,6,7,10]	1. Contralaterally rotates the pelvis at the hip joint[2-4,7,10]

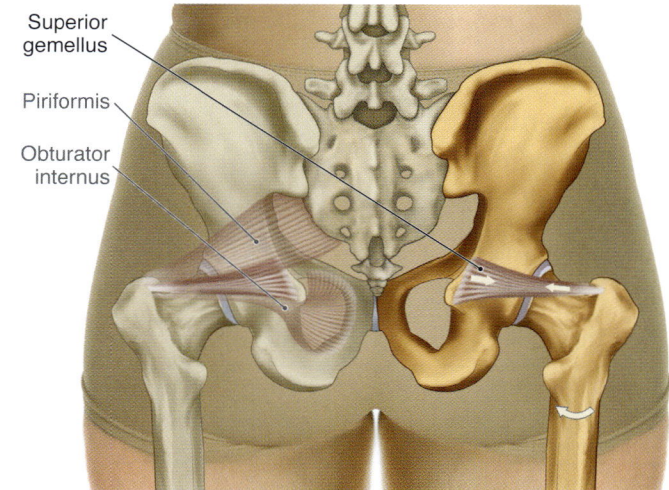

FIGURE 11-136 Posterior view of the superior gemellus bilaterally. The piriformis and obturator internus have been ghosted in on the left.

OBTURATOR INTERNUS (OF DEEP LATERAL ROTATOR GROUP):

Attachments:
- **Internal Surface of the Pelvic Bone Surrounding the Obturator Foramen**
  - the internal surfaces of the margin of the obturator foramen, the obturator membrane, the ischium, the pubis, and the ilium

to the
- **Greater Trochanter of the Femur**
  - the medial surface

Functions:

Major Standard Mover Action	Major Reverse Mover Action
1. Laterally rotates the thigh at the hip joint[1-4,7,10]	1. Contralaterally rotates the pelvis at the hip joint[2-4,7,10]

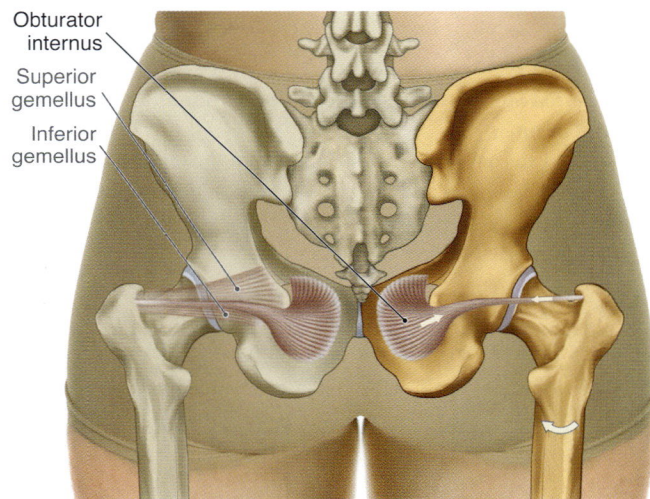

FIGURE 11-137 Posterior view of the obturator internus bilaterally. The superior gemellus and inferior gemellus have been ghosted in on the left.

INFERIOR GEMELLUS (OF DEEP LATERAL ROTATOR GROUP):

Attachments:

- **Ischial Tuberosity**
  - the superior aspect

to the

- **Greater Trochanter of the Femur**
  - the medial surface

Functions:

Major Standard Mover Action	Major Reverse Mover Action
1. Laterally rotates the thigh at the hip joint[1–4,6,7,10]	1. Contralaterally rotates the pelvis at the hip joint[2–4,7,10]

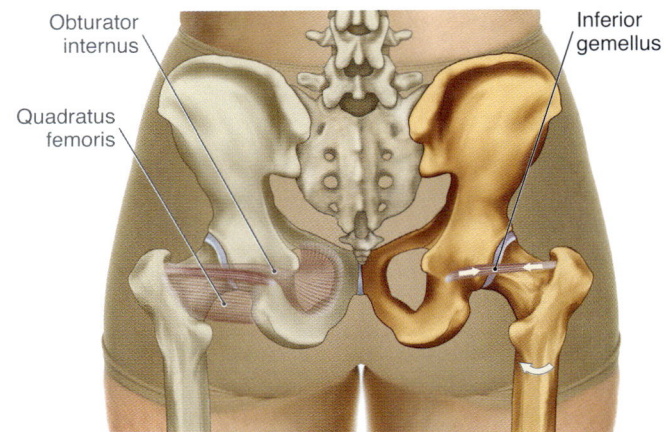

FIGURE 11-138 Posterior view of the inferior gemellus bilaterally. The obturator internus and quadratus femoris have been ghosted in on the left.

OBTURATOR EXTERNUS (OF DEEP LATERAL ROTATOR GROUP):

Attachments:

- **External Surface of the Pelvic Bone Surrounding the Obturator Foramen**
  - the external surfaces of the margin of the obturator foramen on the ischium and the pubis, and the obturator membrane

to the

- **Trochanteric Fossa of the Femur**

Functions:

Major Standard Mover Action	Major Reverse Mover Action
1. Laterally rotates the thigh at the hip joint[1–4,6,7,10]	1. Contralaterally rotates the pelvis at the hip joint[2–4,6,7,10]

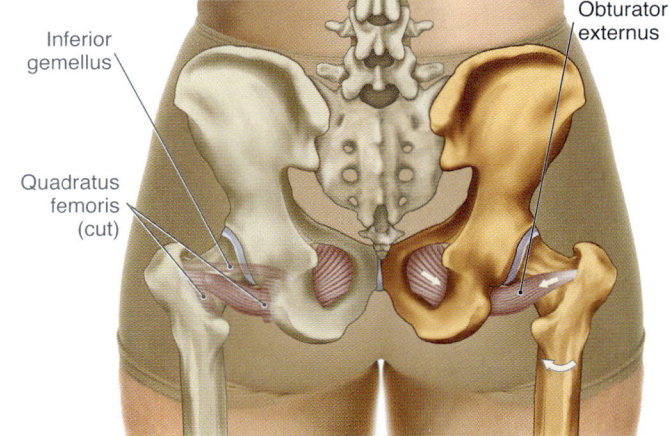

FIGURE 11-139 Posterior view of the obturator externus bilaterally. The inferior gemellus and quadratus femoris (cut) have been ghosted in on the left.

QUADRATUS FEMORIS (OF DEEP LATERAL ROTATOR GROUP):

Attachments:

- **Ischial Tuberosity**
  - the lateral border

to the

- **Intertrochanteric Crest of the Femur**

Functions:

Major Standard Mover Action	Major Reverse Mover Action
1. Laterally rotates the thigh at the hip joint[1–4,6,7,10]	1. Contralaterally rotates the pelvis at the hip joint[2–4,7,10]

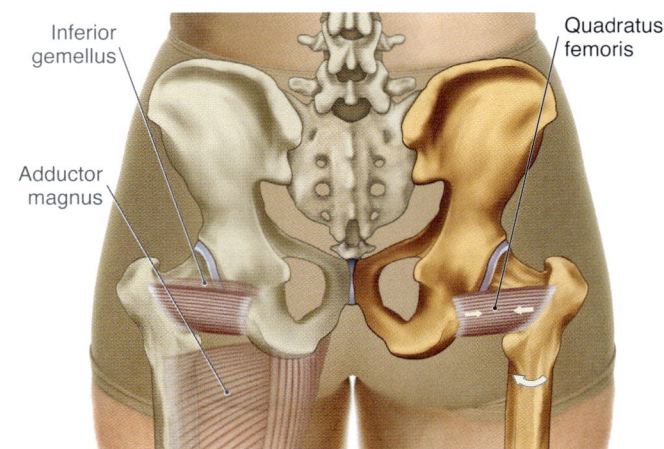

FIGURE 11-140 Posterior view of the quadratus femoris bilaterally. The inferior gemellus and adductor magnus have been ghosted in on the left.

SECTION 11.13   MUSCLES OF THE KNEE JOINT

RECTUS FEMORIS (OF QUADRICEPS FEMORIS GROUP):

Attachments:

- **Anterior Inferior Iliac Spine (AIIS)**
  - and just superior to the brim of the acetabulum

to the

- **Tibial Tuberosity via the Patella and the Patellar Ligament**
  - and the tibial condyles via the retinacular fibers

Functions:

Major Standard Mover Actions	Major Reverse Mover Actions
1. Extends the leg at the knee joint[1–4,6,7,10]	1. Extends the thigh at the knee joint[1–4,6,7]
2. Flexes the thigh at the hip joint[1–4,7,10]	2. Anteriorly tilts the pelvis at the hip joint[1–4,6,7,10]

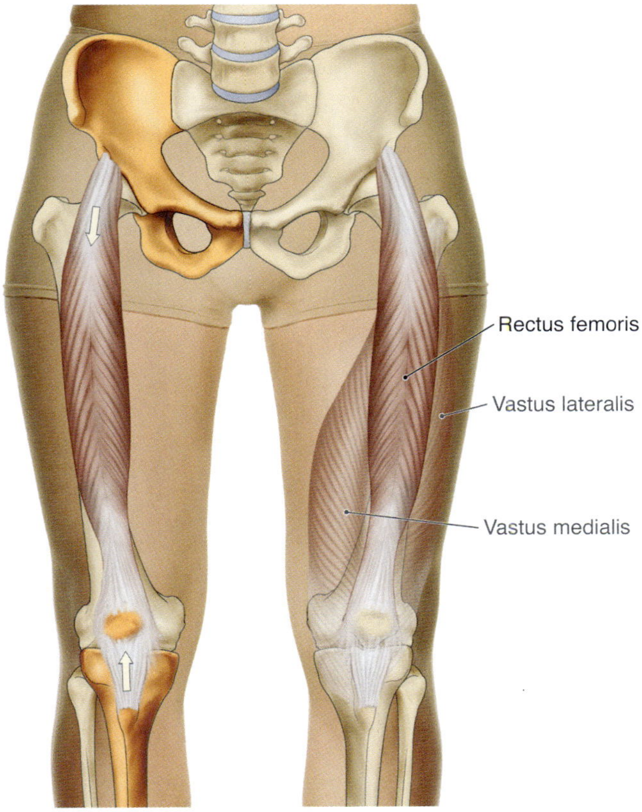

VASTUS LATERALIS (OF QUADRICEPS FEMORIS GROUP):

Attachments:

- **Linea Aspera of the Femur**
  - the lateral lip of the linea aspera of the femur, and the intertrochanteric line and gluteal tuberosity of the femur

to the

- **Tibial Tuberosity via the Patella and the Patellar Ligament**
  - and the tibial condyles via the retinacular fibers

Functions:

Major Standard Mover Action	Major Reverse Mover Action
1. Extends the leg at the knee joint[1–4,6,7,10]	1. Extends the thigh at the knee joint[1–4,6,7,10]

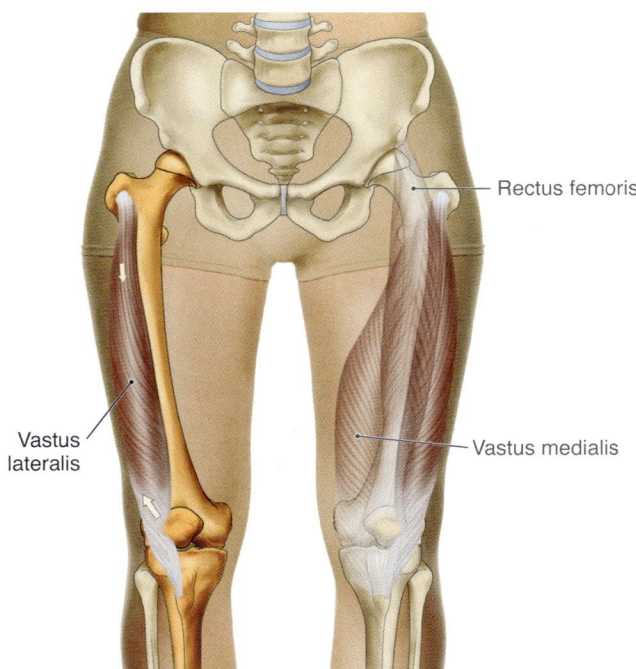

FIGURE 11-142 Anterior view of the vastus lateralis bilaterally. The rest of the quadriceps femoris group has been ghosted in on the left.

FIGURE 11-141 Anterior view of the rectus femoris bilaterally. The rest of the quadriceps femoris group has been ghosted in on the left.

VASTUS MEDIALIS (OF QUADRICEPS FEMORIS GROUP):

Attachments:

- **Linea Aspera of the Femur**
  - the medial lip of the linea aspera, and the intertrochanteric line and the medial supracondylar line of the femur

to the

- **Tibial Tuberosity via the Patella and the Patellar Ligament**
  - and the tibial condyles via the retinacular fibers

Functions:

Major Standard Mover Action	Major Reverse Mover Action
1. Extends the leg at the knee joint[1–4,6,7,10]	1. Extends the thigh at the knee joint[1–4,6,7,10]

VASTUS INTERMEDIUS (OF QUADRICEPS FEMORIS GROUP):

Attachments:

- **Anterior Shaft and Linea Aspera of the Femur**
  - the anterior and lateral surfaces of the femur and the lateral lip of the linea aspera

to the

- **Tibial Tuberosity via the Patella and the Patellar Ligament**
  - and the tibial condyles via the retinacular fibers

Functions:

Major Standard Mover Action	Major Reverse Mover Action
1. Extends the leg at the knee joint[1–4,6,7,10]	1. Extends the thigh at the knee joint[1–4,6,7,10]

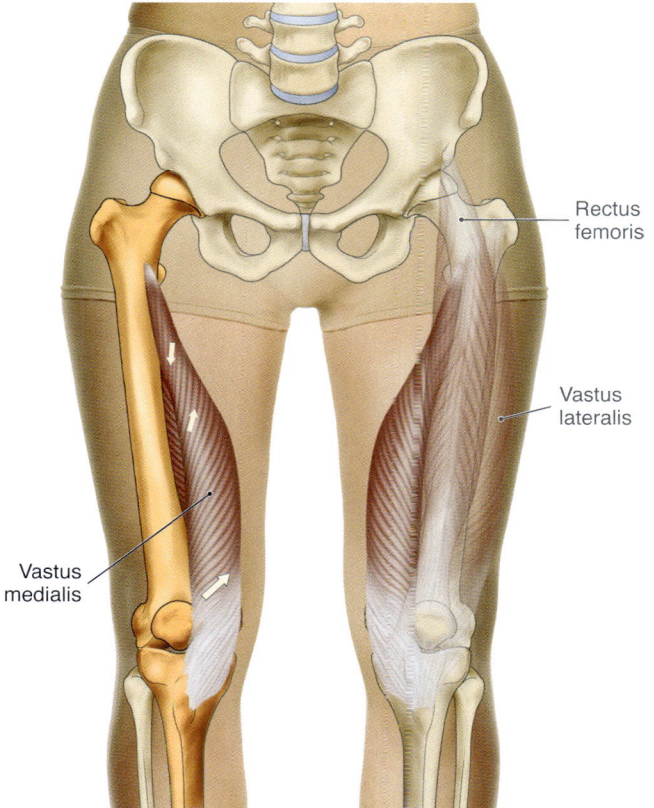

FIGURE 11-143 Anterior view of the vastus medialis bilaterally. The rest of the quadriceps femoris group has been ghosted in on the left.

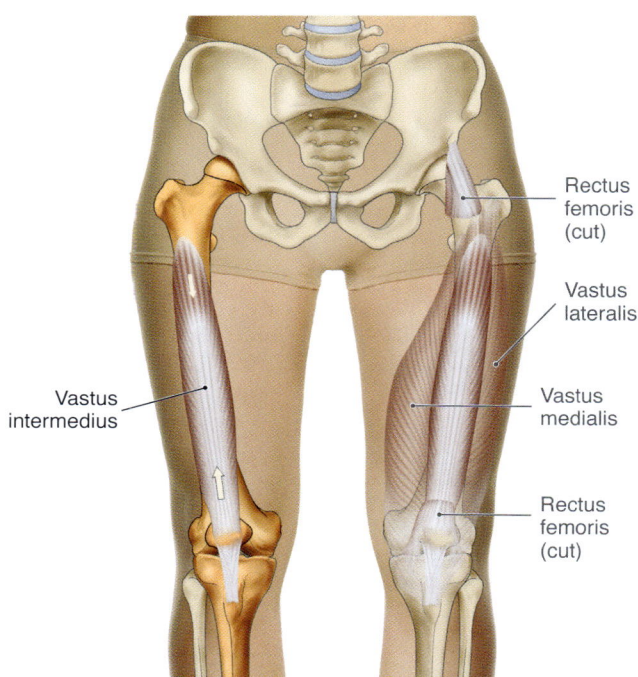

FIGURE 11-144 Anterior view of the vastus intermedius bilaterally. The rest of the quadriceps femoris group has been ghosted in on the left; the rectus femoris is cut.

ARTICULARIS GENUS:

Attachments:
- **Anterior Distal Femoral Shaft**

to the
- **Knee Joint Capsule**

Functions:

Major Standard Mover Action
1. Tenses and pulls the knee joint capsule proximally[1,2,4,6]

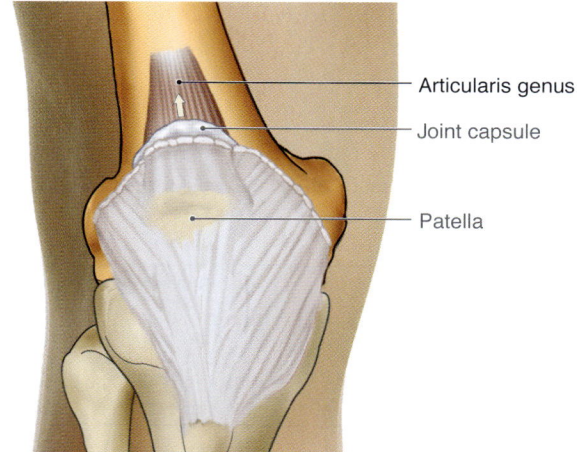

FIGURE 11-145 Anterior view of the right articularis genus.

BICEPS FEMORIS (OF HAMSTRING GROUP):

Attachments:
- **LONG HEAD: Ischial Tuberosity**
  - and the sacrotuberous ligament
- **SHORT HEAD: Linea Aspera**
  - and the lateral supracondylar line of the femur

to the
- **Head of the Fibula**
  - and the lateral tibial condyle

Functions:

Major Standard Mover Actions	Major Reverse Mover Action
1. Flexes the leg at the knee joint[1–4,6,7,10]	
2. Extends the thigh at the hip joint[1–4,6,7,10]	1. Posteriorly tilts the pelvis at the hip joint[1–4,6,7,10]

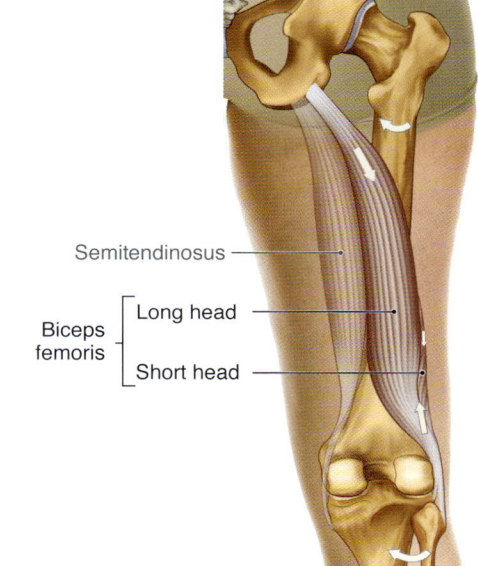

FIGURE 11-146 Posterior view of the right biceps femoris. The semitendinosus has been ghosted in.

SEMITENDINOSUS (OF HAMSTRING GROUP):

Attachments:

- Ischial Tuberosity

to the

- Pes Anserine Tendon (at the Proximal Anteromedial Tibia)

Functions:

Major Standard Mover Actions	Major Reverse Mover Action
1. Flexes the leg at the knee joint[1-4,6,7,10]	
2. Extends the thigh at the hip joint[1-4,6,7,10]	1. Posteriorly tilts the pelvis at the hip joint[1-4,6,7,10]

SEMIMEMBRANOSUS (OF HAMSTRING GROUP):

Attachments:

- Ischial Tuberosity

to the

- Posterior Surface of the Medial Condyle of the Tibia

Functions:

Major Standard Mover Actions	Major Reverse Mover Action
1. Flexes the leg at the knee joint[1-4,6,7,10]	
2. Extends the thigh at the hip joint[1-4,6,7,10]	1. Posteriorly tilts the pelvis at the hip joint[1-4,6,7,10]

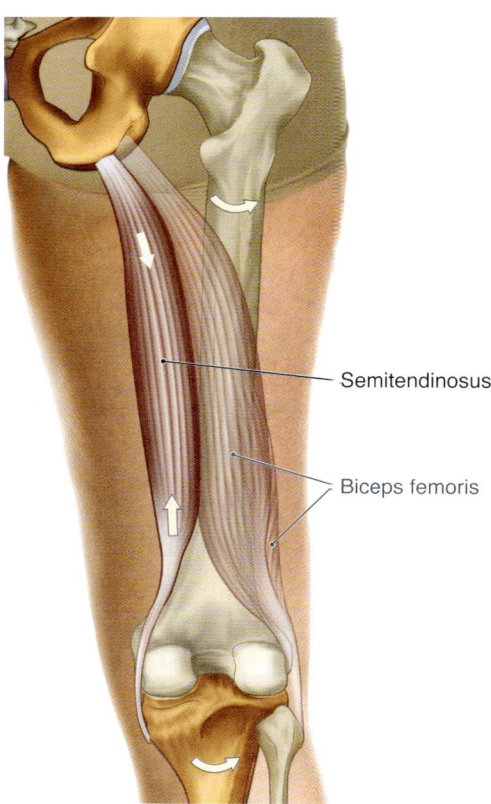

FIGURE 11-147 Posterior view of the right semitendinosus. The biceps femoris has been ghosted in.

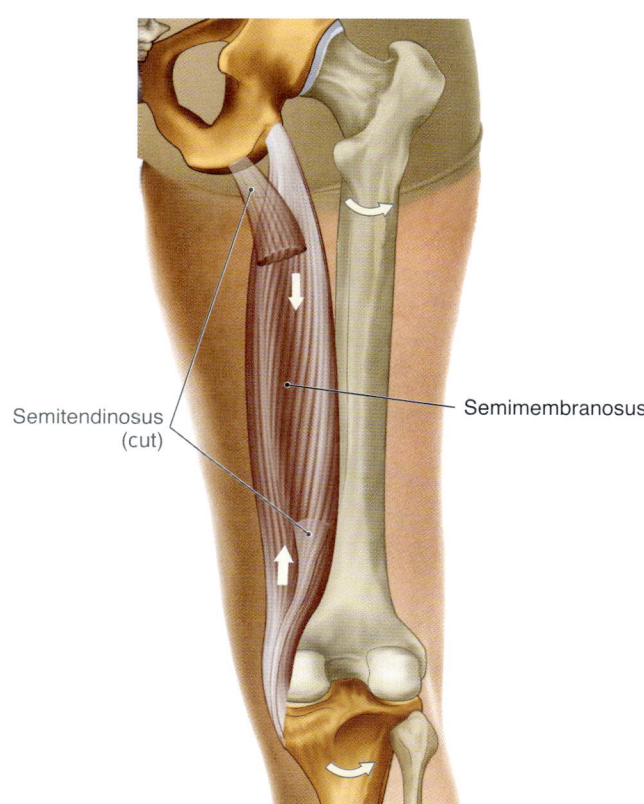

FIGURE 11-148 Posterior view of the right semimembranosus. The proximal and distal tendons of the semitendinosus have been cut and ghosted in.

POPLITEUS:

Attachments:

- **Distal Posterolateral Femur**
  - the lateral surface of the lateral condyle of the femur

to the

- **Proximal Posteromedial Tibia**

Functions:

Major Standard Mover Actions	Major Reverse Mover Action
1. Medially rotates the leg at the knee joint[1–4,6,7,10]	1. Laterally rotates the thigh at the knee joint[1–4,6,7,10]
2. Flexes the leg at the knee joint[2–4,6,7,10]	

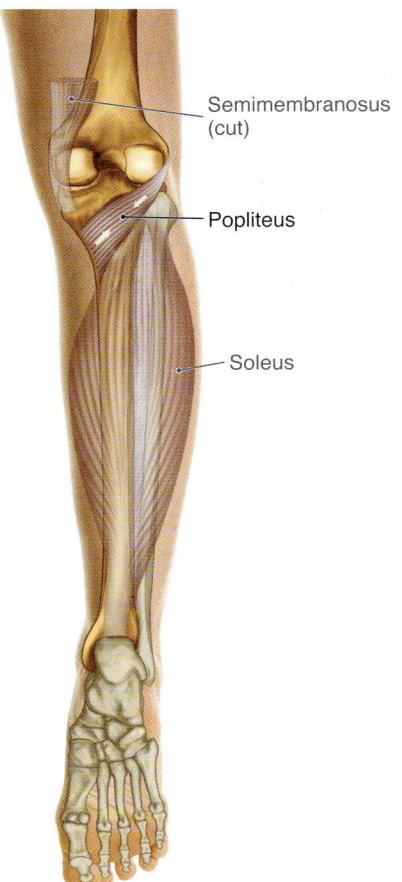

FIGURE 11-149 Posterior view of the right popliteus. The soleus and cut distal tendon of the semimembranosus have been ghosted in.

SECTION 11.14 MUSCLES OF THE ANKLE AND SUBTALAR JOINTS

TIBIALIS ANTERIOR:

Attachments:
- **Anterior Tibia**
  - the lateral tibial condyle, the proximal ⅔ of the anterior tibia, and the proximal ⅔ of the interosseus membrane

to the

- **Medial Foot**
  - the first cuneiform and first metatarsal

Functions:

Major Standard Mover Actions
1. Dorsiflexes the foot at the ankle joint[1–4,6,7,10]
2. Inverts (supinates) the foot at the subtalar joint[1–4,6,7,10]

FIBULARIS TERTIUS:

Attachments:
- **Distal Anterior Fibula**
  - the distal of the anterior fibula and the distal of the interosseus membrane

to the

- **Fifth Metatarsal**
  - the dorsal surface of the base of the fifth metatarsal

Functions:

Major Standard Mover Actions
1. Dorsiflexes the foot at the ankle joint[1–4,6,7,10]
2. Everts (pronates) the foot at the subtalar joint[1–4,6,7,10]

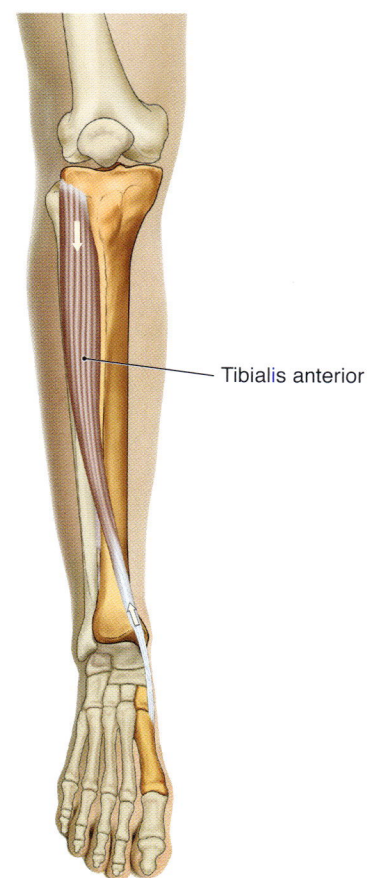

FIGURE 11-150 Anterior view of the right tibialis anterior.

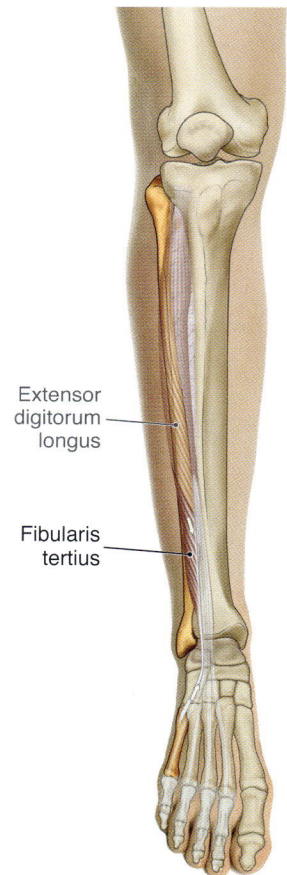

FIGURE 11-151 Anterior view of the right fibularis tertius. The extensor digitorum longus has been ghosted in.

CHAPTER 11 Attachments and Actions of Muscles

FIBULARIS LONGUS:

Attachments:

- **Proximal Lateral Fibula**
  - the head of the fibula and the proximal ½ of the lateral fibula

to the

- **Medial Foot**
  - the first cuneiform and first metatarsal

Functions:

Major Standard Mover Actions
1. Everts (pronates) the foot at the subtalar joint[1-4,6,7,10]
2. Plantarflexes the foot at the ankle joint[1-4,6,7,10]

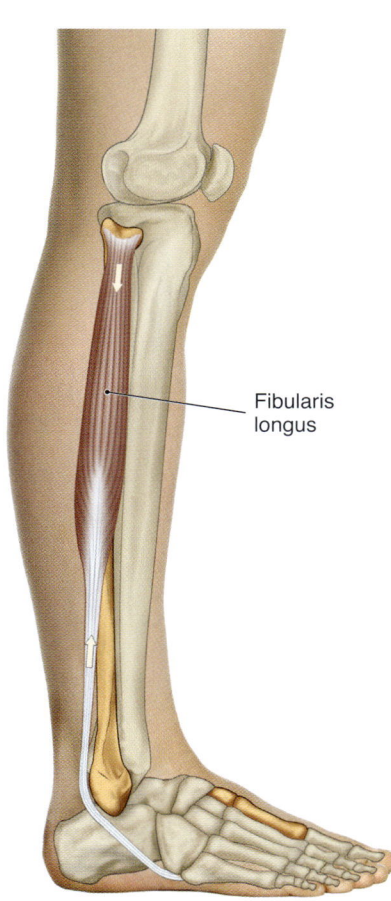

FIGURE 11-152 Lateral view of the right fibularis longus.

FIBULARIS BREVIS:

Attachments:

- **Distal Lateral Fibula**
  - the distal ½ of the lateral fibula

to the

- **Fifth Metatarsal**
  - the lateral side of the base of the fifth metatarsal

Functions:

Major Standard Mover Actions
1. Everts (pronates) the foot at the subtalar joint[1-4,6,7,10]
2. Plantarflexes the foot at the ankle joint[1-4,6,7,10]

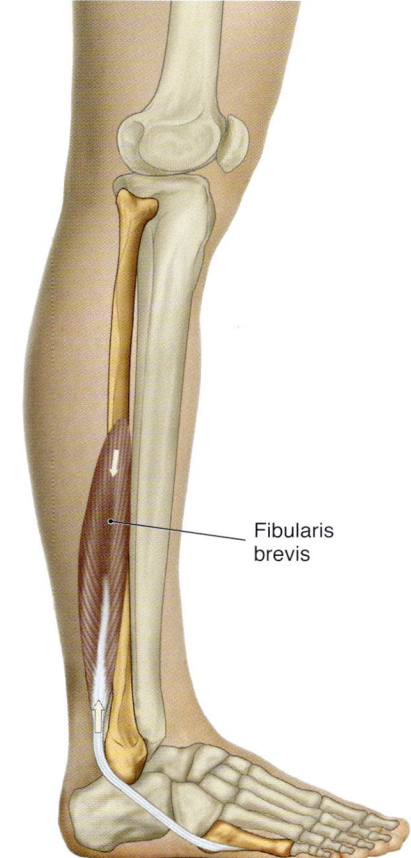

FIGURE 11-153 Lateral view of the right fibularis brevis.

GASTROCNEMIUS (*GASTROCS*) (OF TRICEPS SURAE GROUP):

Attachments:
- **Medial and Lateral Femoral Condyles**
  - and the distal posteromedial femur and the distal posterolateral femur

to the

- **Calcaneus via the Calcaneal (Achilles) Tendon**
  - the posterior surface

Functions:

Major Standard Mover Actions
1. Plantarflexes the foot at the ankle joint[1–4,6,7,10]
2. Flexes the leg at the knee joint[1–4,6,7,10]

SOLEUS (OF TRICEPS SURAE GROUP):

Attachments:
- **Posterior Tibia and Fibula**
  - the soleal line of the tibia and the head and proximal ⅓ of the fibula

to the

- **Calcaneus via the Calcaneal (Achilles) Tendon**
  - the posterior surface

Functions:

Major Standard Mover Action
1. Plantarflexes the foot at the ankle joint[1–4,6,7,10]

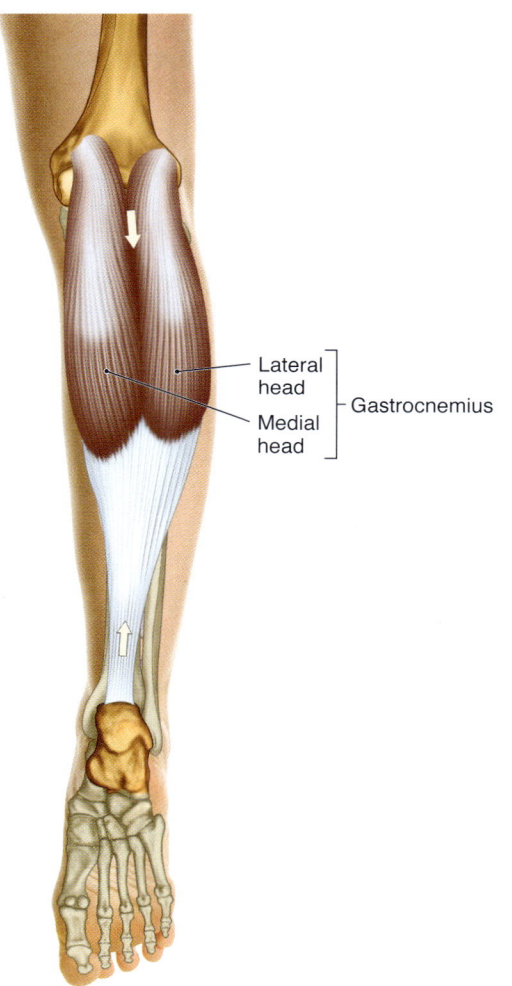

FIGURE 11-154 Posterior view of the right gastrocnemius.

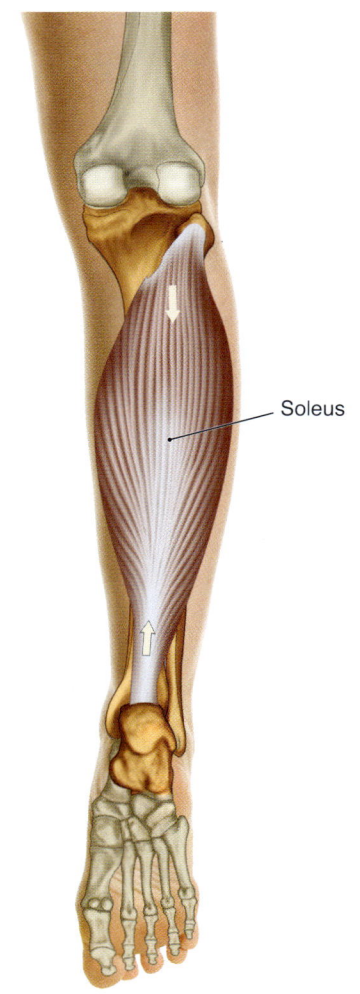

FIGURE 11-155 Posterior view of the right soleus.

PLANTARIS:

Attachments:

- **Distal Posterolateral Femur**
  - the lateral condyle and the distal lateral supracondylar line of the femur

to the

- **Calcaneus**
  - the posterior surface

Functions:

Major Standard Mover Actions
1. Plantarflexes the foot at the ankle joint[1,2,4,6,7,10]
2. Flexes the leg at the knee joint[1,2,4,6,7,10]

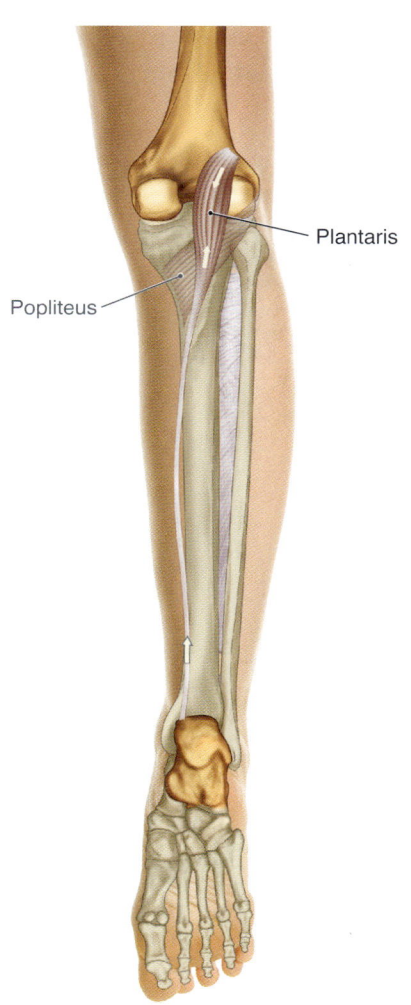

FIGURE 11-156 Posterior view of the right plantaris. The popliteus has been ghosted in.

TIBIALIS POSTERIOR (*TOM* OF *TOM, DICK, AND HARRY* GROUP):

Attachments:

- **Posterior Tibia and Fibula**
  - the proximal ⅔ of the posterior tibia, fibula, and interosseus membrane

to the

- **Navicular Tuberosity**
  - and metatarsals two through four and all the tarsal bones except the talus

Functions:

Major Standard Mover Actions
1. Plantarflexes the foot at the ankle joint[1-4,6,7,10]
2. Inverts (supinates) the foot at the subtalar joint[1-4,6,7,10]

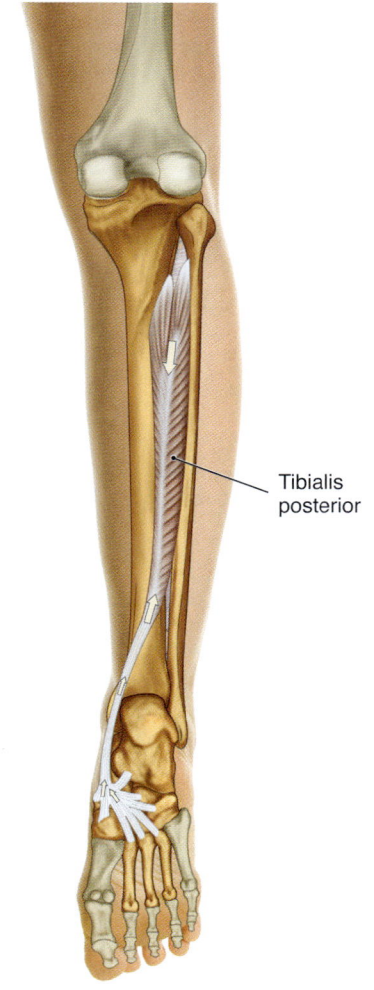

FIGURE 11-157 Posterior view of the right tibialis posterior.

SECTION 11.15 EXTRINSIC MUSCLES OF THE TOE JOINTS

EXTENSOR DIGITORUM LONGUS:

Attachments:
- **Proximal Anterior Fibula**
  - the proximal ⅔ of the fibula, the proximal ⅓ of the interosseus membrane, and the lateral tibial condyle

to the

- **Dorsal Surface of Toes Two through Five**
  - via its dorsal digital expansion onto the dorsal surface of the middle and distal phalanges

Functions:

Major Standard Mover Actions
1. Extends toes two through five at the MTP and IP joints[1–4,6,7,10]
2. Dorsiflexes the foot at the ankle joint[1–4,6,7,10]

IP joints = (proximal and distal) interphalangeal joints; MTP joints = metatarsophalangeal joints

EXTENSOR HALLUCIS LONGUS:

Attachments:
- **Middle Anterior Fibula**
  - the middle ⅓ of the anterior fibula and the middle ⅓ of the interosseus membrane

to the

- **Dorsal Surface of the Big Toe (Toe One)**
  - the distal phalanx

Functions:

Major Standard Mover Actions
1. Extends the big toe (toe one) at the MTP and IP joints[1–4,6,7,10]
2. Dorsiflexes the foot at the ankle joint[1–4,6,7,10]

IP joint = interphalangeal joint; MTP joint = metatarsophalangeal joint

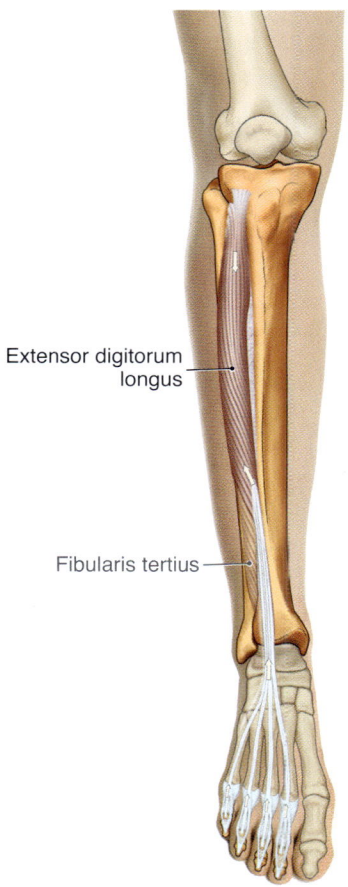

FIGURE 11-158 Anterior view of the right extensor digitorum longus. The fibularis tertius has been ghosted in.

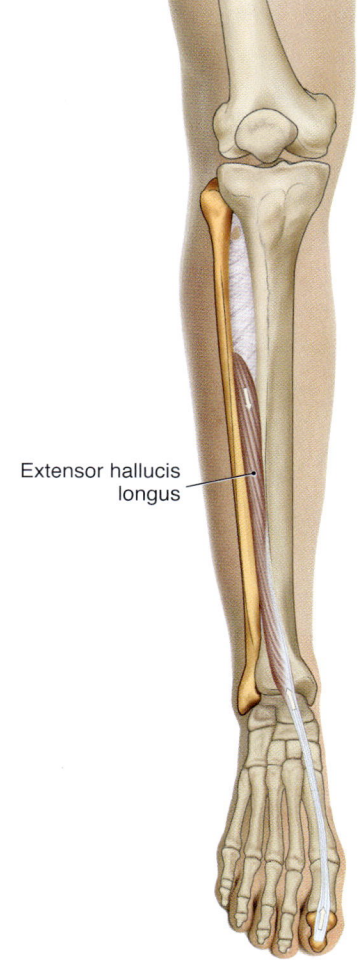

FIGURE 11-159 Anterior view of the right extensor hallucis longus.

FLEXOR DIGITORUM LONGUS (*DICK* OF *TOM*, *DICK* AND *HARRY* GROUP):

Attachments:

- **Middle Posterior Tibia**
  - the middle ⅓ of the posterior tibia

to the

- **Plantar Surface of Toes Two through Five**
  - the distal phalanges

Functions:

Major Standard Mover Actions
1. Flexes toes two through five at the MTP and IP joints[1–4,6,7,10]
2. Plantarflexes the foot at the ankle joint[1–4,6,7,10]
3. Inverts (supinates) the foot at the subtalar joint[2–4,6,7,10]

IP joints = (proximal and distal) interphalangeal joints; MTP joints = metatarsophalangeal joints

FLEXOR HALLUCIS LONGUS (*HARRY* OF *TOM*, *DICK*, AND *HARRY* GROUP):

Attachments:

- **Distal Posterior Fibula**
  - the distal ⅔ of the posterior fibula and the distal ⅔ of the interosseus membrane

to the

- **Plantar Surface of the Big Toe (Toe One)**
  - the distal phalanx

Functions:

Major Standard Mover Actions
1. Flexes the big toe at the MTP and IP joints[1–4,6,7,10]
2. Plantarflexes the foot at the ankle joint[1–4,6,7,10]
3. Inverts (supinates) the foot at the subtalar joint[2–4,6,7,10]

IP joint = interphalangeal joint; MTP joint = metatarsophalangeal joint

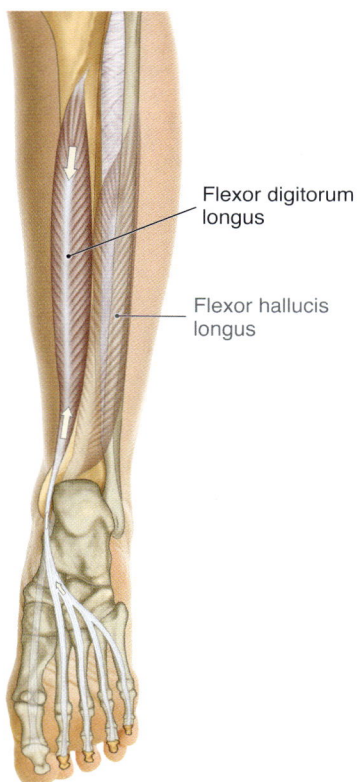

FIGURE 11-160 Posterior view of the right flexor digitorum longus. The flexor hallucis longus has been ghosted in.

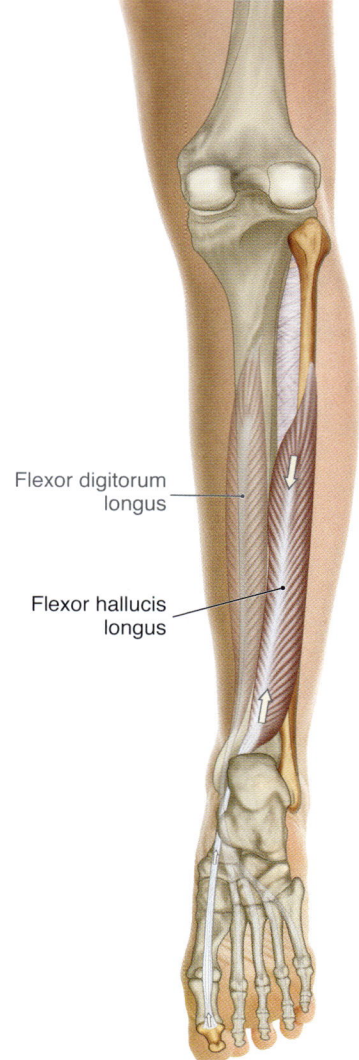

FIGURE 11-161 Posterior view of the right flexor hallucis longus. The flexor digitorum longus has been ghosted in.

SECTION 11.16 INTRINSIC MUSCLES OF THE TOE JOINTS

EXTENSOR DIGITORUM BREVIS:

Attachments:

- **Dorsal Surface of the Calcaneus**

to

- **Toes Two through Four**
  - the lateral side of the distal tendons of the extensor digitorum longus muscle of toes two through four (via the dorsal digital expansion into the middle and distal phalanges)

Functions:

Major Standard Mover Action

1. Extends toes two through four at the MTP, PIP, and DIP joints[1–4,6,7,10]

DIP joints = distal interphalangeal joints; MTP joints = metatarsophalangeal joints; PIP joints = proximal interphalangeal joints

EXTENSOR HALLUCIS BREVIS:

Attachments:

- **Dorsal Surface of the Calcaneus**

to the

- **Dorsal Surface of the Big Toe (Toe One)**
  - the base of the proximal phalanx of the big toe

Functions:

Major Standard Mover Action

1. Extends the big toe at the MTP joint[1–4,7,10]

MTP joint = metatarsophalangeal joint

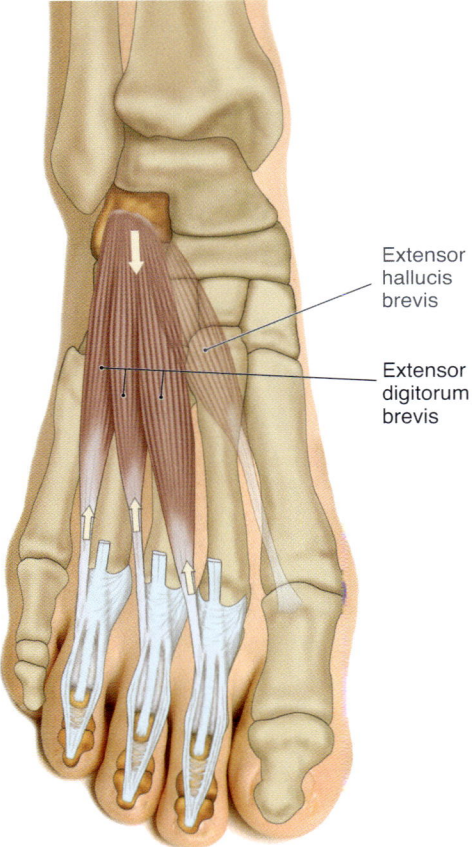

FIGURE 11-162 Dorsal view of the right extensor digitorum brevis. The extensor hallucis brevis has been ghosted in.

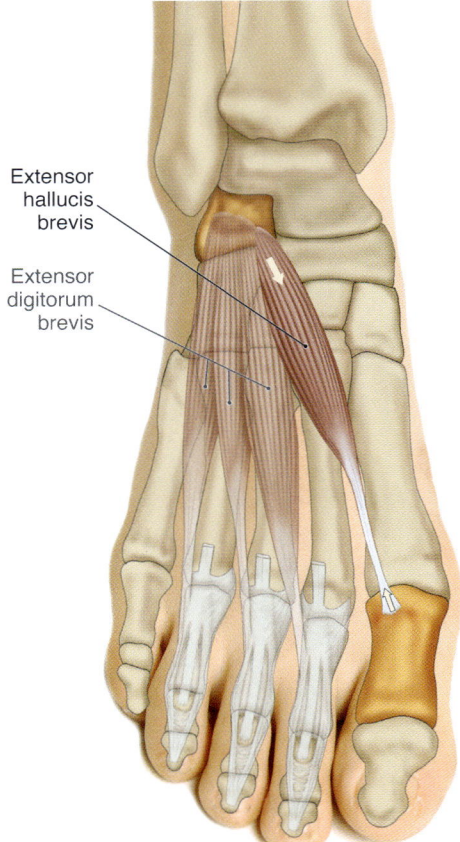

FIGURE 11-163 Dorsal view of the right extensor hallucis brevis. The extensor digitorum brevis has been ghosted in.

ABDUCTOR HALLUCIS:

Attachments:

- **Tuberosity of the Calcaneus**
  - and the flexor retinaculum and plantar fascia

to the

- **Big Toe (Toe One)**
  - the medial plantar side of the base of the proximal phalanx

Functions:

Major Standard Mover Action
1. Abducts the big toe at the MTP joint[1–4,6,7,10]

MTP joint = metatarsophalangeal joint

ABDUCTOR DIGITI MINIMI PEDIS:

Attachments:

- **Tuberosity of the Calcaneus**
  - and the plantar fascia

to the

- **Little Toe (Toe Five)**
  - the lateral plantar side of the base of the proximal phalanx

Functions:

Major Standard Mover Action
1. Abducts the little toe at the MTP joint[1–4,7,10]

MTP joint = metatarsophalangeal joint

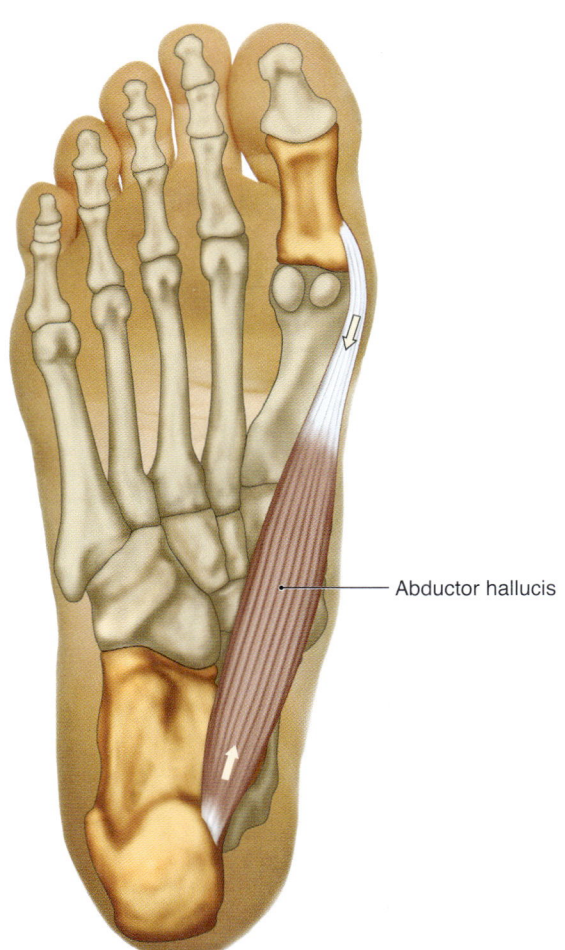

FIGURE 11-164 Plantar view of the right abductor hallucis.

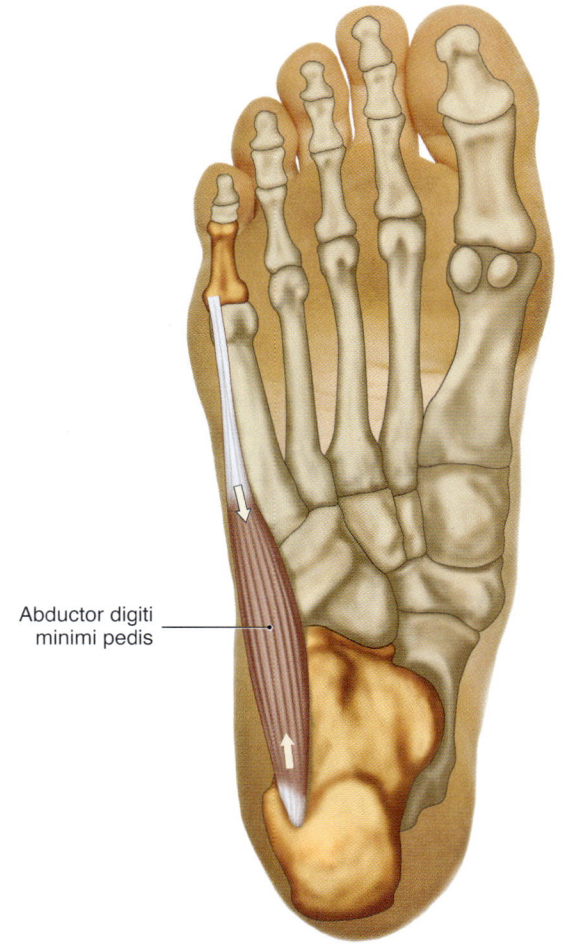

FIGURE 11-165 Plantar view of the right abductor digiti minimi pedis.

FLEXOR DIGITORUM BREVIS:

Attachments:

- Tuberosity of the Calcaneus
  - and the plantar fascia

to

- Toes Two through Five
  - the medial and lateral sides of the middle phalanges

Functions:

Major Standard Mover Action

1. Flexes toes two through five at the MTP and PIP joints[1-4,6,7,10]

MTP joints = metatarsophalangeal joints; PIP joints = proximal interphalangeal joints

QUADRATUS PLANTAE:

Attachments:

- The Calcaneus
  - the medial and lateral sides

to the

- Distal Tendon of the Flexor Digitorum Longus Muscle
  - the lateral margin

Functions:

Major Standard Mover Action

1. Flexes toes two through five at the MTP, PIP, and DIP joints[1,3,4,6,7,10]

DIP joints = distal interphalangeal joints; MTP joints = metatarsophalangeal joints; PIP joints = proximal interphalangeal joints

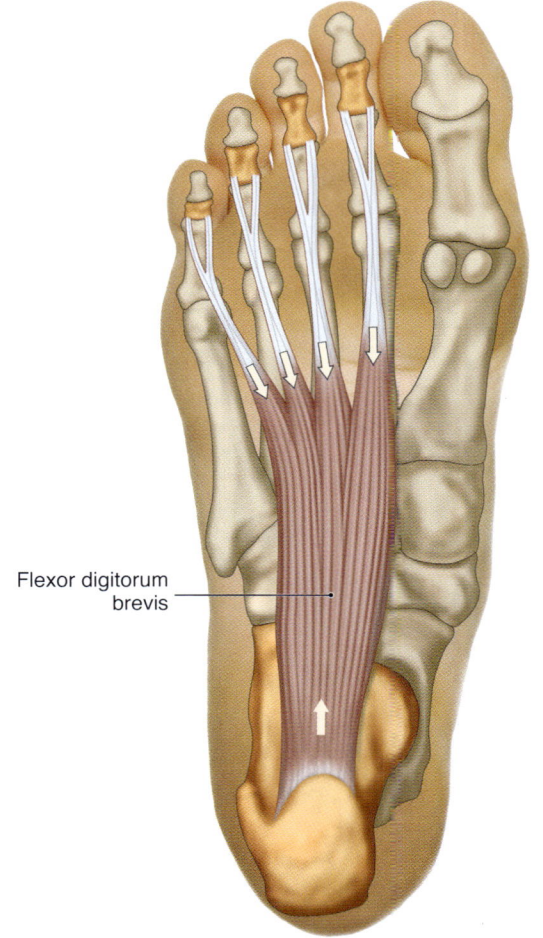

FIGURE 11-166 Plantar view of the right flexor digitorum brevis.

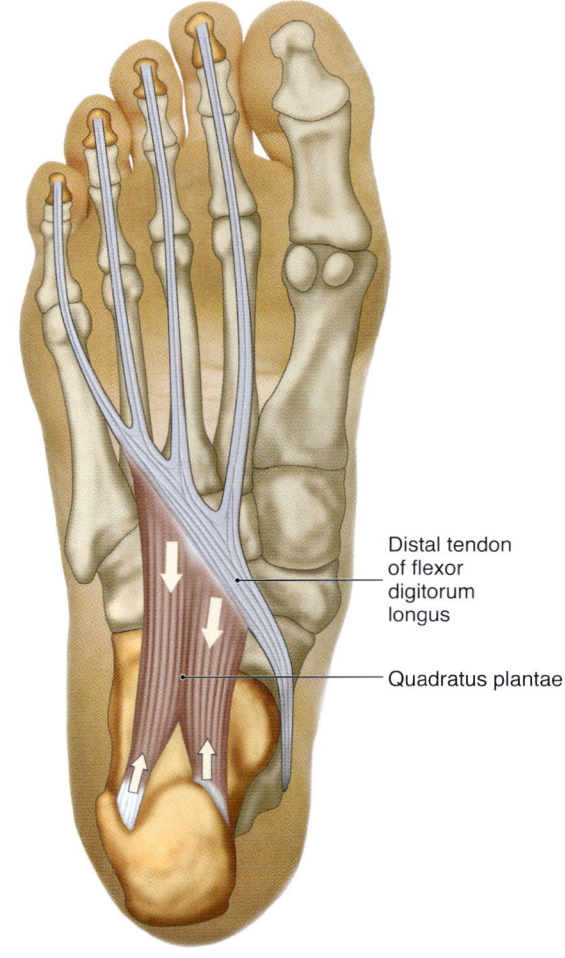

FIGURE 11-167 Plantar view of the right quadratus plantae.

LUMBRICALS PEDIS:

Attachments:

- **The Distal Tendons of the Flexor Digitorum Longus Muscle**
  - **ONE:** medial border of the tendon to toe two
  - **TWO:** adjacent sides of the tendons to toes two and three
  - **THREE:** adjacent sides of the tendons to toes three and four
  - **FOUR:** adjacent sides of the tendons to toes four and five

to the

- **Dorsal Digital Expansion**
  - the medial sides of the extensor digitorum longus tendons, merging into the dorsal digital expansion of toes two through five

Functions:

Major Standard Mover Actions
1. Flex toes two through five at the MTP joints[2–4,6,7,10]
2. Extend toes two through five at the PIP and DIP joints[1,2,4,6,7,10]

DIP joints = distal interphalangeal joints; MTP joints = metatarsophalangeal joints; PIP joints = proximal interphalangeal joints

FLEXOR HALLUCIS BREVIS:

Attachments:

- **Cuboid and the Third Cuneiform**

to the

- **Big Toe (Toe One)**
  - the medial and lateral sides of the plantar surface of the base of the proximal phalanx

Functions:

Major Standard Mover Action
1. Flexes the big toe at the MTP joint[1–4,6,7,10]

MTP joint = metatarsophalangeal joint

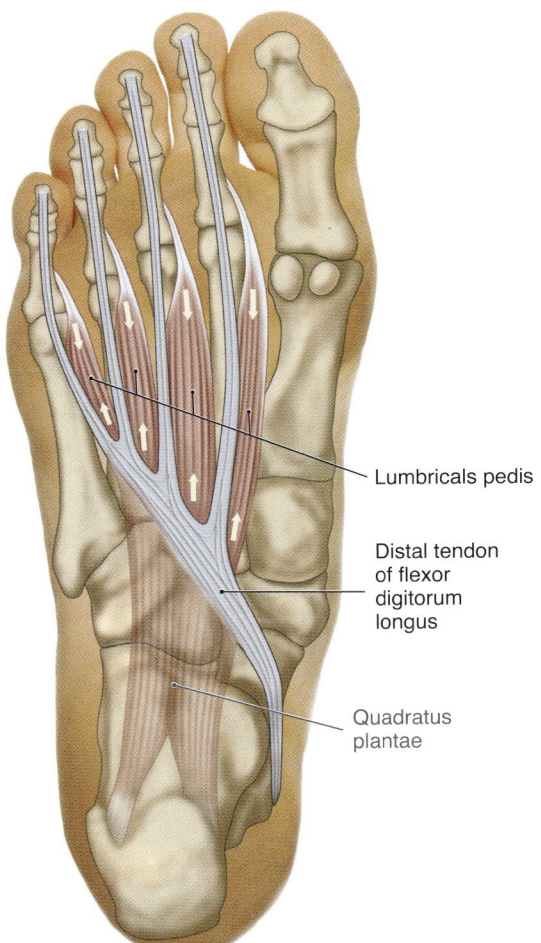

FIGURE 11-168 Plantar view of the right lumbricals pedis. The quadratus plantae has been ghosted in.

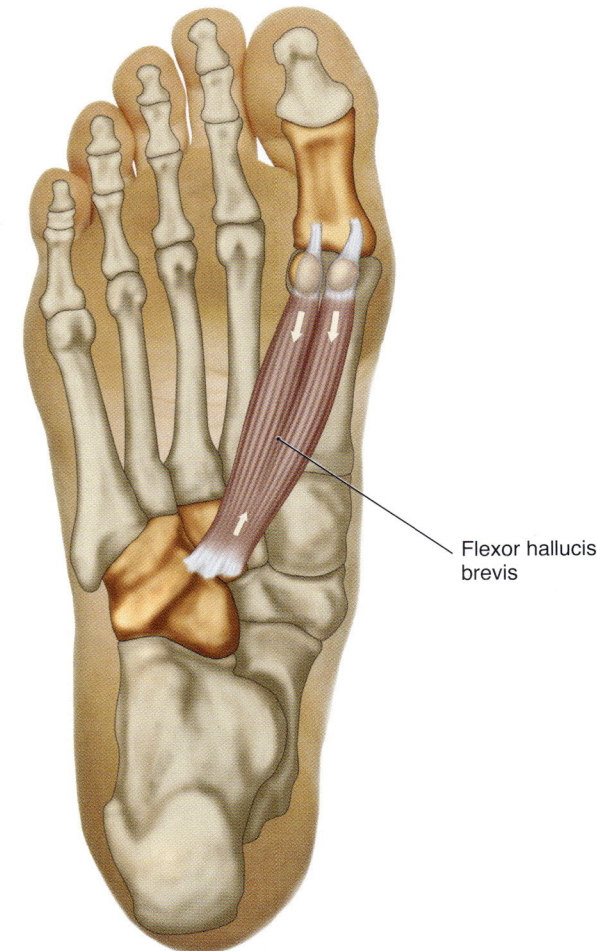

FIGURE 11-169 Plantar view of the right flexor hallucis brevis.

FLEXOR DIGITI MINIMI PEDIS:

Attachments:

- **Fifth Metatarsal**
  - the plantar surface of the base of the fifth metatarsal and the distal tendon of the fibularis longus

to the

- **Little Toe (Toe Five)**
  - the plantar surface of the proximal phalanx

Functions:

Major Standard Mover Action
1. Flexes the little toe at the MTP joint[1–4,7,10]

MTP joint = metatarsophalangeal joint

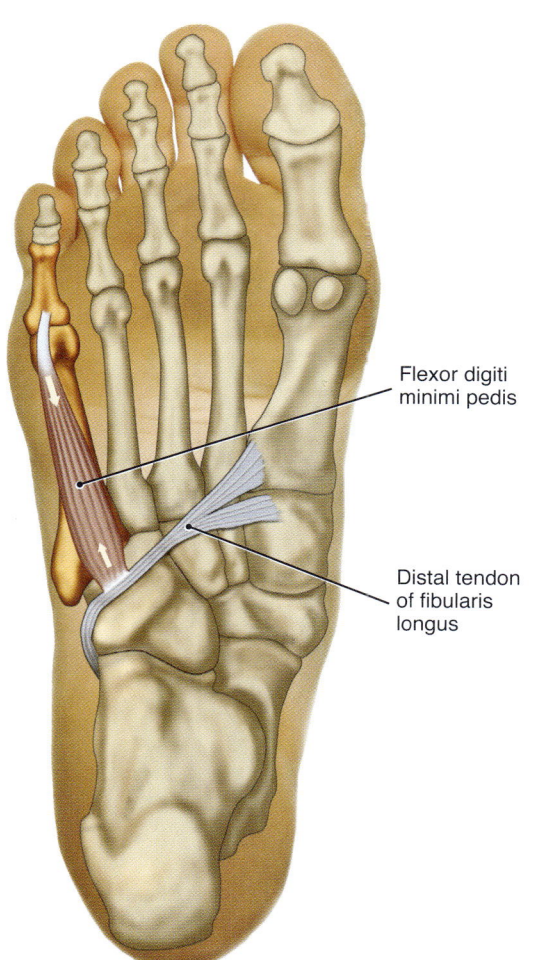

FIGURE 11-170 Plantar view of the right flexor digiti minimi pedis.

ADDUCTOR HALLUCIS:

Attachments:

- **Metatarsals**
  - OBLIQUE HEAD: from the base of metatarsals two through four and the distal tendon of the fibularis longus
  - TRANSVERSE HEAD: arises from the plantar metatarsophalangeal ligaments

to the

- **Big Toe (Toe One)**
  - the lateral side of the base of the proximal phalanx

Functions:

Major Standard Mover Action
1. Adducts the big toe at the MTP joint[2–4,6,7,10]

MTP joint = metatarsophalangeal joint

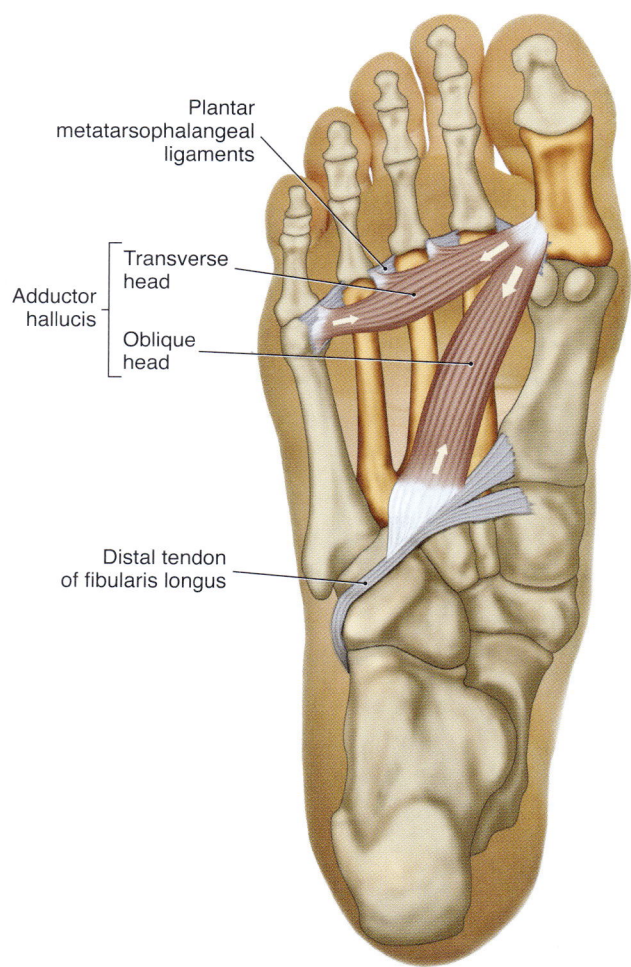

FIGURE 11-171 Plantar view of the right adductor hallucis.

PLANTAR INTEROSSEI:

Attachments:

- **Metatarsals**
  - the medial side (second-toe side) of metatarsals three through five:
    - **ONE:** attaches onto metatarsal three
    - **TWO:** attaches onto metatarsal four
    - **THREE:** attaches onto metatarsal five

to the

- **Second-Toe Sides of the Proximal Phalanges of Toes Three through Five, and the Dorsal Distal Expansion**
  - the bases of the proximal phalanges
    - **ONE:** attaches to toe three
    - **TWO:** attaches to toe four
    - **THREE:** attaches to toe five

Functions:

Major Standard Mover Action
1. Adduct toes three through five at the MTP joints[1,2,4,6,7,10]

MTP joints = metatarsophalangeal joints

DORSAL INTEROSSEI PEDIS:

Attachments:

- **Metatarsals**
  - each one arises from the adjacent sides of two metatarsals:
    - **ONE:** attaches onto metatarsals one and two
    - **TWO:** attaches onto metatarsals two and three
    - **THREE:** attaches onto metatarsals three and four
    - **FOUR:** attaches onto metatarsals four and five

to the

- **Sides of the Phalanges and the Dorsal Digital Expansion**
  - the bases of the proximal phalanges (on the sides away from the center of the second toe)
    - **ONE:** attaches to the medial side of toe number two
    - **TWO:** attaches to the lateral side of toe number two
    - **THREE:** attaches to the lateral side of toe number three
    - **FOUR:** attaches to the lateral side of toe number four

Functions:

Major Standard Mover Action
1. Abduct toes two through four at the MTP joints[1,2,4,6,7,10]

MTP joints = metatarsophalangeal joints

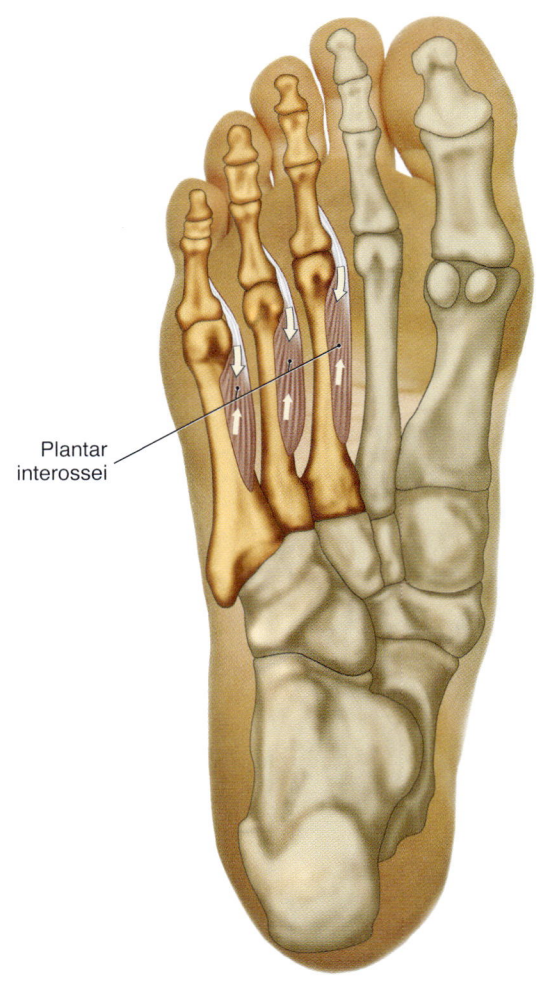

FIGURE 11-172 Plantar view of the right plantar interossei.

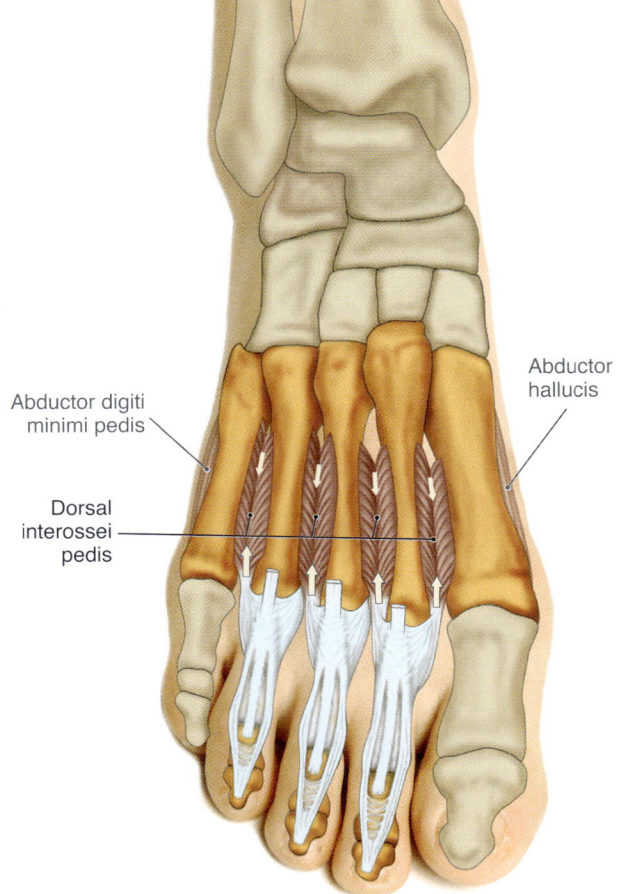

FIGURE 11-173 Dorsal view of the right dorsal interossei pedis. The abductor hallucis and abductor digiti minimi pedis have been ghosted in.

REFERENCES

1. Standring S: Gray's anatomy, ed 40, Melilla, Spain, 2008, Churchill, Livingstone, Elsevier.
2. Neumann DA: Kinesiology of the musculoskeletal system: Foundations for physical rehabilitation, ed 3, St Louis, 2017, Elsevier.
3. Hamilton N, Weimar W, Luttgens K: Kinesiology: Scientific basis of human motion, ed 12, New York, 2012, McGraw-Hill.
4. Oatis CA: Kinesiology: The mechanics and pathomechanics of human movement, Philadelphia, 2004, Lippincott Williams & Wilkins.
5. Simons DG, Travell JG, Simons LS: Travell and Simons' myofascial pain and dysfunction: The trigger point manual; Volume 1: Upper half of body, ed 2, Baltimore, 1999, Williams & Wilkins.
6. Kendall FP, McCreary EK, Provance PG, et al.: Muscles: Testing and function with posture and pain, ed 5, Baltimore, 2005, Lippincott Williams & Wilkins.
7. Levangie PK, Norton CC: Joint structure and function: A comprehensive analysis, ed 5, Philadelphia, 2011, FA Davis.
8. Chaitow L, Delany JW: Clinical applications of neuromuscular techniques; Volume 1: The upper body, Edinburgh, 2000, Churchill Livingstone.
9. Myers TW: Anatomy trains: Myofascial meridians for manual and movement therapists, ed 2, Italy, 2009, Churchill Livingstone.
10. Travell JG, Simons DG: Myofascial pain and dysfunction: The trigger point manual; Volume 2: The lower extremities, Baltimore, 1992, Williams & Wilkins.
11. Kapandji IA: The physiology of the joints: Volume 1: Upper limb, ed 5, Edinburgh, 1983, Churchill Livingstone.
12. Chaitow L, Delany JW: Clinical applications of neuromuscular techniques; Volume 2: The lower body, Edinburgh, 2000, Churchill Livingstone.
13. Fritz S: Mosby's essential sciences for therapeutic massage: Anatomy, physiology, biomechanics, and pathology, ed 4, St Louis, 2013, Elsevier.
14. Son E, Watts T, Quinn Jr FB, et al: Superficial facial musculature [PDF document]. Retrieved from http://www.utmb.edu/otoref/Grnds/facial-plastic-2012-03-29/facial-musc-2012-0329-B.pdf, 2012.
15. Dauzvardis MF, McNulty JA, Espiritu B, et al.: Loyola university medical education network master muscle list. Retrieved from http://www.meddean.luc.edu/lumen/meded/grossanatomy/dissector/mml/, 1998.
16. Comeford M, Mottram S: Kinetic control: The management of uncontrolled movement, Australia, 2012, Churchill Livingstone.
17. Muscolino J: Psoas major function: A biomechanical examination of the psoas major. Massage Therapy Journal, 52(1), 17–31, 2012.
18. Smith LK, Weiss EL, Lehmkuhl LD: Brunnstrom's clinical kinesiology, ed 5, Philadelphia, 1996, FA Davis.
19. Adams JB: Kinesiology [PowerPoint slides]. Retrieved from http://www.kean.edu/~jeadams/docs/Kinesiology/Kines_Power_Points/, 2008.
20. Sahrmann SA: Diagnosis and treatment of movement impairment syndromes. St. Louis, 2002, Mosby, Inc.
21. Simons DG, Travell JG: Travell and Simons' myofascial pain and dysfunction: The trigger point manual; Volume 1: Upper half of body, ed 2, Baltimore, 1999, Williams & Wilkins.

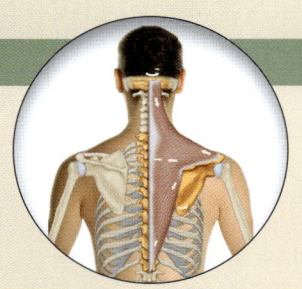

CHAPTER 12
Anatomy and Physiology of Muscle Tissue

CHAPTER OUTLINE

Section 12.1	Skeletal Muscle	Section 12.8	Nervous System Control of Muscle Contraction
Section 12.2	Tissue Components of a Skeletal Muscle	Section 12.9	Motor Unit
Section 12.3	Skeletal Muscle Cells	Section 12.10	All-or-None–Response Law
Section 12.4	Muscular Fascia	Section 12.11	Sarcomere Structure in More Detail
Section 12.5	Microanatomy of Muscle Fiber/Sarcomere Structure	Section 12.12	Sliding Filament Mechanism in More Detail
Section 12.6	Sliding Filament Mechanism	Section 12.13	Red and White Muscle Fibers
Section 12.7	Energy Source for the Sliding Filament Mechanism	Section 12.14	Myofascial Meridians and Tensegrity

CHAPTER OBJECTIVES

After completing this chapter, the student should be able to perform the following:

1. Define the key terms of this chapter and state the meanings of the word origins of this chapter.
2. List the three types of muscular tissue.
3. Describe the characteristics and function of skeletal muscle tissue and skeletal muscle cells.
4. Do the following related to muscular fascia:
   - List the various types of muscular fascia.
   - Describe the structure and function of muscular fascia.
   - State the meaning of the term *myofascial unit*.
5. Describe the structure of a sarcomere.
6. Do the following related to the sliding filament mechanism:
   - Explain the sliding filament mechanism.
   - Explain the relationship between the sliding filament mechanism and the bigger picture of muscle function.
   - Describe how the energy needed for the sliding filament mechanism is supplied.
7. Discuss how the nervous system controls and directs muscle contraction, and describe the structure of the neuromuscular junction.
8. Do the following related to the motor unit:
   - Define *motor unit*.
   - Explain the importance of a motor unit, and explain the differences among motor units.
9. Define the all-or-none–response law, and explain to which structural levels of the muscular system it is applied.
10. Discuss sarcomere structure in detail; list and define the bands of skeletal muscle tissue.
11. Discuss the sliding filament mechanism in detail, and describe the structural and functional characteristics of red slow-twitch and white fast-twitch fibers.
12. Do the following related to myofascial meridians and tensegrity:
    - List and discuss the eleven myofascial meridians.
    - Explain the concepts of myofascial meridian theory and tensegrity and how they apply to the body.

OVERVIEW

The anatomy and physiology of skeletal tissues were addressed in Chapter 3. Before examining the larger kinesiologic concepts of muscle function, this chapter focuses on the anatomy and physiology of a skeletal muscle. The two major tissue types—skeletal muscle tissue and muscular fascia—are examined. Specifically, an understanding of the microanatomy of the sarcomere of a muscle fiber and the sliding filament mechanism are presented; the context of the sliding filament mechanism within the context of the bigger picture of muscle function is then given. Energy sources for muscle contraction and nervous system control of muscle contraction are also covered. The concepts of motor units, the all-or-none–response law, and red slow-twitch versus white fast-twitch fibers are then presented, as well as two sections that offer an in-depth view of the structure of the sarcomere and the sliding filament mechanism. The chapter concludes with an exploration of the concepts of myofascial meridian theory and tensegrity.

KEY TERMS

A-band
Acetylcholine (a-SEET-al-KOL-een)
Acetylcholinesterase (a-SEET-al-KOL-een-EST-er-ace)
Actin filament (AK-tin FIL-a-ment)
Actin filament active site
Actin filament binding site
Actin molecule
Adenosine triphosphate (ATP) (a-DEN-o-SEEN try-FOS-fate)
All-or-none–response law
Anatomy train
Aponeurosis, pl. aponeuroses (AP-o-noo-RO-sis, AP-o-noo-RO-seez)
Cardiac muscle tissue
Connectin (ko-NECK-tin)
Cytoplasmic organelles (SI-to-PLAS-mik OR-gan-els)
Deep fascia (FASH-a)
Easily fatigued fibers
Endomysium, pl. endomysia (EN-do-MICE-ee-um, EN-do-MICE-ee-a)
Energy crisis hypothesis
Epimysium, pl. epimysia (EP-ee-MICE-ee-um, EP-ee-MICE-ee-a)
Fascicles (FAS-si-kuls)
Fasciculus, pl. fasciculi (fas-IK-you-lus, fas-IK-you-lie)
Fast glycolytic (FG) fibers (GLIY-ko-LIT-ik)
Fatigue-resistant fibers
Glycolysis (gliy-KOL-i-sis)
Glycolytic fibers (GLIY-ko-lit-ik)
H-band
Heavy meromyosin (MER-o-MY-o-sin)
Human resting muscle tone (HRMT)
I-band
Innervation (IN-ner-VAY-shun)
Intermediate-twitch fibers
Kreb's cycle (KREBS)
Lactic acid (LAK-tik)
Large fibers
Lateral force transmission
Light meromyosin (MER-o-MY-o-sin)
M-band
M-line
Motor end plate
Motor unit
Muscle cell
Muscle fiber
Muscle memory
Muscular fascia (FASH-a)
Myofascial meridian (MY-o-FASH-al me-RID-ee-an)
Myofascial meridian theory
Myofascial unit (MY-o-FASH-al)
Myofibril (my-o-FIY-bril)
Myoglobin (my-o-GLOBE-in)
Myosin cross-bridge (MY-o-sin)
Myosin filament (MY-o-sin FIL-a-ment)
Myosin head
Myosin tail
Neuromuscular junction (noor-o-MUS-kyu-lar)
Neurotransmitters (noor-o-TRANS-mit-ers)
Organ
Oxidative fibers (OKS-i-DATE-iv)
Oxygen debt
Perimysium, pl. perimysia (per-ee-MICE-ee-um, per-ee-MICE-ee-a)
Phasic fibers (FAZE-ik)
Ratchet theory
Red slow-twitch fibers
Respiration of glucose (res-pi-RAY-shun)
S1 fragment
S2 fragment
Sarcolemma (SAR-ko-lem-ma)
Sarcomere (SAR-ko-meer)
Sarcoplasm (SAR-ko-plazm)
Sarcoplasmic reticulum (SAR-ko-plaz-mik re-TIK-you-lum)
Skeletal muscle tissue (SKEL-i-tal)
Sliding filament mechanism (FIL-a-ment)
Slow oxidative (SO) fibers (OKS-i-DATE-iv)
Small fibers
Smooth muscle tissue
Striated muscle (STRIY-ate-ed)
Synapse (SIN-aps)
Synaptic cleft (sin-AP-tik)
Synaptic gap

Tendon
Tensegrity (ten-SEG-ri-tee)
Titin (TIE-tin)
Tonic fibers
Transverse tubules (TOO-byools)
Trigger points (TrPs)
Tropomyosin molecule (TRO-po-MY-o-sin)
Troponin molecule (tro-PO-nin)
T-tubules (TOO-byools)
Type I fibers
Type II fibers
White fast-twitch fibers
Z-band
Z-line

WORD ORIGINS

- Aer—From Latin *aer,* meaning *air*
- Cardiac—From Latin *cardiacus,* meaning *heart*
- Elle—From Latin *ella,* meaning *little*
- Endo—From Greek *endon,* meaning *within, inner*
- Epi—From Greek *epi,* meaning *on, upon*
- Fasc—From Latin *fascia,* meaning *band, bandage*
- Fibrous—From Latin *fibra,* meaning *fiber*
- Glyco—From Greek *glykys,* meaning *sweet*
- Lysis—From Greek *lysis,* meaning *dissolution, loosening*
- Myo—From Greek *mys,* meaning *muscle*
- Mys—From Latin *mys,* meaning *muscle*
- Peri—From Greek *peri,* meaning *around*
- Sarco—From Greek *sarkos,* meaning *muscle, flesh*

SECTION 12.1 SKELETAL MUSCLE

MUSCLE TISSUE:

- Three types of muscle tissue exist in the human body[1]:
  - **Cardiac muscle tissue**, located in the heart
  - **Smooth muscle tissue**, located in the walls of hollow visceral organs and blood vessels
  - **Skeletal muscle tissue**, located in skeletal muscles
- Skeletal muscle tissue makes up approximately 40% to 45% of total body weight.[1] This chapter, indeed this entire book, deals with skeletal muscle tissue.

CHARACTERISTICS OF SKELETAL MUSCLE:

- Because skeletal muscle tissue exhibits a striated (i.e., banded) appearance under a microscope, it is often called **striated muscle**.[2]
  - Note: Skeletal muscle tissue and cardiac muscle tissue are both striated in appearance under a microscope; smooth muscle tissue is not.[3]
- Skeletal muscle is under voluntary control.[1]
  - Note: Smooth muscle and cardiac muscle tissues are not under voluntary control, at least not typical full voluntary control. Although it is possible via biofeedback to affect the tone of smooth and cardiac muscle, it is not the full voluntary control that we have over skeletal muscles.

SKELETAL MUSCLE—THE BIG PICTURE:

- A skeletal muscle attaches onto two bones, thereby crossing the joint that is located between them.
  - A typical skeletal muscle has two attachments, each onto a bone. However, some skeletal muscles have more than two bony attachments, and some skeletal muscles attach into soft tissue instead of bone.
- The big picture of how a skeletal muscle works is that it can contract, attempting to shorten toward its center. (For a thorough explanation of the bigger picture of how skeletal muscles work, please see Chapter 13.)
- This contraction creates a pulling force on the bony attachments of the muscle.
- If this pulling force is sufficiently strong, one or both of the bones to which the muscle is attached will be pulled toward the center of the muscle.
- Because bones are located within body parts, movement of a bone results in movement of a body part (Figure 12-1).

To better understand the big picture of how muscles create movements of the body, it is necessary to explore and understand the microanatomy and microphysiology of skeletal muscle tissue.

460   PART 4   Myology: Study of the Muscular System

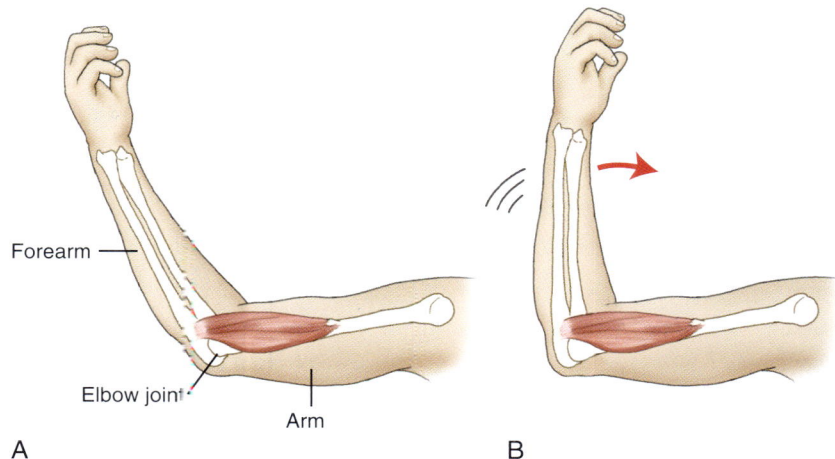

FIGURE 12-1 The "big picture" of muscle contraction. **A,** Muscle attaching from the humerus in the arm to the ulna in the forearm, crossing the elbow joint located between these two bones. When the muscle contracts, it creates a pulling force on the two bones to which it is attached. **B,** This pulling force has resulted in movement of the forearm toward the arm.

SECTION 12.2   TISSUE COMPONENTS OF A SKELETAL MUSCLE

- A skeletal muscle is an organ of the muscular system.
  - Note: By definition, an **organ** is made up of two or more different tissues, all acting together for one function.[4] In the case of a skeletal muscle, that function is to contract and create a pulling force.
- As an organ, a skeletal muscle contains more than one type of tissue. The two major types of tissue found in a skeletal muscle are (1) skeletal muscle tissue and (2) fibrous fascial connective tissue (Figure 12-2).
- Skeletal muscle tissue itself is composed of skeletal muscle cells. These muscle cells are the major structural and functional units of a muscle.[5]
  - They are the major structural units of a muscle in that the majority of a muscle is made up of muscle cells.
  - More important, they are the major functional units of a muscle in that they do the work of a muscle (i.e., the cells contract).
- The fibrous fascia of a muscle provides a structural framework for the muscle by enveloping the muscle tissue.[4]
  - Fibrous fascia wraps around the entire muscle, groups of muscle cells within the muscle, and each individual muscle cell.
- This fibrous fascia also continues beyond the muscle at both ends to create the tendons that attach the muscle to its bony attachment sites.[4] Tendons function to transmit the (tensile) pulling force of the muscle contraction to its attachment sites.
- Skeletal muscles also contain nerves and blood vessels.[6]
- The nerves carry both motor messages from the central nervous system to the muscle that instruct the muscle to contract, and sensory messages from the muscle to the central nervous system that inform the spinal cord and brain as to the state of the muscle.
- The blood vessels bring needed nutrients to the muscle tissue and drain away the waste products of the muscle's metabolism.

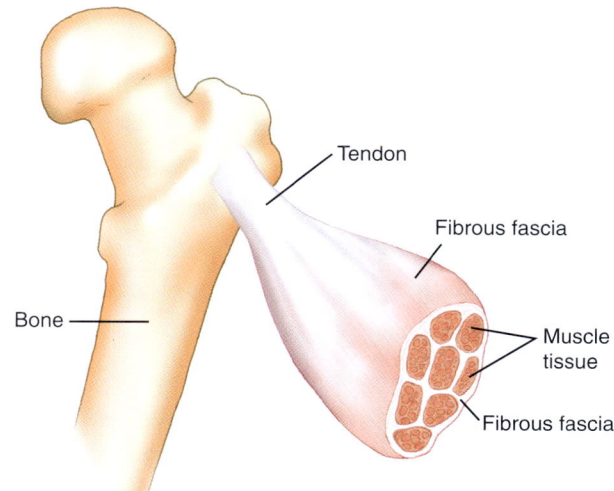

FIGURE 12-2 Cross-section of a muscle attached via its tendon to a bone. On cross-section, we see that the muscle is made up of skeletal muscle tissue and fibrous fascial tissue.

SECTION 12.3   SKELETAL MUSCLE CELLS

As stated, the major structural and functional component of skeletal muscle tissue is the skeletal muscle cell (Figure 12-3).
- Because a skeletal muscle cell has an elongated cylindric shape, a muscle cell can also be called a *muscle fiber* (i.e., the terms **muscle cell** and **muscle fiber** are synonyms).
- Muscle fibers can vary from approximately ½ inch to 20 inches (1 to 50 cm) in length.[7]
- Essentially, a skeletal muscle is made up of many muscle fibers that run lengthwise within the muscle.
- The exact manner in which the muscle fibers run within a muscle can vary and is described as the *architecture* of the muscle fibers. (For more details on muscle fiber architecture, please see Section 17.2.)
- It is rare for muscle fibers to run the entire length of a muscle. Usually they either lay end to end in series or lay parallel and overlap one another within the muscle (Figure 12-4).
- These muscle fibers are organized into bundles known as **fascicles**.[7] A fascicle may contain as many as 200 muscle fibers. (A synonym for fascicle is **fasciculus** [plural: fasciculi].)
- A skeletal muscle is composed of a number of fascicles (Figure 12-5).

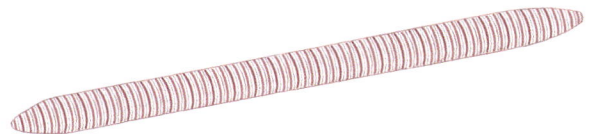

FIGURE 12-3   Individual skeletal muscle fiber (cell). The striated appearance should be noted.

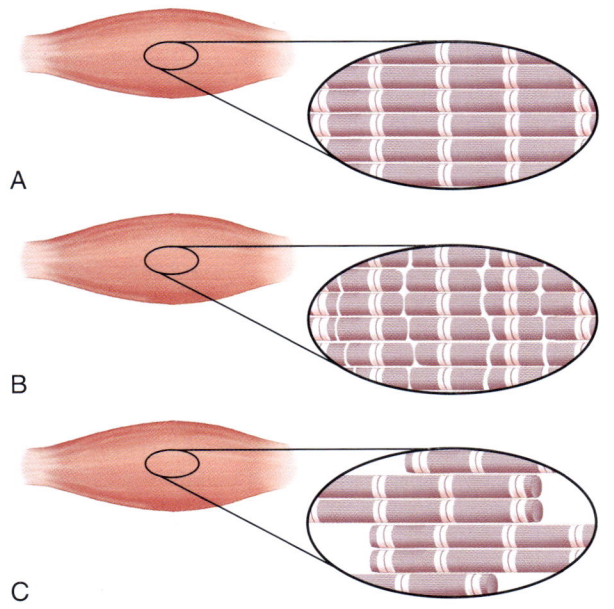

FIGURE 12-4   Various ways in which muscle fibers can be arranged within a muscle. **A,** Long muscle fibers lying parallel and running the length of the muscle. **B,** Shorter muscle fibers lying parallel and arranged end to end within the muscle. **C,** Muscle fibers lying parallel and overlapping.

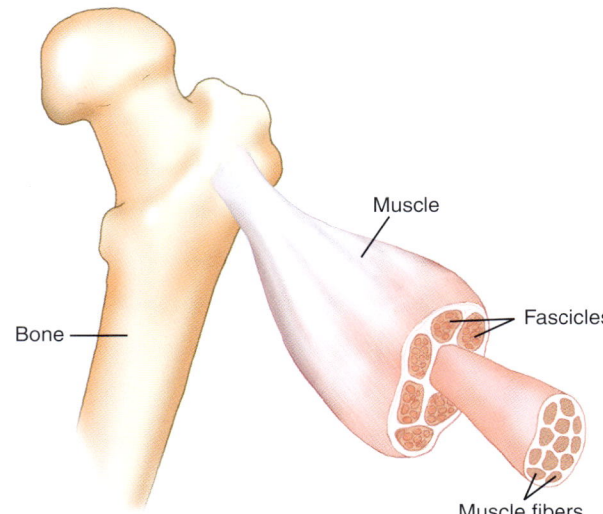

FIGURE 12-5   Cross-section of a muscle attached via its tendon to a bone. On cross-section, we see that the muscle is made up of a number of fascicles. One fascicle has been brought out farther, and we can see that it is longitudinal in length. Each fascicle is a bundle of muscle fibers.

SECTION 12.4 MUSCULAR FASCIA

- The tissue that creates the structural organization of a muscle is the tough fibrous fascia connective tissue that is also known as **muscular fascia** or **deep fascia**[8] (for more on fascia, see Section 4.1).
- The major component of muscular fascia is collagen fibers.[6]
- A small component of elastin fibers also exists in muscular fascia.[6]
- Although all muscular fascia is uniform in its composition, it is given different names depending on its location (Figure 12-6).
- The fibrous fascia that surrounds each individual muscle fiber is called **endomysium**.[3]
- The fibrous fascia that surrounds a group of muscle fibers, dividing the muscle into bundles known as *fascicles*, is called **perimysium**.[3]
- The fibrous fascia that surrounds an entire muscle is called **epimysium**.[3] (*Mys, epi, peri,* and *endo* are all Greek roots. *Mys* refers to muscle; *epi* means *upon; peri* means *around; endo* means *within.*)
- It is important to note that all three of these layers of fibrous fascia blend together and continue beyond the muscle to attach the muscle to a bone. The role of the fascial attachment is to transfer the force of the muscle contraction to the bone.
- These layers of fascia also serve to bind fibers together laterally. The endomysia of adjacent fibers create fascial connections that can serve to transmit the force of contraction laterally from one fiber to the adjacent fibers.[9] In other words, if fibers A and B are adjacent to each other, and fiber A contracts and fiber B does not, the force of contraction of fiber A will be transferred to fiber B, causing a pulling force in fiber B, even though fiber B was not stimulated to contract. This phenomenon is called **lateral force transmission**. Lateral force transmission can also occur between adjacent fascicles of a muscle via their perimysia and has been shown to occur between adjacent muscles via their epimysia. This phenomenon is not negligible. Lateral force transmission between adjacent muscles has been shown to transmit more than 30% of the contractile force from one muscle to the adjacent relaxed muscle.
- If the muscular fascia that attaches the muscle to a bone is round and cordlike, it is called a **tendon**.
- If the muscular fascia is broad and flat, it is called an **aponeurosis**.
  - Regarding their tissue composition, tendons and aponeuroses are identical; they differ only in shape.
- It should also be emphasized that although skeletal muscles usually attach to bones of the skeleton, hence their name, they often attach to other soft tissues of the body as well. One reason to have a broad and flat aponeurosis instead of a cordlike tendon is that an aponeurosis can spread out the force of a muscle's pull on its attachment site; this can allow for the muscle to attach into soft tissue that otherwise would not be able to withstand the concentrated force of a tendon pulling on it.
- Hence the tendons and/or aponeuroses of a muscle are an integral part of the muscle and cannot be divorced from the muscle. Indeed, many texts now refer to a muscle as a **myofascial unit**—*myo* referring to the muscular tissue component, and *fascial* referring to the fibrous fascial component (Box 12-1).

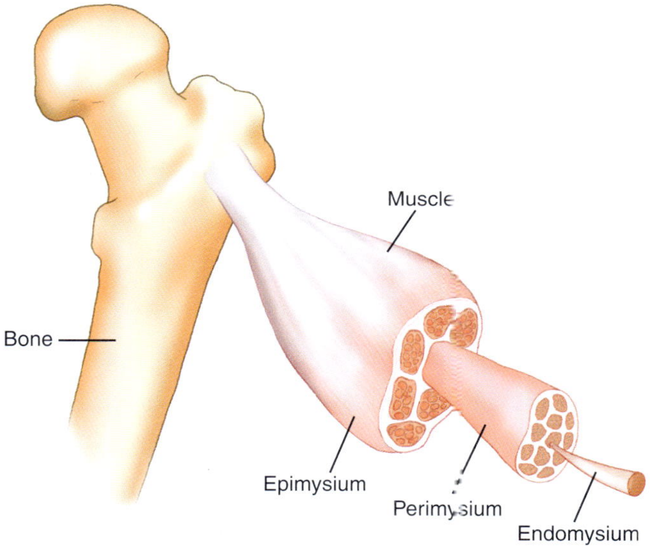

BOX 12-1

There is an interesting application to massage and other manual and movement therapies of the knowledge that the muscular and fascial tissues of a muscle are intimately linked. Many techniques focus on their effect on the muscles; others purport to work solely on the fascial planes of muscles. It is impossible to do any type of manual or movement therapy and not affect both the muscular tissue and the fascial tissue of a muscle!

- In addition to the fact that muscular fascia extends beyond the muscles to become tendons and aponeuroses, it also creates thick intermuscular septa that separate muscles of the body and provide a site of attachment for adjacent muscles.
- Muscular fascia also creates even more expansive thin aponeurotic sheets of fascia that envelop large groups of muscles in the body.
- Another function of these fascial planes of tissue is that they provide pathways for the nerves and blood vessels that innervate and feed nutrients to the muscle fibers[2] (Figure 12-7).

FIGURE 12-6 Organization of muscular fascia within a muscle. Each muscle fiber is surrounded by endomysium; perimysium surrounds a number of muscle fibers, creating groups of fibers known as fascicles. The entire muscle is surrounded by epimysium. All three of these fibrous fascial layers then meld together to create the tendons and/or aponeuroses that attach the muscle to its bony attachments.

CHAPTER 12 Anatomy and Physiology of Muscle Tissue

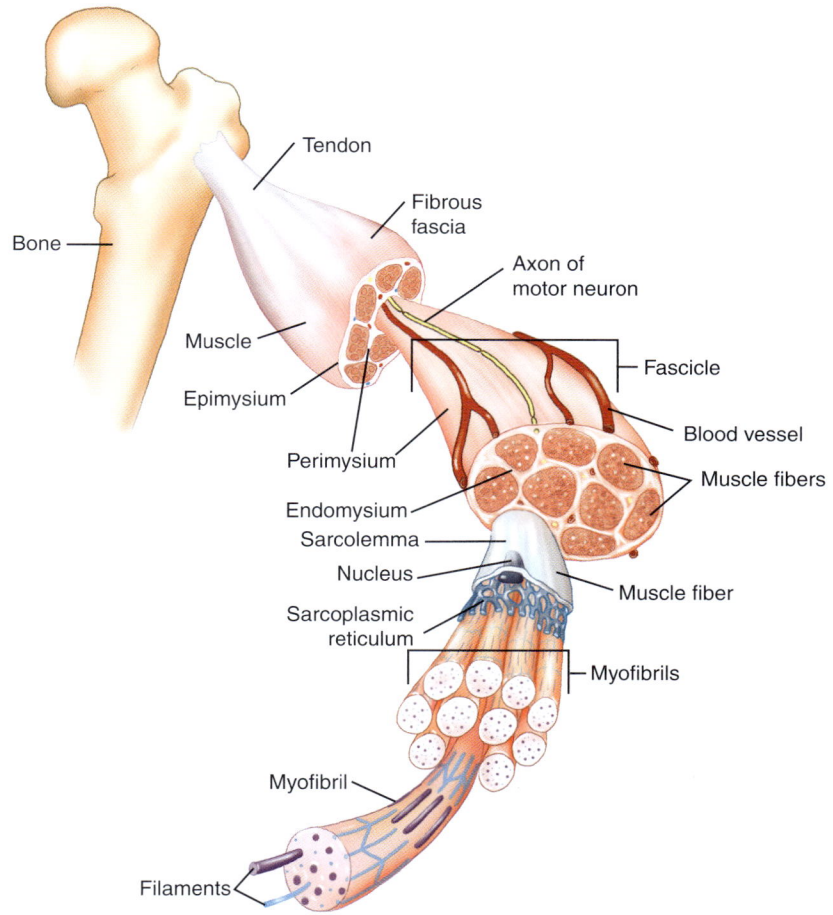

FIGURE 12-7 Interior of a muscle fiber (i.e., muscle cell). Note how the nerves and blood vessels travel along fascial planes.

SECTION 12.5 MICROANATOMY OF MUSCLE FIBER/SARCOMERE STRUCTURE

- Like any other type of cell in the human body, skeletal muscle fibers are enveloped by a cell membrane and contain many **cytoplasmic organelles**.
- However, the names given to many of these cellular structures are slightly different from those given to most of the other types of cells of the body in that the root word *sarco* is often incorporated into the name.
- *Sarco* is the Greek word root denoting flesh (i.e., muscle tissue).
- For example, the cytoplasm of a skeletal muscle fiber is called the **sarcoplasm**; the endoplasmic reticulum is called the **sarcoplasmic reticulum**; and the cell membrane is called the **sarcolemma**.[10]
- Skeletal muscle fibers are unusual in many ways.
- They are multinucleate (they contain many nuclei). This is because each muscle fiber (cell) developed from multiple stem cells grouping together.[2]
- They are rich in mitochondria. Mitochondria create adenosine triphosphate (ATP) molecules aerobically. Because muscle tissue contraction requires a great amount of energy expenditure, multiple mitochondria furnish this energy in the form of ATP molecules.[2]
- And they contain an oxygen-binding molecule called **myoglobin**. Myoglobin is similar to hemoglobin of red blood cells, except that it has an even greater ability to bind oxygen.[4]
- However, the most stunning structural characteristic of skeletal muscle fibers is their tremendous number of cytoplasmic organelles called *myofibrils*. Each **myofibril** is longitudinally oriented within the cytoplasm, running the entire length of the muscle fiber[4] (see Figure 12-7).
- Approximately 1000 myofibrils exist in a muscle fiber.[4]
- Myofibrils are composed of units called **sarcomeres** that are laid end to end from one end of the myofibril to the other end (they also lie side by side).[10]
- Sarcomeres are very short. On average, approximately 10,000 sarcomeres are found per linear inch (approximately 4000 per cm) of myofibril.
- The boundaries of each sarcomere are known as **Z-lines**.[4]

- Within each sarcomere are protein filaments known as *actin* and *myosin*.[9]
- **Actin filaments** are thin, and **myosin filaments** are thick.[10]
- These filaments are arranged in an orderly fashion. Actin filaments are attached to the Z-lines at both ends of a sarcomere. Myosin filaments are not attached to the Z-lines; rather they are located in the center of the sarcomere.
- Skeletal muscle tissue is said to be *striated*; this means that under a microscope it appears to have lines. It is the characteristic pattern of the overlapping of the actin and myosin filaments that creates this striation pattern that skeletal muscle tissue possesses.[2]
- It is also important to note that myosin filaments have globular projections known as *heads*. Each **myosin head** sticks out toward the actin filaments[4] (Figure 12-8).
- It is the sarcomere (of the myofibrils of muscle fibers) that is the actual functional unit of skeletal muscle tissue.
  - That is, sarcomeres perform the essential physiologic function of contraction that makes muscle tissue unique from most all other tissue types of the body.
- Therefore to truly understand the functioning of a muscle, we must examine the function of a sarcomere. If the function of a sarcomere is understood, then the larger picture of musculoskeletal function (i.e., the field of kinesiology) can be better understood.
- The name that is given to this physiologic process of a sarcomere is the *sliding filament mechanism*[5] (Box 12-2).

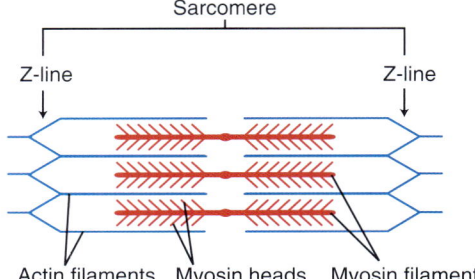

FIGURE 12-8 Structure of a sarcomere. A sarcomere spans from one Z-line to the next Z-line. Sarcomeres contain two types of filaments: (1) actin and (2) myosin. Myosin filaments are the thicker filaments located in the center of the sarcomere. Actin filaments are the thinner filaments attached to the Z-lines. The armlike globular projections, called heads of the myosin filaments, should be noted.

BOX 12-2 Spotlight on the Sliding Filament Mechanism

The knowledge of how the sliding filament mechanism works is essential to understanding the larger picture of how muscles function. Indeed, a clear understanding of concentric, eccentric, and isometric contractions, as well as the principles of trigger point genesis and active insufficiency (among other concepts), is dependent on a fundamental understanding of the sliding filament mechanism. Instead of being merely an abstract study of the microphysiology of muscle cells, the sliding filament mechanism creates the foundation for being able to truly understand (instead of having to memorize) the larger concepts needed to be an effective therapist/trainer/instructor in the musculoskeletal field.

The sliding filament mechanism is often termed the sliding filament theory. It should be noted that the word theory in the field of science is often misunderstood today. In everyday English, the word theory means a guess or conjecture that remains to be proven; it is a fairly weak term that connotes a fair amount of doubt as to whether or not it is true. However, in the field of science, the word theory is a much stronger term (indeed, the word law, which is even stronger, is rarely used). Little doubt exists as to the veracity of the mechanism of the sliding filament theory.

The sliding filament theory is also known as the **ratchet theory**. The name *ratchet theory* denotes the idea of how the myosin's cross-bridges pull on the actin filament in a ratchetlike manner. A ratchet wrench exerts tension on a nut, then lets go of this tension as the wrench is swung back, then exerts tension once again; this cycle is repeated over and over. Similarly, a myosin cross-bridge pulls on the actin filament, exerting tension; then it relaxes by letting go, exerts tension once again, and then relaxes again. This cycle is repeated many times.

SECTION 12.6 SLIDING FILAMENT MECHANISM

- The mechanism that explains how sarcomeres shorten is called the **sliding filament mechanism** because during shortening of a sarcomere, the actin and myosin filaments slide along each other.
- In essence, the mechanism of the sliding filament mechanism is as follows[9] (Figure 12-9):
  1. A message is sent from the nervous system that tells muscle fibers to contract.
  2. This message causes the sarcoplasmic reticulum to release stored calcium into the sarcoplasm (cytoplasm).
  3. These calcium ions attach onto the actin filaments, exposing **actin filament binding sites** (also called **actin filament active sites**).
  4. Myosin heads attach onto these exposed binding sites of the actin filaments, creating cross-bridges between the myosin filament and the actin filaments.
  5. Each **myosin cross-bridge** then bends, creating a pulling force that pulls the actin filaments in toward the center of the sarcomere.

6. These cross-bridges then break, and the myosin heads re-attach onto the next binding sites of the actin filaments, forming new cross-bridges, which then bend, further pulling the actin filaments in toward the center of the sarcomere.[10] (Note: When an illustration of actin and myosin filaments is shown, it is common to simplify and show only one or a few cross-bridges. In reality, thousands of cross-bridges exist between a myosin and multiple actin filaments. When some of these cross-bridges break, others remain attached so that the actin filaments do not slip back.)

7. This process occurs over and over again, as long as the message to contract is given to the muscle by the nervous system.
8. Because the actin filaments are attached to the Z-lines of the sarcomere (i.e., the boundaries of the sarcomere), the Z-lines are pulled in toward the center of the sarcomere.[5]
9. When Z-lines are pulled in toward the center of the sarcomere, the sarcomere shortens[5] (Figure 12-10).
10. To relate this concept to the bigger picture of how a muscle works, it is important to realize that when all the sarcomeres of a myofibril shorten in this manner, the myofibril shortens; when all the myofibrils of a muscle fiber shorten, the muscle fiber shortens. When enough muscle fibers of a muscle shorten, the muscle shortens, exerting a pulling force on its bony attachments. If this pulling force is sufficiently strong, the bones are pulled toward each other, creating movement of the body parts within which the bones are located. Hence via the sliding filament mechanism, muscles can create movement of body parts!

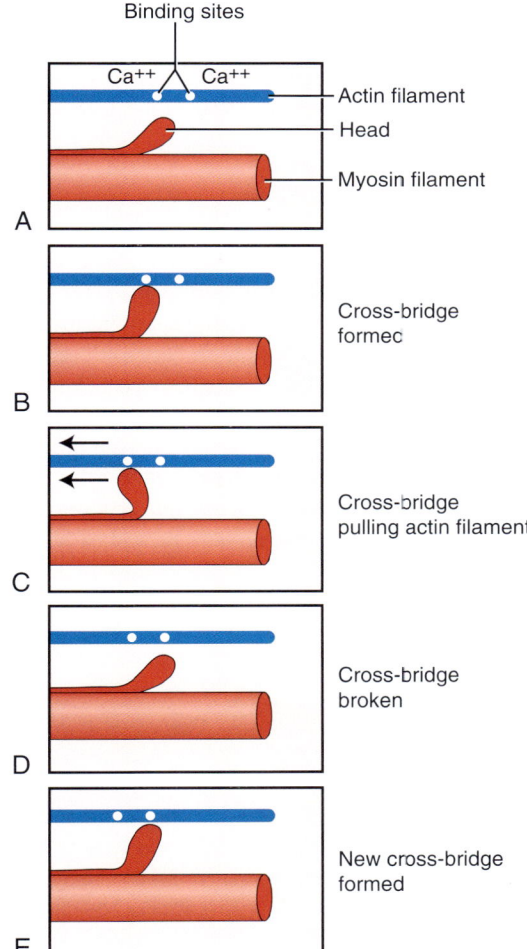

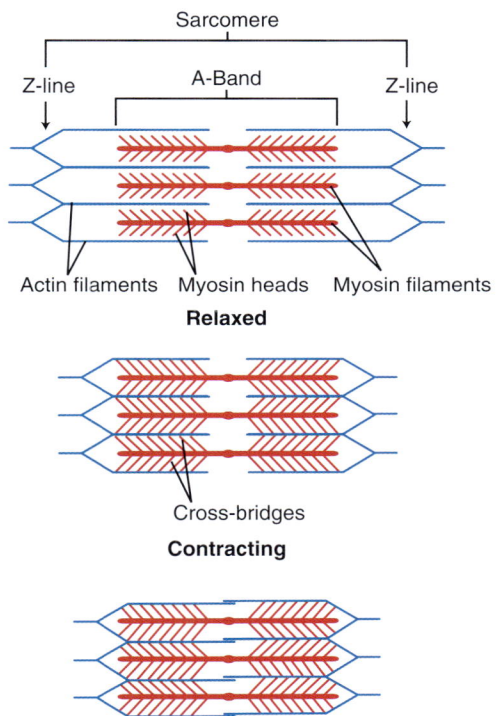

FIGURE 12-9 Steps of the sliding filament mechanism. **A,** Binding sites are exposed because of the presence of calcium ions that have been released by the sarcoplasmic reticulum. **B,** Myosin head forms a cross-bridge by attaching to the actin binding site. **C,** Myosin head bends, pulling the actin filament toward the center of the sarcomere. **D,** Myosin cross-bridge breaks. **E,** Process begins again when the myosin head attaches to another actin binding site.

FIGURE 12-10 Illustration of how the sliding filament mechanism results in a change in length of the sarcomere. From the resting length of a sarcomere when it is relaxed, we see that as the sarcomere begins to contract, it begins to shorten toward its center. When the sarcomere is fully contracted, the sarcomere is at its shortest length.

SECTION 12.7 ENERGY SOURCE FOR THE SLIDING FILAMENT MECHANISM

It is intuitively known that muscle contraction demands a great deal of energy expenditure by the body. We only need to exercise for a short period of time to realize how energy demanding muscle contraction is.

- The energy that drives the sliding filament mechanism comes from **adenosine triphosphate** (ATP) molecules[5] (Box 12-3).
- Two steps of the sliding filament mechanism require the expenditure of energy by ATP molecules[5]:
  1. Energy must be furnished by ATP molecules for myosin-actin cross-bridges to break.
  2. The reuptake of calcium back into the sarcoplasmic reticulum when a muscle contraction is completed also requires energy to be provided by ATP molecules.
- Following is the order of the four steps in which ATP molecules are supplied to provide the energy needed for the sliding filament mechanism[11]:
  1. Stored ATP
  2. Regeneration of ATP from stored creatine phosphate
  3. Regeneration of ATP from anaerobic breakdown of glucose
  4. Regeneration of ATP from aerobic breakdown of glucose
- First, stored ATP molecules within the muscle fiber are used. However, the supply of stored ATP molecules is very small and is soon depleted.[4]
- Therefore the second step is to regenerate more ATP from creatine phosphate molecules that are present and stored in the muscle fiber.[4]
- When the stored creatine phosphate supply is exhausted, ATP must be regenerated from another source, the breakdown of glucose (also called **respiration of glucose**).[4]
- Breakdown of glucose can occur in two ways: (1) aerobically or (2) anaerobically.[4]
- Regeneration of ATP from glucose first occurs anaerobically (without the presence of oxygen) within the sarcoplasm of the cell.
- If a continuing supply of energy is still needed, the muscle fiber gradually transitions to the breakdown of glucose aerobically within the mitochondria (Box 12-4). Aerobic breakdown of glucose within the mitochondria requires oxygen (hence the name *aerobic*) and therefore requires circulation of blood to deliver this oxygen; this increased circulation places a demand on the heart to pump more blood and thereby exercises the heart (see Box 12-4).

OXYGEN DEBT:

- If a person exercises and overcomes the ability of the cardiovascular system to deliver oxygen for the aerobic breakdown of glucose, then the muscle fibers must rely on anaerobic breakdown of glucose to a greater degree. Because anaerobic breakdown of glucose creates lactic acid as a waste product, lactic acid can build up in the muscle fibers. This lactic acid is usually transported to the liver, where it can be converted back to glucose. However,[4] this conversion requires oxygen, and the oxygen needed can be looked at as a debt that the body owes itself. For this reason, the term **oxygen debt** is used to describe this debt of oxygen that is needed to convert the buildup of lactic acid back to glucose. This oxygen debt explains why a person may continue to breathe deeply even after his or her exercise is completed.[4]

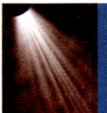

BOX 12-3   Spotlight on ATP

Adenosine triphosphate (ATP) is an adenosine base molecule with three phosphate groups attached. The bonds between the base and the phosphate groups contain energy and can be broken to liberate energy for use by the sliding filament mechanism. Once one of these bonds has been broken, adenosine diphosphate (ADP; adenosine with two phosphate groups) and a free phosphate group result. The ADP can be converted back to ATP for use again by the body. Thus ATP molecules can be likened to rechargeable batteries that provide energy for the processes for metabolism.

Energy provided by ATP is necessary for myosin-actin cross-bridges of the sliding filament mechanism to break. Once the myosin head has disconnected from the actin filament, it can reattach to the actin filament's next binding site and then bend again. Interestingly, the fact that energy is required to break the myosin-actin cross-bridges accounts for rigor mortis, which is the stiffness caused by muscle contractions that occurs shortly after a person dies. Two reasons for these contractions exist: (1) Some of the muscles were in a state of contraction when the person died, and (2) other muscle contractions occur after death because of calcium ions that leak out of the sarcoplasmic reticulum into the sarcoplasm, triggering myosin-actin cross-bridges to occur. However, because the person's metabolism stops after death, no further ATP molecules are created to break these cross-bridges of contraction. Rigor mortis continues until the tissue actually breaks down and the cross-bridges cease to exist.

ATP expenditure is also needed for the reuptake of calcium back into the sarcoplasmic reticulum. This explains the current theory for how **trigger points (TrPs)** form and why they persist. TrPs squeeze blood vessels, thereby diminishing blood flow. Loss of blood flow decreases the delivery of glucose to the muscle cells, resulting in a deficiency of ATP production. This energy shortage results in both a decreased ability to break the cross-bridges that exist and decreased reuptake of the calcium from the sarcoplasm back into the sarcoplasmic reticulum; thus cross-bridges persist in that local area in the form of trigger points. This theory is known as the **energy crisis hypothesis**.[16] (For more detail on the sliding filament mechanism, see Section 12.12.)

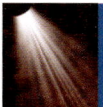

BOX 12-4 Spotlight on Breakdown/Respiration of Glucose

Anaerobic breakdown of glucose is known as **glycolysis** (glyco means sugar; lysis means breakdown). For each molecule of glucose broken down by the process of glycolysis, two adenosine triphosphate (ATP) molecules are formed and the waste product **lactic acid** is created.[11]

Aerobic breakdown of glucose is known as the **Kreb's cycle** (it is also known as the citric acid cycle). The Kreb's cycle creates approximately 36 molecules of adenosine triphosphate (ATP) for each molecule of glucose that is broken down; it is much more efficient than the process of glycolysis. The waste products of the Kreb's cycle are carbon dioxide and water.[11] It is interesting to note that the role of oxygen in the Kreb's cycle is to bond to the carbon atoms that are created when a glucose molecule is broken down; this creates carbon dioxide, which is a gas that can be easily carried away in the bloodstream and eliminated from the body via the lungs. Thus oxygen's role in our bodies is to facilitate the elimination of the carbon atoms.

People often speak of aerobic and anaerobic exercises, which actually refer to the method of the breakdown of glucose to generate ATP for energy for the sliding filament mechanism. Because the body turns to aerobic breakdown of glucose last, aerobic exercises must be, by necessity, exercises that are sustained. For example, a sprint is anaerobic and a marathon is aerobic. It actually takes only 1 to 2 minutes for the energy of an exercise to be primarily delivered via aerobic breakdown of glucose. Of course, once this threshold is reached, it must be sustained for a further period of time for cardiovascular benefits to be gained. Exactly how much longer is optimal is debated.

SECTION 12.8 NERVOUS SYSTEM CONTROL OF MUSCLE CONTRACTION

- A skeletal muscle fiber cannot contract on its own; it must be told to contract by the nervous system.
- Contraction of a skeletal muscle fiber is directed by a message from the central nervous system that travels within a motor neuron that is located within a peripheral nerve. The peripheral spinal nerve that goes out into the periphery and directs the muscle to contract is said to provide **innervation** to the muscle (Figure 12-11).
  - Note regarding neurologic terms: The central nervous system is located in the center of the body; hence the name. It is composed of the brain and the spinal cord. A neuron is a nerve cell; a motor neuron is a motor nerve cell (i.e., a nerve cell that tells muscles to contract). A peripheral nerve is located in the periphery of the body (i.e., not in the center or central nervous system). Spinal nerves that come from the spinal cord and cranial nerves that come from the brain are peripheral nerves. Each peripheral nerve contains many neurons.
- When the motor neuron reaches the muscle fiber, it does not physically attach or connect directly to the muscle fiber. Rather, a small space is located between them that is known as the **synaptic cleft**. A synaptic cleft is also known as a **synaptic gap** or simply a **synapse**.
- The electrical message for contraction that the motor neuron carries causes the motor neuron to release molecules into the synapse. These molecules transmit the neural message for contraction to the muscle fiber; hence they are called **neurotransmitters**.
- Many neurotransmitters exist in the human body. The one that is released between motor neurons and skeletal muscle fibers is **acetylcholine**. When a motor neuron is no longer stimulated to secrete acetylcholine, the acetylcholine that was secreted and is present within the synaptic cleft is removed by the enzyme **acetylcholinesterase**. Once the neurotransmitter acetylcholine is no longer present, the muscle cell is no longer stimulated to contract and can now relax.[4]
- The location where the motor neuron and muscle fiber meet (i.e., junction) is known as the **neuromuscular junction** (Figure 12-12).
- At the neuromuscular junction, the sarcolemma (i.e., cell membrane) of the muscle fiber is specialized to receive the neurotransmitters of the motor neuron and is known as the **motor end plate**.
- These neurotransmitters float through the fluid of the synapse and bind to the motor end plate of the muscle fiber.
- The binding of the neurotransmitters to the motor end plate initiates an electrical impulse to travel along the sarcolemma of the entire muscle fiber. The electrical impulse is then transmitted into the interior of the muscle fiber via the **transverse tubules** (usually called **T-tubules**) of the muscle fiber[2] (Figure 12-13).

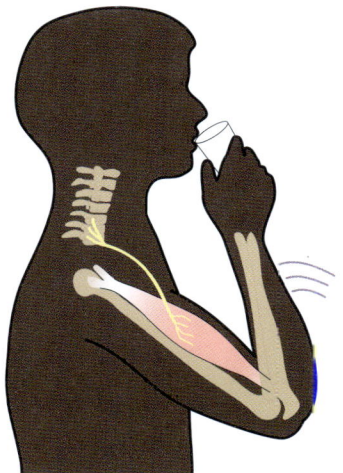

FIGURE 12-11 A person contracting an arm muscle to flex the forearm at the elbow joint to drink a glass of water. The order to contract this muscle occurs within the central nervous system and is then carried within a motor neuron that is located within a peripheral spinal nerve that exits the spinal cord in the cervical spine region. This peripheral spinal nerve is said to innervate this muscle.

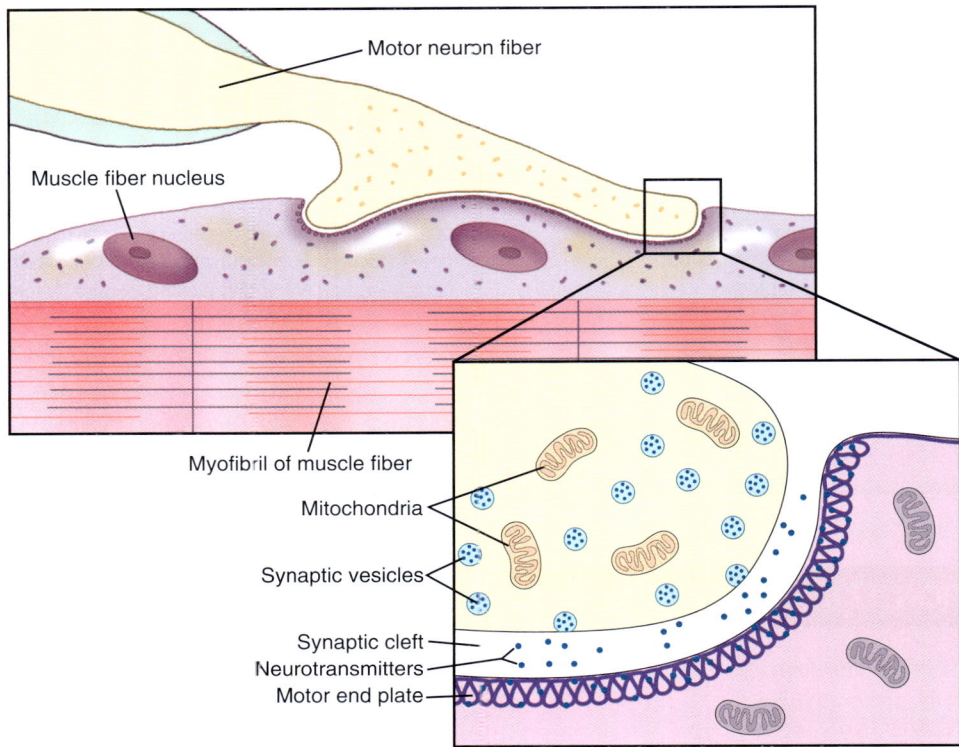

FIGURE 12-12 Neuromuscular junction. We see the synaptic vesicles containing neurotransmitter molecules in the distal end of the motor neuron. These neurotransmitters are released into the synaptic cleft and then bind to the motor end plate of the muscle fiber. (Note: The inset box provides an enlargement.)

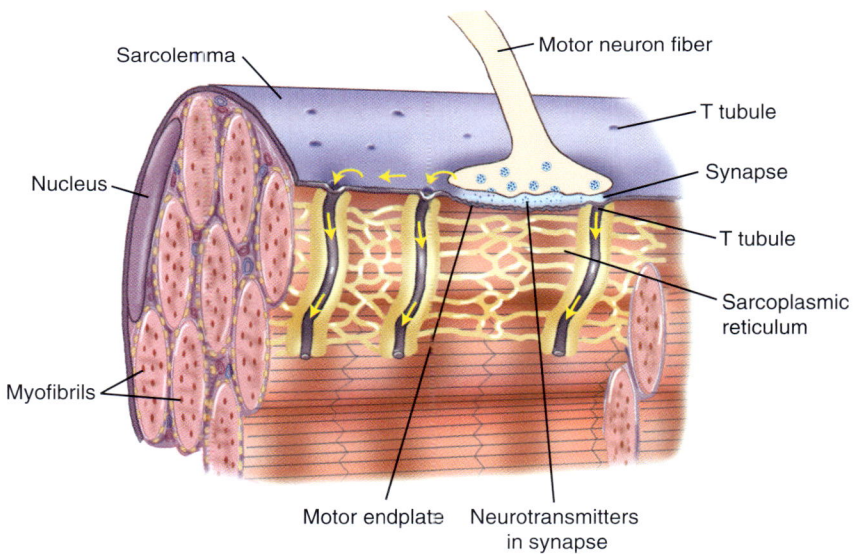

FIGURE 12-13 Binding of the neurotransmitters onto the motor end plate of the muscle fiber initiates an electrical impulse to travel along the sarcolemma of the entire muscle fiber. The electrical impulse is then transmitted into the interior of the muscle fiber via the transverse tubules (T-tubules) of the muscle fiber.

- Once this electrical message to contract has reached the interior of the muscle fiber, it triggers the sliding filament mechanism to begin by causing the release of stored calcium from the sarcoplasmic reticulum into the sarcoplasm. (See the discussion of the sliding filament mechanism in Section 12.6.)
- Motor neurons only carry a message for contraction of the muscle fiber. As long as the motor neuron is stimulating a muscle fiber, calcium will continue to be released from the sarcoplasmic reticulum into the sarcoplasm, which will continue the sliding filament mechanism for contraction, and the muscle fiber will remain in a contracted state.
- If the central nervous system desires a muscle fiber to relax, then a message for contraction is not sent to the muscle. In other words, in the absence of a neural message for contraction, a muscle fiber relaxes (Box 12-5).

- Once a muscle fiber is no longer stimulated to contract, the calcium ions that were released by the sarcoplasmic reticulum are reabsorbed back into the sarcoplasmic reticulum. Now that the calcium is no longer present, the binding sites on actin are no longer available to the myosin heads; thus new cross-bridges cannot be made, and (assuming that already present cross-bridges are released) the sliding filament mechanism no longer occurs. Therefore muscle fiber contraction ceases and the muscle fiber relaxes.
- As previously stated in Section 12.7, reabsorption of calcium back into the sarcoplasmic reticulum is necessary to stop the sliding filament mechanism requires energy expenditure by adenosine triphosphate (ATP).

HUMAN RESTING MUSCLE TONE:

- The statement that a muscle cannot contract on its own without direction from the nervous system is not completely true. It has been found that muscle tissue does have a very low baseline resting muscle tone that is independent of the nervous system's direction. Termed **human resting muscle tone (HRMT)**, this low baseline level of contraction is believed to result from a small but constant presence of calcium ions in the sarcoplasm. Their presence exposes a small number of active sites on actin filaments that are then attached onto by myosin heads, creating cross-bridges and therefore contraction. HRMT has been found to create a contractile force that is approximately 1% of the maximum contractile force of the muscle, and is believed to be important for postural stability. Note: The term *human resting muscle tone* should not be confused with the term *resting tone* (see Box 19-1 in Section 19.2), which refers to the tone of a muscle when it is at rest, and is directed by the nervous system as a result of the *muscle memory* of the gamma motor nervous system[12] (see Box 19-7 in Section 19.6).

BOX 12-5

It is important to emphasize that a muscle fiber does not contract on its own. Furthermore, it has no stored pattern or memory of how or when to contract. The term **muscle memory**, used so prevalently in the fields of manual and movement therapies and exercise, describes the very important concept of the memory pattern of muscle contractions that exists in the body. However, muscle memory resides in the nervous system, not within the muscle tissue itself (more specifically, muscle memory resides in the gamma motor system; see Section 19.6). A muscle that has lost its innervation loses its ability to contract (unless electricity is applied to it from an outside source, such as from physical therapy equipment).

SECTION 12.9 MOTOR UNIT

- A **motor unit** is defined as "one motor neuron and all the muscle fibers that it controls" (i.e., with which it synapses).
- When a motor neuron reaches a muscle, it branches numerous times to synapse with a number of muscle fibers. In this manner, a motor neuron actually controls a number of muscle fibers (Figure 12-14).
- It is interesting to note that one motor unit usually has muscle fibers that are located in a number of different fascicles; in other words, motor units have fibers that are somewhat spread throughout the muscle and are not restricted to fascicular organization.
- This branching is important because skeletal muscle fibers cannot pass the message to contract from one to another. Instead, each individual muscle fiber must be told to contract directly by the motor neuron.
- All motor units are similar in that they have one motor neuron. The distinguishing factor that determines the size of a motor unit is the number of branches and therefore the number of muscle fibers that one motor neuron controls; this varies from as few as two or three to as many as 2000.[10] The average number of fibers in a motor unit is 100 to 200.
- Smaller motor units create contraction of a smaller number of muscle fibers and therefore create smaller, finer, more precise actions.[4]
  - Therefore smaller motor units exist in locations where very fine and precise body movements are needed. The smallest motor units exist in the muscles that move the eyeball (i.e., extraocular muscles).
- Larger motor units create a contraction of a greater number of muscle fibers and therefore create larger, grosser, more powerful actions.[4]
  - Therefore larger motor units tend to exist where larger movements are needed and finer precise movements are not necessary. Larger motor units exist in such muscles as the gluteus maximus and gastrocnemius. (For information on the types of muscle fibers that are found in smaller versus larger motor units, see Section 12.13. For more details on how and when motor units are recruited to contract, see Section 17.1.)
- Generally a muscle has a mixture of motor units; some are small and some are large.

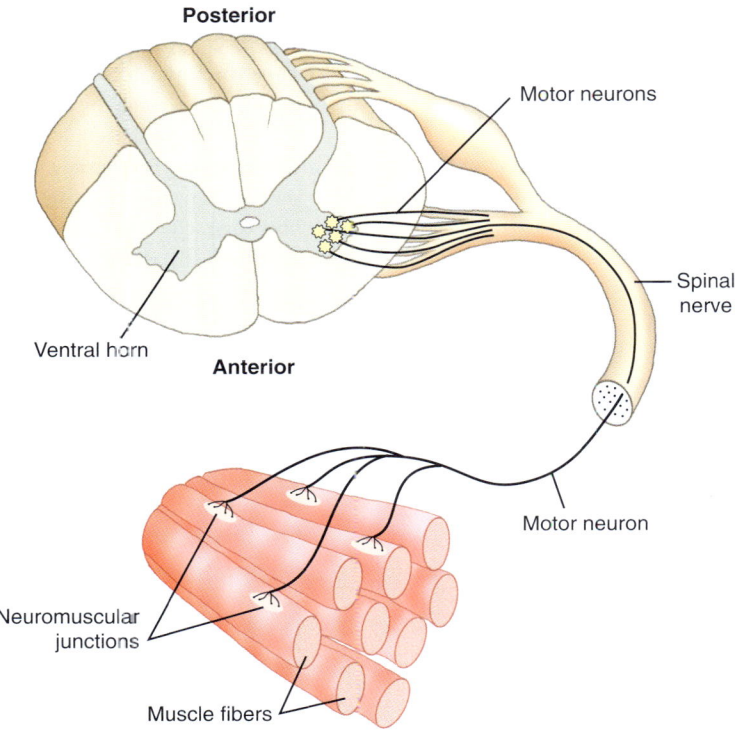

FIGURE 12-14 Small motor unit containing four muscle fibers. A motor neuron is shown exiting the spinal cord and traveling through a spinal nerve and innervating four muscle fibers of a muscle.

SECTION 12.10 ALL-OR-NONE–RESPONSE LAW

- When a message for contraction is sent from the nervous system to a muscle fiber, that message instructs the muscle fiber to contract completely (i.e., 100%). If no message is sent, then the muscle fiber relaxes completely (i.e., 0% contraction).[10]
- Therefore a muscle fiber contraction is an all-or-nothing mechanism, and this concept is called the **all-or-none–response law**.
- If we understand how muscle tissue is innervated by the nervous system, then it is easy to apply the all-or-none–response law to muscle tissue.
  - The all-or-none–response law applies to the sarcomere, the myofibril, the muscle fiber, and the motor unit, because all these structural levels of muscle tissue are innervated by a single motor neuron that either carries the message to contract or does not carry the message to contract.
  - However, the all-or-none–response law does not apply to an entire skeletal muscle. A skeletal muscle can have partial contractions.
  - A skeletal muscle has a number of motor units within it; some of these motor units may be told to contract by their motor neurons, whereas other motor units within the muscle may be relaxed because their motor neurons are not stimulating them to contract at that time.
  - Therefore an entire skeletal muscle can have partial contractions because the nervous system can order some motor units to contract while others are relaxed. In this manner the nervous system can control the degree of contraction of a muscle. By having the ability to control the degree of contraction, a person can generate just the right amount of force needed for each particular situation. For example, if a person wants to do a bicep curl and lift a 5-lb weight, a partial contraction of the biceps brachii muscle is needed. If however, the person wants to do a bicep curl and lift a 15-lb weight, a stronger partial contraction by the biceps brachii is needed. Again, a partial contraction of a muscle occurs by having some of the motor units of the muscle contract completely and other motor units of the muscle not contract at all (Figure 12-15). In other words, more motor units will contract to lift the 15-lb weight than the 5-lb weight.

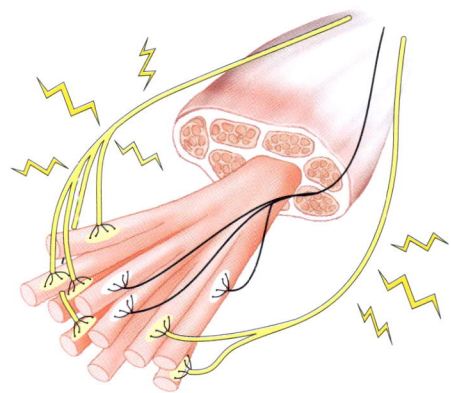

FIGURE 12-15 Illustration of the idea that a muscle contains multiple motor units and that some may contract while others are relaxed. In this figure, two motor units (yellow) are contracting, while the other motor unit (black) is relaxed.

SECTION 12.11 SARCOMERE STRUCTURE IN MORE DETAIL

- A myofibril of a muscle fiber is made up of many sarcomeres that are arranged both next to one another and also end to end along the length of the sarcomere.
- Each sarcomere is made up of actin and myosin filaments. These filaments are arranged in a hexangular fashion so that a myosin filament is located in the center of the sarcomere and six actin filaments are located around each end of the myosin filament, partially overlapping it (Figure 12-16).
- This consistent pattern of overlapping filaments within the sarcomeres gives myofibrils a banded striated appearance. These bands are designated with letters (Figure 12-17, A).
- Sarcomeres also contain very large molecules of a protein called titin.
- The two main bands of a sarcomere are the A-band and the I-band.
- The letters *A* in A-band and *I* in I-band stand for *anisotropic* and *isotropic,* which are optical terms that describe how light is affected when this tissue is viewed under a microscope.[9]
  - The **A-band** is dark and is defined by the presence of myosin. Because myosin is in the center of a sarcomere, the A-band is located in the center of the sarcomere. Note: Within the A-band, a region exists where only myosin is located (H-band), and a region exists where myosin and actin are located.
  - The **I-band** is light and is defined by where only actin filaments are located. Note that the I-band is partially within one sarcomere and partially located within the adjacent sarcomere.
- Again, these alternating dark and light bands give skeletal muscle its striated appearance (see Figure 12-17, B and C).
- Smaller bands are also located within these larger bands[5]:
  - The **H-band** is the region of the A-band that contains only myosin.
  - The **M-band** (usually referred to as the **M-line**) is within the H-band (which in turn is located within the A-band) at the center of the myosin molecule.
  - The **Z-band**, usually referred to as the *Z-line,* is at the center of the I-band. Remember that the Z-line is the border between two adjacent sarcomeres.

MYOSIN FILAMENT IN MORE DETAIL:

- A myosin filament is actually made up of many myosin molecules that are bound together (Figure 12-18, A). Each individual myosin molecule has a shape that resembles a golf club[4] (Figure 12-18, B).
- These myosin molecules are arranged such that half of them have their heads sticking out at one end of the sarcomere and the other half of them have their heads sticking out at the other end of the sarcomere.
- Each myosin molecule is composed of two main parts: (1) the **myosin tail** and (2) the myosin head.
- The tail is the main length of the myosin molecule.
- The tail of a myosin molecule is called the **light meromyosin** component.[10]
- The head is the part that sticks out to attach onto the actin filament, forming the actin-myosin cross-bridge.

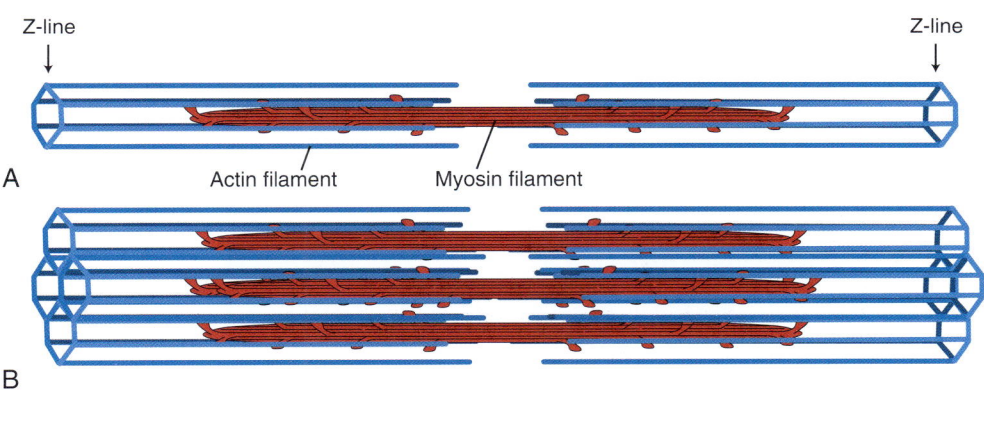

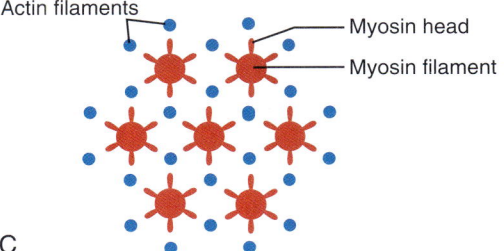

FIGURE 12-16 **A,** One myosin filament surrounded by six actin filaments at each end. **B,** How multiple sarcomeres that lay next to one another are arranged. **C,** Cross-section of a sarcomere showing that each myosin filament is surrounded by six actin filaments.

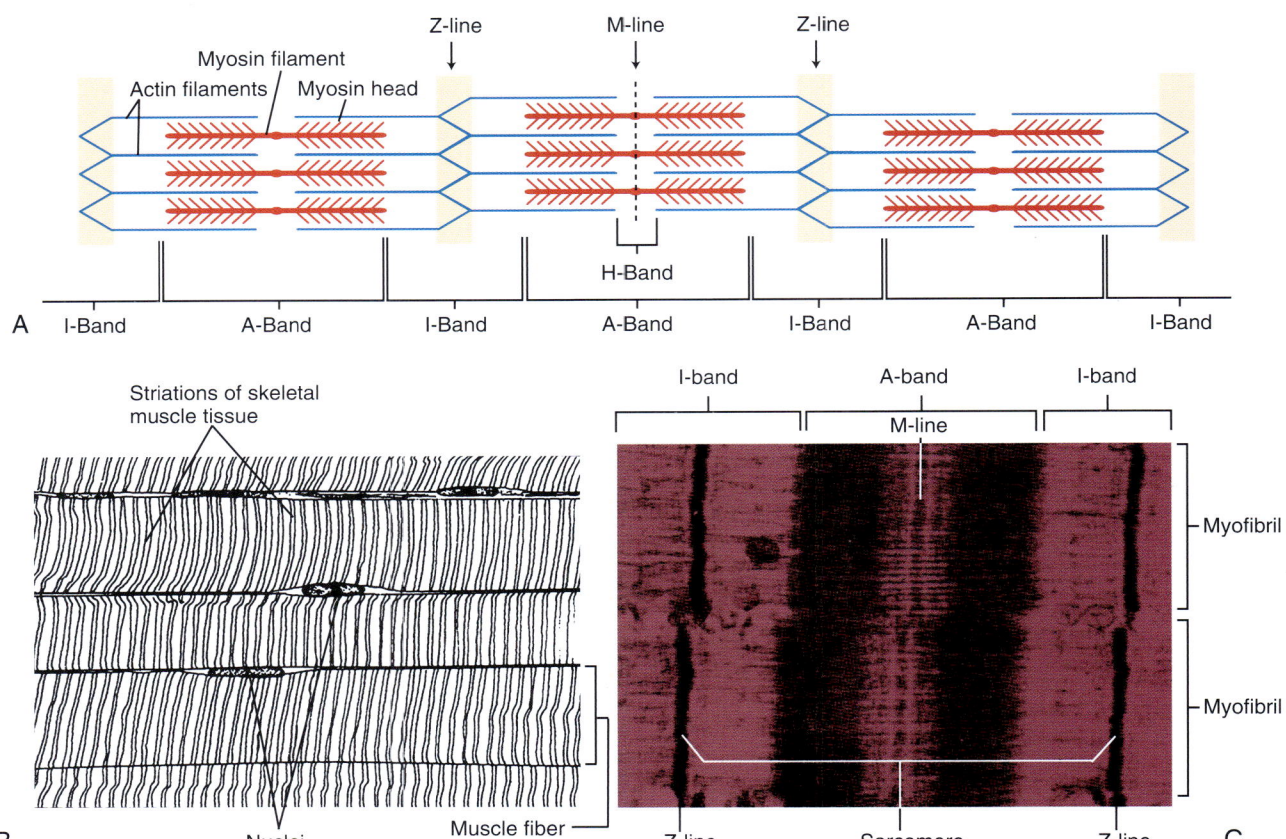

FIGURE 12-17 **A,** Three sarcomeres laid end to end. The consistent overlapping of actin and myosin filaments creates bands of striations that are named with letters. The two major bands are the A-band (where actin and myosin overlap) and the I-band (where only actin is present). **B,** Sketch of photomicrograph of skeletal muscle tissue that demonstrates the striated appearance. **C,** Same view as in B but at greater magnification in an electron micrograph. The A-band and I-bands are easy to see and identify. (*B and C,* From Thibodeau GA, Patton KT: *Anatomy and physiology,* ed 5, St Louis, 2003, Mosby.)

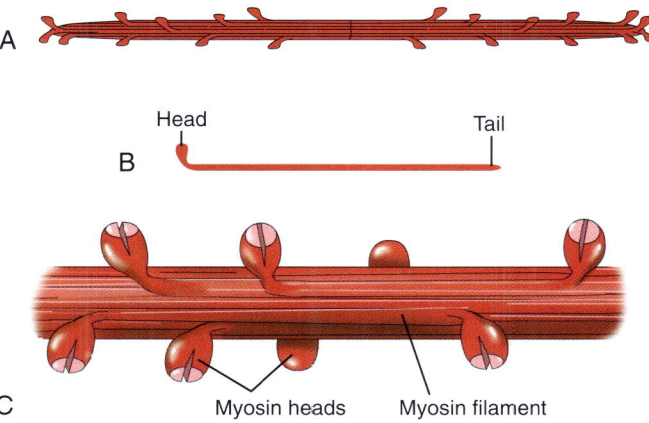

FIGURE 12-18 **A,** Myosin filament made up of many myosin molecules. **B,** One myosin molecule. **C,** Close-up of a myosin filament.

CHAPTER 12 Anatomy and Physiology of Muscle Tissue

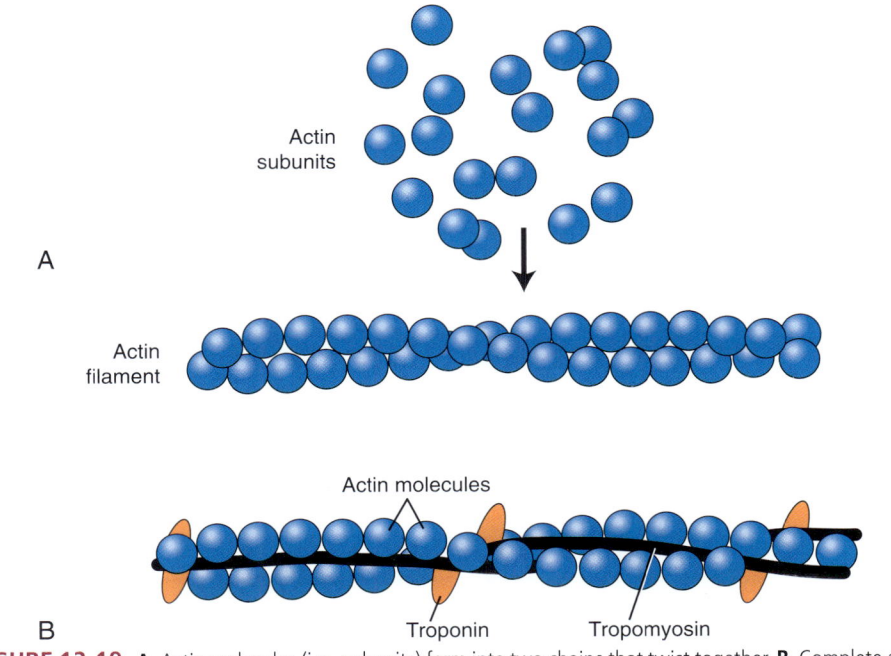

FIGURE 12-19 A, Actin molecules (i.e., subunits) form into two chains that twist together. **B,** Complete actin filament composed of actin molecules, tropomyosin, and troponin molecules.

- The head (actin-myosin cross-bridge) is called the **heavy meromyosin** component.[10] It is actually composed of two subcomponents: (1) the head (also known as the **S1 fragment**) and (2) the neck (also known as the **S2 fragment**). Although a number of differences exist between the different types of muscle fibers (see Section 12.13 for details), the largest difference seems to occur in the cross-bridge of myosin filaments.

ACTIN FILAMENT IN MORE DETAIL:

- An actin filament is made up of three separate protein molecules: (1) actin, (2) troponin, and (3) tropomyosin.[10]
- The bulk of the actin filament is composed of many small spheric **actin molecules** that are strung together like beads, forming two strands that twist around each other[4] (Figure 12-19, *A*).
  - Each actin molecule is a binding site to which a myosin cross-bridge can attach. However, these binding sites are not normally *exposed*.

- Attached to these strands of actin molecules are troponin and tropomyosin molecules[4] (Figure 12-19, *B*).
  - **Tropomyosin molecules** normally block the binding sites of actin from being exposed (and bound to by myosin's heads).[4]
  - When calcium ions attach to the **troponin molecules** of the actin filament, the troponin molecules move the tropomyosin molecules out of the way so that the binding (active) sites of actin are exposed. This allows for the formation of cross-bridges (i.e., contraction).[11]

TITIN:

- Sarcomeres also contain a protein called *titin* (Figure 12-20). **Titin** is the largest protein in the human body[5] (containing approximately 27,000 amino acids) and forms much of the cytoskeletal framework for the sarcomere, connecting the myosin filament to the Z-line. For this reason, titin is also sometimes referred to as **connectin**.[4] Just as there are six actin filaments

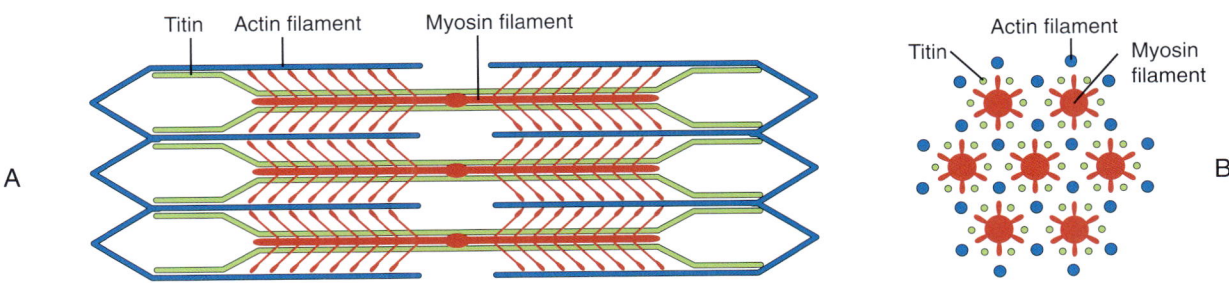

FIGURE 12-20 Titin. Titin is a large protein molecule located within the sarcomere of muscle tissue. Each titin molecule runs half the length of the sarcomere, connecting from the myosin filament at the M-line in the center of the sarcomere to the Z-line at the border of the sarcomere.

that surround each side of the myosin filament, there are six titin molecules that attach to each side of the myosin filament (see Figure 12-20, B).

○ More specifically, each titin molecule runs half the length of the sarcomere, connecting from the myosin filament at the M-line in the center of the sarcomere to the Z-line at the border of the sarcomere. Therefore, titin is found in both the A-band and the I-band regions of the sarcomere (see Figure 12-17, A). As the titin enters the I-band region, it lies next to the actin filament on its way to the Z-line.[4]

○ Of particular significance is a portion of the titin molecule located in the I-band region that is called the *PEVK section* (P, E, V, and K are the one-letter abbreviations for the amino acids proline, glutamate, valine, and lysine, which make up the majority of this section). The PEVK section is functionally of great importance because it is extremely extensible and elastic. In fact, it is this region of titin that is now proposed to be primarily responsible for the elasticity, and therefore passive tension, of extended muscle/myofascial tissue.[5] This means that the springy end-feel of a stretched muscle (absent bony and ligamentous abnormalities) that is sensed by the manual/movement therapist might be caused by titin. In this regard, we may "feel" titin when stretching and assessing muscle length.[13]

○ Some sources have posited that titin may also be responsible for chronic muscle stiffness that is felt with activities. This increased stiffness may result from increased connections (i.e., adhesions) between titin and the myosin filament, or perhaps even between titin and the actin filaments. Classically, muscle stiffness has been considered to be caused by two factors: active contraction via the sliding filament mechanism, and fascial adhesions. Adding titin as a possible causative agent of passive tension may have important implications for treatment and would be of particular importance to manual and movement therapists.[13]

SECTION 12.12 SLIDING FILAMENT MECHANISM IN MORE DETAIL

○ In more detail, the steps of the sliding filament mechanism occur as follows (Figure 12-21):[10]

1. When we will a contraction of a muscle, a message commanding this to occur originates in our brain. This message travels as an electrical impulse within our central nervous system.
2. This electrical impulse then travels out into the periphery in a motor neuron of a peripheral nerve to go to the skeletal muscle. (The peripheral nerve can be a cranial nerve or a spinal nerve, and this message may be carried in many motor neurons—in other words, one motor neuron for each motor unit that is directed to contract).
3. When the impulse gets to the end of the motor neuron, the motor neuron secretes its neurotransmitters (i.e., acetylcholine) into the synaptic cleft at the neuromuscular junction (see Figure 12-12).
4. These neurotransmitters float across the synaptic cleft and bind to the motor end plate of the muscle fiber (see Figure 12-12).
5. The binding of these neurotransmitters onto the motor end plate causes an electrical impulse on the muscle fiber that travels along the muscle fiber's cell membrane (see Figure 10-13).
6. This electrical impulse is transmitted into the interior of the muscle fiber by the T-tubules (transverse tubules) (see Figure 12-13).
7. When this electrical impulse reaches the interior, it causes the sarcoplasmic reticulum of the muscle fiber to release stored calcium ions into the sarcoplasm.
8. These calcium ions then bind onto troponin molecules of the actin filament.
9. This causes a structural change, causing the tropomyosin molecules of the actin filament to move.
10. When the tropomyosin molecules move, the binding sites of the actin filament (the actual actin molecules themselves) become exposed.
11. Heads of the myosin filament attach onto the binding sites of the actin filament, creating cross-bridges. These cross-bridges then bend, pulling the actin filament in toward the center of the sarcomere (see Figure 12-9).
12. If no ATP is present, this cross-bridge bond will stay in place and no further sliding of the filament will occur.
13. When ATP is present, the following sequence occurs: the cross-bridge between the myosin and actin breaks, and the myosin head attaches onto the next binding site on the actin molecule, forming a new cross-bridge. This new cross-bridge bends and pulls the actin filament in toward the center of the sarcomere (see Figure 12-9).
14. This process in step 13 will continue to occur as long as ATP molecules are present to initiate the breakage, reattachment, and bending of the myosin cross-bridge.
15. In this manner, the sarcomeres of the innervated muscle fibers will contract to 100% of their ability.
16. When the nervous system message is no longer sent, neurotransmitters will no longer be released into the synapse. The neurotransmitters that were present are either broken down or are reabsorbed back into the motor neuron.
17. Without the presence of neurotransmitters in the synapse, no impulse is sent into the interior of the muscle fiber, and calcium ions are no longer released from the sarcoplasmic reticulum.
18. Calcium that was present in the sarcoplasm is reabsorbed into the sarcoplasmic reticulum by the expenditure of energy by ATP molecules.
19. As the concentration of calcium drops, calcium will no longer be available to bind to troponin. Without calcium bound to it, troponin will no longer keep the tropomyosin from blocking the binding sites of the actin filament, and the actin binding sites will be blocked once again. Therefore cross-bridges will no longer be made, and the sliding of filaments will no longer occur.

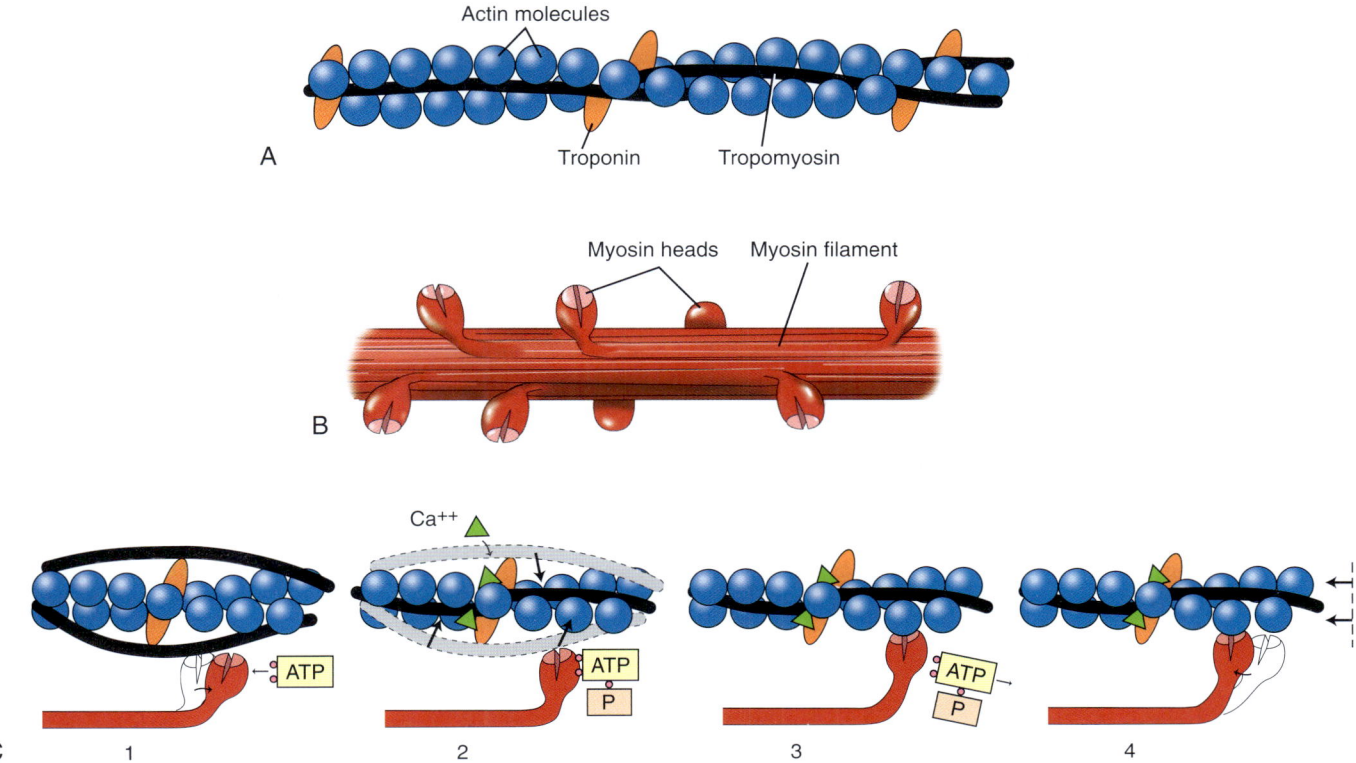

FIGURE 12-21 A, Structure of an actin filament; it is composed of actin, tropomyosin, and troponin molecules. **B,** Structure of a myosin filament. The heads stick out and can form cross-bridges by attaching to the binding sites of the actin filament when calcium is present. **C,** Steps of how the myosin-actin cross-bridges are formed and broken. In step 1, when an adenosine triphosphate (ATP) molecule attaches to the myosin head, the myosin head moves into its resting position. Step 2 shows calcium binding to the troponin molecule of the actin filament, causing the tropomyosin molecule to move out of the way and exposing the binding site of the actin filament. Step 3 shows the myosin head now attaching to the exposed binding site of the actin filament, forming the cross-bridge (and the ATP molecule is released from the myosin head). Step 4 shows the myosin head bend, pulling the actin filament in toward the center of the sarcomere (hence the sliding filament mechanism). (Note: The myosin head will remain bound to the actin filament in this position until another ATP molecule binds to the myosin head, breaking the cross-bridge and causing the myosin head to move back to its resting position.)

- The big picture of the sliding filament mechanism must not be lost! The entire point of this process is that if actin filaments slide along myosin filaments in toward the center of the sarcomere, then the Z-lines that the actin filaments attach to will be pulled in toward the center of the sarcomere and the sarcomere will shorten.
- The sliding filament mechanism is called the sliding *filament* mechanism, not the sliding actin mechanism. Given that sarcomeres are laid end to end, it is not possible for actin filaments to do all the sliding and for myosin filaments to always be fixed in place. If the actin filaments of two adjacent sarcomeres were to both shorten toward their respective centers, the Z-line that is common to them would have to rupture. Instead, myosin filaments can also slide along actin filaments. This can be pictured by thinking of a muscle contraction with one end of the muscle fixed as it contracts. The Z-line of the very last sarcomere of the muscle will be fixed and would not allow the actin filament to slide away from it toward the center of the sarcomere. Instead, when the cross-bridges pull, because the Z-line and its actin filament are fixed, the myosin filament will slide along the fixed actin filament in the direction of the fixed attachment of the muscle (this could be looked at as being conceptually similar to the idea of a reverse action of a muscle). The result is the same in that the sarcomere shortens. The adjacent sarcomere will then be pulled toward that sarcomere, and the same filament sliding pattern would occur in that sarcomere, as well as every successive sarcomere within the muscle.
- Because myofibrils are made up of sarcomeres laid end to end, when sarcomeres shorten, the myofibril shortens.
- Because a muscle fiber is made up of myofibrils, when myofibrils shorten, the muscle fiber shortens.
- Because a muscle is made up of many muscle fibers, when enough muscle fibers shorten, the muscle shortens in toward its center.
- Because the muscle is attached to two bones via its tendons, if this pulling force toward the center of the muscle is sufficient, the bones that the muscle attaches to will be pulled toward each other.
- Because bones are within body parts, movement of parts of our body can occur!
- In this manner, the sliding filament mechanism creates the force of a muscle contraction that creates movement of our body. The different types of muscle contractions (concentric, eccentric, and isometric) will be discussed in Chapter 14.

SECTION 12.13   RED AND WHITE MUSCLE FIBERS

- Up until now, we have spoken about muscle fibers as if they were all identical. This is not true.
- Generally two types of muscle fibers exist: (1) red fibers and (2) white fibers.[4]
- Red fibers are also known as *red slow-twitch fibers;* white fibers are also known as *white fast-twitch fibers* (Box 12-6).
- Red and white fibers are analogous to dark and white meat in chicken or turkey. Dark meat of a chicken or turkey is muscle primarily composed of red fibers; white meat is muscle primarily composed of white fibers.
- An intermediate category of fibers that falls between the other two does exist. The muscle fibers of this category are often termed **intermediate-twitch fibers**.[4]
- **Red slow-twitch fibers** are so named because they are red and slow to contract.
    - The reason that red fibers are red is that they have a rich blood supply.[4]
    - They are termed *slow-twitch* because they are slow to contract from the instant that they receive the impulse to contract from the nervous system.
    - They take approximately 1/10 of a second to reach maximum tension.[11]
    - Red slow-twitch fibers are usually small in size.
- **White fast-twitch fibers** are so named because they are white and contract relatively fast.
    - The reason that white fibers are white is that they do not have a rich blood supply.[4]
    - They are termed *fast-twitch* because they contract quickly when they are directed to contract by the nervous system.
    - They take approximately 1/20 of a second to reach maximum tension.[11]
    - White fast-twitch fibers are usually large in size.
- Within a muscle, motor units are homogeneous—that is, a motor unit has either all red slow-twitch fibers or all white fast-twitch fibers.[11]
- Small motor units are composed of red slow-twitch fibers; large motor units are composed of white fast-twitch fibers.[11]
- Smaller motor units composed of red muscle fibers are innervated by smaller-diameter motor neurons that carry the direction to contract at a slower rate from the central nervous system than the larger diameter motor neurons that innervate the larger motor units composed of white fibers. This is another factor that accounts for the relative speed with which the different types of muscle fibers contract.[11]
- Every muscle of the human body has a mixture of red and white fibers.
    - The percentage of this mixture will vary from one muscle to another muscle within one person's body.
    - Furthermore, from one person to another person, the percentage of this mixture for the same muscle can also vary.
    - For the most part, the ratio of red and white fibers in our bodies is genetically determined. However, the intermediate class of fibers mentioned previously has the ability to convert and attain the characteristics of red slow-twitch or fast white-twitch fibers.[11]
- Note: Numerous terms describe the different types of muscle fibers. The names are based on describing different aspects of the fibers' anatomy or physiology. Beyond being described as *red slow-twitch* and *white fast-twitch,* these fibers are also described as being **Type I fibers** and **Type II fibers**, **oxidative fibers** and **glycolytic fibers**, **small fibers** and **large fibers**, **fatigue-resistant fibers** and **easily fatigued fibers**, and **tonic fibers** and **phasic fibers**, respectively. Furthermore, these terms are often combined together to create categories such as **slow oxidative (SO) fibers** and **fast glycolytic (FG) fibers**, among others.[13] Unfortunately, all of these terms are used widely, so it is important that the student be at least somewhat familiar with them.
- Generally, red slow-twitch fibers contract slowly and do not create very powerful contractions, but they are able to hold their contraction for long periods of time. As a result, they are often more plentiful in muscles that must exhibit endurance and hold contractions for long periods of time, such as deeper postural stabilization muscles.[4]

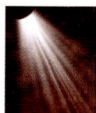

BOX 12-6   Spotlight on Muscle Type and Breakdown of Glucose

The speed of contraction of a muscle fiber is primarily based on its method of adenosine triphosphate (ATP) formation from glucose. Red fibers rely primarily on the slower process of aerobic respiration of glucose via the Kreb's cycle in the mitochondria—thus the need for the greater blood supply to provide the oxygen needed for this pathway. Because aerobic respiration of glucose yields 36 ATPs per glucose molecule that is broken down, red slow-twitch fibers are ideally suited for endurance activities. White fibers rely primarily on the faster process of anaerobic respiration of glucose in the sarcoplasm via glycolysis—thus a lesser need for an oxygen-carrying blood supply. Because anaerobic respiration of glucose produces only two ATPs per glucose molecule that is broken down, white fast-twitch fibers are easily fatigued and are best suited for activities that require short bursts of maximal effort. Hence the relationship between red fibers and white fibers and aerobic and anaerobic activities stems from the blood supply and method of glucose breakdown. An analogy could be made between muscle fiber type and the classic story of the long-distance tortoise and the sprinter hare.

- Generally, white fast-twitch fibers are able to generate faster, more powerful contractions, but they fatigue easily. Therefore they are usually more plentiful in muscles that need to create fast powerful movements but do not have to hold that contraction for a long period of time, such as superficial mobility muscles (Box 12-7). (For more on postural stabilization versus mobility muscles, see Chapter 15, especially Section 15.6.)
  - For example, the soleus, which is more concerned with postural stabilization of the ankle joint, generally contains approximately 67% red fibers and 33% white fibers,[9] whereas the gastrocnemius, which is more concerned with creating movement at the ankle joint, generally contains approximately 50% red fibers and 50% white fibers.[11]

> **BOX 12-7**
>
> Given that the percentage of red versus white fibers varies from individual to individual and that these differences seem to be genetically determined, a natural conclusion is that although every person can improve at any sport with practice, based on our genetic differences of red/white muscle fiber concentrations, each person may have an inborn predisposition to excel at certain types of sports. For example, individuals with a greater concentration of red slow-twitch fibers are naturally suited for endurance activities such as long distance running, whereas individuals with a greater concentration of white fast-twitch fibers are naturally suited for sports that require short bursts of maximal energy such as sprinting.

SECTION 12.14 MYOFASCIAL MERIDIANS AND TENSEGRITY

- When a student is first exposed to the study of kinesiology, it is customary to begin by learning the components of the musculoskeletal system separately. Thus we approach the study of kinesiology by first learning each of the individual bones and muscles of the human body as separate entities. We even separate the muscles from their fascial tissues, describing the muscle fibers as distinct from the endomysial, perimysial, and epimysial fascial wrappings and separating the muscle belly from its fascial tendons/aponeuroses.
- Although this approach of breaking a whole into its parts may be useful and even necessary for the beginning student, it is crucially important that, once the important job of learning these separate components has been accomplished, the student begin the even more important job of putting the pieces back together into the whole.
- After all, a muscle and its fascial tissues are one unit that cannot really be structurally or functionally separated.[6] Indeed, the term *myofascial unit*, which describes this idea of the unity of a muscle and its fascial tissues, is gaining popularity. Furthermore, even myofascial units (i.e., muscles) are not truly separate units that act in isolation from one another. Rather they belong to functional groups, the members of each group sharing a common joint action. These individual functional groups of muscles then coordinate together on an even larger stage to create body-wide movement patterns. For more detail on functional groups of muscles, see Chapter 15.
- To this picture, fascial ligaments, joint capsules, bursae, tendon sheaths, and articular and fibrous cartilage must be added, creating a myofascial-skeletal system. In addition, because this system cannot function without direction from the nervous system, the nervous system must be included as well, creating a neuro-myo-fascial-skeletal system that functions seamlessly.
- The concept of myofascial meridians is another way of looking at the structural and functional interconnectedness of this neuro-myo-fascial-skeletal system. **Myofascial meridian theory** puts forth the concept that muscles operate within continuous lines of fascia that span across the body. Most notable for advancing this view is author Tom Myers. In his book *Anatomy Trains*, Myers defines a **myofascial meridian** (also known as an **anatomy train**) as a traceable continuum within the body of muscles embedded within fascial webbing (for more on fascia and the fascial web, see Sections 4.1 through 4.3). In effect, the muscles of a myofascial meridian are connected by the fibrous fascia connective tissue and act together synergistically, transmitting tension and movement through the meridian by means of their contractions[14] (Figure 12-22).
- Myers has codified this interpretation of the myofascial system of the body into eleven major myofascial meridians (Figure 12-23). The eleven myofascial meridians are as follows[14]:
  - Superficial back line
  - Superficial front line
  - Lateral line
  - Spiral line
  - Superficial front arm line
  - Deep front arm line
  - Superficial back arm line
  - Deep back arm line
  - Back functional line
  - Front functional line
  - Deep front line

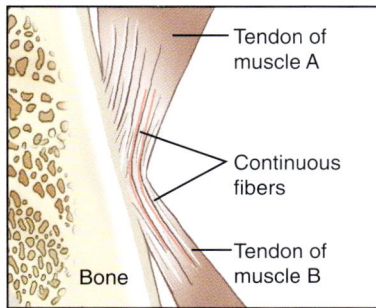

FIGURE 12-22 Myofascial meridian continuity. When a muscle's tendon attaches onto a bone, although most of its fibers usually do attach onto the bone itself, some of its fibers are continuous with the fascial fibers of an adjacent muscle's tendon.

Text continued on page 481

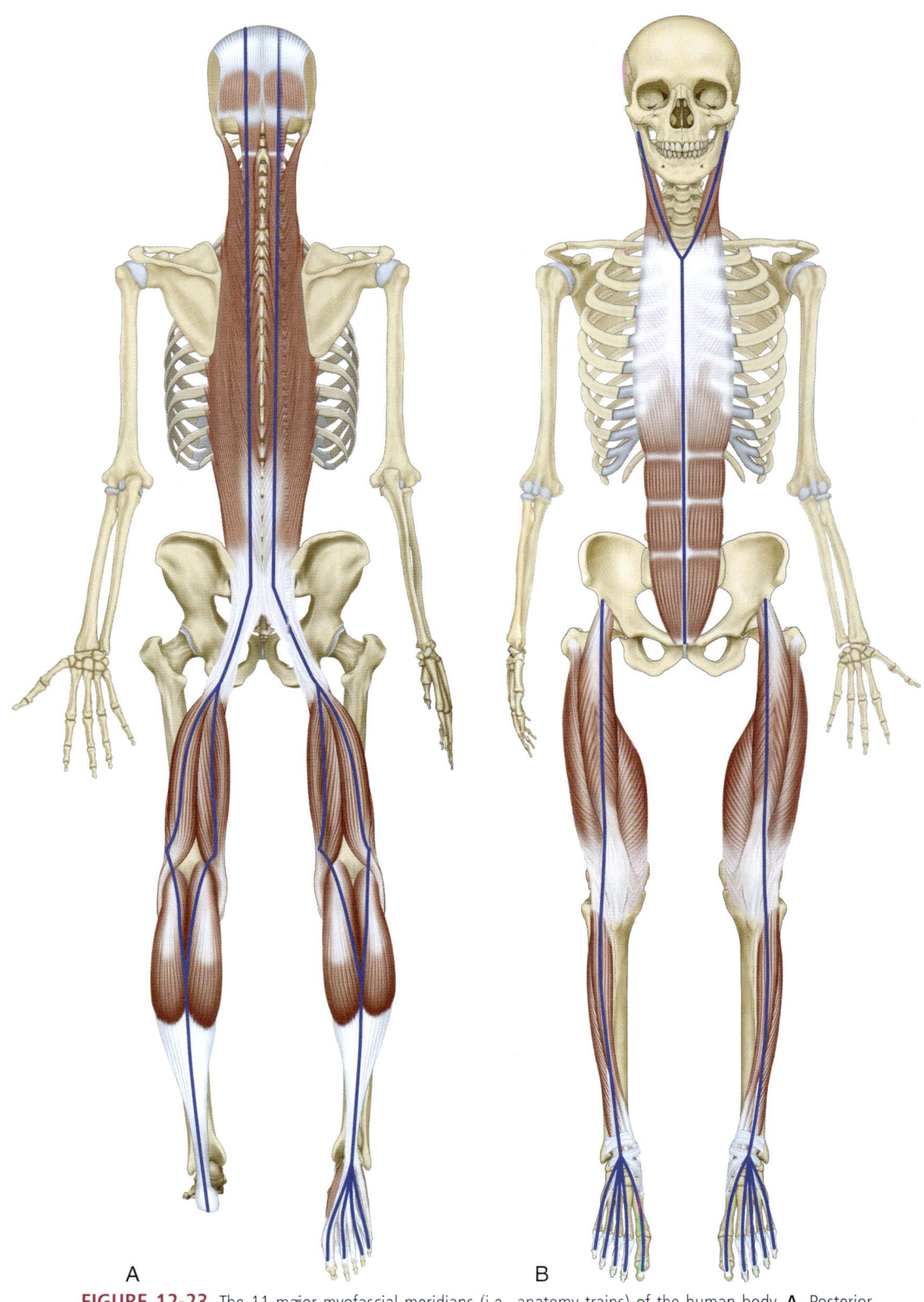

FIGURE 12-23 The 11 major myofascial meridians (i.e., anatomy trains) of the human body. **A,** Posterior view of the superficial back line. **B,** Anterior view of the superficial front line. *(Modeled from Myers TW:* Anatomy trains: myofascial meridians for manual & movement therapists, *ed 3, Edinburgh, 2014, Churchill Livingstone, Elsevier.)*

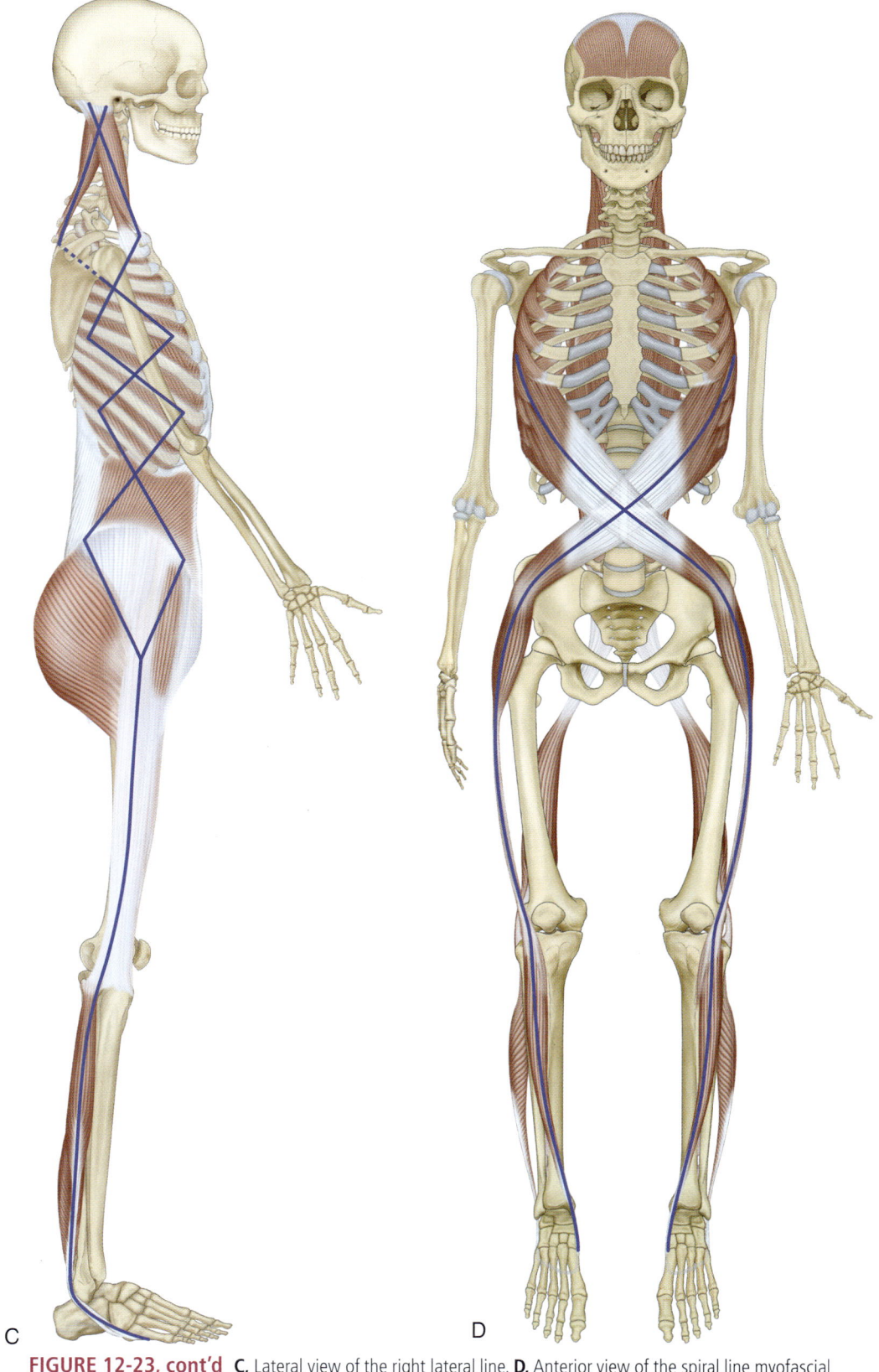

FIGURE 12-23, cont'd **C,** Lateral view of the right lateral line. **D,** Anterior view of the spiral line myofascial meridian.

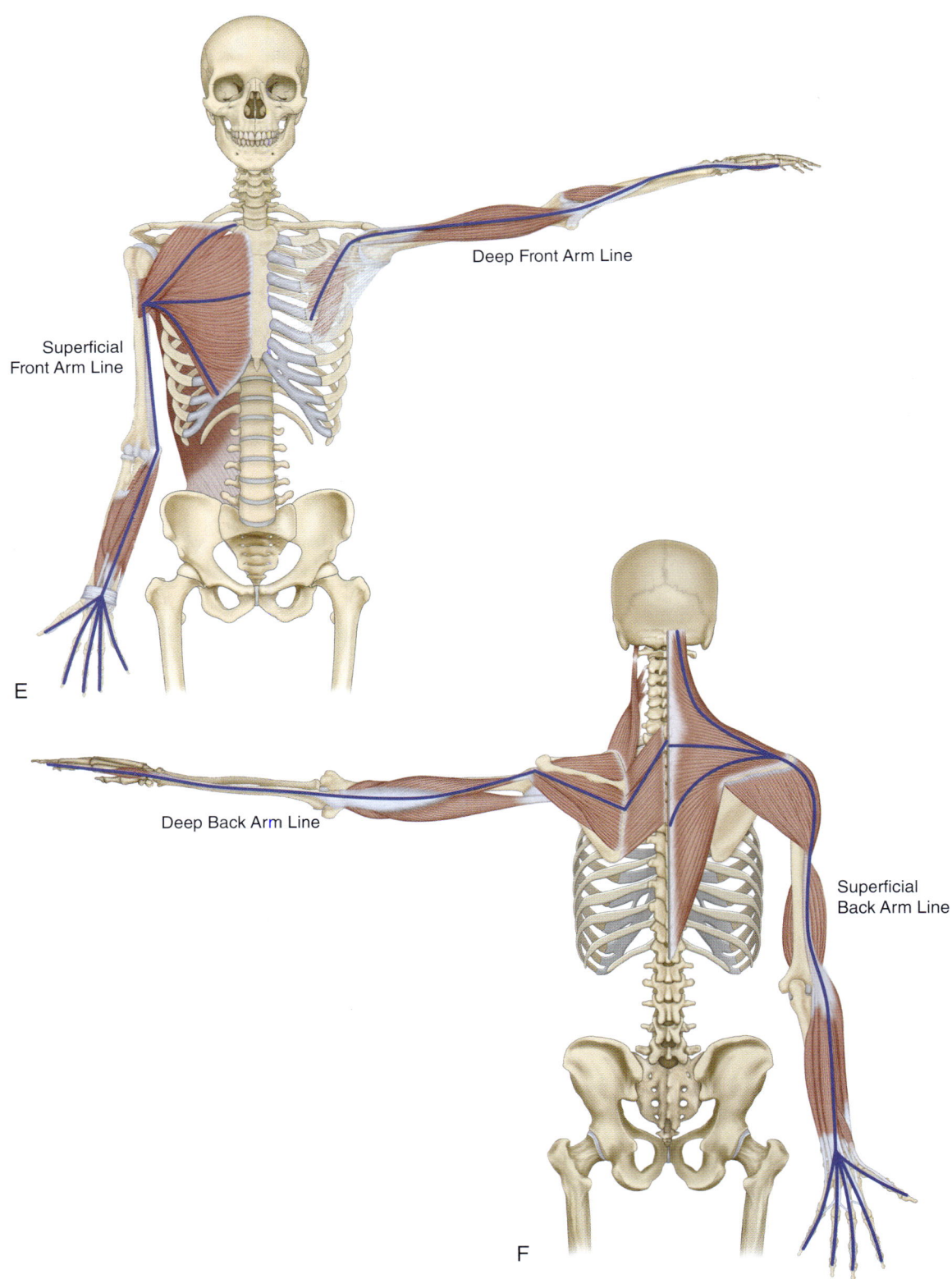

FIGURE 12-23, cont'd **E,** Anterior view of the superficial and deep front arm lines. **F,** Posterior view of the superficial and deep back arm lines.

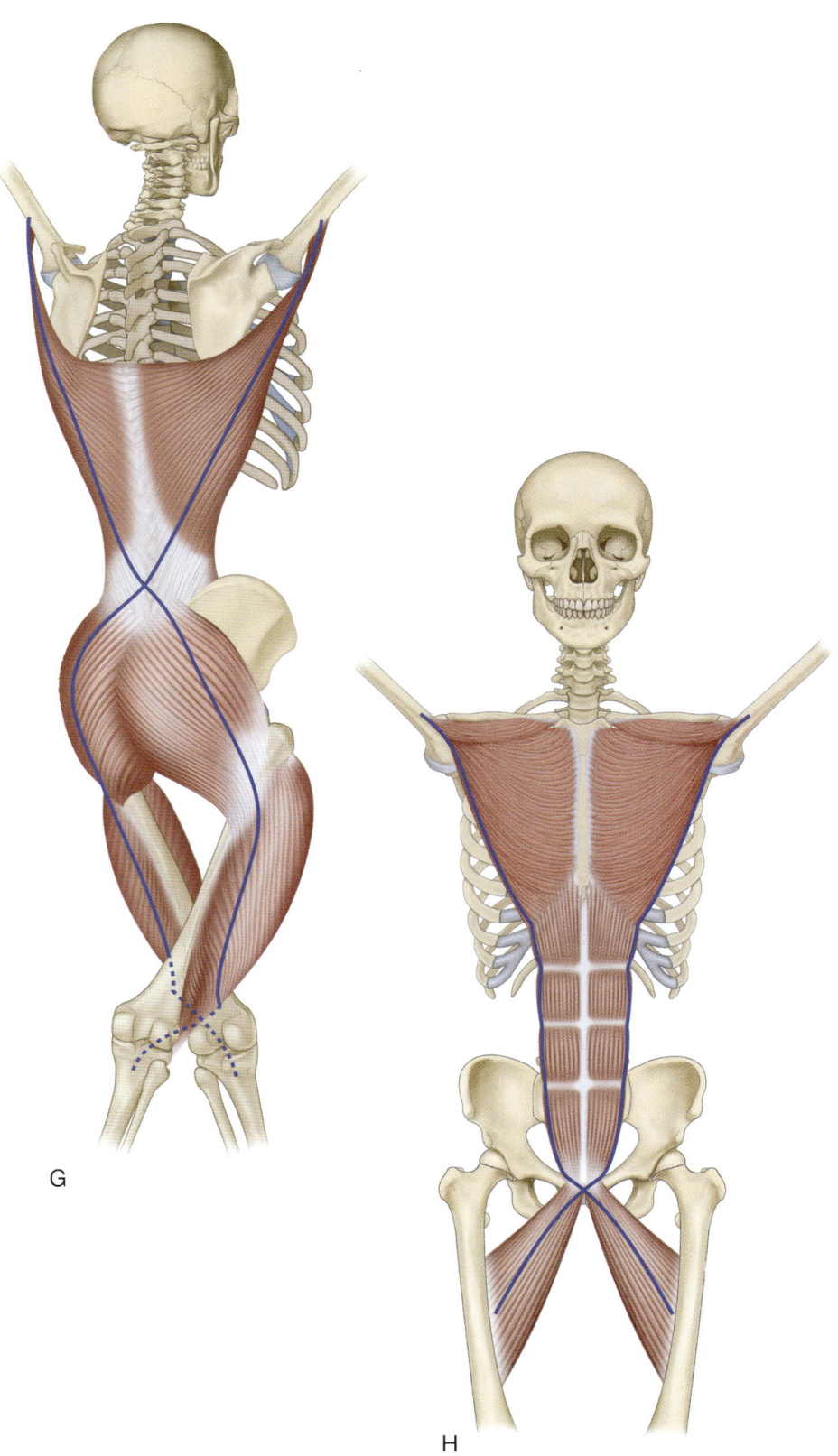

FIGURE 12-23, cont'd **G**, Posterolateral view of the back functional line. **H**, Anterior view of the front functional line.

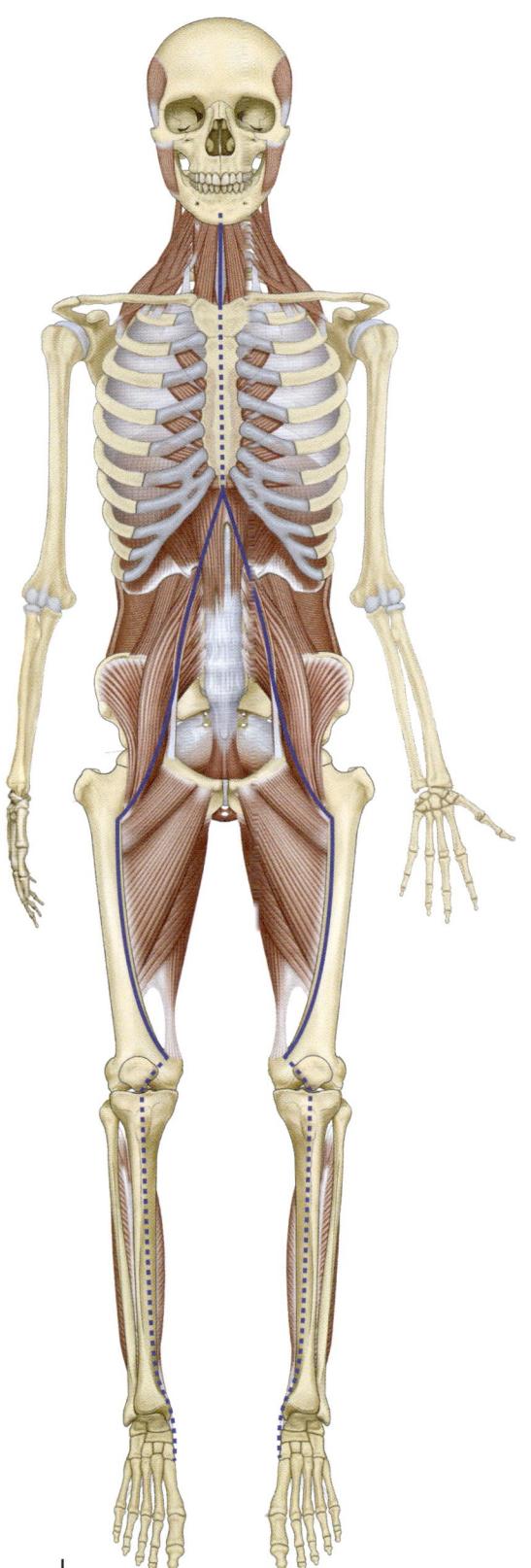

FIGURE 12-23, cont'd I, Anterior view of the deep front line.

- The importance of myofascial meridian theory is manyfold:[14]
  - First, it places muscles into larger structural and functional patterns that help to explain patterns of strain and movement within the body. Figure 12-24 illustrates an example of a line of strain/movement within the body. We see that when a monkey hangs from a branch, a continuum of muscles must synergistically work, beginning in the upper extremity and ending in the opposite-side lower extremity. This myofascial continuum is an example of a structural and functional myofascial meridian. Thus myofascial meridian theory helps the kinesiologist understand the patterns of muscle contraction within the body.
  - Second, myofascial meridian theory creates a model that explains how forces placed on the body at one site can cause somewhat far-reaching effects in distant sites of the body. For example, in Figure 12-25 we see a dissection of the myofascial tissues that comprise the superficial back line myofascial meridian. If tension develops at one point along this line, say in the

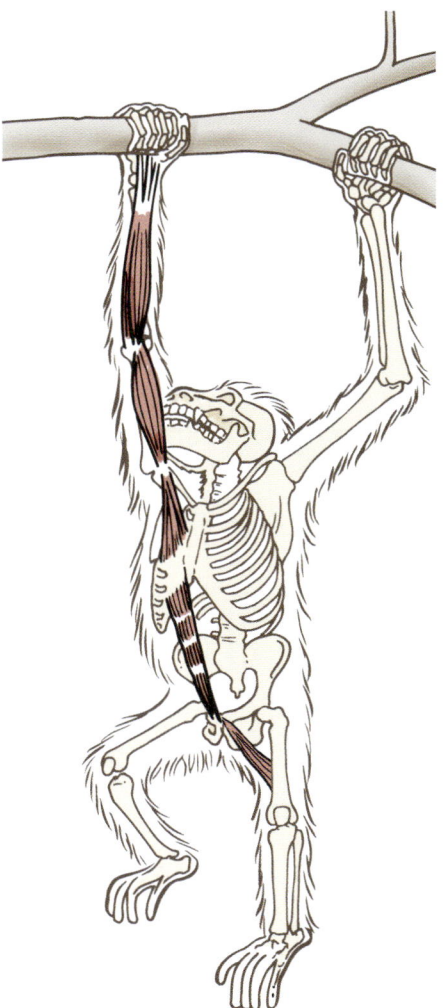

FIGURE 12-24 In this illustration we see that when a monkey is hanging from a branch, a chain of muscles must work in concert with one another and contract. A chain of muscles transmitting force across the body is a myofascial meridian. *(Modified from Myers TW: Anatomy trains: myofascial meridians for manual and movement therapists, ed 3, Edinburgh, 2014, Churchill Livingstone.)*

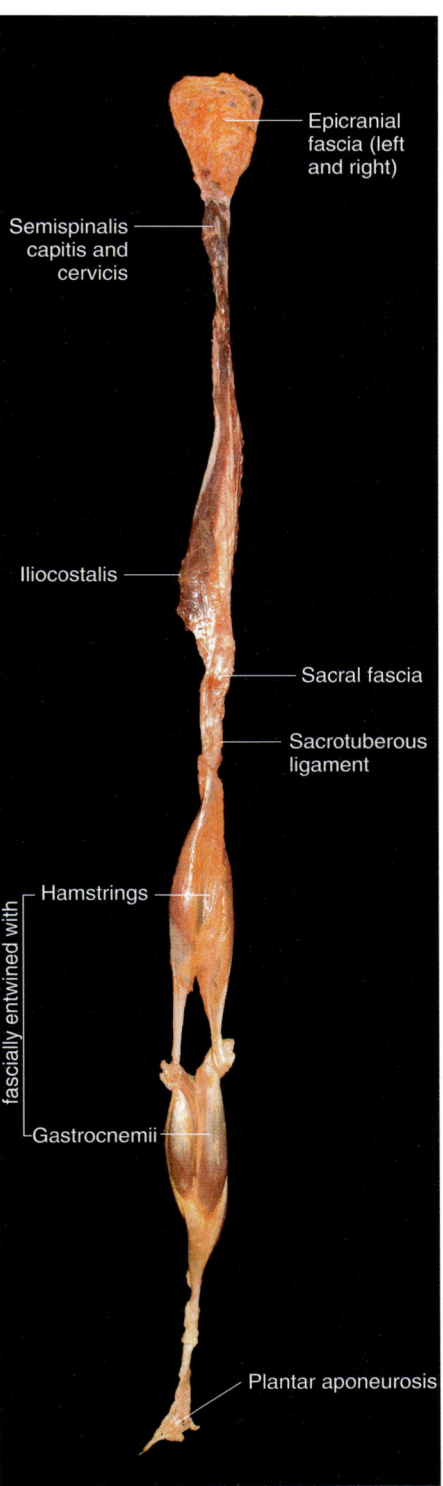

FIGURE 12-25 A dissection of the superficial back line myofascial meridian of the body. Conceptually, if a strain occurs at one point along this myofascial meridian, effects of that strain could be felt in distant locations along the myofascial meridian. *(Courtesy Thomas W. Myers. In Myers TW: Anatomy trains: myofascial meridians for manual and movement therapists, ed 3, Edinburgh, 2014, Churchill Livingstone.)*

gastrocnemius muscle, that tension could be transmitted up the line through the hamstrings to the ischial tuberosity attachment, through the sacrotuberous ligament to the sacrum, up through the thoracolumbar fascia and erector spinae musculature (iliocostalis) and transversospinalis (semispinalis) musculature to the occiput, and from the occiput into the epicranial myofascia (occipitalis muscle, galea aponeurotica, and frontalis muscle) to the frontal region of the head. Therefore by the concept of strain moving along myofascial meridians, a person with excessive tightness in their gastrocnemius may experience an effect of that strain in the head, perhaps manifesting as a headache.

- The repercussions of this are important for every therapist, instructor, or trainer who works in a clinical or rehabilitative setting. The actual codification of eleven major myofascial meridians offers a blueprint with which the therapist/trainer can begin to address these patterns of strain and injury throughout the body (Box 12-8).
- The third importance of the myofascial meridian theory relates to the concept of *tensegrity*.

BOX 12-8 Spotlight on the Application of Myofascial Meridians

Given the connective nature of myofascial tissues, the concept of connectiveness and continuity of the myofascial tissues of the body cannot be disputed. Working with the myofascial meridians that Myers has mapped out, a force placed on any one point of a myofascial meridian can be transmitted along the myofascial meridian to distant sites in the body. For example, a tight gastrocnemius muscle in the leg could conceivably cause a tension (pulling) force that is transmitted and felt all the way to the galea aponeurotica of the scalp in the head. However, it is likely that the magnitude of this transmitted force of the tight gastrocnemius will lessen as the distance from the gastrocnemius increases. This is especially true if the myofascial tissues are loose between the gastrocnemius and the head, because if the myofascial tissues of the posterior thigh, buttock, trunk, and/or neck are loose, then the pulling force of a tight gastrocnemius muscle would be absorbed long before it could be transmitted to the head. Thus even though a strain/tension at the gastrocnemius can lead to this strain being transmitted to the hamstrings, erector spinae, and transversospinalis and on to the galea aponeurotica of the scalp, the intensity of the effects of this strain will likely lessen as we move along the myofascial meridian from the gastrocnemius toward the head. On the other hand, if all the tissues of the myofascial meridian are tight, then the effects of a tight gastrocnemius will be immediately transmitted and felt in the galea aponeurotica of the head. Myofascial meridian theory is of undeniable value to the field of bodywork; however, its actual clinical importance with clients should be evaluated by the manual/movement therapist on a case-by-case basis.

TENSEGRITY:

- The concept of **tensegrity** relates to how the structural integrity and support of the body are created.[15]
- The classic view of the body is that it is a compression structure made up of a number of parts, each one stacked on another and bearing weight down through the body parts below. Thus the weight-bearing compression force of the head rests on the neck; the weight of the head and neck rests on the trunk; the weight of the head, neck, and trunk rests on the pelvis; and so forth, all the way down to the feet (Figure 12-26).
- Thus the structural integrity of the body is dependent on compression forces, similar to a brick wall in which the structural integrity of the brick wall is dependent on the proper position of each brick on the bricks below so that the weight of each brick can be transmitted through the bricks below.[14]
- However, myofascial meridian theory, which views the musculoskeletal body as having continuous lines of pull created by muscles linked to one another in a web or network of fascia, offers another way to view the structural integrity of the body. Myofascial meridian theory looks at the lines of tension created by these myofascial meridians as being largely responsible for the structural integrity of the body. In this view, the proper posture and balancing of the bones of the skeleton are largely caused by the tensile forces created by muscles within myofascial meridians that act on the skeleton.[14]
- The concept of structural integrity coming from tensile forces is termed *tensegrity*. The advantage of a tensegrity structure compared with a compression structure is that tensegrity structures are more resilient because stresses/forces that are applied

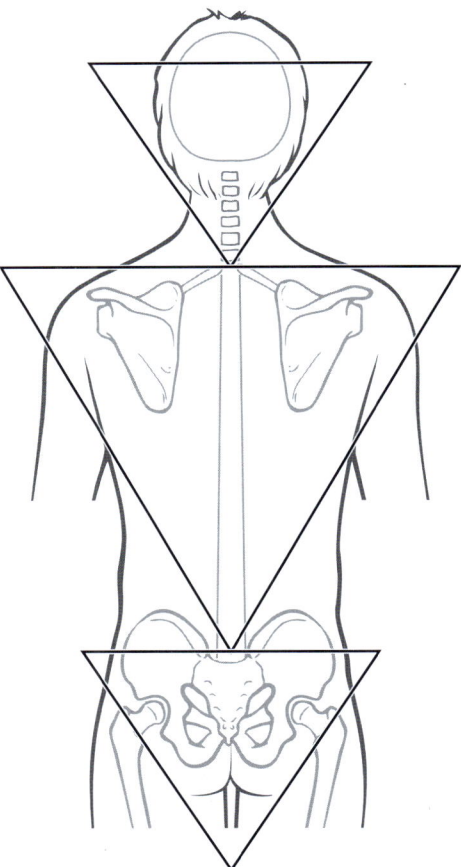

FIGURE 12-26 Typical view of the body as being a compression structure in which the structural integrity and support of the body are determined by the compressive weight-bearing forces transmitted through the body parts. *(Modeled from Cailliet R: Soft tissue pain and disability, Philadelphia, 1997, FA Davis.)*

to them are more efficiently transmitted throughout the structure, spreading out and diminishing their effect. Thus no one region of the skeleton bears the entire load of a stress. If a force is applied to a bone at any specific point along the skeleton, that force will be transmitted throughout the body along myofascial meridians, diminishing its effect at the local site of application.[15]
- The term *tensegrity* comes from the phrase *tension integrity* and was first used by designer R. Buckminster Fuller, an American engineer and inventor.
- For example, a force applied to any vertebral level of the lumbar spine, say L3, will have that force dissipated by tensile forces that will spread to the entire spine, head, arms, pelvis, and thighs via muscular attachments of such muscles as the erector spinae group, transversospinalis group, psoas major, and latissimus dorsi muscles. Then the fascial attachments of these muscles to other muscles will continue to spread the effects of the force to every other part of the body. The result will be that much of the force that was placed on L3 will be spread to other areas of the body, lessening the deleterious effect and likelihood of injury to L3.
- In reality, neither view is entirely exclusive of the other; the structural integrity of the body is dependent on both tensile and compressive forces.[14]
  - The bones of the skeleton are compression members that do derive some of their structural stability from being stacked on one another and bearing weight down through the skeleton below.
  - However, much of the structural stability of the skeleton also comes from myofascial tensile forces attaching and spanning from one bone to every other bone of the body (Figure 12-27).
- Describing the body as having both compression integrity and tensile integrity (tensegrity), Myers describes the bones as being compression members that are like "islands, floating in a sea of continuous tension." (Myers TW: *Anatomy trains: myofascial meridians for manual and movement therapists*, ed 3, Edinburgh, 2014, Churchill Livingstone.)

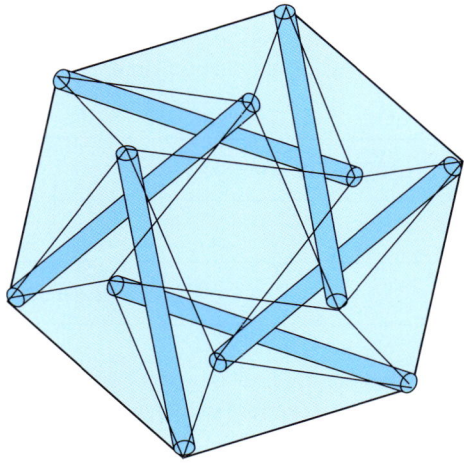

FIGURE 12-27 Classic tensegrity structure composed of dowels that are compression members suspended via rubber bands, which are the tension elements. The analogy to the human body is that our bones, which are compression elements, are largely suspended by our myofascial meridians of soft tissue, which are our tension elements. *(From Fritz S: Mosby's fundamentals of therapeutic massage, ed 5, St Louis, 2013, Mosby.)*

REVIEW QUESTIONS

evolve Answers to the following review questions appear on the Evolve website accompanying this book at: http://evolve.elsevier.com/Muscolino/kinesiology/.

1. Describe the big picture function of a muscle contraction.

2. What are the two major tissue types found in a skeletal muscle?

3. What is a synonym for the term *muscle cell*?

4. What is the term given to a bundle of muscle fibers?

5. What is the name given to the muscular fascia that surrounds an entire muscle?

6. What is the difference between a tendon and an aponeurosis?

7. What are myofibrils?

8. Describe the structure of a sarcomere.

9. Describe the steps of the sliding filament mechanism.

10. In order, what are the four sources of energy for the sliding filament mechanism within a muscle cell?

11. Regarding nervous system control of muscle contraction, what is the role of neurotransmitters?

12. Describe the concept of muscle memory.

13. Define *motor unit*.

14. Define and give an example of the all-or-none–response law.

15. What is the A-band of skeletal muscle tissue?

16. What is the role of troponin molecules?

17. Describe the difference between red slow-twitch and white fast-twitch fibers.

18. Which type of muscle fibers predominate in postural stabilization muscles?

19. Define *myofascial meridian*.

20. What is the difference between the concepts of tensegrity and compression integrity?

21. Apply the concepts of myofascial meridian theory and tensegrity to manual and movement therapy.

REFERENCES

1. Watkins J: Structure and function of the musculoskeletal system, Champaign, IL, 1999, Human Kinetics.
2. MacIntosh BR, Gardiner PF, McComas AJ: Skeletal muscle: Form and function, ed 2, Champaign, IL, 2006, Human Kinetics.
3. Palastanga N, Field D, Soames R: Anatomy and human movement: Structure and function, ed 4, Oxford, 2002, Butterworth-Heinmann.
4. Thibodeau GA, Paton KT: Anatomy & physiology, ed 5, St Louis, 2003, Mosby.
5. Nordin M, Frankel VH: Basic biomechanics of the musculoskeletal system, ed 3, Baltimore, 2001, Lippincott Williams & Wilkins.
6. Neumann DA: Kinesiology of the musculoskeletal system: Foundations for physical rehabilitation, ed 3, St Louis, 2017, Elsevier.
7. Hamilton N, Weimar W, Luttgens K: Kinesiology: Scientific basis of human motion, ed 12, New York, 2012, McGraw Hill.
8. Paoletti S: The fascia: Anatomy, dysfunction & treatment, Seattle, 2006, Eastland Press.
9. Levangie PK, Norkin CC: joint structure and function: A comprehensive analysis, ed 5, Philadelphia, 2011, FA Davis.
10. Smith LK, Weiss EL, Lehmkuhl LO: Brunstrom's clinical kinesiology, ed 5, Philadelphia, 1996, FA Davis.
11. Kenney WL, Wilmore JH, Castill DL: Physiology of sport and exercise, ed 5, Champaign, IL, 2012, Human Kinetics.
12. Masi AT, Nair K, Evans T, et al: Clinical, biomechanical, and physiological translational interpretations of human resting myofascial tone or tension. International Journal of Therapeutic Massage & Bodywork 3(4):16-28, 2010.
13. Lieber RL: Skeletal muscle, structure, function, & plasticity: The physiological basis of rehabilitation, ed 2, Baltimore, 2002, Lippincott Williams & Wilkins.
14. Myers TW: Anatomy trains: Myofascial meridians for manual & movement therapists, ed 3, Italy, 2014, Churchill Livingstone Elsevier.
15. Page P, Frank CC, Lardner R: Assessment and treatment of muscle imbalance: The Janda approach, Champaign, IL, 2010, Human Kinetics.
16. Simons DG, Travell JG, Simons LS: Travell & Simons' myofascial pain and dysfunction: The trigger point manual: Volume 1: Upper half of body, ed 2, Baltimore, 1999, Williams & Wilkins.

CHAPTER 13
How Muscles Function: the Big Picture

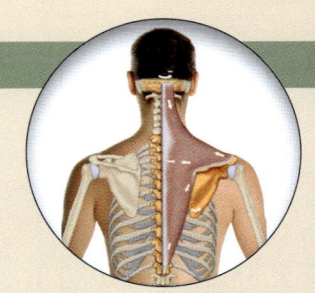

CHAPTER OUTLINE

Section 13.1	"Big Picture" of Muscle Structure and Function	Section 13.6	Functional Group Approach to Learning Muscle Actions
Section 13.2	What Happens When a Muscle Contracts and Shortens?	Section 13.7	Determining Functional Groups
		Section 13.8	Off-Axis Attachment Method for Determining Rotation Actions
Section 13.3	Five-Step Approach to Learning Muscles	Section 13.9	Transferring the Force of a Muscle's Contraction to Another Joint
Section 13.4	Rubber Band Exercise		
Section 13.5	Lines of Pull of a Muscle	Section 13.10	Muscle Actions That Change

CHAPTER OBJECTIVES

After completing this chapter, the student should be able to perform the following:

1. Define the key terms of this chapter and state the meanings of the word origins of this chapter.
2. Do the following related to muscle structure and function:
   - Explain the "big picture" of how a muscle creates motion of a body part at a joint.
   - Define and relate the terms *concentric contraction* and *mover* to the big picture of how a muscle creates joint motion.
3. Do the following related to the contraction and shortening of a muscle:
   - Explain why a muscle that contracts either succeeds or does not succeed in shortening toward the middle.
   - Using the terms *fixed* and *mobile*, describe and give an example of each of the three scenarios that can occur when a muscle concentrically contracts (i.e., contracts and shortens).
   - List what three things must be stated to fully describe a joint action.
   - Describe and give an example of a *reverse action*.
   - Explain what factors determine which attachment of a muscle moves when a muscle concentrically contracts.
4. Do the following related to the five-step approach to learning muscles:
   - List and explain the importance of each of the steps of the five-step approach to learning muscles.
   - State the three questions that should be asked in Step 3.
   - Describe the importance of understanding the direction of fibers and/or the line of pull of a muscle relative to the joint that it crosses.
5. Describe how to use the *rubber band exercise* to help learn the action(s) of a muscle.
6. Explain the importance (relative to determining the possible actions of a muscle) of evaluating each of the following four scenarios: (1) if a muscle with one line of pull has that one line of pull in a cardinal plane; (2) if a muscle with one line of pull has that one line pull in an oblique plane; (3) if a muscle has more than one line of pull; and (4) if a muscle is a one-joint muscle or a multijoint muscle. In addition, explain how a muscle that has more than one action can contract, and yet only one or some of its actions occur.
7. Explain how understanding functional mover groups of muscles can help one learn the actions of muscles, as well as determine functional groups.
8. Describe the meanings of the terms *on-axis* and *off-axis*, and explain how the *off-axis attachment* method can be used to determine a muscle's rotation action. Furthermore, state how one can determine the long axis of a bone.

9. Discuss transferring the force of a muscle's contraction to another joint, and give an example of and explain how a muscle can create an action at a joint that it does not cross.

10. Discuss how muscle actions change, and give an example of and explain how a muscle's action can change when the position of the body changes.

OVERVIEW

This chapter has two major thrusts: it explores the "big picture" of how muscles function concentrically (i.e., contracting and shortening) to create joint actions, and it offers easy methods that can be used by the student to learn muscles. Regarding muscle concentric contraction function, this chapter explores the idea of fixed versus mobile attachments of a muscle and introduces the concept of a muscle's reverse action(s). Included in this discussion is an exploration of the lines of pull of a muscle and how they affect the possible actions of the muscle. Other, more advanced topics such as how a muscle can transfer the force of its contraction to another joint that it does not cross and how a muscle's actions can change with a change in joint position are also explored. Regarding learning muscles, a five-step approach to learning muscles is presented in this chapter. This five-step approach breaks the process of learning the attachments and actions of a muscle into five easy and logical steps. Particularly important is step 3, which shows how to figure out what the actions of a muscle are instead of having to memorize them. Specifically for the rotation actions of a muscle, the *off-axis attachment* method is explained. For kinesthetic learners, a *rubber band exercise* is given to further facilitate learning muscles. Continuing the process of learning muscles, a functional group approach is then given that greatly decreases the amount of time necessary to learn the actions of muscles.

KEY TERMS

Anatomic action
Concentric contraction (con-SEN-trik)
Fixator
Fixed attachment
Functional group
Functional mover group
Long axis (AK-sis)
Mobile attachment
Mover

Multijoint muscle
Off-axis
Off-axis attachment method
On-axis
One-joint muscle
Reverse action
Stabilized attachment
Stabilizer

WORD ORIGINS

- Concentric—From Latin *con*, meaning *together* or *with*, and *centrum*, meaning *center*
- Fix—From Latin *fixus*, meaning *fastened*
- Mobile—From Latin *mobilis*, meaning *movable, mobile*
- Multi—From Latin *multus*, meaning *many, much*
- Stabilize—From Latin *stabilis*, meaning *not moving, fixed*

SECTION 13.1 "BIG PICTURE" OF MUSCLE STRUCTURE AND FUNCTION

- A muscle attaches, via its tendons, from one bone to another bone. In so doing, a muscle crosses the joint that is located between the two bones (Figure 13-1).
- When a muscle contracts, it creates a pulling force on its attachments that attempts to pull them toward each other. In other words, this pulling force attempts to shorten the muscle toward its center. To understand how a muscle creates a pulling force, it is necessary to understand the sliding filament mechanism (see Sections 12.6 and 12.12).
- If the muscle is successful in shortening toward its center, then one or both of the bones to which it is attached will have to move (Figure 13-2).
- Because the bony attachments of the muscle are within body parts, if the muscle moves a bone, then the body part that the bone is within is moved. In this way, muscles can cause movement of parts of the body.

- When a muscle contracts and shortens as described here, this type of contraction is called a **concentric contraction**, and the muscle that is concentrically contracting is called a **mover**.[1]
- Note: A muscle can contract and not shorten! A muscle contraction that does not result in shortening is called an *eccentric contraction* or *isometric contraction*.[2] (For more information on eccentric and isometric contractions, see Chapter 14.)
- It is worth noting that whether or not a muscle is successful in shortening toward its center is determined by the strength of the pulling force of the muscle compared with the force necessary to actually move one or both body parts to which the muscle is attached.
- The force necessary to move a body part is usually the force necessary to move the weight of the body part. However, other forces may be involved.

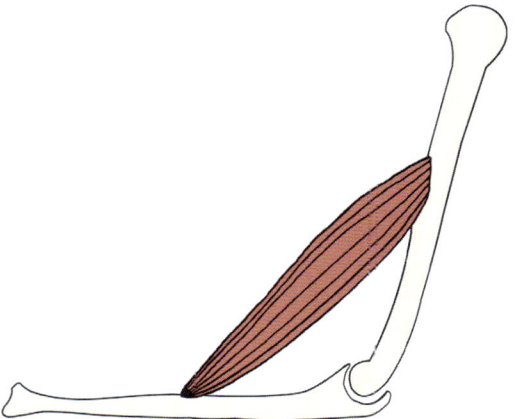

FIGURE 13-1 A generic muscle is shown; it attaches from one bone to another bone and crosses the joint that is located between them. *(From Muscolino JE: The muscular system manual: the skeletal muscles of the human body, ed 4, St Louis, 2017, Mosby.)*

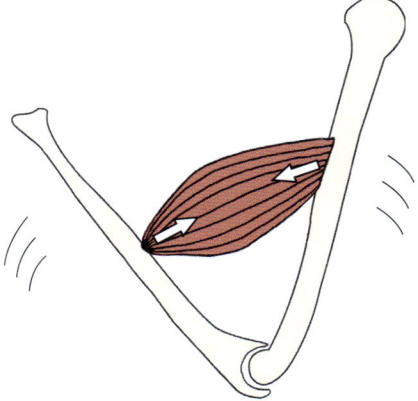

FIGURE 13-2 Muscle shown contracting and shortening (i.e., a concentric contraction). For a muscle to shorten, one or both of the bones to which it is attached must move toward each other. *(From Muscolino JE: The muscular system manual: the skeletal muscles of the human body, ed 4, St Louis, 2017, Mosby.)*

SECTION 13.2   WHAT HAPPENS WHEN A MUSCLE CONTRACTS AND SHORTENS?

- Assuming that a muscle contracts with sufficient strength to shorten toward its center (i.e., concentrically contract), it is helpful to look at the possible scenarios that can occur. (For more information on concentric contractions, see Sections 14.1 to 14.4.)
- If we call one of the attachments of the muscle *Bone A* and the other attachment of the muscle *Bone B,* then we see that three possible scenarios exist[3] (Figure 13-3):
  1. *Bone A* will be pulled toward *Bone B.*
  2. *Bone B* will be pulled toward *Bone A.*
  3. Both *Bone A* and *Bone B* will be pulled toward each other.
- Essentially, when a muscle contracts, its freest attachment moves.
- If an attachment of the muscle moves, it is said to be the mobile attachment. If an attachment of the muscle does not move, it is said to be the **fixed attachment** or **stabilized attachment**.[4]

- Note: We usually think of a typical muscle as having two attachments and a typical muscle contraction as having one of its attachments fixed and its other attachment mobile. However, it is possible for a muscle to contract and have both of its attachments mobile, as seen in Figure 13-3, *C*. It is also possible for a muscle to contract and have both of its attachments fixed (as occurs during isometric contractions). (For more on this see Chapter 14.)
- When a muscle contracts and one of its attachments moves, the muscle creates a joint action. To fully describe this joint action, we must state three things[5]:
  1. The type of motion that has occurred
  2. The name of the body part that has moved
  3. The name of the joint where the movement has occurred

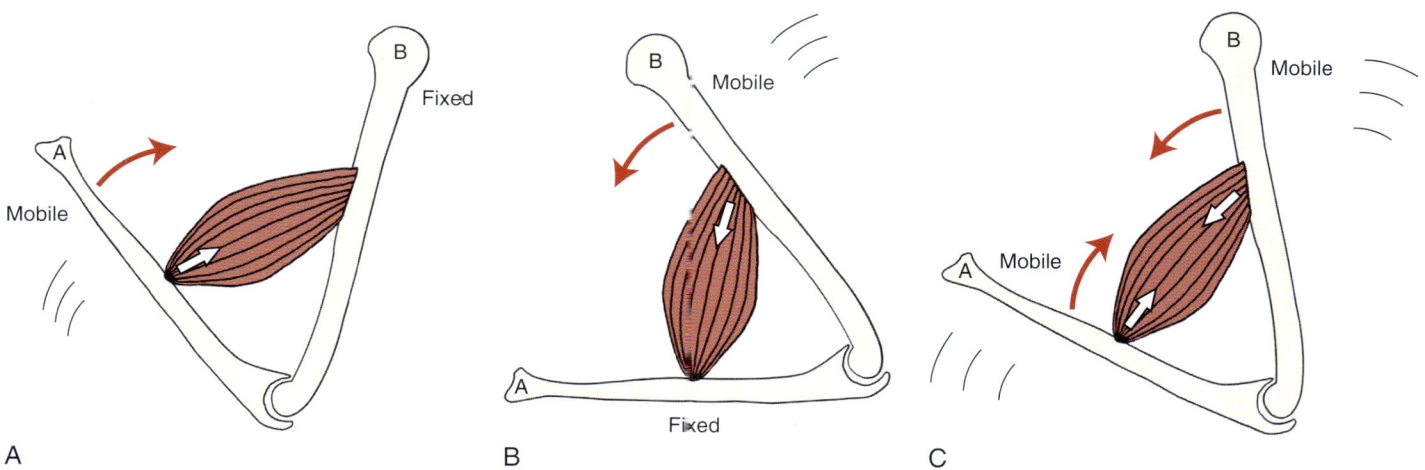

FIGURE 13-3 The three scenarios of a muscle contracting and shortening. If the attachment moves, it is said to be the mobile attachment; if the attachment does not move, it is said to be the fixed attachment. In **A,** bone A moves toward bone B. In **B,** bone B moves toward bone A. In **C,** bone A and bone B both move toward each other. *(From Muscolino JE: The muscular system manual: the skeletal muscles of the human body, ed 4, St Louis, 2017, Mosby.)*

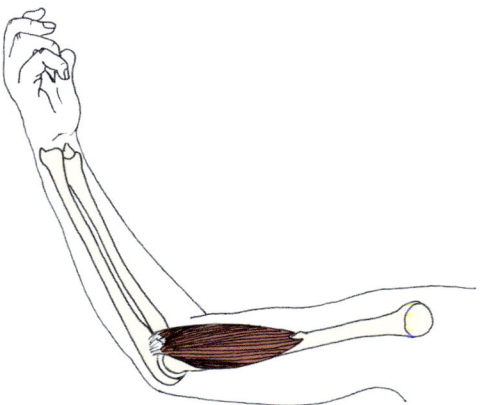

FIGURE 13-4 The right brachialis muscle at rest (medial view). The brachialis attaches from the humerus of the arm to the ulna of the forearm and crosses the elbow joint located between the arm and forearm. *(From Muscolino JE: The muscular system manual: the skeletal muscles of the human body, ed 4, St Louis, 2017, Mosby.)*

As an example to illustrate these concepts, it is helpful to look at the brachialis muscle. One attachment of the brachialis is onto the humerus of the arm, and the other attachment is onto the ulna of the forearm. In attaching to the arm and the forearm, the brachialis crosses the elbow joint that is located between these two body parts (Figure 13-4).

When the brachialis contracts, it attempts to shorten toward its center by exerting a pulling force on the forearm and the arm.

- Scenario 1: The usual result of the brachialis contracting is that the forearm will be pulled toward the arm. This is because the forearm is lighter than the arm and therefore would be more likely to move before the arm would. (In addition, if the arm were to move, the trunk would have to move as well, which makes it even less likely that the arm will be the attachment that moves.) To fully describe this action, we call it *flexion of the forearm at the elbow joint*, because the forearm is the body part that has moved and the elbow joint has flexed (Figure 13-5, *A*). In this scenario the arm is the attachment that is fixed and the forearm is the attachment that is mobile.
- Scenario 2: However, it is possible for the arm to move toward the forearm. If the forearm were to be fixed in place, perhaps because the hand is holding onto an immovable object, then the arm would have to move instead. This action is called *flexion of the arm at the elbow joint* because the arm is the body part that has moved and the elbow joint has flexed (Figure 13-5, *B*). In this scenario the forearm is the attachment that is fixed and the arm is the attachment that is mobile. This scenario can be called a **reverse action**, because the attachment that is usually fixed, the arm, is now mobile, and the attachment that is usually mobile, the forearm, is now fixed.[6] (Reverse actions are covered in more detail in Section 6.29.)
- Scenario 3: Because the contraction of the brachialis exerts a pulling force on the forearm and the arm, it is possible for both of these bones to move. When this occurs, two actions take place: (1) flexion of the forearm at the elbow joint, and (2) flexion of the arm at the elbow joint (Figure 13-5, *C*). In this case both bones are mobile and neither one is fixed.
- It is important to realize that the brachialis does not intend or choose which attachment will move or if both attachments will move.
- When a muscle contracts, it merely exerts a pulling force toward its center. Which attachment moves is determined by other factors. The relative weight of the body parts is the most common factor.
- However, another common determinant is when the central nervous system directs another muscle in the body to contract, which may stop or "fix" one of the attachments of the mover muscle. If this occurs, this second muscle that contracts to fix a body part would be called a **fixator** or **stabilizer** muscle.[7] (For more information on fixator [stabilizer] muscles, see Sections 15.5 and 15.6.)
- It follows that if a muscle does successfully shorten, and one attachment is fixed, then the other attachment must be mobile.

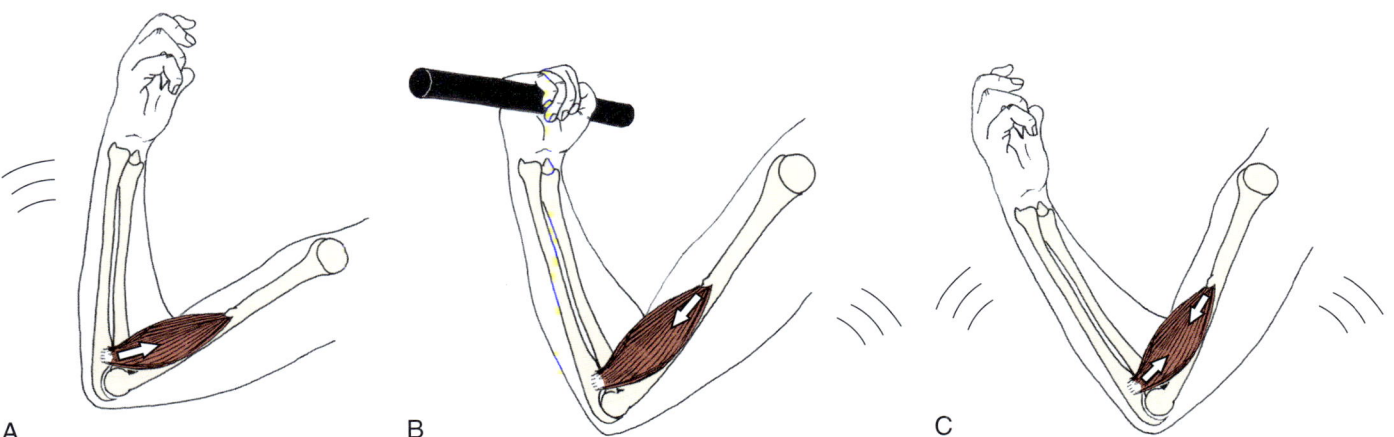

FIGURE 13-5 The three scenarios that can result from a shortening (i.e., concentric) contraction of the brachialis muscle. **A,** Flexion of the forearm at the elbow joint. The arm is fixed, and the forearm is mobile, moving toward the arm. **B,** Flexion of the arm at the elbow joint. The forearm is fixed (the hand is holding onto an immovable bar), and the arm is mobile, moving toward the forearm. **C,** Flexion of the forearm and the arm at the elbow joint. Neither attachment is fixed. Both attachments are mobile, moving toward each other. *(From Muscolino JE: The muscular system manual: the skeletal muscles of the human body, ed 4, St Louis, 2017, Mosby.)*

SECTION 13.3 FIVE-STEP APPROACH TO LEARNING MUSCLES

- Essentially, to learn about muscles, two major aspects must be learned: (1) the attachments of the muscle and (2) the actions of the muscle.
- Generally speaking, the attachments of a muscle must be memorized. However, times exist when clues are given about the attachments by the muscle's name.[4]
  - For example, the name *coracobrachialis* tells us that this muscle has one attachment on the coracoid process of the scapula and that its other attachment is on the brachium (i.e., the humerus).
  - Similarly, the name *zygomaticus major* tells us that this muscle attaches onto the zygomatic bone (and that it is bigger than another muscle called the *zygomaticus minor*).
- Unlike muscle attachments, muscle actions do not have to be memorized. Instead, through an understanding of the simple concept that a muscle pulls at its attachments to move a body part, the action or actions of a muscle can be reasoned out.

FIVE-STEP APPROACH TO LEARNING MUSCLES:

When a student is first confronted with having to study and learn about a muscle, the following five-step approach is recommended:
- Step 1: Look at the name of the muscle to see if it gives you any "free information" that saves you from having to memorize attachments or actions of the muscle.
- Step 2: Learn the general location of the muscle well enough to be able to visualize the muscle on your body. At this point, you need only know it well enough to know:
  - What joint it crosses
  - Where it crosses the joint
  - How it crosses the joint (i.e., the direction in which its fibers are running)
- Step 3: Use this general knowledge of the muscle's location (step 2) to figure out its actions.
- Step 4: Go back and learn (memorize, if necessary) the specific attachments of the muscle.
- Step 5: Now look at the relationship of this muscle to other muscles (and other soft tissue structures) of the body. Look at the following: Is this muscle superficial or deep? In addition, what other muscles (and other soft tissue structures) are located near this muscle?

Figuring out a Muscle's Actions (Step 3 in Detail):

- Once you have a general familiarity with a muscle's location on the body, then it is time to begin the process of reasoning out the actions of the muscle. The most important thing that you must look at is the following:
  - The direction of the muscle fibers relative to the joint that it crosses
  By doing this, you can see the following:
  - The line of pull of the muscle relative to the joint. (When a muscle contracts, it creates a *pulling* force. It is this pulling force that can create motion—in other words, joint actions. Note: Muscles do not push, they *pull*!)
- This line of pull will determine the actions of the muscle[6] (i.e., how the contraction of the muscle will cause the body parts to move at that joint).
- The best approach is to ask the following three questions:
  1. What joint does the muscle cross?
  2. Where does the muscle cross the joint?
  3. How does the muscle cross the joint?

Question 1—What Joint Does the Muscle Cross?

- The first question to ask and answer in figuring out the action(s) of a muscle is to simply know what joint it crosses.
- The following rule applies: If a muscle crosses a joint, then it can have an action at that joint.[5] (Note: This, of course, assumes that the joint is healthy and allows movement to occur.)
  - For example, if we look at the coracobrachialis, knowing that it crosses the glenohumeral (GH) joint tells us that it must have an action at the GH joint.
  - We may not know what the exact action of the coracobrachialis is yet, but at least we now know at what joint it has its actions.
  - To figure out exactly what these actions are, we need to look at questions 2 and 3.
- Note: It is worth pointing out that the converse of the rule about a muscle having the ability to create movement (i.e., an action) at a joint that it crosses is also true. In other words, if a muscle does not cross a joint, then it cannot have an action at that joint. However, this rule is not 100% accurate. Sometimes the force of a muscle can be transferred to another joint, even if the muscle does not cross that joint.[5] (For more on this concept, see Section 13.9.)

Questions 2 and 3—Where Does the Muscle Cross the Joint? How Does the Muscle Cross the Joint?

- Questions 2 and 3 must be looked at together.
- The *where* of a muscle crossing a joint is whether it crosses the joint anteriorly, posteriorly, medially, or laterally.
- It is helpful to place a muscle into one of these broad groups because the following general rules apply: muscles that cross a joint anteriorly will usually flex a body part at that joint, and muscles that cross a joint posteriorly will usually extend a body part at that joint; muscles that cross a joint laterally will usually abduct or laterally flex a body part at that joint, and muscles that cross a joint medially will usually adduct a body part at that joint.[6]
  - Notes: (1) Flexion is nearly always an anterior movement of a body part, and extension is nearly always a posterior movement of a body part. However, from the knee joint and farther distal, flexion is a posterior movement and extension is an anterior movement of the body part. (2) Abduction occurs at joints of the appendicular skeleton; lateral flexion occurs at joints of the axial skeleton.

- The *how* of a muscle crossing a joint is whether it crosses the joint with its fibers running vertically or horizontally. This is also very important.
  - To illustrate this idea, we will look at the pectoralis major muscle. The pectoralis major has two parts: (1) a clavicular head and (2) a sternocostal head. The *where* of these two heads of the pectoralis major crossing the GH joint is the same (i.e., they both cross the GH joint anteriorly). However, the *how* of these two heads crossing the GH joint is very different. The clavicular head crosses the GH joint with its fibers running primarily vertically; therefore it flexes the arm at the GH joint (because it pulls the arm upward in the sagittal plane, which is termed *flexion*). However, the sternocostal head crosses the GH joint with its fibers running horizontally; therefore it adducts the arm at the GH joint (because it pulls the arm from lateral to medial in the frontal plane, which is termed *adduction*).[5]
- With a muscle that has a horizontal direction to its fibers, another factor must be considered when looking at *how* this muscle crosses the joint (i.e., whether the muscle attaches to the first place on the bone that it reaches, or whether the muscle wraps around the bone before attaching to it). Muscles that run horizontally (in the transverse plane) and wrap around the bone before attaching to it create a rotation action when they contract and pull on the attachment.[5]
  - For example, the sternocostal head of the pectoralis major does not attach to the first point on the humerus that it reaches. Instead it continues to wrap around the shaft of the humerus to attach onto the lateral lip of the bicipital groove of the humerus. When the sternocostal head pulls, it medially rotates the arm at the GH joint (in addition to its other actions).
- In essence, by asking the three questions of step 3 of the five-step approach to learning muscles (What joint does a muscle cross? Where does the muscle cross the joint? How does the muscle cross the joint?), we are trying to determine the direction of the muscle fibers relative to the joint. Determining this will give us the line of pull of the muscle relative to the joint, and that will give us the actions of the muscle—saving us the trouble of having to memorize this information!

SECTION 13.4 RUBBER BAND EXERCISE

VISUAL AND KINESTHETIC EXERCISE FOR LEARNING A MUSCLE'S ACTIONS:

Rubber Band Exercise:

- An excellent method for learning the actions of a muscle is to place a large colorful rubber band (or large colorful shoelace or string) on your body, or the body of a partner, in the same location that the muscle you are studying is located.
- Hold one end of the rubber band at one of the attachment sites of the muscle, and hold the other end of the rubber band at the other attachment site of the muscle.
- Make sure that you have the rubber band running/oriented in the same direction as the direction of the fibers of the muscle. If it is not uncomfortable, you may even loop or tie the rubber band (or shoelace) around the body parts that are the attachments of the muscle.
- Once you have the rubber band in place, pull one of the ends of the rubber band toward the other attachment of the rubber band to see the action that the rubber band/muscle has on that body part's attachment. Once done, return the attachment of the rubber band to where it began and repeat this exercise for the other end of the rubber band to see the action that the rubber band/muscle has on the other attachment of the muscle (Box 13-1).
- By placing the rubber band on your body or your partner's body, you are simulating the direction of the muscle's fibers relative to the joint that it crosses.
- By pulling either end of the rubber band toward the center, you are simulating the line of pull of the muscle relative to the joint that it crosses. The resultant movements that occur are the actions that the muscle would have. This is an excellent exercise both to visually see the actions of a muscle and to kinesthetically experience the actions of a muscle.

 BOX 13-1

When doing the rubber band exercise, it is extremely important that the attachment of the rubber band that you are pulling is pulled exactly toward the other attachment and in no other direction. In other words, your line of pull should be exactly the same as the line of pull of the muscle (which is essentially determined by the direction of the fibers of the muscle).

When doing the rubber band exercise, the attachment of the muscle that you are pulling would be the mobile attachment in that scenario; the end that you do not move is the fixed attachment in that scenario. Furthermore, by doing this exercise twice (i.e., by then repeating it by reversing which attachment you hold fixed and which one you pull and move), you are simulating the standard action and the reverse action of the muscle.

- This exercise can be used to learn all muscle actions and can be especially helpful for determining actions that may be a little more difficult to visualize, such as rotation actions.
- Note: The use of a large colorful rubber band is more helpful than a shoelace or string, because when you stretch out a rubber band and place it in the location that a muscle would be, the natural elasticity of a rubber band creates a pull on the attachment sites that nicely simulates the pull of a muscle on its attachments when it contracts.
- If you can, you should work with a partner to do this exercise. Have your partner hold one of the "attachments" of the rubber band while you hold the other "attachment." This leaves one of your hands free to pull one of the rubber band attachment sites toward the center.
- A further note of caution: If you are using a rubber band, be careful that you do not accidentally let go and have the rubber band hit you or your partner. For this reason, it would be preferable to use a shoelace or string instead of a rubber band when working near the face.

SECTION 13.5 LINES OF PULL OF A MUSCLE

- Because the line of pull of a muscle relative to the joint it crosses determines the actions that it has, it is extremely important to fully understand the line or lines of pull of a muscle[6] (Box 13-2).

BOX 13-2

For each scenario that is presented in this section with regard to a line of pull of a muscle and the resultant action that the muscle has, we are not considering the reverse action of a muscle. Given that a reverse action is always theoretically possible for every named standard action of a muscle, the complementary reverse action always exists.

- It is helpful to examine four scenarios regarding a muscle and its line or lines of pull:
  - Scenario 1: A muscle with one line of pull in a cardinal plane
  - Scenario 2: A muscle with one line of pull in an oblique plane
  - Scenario 3: A muscle that has more than one line of pull
  - Scenario 4: A muscle that crosses more than one joint

SCENARIO 1—A MUSCLE WITH ONE LINE OF PULL IN A CARDINAL PLANE:

- If a muscle has one line of pull and that line of pull lies perfectly in a cardinal plane, then that muscle will have one action (plus the reverse action of that action).
- A perfect example is the brachialis muscle. The brachialis crosses the elbow joint anteriorly with a vertical direction to its fibers. All of its fibers are essentially running parallel to one another and are oriented in the sagittal plane. Therefore the brachialis has one action, namely flexion of the forearm at the elbow joint[5] (as well as its reverse action of flexion of the arm at the elbow joint). The brachialis's line of pull is in the sagittal plane; therefore the action that it creates must be in the sagittal plane, and that action is flexion (Figure 13-6).

SCENARIO 2—A MUSCLE WITH ONE LINE OF PULL IN AN OBLIQUE PLANE:

- If a muscle has one line of pull, but that line of pull is in an oblique plane, then the muscle will create movement in that oblique plane. However, when this movement is named, no name for oblique plane movement exists. Instead this movement has to be broken up into names for its component cardinal plane actions. (The concept of naming oblique plane motions is covered in Section 6.28.)
  - An excellent example is the coracobrachialis. The coracobrachialis has a line of pull that is in an oblique plane. That oblique plane is a combination of sagittal and frontal cardinal planes. When the coracobrachialis pulls, it pulls the arm diagonally in a direction that is both anterior and medial at the same time. However, no one name for this oblique plane motion exists. To name this one motion that would occur, we must break it up into its component cardinal plane actions of flexion in the sagittal plane and adduction in the frontal plane. Therefore even though the muscle actually creates only one movement in an oblique plane, we describe it as having two cardinal plane actions[1] (Figure 13-7). (To understand how an oblique plane muscle can create only one of its cardinal plane actions, see Section 15.4.)
- For this reason, a muscle that has one line of pull can be said to have more than one cardinal plane action if that muscle's line of pull is oriented within an oblique plane. Of course, for each of its actions, a reverse action is theoretically possible.

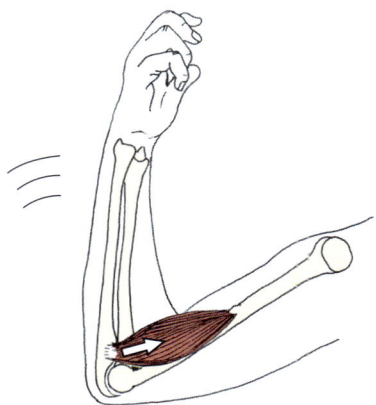

FIGURE 13-6 The brachialis muscle has one line of pull to its fibers, and that line of pull is located within the sagittal plane; therefore the brachialis can flex the elbow joint. (Note: Flexion of the forearm at the elbow joint is its standard action; flexion of the arm at the elbow joint would be the complementary reverse action.) *(From Muscolino JE: The muscular system manual: the skeletal muscles of the human body, ed 4, St Louis, 2017, Mosby.)*

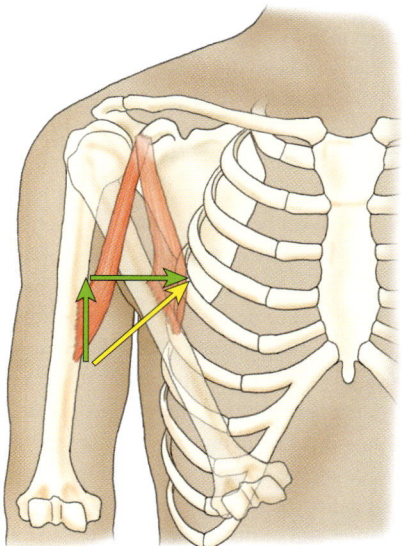

FIGURE 13-7 Illustration of the motion that is caused when the coracobrachialis contracts (with the scapula fixed and the humerus mobile). This one oblique plane motion (*yellow arrow*) must be broken down into its two cardinal plane actions (*green arrows*) when the joint actions of the coracobrachialis are discussed. Hence the coracobrachialis can flex the arm in the sagittal plane and adduct the arm in the frontal plane (all at the glenohumeral joint).

SCENARIO 3—A MUSCLE THAT HAS MORE THAN ONE LINE OF PULL:

- If a muscle has more than one line of pull, then we apply the same logic that was used in scenarios 1 and 2 to this muscle.
- For each line of pull that is oriented perfectly in a cardinal plane, there will be one action possible (along with the corresponding reverse action).
- For each oblique plane line of pull, the movement that occurs in that oblique plane can be broken up into its separate cardinal plane components (with their corresponding reverse actions).
  - An example is the gluteus medius. The gluteus medius has posterior fibers, middle fibers, and anterior fibers, each with a different line of pull on the femur at the hip joint. The posterior fibers pull in an oblique plane; the cardinal plane components of this oblique plane are extension in the sagittal plane, abduction in the frontal plane, and lateral rotation in the transverse plane. The anterior fibers also pull in an oblique plane; their cardinal plane components are flexion in the sagittal plane, abduction in the frontal plane, and medial rotation in the transverse plane. However, the middle fibers are oriented perfectly in the frontal plane; therefore their only action is abduction in the frontal plane.[5] In this example, the posterior and anterior fibers fit scenario 2 (one line of pull in an oblique plane), and the middle fibers fit scenario 1 (one line of pull in a cardinal plane) (Figure 13-8). (Note: The reverse actions of the gluteus medius are movements of the pelvis toward the thigh at the hip joint.)

SCENARIO 4—A MUSCLE THAT CROSSES MORE THAN ONE JOINT:

- If a muscle crosses only one joint, it is termed a **one-joint muscle**; if a muscle crosses more than one joint, it is termed a **multijoint muscle**.
- If a muscle is a multijoint muscle, then the reasoning that is applied at one joint for each line of pull that the muscle has is applied at each joint that the muscle crosses.
- Many multijoint muscles exist in the human body.
- Examples include the following:
  - The rectus femoris of the quadriceps femoris group crosses the knee and hip joints with one line of pull. Therefore it can extend the leg at the knee joint in the sagittal plane, and it can flex the thigh at the hip joint in the sagittal plane[5] (as well as create the corresponding reverse actions) (Figure 13-9, A).
  - The flexor carpi ulnaris crosses the elbow joint with one line of pull in a cardinal plane and crosses the wrist joint with one line of pull in an oblique plane. Therefore it can flex the forearm at the elbow joint in the sagittal plane, and it can flex and ulnar deviate (i.e., adduct) the hand at the wrist joint in the sagittal and frontal planes, respectively[5] (as well as create the corresponding reverse actions) (Figure 13-9, B).

CAN A MUSCLE CHOOSE WHICH OF ITS ACTIONS WILL OCCUR?

- No. Muscles are basically machines that contract when they are ordered to contract by the nervous system (Box 13-3). If a muscle contracts, then whichever motor units are ordered to contract have every muscle fiber within them contract and attempt to shorten.[8] (For more on this concept, see the discussion of the all-or-none–response law in Section 12.10.) Whatever line of pull these fibers lie within will have a pulling force created that will pull on the attachments of the muscle. When a muscle has only one line of pull, it must attempt to create every action that would occur from that one line of pull. Only muscles that have more than one line of pull can attempt to create certain actions and not other actions. This occurs when the central nervous system directs to contract motor units that lie within only one line of pull of the muscle (and does not direct to contract motor units that lie within

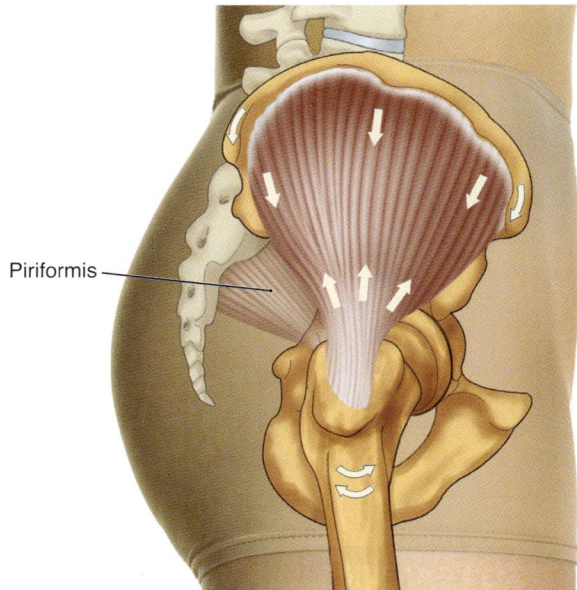

FIGURE 13-8 Gluteus medius muscle. The gluteus medius has posterior fibers and anterior fibers that are each oriented in an oblique plane; therefore these fibers have an action in each of the component cardinal planes that the oblique plane is within. The middle fibers of the gluteus medius are oriented directly in a cardinal plane; hence they have only one action within that cardinal plane. (Of course, for any action that a muscle possesses, a reverse action is always theoretically possible. In the case of the gluteus medius, the reverse action would be movement of the pelvis toward the thigh at the hip joint instead of movement of the thigh toward the pelvis at the hip joint.) *(From Muscolino JE: The muscular system manual: the skeletal muscles of the human body, ed 4, St Louis, 2017, Mosby.)*

BOX 13-3

I spend most of my time reading about, studying, working on, teaching, and writing about muscles. As much as I love the muscular system, I often tell my students that muscles are dumb machines. They do not know what actions they are or are not creating; they do not intend anything. They simply contract when they are ordered to by the central nervous system. The movements that they make and the patterns of those movements are ultimately determined by the nervous system. Muscle contraction, muscle coordination, muscle patterning, muscle armoring, and muscle memory all reside in the nervous system. (For more information on how certain actions of muscles can occur and not others, see Section 15.4. For more on the nervous system control of the muscular system, see Chapter 19.)

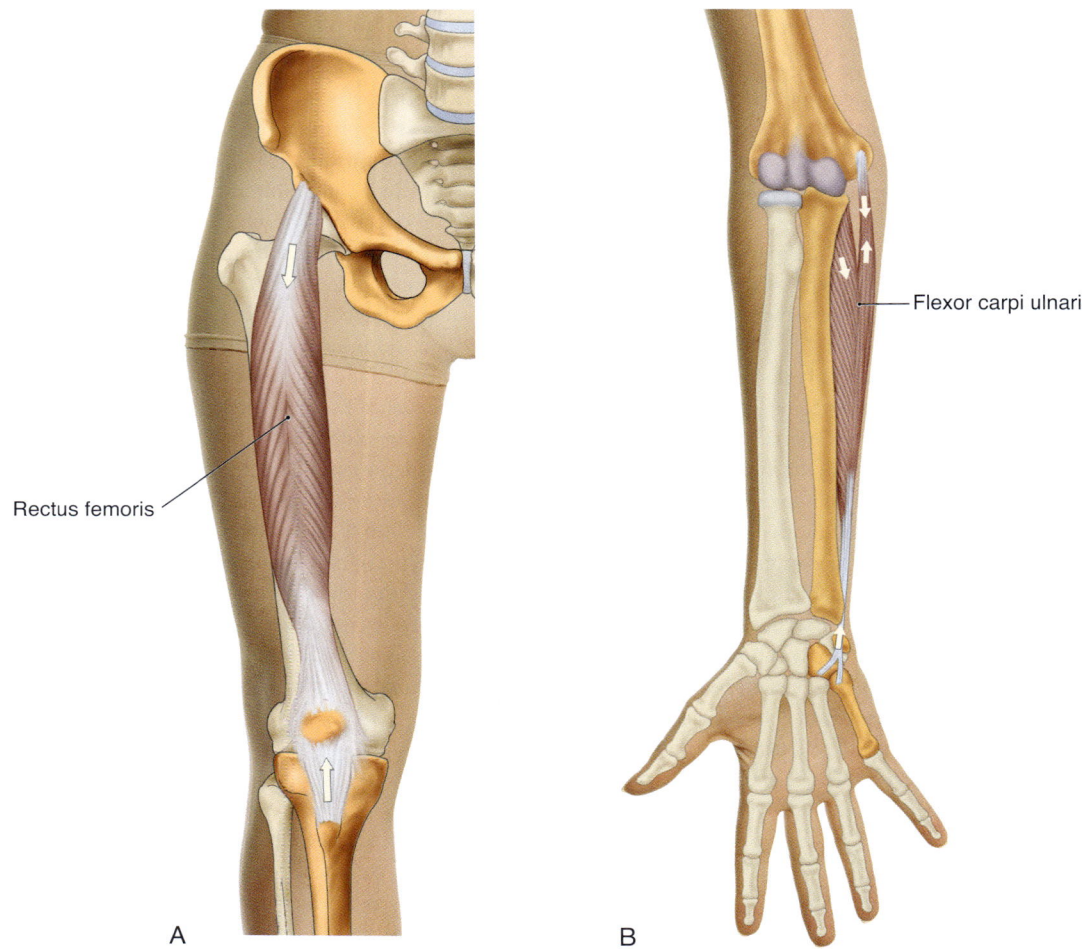

FIGURE 13-9 Whenever a muscle crosses more than one joint (i.e., is a multijoint muscle), it can create movement at each of the joints that it crosses. **A,** Rectus femoris (of the quadriceps femoris group), which crosses both the hip and knee joints. **B,** Flexor carpi ulnaris, which crosses the elbow joint and also crosses the wrist joint. *(From Muscolino JE: The muscular system manual: the skeletal muscles of the human body, ed 4, St Louis, 2017, Mosby.)*

other lines of pull). An example is the trapezius. It has three parts: (1) upper, (2) middle, and (3) lower. Each part has its own line of pull. The upper trapezius can be ordered to contract without the middle or lower parts being ordered to contract. In this manner, a muscle with more than one line of pull can attempt to create some of its actions and not others.[5] Other examples of muscles with more than one line of pull are the deltoid and gluteus medius.

Therefore we can state the following two rules:
- A muscle with one line of pull attempts to create every one of its actions when it contracts.
- A muscle with more than one line of pull does not necessarily attempt to create every one of its actions when it contracts. It may attempt to create the action(s) of one of its lines of pull but not the action(s) of another of its lines of pull.

SECTION 13.6 FUNCTIONAL GROUP APPROACH TO LEARNING MUSCLE ACTIONS

- The best method for approaching and learning each action of a new muscle that you first encounter is to use the reasoning of step 3 of the five-step approach. For each aspect of the direction of fibers for a muscle, you apply the questions of *where* and *how* the muscle crosses the joint. This reasoning is solid and will lead you to reason out all actions of the muscle that is being studied.
- However, it can be very repetitive and time-consuming as you apply this method to muscle after muscle after muscle that all cross the same joint in the same manner.

- Therefore, once you are very comfortable with applying the questions of step 3 for learning the actions of each muscle individually, it is recommended that you begin to use your understanding of how muscles function and apply it on a larger scale.
- Instead of looking at each muscle individually and going through all of the questions of step 3 for that muscle, take a step back and look at the broad functional groups of muscles at each joint.
- A muscle belongs to a **functional group** if it shares the same function (e.g., joint action) as the other members of the functional

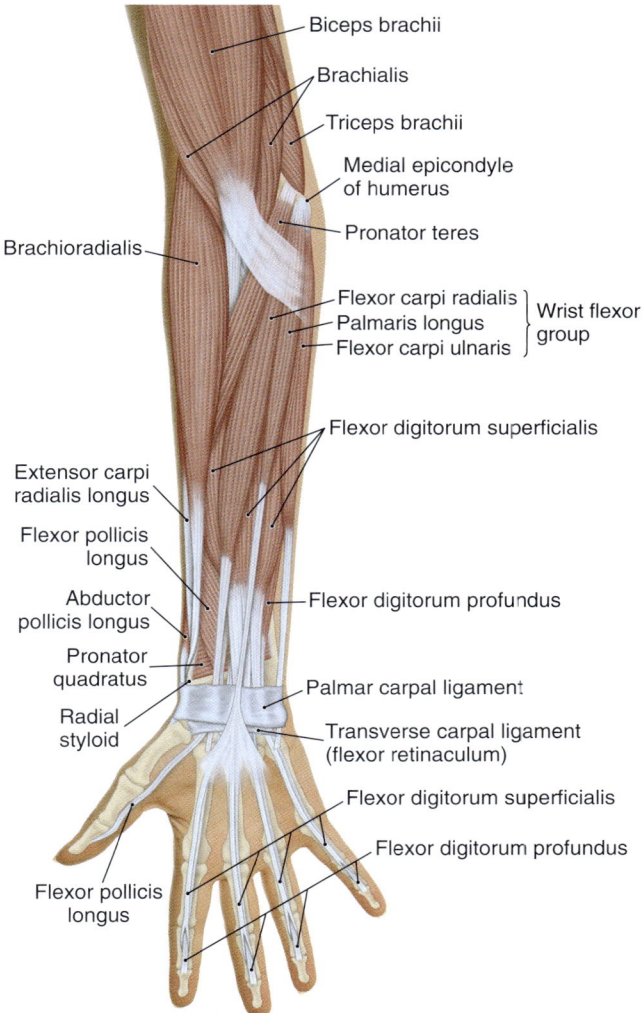

FIGURE 13-10 Anterior view of the elbow joint region. All muscles that cross the elbow joint anteriorly belong to the functional mover group of elbow joint flexors. *(From Muscolino JE:* The muscular system manual: the skeletal muscles of the human body, *ed 4, St Louis, 2017, Mosby.)*

group.[5] The type of functional group that is being referred to in this section is a **functional mover group** (i.e., all the muscles in a group create the same joint action when they concentrically contract). Muscles can also be functionally grouped in roles other than as movers of a joint action. (For more on the various roles of muscles, see Chapter 15.)

❍ For example, instead of individually using the questions of step 3 to learn that the brachialis flexes the forearm at the elbow joint, and then that the biceps brachii flexes the forearm at the elbow joint, and then that the pronator teres flexes the forearm at the elbow joint, and also the flexor carpi radialis, palmaris longus, and so forth, it is a simpler and more elegant approach to look at the functional group of muscles that all flex the elbow joint.

❍ In other words, the bigger picture is to see that *all muscles* that cross the elbow joint anteriorly flex the forearm at the elbow joint. Looking at the body this way, when you encounter yet another muscle that crosses the elbow joint anteriorly, you can automatically place it into the group of forearm flexors at the elbow joint (Figure 13-10).

❍ For each joint of the human body, look for the functional groups of movers. In the case of the elbow joint, because it is a pure hinge, uniaxial joint, it is very simple. Only two functional mover groups exist: (1) anterior muscles that flex and (2) posterior muscles that extend.

❍ Triaxial joints such as the shoulder or hip joint will have more functional mover groups[5] (flexors, extensors, abductors, adductors, medial rotators, and lateral rotators), but the concept will always be the same. Once you clearly see this concept, learning the actions of muscles of the body can be greatly simplified and streamlined. (Guidelines to determine the functional group to which a muscle belongs are given in Section 13.7.)

REMINDER ABOUT REVERSE ACTIONS:

Remember that the reverse actions of a muscle are always possible,[5] even if they have not been specifically listed in this book! (For more information on reverse actions, see Section 6.29.) So, each muscle that flexes the forearm at the elbow joint can also flex the arm at the elbow joint.

SECTION 13.7 DETERMINING FUNCTIONAL GROUPS

Understanding actions of muscles from a functional group approach is the most efficient and elegant method to learn the actions of the muscles of the body.
- The muscles of a functional mover group are grouped together because they all share the same joint action. If their joint action is the same, then their line of pull relative to that joint must be the same. Therefore it stands to reason that a functional group can also be looked at as a structural group (i.e., the muscles of a functional group are located together).
- Generally, certain guidelines can be stated regarding the location of functional groups of muscles.
  - Note: The general rules presented for learning functional mover groups of muscles are not hard and fast. They are better looked at as guidelines, because exceptions to these rules exist. For example, across the ankle joint, frontal plane functional groups are named as *everters* and *inverters*, not *abductors* and *adductors*. Another example is the saddle joint of the thumb, where flexion and extension occur in the frontal plane and abduction and adduction occur in the sagittal plane. Occasional exceptions aside, these general rules or guidelines are extremely valuable!

SAGITTAL PLANE:

- All groups of muscles that cross a joint in the sagittal plane can perform either flexion or extension[3] (Figure 13-11).
  - If the muscles cross the joint anteriorly, they perform flexion (except for the knee joint and farther distal).
  - If the muscles cross the joint posteriorly, they perform extension (except for the knee joint and farther distal).

FRONTAL PLANE:

- All groups of muscles that cross a joint in the frontal plane can perform either right lateral flexion/left lateral flexion or abduction/adduction[3] (Figure 13-12).
  - If the body part being moved is an axial body part, then the muscles perform lateral flexion to the same side (i.e., muscles on the right side of the body perform right lateral flexion; muscles on the left side of the body perform left lateral flexion).
  - If the body part being moved is an appendicular body part, then the muscles perform abduction if they cross on the lateral side of the joint, and the muscles perform adduction if they cross on the medial side of the joint.

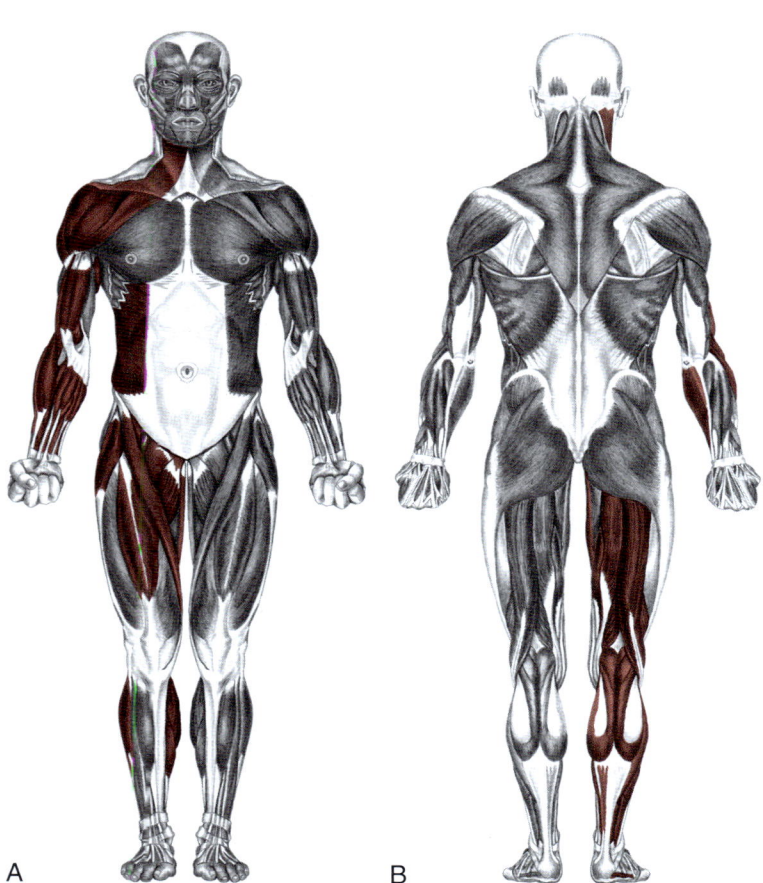

FIGURE 13-11 A, Anterior view of the musculature of the body. **B,** Posterior view of the musculature of the body. The flexor functional mover groups are colored red on the right side of the body. The flexor muscles are generally located anteriorly (except for the knee joint and farther distal).

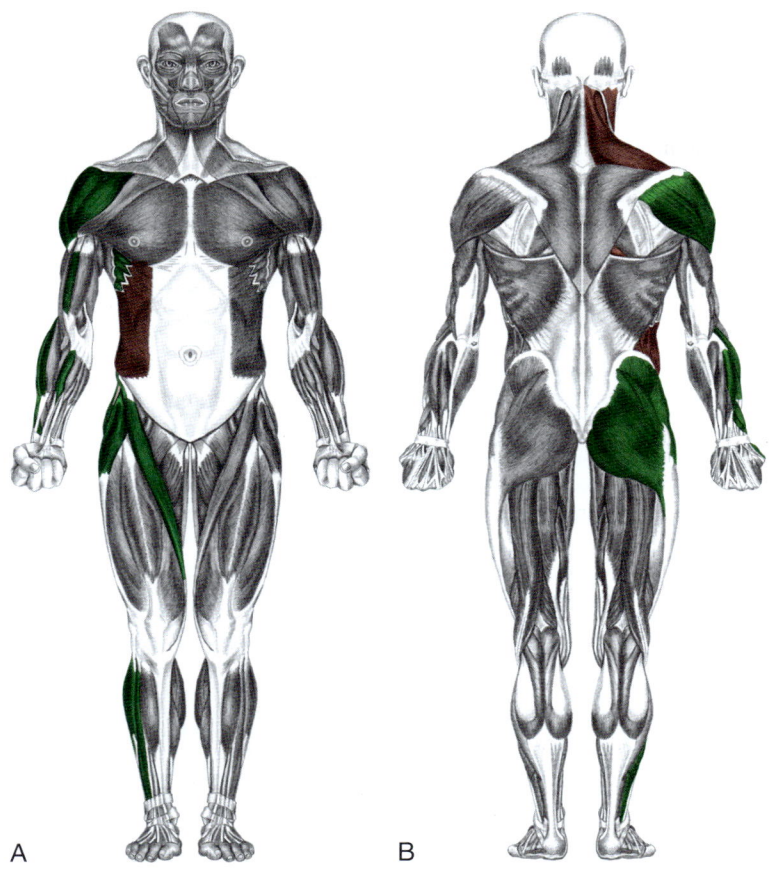

FIGURE 13-12 A, Anterior view of the musculature of the body. **B,** Posterior view of the musculature of the body. The muscles of the lateral flexor functional mover groups (for axial body joints) are colored red, and the muscles of the abductor functional mover groups (for appendicular body joints) are colored green on the right side of the body. (Note: The muscles of these functional groups are generally located laterally.)

TRANSVERSE PLANE:

- Transverse plane actions are slightly more difficult to determine because the muscles of a transverse plane functional mover group are not necessarily located together in one structural group (as are the muscles of the sagittal and frontal plane functional mover groups).
  - For example, the right splenius capitis and the left sternocleidomastoid both perform right rotation of the neck (and head) at the spinal joints. However, even though these two muscles share the same joint action and are therefore in the same functional group, they are not located together. The right splenius capitis is in the right side of the neck, and the left sternocleidomastoid is in the left side of the neck; furthermore, the splenius capitis is located posteriorly, and the sternocleidomastoid is located primarily anteriorly.
- Functional groups of the transverse plane perform rotation.[3]
  - If the body part being moved is an axial body part, then the muscles perform right rotation or left rotation.
  - If the body part being moved is an appendicular body part, then the muscles perform lateral rotation or medial rotation.
- An easy method to determine the transverse plane rotation action of a muscle to place it into its functional mover group is to look at the manner in which the muscle *wraps around* the body part to which it attaches. (Another method to determine rotation actions that is technically more exacting is called the *off-axis attachment* method,[9] presented in Section 13.8.)
  - For example, the right splenius capitis and the left sternocleidomastoid both have the same action of right rotation because they both wrap around the neck region in the same manner (Figure 13-13, *A*).
  - The right pectoralis major and the right latissimus dorsi have the same action of the medial rotation of the right arm at the glenohumeral joint because they both wrap around the humerus in the same manner (Figure 13-13, *B*).
- When trying to see the manner in which a muscle wraps, it is usually best to visualize the muscle from a superior (or proximal) perspective, as in Figures 13-13, *A* and *B*.

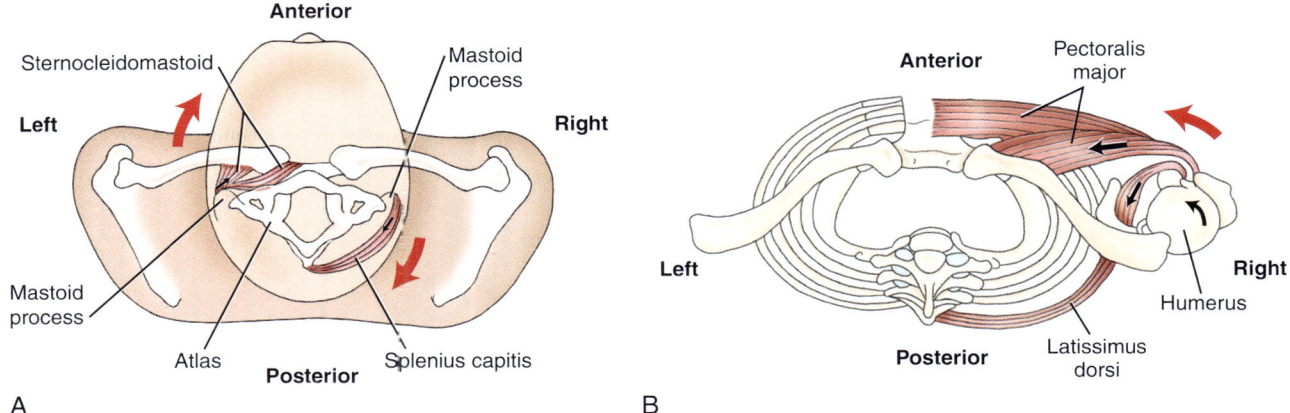

FIGURE 13-13 **A,** Superior view of the right splenius capitis and left sternocleidomastoid muscles. Even though one of these muscles is posterior and on the right side and the other is primarily anterior and on the left side, they both have the same action of right rotation of the neck and head at the spinal joints. This is because they both wrap around the neck/head in the same direction. **B,** Superior view of the right pectoralis major and right latissimus dorsi. Because they both wrap around the humerus in the same direction, they are both able to medially rotate the arm at the glenohumeral joint. As can be seen in these two examples, unlike other functional groups of movers, muscles of the same mover functional rotation group are often not located together in the same structural group location.

SECTION 13.8 OFF-AXIS ATTACHMENT METHOD FOR DETERMINING ROTATION ACTIONS

- Seeing how the direction of a muscle's fibers *wrap* around the bone to which it attaches is a convenient visual method for determining the transverse plane rotation action of a muscle.[9]
- However, another method can be used to determine rotation actions that might be a little more challenging to visualize at first;

but once the rotation is visualized and understood, this method is a more accurate and elegant method to use. This method is called the **off-axis attachment method**.

- Figure 13-14, *A* illustrates a side view of a muscle that crosses from one bone (labeled *fixed*) to another bone (labeled *mobile*).

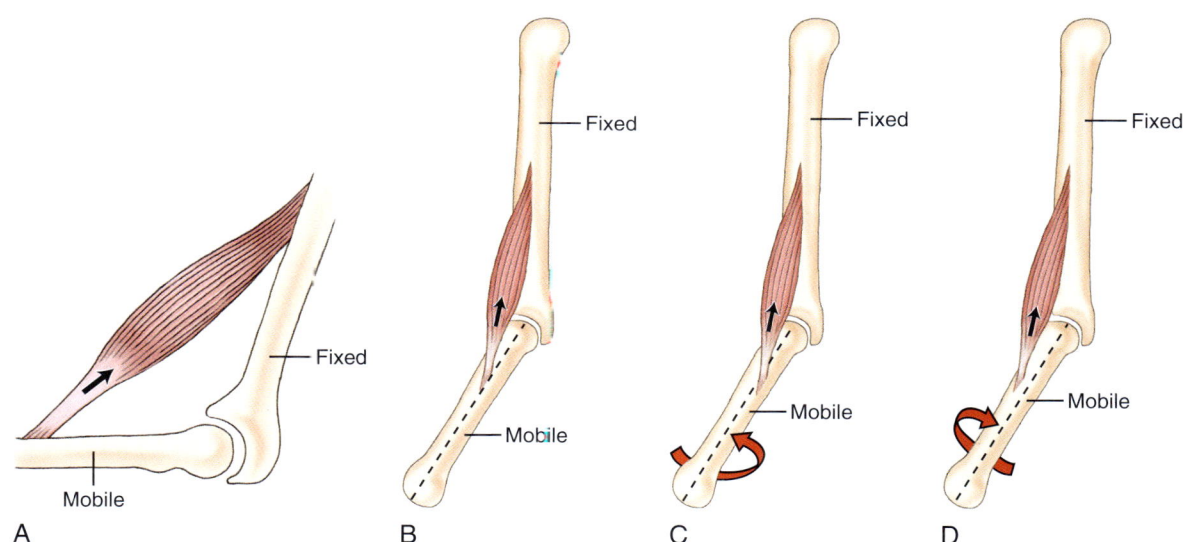

FIGURE 13-14 A, Side view of a muscle that attaches from one bone to another. When this muscle contracts and shortens, the mobile bone will be moved toward the fixed bone. **B to D,** Oblique views of muscles that cross from the same fixed bone to the same mobile bone. (Note: In all cases a dashed line indicates the long axis of the mobile bone.) The muscle in **B** attaches on-axis; therefore it produces no rotation action of the mobile bone. The muscles in **C** and **D** attach off-axis; therefore they can produce a rotation action of the mobile bone. The red arrows indicate these rotation actions. (Note: The muscles, bones, and joint illustrated in **A** to **D** are hypothetical; they are not meant to represent any specific structures of the body.)

It is fairly intuitive to see that this muscle will move the mobile bone toward the fixed bone. However, to determine whether this muscle can create a rotation motion requires that we see exactly where the muscle attaches onto this mobile bone; more specifically, we need to see whether the muscle attaches *on-axis* or *off-axis*.

○ Figure 13-14, *B* is an oblique view that illustrates a hypothetical muscle that attaches onto the mobile bone **on-axis** (i.e., directly over the long axis of the mobile bone represented by the dashed line). When this muscle contracts and shortens, even though the mobile bone will be moved toward the fixed bone, no rotation of the mobile bone will occur because the muscle attaches on-axis (i.e., it does not wrap around to attach onto the bone to either side of the axis). Figure 13-14, *C* is an oblique view of another hypothetical muscle that attaches onto the mobile bone; however, this muscle attaches **off-axis** (i.e., it wraps around the bone to attach off to the side of the long axis of the mobile bone). When this muscle contracts and shortens, it can move the mobile bone toward the fixed bone; it can also rotate the mobile bone as demonstrated by the red arrow. Figure 13-14, *D* shows a similar muscle attaching onto the mobile bone off-axis to the other side and shows the rotation that this muscle would produce when contracting and shortening. (Note: The two muscles in Figure 13-14, *C* and *D* attach off-axis on the opposite sides of the long axis from each other; therefore they produce rotation actions that are opposite to each other.)

○ Using the *off-axis attachment method* to determine the rotation action of a muscle necessitates that one visualize the long axis of a bone. If a muscle attaches onto the bone on-axis (i.e., such that its attachment is directly over the axis), it has no possible rotation action. However, if it attaches onto the bone off-axis (i.e., off the axis to either side), it can create a rotation action (Box 13-4).

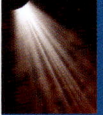

BOX 13-4 Spotlight on Determining the Long Axis of a Bone

It is the long axis (also known as the longitudinal axis) of a bone that needs to be visualized to determine rotation actions of a muscle. The long axis of a bone is a straight line that runs from the center of the articular surface of the bone at one end to the center of the articular surface of the bone at the other end (i.e., from the center of the joint at one end to the center of the joint at the other end). This long axis usually runs through the shaft of the bone itself, as seen in Figures 13-14, *B* to *D*; however, depending on the shape of the bone, it may not. For example, the long axis of the femur is a straight line that connects the center of the hip and knee joints; as a result, the femur's long axis lies outside the shaft of the femur (see accompanying figure). The location of this long axis is important in determining the rotation actions of muscles that attach onto the femur.

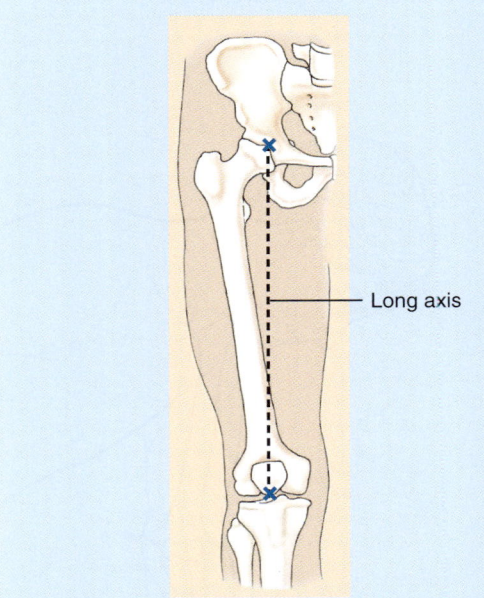

SECTION 13.9 TRANSFERRING THE FORCE OF A MUSCLE'S CONTRACTION TO ANOTHER JOINT

In Section 13.3, we stated two rules about muscle contractions:
○ Rule 1: If a muscle crosses a joint, it can have an action at that joint[5] (if the joint allows movement along the line of pull of the muscle).
○ Rule 2: If a muscle does not cross a joint, it cannot have an action at that joint.
○ Although rule 1 is true, rule 2 is usually, but not always, true. Sometimes the force of a muscle's contraction can be transferred to a joint that the muscle does not cross.[5]
○ An example of this is lateral rotation of the arm at the glenohumeral (GH) joint with the distal end of the upper extremity fixed (i.e., closed-chain). Usually when the lateral rotators of the arm contract, the humerus rotates laterally relative to the scapula at the GH joint, and the bones of the forearm and hand "go along for the ride," maintaining their relative positions to each other. (Note: For an explanation of the distinction between true joint movement and *going along for the ride*, see Section 1.6.) However, when the distal end of the upper extremity is fixed, the hand cannot go along for the ride; and because the hand is fixed, the radius is also fixed and cannot move (with regard to rotation motion, because the wrist joint does not allow rotation). In this scenario, when the lateral

rotators of the humerus contract and shorten, the humerus laterally rotates. Because the elbow joint does not allow rotation, this rotation force is transferred to the ulna, which then *rotates laterally* relative to the fixed radius. This motion causes the ulna to cross over the radius. When the ulna and radius cross, the motion is defined as pronation of the forearm. Although it is possible for pronators of the forearm to create this action of forearm pronation, in this instance the force for forearm pronation came from lateral rotators of the humerus at the GH joint (whose force was transferred to the radioulnar joints). Hence, even though these lateral rotator muscles of the GH joint do not cross the radioulnar joints, they were able to create radioulnar joint motion because the force of their contraction was transferred to the radioulnar joints (Figure 13-15). (Note: This concept could work in the reverse manner. If pronation musculature [e.g., pronator quadratus] were to contract, the force would transfer across the elbow joint to the humerus, causing lateral rotation of the humerus at the GH joint.)

○ Note: Whenever the distal end of an extremity is fixed, the activity is termed a *closed-chain* activity. An open-chain activity is one wherein the distal end of the extremity is free to move.[5] With pronation of the forearm, the radius is usually considered to move and cross over a fixed ulna. When the radius is fixed and the ulna is mobile, moving and crossing over the radius, it is still defined as pronation; however, it is an example of a reverse action in which the ulna moves instead of the radius (at the radioulnar joints).
○ Another example of the force of a muscle being transferred to a joint that it does not cross is contraction of shoulder joint adductor muscles with the distal end of the upper extremity fixed. In this scenario movement of the humerus is transferred across the elbow joint to create extension of the forearm at the elbow joint (Figure 13-16).
○ The force of a muscle's contraction is often transferred to another joint in the human body. This force transference usually occurs when the distal end of an extremity is fixed and does not allow

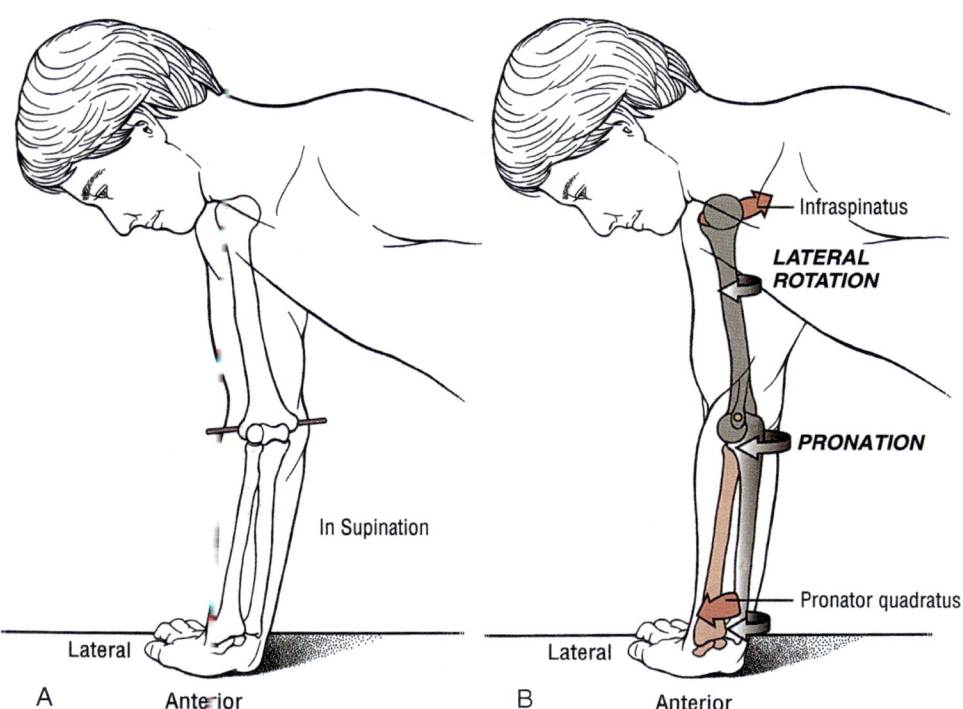

FIGURE 13-15 **A,** Person whose glenohumeral (GH) joint is medially rotated; forearm is supinated. (Note: The bones of the forearm are parallel to each other, and hand is fixed to a table top.) **B,** Person contracts the lateral rotator musculature of the GH joint (e.g., infraspinatus). When this occurs, the humerus laterally rotates at the GH joint relative to the scapula. Because the elbow joint does not allow rotation, the ulna moves along with the humerus and rotates laterally relative to the fixed radius. (Because the hand is fixed, the radius is unable to rotate because the wrist joint [i.e., the radiocarpal joint] does not allow rotation motions; therefore the radius is fixed relative to the hand.) This motion creates pronation at the radioulnar joints. In this scenario the force of GH lateral rotator muscles has been transferred to the radioulnar joints. This illustrates an example of a muscle that does not cross a joint but is able to create motion at that joint. *(Modified from Neumann DA: Kinesiology of the musculoskeletal system: foundations for physical rehabilitation, ed 2, St Louis, 2010, Mosby.)*

CHAPTER 13 How Muscles Function: the Big Picture

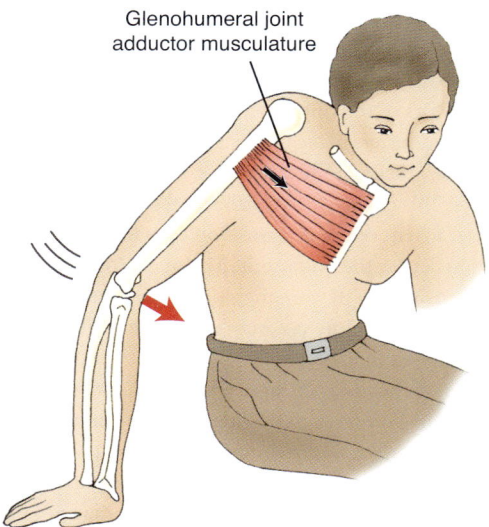

FIGURE 13-16 Person who is seated with the elbow joint partially flexed and the hand fixed to a tabletop. This person is contracting the shoulder joint adductor muscles. Because the hand is fixed, the distal forearm is also fixed and unable to "go along for the ride" with the humerus. As a result, when the humerus is pulled into adduction by the glenohumeral adductor musculature, the proximal end of the forearm is pulled medially but the distal end of the forearm stays fixed. This results in elbow joint extension.

for free motion of the distal body part (closed-chain). As a result, when the distal attachment of the contracting muscle moves, it forces motion to occur at another joint—in other words, its force is transferred to another joint that it does not cross.[4]

❍ Note: Transferring the force of a muscle contraction to another joint that the muscle does not cross is not the same as another body part simply *going along for the ride*. When other body parts go along for the ride, they always maintain their relative position to each other at the other joints that were not crossed by the contracting muscle; the only relative joint position change is at the joint that is crossed by the muscle that contracted. When the force of a muscle's contraction is transferred to another joint, a change in the relative position of body parts takes place at the other joint that is not crossed by the muscle that contracted. (To better visualize this, see Figures 13-15 and 13-16.)

❍ Many other scenarios exist in which the force of a muscle's contraction is transferred to a joint that it does not cross. One is the ability of the hamstrings to extend the knee joint in a person who is standing with the feet fixed to the ground; another is the lateral rotation force of the gluteus maximus causing the feet to supinate/invert at the subtalar tarsal joint if a person is standing with the feet fixed to the ground; and yet another is the ability of the ankle plantarflexors to create extension at the metatarsophalangeal joints when a person is standing. Try these scenarios for yourself.

SECTION 13.10 MUSCLE ACTIONS THAT CHANGE

CAN A MUSCLE'S ACTION CHANGE?

❍ Yes. A muscle's action is dependent on its line of pull *relative* to the joint that it crosses; therefore if the relationship of the muscle's line of pull to the joint changes, the muscle's action changes. This relationship can change if the position of the joint changes.[5]

❍ Some kinesiologists use the term **anatomic action** of a muscle to describe a muscle's action when the body is in anatomic position. This verbiage implicitly recognizes that a muscle's action on the body when the body is not in anatomic position may well be different from the action of the muscle when the body is in anatomic position.

❍ Example 1: Clavicular head of the pectoralis major
  ❍ The clavicular head of the pectoralis major is considered to be an adductor of the arm at the glenohumeral (GH) joint. This is because its line of pull is from medial to lateral, below the center of the GH joint.
  ❍ However, if the arm is abducted to approximately 100 degrees or more, the orientation of the clavicular head of the pectoralis major relative to the GH joint changes from being below the center of the joint to being above the center of the joint (Figure 13-17). Like any muscle that crosses above the center of the GH joint (e.g., deltoid, supraspinatus), the clavicular head of the pectoralis major can now abduct the arm at the GH joint.[10]
  ❍ It stands to reason that if the line of pull relative to the joint changes, the action of the muscle changes. In anatomic

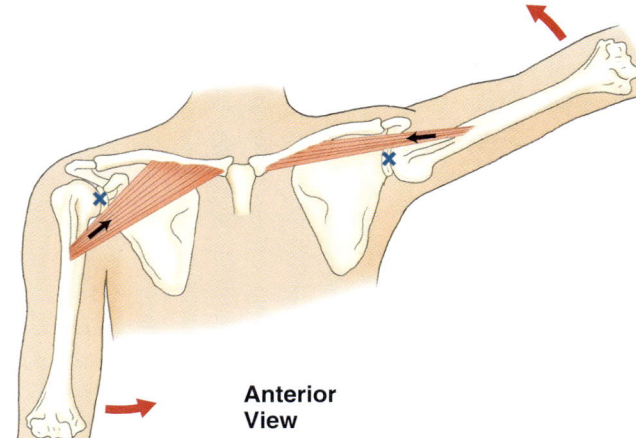

FIGURE 13-17 Orientation of the fibers of the clavicular head of the pectoralis major to the glenohumeral (GH) joint when the GH joint is in two different positions. Person's right arm is in anatomic position, and we see that the clavicular head of the pectoralis major is located below the center of the joint. In this position, given the direction of fibers relative to the joint, the clavicular head of the pectoralis major has the ability to adduct the arm at the GH joint. The person's left arm is abducted approximately 100 degrees at the GH joint. In this position the clavicular head of the pectoralis major is now located above the center of the joint. Given the direction of fibers relative to the joint, the clavicular head of the pectoralis major now has the ability to abduct the arm at the GH joint. (Note: The center of the shoulder joint on both sides is indicated by an X.)

position, the clavicular head of the pectoralis major is an adductor of the arm at the GH joint. However, with the arm abducted to 100 degrees or more, the clavicular head of the pectoralis major changes to become an abductor.
- More specifically, a muscle's action is dependent on its line of pull relative to the *axis of motion* of the joint that it crosses. In Figure 13-17, the 'x', representing the "center of the joint" more specifically represents the anteroposterior axis for frontal plane motion.
- Note: This change in action becomes very useful. As the supraspinatus and deltoid muscles become functionally weaker with the arm in a great deal of abduction, the pectoralis major steps in to become an additional abductor, adding strength to this joint action.
- Example 2: Adductor longus
  - The adductor longus is considered to be a flexor (in addition to being an adductor) of the thigh at the hip joint, because it passes anteriorly to the hip joint with a vertical direction to its fibers. All flexors of the thigh have their lines of pull anterior to the hip joint (Figure 13-18, *B*). However, when the thigh is first flexed to approximately 60 degrees or more, the line of pull of the adductor longus lies posterior to the hip joint and the adductor longus becomes an extensor of the thigh at the hip joint (Figure 13-18, *A*). Except for the posterior head of the adductor magnus, which is always an extensor at the hip joint, this change in action is true for the other adductors of the thigh at the hip joint.[3] (Note: The *members of the adductors of the thigh group* are the pectineus, adductor longus, gracilis, adductor brevis, and adductor magnus.)
  - Note: This change in action becomes very useful. While running, when we are in a position of extension, the adductors aid in flexing the thigh at the hip joint. However, when we are in a position of flexion, they aid in extending the thigh at the hip joint. This dual use may also explain why these muscles are so often injured.
- A muscle's action often changes when its line of pull relative to the joint changes[3] (because of a change in the position of the joint).
- For this reason, a certain amount of flexibility is needed when learning the actions of muscles. If one memorizes that a certain muscle does a certain action, it may or may not be true depending on the position of the joint. This is another reason why memorizing muscle actions is not recommended.
- Being able to reason a muscle's actions from its line of pull requires less brain memory, allows for a deeper and easier understanding of muscles' actions, and facilitates a better clinical application of this information!

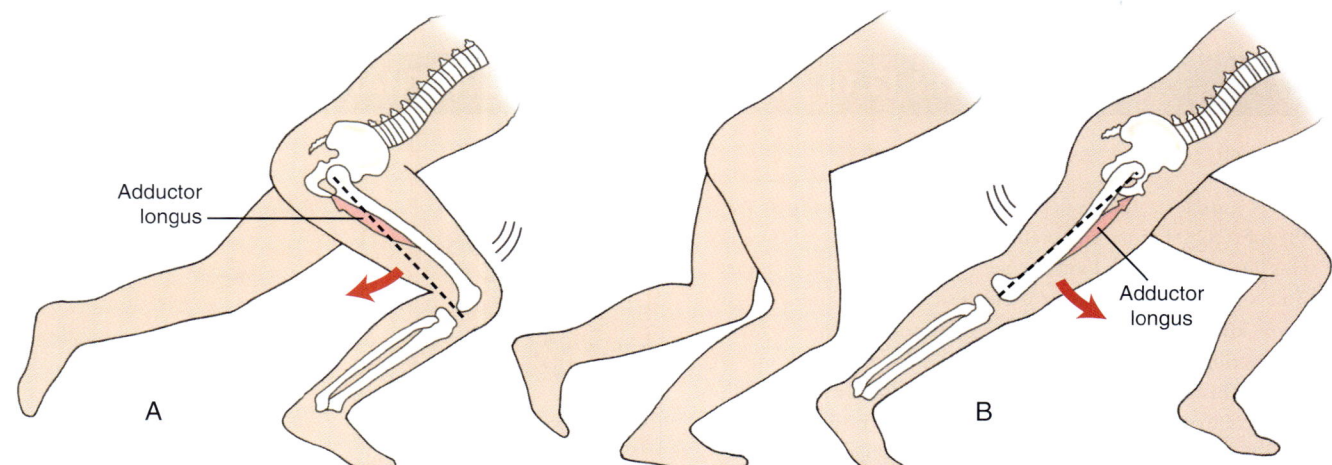

FIGURE 13-18 Illustration of a person who is running. **A,** Person's right thigh is in a position of flexion and is now being extended at the hip joint, helping to propel him forward. We see that the adductor longus assists in extending the thigh at the hip joint because in this position, the adductor longus is located posterior to the joint. **B,** Person's right thigh is in a position of extension and is now beginning to flex at the hip joint. In this position the adductor longus is now located anterior to the joint, so it is able to assist in flexing the thigh at the hip joint. (Note: In both figures the dashed line represents the axis for motion of the thigh at the hip joint.) *(Modeled from Neumann DA: Kinesiology of the musculoskeletal system: foundations for physical rehabilitation, ed 2, St Louis, 2010, Mosby.)*

REVIEW QUESTIONS

Answers to the following review questions appear on the Evolve website accompanying this book at: http://evolve.elsevier.com/Muscolino/kinesiology/.

1. When a muscle contracts, does it always succeed in shortening?

2. What is the name given to a shortening contraction of a muscle?

3. What are the three possible scenarios that can occur when a muscle contracts and shortens?

4. What is the name given to the attachment of a muscle that moves and to the attachment of a muscle that does not move?

5. Describe and give an example of a *reverse action*.

6. What are the five steps of the five-step approach to learning muscles?

7. What are the questions that must be asked and answered in step 3 of the five-step approach to learning muscles?

8. What determines the action(s) of a muscle?

9. Other than the reverse action(s), how many actions will a muscle have if it is has one line of pull and that line of pull is oriented within a cardinal plane?

10. How does one determine the action(s) of a muscle that has its line of pull within an oblique plane?

11. Can a multijoint muscle create movement at every one of the joints that it crosses?

12. What is the importance of using the *functional group approach* to learning muscles?

13. Give an example of a muscle that has more than one line of pull.

14. Muscles that belong to a flexor functional mover group are usually located in what plane?

15. Muscles that belong to an abductor functional mover group are usually located in what plane?

16. Muscles that belong to a rotation functional mover group are usually located in what plane?

17. How is the long axis of a bone determined?

18. Describe how the off-axis attachment method is used to determine the rotation action of a muscle.

19. Give an example of and explain how a muscle can create a joint action at a joint that it does not cross.

20. Give an example of and explain how a muscle can change its action at a joint based on a change in the position of that joint.

REFERENCES

1. Palastanga N, Field D, Soames R: Anatomy and human movement, ed 4, Oxford, 2002, Butterworth-Heinemann.
2. Nordin M, Frankel VH: Basic biomechanics of the musculoskeletal system, ed 3, Baltimore, 2001, Lippincott Williams & Wilkins.
3. Smith LK, Weiss EL, Lehmkuhl LO: Brunstrom's clinical kinesiology, ed 5, Philadelphia, 1996, FA Davis.
4. Thibodeau GA, Patton KT: Anatomy & physiology, ed 5, St Louis, 2003, Mosby.
5. Neumann DA: Kinesiology of the musculoskeletal system: Foundations for physical rehabilitation, ed 3, St Louis, 2017, Elsevier.
6. Levangie PK, Norkin CC: Joint structure and function: A comprehensive analysis, ed 5, Philadelphia, 2011, FA Davis.
7. Hamill J, Knutzen KM: Biomechanical basis of human movement, ed 12, Baltimore, 2003, Lippincott Williams & Wilkins.
8. Watkins J: Structure and function of the musculoskeletal system, Champaign, IL, 1999, Human Kinetics.
9. Enoka RM: Neuromechanics of human movement, ed 3, Champaign, IL, 2002, Human Kinetics.
10. Muscolino JE: The muscular system manual: The skeletal muscles of the human body, ed 4, St Louis, 2017, Elsevier.

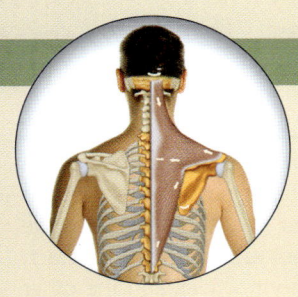

CHAPTER 14

Types of Muscle Contractions

CHAPTER OUTLINE

Section 14.1	Overview of the Types of Muscle Contractions	Section 14.4	Concentric Contractions in More Detail
Section 14.2	Concentric, Eccentric, and Isometric Contraction Examples	Section 14.5	Eccentric Contractions in More Detail
		Section 14.6	Isometric Contractions in More Detail
Section 14.3	Relating Muscle Contraction and the Sliding Filament Mechanism	Section 14.7	Movement versus Stabilization

CHAPTER OBJECTIVES

After completing this chapter, the student should be able to perform the following:

1. Define the key terms of this chapter and state the meanings of the word origins of this chapter.
2. Do the following related to the types of muscle contractions:
   ○ State, define, and give examples of the three types of muscle contractions (concentric, eccentric, and isometric).
   ○ Describe the relationship among the force of a muscle's contraction, the force of resistance to the muscle's contraction, and which type of muscle contraction results.
   ○ Define and give an example of a resistance exercise.
3. Do the following relating to muscle contraction and the sliding filament mechanism:
   ○ Relate the sliding filament mechanism to each of the three types of muscle contractions.
   ○ Give a brief review of muscle structure, the nervous system's control of a muscle, and the sliding filament mechanism.
   ○ Define the terms *muscle contraction, tension,* and *tone.*
4. Do the following related to concentric contractions:
   ○ List and describe the three scenarios in which a concentric contraction occurs.
   ○ Describe the relationship between gravity and concentric contractions.
   ○ Define the term *gravity neutral*, and describe its relationship to concentric contractions.
   ○ Relate the analogy of the motor and brakes of a car to concentric contractions.
5. Do the following related to eccentric contractions:
   ○ List and describe the three scenarios in which an eccentric contraction occurs.
   ○ Define, describe, and give an example of internal forces and external forces.
   ○ Describe the relationship between gravity and eccentric contractions.
   ○ State the most usual circumstance in which an eccentric contraction occurs.
   ○ Relate the analogy of the motor and brakes of a car to eccentric contractions.
6. Do the following related to isometric contractions:
   ○ List and describe the two scenarios in which an isometric contraction occurs.
   ○ Describe the relationship between gravity and isometric contractions.
7. Do the following related to movement versus stabilization:
   ○ Explain how a muscle can create, modify, or stop movement.
   ○ Describe the relationship between joint mobility and stability.

OVERVIEW

Most textbooks and classes that teach the actions of the muscles of the body teach the concentric actions of the muscles. That is, they teach the action(s) that a muscle will create if it contracts and shortens. Therefore when the student learns the actions of a particular muscle, the student learns the shortening concentric actions of that muscle. Nothing is inherently wrong with this approach to teaching muscles. Indeed, for beginning students, this simple and concrete approach to muscle contractions and actions is probably best. However, the one thing that must be kept in mind is that a muscle does not have to shorten when it contracts; in fact, the role of most muscle contractions in the human body is not to shorten and contract. This chapter examines concentric contractions and the other types of contractions that a muscle can have. Chapter 15 then continues to examine the various roles that muscles have in movement patterns when they contract in these ways.

KEY TERMS

Action in question
Antagonist (an-TAG-o-nist)
Aqua therapy (Ah-kwa)
Concentric contraction (con-SEN-trik)
Eccentric contraction (e-SEN-trik)
External force
Fix
Fixator (FIKS-ay-tor)
Gravity
Gravity neutral
Internal force

Isometric contraction (ICE-o-MET-rik)
Mover
Muscle contraction
Negative contraction
Resistance exercises
Resistance force
Stabilize
Stabilizer
Tension
Tone
Weight

WORD ORIGINS

- Antagonist—From Greek *anti*, meaning *against, opposite*, and *agon*, meaning *a fight, a contest*
- Concentric—From Latin *con*, meaning *together, with*, and *centrum*, meaning *center*
- Eccentric—From Greek *ek*, meaning *out of, away from*, and Greek *kentron* (or Latin *centrum*), meaning *center*
- Fix—From Latin *fixus*, meaning *fastened*
- Isometric—From Greek *isos*, meaning *equal*, and *metrikos*, meaning *measure*
- Stabilize—From Latin *stabilis*, meaning *not moving, fixed*
- Tension—From Latin *tensio*, meaning *to stretch*
- Tone—From Latin *tonus*, meaning *a stretching, tone*

SECTION 14.1 OVERVIEW OF THE TYPES OF MUSCLE CONTRACTIONS

In Chapter 13 we went through a brief sketch of the big picture of learning how muscles function. It was explained that when a muscle is directed to contract by the nervous system, the muscle attempts to shorten toward its center.

- Whether or not a muscle is successful in shortening toward its center is determined by the strength of the pulling force of the muscle compared with the force necessary to actually move one or both body parts to which the muscle is attached.[1]
- The force necessary to move a body part is usually the force necessary to move the weight of the body part. For example, when the brachialis muscle contracts, for it to be able to successfully shorten and flex the elbow joint, it will have to generate enough force to be able to move the weight of either the forearm or the arm. The weight of the forearm or the arm would be the force that is resistant to the brachialis contracting and successfully shortening. If the force of the muscle's contraction is greater than the resistance to the muscle's contraction, the muscle will successfully shorten.
- This type of contraction wherein a muscle contracts and shortens is called a **concentric contraction**.[1] Furthermore, because the concentrically contracting muscle generates the force that moves a body part to create the joint action that is occurring, it is termed the **mover**.[2] Simply put, the mover creates the movement! Note: The joint action that is occurring is usually termed the **action in question**.
- The force that opposes this action of the mover is the **resistance force**. The resistance force in this scenario is an **antagonist** to the action that is occurring.[2] The force of an antagonist is opposite to the action that is occurring (hence the term *antagonist*) (Figure 14-1).

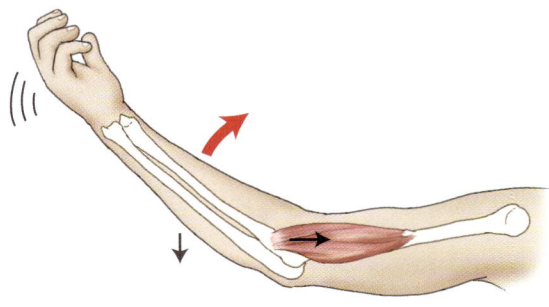

FIGURE 14-1 Medial view of the brachialis muscle. In this example, we are considering the arm to be fixed and the forearm to potentially be mobile. The arrow within the brachialis shows the line of pull of the muscle. For the brachialis to contract and successfully shorten, the force of its contraction would have to move the forearm up toward the arm. The red curved arrow above the forearm represents the strength and direction of pull of the brachialis acting on the forearm; the straight brown arrow drawn downward from the forearm represents the strength and direction of pull of gravity acting on the forearm (i.e., the weight of the forearm), resisting the pull of the brachialis. When the force of the contraction of the brachialis is greater than the force of the weight of the forearm (i.e., the resistance force) as represented by the relative sizes of the arrows, the brachialis will successfully shorten and move the forearm toward the arm, as seen in this figure. In this scenario, the brachialis concentrically contracted and would be termed the mover of flexion of the forearm at the elbow joint.

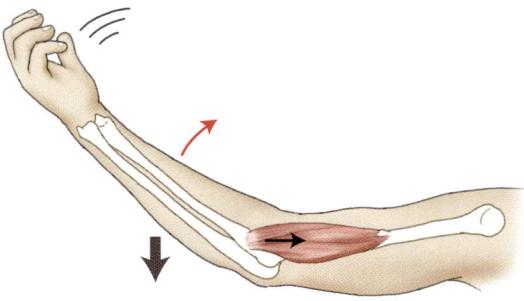

FIGURE 14-2 Medial view of the brachialis muscle pictured in Figure 14-1. However, in this scenario the force of the contraction of the brachialis is less than the resistance force of the weight of the forearm. Because the force of the weight of the forearm is greater than the force of the brachialis's contraction, the forearm extends with gravity, causing the brachialis to lengthen. This scenario illustrates an eccentric contraction of the brachialis because it is contracting and lengthening. The mover is gravity, and the brachialis is an antagonist.

- If the force of the muscle's contraction is less than the resistance to the muscle's contraction (or put another way, if the force of the antagonist is greater than the force of the muscle), the muscle will lengthen instead of shorten.
- This type of contraction is called an *eccentric contraction*. An **eccentric contraction** occurs when a muscle contracts and lengthens[1] (Figure 14-2; Box 14-1).
- When this situation occurs, the resistance force (i.e., the weight of the body part) creates the action that is occurring and is now termed *the mover*, and the muscle that is eccentrically lengthening is now called *the antagonist*.
- If the force of the muscle's contraction is exactly equal to the resistance force, then the muscle will neither shorten nor lengthen.
- This type of contraction is called an *isometric contraction*. An **isometric contraction** is one wherein the muscle contracts and stays the same length.[3]

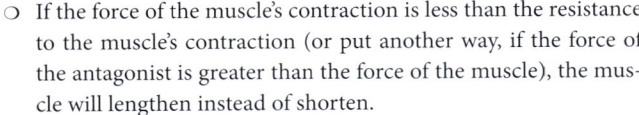

BOX 14-1 Spotlight on the Resistance to a Muscle's Contraction

The force of resistance that a muscle must overcome to be able to contract and shorten is usually the weight of the body part of one (or both) of the attachments of the muscle. However, when one body part moves, other body parts must often be moved with it. For example, for the brachialis muscle to contract, shorten, and move the forearm at the elbow joint, the hand must be moved as well. Therefore the contraction of the brachialis must be sufficiently strong to move the weight of the forearm and the hand together. If the brachialis is to create the reverse action and move the arm attachment instead of the forearm attachment at the elbow joint, then its contraction must be sufficiently strong to move not only the weight of the arm but also the weight of the entire trunk, because the arm cannot move without the trunk "going along for the ride."

Often, other factors affect the resistance to a muscle's contraction. When exercises are done with weights, the force of the muscle contraction must be strong enough to move the weight of the body part plus the weight that has been added. In addition, certain exercises incorporate other forms of added resistance. For example, the resistance of springs, rubber tubing, or large rubber bands is often used. In fact, these exercises are often called **resistance exercises** because they add to the force of resistance against which the contracting muscle must work.[12] Whether weights are used or other forms of additional resistance are used, if a muscle is to contract and successfully shorten when doing resistance exercises, the muscle must contract with greater force to overcome the greater resistance force that it encounters (Figure 14-3).

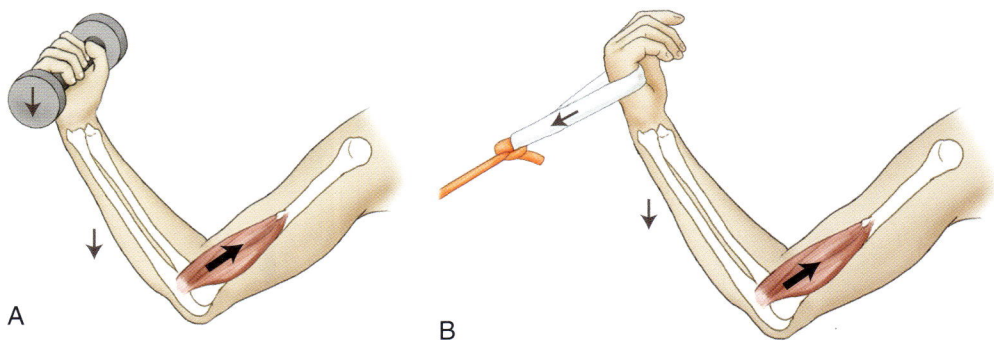

FIGURE 14-3 Two examples of resistance exercises. **A,** Added resistance to flexion of the forearm at the elbow joint is provided by a weight held in the person's hand. **B,** Added resistance is provided by the rubber tubing that must be stretched for the person to be able to flex the forearm at the elbow joint.

- In this case no movement of a body part at the joint occurs; therefore no joint action occurs (Figure 14-4).
- Because no joint action occurs, the muscle that is isometrically contracting is neither a mover nor an antagonist. (For more information on concentric, eccentric, and isometric contractions, see Sections 14.4 to 14.6. For more information on the roles of muscles as movers and antagonists, see Sections 15.1 and 15.2.)
- There are times when it is desirable to reduce the force of resistance that a muscle must work against. For example, if exercises are done in water, the buoyancy of the water may support the body part being moved and would decrease the resistance force to the muscle's contraction.[4] For this reason, exercise in pools (i.e., **aqua therapy**) is often recommended for clients who have recently sustained an injury and are beginning a rehabilitation program, because it provides a gentle way to begin strengthening exercises.

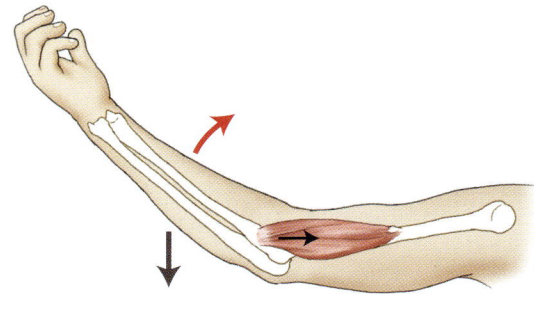

FIGURE 14-4 Medial view of the brachialis muscle pictured in Figures 14-1 and 14-2. In this scenario, the force of the contraction of the brachialis is exactly equal to the resistance force of the weight of the forearm (and hand). Because these two forces are exactly matched, the brachialis does not succeed in shortening and flexing the forearm, nor does gravity succeed in lengthening the brachialis and extending the forearm. This scenario illustrates an isometric contraction of the brachialis because it is contracting and staying the same length.

SECTION 14.2 CONCENTRIC, ECCENTRIC, AND ISOMETRIC CONTRACTION EXAMPLES

Following are examples of concentric, eccentric, and isometric contractions.

- Figure 14-5 shows a person who is first abducting the arm at the glenohumeral (GH) joint, then adducting the arm at the GH joint, and then holding the arm in a static position of abduction at the GH joint.

In Figure 14-5, *A* he is abducting his arm at the GH joint. To accomplish this, he is concentrically shortening the abductor musculature of his GH joint. As this musculature shortens, the arm is lifted up into the air in the frontal plane (i.e., it abducts).

In Figure 14-5, *B* he is adducting his arm at the GH joint (from a *higher* position of abduction). To adduct the arm at the GH joint, the abductor musculature must lengthen. However, because gravity is adducting the arm, his abductor musculature contracts as it lengthens, creating an upward force of abduction of the arm that slows down the movement of adduction created by gravity.

This slowing down of gravity is necessary to prevent gravity from slamming his arm/forearm/hand into the side of his body. The abduction force of his musculature must be less powerful than the force of gravity so that adduction of the arm continues to occur (but is slowed down). In this scenario the abductor musculature is lengthening as it contracts; therefore it is eccentrically contracting.

In Figure 14-5, *C* we see that he is holding his arm statically in a position of abduction. In this scenario his abductor musculature is contracting with exactly the same amount of upward force as the downward force of gravity. Therefore the arm neither moves up into further abduction nor falls down into adduction. Because no joint action is occurring, the musculature of the joint does not change in length. In this scenario the abductor musculature is staying the same length as it contracts; therefore it is isometrically contracting.

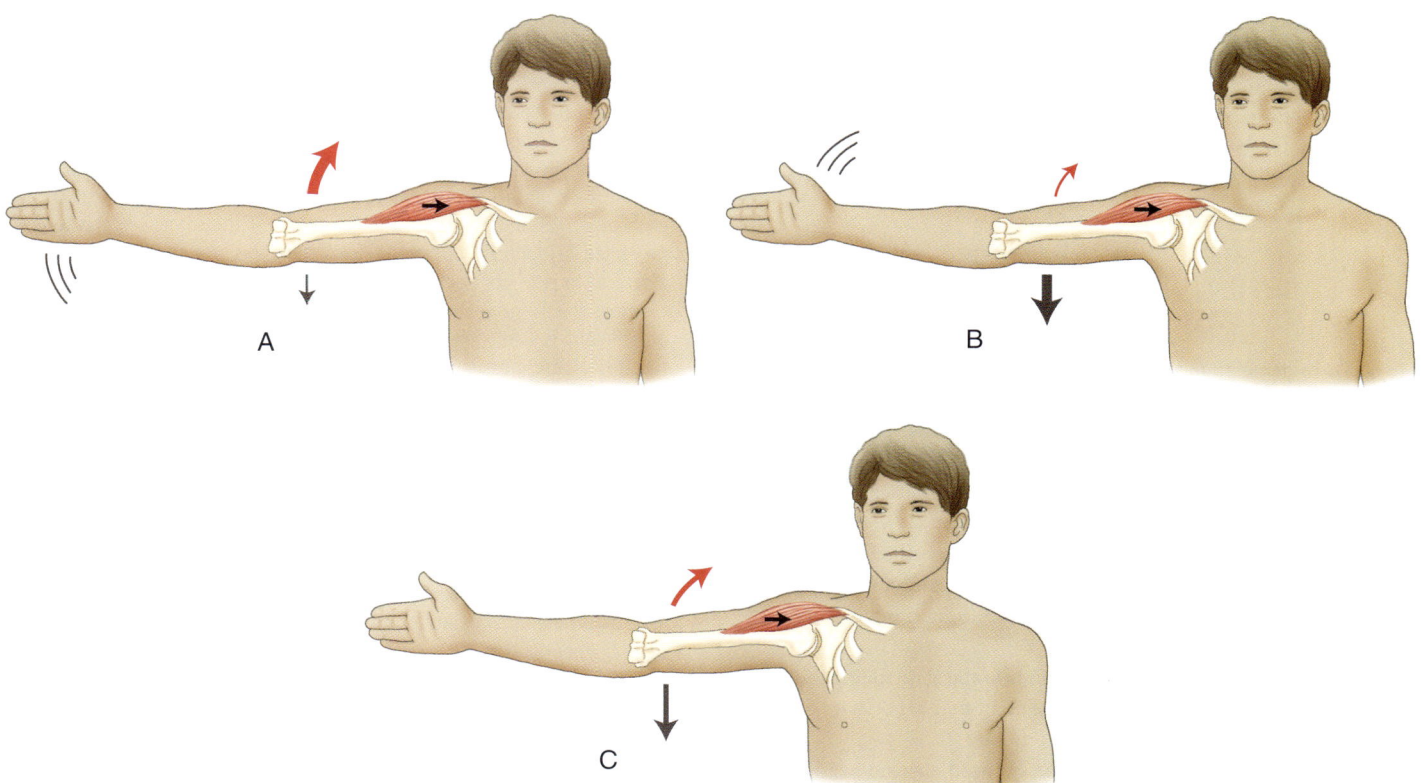

FIGURE 14-5 A, Person abducting the right arm at the glenohumeral (GH) joint against the force of gravity; this force of abduction is created by concentric contraction of the abductor musculature. **B,** Same person adducting the arm at the GH joint. In this case gravity is the mover force that creates adduction, but the abductor musculature is eccentrically contracting to slow down the force of gravity. **C,** Person statically holding the arm in a position of abduction. In this case the abductor musculature is isometrically contracting, equaling the force of gravity so that no motion occurs.

SECTION 14.3 RELATING MUSCLE CONTRACTION AND THE SLIDING FILAMENT MECHANISM

Section 14.1 began with the assumption that when a muscle contracts, it attempts to shorten toward its center. To understand the concept of muscle contraction more fully, muscle structure and the sliding filament mechanism must first be understood. To accomplish this, a brief review of muscle structure, nervous system control, and the sliding filament mechanism is helpful.

BRIEF REVIEW OF MUSCLE STRUCTURE:

- A muscle is an organ that attaches from one bone to another (via its tendons), thereby crossing the joint that is located between the two bones.[5]
- A muscle is composed of thousands of muscle fibers that generally run longitudinally within the muscle.
- Each muscle fiber is composed of many myofibrils that run longitudinally within the muscle fiber.
- Each myofibril is composed of thousands of sarcomeres that are laid side by side and end to end.
- Each sarcomere is composed of actin and myosin filaments.
  - Each sarcomere has a myosin filament located at its center.
  - Actin filaments are located on both sides of the myosin filament and are attached to the Z-lines, which are the boundaries of the sarcomere.

BRIEF REVIEW OF NERVOUS SYSTEM CONTROL OF A MUSCLE:

- A muscle is innervated by a motor nerve from the nervous system.[6]
- When a signal for contraction is sent to a muscle by the central nervous system, this signal is sent through neurons (i.e., nerve cells) located within a peripheral nerve.
- Each neuron that carries the message for contraction splits to innervate a number of muscle fibers.
- One motor neuron and all the muscle fibers that it controls are defined as a motor unit.

- A contraction message that is sent to any one muscle fiber of a motor unit is sent to every muscle fiber of that motor unit.
- At the muscle fiber, the message to contract from the neuron is carried into the interior of the muscle fiber and given to every sarcomere of every myofibril of the muscle fiber.
- The sliding filament mechanism explains how each sarcomere of a muscle fiber contracts.

BRIEF REVIEW OF THE SLIDING FILAMENT MECHANISM:

- As its name implies, the sliding filament mechanism explains how actin and myosin filaments slide along each other. (For more details on the sliding filament mechanism, see Sections 12.6 and 12.12.)[1]
- When a muscle contraction is desired, the central nervous system sends a message for contraction to the muscle that is to be contracted.
  - When this message for contraction enters the interior of the muscle fiber, it causes calcium that is stored in the sarcoplasmic reticulum to be released into the sarcoplasm of the muscle fiber.
  - Calcium in the sarcoplasm binds to the actin filaments, causing a structural change in the actin that exposes its binding (active) sites.
  - When actin's binding sites are exposed, myosin heads attach to them, creating cross-bridges.
  - These cross-bridges bend, attempting to pull the actin filaments in toward the center of the sarcomere.
  - The attempted bending of the cross-bridges causes a pulling force on the actin filaments.
  - Because actin filaments are attached to Z-lines, this pulling force is transferred to the Z-lines.
  - Thus a pulling force toward the center of the sarcomere is exerted on the Z-lines of a sarcomere.
  - It is the formation of the cross-bridges between the myosin and actin filaments and the pulling force that they exert that defines a **muscle contraction**. In other words, when cross-bridges form and create a pulling force toward the center of the sarcomeres, the muscle is defined as contracting.[7]
- What happens after this step determines the type of contraction that will occur.
- As we have seen, three types of contractions exist[7]: (1) concentric, (2) eccentric, and (3) isometric.

Scenario One—Concentric Contraction:

- If the bending force of the myosin cross-bridges is successful in pulling the actin filaments in toward the center, the Z-lines are drawn toward the center of the sarcomere and the sarcomere shortens.[7]
- Because this message for contraction is given to every sarcomere of the muscle fiber, if one sarcomere succeeds in shortening, every sarcomere will succeed in shortening and the entire muscle fiber will shorten (Box 14-2).
- Because the message for contraction is given to every muscle fiber of a motor unit, every muscle fiber of that motor unit will shorten.
- If enough muscle fibers of a muscle shorten, the entire muscle shortens toward its center.

BOX 14-2

Picturing one sarcomere shortening is fairly simple. Both actin filaments come in toward the center, bringing their Z-line attachments with them. However, some students have a difficult time picturing how two or more consecutive sarcomeres that are located next to each other can all shorten at the same time if the same Z-line is to be pulled in opposite directions. To picture this, we should look at a typical muscle contraction in which one attachment of the muscle stays fixed. The Z-line of the sarcomere located next to the fixed attachment is itself fixed and cannot move, so the other Z-line of that sarcomere must move toward the fixed Z-line. When this mobile Z-line moves toward the fixed one, the next sarcomere must move as a whole toward the fixed attachment. In addition, this sarcomere will also shorten toward its own center as it moves toward the fixed attachment of the muscle. In reality, what is happening is that the myosin filament on the fixed attachment side of each sarcomere is actually sliding toward the actin filament on that side. For this reason, the sliding filament mechanism is called the sliding filament mechanism, not the sliding actin filament mechanism. Either filament can slide along the other when the cross-bridges between the myosin and actin filaments bend.

- When the entire muscle shortens toward its center, it pulls on its attachments such that one or both of its attachments will be pulled toward the center of the muscle.
- Because muscle attachments are on bones, and bones are within body parts, the body parts that the muscle attachments are within will be moved toward each other.
- This type of a contraction in which the muscle succeeds in shortening is called a *concentric contraction*. A concentric contraction is a shortening contraction.
- As explained in Section 13.2, a concentrically contracting muscle may shorten by moving either one or both of its attachments toward the center of the muscle (i.e., toward each other). (See Figure 14-5, *A* for an example of a concentric contraction.)
- Note: The term "concentric" literally means "with center;" hence the muscle is bringing their attachment(s) toward the center, and thereby shortening.
- Note: The foregoing explanation is how the concept of muscle contraction is usually explained. However, this scenario applies only to a shortening concentric contraction, and a muscle does not necessarily shorten when it contracts.

Scenario Two—Eccentric Contraction:

- If the force of resistance to the muscle shortening is greater than the force of the muscle contraction, then the myosin cross-bridges will not be successful in bending and pulling the actin filaments in toward the center, and the sarcomeres will not shorten.[1] If the sarcomeres do not shorten, the muscle will not shorten. In fact, because the force of the resistance is greater than the muscle contraction force, the resistance force will actually pull the actin filaments away from the center of the sarcomere and each sarcomere will lengthen.
- If all of the sarcomeres (in the myofibrils of the muscle fibers of the motor unit) lengthen, the entire muscle will lengthen.

- A lengthening of the muscle results in the attachments of the muscle moving farther from each other.
- Because muscle attachments are on bones, and bones are within body parts, the body parts that the muscle attachments are within will move farther from each other.
- This type of a contraction in which the muscle lengthens is called an *eccentric contraction*. An eccentric contraction is a lengthening contraction. (See Figure 14-5, *B* for an example of an eccentric contraction.)

Scenario Three—Isometric Contraction:

- If the force of the muscle's contraction is exactly equal to the force of the resistance to the muscle's contraction, then the myosin cross-bridges will not be able to bend and pull the actin in toward the center of the sarcomere; therefore the sarcomeres of the muscle will not shorten. However, the isometric contraction will generate enough strength to oppose any resistance force that would lengthen the sarcomeres. Therefore the sarcomeres neither shorten nor lengthen; rather they remain the same length.[3]
- If the sarcomeres remain the same length, then the muscle will remain the same length and the attachments and body parts will not move.
- This type of a contraction in which the muscle stays the same length is called an *isometric contraction*. (See Figure 14-5, *C* for an example of an isometric contraction.)

CONCLUSION:

- What defines a muscle as contracting is the fact that myosin cross-bridges are grabbing actin filaments, *attempting* to bend and pull the actin filaments toward the center of the sarcomere.[8] This creates the tension or pulling force toward the center of the sarcomere that defines contraction! Extrapolating this idea to an entire muscle, it can be stated that it is the tension or pulling force of the muscle toward its center that defines a muscle as contracting.

- The term **tension** is defined as a pulling force; tensile forces are pulling forces. Because muscles only pull (they do not push), muscles create tensile forces in the body. In all three types of muscle contractions, what defines a muscle as contracting is not the length change of the muscle; when a muscle contracts, it may shorten, lengthen, or stay the same length.[2] A muscle is defined as contracting when it generates a *pulling force* toward its center!
- The term **tone** is often used to describe when a muscle is contracting (i.e., when it is generating tension). Using the term *tone*, the following can be said:
  - A concentric contraction is when a muscle shortens with tone.
  - An eccentric contraction is when a muscle lengthens with tone.
  - An isometric contraction is when a muscle stays the same length with tone.
- Hence three types of muscle contractions exist: (1) concentric, (2) eccentric, and (3) isometric.[3]
  - The term *concentric* means *toward the center;* a concentric contraction is one in which the muscle moves toward its center. The term *eccentric* means *away from the center;* an eccentric contraction is one in which the muscle moves away from its center. The term *isometric* means *same length;* an isometric contraction is one in which the muscle stays the same length.
- A concentric contraction occurs when the force of the muscle's contraction is greater than the force of resistance to movement.
  - A concentric contraction is a shortening contraction.
- A lengthening eccentric contraction occurs when the force of the muscle's contraction is less than the force of resistance to movement.
  - An eccentric contraction is a lengthening contraction.
- An isometric contraction occurs when the force of the muscle's contraction is equal to the force of the resistance to movement.
  - An isometric contraction is one in which the muscle contracts and stays the same length.

SECTION 14.4 CONCENTRIC CONTRACTIONS IN MORE DETAIL

CONCENTRIC CONTRACTIONS—SHORTENING CONTRACTIONS:

- Concentric contractions are the type of contractions that are usually taught to beginning students of kinesiology when the actions of muscles are taught. Therefore it is usually not hard for students to understand concentric contractions when they occur in the body.
- A concentric contraction is defined as a shortening contraction[9] (i.e., a muscle contracts and shortens).
- If the muscle shortens, then the attachments of the muscle must come closer together[10] (i.e., the muscle shortens toward its center and pulls the attachments toward each other).
- As discussed in Section 13.2, either attachment can move toward the other, or both attachments can move toward each other.

- Usually the lighter (i.e., more mobile, less fixed) attachment does the moving because it is less resistant to moving.

WHEN DO CONCENTRIC CONTRACTIONS OCCUR?

- Concentric contractions occur in our body when the force of the concentric contraction is needed to move a body part. Because concentric contractions create movement, a muscle that concentrically contracts is called a *mover*.[2] (For more information on the role of movers, see Section 15.1.)
- These concentric contractions can occur in the following three scenarios.
- Note: Another factor to consider when looking at the three scenarios of a concentric contraction is if an additional

resistance force exists beyond the weight of the body part (i.e., beyond the force of gravity). An additional resistance force may exist whether the movement is vertically upward, horizontal, or vertically downward.[6] (For more on resistance forces, see Section 14.1, Figure 14-3.) The following three scenarios are based on gravity being the only resistance force to movement.

Scenario 1—Against Gravity ("Vertically Upward"):

- A concentric contraction is necessary whenever a body part is being lifted upward (i.e., when the motion is against gravity) (Figure 14-6, *A*).
- Simply put, if gravity is not lifting our body part upward (which it cannot do, because gravity only pulls downward), then a muscle in our body must be generating the force that is creating this upward movement. In this scenario the concentric contraction of the muscle is generating more upward force on the body part than the downward force that gravity is exerting on the body part, in other words, the weight of the body part (Box 14-3).

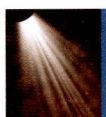

BOX 14-3 Spotlight on Gravity

Gravity is, by definition, a force that pulls downward. More specifically, gravity is the force caused by the mutual attraction of all physical matter (i.e., the mass of objects). Because the largest physical mass in the world is the earth itself, we feel the force of gravity pulling us toward the earth (i.e., downward). The force that gravity exerts on the mass of an object is then defined as the **weight** of that object.

When a concentric contraction creates a force to lift a body part up against gravity, it must lift the weight of the body part that is being moved; it must also move whatever other body part(s) is/are going along for the ride. For example, if the deltoid lifts the arm at the shoulder joint up into abduction, it must contract sufficiently to lift the arm and the forearm and hand, because these two body parts go along for the ride.

Scenario 2—Gravity Neutral ("Horizontal"):

- A concentric contraction is necessary whenever a body part is being moved horizontally (i.e., when the motion is **gravity neutral**). A gravity-neutral motion is one in which gravity neither resists the motion nor aids it (because the body part is not being lifted up or down) (see Figure 14-6, *B*).
  - Again, if gravity is not creating the movement, then our concentrically contracting muscle must be creating it. In this scenario because gravity is not opposing our muscle's movement of the body part, less force is usually required by our muscle's concentric contraction to move the body part.
- These horizontal gravity-neutral motions are often rotation movements, because rotations usually occur in the transverse plane, which is a horizontal plane. Rotation actions are defined as occurring in the transverse plane in anatomic position. However, we do not always initiate all joint actions from anatomic position. Therefore not all rotation actions necessarily occur horizontal to the ground (i.e., gravity neutral).

Scenario 3—With Gravity ("Vertically Downward"):

- A concentric contraction is necessary whenever a body part is moving downward and we want the body part to move *faster* than gravity would move it (see Figure 14-6, *C*).
  - Because gravity constantly supplies a downward force, whenever we want to move a body part downward, we can have a free ride and let gravity create this movement of the body part. Therefore no muscle contraction is necessary for the body part to move downward. However, if we want the body part to move downward *faster* than gravity would move it, then we have to concentrically contract muscles that add to the downward force of gravity.
  - The key aspect to understand when a muscle concentrically contracts to aid gravity's movement of a body part downward is to realize that we want to move the body part *faster* than gravity would move us. This is very common when strong exertions are desired such as in sports. For example, when bringing a golf club down to hit a golf ball, gravity alone would accomplish this task—but not with sufficient force to move the golf ball very far. Therefore we aid the force of gravity with concentric contractions of our musculature that move the golf club faster. (However, when we do not need a fast downward movement of a body part, we usually look to slow the force of gravity with eccentric muscular contractions that are antagonistic to the force of gravity.)
  - In this discussion of a vertical downward movement (as in the other two scenarios), it was assumed that gravity was the only external force that existed. However, if other forces are present, the contraction of our musculature might change. For example, if another resistance force exists that resists the downward motion of the body part (and this force is greater than the force of gravity), then a concentric contraction would be necessary to move the body part downward (Figure 14-6, *D*).

ANALOGY TO DRIVING A CAR:

- A good analogy to facilitate the understanding of why and when concentric contractions occur is to compare the motor of a car to a concentrically contracting muscle.
- Just as a concentrically contracting muscle creates a force to move a body part, the motor of a car creates a force to move the car. We can draw this analogy of a motor powering the movement of a car to the three scenarios that we just discussed when concentric contractions occur.

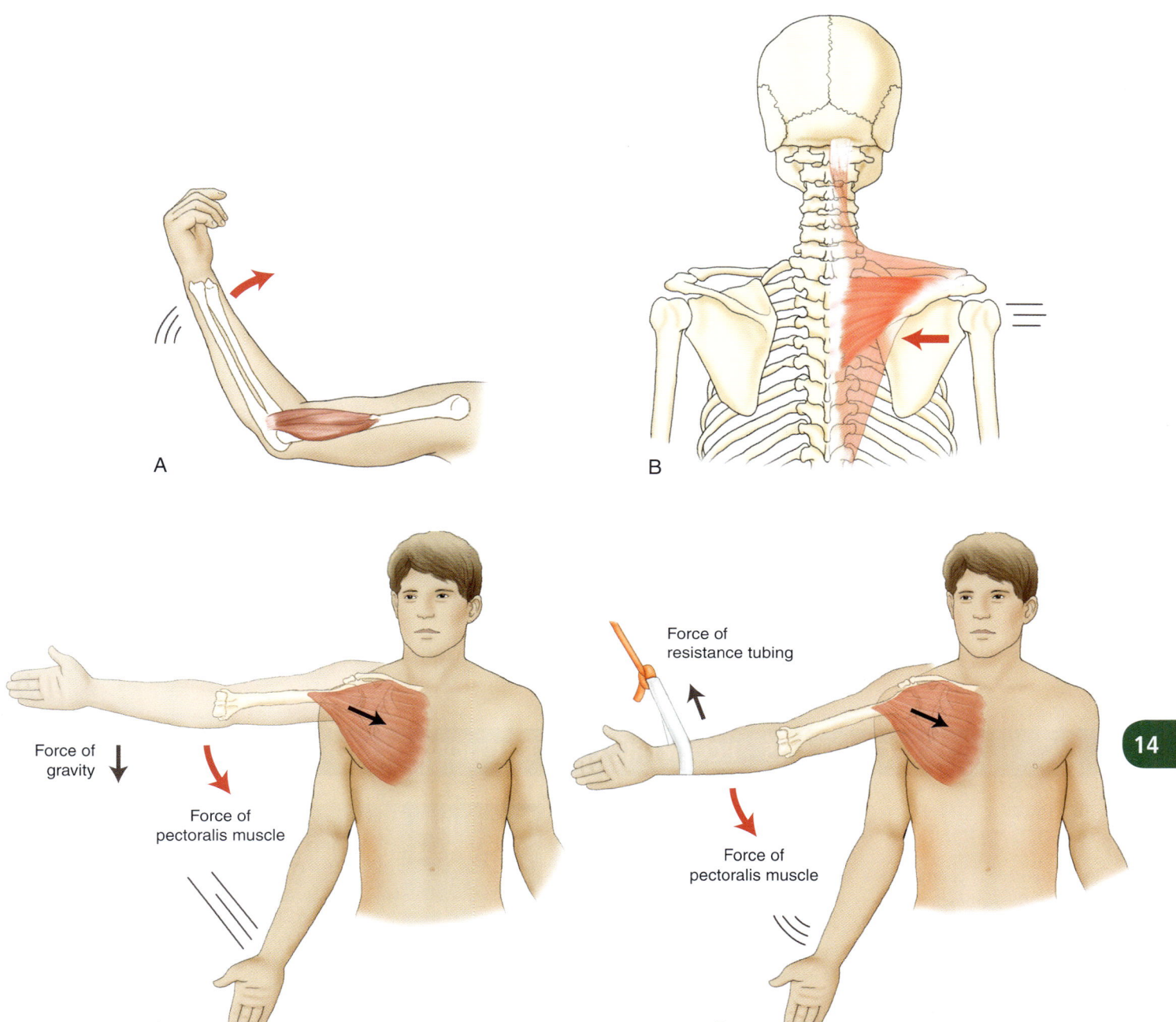

FIGURE 14-6 Concentric contractions. **A,** Forearm flexing at the elbow joint. This motion is vertically upward, against gravity; therefore the forearm flexor muscles must contract concentrically as movers to create this motion. The brachialis is seen contracting in this figure; however, any forearm flexor might concentrically contract to create this motion. **B,** Scapula retracting at the scapulocostal joint. This motion is horizontal and gravity neutral; therefore the muscles of scapular retraction must concentrically contract as movers to create this motion. The trapezius (and especially the middle trapezius) is seen contracting in this figure; however, any scapular retractor might concentrically contract to create this motion. **C,** The arm adducting at the glenohumeral (GH) joint. This motion is downward so gravity is the mover; therefore no muscles need to concentrically contract to create this motion. However, if we want to adduct the arm faster than would happen by gravity, GH adductors can contract concentrically as movers to add to the force of gravity and increase the speed of this action. The pectoralis major is seen contracting in this figure; however, any arm adductor might concentrically contract to create this motion. **D,** Same scenario as in C, but this time the person is adducting the arm against the resistance of rubber tubing. Therefore even though this motion is downward and aided by gravity, because of the resistance of the tubing, GH adductors must concentrically contract to overcome the resistance and adduct the arm at the GH joint.

516 PART 4 Myology: Study of the Muscular System

- Scenario 1: If we are driving a car uphill (i.e., against gravity), we step on the gas to make the motor of the car power the car up the hill (Figure 14-7, *A*).
- Scenario 2: If we are driving a car on a level surface (i.e., gravity neutral), we step on the gas to make the motor power the car to go forward (Figure 14-7, *B*).
- Scenario 3: If we are driving a car downhill (i.e., with gravity), and we want to drive *faster* than gravity would bring us down the hill, we step on the gas to make the motor power the car down the hill faster than coasting by gravity would create (Figure 14-7, *C*).

CONCLUSION:

- Concentric contractions occur to move a body part in three scenarios:
  - Scenario 1: Vertically upward (i.e., against gravity)
  - Scenario 2: Horizontally (i.e., gravity neutral)
  - Scenario 3: Vertically downward (i.e., to move faster than gravity would move us)

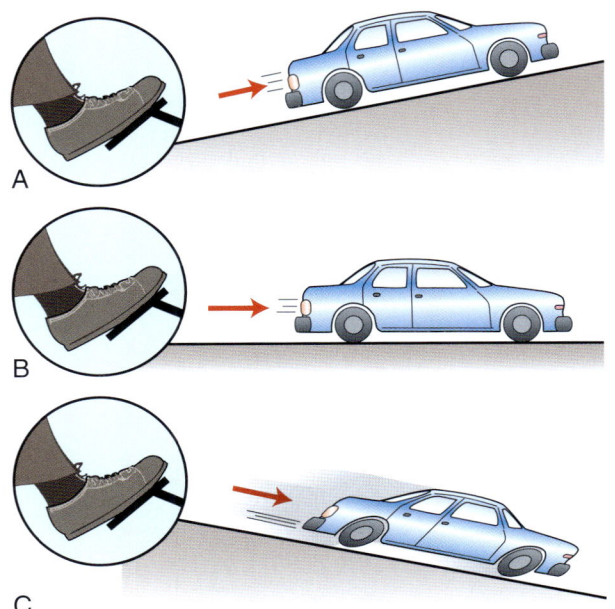

FIGURE 14-7 Illustration of the idea of the motor of a car being necessary to power the car in three scenarios. **A**, Car moving uphill. **B**, Car moving on level ground. **C**, Car moving downhill (faster than coasting with gravity). The concept of the motor powering the car to move in these three scenarios can be compared with a muscle concentrically contracting to move a body part and creating a joint action in three scenarios of movement: (1) vertically upward against gravity; (2) on level ground (i.e., gravity neutral); and (3) vertically downward, but faster than gravity would create.

SECTION 14.5 ECCENTRIC CONTRACTIONS IN MORE DETAIL

ECCENTRIC CONTRACTIONS—LENGTHENING CONTRACTIONS:

- An eccentric contraction is defined as a lengthening contraction[9] (i.e., a muscle contracts and lengthens).
- Note: Just because a muscle is lengthening, it does not mean that it is eccentrically contracting! A muscle can lengthen when it is relaxed (e.g., when a person stretches). A muscle can also lengthen while it is contracting (i.e., when myosin filament heads are grabbing actin filaments). Lengthening while contracting is defined as an eccentric contraction. It is important to distinguish between these two instances of a muscle lengthening!
- If a muscle is lengthening, then its attachments are moving away from each other.[10]
- This means that instead of the myosin heads succeeding in pulling the actin filaments toward the center of the sarcomere, the resistance force to contraction is greater than the contraction force and the myosin heads are actually stretched in the opposite direction. Consequently, the actin filaments are pulled away from the center of the sarcomere and the sarcomeres lengthen (Figure 14-8).
- Movement of a muscle's attachments away from each other is usually not caused by muscle contractions within our body; rather, it is usually caused by an external resistance force. An external force is a force that is generated external to—in other words, outside of—our body (Box 14-4). The movement

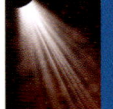

BOX 14-4 Spotlight on Internal and External Forces

An **internal force** is a force that originates inside our body; internal forces are created primarily by our muscles. An **external force** is any force that originates outside our body.[6] Gravity is the most common external force that acts on our body, but it is not the only one. By virtue of being an external force, it is not a force that we directly can control. When we move our body with muscular contractions (i.e., internal forces), we can speed up or slow down the movement by altering the command from the nervous system to the muscles. External forces, however, do not respond to our commands. For that reason, the movements that they create usually need to be modified or controlled by our muscular internal forces. These muscular internal forces modify/control the external forces acting on our body by opposing them—similar to how a brake controls the movement of a car. The muscles that do this braking eccentrically contract, allowing the motion by the external force to occur, but slowing it down as is necessary. Other examples of external forces that may act on the body are springs, rubber tubing (see Figure 14-3, *B*), and bands that pull on the body during strengthening and rehabilitative exercising. Other examples include a strong wind, an ocean wave, wrestling with another person, or even the jostling of a subway train.

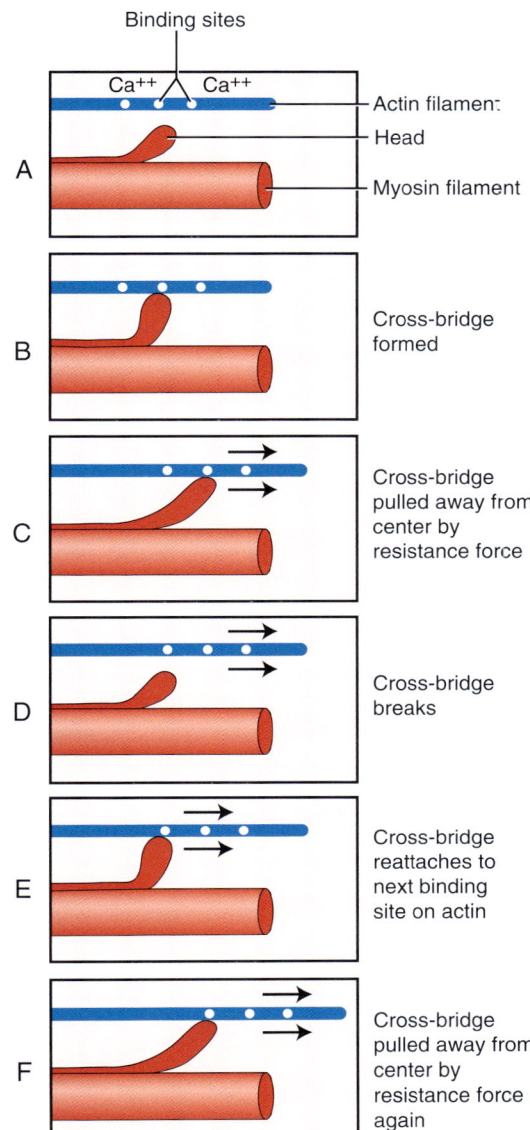

FIGURE 14-8 During an eccentric contraction, instead of the myosin heads bending toward the center of the sarcomere, they are overpowered by the resistance force to contraction and they are bent in the other direction. As a result, the actin filaments slide away from the center and the sarcomere lengthens.

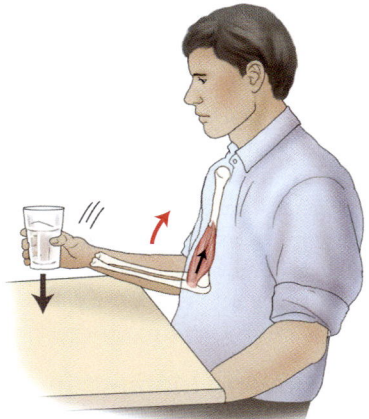

FIGURE 14-9 Person is lowering a glass of water to a tabletop. The joint action that is occurring is extension of the forearm at the elbow joint and is caused by gravity (therefore gravity is the mover in this scenario). However, without control from our muscular system, gravity would cause the glass to come crashing down to the table and break. Therefore a flexor of the forearm must eccentrically contract and lengthen (as an antagonist) to contract to oppose the elbow joint extension force that is being caused by gravity (the brachialis has been drawn in this illustration as our elbow joint flexor). The brachialis must contract with less force than gravity so that gravity in effect "wins" and succeeds in lowering the glass to the table; however, the brachialis acts as a brake on gravity, resulting in the glass being lowered more slowly.

of a body part created by this external force is slowed down by an eccentric contraction of a muscle.
- The eccentrically contracting muscle slows down the movement of the body part caused by the external force because it has an action that is opposite to the action of the external force[7] (Figure 14-9).
- Because a muscle that is eccentrically contracting creates a force that is opposite to the joint action that is occurring, an eccentrically contracting muscle must, by definition, act as an antagonist.[7] (For more information on the role of antagonists, see Section 15.2).
- Note: An eccentric contraction is sometimes called a **negative contraction**, perhaps because an eccentric contraction opposes (i.e., *negates*) the force that is creating the action that is occurring.[2]

WHEN DO ECCENTRIC CONTRACTIONS OCCUR?

- Eccentric contractions usually occur in our body when the force of the eccentric contraction is needed to slow down a movement caused by gravity or some other external force.[3]
- These eccentric contractions can occur in the following three scenarios.
  - Note: Another factor to consider when looking at the possible ways that a muscle might eccentrically contract is the presence of other external resistance forces. A muscle often needs to contract to slow down other external forces that are acting on the body, whether the direction of movement that is being slowed is vertically upward, horizontal, or vertically downward.[6] External forces providing resistance such as springs, rubber tubing, and bands are often used when exercising. The following three scenarios are based on gravity being the only resistance force to movement.

Scenario 1—"Slowing Gravity's Vertical Downward Motion":

- When gravity creates a downward movement of a body part, it is necessary for the eccentrically contracting muscle to create an upward force that is opposite the downward force of gravity, slowing gravity's movement of the body part.
- The reason to slow down the movement caused by gravity is that gravity knows only one speed; if it is not slowed down, then the body part would crash into whatever surface stops it, possibly causing injury (see Figure 14-9).

Scenario 2—"Slowing Momentum of a Horizontal Motion":

- Eccentric contractions also occur to slow down the movement of a body part when it is moving horizontally. Horizontal motion is gravity neutral (i.e., gravity neither adds to this motion nor resists this motion). In the case where a body part is moving horizontally because of a previous muscular contraction, if the muscle that initiated that movement were to relax, momentum would keep the body part moving farther than we might want. If we want to slow it down, then we can eccentrically contract a muscle that does the opposite action of the horizontal movement that is occurring (Figure 14-10, A).

Scenario 3—"Slowing Momentum of a Vertical Upward Motion":

- Eccentric contractions can also occur to slow down the movement of a body part when it is moving upward (i.e., against gravity). In the case where a body part is moving upward quickly because of a previous muscular contraction, if the muscle that initiated that movement were to relax, gravity would eventually slow down the upward movement of the body part. However, if we want to slow it down more rapidly than the force of gravity would, then we can eccentrically contract a muscle that does the opposite action of the upward movement of the body part that is occurring (see Figure 14-10, B).

ANALOGY TO DRIVING A CAR:

- A good analogy to facilitate the understanding of why and when eccentric contractions occur is to compare the brakes of a car with an eccentrically contracting muscle.
- Just as an eccentrically contracting muscle creates a force to slow down movement of a body part, the brakes of a car create a force to slow down the movement of the car. We can draw this analogy of the brakes of a car to the three scenarios that we just discussed for when eccentric contractions occur.
  - Scenario 1: If we are driving a car downhill (i.e., with gravity) and we do not want the car to gain too much speed because of the force of gravity, then we must step on the brakes to control the car's speed downhill (to slow the downward movement of the car) (Figure 14-11, A).
  - Scenario 2: If we are driving a car on a level surface (i.e., gravity neutral) and the car has momentum because we have already pressed on the gas to go fast, then we can press on the brakes to slow the movement of the car (Figure 14-11, B).
  - Scenario 3: If we are driving a car uphill (i.e., against gravity) and we need to slow down faster than we would if gravity were to slow us down, then we can press on the brakes to more quickly slow the movement of the car uphill (Figure 14-11, C).

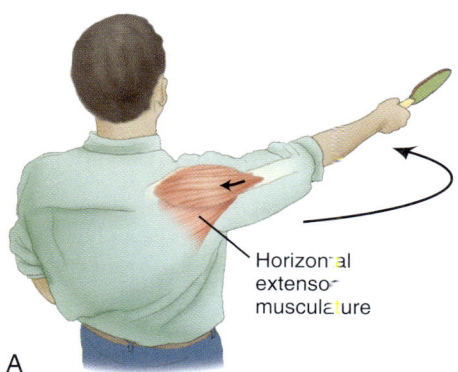

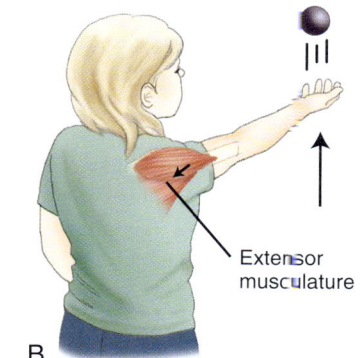

FIGURE 14-10 Eccentric contractions. **A,** Person who has just hit a ping-pong ball with a forehand stroke by horizontally flexing the arm at the shoulder joint. After having initiated the stroke with muscular force, movement of the stroke continues with momentum. Toward the end of the stroke, the person eccentrically contracts the muscles that do the opposite action of the stroke (i.e., horizontal extension) to slow down the motion of the arm, preventing it from moving too far. **B,** Person who has just thrown a ball up into the air by flexing the arm at the shoulder joint. This motion was initiated by muscular contraction. After release of the ball, this upward motion of flexion of the arm is slowed down by an eccentric contraction of muscles on the other side of the joint (i.e., the antagonistic shoulder extensors).

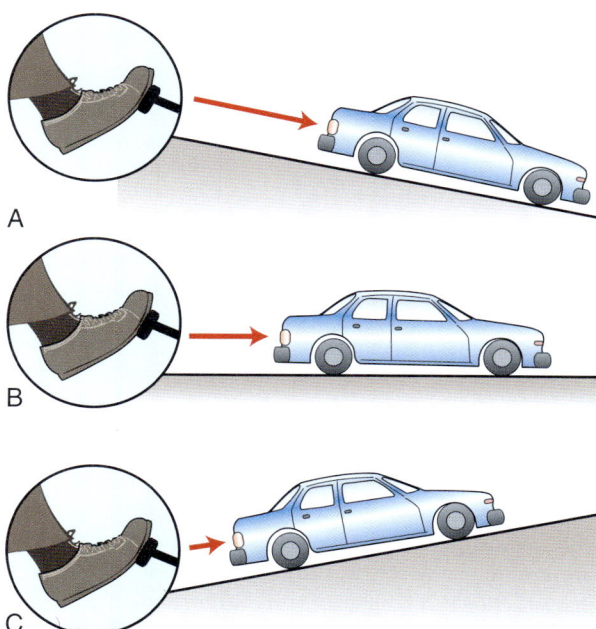

FIGURE 14-11 Illustration of the brakes of a car being necessary to slow down the movement of the car in three scenarios. **A,** Car moving downhill and slowing down. **B,** Car moving on level ground and slowing down. **C,** Car moving uphill and slowing down (slowing down more quickly than it would if just gravity were to slow it down). The concept of the brakes slowing the movement of a car in these three scenarios can illustrate the concept of a muscle eccentrically contracting to slow the motion of a joint action that is occurring vertically downward with gravity, on level ground (i.e., gravity neutral), and vertically upward (but slowing the joint action more quickly than gravity alone would have done.)

CONCLUSION:

- Eccentric contractions occur to slow movement of a body part in three scenarios:
  - Scenario 1: To slow vertically downward motion (i.e., to slow gravity's downward motion of the body part).
  - Scenario 2: To slow horizontal motion (i.e., gravity is neutral, but momentum must be slowed down).
  - Scenario 3: To slow vertically upward motion (i.e., to slow the upward motion of momentum more quickly than gravity alone would).
  - Note: Of the possible ways in which a muscle eccentrically contracts, the most common example is to slow downward movement of a body part resulting from the force of gravity!

SECTION 14.6 ISOMETRIC CONTRACTIONS IN MORE DETAIL

ISOMETRIC CONTRACTIONS—SAME LENGTH CONTRACTIONS:

- An isometric contraction is defined as a contraction in which the muscle stays the same length (i.e., the muscle contracts and stays the same length).[9]
- If a muscle contracts and stays the same length, then there must be an opposing force (of resistance) that is also acting on the body part that keeps the body part from moving and therefore stops the muscle from being able to shorten.[6]
- This other force could be any external force such as gravity or could be an internal force created by another muscle in our own body.[6]
- The force by our isometrically contracting muscle and the opposing force must be exactly the same strength (i.e., their forces balance each other out). Hence neither one succeeds in moving the body part.
- A nice analogy to better see and understand isometric contractions is to think of a tug-of-war wherein both sides are pulling on the rope with exactly the same force and as a result no movement occurs (i.e., neither side is pulled toward the other).
- Isometric contractions are very easy to recognize because a muscle is contracting and its length is not changing; hence the muscle's attachments are not moving—in other words, whatever body part it is acting on is staying still (Box 14-5).

BOX 14-5

There is an interesting example of isometric muscle contraction in which joint motion occurs. When a two-joint muscle (i.e., a muscle that crosses two joints) contracts, it can shorten across one joint that it crosses and lengthen across the other, the net result being that the muscle stays the same length overall but motion has occurred at both joints that it crosses. For example, the rectus femoris can shorten across the hip joint, causing flexion of the thigh at the hip joint, while at the same time lengthening across the knee joint, allowing the knee joint to flex. (Interestingly, at the same time, a hamstring muscle could have been shortening across the knee joint, causing flexion of the knee joint, while at the same time lengthening across the hip joint, allowing the hip joint to flex.)

- Because the body part is staying still, no joint action is occurring. Because no joint movement occurs, when we start assigning roles to muscles, no mover or antagonist is named because these terms are defined relative to a movement of a body part at a joint. Instead, we simply have two equally strong forces acting on a body part to hold it still; these forces are usually called *fixator forces*[7] (i.e., stabilizer forces). (See Sections 15.5 and 15.6 for more on this muscle role.)

WHEN DO ISOMETRIC CONTRACTIONS OCCUR?

- Isometric contractions occur in our body when the force of the isometric contraction is needed to stop a body part from moving.[3] When an isometric contraction acts to hold a body part in position, that body part is said to be *fixed* or *stabilized*. (For more information on these terms, see Sections 15.5 and 15.6.)
- These isometric contractions can be divided into two scenarios.

Scenario 1—Against Gravity ("Holding a Body Part Up"):

- The isometrically contracting muscle opposes gravity. This occurs whenever a body part is being held up against gravity (i.e., when the body part would fall because of gravity if the muscle were not isometrically contracting) (Figure 14-12, *A*).

Scenario 2—Against Any Force Other Than Gravity ("Holding a Body Part in Position"):

- The isometrically contracting muscle opposes any force other than gravity. This occurs whenever a body part is being held in its position against any force other than gravity (i.e., when the body part would move in some direction if our isometrically contracting muscle were not contracting). This other force could come from another muscle contracting within the body and acting on a body part. This other force could also be the result of an external force such as the springs/pulleys of an exercise machine or the elastic pulling force of a stretched rubber tubing or band used for exercising. Other examples of external forces might be another person acting on our body, a strong wind, or a wave in the ocean (see Figure 14-12, *B*).

CONCLUSION:

- Isometric contractions occur to hold still (i.e., fix or stabilize a body part). Isometric contractions can be divided into two scenarios:
  - Scenario 1: To statically hold a body part up in position against gravity
  - Scenario 2: To statically hold a body part in position against any force other than gravity

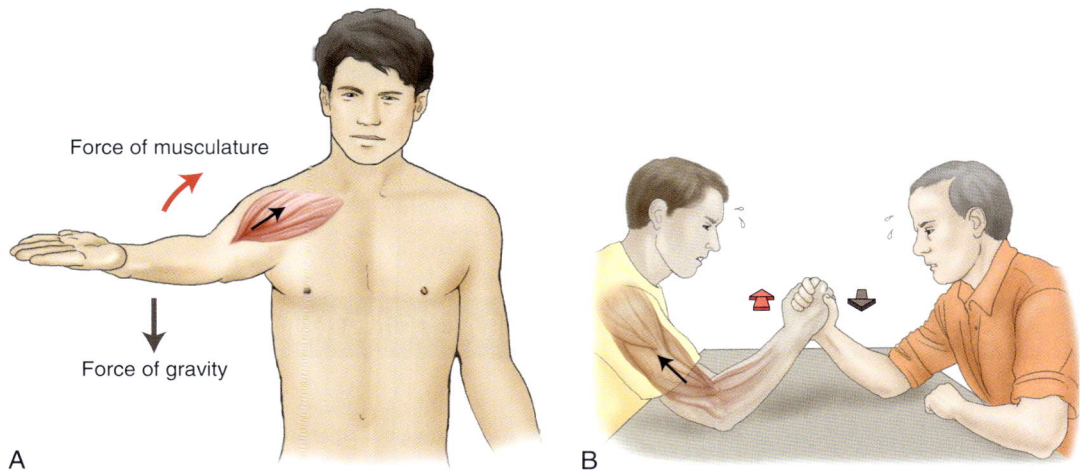

FIGURE 14-12 Isometric contractions. **A,** Person holding the arm in a position of flexion. To accomplish this, the shoulder joint flexor musculature must isometrically contract with enough force to equal the force of gravity (which is pulling the arm down toward extension). **B,** Person arm wrestling with another individual. In this case the force of the person's isometric contraction is exactly equal to the opposing force from the other individual; hence neither force is capable of moving a body part, and the part remains statically still. In both cases the person's musculature contracts and does not shorten (nor lengthen), but rather it remains the same length; therefore it is isometrically contracting.

SECTION 14.7   MOVEMENT VERSUS STABILIZATION

- With a better understanding of the concept of muscle contraction, we see that what defines a muscle as contracting is not that it shortens but rather that it generates a pulling force (Box 14-6).

 BOX 14-6

When a muscle is said to contract, we can confidently state that it is generating a pulling force toward its center. However, we cannot state anything about its length unless we see the particular scenario to know all the other forces that are also acting on the body parts in question. A contracting muscle may successfully shorten, or it may lengthen, or it may stay the same length, depending on the interaction of the force of that muscle's contraction with the other forces, both internal and external, that are present.

- Looking at the result of the muscle's contraction, we see the following:
  - A concentric contraction *creates movement*.
  - An eccentric contraction *modifies movement* that is being created by another force (often gravity).
  - An isometric contraction *stops movement* by creating a force that is equal to and therefore balances out an opposing force on a body part.
  - Although both concentric and eccentric contractions are involved with creating/modifying movement of a body part at a joint, isometric contractions are not. In fact, the purpose of an isometric contraction is to stop movement altogether.
- In Section 6.1, an overview of the roles of the parts of the musculoskeletal system was presented as the following:
  - Joints, being passive, allow movement.
  - Ligaments, holding bones together, limit movement at a joint (by limiting the end range motion at the joint).
  - Muscles (having the ability to contract and create a pulling force) can create movement.
- Although this overview is not wrong, we can see that it is a bit simplistic and incomplete because even though a muscle can create a force that can cause or modify movement of a body part at a joint, it can also create a force that can stop movement of a body part at a joint.
- Whenever a body part is stopped from moving and held still, it is said to be fixed or stabilized. Therefore a muscle that contracts to create a force that holds a body part in a static position is said to **fix** or **stabilize** that body part.[11]
  - When a muscle acts to fix a body part in place (i.e., stabilize it), that muscle can be termed a **fixator** (i.e., **stabilizer**) muscle. (For more on fixator [i.e., stabilizer] muscles, see Section 15.5.)
- Isometric muscle contractions act to fix or stabilize body parts.
- The concept of joint stabilization is extremely important. Often, forces that act on body parts create joint movements that are undesired. Isometric contractions act to stop these undesired movements, thereby stabilizing the joint.[6]
- Therefore when thinking of muscle contractions, we should keep in mind that they can act to create movement or they

can act to create stability. For more on the concept of muscle contraction and stability, see Section 15.5 on the role of fixator (i.e., stabilizer) muscles and Section 15.6 on core stability.
- Although joints exist to allow movement, they also must be sufficiently stable to remain healthy. An antagonistic relationship exists between joint mobility and joint stability: the more mobile a joint is, the less stable it is; the more stable a joint is, the less mobile it is.[10] (For more on joint mobility/stability, see Section 7.3.)
  - Each joint of the body must find its balance between mobility and stability.
  - Muscles can create forces that increase the mobility of a joint or increase the stability of a joint.

REVIEW QUESTIONS

evolve *Answers to the following review questions appear on the Evolve website accompanying this book at:*
http://evolve.elsevier.com/Muscolino/kinesiology/.

1. What are the three types of muscle contractions?

2. What is the name given to a muscle that concentrically contracts?

3. What is the name given to the force that a concentrically contracting muscle must work against?

4. What type of contraction occurs when a muscle contracts and shortens?

5. What type of contraction occurs when a muscle contracts and lengthens?

6. What type of contraction occurs when a muscle contracts and stays the same length?

7. Give an example of a resistance exercise.

8. What defines a muscle contraction?

9. What type of force is a tensile force?

10. Do muscles pull or push when they contract?

11. What does the term *gravity neutral* mean?

12. What type of muscle contraction is necessary for a person to flex the arm at the shoulder joint from anatomic position?

13. What type of muscle contraction is necessary for a person to slowly adduct the arm from a position of 90 degrees of abduction (at the shoulder joint) to anatomic position?

14. What type of muscle contraction is necessary for a person in anatomic position to rotate the neck to the right at the spinal joints?

15. What type of muscle contraction is necessary for a person (otherwise in anatomic position) to hold the left thigh in 30 degrees of abduction at the hip joint?

16. What is the most common scenario in which a muscle eccentrically contracts?

17. Why might a person contract mover muscles for a joint action that brings a body part downward?

18. Give one example each of an internal force and an external force.

19. Which type of muscle contraction stops movement from occurring?

20. Which type of muscle contraction fixes (i.e., stabilizes) a body part in position?

21. What is the relationship between joint mobility and joint stability?

REFERENCES

1. Lieber RL: Skeletal muscle, structure, function, & plasticity: The physiological basis of rehabilitation, ed 2, Baltimore, 2002, Lippincott Williams & Wilkins.
2. Levangie PK, Norkin CC: Joint structure and function: A comprehensive analysis, ed 5, Philadelphia, 2011, FA Davis.
3. Nordin M, Frankel VH: Basic biomechanics of the musculoskeletal system, ed 3, Baltimore, 2001, Lippincott Williams & Wilkins.
4. McGinnis PM: Biomechanics of sport and exercise, ed 3, Champaign, IL, 2013, Human Kinetics.
5. MacIntosh BR, Gardiner PF, McComas AJ: Skeletal muscle: Form and function, ed 2, Champaign, 2006, Human Kinetics.
6. Neumann DA: Kinesiology of the musculoskeletal system: Foundations for physical rehabilitation, ed 3, St Louis, 2017, Elsevier.
7. Smith LK, Weiss EL, Lehmkuhl LO: Brunstrom's clinical kinesiology, ed 5, Philadelphia, 1996, FA Davis.
8. Enoka RM: Neuromechanics of human movement, ed 3, Champaign, IL, 2002, Human Kinetics.
9. Palastanga N, Field D, Soames R: Anatomy and human movement, ed 4, Oxford, 2002, Butterworth-Heinemann.
10. Oatis CA: Kinesiology: The mechanics and pathomechanics of human movement, Philadelphia, 2004, Lippincott Williams & Wilkins.
11. Hall SJ: Basic biomechanics, ed 6, New York, 2012, McGraw Hill.
12. Kenney WL, Wilmore JH, Castill DL: Physiology of sport and exercise, ed 5, Champaign, 2012, Human Kinetics.

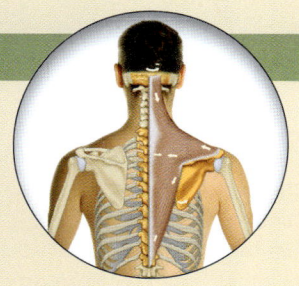

CHAPTER 15
Roles of Muscles

CHAPTER OUTLINE

Section 15.1	Mover Muscles	Section 15.7	Neutralizer Muscles
Section 15.2	Antagonist Muscles	Section 15.8	Step-by-Step Method for Determining Fixators and Neutralizers
Section 15.3	Determining the "Muscle That Is Working"		
Section 15.4	Stopping Unwanted Actions of the "Muscle That Is Working"	Section 15.9	Support Muscles
		Section 15.10	Synergists
Section 15.5	Fixator/Stabilizer Muscles	Section 15.11	Coordinating Muscle Roles
Section 15.6	Concept of Fixation and Core Stabilization	Section 15.12	Coupled Actions

CHAPTER OBJECTIVES

After completing this chapter, the student should be able to perform the following:

1. Define the key terms of this chapter and state the meaning of the word origins of this chapter.
2. Do the following related to mover muscles:
   - List and define the six major roles that a muscle may have when contracting.
   - Describe the relationship between the role that a muscle plays and the *action in question*.
3. Do the following related to antagonist muscles:
   - Compare and contrast the roles of mover and antagonist.
   - Describe the relationship between gravity and joint actions.
   - Discuss the concept of co-contraction.
   - Explain the application of tight antagonists to restricted joint motion.
4. State the *muscle that is working* during the action in question, and discuss the role of gravity in the action in question.
5. Describe the general concept of the relationship between fixators and neutralizers and the muscle that is working.
6. Do the following related to fixator and neutralizer muscles:
   - Compare and contrast the roles of fixator and neutralizer muscles.
   - Discuss the concept of fixation and core stabilization.
   - Give an example of a fixator and a neutralizer relative to a specific joint action (i.e., the action in question).
7. State the step-by-step method for determining fixators and neutralizers relative to a specific joint action (i.e., the action in question).
8. Describe the role of a support muscle.
9. Do the following related to synergists:
   - Explain the two ways in which a synergist can be defined.
   - Compare and contrast synergists and antagonists for a given joint action.
10. Do the following related to coordinating muscle roles:
    - Explain the concept of coordination as it relates to the roles of muscles.
    - Describe the possible clinical effects of isometric contractions.
    - Define and give an example of a second-order fixator.
    - Explain why it is difficult to isolate a specific muscle contraction; furthermore, explain and give an example of how muscle contractions tend to spread through the body.
11. Discuss and give an example of the concept of coupled actions in the body.

OVERVIEW

When muscles contract in our body to contribute to movement patterns, these muscles may have different roles. (The concepts of concentric contractions of movers and eccentric contractions of antagonists were briefly mentioned in Chapter 14.) However, of all the muscle contractions that are occurring in the body at any given time, most muscles are not contracting concentrically as movers or eccentrically as antagonists but rather fulfilling other roles. The names of these roles are assigned relative to the specific joint action that is occurring. We term this joint action that is occurring the *action in question*. Given that any muscle that contracts may be used, overused, and injured, it is critically important for manual and movement therapists and fitness trainers to understand the various roles in which a muscle may contract and potentially be injured.

Of course, most of the time as a part of larger movement patterns, we perform multiple joint actions at the same time. However, to simplify our ability to determine which muscles are working in which roles, it is helpful to break more complicated movement patterns into specific joint actions and then determine the roles in which the muscles in our body are working relative to each specific action in question.

Muscles have six major roles when they contract[1]:

1. Mover—A mover is a muscle (or other force) that can do the action in question.
2. Antagonist—An antagonist is a muscle (or other force) that can do the opposite action of the action in question.
3. Fixator (also known as *stabilizer*)—A fixator is a muscle (or other force) that can stop an unwanted action at the fixed attachment of the muscle that is working.
4. Neutralizer—A neutralizer is a muscle (or other force) that can stop an unwanted action at the mobile attachment of the muscle that is working.
5. Support—A support muscle is a muscle that can hold another part of the body in position while the action in question is occurring.
6. Synergist—A synergist is a muscle (or other force) that works with a muscle that is contracting.

KEY TERMS

Action in question
Agonist (AG-o-nist)
Antagonist (an-TAG-o-nist)
Assistant mover
Co-contraction
Contralateral muscle (CON-tra-LAT-er-al)
Coordination
Core stabilizers
Coupled action
Fixator (FIKS-ay-tor)
Force-couple
Ischemia (is-KEEM-ee-a)
Mobility muscles
Mover
Muscle role
Muscle that is working

Mutual neutralizers
Neutralizer
Phasic muscles (FAZE-ik)
Pilates method (pi-LAH-tees)
Postural stabilization muscles
Powerhouse
Prime antagonist (an-TAG-o-nist)
Prime mover
Prime mover group
Productive antagonism
Scapulohumeral rhythm (SKAP-you-lo-HUME-er-al)
Second-order fixator (FIKS-ay-tor)
Stabilizer
Support muscle
Synergist (SIN-er-gist)
Tonic muscles (TON-ik)

WORD ORIGINS

- Agonist—From Greek *agon*, meaning *a contest*
- Antagonist—From Greek *anti*, meaning *against, opposite*, and Greek *agon*, meaning *a contest*
- Contralateral—From Latin *contra*, meaning *opposed, against*, and *latus*, meaning *side*
- Coordination—From Latin *co*, meaning *together*, and *ordinare*, meaning *to order, to arrange*
- Ischemia—From Greek *ischo*, meaning *to keep back*, and *haima*, meaning *blood*
- Prime—From Latin *primus*, meaning *first*
- Synergist—From Greek *syn*, meaning *together*, and *ergon*, meaning *to work*

SECTION 15.1 MOVER MUSCLES

- A **mover** is a muscle (or other force) that can do the **action in question**.[1]
- The *action in question* is the term that is used to describe whatever specific joint action is occurring that we are examining. Assigning muscles the role of mover (and all other roles) is always done relative to the role that they play *relative to the action in question*.
- By definition, mover muscles shorten when the action in question occurs.
- A mover is called a *mover* because it can create the movement of the action in question (i.e., it can *move* the body part during this joint action). This movement occurs because when a mover contracts, it concentrically contracts, thereby shortening and causing one or both of its attachments to move.[2] It is this movement of an attachment that is the action in question.
- Students sometimes ask the following: What happens if the mover muscle contracts but does not concentrically contract? If a muscle contracts but does not concentrically contract, then it is not a mover. It is the shortening of the concentric contraction of a muscle that creates the movement and defines the muscle as the mover. If the muscle is eccentrically contracting, then another joint action is occurring and this muscle is not creating it; and it cannot be the mover if it does not create the movement. Similarly, if the muscle is isometrically contracting instead of concentrically contracting, no joint action is occurring at all, because the muscle is not changing its length. Again, the muscle cannot be a mover (in this case because no movement is occurring). A contracting muscle must be concentrically contracting to be a mover. (For more information on concentric, eccentric, and isometric contractions, see Chapter 14.)
- A mover muscle can shorten in two ways:
  1. It can concentrically contract and shorten, generating the force that creates the action in question.
  2. It can be relaxed and shorten, in effect slackening because its attachments are brought closer together as the joint action is created by another mover force.
- For almost every joint action that is possible in the human body, a functional group of movers can contract to create it[3] (Box 15-1).

- Just because a group of movers exists does not mean that every muscle of that group necessarily contracts every time the action in question occurs. It is entirely possible for one or a few muscles of a mover group to contract and create the action in question while the rest of the muscles of the mover group are relaxed when the action in question is occurring.[4]
- If a mild force is needed to create the action in question, one or a few of the movers is/are recruited to contract; if a stronger force is needed, a greater number of movers are recruited to contract.
- Within each functional group of movers, usually one muscle is the most powerful at performing the action in question. This most powerful mover is called the **prime mover**.
- If a number of muscles are equally strong at performing the action in question, they are sometimes called the **prime mover group**.
- Some sources define any mover other than the prime mover (or any muscle not a member of the prime mover group) as an **assistant mover**.[5]
- A mover is also known as an **agonist**.[6]
- The role of mover is the most commonly known role of a contracting muscle. When students are first taught muscles, the actions that are taught for each muscle studied are its mover concentric contraction actions. And when we speak of learning the functional groups of muscles (as was discussed in Section 15.1), unless the context is made otherwise clear, it is usually assumed that we are speaking of learning the functional groups of mover muscles. However, muscles may act in roles other than mover; therefore other functional groups exist. This chapter examines these other functional groups of muscles.
- Although we usually think of actions as occurring because of a muscle contraction, any force can cause the action in question to occur. For this reason, the definition of a mover is a muscle *(or other force)* that can create the action in question. The most common *other force* that can be a mover force is gravity.
  - Any joint action that moves downward is aided by gravity. Therefore in any downward movement, gravity is a mover.[3]

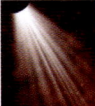

BOX 15-1   Spotlight on Force-Couples

Two or more muscles can have lines of pull that are in different linear directions yet create the same axial joint motion; these muscles form what is called a muscular **force-couple**.[7] For example, the rectus abdominis pulls superiorly on the pelvis, and the biceps femoris of the hamstring group pulls inferiorly on the pelvis; yet both muscles form a force-couple that creates posterior tilt of the pelvis. Another example is the right sternocleidomastoid, which pulls the anterior head/neck to the left, and the left splenius capitis, which pulls the posterior head/neck to the right, yet they both form a force-couple that creates left rotation of the head and neck at the spinal joints. Therefore, even though the muscles of a force-couple may have different linear lines of pull, they are synergistic in that they are movers of the same axial joint action.

- If gravity is the mover, then our muscle movers will usually be relaxed because another force is creating the joint action for them.
- Figure 15-1 demonstrates three examples of movers. In all three scenarios, whatever force can do the action in question is a mover. However, not every mover is necessarily working (see Figure 15-1).

ESSENTIAL FACTS:

- A mover is a muscle (or other force) that can do the action in question.
- By definition, during the action in question, mover muscles shorten.
- By definition, when a mover muscle contracts, it contracts concentrically.

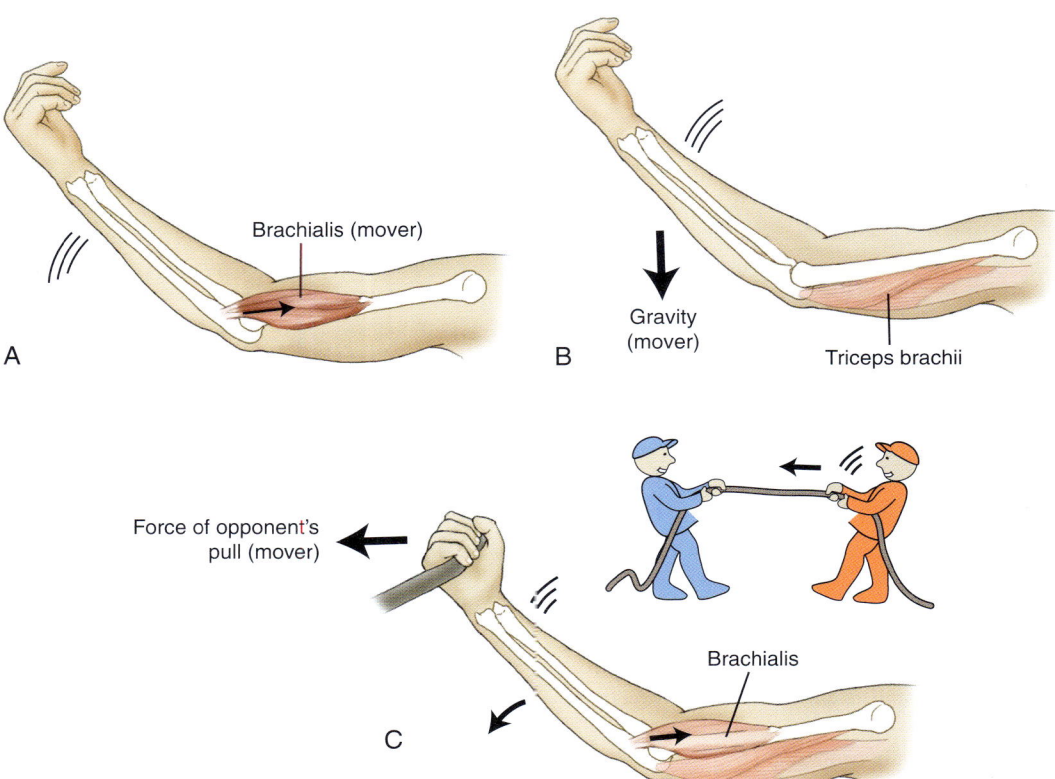

FIGURE 15-1 Three examples of movers. **A,** The forearm flexing at the elbow joint. Because this motion is upward, a muscle must generate the force to create this movement. In this scenario the brachialis is shown as the mover. **B,** Forearm extending at the elbow joint. Because this motion is downward, gravity is capable of bringing the forearm downward; therefore no muscle needs to contract in this case. In this scenario, gravity is the mover. **C,** A person's forearm being pulled into extension at the elbow joint while playing tug-of-war. In this scenario the force of the opponent's pull is the mover force that is creating the action in question, namely extension of the forearm at the elbow joint.

SECTION 15.2 ANTAGONIST MUSCLES

- An **antagonist** is a muscle (or other force) that can perform the opposite action of the action in question.[1]
- By definition, antagonists lengthen when the action in question occurs.
- An antagonist can lengthen in two ways:
  1. It can eccentrically contract and lengthen, generating a braking force on the action in question.[7] (For more information on eccentric contractions, see Sections 14.1, 14.2, and 14.5.)
  2. It can be relaxed and lengthen, allowing the action in question to occur.
- When an antagonist lengthens, it lengthens because the joint action that is occurring (the action in question) is causing the two attachments of the antagonist muscle to move away from each other (either one or both attachments of the antagonist could be moving). If the attachments of the antagonist are moving away from each other, then the joint action that is occurring must be the opposite action from the joint action that the antagonist muscle would perform if it were to shorten. Thus an antagonist can perform the opposite action of the action in question (Box 15-2).
  - For example, if the action that is occurring is protraction of the scapula at the scapulocostal (ScC) joint, then the scapula is moving anteriorly. An antagonist to this action is the rhomboids, and as the scapula protracts, the attachments of the rhomboids are moving farther from each other (i.e., the scapula is moving away from the spine). If the rhomboids were to concentrically contract, they would cause the opposite action of this action in question (i.e., they would cause retraction of the scapula at the ScC joint).
- Because an antagonist is usually located on the opposite side of the joint from the mover muscle(s) that can create the action in question, an antagonist is sometimes called a **contralateral muscle** (the term *contralateral* literally means *opposite side*).
- Usually for any joint action there will be a group of antagonists that can perform the opposite action of the action in question. Among the muscles of the antagonist group, the antagonist that is most powerful at opposing the action in question is called the **prime antagonist**.
- Although we usually think of antagonists as being muscles, any force can oppose the action in question. For this reason, the definition of an antagonist is *a muscle (or other force) that can perform the opposite action of the action in question*. The most common *other force* that can be an antagonist is gravity.
  - Any joint action that moves upward is opposed by gravity. Therefore in any upward movement, gravity is an antagonist.
- When a mover contracts and shortens, creating a joint motion, the antagonist must lengthen. If this lengthening is sufficient, the antagonist will stretch. Like a rubber band that is stretched, a passive elastic recoil tension force will build up in the stretched antagonist. If the mover is relaxed and the antagonist is now contracted, the passive tension force that is built up within the antagonist will augment the force of the antagonist's active contraction, creating a stronger force by the muscle. Given the benefit of this passive tension force, this phenomenon has been termed **productive antagonism**.[3]
  - The term *productive antagonism* was coined by Don Neumann, PT, PhD. For more on this concept, please see his textbook *Kinesiology of the Musculoskeletal System*, second edition (2010, Elsevier).

DETERMINING HOW AN ANTAGONIST LENGTHENS:

- It is critically important to realize that whenever a joint action occurs, the antagonist muscles must lengthen.
- However, as previously stated, an antagonist can lengthen in two manners:
  1. It can eccentrically contract and lengthen, allowing the action in question to occur, but also creating a braking force upon it (i.e., slowing the action in question).
  2. It can be relaxed and lengthen, allowing the action in question to occur.
- To determine how an antagonist lengthens (i.e., whether it is relaxed or eccentrically contracting), we need to look at whether the action in question needs to be slowed down in some manner.

BOX 15-2 Spotlight on What an Antagonist Is Antagonistic To

The name *antagonist* literally means antiagonist (i.e., antimover); therefore many people assume that the definition of an antagonist is that it performs the opposite action of the mover (i.e., it opposes the mover). Although the antagonist can oppose the action in question that is performed by the mover, the mover may have other actions that the antagonist cannot oppose. For this reason, it is always best to remember that an antagonist is defined as being able to do the opposite action *of the action in question*. For example, if the action in question is elevation of the scapula at the scapulocostal (ScC) joint and we choose to consider the upper trapezius as our mover (because it can perform elevation of the scapula), then the lower trapezius would be an antagonist because it can perform depression of the scapula at the ScC joint (i.e., the action that is opposite the action in question). Is the lower trapezius an antagonist to the upper trapezius? It is, only relative to the action of elevation of the scapula. The upper trapezius can also retract the scapula, as can the lower trapezius. With regard to the mover's action of retraction of the scapula, it should be noted that not only does the lower trapezius not perform the opposite action (protraction), but it can actually help the upper trapezius perform retraction. Therefore when we look at the action in question as being retraction of the scapula, the upper trapezius and lower trapezius are synergistic to each other (i.e., they perform the same action). For this reason, it is best to avoid saying that a muscle is or is not an antagonist to another muscle; rather it is or is not an antagonist to a specific joint action (i.e., the action in question).

- Generally, when the mover force is gravity or any other external force that we cannot directly control, we need to slow the joint action to keep our body part from crashing to the ground (or crashing against some other surface).
  - Therefore when gravity or some other external force is the mover, our antagonists usually eccentrically contract and lengthen.
  - By far, the most common scenario of a muscle being an antagonist is when it eccentrically contracts to slow a joint action that is caused by gravity—in other words a joint action in which gravity is the mover.
- However, when one of our muscles provides the mover force (i.e., it is creating the action in question), no need exists to slow it down with our antagonistic muscles. If we feel that our mover muscle is causing the action in question to occur too rapidly and that our body part that is moving will crash into something, we can simply command the mover muscle itself to not contract as hard, and the joint action will slow.
  - Therefore when one of our muscles is the mover, our antagonists usually relax and lengthen.[2]

- If the mover muscles and the antagonist muscles do contract at the same time, it is called **co-contraction**[2] (Box 15-3).
- Figure 15-2 demonstrates three examples of antagonists. In all three scenarios, whatever force can do the opposite action of the action in question is an antagonist.
- As with muscles of a mover group, it should be remembered that not every muscle of an antagonist group is necessarily working during a specific action in question.

ESSENTIAL FACTS:

- An antagonist is a muscle (or other force) that can perform the opposite action of the action in question.
- By definition, during the action in question, antagonist muscles lengthen.
- By definition, when an antagonist muscle contracts, it contracts eccentrically.
- The most common scenario in which a muscle acts as an antagonist is when a muscle eccentrically contracts to slow down a joint action that is caused by gravity.

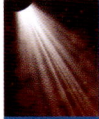

BOX 15-3 Spotlight on Co-Contraction

Many new students of kinesiology assume that whenever a mover muscle concentrically contracts and shortens, the antagonist muscle eccentrically contracts and lengthens. This is not the case. Antagonists need to be relaxed and lengthen when mover muscles contract; otherwise the antagonists are fighting the movers. When both mover and antagonist muscles do contract at the same time, it is called co-contraction. Co-contraction is not generally considered to be healthy. An analogy would be to press on the gas and the brake of a car at the same time when driving (in this analogy, the mover muscles are the gas and the antagonist muscles are the brake). Just as this would wear out the engine and brakes of the car, co-contraction would fatigue and may eventually injure the mover and antagonist muscles of our body, as well as the joint being acted upon.

An interesting application of this principle to bodywork is when a new manual therapist is doing bodywork and is afraid of using too much pressure for fear of hurting the client. To deliver pressure, the therapist contracts the extensors of the elbow joint; however, at the same time the therapist is subconsciously contracting the flexors of the elbow joint to hold back from exerting too much pressure. This creates a situation in which the therapist both is ineffectual in delivering pressure to the client and is in danger of eventually hurting himself or herself.

Notes:
1. It should be emphasized that co-contraction is defined as the mover and antagonist muscles contracting at the same time. A contraction of the mover to initiate a contraction and then a contraction of the antagonist to slow down the momentum of that motion after the mover has relaxed form a sequence of muscle contractions that often occurs in the body and is not co-contraction.
2. If a co-contraction occurs in which the mover and antagonist muscles contract with the same force, then their forces will balance out and no joint action will occur. If no joint action occurs, then by definition these muscles are not defined as movers and antagonists. Rather, they are isometrically contracting opposed muscles.
3. Some kinesiologists believe that co-contraction is a necessary and natural occurrence when we are first learning a new sport or kinesthetic skill. They believe that as we refine and perfect this new skill, we gradually learn to lessen and eliminate the amount of our co-contraction. Therefore part of becoming more efficient, graceful, and coordinated is to learn to lessen the amount that we fight ourselves by co-contracting our muscles.
4. Although co-contraction is inefficient with regard to the production of movement, when stabilization of a body part is needed, co-contraction is desirable and often occurs (for more on stabilization, see Section 15.6).

CHAPTER 15 Roles of Muscles 529

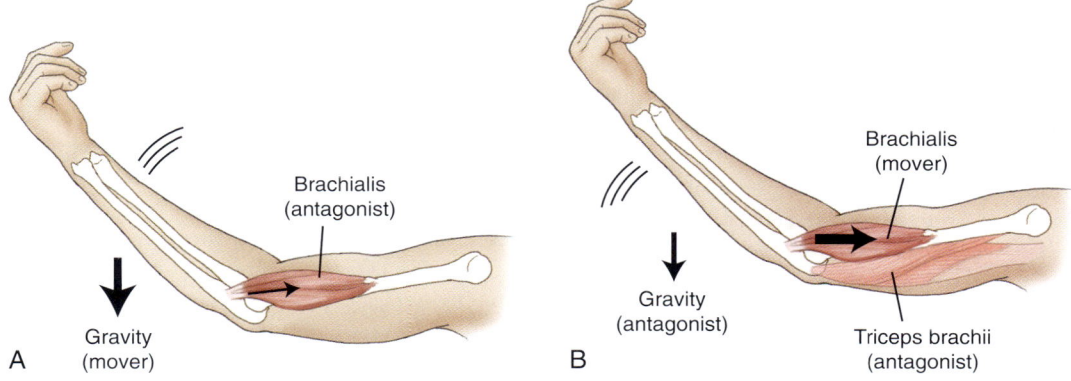

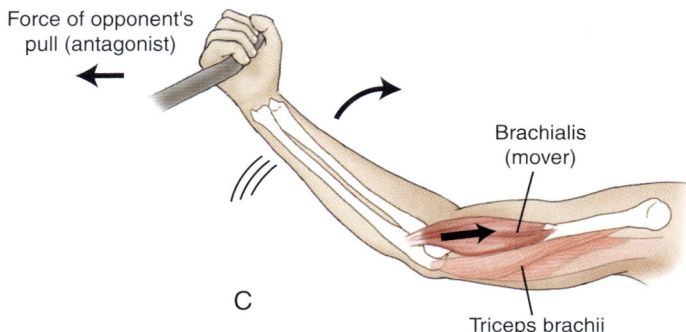

FIGURE 15-2 Three examples of antagonists. **A,** Forearm is extending at the elbow joint. Because this motion is downward, gravity is the mover that moves the forearm downward into extension. The brachialis (an elbow joint flexor) is shown eccentrically contracting to slow down the extension of the forearm; therefore the brachialis is an antagonist. **B,** Forearm flexing at the elbow joint because of the contraction of the brachialis (i.e., the mover). Because this action is upward, gravity is an antagonist, because it exerts a force of extension of the forearm at the elbow joint. **C,** Elbow joint of a person playing tug-of-war. The force of the brachialis is the mover force that is pulling the person's forearm into flexion at the elbow joint. In this case the force of the opponent's pull is an antagonist, because it is opposing the action in question (which is flexion of the forearm at the elbow joint).

SECTION 15.3 DETERMINING THE "MUSCLE THAT IS WORKING"

- As explained in Sections 15.1 and 15.2, mover muscles and antagonist muscles do not usually co-contract (contract at the same time) when a joint action is occurring.
  - If the movers are contracting, the antagonists are usually relaxing.
  - If the antagonists are contracting, the movers are usually relaxing.
- As a rule, either a mover *or* an antagonist contracts during the action in question (or if more force is necessary, a group of movers *or* a group of antagonists contracts during the action in question).
- Whichever muscle does contract during the action in question is called the **muscle that is working**.
- To determine which functional group (i.e., movers or antagonists) is contracting (i.e., working), we need to look at what force is creating the action in question.

ROLE OF GRAVITY IN THE ACTION IN QUESTION:

- Assuming that no other external forces are involved, the easiest way to determine what force is creating the action in question is to determine gravity's role with relation to the action in question.
- Gravity's force pulls downward.
- Therefore simply look at whether the action in question involves a downward, upward, or horizontal movement of a body part.
- Following are the three possible scenarios:
  1. Upward movement: If the joint action involves upward movement of a body part, then gravity cannot be causing it; therefore the mover muscles must be concentrically contracting to cause it.
     - Therefore the movers are concentrically contracting (i.e., working) in this scenario, and the antagonists are relaxed.

530　PART 4　Myology: Study of the Muscular System

2. **Horizontal movement:** If the joint action is neither up nor down, in other words, it is horizontal, then the force of gravity is neutral and is not involved. If gravity is not involved, then it cannot cause the action in question to occur; therefore the mover muscles must be concentrically contracting to cause it.
   ○ Therefore the movers are concentrically contracting (i.e., working), and the antagonists are relaxed.
3. **Downward movement:** If the joint action involves downward movement of the body part, then gravity causes it and the mover muscles do not need to contract. They can relax and let gravity create the motion; in effect, they get a free ride.
   ○ However, to control the downward motion caused by gravity, the antagonist muscles most likely will eccentrically contract to slow the force of gravity.
   ○ Therefore the antagonists are eccentrically contracting (i.e., working) in this scenario, and the movers are relaxed.

ESSENTIAL FACTS:

○ We can state the following three general rules for our muscle movers and antagonists:
  1. With upward movements, movers work and antagonists relax.
  2. With horizontal movements, movers work and antagonists relax.
  3. With downward movements, antagonists work and movers relax.
○ Figure 15-3 illustrates the three general rules for when movers versus antagonists contract.
○ Of course, for every rule an exception exists: If we desire a downward movement that is faster than gravity alone would create, we can supplement the force of gravity with the contraction force of our muscle movers. The antagonists would not work, because we do not want to slow down the movement. Therefore in this scenario our muscle movers would be working and our antagonist muscles would be relaxed. An example is a downward golf swing.

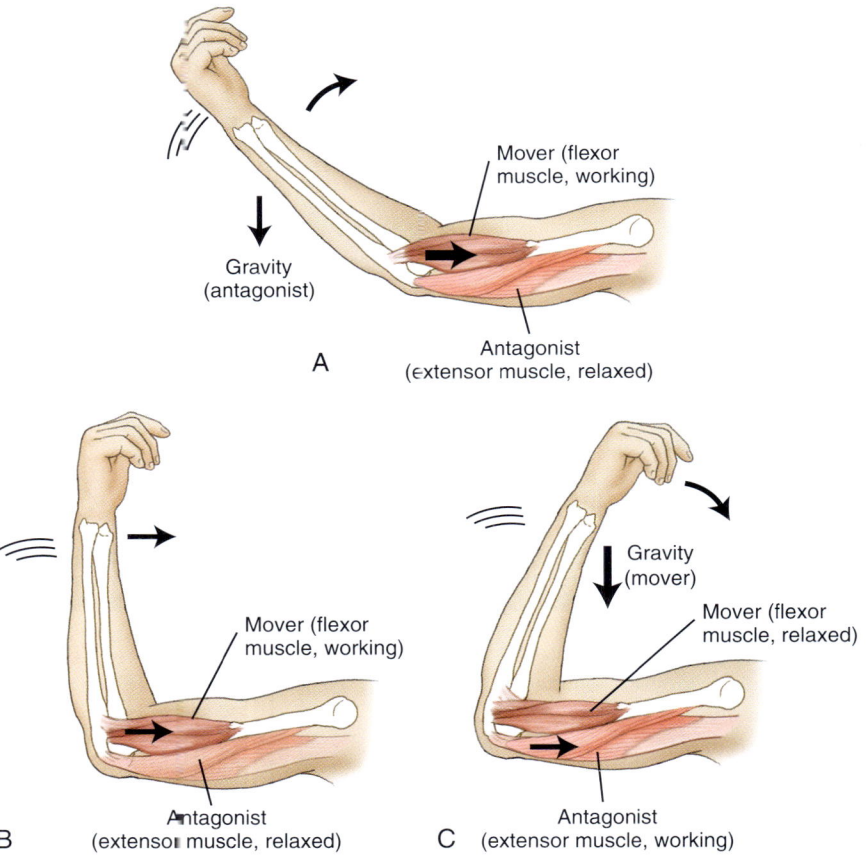

FIGURE 15-3 Three instances of a person flexing the forearm at the elbow joint. **A** and **B,** Forearm moves in an upward and horizontal direction, respectively. In both of these cases the movers of flexion at the elbow joint must work (i.e., concentrically contract) to create this action. In both of these cases the antagonists are relaxed, allowing the action to occur. (Note: In *A*, gravity is an antagonist; in *B*, gravity is neutral.) **C,** Forearm moves in a downward direction. In this instance, gravity is the mover of elbow joint flexion, so the muscular movers of flexion are relaxed; the extensors of the elbow joint are antagonists, working (i.e., eccentrically contracting) to slow the flexion of the forearm.

SECTION 15.4 STOPPING UNWANTED ACTIONS OF THE "MUSCLE THAT IS WORKING"

- A muscle that is working is a muscle that is contracting when the action in question is occurring.
- In Section 15.3, we learned how to figure out whether it is the mover group or antagonist group that works.
- Now that we know which group is working, we must look at another factor. That is, during the action in question, are there any unwanted actions of the muscle that is working that need to be canceled out?

EXAMPLE OF STOPPING AN UNWANTED ACTION:

- To understand this concept, it is helpful to look at the example of flexion of the fingers to make a fist. (Note: Flexion of fingers #2 through #5 occurs at the metacarpophalangeal [MCP] and interphalangeal [IP] joints.)
- If our upper extremity is in a position such that flexing the fingers is an upward motion, gravity cannot be the mover. This means we need a muscle mover to concentrically contract to do flexion of the fingers. Therefore movers are working (i.e., contracting), and antagonists are relaxed.
- Two movers can flex the fingers: (1) the flexor digitorum superficialis (FDS) and (2) the flexor digitorum profundus (FDP). We could choose either one, but for this example it will be helpful to consider the FDS. Therefore our action in question is flexion of the fingers, and our muscle that is working (i.e., the FDS) is the mover.
- As soon as the FDS flexes the fingers (the action in question), a fist is made. This means we are done, right?
- No, because if the only joint action that we want is flexion of the fingers, then we have a problem. This is because when the FDS contracts, it will attempt to create every one of its actions. (Note: The FDS has only one line of pull that crosses multiple joints. A muscle with one line of pull cannot intend only one of its actions to occur. When a muscle with one line of pull contracts, it attempts to create every action along that line of pull [see Section 13.5].)
- The FDS can also flex the hand at the wrist joint. Flexion of the hand at the wrist joint is an unwanted action of our muscle that is working (i.e., our contracting mover, the FDS).
- Whenever our *working* muscle has an unwanted action, then that unwanted action has to be stopped.
- In this scenario it is the job of an extensor of the hand at the wrist joint to contract and stop flexion of the hand at the wrist joint. Palpate the common extensor tendon region near the lateral epicondyle of the humerus while making a fist, and a contraction will clearly be felt to occur when flexing fingers to make a fist.
- Theoretically, any extensor of the hand at the wrist joint could stop the flexor digitorum superficialis (FDS) from flexing the hand at the wrist joint. However, the extensor carpi radialis brevis is the wrist joint extensor that is usually chosen by the central nervous system for this task.[8]
- How? When the extensor carpi radialis brevis contracts, it creates a force of extension of the hand at the wrist joint that stops the FDS from flexing the hand at the wrist joint. (Note: The FDS also crosses the elbow joint and could cause flexion of the forearm at the elbow joint. Theoretically, this is another unwanted action that would have to be stopped.)
- What role does the extensor carpi radialis brevis play? It cannot create the action in question (i.e., flexion of the fingers); therefore it is not a mover. It cannot perform the opposite action of the action in question (i.e., extension of the fingers); therefore it is not an antagonist. In this scenario the role in which the extensor carpi radialis brevis functions is as a fixator (stabilizer) muscle (Box 15-4).
- Two types of muscle roles serve to stop unwanted actions of the muscle that is working. One is fixator, as exemplified in the previously discussed scenario; the other is neutralizer.

BOX 15-4

In the scenario of flexing the fingers and making a fist, the extensor carpi radialis brevis acts as a fixator muscle. An interesting clinical application arises from this example. Tennis elbow (also known as lateral epicondylitis or lateral epicondylosis) is overuse/misuse of the muscles of the common extensor belly/tendon. Although the cause of tennis elbow is usually blamed on overuse of the wrist extensor muscles as movers (e.g., the client is extending the hand at the wrist joint when executing a backhand stroke while playing tennis), another major aggravating factor of tennis elbow is the contraction of wrist extensors as fixators every time that the finger flexor muscles contract to make a fist or hold something. This means that every moment that the person holds and grips the tennis racquet, or for that matter grasps a doorknob to open a door, grips a steering wheel, or simply holds a pen, the condition of tennis elbow is aggravated!

FIXATORS AND NEUTRALIZERS:

- Fixators and neutralizers are similar in that they both stop unwanted actions of the muscle that is working.[6] (Again, the muscle that is working is either a mover concentrically contracting or an antagonist eccentrically contracting.)
- Fixators and neutralizers are different in that the fixator stops an unwanted action at the *fixed attachment* of the muscle that is working; the neutralizer stops an unwanted action at the *mobile attachment* of the muscle that is working.[1]
- Note: Not every contracting muscle has one fixed attachment and one mobile attachment. It is possible for a muscle to contract and move both of its attachments, in which case both attachments are mobile and no fixed attachment exists. It is also possible for a muscle to contract isometrically and have both attachments stay fixed, in which case no mobile attachment exists. Furthermore, some muscles have more than two attachments. Viewing a muscle as having two attachments (with one attachment fixed and one attachment mobile when it contracts) is the typical scenario.

The roles of fixators and neutralizers are explored in more detail in the next four sections (15.5 through 15.8).

MUSCLE THAT IS WORKING:

- In our scenario of flexing fingers to make a fist, the muscle that is working is the concentrically contracting mover, the FDS.
- However, as we have learned, movers do not always contract. Sometimes they are relaxed, and it is the antagonist group that is working. Just like a mover that is working, when an antagonist is working, it can also create a pulling force that would create unwanted actions. When this occurs, unwanted actions of the antagonist would need to be stopped just as the unwanted actions of a mover would have to be stopped.
- Therefore the muscle that is working could either be a concentrically contracting mover or an eccentrically contracting antagonist.

ESSENTIAL FACTS:

- The muscle that is working is the muscle that is contracting. It is either a concentrically contracting mover or an eccentrically contracting antagonist.
- Fixators and neutralizers are similar in that they both stop unwanted actions that would occur because of the contraction of the muscle that is working.
- Fixators and neutralizers differ in that fixators stop unwanted actions that would occur at the *fixed* attachment of the muscle that is working; neutralizers stop unwanted actions that would occur at the *mobile* attachment of the muscle that is working.
- Fixators are also known as stabilizers.

SECTION 15.5 FIXATOR/STABILIZER MUSCLES

- A **fixator** is a muscle (or other force) that can stop an unwanted action at the fixed attachment of the muscle that is working.[1]
- A fixator is also known as a **stabilizer**.[1]
- We have seen that whether it is the mover or the antagonist that is contracting during our desired action in question, this muscle that is working can cause other joint actions to occur. These other joint actions may be unwanted, and therefore they need to be stopped. The role of a fixator is to stop these unwanted actions that occur at the *fixed attachment* of the muscle that is working.
- This is why the fixator is so named; it "fixes" one attachment in place so that it does not move.
- To determine which attachment of the working muscle is fixed, simply look at the action in question that is occurring. Whichever body part is named as moving is the mobile attachment; whichever body part is not moving is the fixed attachment.
  - For example, if the right levator scapulae is contracting and creating right lateral flexion of the neck at the spinal joints, then the mobile attachment is the neck (because it is moving) and the fixed attachment is the scapula (because it is not moving).
- Fixator muscles fix a body part by creating a contraction force that is equal in strength but opposite in direction to the force of the unwanted action of the muscle that is working. Because the fixator does this, the attachment that is being pulled on by both the muscle that is working and the fixator muscle cannot move in either direction.[1] (Note: In the example of making a fist in Section 15.4, the muscle that performed extension of the hand at the wrist created an extension force on the hand that was equal in strength [but opposite in direction] to the force of flexion of the hand at the wrist joint that the FDS created.)
- Because the attachment is fixed by the fixator muscle, the attachment does not move. If the attachment does not move, the fixator muscle does not change its length. Therefore fixator muscles isometrically contract when they fix body parts in place. Figures 15-4 to 15-6 provide examples of fixators.
- In Figure 15-4, we see a posterior view of the right levator scapulae muscle. If the levator scapulae muscle is the only muscle that contracts, it will create a pulling force on both the scapula and the neck. If we want only the neck to move, the actions of the right levator scapulae on the scapula have to be cancelled out (i.e., the scapula would have to be fixed so that it does not move).

Figure 15-4, *A* shows the right levator scapulae elevating the scapula at the scapulocostal (ScC) joint and also moving the neck at the spinal joints (the neck is being right laterally flexed, extended, and rotated to the right); hence both attachments of the levator scapulae are mobile. Figure 15-4, *B* shows the right lower trapezius contracting at the same time. The lower trapezius creates a force of depression on the scapula at the ScC joint that stops the scapula from elevating; therefore the scapula is fixed in place and only the neck moves. In this scenario the right lower trapezius is a fixator that cancels out an unwanted action (i.e., elevation of the right scapula) at the fixed attachment of the right levator scapulae.

- Note: Any muscle that can perform depression of the right scapula at the ScC joint would be a fixator in this scenario. The right lower trapezius shown in Figure 15-4 is simply the one chosen to illustrate this concept.
- Figure 15-5 is a lateral view of the right upper extremity with a weight in the hand. When the person does a bicep curl (i.e., flexes the forearm at the elbow joint) to lift the weight, the biceps brachii would also create a pulling force on the arm that would cause flexion of the arm at the glenohumeral (GH) joint. If we want just the forearm to move and not the arm, then the arm would have to be fixed from moving. The arm is fixed in place by a contraction of the posterior deltoid. In this scenario the posterior deltoid is a fixator, because it creates a force of extension of the arm at the GH joint that stops the biceps brachii from flexing the arm at the GH joint. (Note: Any muscle that performs extension of the right arm at the GH joint would be a fixator in this scenario. The posterior deltoid is the muscle that we happened to show in Figure 15-5 to illustrate this concept.)
- If the person were to be lowering the weight (i.e., extending the forearm at the elbow joint), gravity would be the mover and the biceps brachii would become an eccentrically contracting antagonist that would still create a flexion force on the arm at the GH joint. In this scenario the posterior deltoid would still contract as a fixator to keep the arm fixed.
- Whether the muscle that is working (i.e., the biceps brachii) is working as a mover or as an antagonist, a fixator muscle functions to cancel out its unwanted action at the attachment that is fixed. (Note: The biceps brachii can create other joint actions that would also need to be fixed from occurring.) They have

CHAPTER 15   Roles of Muscles   533

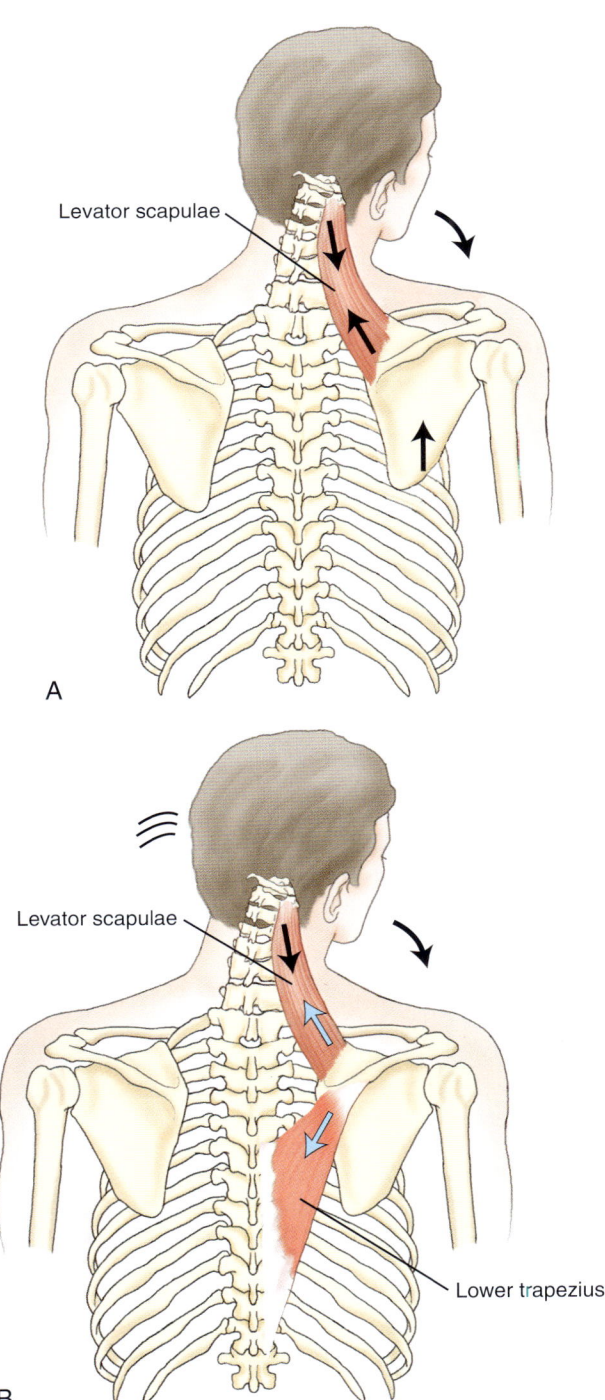

FIGURE 15-4 A, Right levator scapulae muscle contracts and creates a pulling force that moves both the scapula and the neck. **B,** Right lower trapezius is seen to contract as a fixator of the scapula by creating a force of depression on the scapula at the scapulocostal (ScC) joint that stops the levator scapulae from elevating the scapula. Because the right lower trapezius stops the scapula from moving (i.e., it fixes the scapula), the right lower trapezius is a fixator.

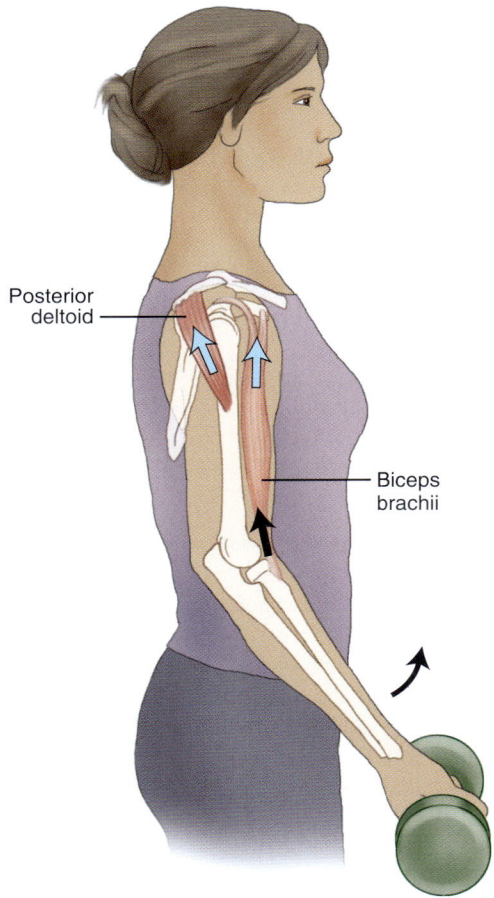

FIGURE 15-5 Right biceps brachii muscle contracts and creates a pulling force that could move both the forearm and the arm. The right posterior deltoid acts as a fixator of the arm by creating a force of extension on the arm at the GH joint that stops the biceps brachii from flexing the arm at the GH joint. Because the arm cannot move, it is fixed.

not been considered here; they were omitted to simplify the example. The biceps brachii can also supinate the forearm at the radioulnar (RU) joints, abduct and adduct the arm at the GH joint, and also move the scapula at the shoulder and ScC joints (this scapular motion is a reverse action if the forearm and arm are held fixed and the biceps brachii concentrically contracts).

○ Note: When we speak of a fixator working at the fixed attachment of the muscle that is working, we use the word *attachment* loosely. What is really being referred to is any *body part* that needs to be held fixed when the muscle contracts. For example, in Figure 15-5, the arm needs to be fixed when the biceps brachii contracts. However, the biceps brachii does not actually attach onto the humerus of the arm; it attaches to the scapula and the forearm. However, because the biceps brachii crosses the shoulder joint and would cause movement of the arm, the arm needs to be fixed.

○ Figure 15-6 is a lateral view of the tensor fasciae latae muscle. When it contracts, it could potentially move both the thigh at the hip joint and the pelvis at the hip joint. If we want just the thigh to move, the pelvis must be fixed. For the pelvis to be fixed from moving, we see that the rectus abdominis is contracting as a fixator. The rectus abdominis creates a force of posterior tilt

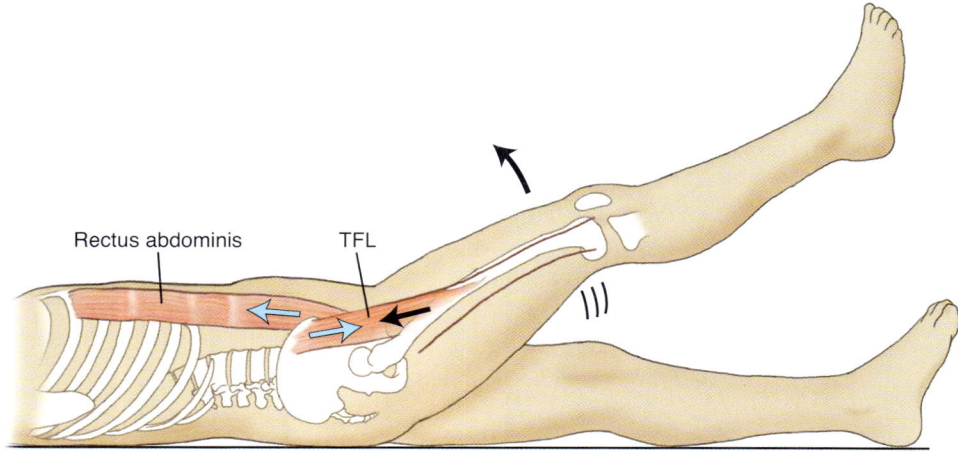

FIGURE 15-6 Right tensor fasciae latae (TFL) muscle contracts and creates a pulling force that could move both the thigh and the pelvis. The rectus abdominis acts as a fixator of the pelvis by creating a force of posterior tilt on the pelvis that stops the TFL from anteriorly tilting the pelvis. Because the pelvis cannot move, it is fixed. *(Modeled from Neumann DA: Kinesiology of the musculoskeletal system: foundations for physical rehabilitation, ed 2, St Louis, 2010, Mosby.)*

of the pelvis; this stops the tensor fasciae latae from anteriorly tilting the pelvis.
○ Any muscle that can perform posterior tilt of the pelvis would be a possible fixator in this scenario.
○ In these examples of fixators it is important to emphasize that, similar to the idea that many possible movers or antagonists can contract when a joint action occurs, many possible fixators can contract to fix the fixed attachment of the muscle that is working. For example, in Figure 15-5, we showed the posterior deltoid as the fixator. Theoretically, we could have chosen any extensor of the arm at the GH joint, such as the latissimus dorsi, the teres major, or the long head of the triceps brachii. However, cases exist in which the contraction of a certain fixator might make more sense than another. For example, in Figure 15-5, contraction of the long head of the triceps brachii would not be an efficient fixator because it is also an antagonist to the action in question (i.e., it extends the forearm at the elbow joint that opposes flexion of the forearm to lift the weight). Therefore even though the long head of the triceps brachii would accomplish its fixation task, it would also oppose the action that we do want. It is more likely that the body would choose the posterior deltoid or the teres major instead.
○ Just as movers and antagonists are not always muscles, fixator forces do not always need to be muscles. Any external force can be a fixator. In fact, the external force of gravity is an extremely common fixation force.[3]
○ For example, when the brachialis contracts and the forearm flexes at the elbow joint instead of the reverse action of the arm flexing at the elbow joint, the reason the forearm tends to move instead of the arm is that the forearm is lighter than the arm (plus if the arm moved, the weight of the trunk would also have to be moved, because the trunk would have to move with the arm). Weight is a factor of the force of gravity. Therefore gravity acts as a fixator, fixing the arm so that the forearm moves instead.
○ Figures 15-4 to 15-6 are three examples of fixators working. Given that a reverse action of a muscle is always theoretically possible, theoretically a fixator force always exists in every instance of a *working* muscle that contracts; the fixator force is working to hold one attachment fixed and stop the reverse action from occurring. The examples in Figures 15-4 to 15-6 were chosen because they are a relatively straightforward way to help the new student understand the concept of fixators. Seeing the fixator in some scenarios can be more challenging than seeing it in others.
○ The concept of the terminology system of naming the heavier more proximal attachment of a muscle as the *origin* and naming the lighter more distal attachment as the *insertion* is primarily based on the heavier proximal attachment being relatively less likely to move than the lighter distal attachment. In other words, the force of gravity acts as a fixator force that tends to stop movement of the heavier proximal attachment of the muscle.
○ In the terminology system of origin and insertion, fixator muscles work at the origin (Box 15-5).

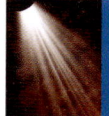

BOX 15-5 Spotlight on Reverse Actions

The use of the term *reverse action* is also based on the concept of the fixation force of gravity. A reverse action describes when the proximal attachment (which is less likely to move because of the fixation force of gravity) moves instead of the distal attachment (which would be more likely to move because less fixation force by gravity exists). When this occurs, a reverse action is said to occur and the origin and insertion of the muscle switch. That is, what is usually called the origin is now the insertion because it moves, and what is usually called the insertion is now the origin because it stays fixed. If the origin of a muscle is strictly defined as the attachment that does not move (whether it is the heavier proximal one or the lighter distal one), then we can say that fixators always work at the origin of a muscle.

ESSENTIAL FACTS:

○ A fixator is a muscle (or other force) that can stop an unwanted action at the fixed attachment of the muscle that is working.
○ Fixators are also known as *stabilizers*.
○ By definition, when a fixator muscle contracts, it contracts isometrically.
○ In the terminology system of origin/insertion, fixator muscles work at the origin.

SECTION 15.6 CONCEPT OF FIXATION AND CORE STABILIZATION

- Muscles in the body are often divided into two general categories:
  1. Mobility muscles
  2. Postural stabilization muscles

MOBILITY MUSCLES:

- **Mobility muscles** tend to be larger, longer, more superficial muscles.[3]
- These muscles are important primarily for their ability to concentrically contract and create large joint movements.
- Therefore during any particular action in question, the mobility muscles would tend to be the movers of the joint action.
- Although antagonists do not *create* motion, they do act to modify motion that is created by other mover forces such as gravity. In that role, antagonist muscles can also be considered to be mobility muscles.
- Mobility muscles tend to be composed of a greater percentage of white fiber fast-twitch motor units. This fiber type is best suited for motions that need to occur but are not held for long periods of time.[2]
- Mobility muscles are often called **phasic muscles**.[9]

POSTURAL STABILIZATION MUSCLES:

- **Postural stabilization muscles** tend to be smaller, deeper muscles that are located close to joints.[3]
- These muscles are important primarily for their ability to isometrically contract and hold the posture of joints fixed while mobility muscles perform their actions.
- Therefore during any particular action in question, the postural stabilization muscles would be the fixators (remember that the term *fixator* is synonymous with the term *stabilizer*), stopping unwanted movement of the fixed attachments of the muscles that are working.
- Postural stabilization muscles tend to be composed of a greater percentage of red fiber slow-twitch motor units. This fiber type is best suited for endurance contractions that need to occur to hold a muscle attachment fixed for longer periods of time.[2]
- Because more proximal attachments usually need to stay fixed as more distal attachments are moved, postural stabilizer muscles

BOX 15-6

Smaller, deeper postural stabilizer muscles have often been overlooked by people who exercise and work out. Perhaps one of the reasons is that they are smaller and deeper and do not directly show when a person tones the body. Furthermore, because they do not directly contribute appreciable strength to the joint action that is occurring, it is easy to discount them. However, these underappreciated muscles may very well be more important to the health and efficiency of the body than the larger, more visible mobility muscles. When exercising, it is important to work the smaller, deeper core stabilization muscles, as well the larger, more superficial mobility muscles.

BOX 15-7

One of the major tenets of the **Pilates method** of body conditioning (developed by Joseph Pilates) is to strengthen what is referred to as the **powerhouse** of the body. Essentially, the powerhouse equates to the core of the body. Through exercises that are primarily designed to isometrically tone the core powerhouse muscles and to create efficient coordination of these postural stabilization powerhouse muscles with mobility muscles, Pilates creates a stronger, healthier, more efficient body.

are often referred to as **core stabilizers**—the term *core* referring to the proximal core of the body (i.e., the axial body and pelvis).
- When a number of muscles are ordered to contract for a particular joint motion, there is usually an order to the contraction of the muscles, some being ordered to contract slightly earlier than others. Generally, postural stabilization muscles tend to be engaged to contract slightly earlier than mobility muscles so that the joint is stabilized before powerful muscle contraction forces are placed on it (Box 15-6).
- Postural stabilization muscles are often termed **tonic muscles**.[9]
- This concept of core stabilization (Box 15-7) is crucial to the functioning and health of the body for two reasons[10]:
  1. Core stabilization creates stronger and more efficient movements.
  2. Core stabilization is important for the health of the spine.

HOW DOES CORE STABILIZATION CREATE STRONGER AND MORE EFFICIENT MOVEMENTS OF OUR BODY?

- Whenever a muscle concentrically contracts, it pulls toward its center and exerts a pulling force on both of its attachments. If we desire one of the attachments to move powerfully and efficiently, then the other attachment must stay fixed, because any part of the pulling force of the muscle that is allowed to move the attachment that is supposed to stay fixed will diminish the strength of the pulling force on the mobile attachment that we want to move. This will lessen the strength and efficiency of the joint movement. Because we often want to move our extremities relative to our axial body, it is essential that we stabilize our core axial body so that all the strength of the muscle's contraction goes toward moving the body parts of the upper and/or lower extremities and is not lost on unwanted movement of our core.
- For example, if we contract hip flexor musculature with the intention of flexing the thigh at the hip joint while exercising, then any anterior tilt of the pelvis that is allowed to occur by this *hip flexor* musculature will decrease the strength with which our thigh can move into flexion (hip flexor musculature is also pelvic anterior tilt musculature). Therefore strong abdominals help to hold the pelvis posturally stabilized (i.e., fixed) so that the thigh may move more powerfully and efficiently. In this scenario, abdominals are acting as postural stabilizer muscles (Figure 15-7).

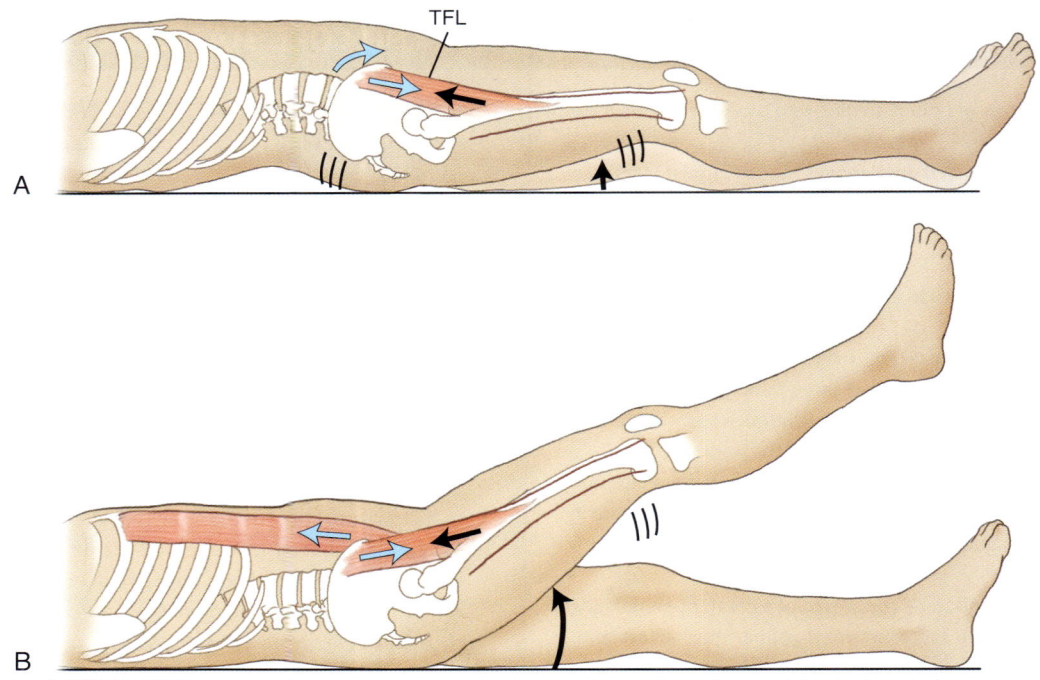

FIGURE 15-7 A, Tensor fasciae latae (TFL) contracting and creating both flexion of the thigh at the hip joint and anterior tilt of the pelvis at the hip joint. **B,** Pelvis is fixed by the rectus abdominis. Because some of the pulling force of the TFL's contraction went toward moving the pelvis in A, the thigh does not flex as much as it does in B, when all the pulling force went toward moving the thigh. *(Modeled from Neumann DA: Kinesiology of the musculoskeletal system: foundations for physical rehabilitation, ed 2, St Louis, 2010, Mosby.)*

HOW DOES CORE STABILIZATION CREATE A HEALTHIER SPINE?

- Apart from the concept of strength and efficiency, core stabilization can help to maintain a healthier spine by diminishing unwanted excessive motions of the spine. Excessive use of a joint in time leads to overuse, misuse, and abuse; the result would be a degenerated osteoarthritic spine.[3]
- For example, if we intend to move our arm into flexion or abduction, both of which require the coupled action of upward rotation of the scapula at the scapulocostal (ScC) joint, a pull will be exerted on the spine as the upper trapezius contracts (as an upward rotator of the scapula at the ScC joint). (Note: For information on the coupled actions of the arm and shoulder girdle, see Section 10.6.) If the smaller deeper postural stabilizer muscles of the vertebrae of the spine do not contract to hold the position of the vertebrae fixed, the vertebrae will be moved with these movements of the arm. When we think of how often the arm is lifted forward and/or to the side (i.e., flexion and/or abduction) during activities of daily life, let alone sports activities, the accumulation of stress that would be placed on the spine by these repetitive motions would eventually create degenerative osteoarthritic changes. The smaller deeper spinal muscles such as the multifidus, rotatores, interspinales, and intertransversarii are crucial to posturally stabilizing (i.e., fixing) the core (i.e., the spine in scenarios such as this) (Figure 15-8).
- Although it can be helpful to examine the muscles of the body in their roles as mobility muscles and postural stabilizer muscles, it is important to keep in mind that these two groups of muscles must always work together. The proper coordination of these two roles is essential for efficient motion and stability of the body!

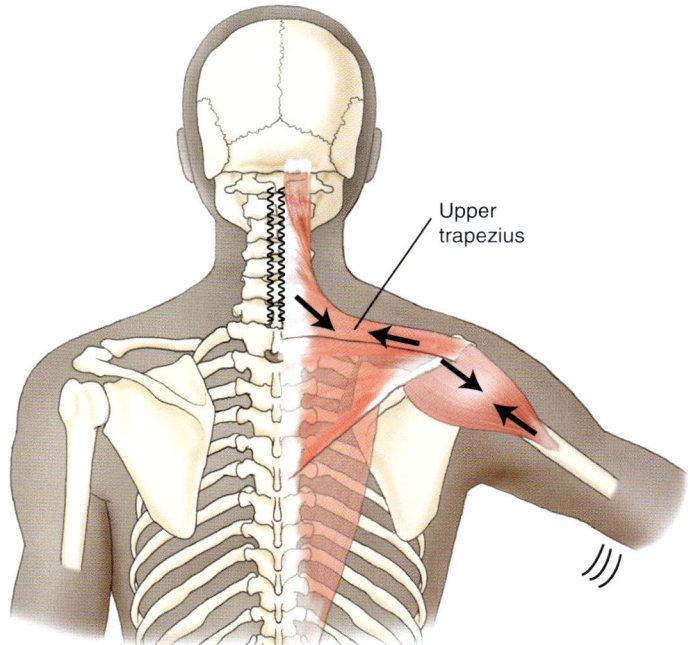

FIGURE 15-8 A person lifts the right arm up into abduction at the glenohumeral joint. This action requires the coupled action of upward rotation of the scapula at the scapulocostal (ScC) joint; the right upper trapezius is seen contracting to create this coupled action. We also see that the upper trapezius creates a pulling force on its spinal attachment. If the vertebrae are not well stabilized (i.e., fixed), then the vertebrae will be moved every time the arm abducts. These repetitive motions can lead to degenerative osteoarthritic changes of the spine over time.

CHAPTER 15 Roles of Muscles

SECTION 15.7 NEUTRALIZER MUSCLES

- A **neutralizer** is a muscle (or other force) that can stop an unwanted action at the mobile attachment of the muscle that is working.[1]
- We have seen that whether a mover or antagonist contracts during our desired action in question, it can cause other joint actions to occur. These other joint actions may be unwanted and therefore need to be stopped.
- The role of a neutralizer is to stop these unwanted actions that occur at the *mobile attachment* of the muscle that is working.[1]
- To determine which attachment of the working muscle is mobile, simply look at the action in question that is occurring. Whichever body part is moving during the action in question is the mobile attachment.
  - For example, if the right levator scapulae is contracting and creating right lateral flexion of the neck at the spinal joints, then the mobile attachment is the neck because it is moving (and the fixed attachment is the scapula because it is not moving).
- When the muscle that is working contracts and creates a desired action of the mobile attachment, that desired action occurs within one of the three cardinal planes. However, the muscle that is contracting might also create an unwanted motion of the mobile attachment in another plane. It is the unwanted action that occurs in this other plane that is stopped by a neutralizer muscle.
- Three cardinal planes (sagittal, frontal, and transverse) exist. Assuming that the *desired* action occurs in one of those three planes, then there could be one or two *unwanted* actions that would occur in one or both of the other two planes that a neutralizer muscle or neutralizer muscles would have to stop.
- Neutralizer muscles stop an unwanted action of a mobile body part by creating a contraction force that is equal in strength but opposite in direction to the force of the unwanted action of the muscle that is working.[1] By doing this, the neutralizer muscle stops the mobile attachment's unwanted action within that plane.
- Because the mobile attachment does not move within that plane, the neutralizer muscle does not change its length within that plane; therefore some sources state that neutralizers isometrically contract. However, the neutralizer muscle may change its length within another plane; this means it does not necessarily stay the same length and therefore does not necessarily contract isometrically.
- If a neutralizer muscle is neutralizing an unwanted action of a mover, even though it does not change its length in the plane of the action that it is stopping, it may shorten in the plane of the motion that is occurring at the mobile attachment of the mover. In this case the neutralizer can concentrically contract and shorten. If the neutralizer muscle is neutralizing an unwanted action of an antagonist instead (remember, the muscle that is working can be an antagonist), the same reasoning applies, except that now the neutralizer might be eccentrically contracting and lengthening overall.

Figures 15-9 and 15-10 provide examples of neutralizers.

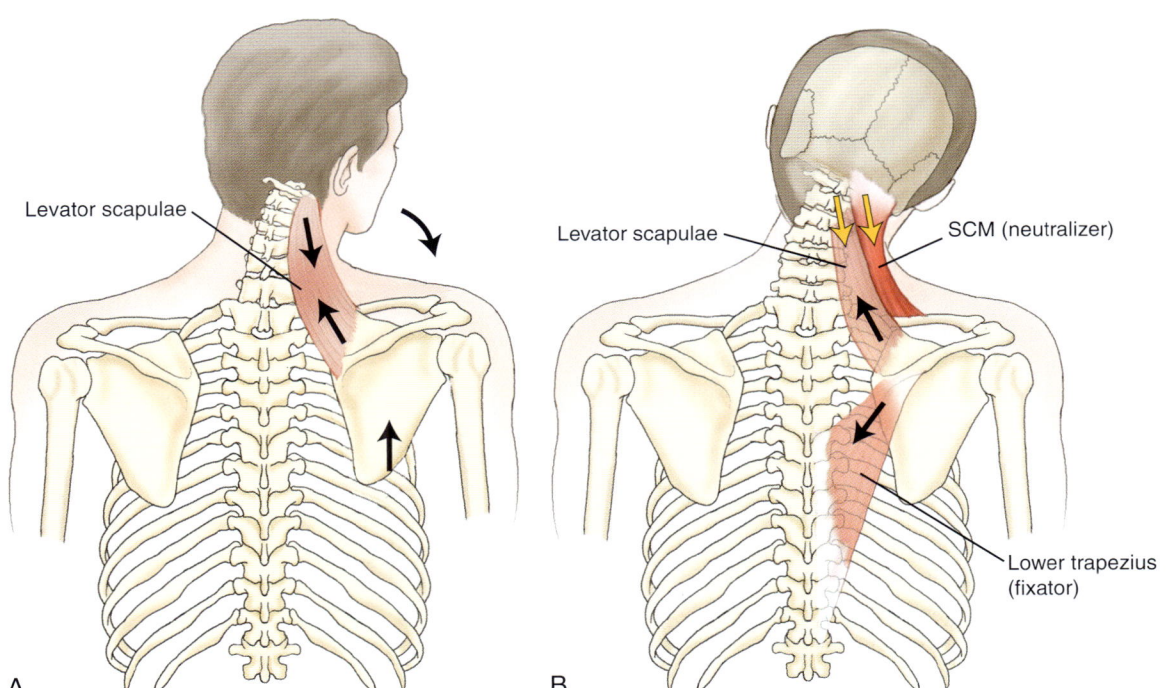

FIGURE 15-9 A, Right levator scapulae muscle is contracting and moving the neck into right lateral flexion, extension, and right rotation. **B,** Right sternocleidomastoid (SCM) is also contracting. The right SCM is a neutralizer of the neck, because it creates a force of flexion on the neck at the spinal joints that stops the right levator scapulae from extending the neck, and it creates a force of left rotation of the neck at the spinal joints that stops the right levator scapulae from rotating the neck to the right. (Note: In *B,* the right lower trapezius is also seen contracting as a fixator.)

538   PART 4   Myology: Study of the Muscular System

right sternocleidomastoid happened to be a neutralizer for both of them. We could have chosen two separate neutralizers, one for each of these two actions. Any muscle that could perform flexion of the neck at the spinal joints and any muscle that could perform left rotation of the neck at the spinal joints would potentially be a neutralizer in this example.

- In Figure 15-10, we see an anteromedial view of the right biceps brachii muscle. In this illustration, the right biceps brachii is contracting, and the only joint action that is occurring is flexion of the forearm at the elbow joint. (Note: We are considering the arm to be fixed in this scenario; see Section 15.5, Figure 15-5.) However, the biceps brachii can also supinate the forearm (at the radioulnar [RU] joints), which is its mobile attachment. If supination is not canceled out (i.e., neutralized), it would occur. Although any pronator could do this, the pronator teres is shown in Figure 15-10 as the neutralizer. By creating a force of pronation of the forearm at the RU joints, the pronator teres stops the biceps brachii from supinating the forearm at the RU joints; therefore the pronator teres is a neutralizer.
- In Figure 15-11, the right upper trapezius and left upper trapezius muscles contract as movers to extend the neck and head at the spinal joints (in the sagittal plane). However, they would also create unwanted actions in the frontal and transverse planes as well. These unwanted actions do not occur because each upper trapezius cancels out these unwanted actions of the other upper trapezius. In the frontal plane the right lateral flexion of the right upper trapezius is neutralized by the left lateral

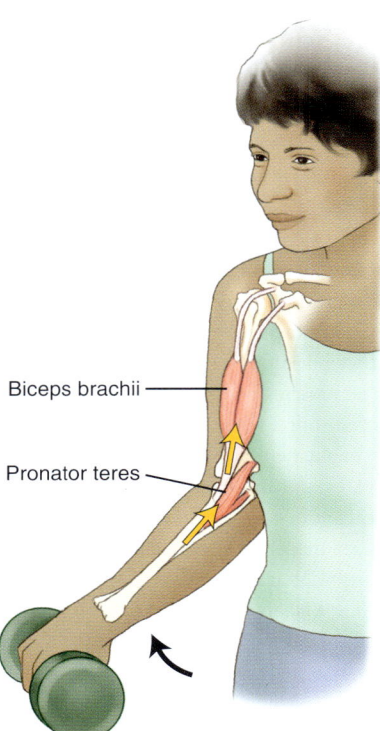

FIGURE 15-10 Biceps brachii is contracting as a mover of flexion of the forearm at the elbow joint; therefore the forearm is its mobile attachment. The biceps brachii should also supinate the forearm (at the radioulnar [RU] joints) because this is another one of its actions. In this illustration, the pronator teres is a neutralizer, because it creates a force of pronation of the forearm at the RU joints that cancels out supination of the forearm at the RU joints by the biceps brachii.

- In Figure 15-9, *A* we see a posterior view of the right levator scapulae muscle. In this illustration, the right levator scapulae is contracting and causing the neck to right laterally flex, extend, and rotate to the right (note: the scapula would also move if not fixed by a fixator, as was explained in Section 15-5, Figure 15-4). If we want the neck to only right laterally flex, then the other two actions of the right levator scapulae must be stopped. In Figure 15-9, *B* we see that the right sternocleidomastoid (SCM) is contracting as a neutralizer to stop these other two undesired actions of the right levator scapulae. The right SCM creates a force of flexion of the neck that cancels out the extension force of the right levator scapulae; and the right SCM creates a force of left rotation of the neck that cancels out the right rotation force of the right levator scapulae. As a result, the neck can only right laterally flex at the spinal joints. In this scenario, the right SCM is a neutralizer because it cancels out unwanted actions at the mobile attachment of the muscle that is contracting, the right levator scapulae. (Note: The right lower trapezius acting as a fixator is also seen.)
- Note: To be a neutralizer, a muscle need cancel only one unwanted action of the muscle that is working. In the example in Figure 15-9, there happened to be two unwanted actions at the mobile attachment of the muscle that was working, and the

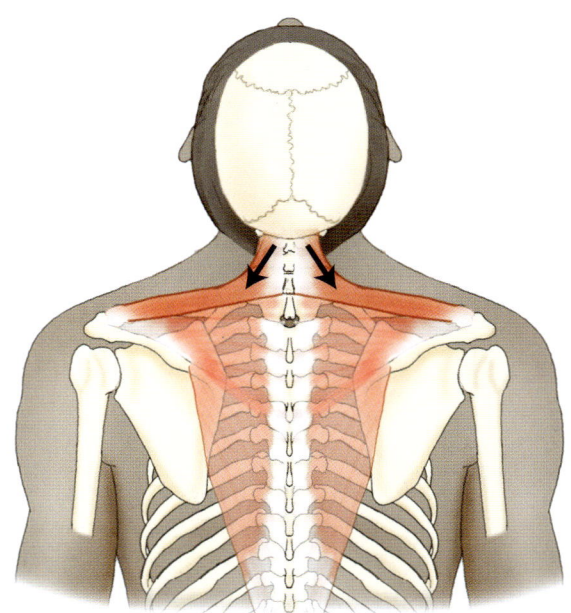

FIGURE 15-11 Right and left upper trapezius muscles are both contracting to cause the action in question (i.e., extension of the head and neck at the spinal joint); therefore they are both movers. They also both act as neutralizers, canceling out each other's frontal and transverse plane actions (i.e., lateral flexion and rotation actions) of the head and neck at the spinal joints.

flexion of the left upper trapezius; and the left lateral flexion of the left upper trapezius is neutralized by the right lateral flexion of the right upper trapezius. In the transverse plane the left rotation of the right upper trapezius is neutralized by the right rotation of the left upper trapezius; and the right rotation of the left upper trapezius is neutralized by the left rotation of the right upper trapezius. Therefore these two movers act as neutralizers of each other's unwanted actions, and only the desired action of pure extension of the head and neck at the spinal joints results.

- In these examples of neutralizers, it is important to emphasize that similar to the idea that many possible movers, antagonists, or fixators can contract when a joint action occurs, there may be many possible neutralizers that will contract as well. In Figure 15-10, we showed the pronator teres as the neutralizer. Theoretically, we could have chosen a different pronator of the forearm at the RU joints, such as the pronator quadratus.
- It should also be recognized that a neutralizer is not always present in every given scenario. If no undesired action at the mobile attachment of the muscle that is working takes place, then there will not be a neutralizer. For example, if the muscle that is working is creating the action in question at a uniaxial joint, then no undesired actions are possible.
- Just as movers, antagonists, and fixators are not always muscles, neutralizer forces do not always need to be muscles. Any external force such as gravity can be a neutralizer.
  - For example, when a person is in anatomic position and the anterior deltoid contracts, causing the arm to medially rotate at the shoulder joint but not abduct and/or flex (its other two actions), part of the reason is that to abduct or flex, the arm would have to be lifted up against the force of gravity. In this instance, with a weak contraction by the anterior deltoid, gravity would tend to stop (i.e., neutralize) these upward motions of the arm of abduction and flexion. Of course, if the contraction of the anterior deltoid were strong enough, enough force would be generated to move the arm upward into abduction and/or flexion; with this stronger contraction of the anterior deltoid, neutralizer muscles would then have to be recruited to fully stop these actions if they were unwanted.
- If the insertion is strictly defined as the attachment of a muscle that does move (regardless of which attachment it is [i.e., the lighter distal one that usually does move or the heavier proximal one that usually does not move]), then we can say that neutralizers always work at the insertion of a muscle.

MUTUAL NEUTRALIZERS:

- Two muscles that are both movers (or both antagonists) of the action in question and neutralize each other's unwanted actions are called **mutual neutralizers**.[10] Mutual neutralizers are actually very common. In every pair (right and left sided) of axial body muscles (e.g., right and left trapezius, right and left sternocleidomastoid), the muscles act as mutual neutralizers to each other when they both contract. They cancel out whatever frontal and/or transverse plane motions they each have, and the result is a pure sagittal plane motion (either flexion or extension depending on the muscle) (see Figure 15-11). Although this is the most common example, a set of mutual neutralizers does not have to consist of the same pair of muscles. Another example is the TFL and sartorius. Although they are both movers of flexion of the thigh at the hip joint in the sagittal plane, they cancel out each other's transverse plane motions (the TFL is a medial rotator of the thigh at the hip joint, and the sartorius is a lateral rotator of the thigh at the hip joint).

ESSENTIAL FACTS:

- A neutralizer is a muscle (or other force) that can stop an unwanted action at the mobile attachment of the muscle that is working.
- In the terminology system of origin/insertion, neutralizer muscles work at the insertion.

SECTION 15.8 STEP-BY-STEP METHOD FOR DETERMINING FIXATORS AND NEUTRALIZERS

- Once the concept of how fixator and neutralizer muscles work in the body is fully understood, figuring out possible fixators and neutralizers can be reasoned out; however, like all aspects of knowledge, getting to the point of *full* understanding is a work in progress as we gradually see things in increasing layers of depth and clarity. For some students, determining fixators and neutralizers takes a little more time. For that reason, the following rubric is offered. This rubric gives a step-by-step method for determining the fixators and neutralizers in any given scenario.
- To demonstrate the steps of this rubric, it is helpful to look at the following scenario: The right levator scapulae is contracting, and only right lateral flexion of the neck at the spinal joints is occurring (Figure 15-12; Box 15-8).
- Based on the steps of the rubric, the right lower trapezius was chosen as a fixator and the right sternocleidomastoid was chosen as a neutralizer (as used as examples in Section 15.5, Figure 15-4, and Section 15.7, Figure 15-9, respectively). Again, it is important to emphasize that other possible fixators and neutralizers could have been chosen. In addition, the right sternocleidomastoid happened to work as a neutralizer for both undesired actions of the mover at the mobile attachment (we could have chosen two different neutralizers instead, as long as they opposed the actions that needed to be cancelled at the mobile attachment). The exact fixators and neutralizers that the body chooses will vary from individual to individual and will also vary based on the needed strength of the fixators and neutralizers.

540 PART 4 Myology: Study of the Muscular System

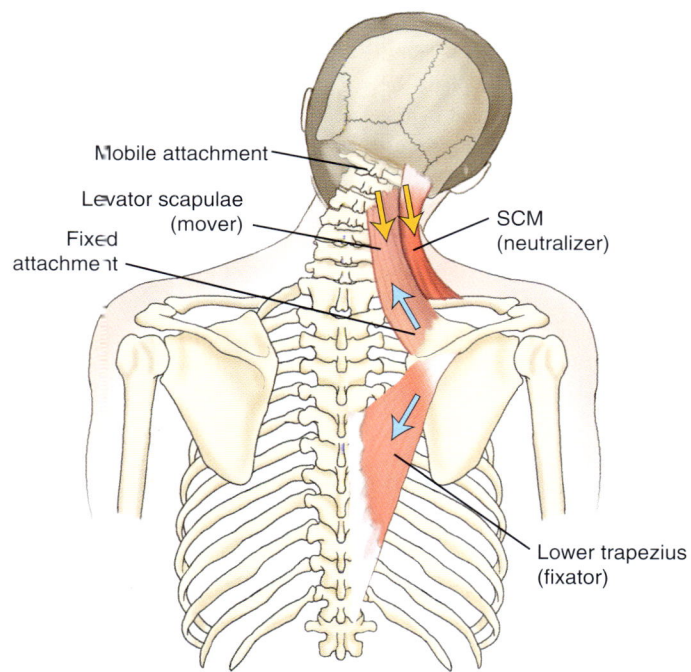

FIGURE 15-12 Right levator scapulae is contracting, and the only joint action that is occurring is right lateral flexion of the neck at the spinal joints. In this scenario the right lower trapezius is a fixator, stopping the right levator scapulae from elevating the right scapula at the scapulocostal joint, and the right sternocleidomastoid is a neutralizer, stopping the right levator scapulae from both extending the neck and rotating it to the right at the spinal joints.

BOX 15-8 Steps of the Rubric to Determine Fixators and Neutralizers (Using the Example Given in Figure 15-12)

Step 1: Determine the action in question:
- Right lateral flexion of the neck at the spinal joints

Step 2: Determine the muscle that is working and its role:
- Right levator scapulae; it is a mover

Step 3: Determine which attachment is the fixed attachment and which attachment is the mobile attachment (mobile attachment is whichever attachment is moving in the action in question):
- Fixed attachment: scapula
- Mobile attachment: neck

Step 4: List all actions of the muscle that is working (i.e., the right levator scapulae), and state whether each action is the desired action or an undesired action; furthermore, state if the undesired actions occur at the fixed or mobile attachment and what muscle role stops each undesired action:
- Right lateral flexion of the neck at the spinal joints (desired action—do not stop)
- Elevation of the right scapula at the scapulocostal (ScC) joint (undesired action at the fixed attachment—stop with a fixator)
- Extension of the neck at the spinal joints (undesired action at the mobile attachment—stop with a neutralizer)
- Right rotation of the neck at the spinal joints (undesired action at the mobile attachment—stop with a neutralizer)

Step 5: Determine the action of each fixator at the fixed attachment (i.e., the scapula); it will be the opposite action of the undesired action at the fixed attachment:
- Depression of the right scapula at the ScC joint

Step 6: Choose a muscle that can do the action determined for each fixator:
- Right lower trapezius (any muscle that performs depression of the right scapula is a fixator)

Step 7: Determine the action of each neutralizer at the mobile attachment (i.e., the neck). It will be the opposite action of the undesired action at the mobile attachment:
- Flexion of the neck at the spinal joints
- Left rotation of the neck at the spinal joints

Step 8: Choose a muscle that can do the action determined for each neutralizer:
- Right sternocleidomastoid (any muscle that performs flexion of neck is a neutralizer)
- Right sternocleidomastoid (any muscle that performs left rotation of neck is a neutralizer)

SECTION 15.9 SUPPORT MUSCLES

- A **support muscle** is a muscle (or other force) that can hold another part of the body in position while the action in question is occurring.[10]
- Unlike movers, antagonists, fixators, and neutralizers, support muscles do not work directly at the site of the action in question.
- The role of a support muscle is to hold *another* body part in position while the action in question is occurring. Therefore support muscles often work far from the joint where the action in question is occurring.
- Support muscles usually work against gravity, in other words, they keep a body part from falling down.[10]
- They do this by creating a contraction force that is equal in strength but opposite in direction to the force that gravity exerts on that body part. Because they do this, the body part that is being pulled downward by gravity does not fall (and the support muscle does not contract so hard that the body part is moved upward, either).
- Because the body part is held in place by the support muscle, it does not move. If the body part does not move, the support muscle does not change its length. Therefore support muscles isometrically contract when they hold body parts in place. Figures 15-13 and 15-14 provide examples of support muscles.
- In Figure 15-13, we see a person holding a heavy weight in her right hand at the side of her body. The action in question is flexion of the right forearm at the elbow joint as she does a bicep curl. However, given the presence of this heavy weight on her right side, her trunk would be pulled to the right and fall into right lateral flexion at the spinal joints if it were not for the isometric contraction of her left paraspinal musculature. The left paraspinal musculature creates a force of left lateral flexion that counters gravity's force of right lateral flexion on the trunk. The left paraspinal musculature supports and holds the trunk in position while the action in question (i.e., flexion of the right forearm) occurs elsewhere; therefore the left paraspinal musculature is a support muscle in this scenario.
- Figure 15-14 shows a person typing at a keyboard. The action in question is the motion of the fingers as they hit the keys. However, in this position, notice that the person has his arms abducted at the glenohumeral (GH) joints away from his body. This requires his arm abductor musculature to isometrically contract to hold this position of arm abduction so that his arms do not fall into adduction. These arm abductors are support muscles because they support the arms in position while the action in question (occurring at the fingers) is being carried out. (Note: This scenario illustrates an example of someone who has poor ergonomic posture and as a result stresses his musculature, in this case his muscles of arm abduction at the GH joint. If this person were to relax and let his arms rest at his sides, his posture and health would be improved.)
- In these examples of support muscles it is important to note that, similar to the idea that many possible movers or antagonists can contract when a joint action occurs, many possible support muscles can contract to hold another body part in position. For example, in Figure 15-13, we showed the left paraspinal musculature as the support muscle. Theoretically, we could have

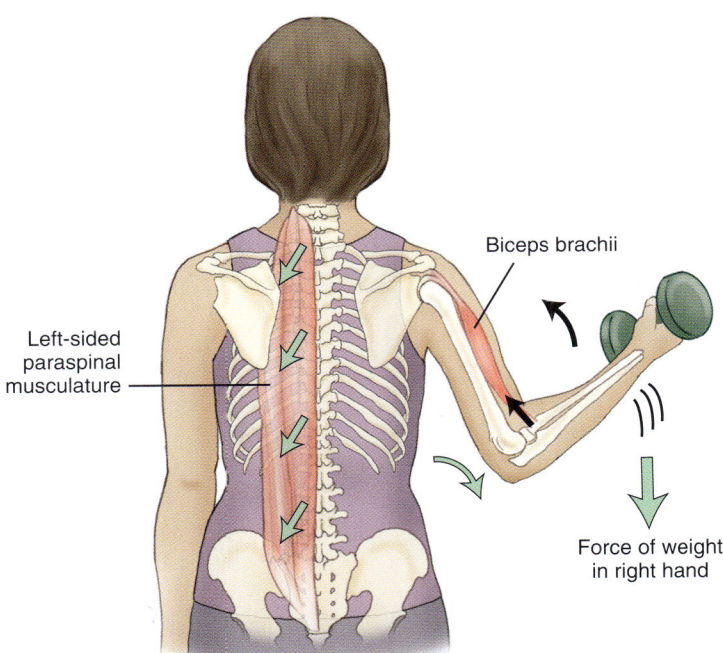

FIGURE 15-13 As this person lifts a weight out to the right side of the body, the presence of the heavy weight on her right side creates a force that would pull her trunk into right lateral flexion at the spinal joints. Muscles of left lateral flexion of the trunk (the left paraspinal musculature is shown) contract isometrically as support muscles to hold the trunk in position so that it does not fall into right lateral flexion.

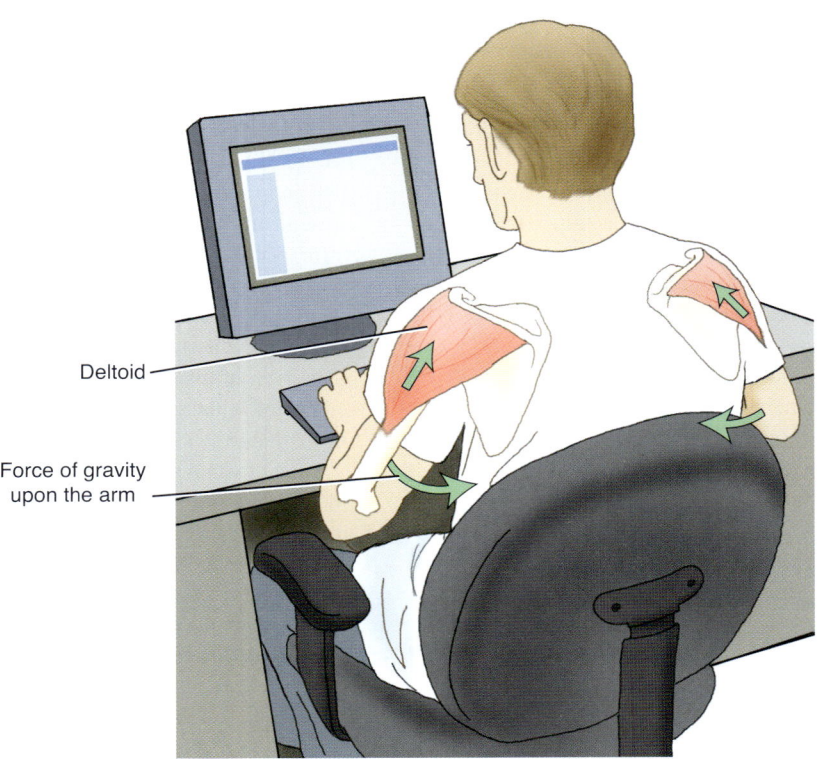

FIGURE 15-14 Person typing at a keyboard with the arms in a position of abduction. The abductor musculature of the glenohumeral joints are support muscles in this scenario because they isometrically contract to support and hold the arms abducted against gravity as the action in question (i.e., finger motion on the keyboard) occurs elsewhere.

chosen any left lateral flexor of the trunk at the spinal joints as the support muscle.
○ Support muscles are often overlooked because the focus of the activity is elsewhere. As a result, the client may have no idea that support muscles are being tremendously overworked and irritated (Box 15-9).

 BOX 15-9

Clinically, it is easy for the therapist/trainer to overlook an overused/abused support muscle. When we ask the client what activity he or she is engaging in that causes pain, unless we ask the client to actually show or explain the position of the entire body when the activity is done, we may miss the patterns of use of support muscles distant from the site of the activity itself. Clinically, support muscles usually stop body parts from letting gravity pull them down. This means that if one looks at the posture of the body with relation to gravity, any unbalanced body part that should fall because of gravity, yet is not falling, must be supported by muscular activity. The support musculature responsible for this should be evaluated. (See Sections 20.1 to 20.7 on posture for more on this topic.)

○ Just as movers, antagonists, fixators, and neutralizers are not always muscles, support forces do not always need to be muscles. Any external force that helps to hold a body part in position could be termed a *support*.
○ For example, a male ballet dancer who holds a ballerina in position during a dance performance would be a support force. External objects may also act as a support. For example, the headrest of a car, which supports the head of the driver as he or she leans the head back against it, is a support.

ESSENTIAL FACTS:

○ A support muscle is a muscle (or other force) that can hold another part of the body in position while the action in question is occurring.
○ Support muscles do not work directly at the joint where the action in question is occurring; they work on another body part at a distant joint.
○ Support muscles usually oppose the force of gravity on a body part.
○ By definition, when a support muscle contracts, it contracts isometrically.

SECTION 15.10 SYNERGISTS

- A **synergist** is a muscle (or other force) that *works with* a muscle that is contracting.[10]
- The word *synergist* literally means to *work with: syn* means *with; erg* means *work*.
- The term *synergist* can be defined two different ways.[1]
  1. Defined broadly, a synergist is any muscle other than the prime mover (or prime antagonist) that works (i.e., contracts) to help the joint action in question occur.
     - By this definition, a synergist could be any other mover or antagonist (whichever group is working), as well as any fixator, neutralizer, or support muscle.
  2. Defined narrowly, a synergist is any mover that contracts other than the prime mover or any antagonist that contracts other than the prime antagonist.
     - For example, because the iliopsoas is the prime mover of flexion of the thigh at the hip joint, when the thigh is flexing at the hip joint, any other flexor of the thigh at the hip joint that contracts to help create this joint action (e.g., tensor fasciae latae, rectus femoris) would be a synergist.
- When determining that a muscle is a synergist, it is important to always keep in mind that this term, like all the other terms for muscle roles, is relative to a particular joint action (i.e., the action in question).
- Confusion often arises when people describe a muscle as being a synergist (i.e., synergistic) to another muscle. It is more accurate to say that these two muscles are synergistic with regard to a particular joint action.
- The same concept is true for the term *antagonist*. An antagonist is antagonistic to a specific joint action, not to another muscle generally. The following two examples illustrate this point.

SYNERGIST/ANTAGONIST—EXAMPLE 1:
Biceps Brachii and Pronator Teres:
- Would the biceps brachii and the pronator teres be considered synergistic or antagonistic to each other (Figure 15-15, *A*)?
- The biceps brachii and the pronator teres both flex the forearm at the elbow joint in the sagittal plane; therefore they are

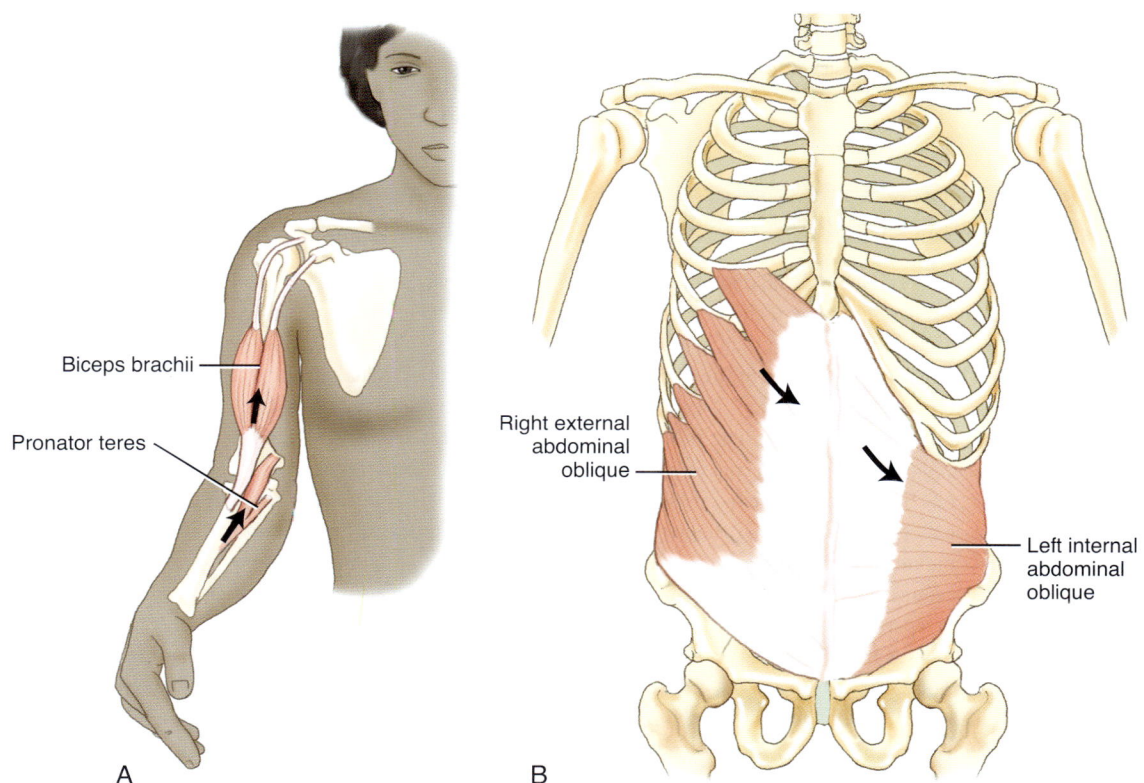

FIGURE 15-15 Illustration of the concept that two muscles are inherently neither synergistic nor antagonistic to each other. Being synergistic or antagonistic is determined relative to a specific plane of motion. **A,** Biceps brachii and pronator teres muscles. With respect to sagittal plane motion at the elbow joint, these two muscles are synergistic to each other, because they both flex the forearm at the elbow joint. However, with respect to transverse plane motion at the radioulnar (RU) joints, these two muscles are antagonistic to each other, because the biceps brachii performs supination and the pronator teres performs pronation. **B,** Right external abdominal oblique and left internal abdominal oblique muscles. With respect to sagittal and transverse plane motions at the spinal joints, these muscles are synergistic to each other, because they both flex and left rotate the trunk at the spinal joints. However, with respect to frontal plane motion at the spinal joints, these two muscles are antagonistic to each other, because the right external abdominal oblique performs right lateral flexion and the left internal abdominal oblique performs left lateral flexion of the trunk at the spinal joints.

synergists. However, the biceps brachii supinates the forearm at the radioulnar (RU) joints in the transverse plane, whereas the pronator teres pronates the forearm at the RU joints in the transverse plane; therefore they are antagonists.

○ For this reason, asking whether any two muscles are synergists or antagonists is not a valid question *unless we specify which action we are considering*. Two muscles may be synergistic with regard to one action in one plane, yet antagonistic with regard to another action in another plane.

SYNERGIST/ANTAGONIST—EXAMPLE 2:
Right External Abdominal Oblique and Left Internal Abdominal Oblique:

○ Would the right external abdominal oblique and the left internal abdominal oblique be considered synergistic or antagonistic to each other (see Figure 15-15, *B*)?

○ The right external abdominal oblique and the left internal abdominal oblique both flex the trunk at the spinal joints in the sagittal plane; therefore with respect to sagittal plane motion, they are synergistic to each other.

○ The right external abdominal oblique performs right lateral flexion of the trunk in the frontal plane, whereas the left internal abdominal oblique performs left lateral flexion of the trunk in the frontal plane. Therefore with respect to frontal plane motion, they are antagonistic to each other.

○ The right external abdominal oblique, being a contralateral rotator, performs left rotation of the trunk in the transverse plane; the left internal abdominal oblique, being an ipsilateral rotator, also performs left rotation of the trunk in the transverse plane. Therefore with respect to transverse plane motion, these two muscles are synergistic to each other.

○ As we can see, the right external abdominal oblique and the left internal abdominal oblique are inherently neither synergistic nor antagonistic to each other. Rather, they can only be considered to be synergistic or antagonistic to each other with respect to a specific joint action within a particular plane.

○ As with all roles of muscles, the roles of synergist and antagonist are relative to the action in question.

ESSENTIAL FACTS:

○ A synergist is a muscle (or other force) that *works with* the muscle that is contracting.

○ Defined broadly, a synergist is any muscle other than the prime mover (or prime antagonist) that works (i.e., contracts) to help the joint action in question occur.

○ Defined narrowly, a synergist is any mover that contracts other than the prime mover or any antagonist that contracts other than the prime antagonist.

SECTION 15.11   COORDINATING MUSCLE ROLES

○ Beginning kinesiology students often approach a joint action of the body with the question "What muscle performs this action?" This question presupposes that one specific muscle is responsible for each specific joint action that can occur in the body. Yet, as we can see, muscles rarely act in isolation.

○ First, among a functional group of movers, a number of muscles may contract for any given joint action. Depending on the strength needed for the contraction, one or more of them may contract.

○ If gravity or some other outside force is creating the action in question, then most likely the movers are not working, and it is the functional group of antagonists that is working to slow down and control the joint action. Depending on the antagonistic force needed, one or more antagonists will be ordered to contract.

○ For either functional group that is working, movers or antagonists, it is likely that the other attachment of each of the working muscles will need to be fixed for every unwanted action that would occur there. This will require functional groups of fixators to become involved and contract, and within each fixator group, a number of muscles can be ordered to contract.

○ In addition, for every unwanted action at the mobile attachment of each muscle that is working, functional groups of neutralizers would also have to be ordered to contract, and many of these can be ordered to work.

○ Beyond this, functional groups of support muscles are likely to be working elsewhere in the body to hold the posture of the body parts against gravity.

○ Thus we have muscles potentially contracting in five major roles[10]: (1) movers, (2) antagonists, (3) fixators, (4) neutralizers, and (5) support muscles.

○ Remember that a **muscle role** is defined as the role that the muscle plays relative to the action in question.[10]

○ A sixth term to describe a muscle role is *synergist*. (For more information on synergists, see Section 15.10.)

○ All of this is necessary for one simple joint action. When coupled actions or more complex movement patterns need to be executed simultaneously, the complexity of the co-ordering of all the muscles that must work seamlessly is multiplied many times.

  ○ It is the complexity of this co-ordering of muscles that defines coordination in the body. **Coordination** is defined as the co-ordering of muscles in the body in their various roles to create smooth and efficient movement.[4]

  ○ It is for this reason that humans spend years and decades becoming coordinated. In addition, when we consider dance and athletic performances at a higher level, we can spend our entire lives learning to master the most efficient coordination of the muscles involved.

○ A science exists to the kinesiology of our body, and this chapter provides the understanding and tools to help determine what muscles might be contracting, as well as when and for what reasons. However, we should never lose sight of the fact that an art also exists to the kinesiology of our body. The exact co-ordering

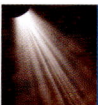

BOX 15-10 Spotlight on the Clinical Effects of Isometric Contractions

When it comes to clinical importance, the isometric contractions of fixators and support muscles are often more important than the concentric and eccentric contractions of movers, antagonists, and neutralizers. This is because of the effect of muscle contractions on blood supply. The strength of the heart's contraction is responsible for arterial circulation of blood to bring nutrients out to the tissues of the body. However, the heart is not able to pump the venous blood containing the waste products of metabolism from the tissues back to the heart. Instead, veins are dependent on muscle contractions to propel their blood back toward the heart. For this purpose, veins have thin collapsible walls with unidirectional valves that help to propel blood toward the heart when muscle contractions collapse them. Therefore alternating contractions and relaxation that naturally occur with concentric and eccentric contractions are necessary and valuable for venous circulation to eliminate the waste products of metabolism from the tissues. However, isometric contractions, by virtue of being sustained, close off these collapsible veins and keep them closed off for the entire length of the time that the isometric contraction is held, resulting in an interruption of venous blood circulation. This results in a buildup of toxic waste products in the tissues. The presence of these substances irritates the nerves in the region, which often results in further tightening of the muscles of the region via the pain-spasm-pain cycle (see Section 19.10). Furthermore, if the strength of the isometric contraction is great enough, even the arterial supply could be closed off, resulting in a loss of nutrients and further irritation to the tissue of the body that is fed by these arteries (loss of arterial blood supply is called **ischemia**). Therefore, based on the irritation to the muscles and other local tissues caused by the waste products of metabolism, and the possible ischemia, the clinical effects of sustained isometric contractions tend to be more important than the clinical effects of concentric and eccentric contractions. This is one more reason to look beyond the contractions of movers and antagonists and see the contractions of muscles in their other roles!

---

of muscles that may occur for any specific joint action or more complex movement pattern will vary from individual to individual. It is this diversity that accounts for the many ways that we may walk, talk, dance, run, play tennis, or create every other movement pattern that exists. Although certain patterns of coordination may be more efficient than others, no one exact pattern of coordinating muscles is right or wrong. Each person's coordination pattern is unique.

❍ From a clinical point of view, we must always remember that muscles that perform the actions that we learned when we first learned muscle actions (i.e., concentric shortening contractions of movers) are not the only muscles that work in our body. Unfortunately, initially learning muscles' actions only as concentric contractions tends to foster the rigid idea that muscles only shorten as movers when they contract. In reality, many other functional groups other than movers work in our body when we are physically active. Every muscle that works, regardless of its role in the movement, is a muscle that contracts and is used. In addition, if this same muscle is overused, it can become unhealthy and injured. Only when we have the ability to see beyond mover actions of muscles and realize the many roles that muscles can play in movement patterns will we be able to have the critical reasoning needed to be able to work effectively with clients in clinical and rehabilitative settings (Box 15-10). Figures 15-16 and 15-17 provide examples of the coordination of the many roles that muscles play in a joint action.

❍ Figure 15-16 shows the example that has been used throughout this chapter of a person doing a bicep curl at the right elbow joint. In this scenario the action in question is flexion of the right forearm at the elbow joint, and we see an example of each of the five muscle roles relative to this joint action.
  ❍ Mover: The biceps brachii is contracting as a mover to create flexion of the forearm at the elbow joint.
  ❍ Antagonist: If the weight were being lowered (i.e., the action was extension of the forearm at the elbow joint), then gravity would be the mover and the biceps brachii would eccentrically contract as an antagonist.
  ❍ Fixator: The posterior deltoid acts as a fixator, creating a force of extension of the arm at the glenohumeral (GH) joint, which stops the biceps brachii from flexing the arm at the GH joint (Box 15-11).

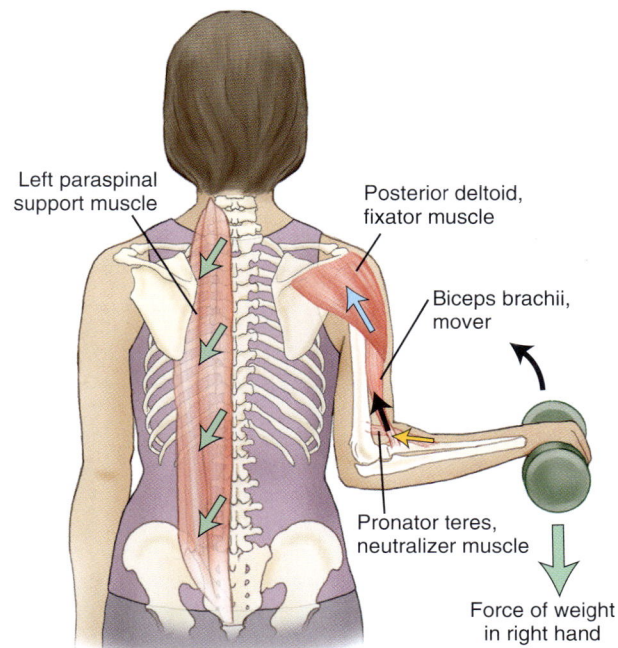

FIGURE 15-16 Person carrying out a simple joint action (i.e., flexion of the forearm at the elbow joint to do a bicep curl). The biceps brachii is seen as the mover of flexion of the forearm at the elbow joint (if the weight were being lowered, the biceps brachii would act as an antagonist instead). The posterior deltoid acts as a fixator of the arm at the GH joint. The pronator teres acts as a neutralizer of the forearm at the radioulnar (RU) joints. The left paraspinal musculature acts as a support muscle, holding the trunk in place.

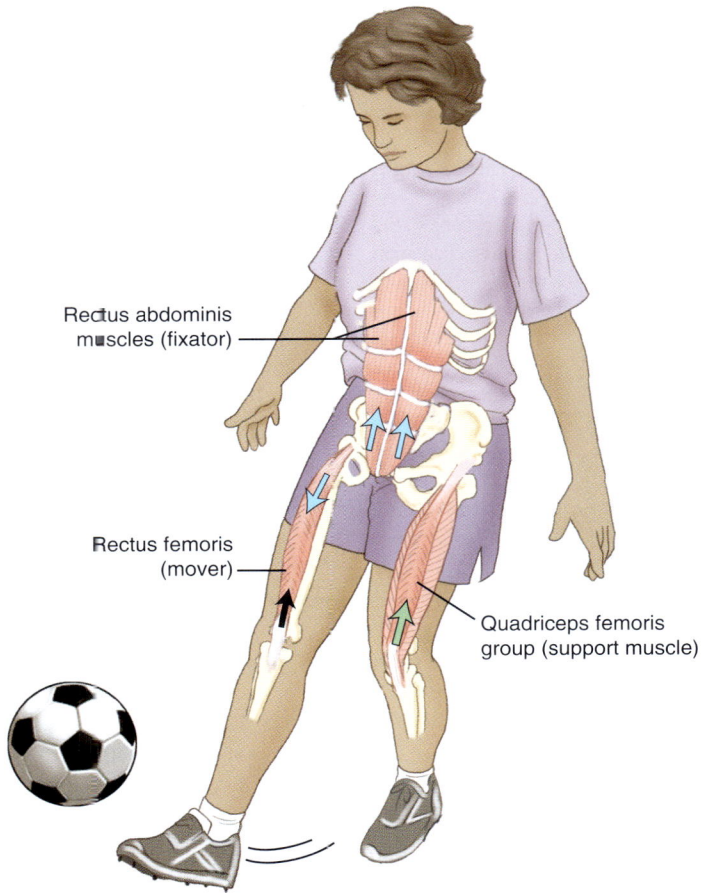

FIGURE 15-17 Person performing flexion of the right thigh at the hip joint to kick a soccer ball. The right rectus femoris of the quadriceps femoris group is seen as the mover of flexion of the right thigh at the hip joint. The rectus abdominis acts as a fixator of the pelvis. Because the rectus femoris has no undesired action on the thigh at the hip joint, no neutralizer exists. The left quadriceps femoris group acts as a support muscle, holding the left knee joint extended against the force of gravity that would otherwise flex it, causing the person to fall.

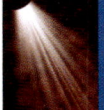 **BOX 15-11** **Spotlight on Second-Order Fixators**

Although a fixator stops the unwanted motion of the fixed attachment of a mover or antagonist (whichever one is working in that scenario), a **second-order fixator** is a fixator that contracts to fix an attachment of a fixator or neutralizer during a joint action.

Figure 15-16 illustrates muscles acting in all five roles relative to the action in question. However, even more muscles would be ordered to contract than are shown in Figure 15-16. For example, because the right posterior deltoid contracts as a fixator to stop the unwanted flexion of the arm, the pull of the right posterior deltoid on the scapula would cause downward rotation of the scapula at the scapulocostal (ScC) joint. We do not want this to occur, so the scapula would have to be fixed by a muscle that performs upward rotation; the muscle that does this is a fixator. However, because it is a fixator of a fixator, it is called a second-order fixator. To continue along this line of reasoning, if the upward rotator second-order fixator chosen by the body to contract is the right upper trapezius, then its other attachment on the head and neck may have to be fixed from extending, right laterally flexing, and left rotating by other second-order fixators. (Perhaps a better term would be third-order fixator!) If instead of the upper trapezius, the serratus anterior had contracted as the upward rotator second-order fixator, then its action of protraction of the scapula may have had to be stopped from occurring by another second-order fixator that in this case retracts the scapula. Furthermore, when the right posterior deltoid contracts as our fixator, it would have also created a force of abduction and lateral rotation on the arm at the glenohumeral joint; second-order fixators (that can perform adduction and/or medial rotation of the arm) might have to contract to stop the arm from performing these actions.

To kinesthetically experience this yourself, place a heavy weight in your right hand and slowly palpate each of the muscles mentioned in the caption for Figure 15-16, as well as the muscles mentioned in this Spotlight box; you will probably be able to feel their contractions. The domino effect of muscle contractions that occurs through the body can be truly amazing! It makes one realize how silly it can be when we hear people in the fields of health and sports training talk about isolating a muscle when exercising.

- Neutralizer: The pronator teres acts as a neutralizer, creating a force of pronation of the forearm at the RU joints, which stops the biceps brachii from supinating the forearm at the RU joints.
- Support: The left paraspinal musculature acts as a support muscle, creating a force of left lateral flexion of the trunk at the spinal joints, which stops the trunk from falling into right lateral flexion because of the weight being held in the right hand.
○ Figure 15-17 shows a person kicking a soccer ball with her right foot. In this scenario the action in question is flexion of the right thigh at the hip joint.
- Mover: The rectus femoris is contracting as a mover to create flexion of the thigh at the hip joint.
- Fixator: The rectus abdominis acts as a fixator, creating a force of posterior tilt of the pelvis, which stops the rectus femoris from anteriorly tilting the pelvis.
- Neutralizer: If the rectus femoris is the mover that contracts, there will be no neutralizer because the rectus femoris has no other action on the thigh at the hip joint. (Note: If a different mover such as the right iliopsoas or one of the right-sided adductors of the thigh at the hip joint contracts, then there would be other undesired actions of the thigh at the hip joint that would need to be neutralized.)
- Support: The left quadriceps femoris group acts as a support muscle, creating a force of extension of the left knee joint, preventing the left knee joint from flexing and the person falling to the ground.
○ As we can see from these examples, the contractions of muscles leapfrog through the body like the ripples of a stone thrown into a pond. Certainly as the contractions become more distant from the original contraction of the concentrically contracting mover or eccentrically contracting antagonist (whichever is the muscle that is working), the strength of these contractions diminishes. However, they do occur and in injured clients may be functionally important to their health! To fully explore all the contractions that would occur, one must examine every line of pull in every plane of every muscle that is contracting!
○ It must be emphasized that the particular set of muscles that contracts in any given movement pattern can vary greatly from one person to another and from one circumstance to another.
○ Each person has his or her own coordination pattern that has been learned through his or her lifetime. The change of even one mover for a joint action can have ripple effects that change which fixators and neutralizers then have to contract, which then changes which second-order fixators have to contract, and so forth.
○ Furthermore, the strength needed for a contraction and the position of the body during a joint action can alter muscle contraction patterns.
- Depending on the force of contraction needed for a specific joint action, more or fewer movers (or antagonists) might need to contract. This would then affect the coordination pattern of fixators and neutralizers. For example, lifting a 10-lb weight instead of a 5-lb weight might trigger an entirely different pattern of coordinating muscles.
- Furthermore, if the body is in a different position while performing the joint action, the role of gravity might change, triggering a different pattern of coordinating muscles.

SECTION 15.12 COUPLED ACTIONS

○ Although we often choose to direct multiple specific joint actions to occur as part of more complex movement patterns, sometimes two joint actions *must* occur together (i.e., one joint action cannot occur unless the second joint action also occurs at the same time).
○ Two separate joint actions that must occur simultaneously are called **coupled actions** because they exist as a couple[11] (Box 15-12).
○ We do not consciously direct a coupled second action; rather, it is automatically ordered subconsciously by our nervous system when we order the first joint action to occur.
○ Coupled actions are different from a muscle that has more than one action at a joint; they are also different from a multijoint muscle that has actions at more than one joint.
○ Coupled actions are separate actions that are caused by separate movers.
○ The best examples of coupled actions in the human body are the coupled actions of the arm and shoulder girdle. These actions couple together, because for full excursion of the humerus to occur, the shoulder girdle must move as well. The coupled actions of the arm and shoulder girdle are usually referred to as **scapulohumeral rhythm** because a rhythm exists to the movement between the humerus and the scapula.[3] (Note: For a more detailed exploration of scapulohumeral rhythm, see Section 10.6.) Coupled actions of the thigh and the pelvic girdle are also common. Just as the shoulder girdle must move to allow for a fuller excursion of the humerus, motion of the pelvic girdle must occur to allow for a fuller excursion of the femur. This coupling is usually referred to as *femoropelvic rhythm*. (For information on femoropelvic rhythm, see Section 9.11.)
○ The classic example of coupled actions that has been most extensively studied involves abduction of the arm coupled with shoulder girdle actions.
○ Figure 15-18, *A* illustrates an arm that is abducted 180 degrees *relative to the rest of the body*. Normally, we assume that arm abduction occurs relative to the scapula at the glenohumeral (GH) joint. However, in Figure 15-18, *A* we see that of these 180 degrees of arm abduction, only 120 degrees were movement of the humerus relative to the scapula at the GH joint; the remaining 60 degrees were the result of upward rotation of the scapula relative to the ribcage at the scapulocostal (ScC) joint[3] (Box 15-12). This scapular action is coupled with the humeral action of abduction, because otherwise the head of the humerus would bang into the acromion process of the scapula, both limiting overall humeral range of motion and causing

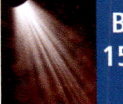

BOX 15-12 Spotlight on Movement Patterns

The concept of coupled actions points to the larger picture of how the muscular system works. When the brain directs muscular activity, it does not think in terms of directing specific joint actions to occur or even directing specific muscles to contract. Rather, the brain thinks in terms of movement patterns to achieve a desired position of the body. For example, if we want to reach a book that is up on a high shelf, the brain does not think of creating abduction of the arm at the GH joint or any other specific joint action. Instead, its only goal is create whatever coordinated movement pattern is necessary to bring the hand to this elevated position, and whatever muscular contractions are necessary to create this will be directed to occur. Therefore muscles that abduct the arm at the GH joint will be ordered to contract, along with scapular and clavicular muscles that upwardly rotate the shoulder girdle to further the ability of the hand to reach this elevated position. In addition, muscles of the elbow, wrist, and finger joints will also be ordered to contract. Beyond the upper extremity, muscular activity throughout the contralateral upper extremity, lower extremities, and axial body will also be recruited to aid in raising the hand higher. Ordering each of these specific muscular contractions is not consciously thought of; rather, they happen automatically as a part of the larger movement pattern with the intended goal of bringing the hand higher. Furthermore, if for some reason one body part cannot be moved as a part of this set of movements (perhaps because of an injury), another body part will automatically be recruited by the brain to compensate for this loss. For example, if the arm cannot abduct, muscles that elevate the scapula and clavicle might be directed to contract in an attempt to raise the hand higher. In short, the essence of neural control of the muscular system is that the brain does not talk to specific muscles per se; rather it thinks in larger movement patterns and talks to motor units of multiple muscles throughout the body to achieve whatever larger movement patterns are desired!

impingement of the rotator cuff tendon and subacromial bursa. Figure 15-18, *B* illustrates the mover muscles that work in this circumstance: The deltoid is the mover of abduction of the arm at the GH joint, and the upper trapezius and lower trapezius are movers of upward rotation of the scapula at the ScC joint. We do not consciously choose to contract the trapezius in this circumstance; its contraction is automatically ordered by the nervous system to couple with the deltoid's action of abduction of the arm at the GH joint. (Note: Only these movers of arm abduction and scapula upward rotation have been shown; the various fixators and neutralizers as well as other possible movers that would need to contract during this coordination pattern are not shown.)

- Note: The scapular upward rotation that couples with humeral abduction also involves coupled actions of clavicular elevation and upward rotation. Overall, for the arm to abduct, coupled actions of the humerus, scapula, and clavicle must occur at the GH, ScC, sternoclavicular, and acromioclavicular joints[3]! See Section 10.6 for more information on the coupled actions of the arm and shoulder girdle.

ESSENTIAL FACTS:

- Two separate joint actions that must occur simultaneously are called *coupled actions*.
- Coupled actions are separate joint actions that are caused by separate movers.

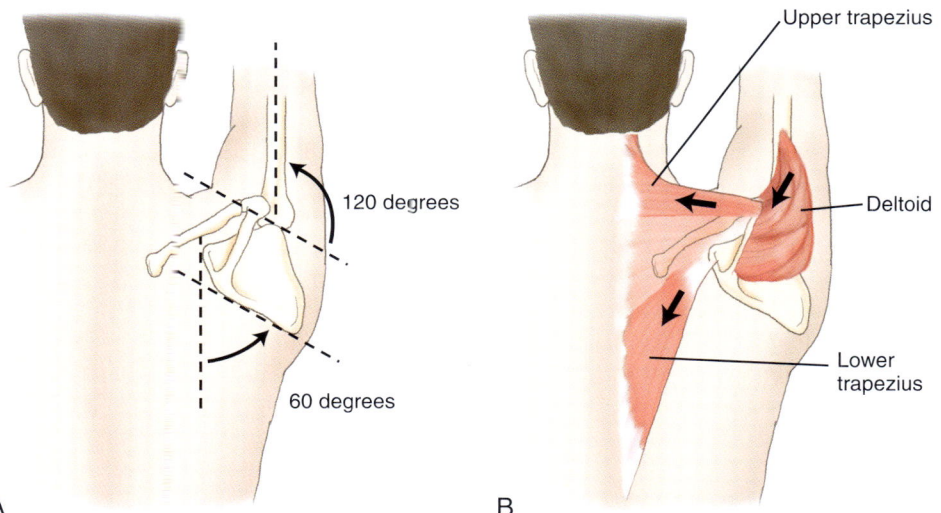

FIGURE 15-18 Illustration of the concept of coupled actions in the body. **A,** Figure shows that 180 degrees of abduction of the arm relative to the trunk is actually made up of two separate coupled joint actions: (1) humeral motion at the glenohumeral (GH) joint and (2) scapular motion at the scapulocostal (ScC) joint. **B,** Two separate movers must independently contract to create these two coupled actions: (1) the deltoid is the mover of abduction of the arm at the GH joint, and (2) the upper trapezius and lower trapezius are the movers of upward rotation of the scapula at the ScC joint.

REVIEW QUESTIONS

Answers to the following review questions appear on the Evolve website accompanying this book at: http://evolve.elsevier.com/Muscolino/kinesiology/.

1. What are the six major roles in which a muscle can contract during a joint action?

2. What is the definition of a *mover*?

3. When a joint action occurs, what happens to the length of a mover?

4. Do mover muscles always contract when a joint action occurs?

5. What is the definition of an *antagonist*?

6. When a joint action occurs, what happens to the length of an antagonist?

7. Do antagonist muscles always contract when a joint action occurs?

8. What is the most common external force that can be a mover or an antagonist?

9. Define co-contraction.

10. What is the definition of a *fixator*?

11. What is the definition of a *neutralizer*?

12. What do fixators and neutralizers have in common? What is the difference between a fixator and a neutralizer?

13. What is the importance of core stabilization, and what effect does it have on our health?

14. What is the difference between postural stabilization muscles and mobility muscles?

15. What is the definition of a support muscle?

16. What are two ways in which a synergist can be defined?

17. Define the term *coordination*, and describe its application to the concept of muscle roles.

18. Explain why isometric contractions are more likely to diminish venous return of blood to the heart and also cause ischemia of tissues.

19. What is the difference between a regular fixator (i.e., first-order fixator) and a second-order fixator?

20. Give an example of a coupled action in the human body.

21. State a specific joint action (and the position that the body is in when performing this action), and give an example of a mover, antagonist, fixator, neutralizer, and support muscle for this action; furthermore, state whether it is the mover group or the antagonist group that is working in this scenario.

REFERENCES

1. McGinnis PM: Biomechanics of sport and exercise, ed 2, Champaign, IL, 2005, Human Kinetics.
2. Levangie PK, Norkin CC: Joint structure and function: A comprehensive analysis, ed 5, Philadelphia, 2011, FA Davis.
3. Neumann DA: Kinesiology of the musculoskeletal system: Foundations for physical rehabilitation, ed 3, St Louis, 2017, Elsevier.
4. Enoka RM: Neuromechanics of human movement, ed 3, Champaign, IL, 2002, Human Kinetics.
5. Watkins J: Fundamental biomechanics of sport and exercise, Abingdon, 2014, Routledge.
6. Smith LK, Weiss EL, Lehmkuhl LO: Brunnstrom's clinical kinesiology, ed 5, Philadelphia, 1996, FA Davis.
7. Hall SJ: Basic biomechanics, ed 6, New York, 2012, McGraw Hill.
8. Muscolino JE: The muscular system manual: The skeletal muscles of the human body, ed 4, St Louis, 2017, Elsevier.
9. Page P, Frank CC, Lardner R: Assessment and treatment of muscle imbalance: The Janda approach, Champaign, IL, 2010, Human Kinetics.
10. Hamilton N, Weimar W, Luttgens K: Kinesiology: Scientific basis of human motion, ed 12, New York, 2012, McGraw Hill.
11. Oatis CA: Kinesiology: The mechanics and pathomechanics of human movement, Philadelphia, 2004, Lippincott Williams & Wilkins.

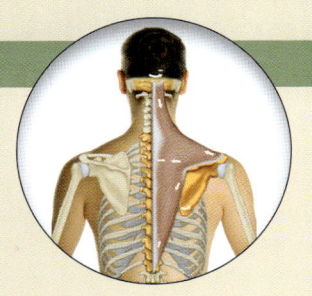

CHAPTER 16

Types of Joint Motion and Musculoskeletal Assessment

CHAPTER OUTLINE

Section 16.1	Active versus Passive Range of Motion	Section 16.4	Muscle Palpation
Section 16.2	Resisted Motion/Manual Resistance	Section 16.5	Do We Treat Movers or Antagonists?
Section 16.3	Musculoskeletal Assessment: Muscle or Joint?	Section 16.6	Do We Treat Signs or Symptoms?
		Section 16.7	Understanding Research

CHAPTER OBJECTIVES

After completing this chapter, the student should be able to perform the following:

1. Define the key terms of this chapter and state the meanings of the word origins of this chapter.
2. Do the following related to active versus passive range of motion:
   - Define, discuss, and give an example of passive and active range of motion of joints.
   - Define and discuss the relationship of joint play and joint adjustments.
   - Define and discuss ballistic motion and explain why ballistic motions occur in the body.
   - Define and discuss the concept of *end-feel*.
3. Define, discuss, and give an example of resisted motion in the body.
4. Explain how active range of motion, passive range of motion, and manual resistance can be used as test procedures to assess musculoskeletal soft tissue conditions.
5. List the five major guidelines as well as the additional guidelines for palpating muscles; furthermore, explain the importance of each of these guidelines, and apply them to a muscle palpation.
6. Explain the importance of assessing and treating tight antagonists of a joint motion.
7. Do the following related to signs and symptoms:
   - Define the terms *signs* and *symptoms*.
   - Discuss the importance of signs and symptoms in the assessment and treatment of a client.
   - Make and explain an analogy between the concept of signs/symptoms and a glass of water that overflows.
8. List and describe the six major sections of a research article.

OVERVIEW

The last few chapters have explored the various ways in which muscles can contract, and the various roles that muscles have when a joint action is occurring. We will now begin to investigate the different types of motion that can occur (i.e., active versus passive) when a joint action occurs. We will then use the understanding of these types of motion, along with resisted isometric contraction, to learn how to assess musculoskeletal soft tissue injuries. Continuing with assessment techniques, methods of muscle palpation are given. There is a discussion of the types of problems that manual and exercise therapists most commonly treat. And, finally, the chapter concludes with an examination of the importance of research and the *anatomy of a research article*.

KEY TERMS

Abstract	Metastudy
Active range of motion	Methods section
Antagonist soft tissue	Muscle-bound
Assessment	Muscle spasm end-feel
Ballistic motion	Myo-fascio-skeletal system
Blind	Neuro-myo-fascio-skeletal system
Bone-to-bone end-feel	Orthopedic test procedures
Control group	Parameter
Criterion (plural: criteria)	Passive range of motion
Diagnosis (DYE-ag-NO-sis)	Placebo
Discussion section	Population
Double blind	Random sample
Empty end-feel	References section
End-feel	Resisted motion
Evidence-based	Results section
Exclusion criteria	Signs
False-negative result	Soft end-feel
False-positive result	Soft tissue approximation end-feel
Firm end-feel	Soft tissue stretch end-feel
Grade IV joint mobilization	Sprain
Grade V joint mobilization	Springy-block end-feel
Hypothesis	Standard deviation
Inclusion criteria	Strain
Introduction section	Symptoms
Joint mouse	Target muscle
Joint play	Tendinitis
Manual resistance	Test procedure
Mean	Treatment group
Median	

WORD ORIGINS

- Active—From Latin *actus*, meaning *to do*
- Assess—From Latin *assideo*, meaning *to assist in judging*
- Ballistic—From Greek *ballein*, meaning *to throw*
- Diagnosis—From Greek *diagnosis*, meaning *a decision, discernment*
- Orthopedic—From Greek *orthos*, meaning *correct*, and *paid*, meaning *child*
- Passive—From Latin *passivus*, meaning *permits, endures*
- Sign—From Latin *signum*, meaning *a sign, mark, warning*
- Sprain—From Old French *espraindre*, meaning *to twist*
- Strain—From Latin *stringere* meaning *to draw tight*
- Symptom—From Greek *symptoma*, meaning *an occurrence*

SECTION 16.1 ACTIVE VERSUS PASSIVE RANGE OF MOTION

- Two types of range of motion (ROM) can occur at a joint[1] (Figure 16-1):
  1. **Active range of motion** is defined as joint motion that is created by the mover muscles of that joint.
  2. **Passive range of motion** is defined as joint motion that is created by a force other than the mover muscles of that joint.
- The therapist does not have a role in performing active ROM of the client.

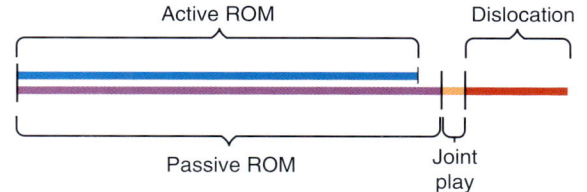

FIGURE 16-1 Schematic illustration of the relationship of the ranges of motion of a typical healthy joint.

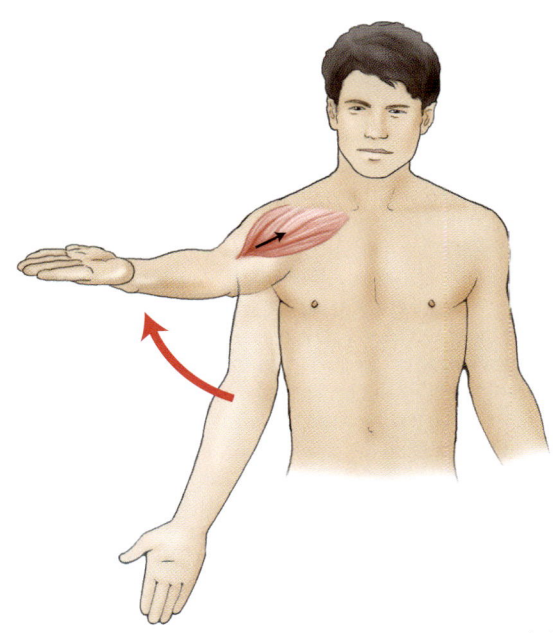

FIGURE 16-2 Active joint motion in which a person is actively flexing the right arm at the shoulder (glenohumeral [GH]) joint. This motion is defined as active, because the mover muscles of that joint (i.e., flexors of the right arm at the GH joint) are creating it.

- Because active motion is created by the mover muscles of the client's joint that is moving, active ROM must be done by the client. Figure 16-2 illustrates an example of active joint motion.
- Passive ROM is usually slightly greater than active ROM.[2]
- Beyond passive ROM is a small amount of nonaxial gliding motion called **joint play**. Joint play is a passive motion because it cannot be created by the mover muscles of the joint[2] (Box 16-1).
- The therapist can have a role in performing passive ROM of the client.
  - Because the mover muscles of the joint that is being moved are not creating the joint motion, another force must do this; the force to move the joint in passive motion can be created by the therapist.
  - However, it is important to realize that passive ROM of a client's joint can be done without the assistance of a therapist or trainer; a client can do passive ROM by himself or herself. This can be accomplished by the client using muscles of one part of the body to create passive motion at another joint of the body. Because the mover muscles of the joint that is being moved are relaxed and passive, this motion is defined as passive ROM. Figure 16-3 illustrates two examples of passive joint motion: one in which the therapist performs the passive motion of the client's joint and another in which the client performs passive range of motion alone.
- Knowledge of active and passive motion can be helpful in assessing and treating clients. (For more details on using active and passive range of motion to assess and treat clients, see Section 16.3.)
- Beyond joint play is dislocation.

BALLISTIC MOTION:

- Whenever a joint motion is begun actively by the client and then is completed passively by momentum, it is called a **ballistic motion**.[3]
- Most motions of the body are ballistic because ballistic motions are very efficient. A ballistic motion allows the muscles that actively contracted to initiate the joint motion to relax while momentum completes the motion. The normal swing of our lower and upper extremities when walking is a good example of ballistic motion. If these motions were not done in a ballistic manner, then our muscles would have to actively contract during the entire range of motion of the lower and upper extremities (the military *goose-step* march is done in this manner). Another good example of a ballistic motion is the swing of a tennis racquet or a golf club. A strong active contraction of the muscles of the joint is necessary to begin the motion; natural passive momentum then completes the swing, allowing our muscles to relax.

END-FEEL:

- When evaluating joint motion, it is also important to feel for and assess the quality of motion at the end of a joint's passive range of motion; this is called **end-feel**.[4] This quality can alert the therapist or trainer to whether the joint is normal and healthy or pathologic.
- There are six major qualities of end-feel. They are soft tissue stretch, soft tissue approximation, bone-to-bone, muscle spasm, springy-block, and empty.
  - **Soft tissue stretch end-feel** occurs when the stretch of the soft tissue of a joint limits its motion. If the soft tissue limiting the motion is muscle, it is often described as **soft end-feel** because muscle tissue is fairly elastic. If the soft tissue limiting the motion is ligament, it is often described as **firm end-feel** because ligamentous tissue is less elastic and yielding than muscle tissue. Although firmer, there is still a slight elastic springiness or bounce to a ligament's firm end-feel. An example of soft end-feel is lateral rotation of the arm at the shoulder joint (limited by medial rotation musculature). An example of firm end-feel is extension of the knee joint (limited by the cruciate ligaments). Soft tissue stretch end-feel is usually indicative of a healthy joint.
  - **Soft tissue approximation end-feel** occurs when the motion ends because of the compression of superficial soft tissues between the two body parts moving at the joint. The classic example of soft-tissue approximation end-feel is flexion of the elbow joint. Soft-tissue approximation end-feel does not indicate a pathologic joint. However, when it occurs in a joint that does not usually have soft tissue approximation end-feel, it may indicate that a client has increased fat deposition because of excessive caloric intake. It may also indicate that a client has built up muscle mass by strengthening exercise; in this instance, the client is often described as being **muscle-bound**.
  - **Bone-to-bone end-feel** occurs when joint motion ends with the two bones of the joint meeting each other. The classic example of bone-to-bone end-feel is extension of the radioulnar (elbow) joint. Bone-to-bone end-feel at a joint that should not have it is an indication of a joint that has undergone pathologic degenerative (osteoarthritic) changes.

BOX 16-1 Spotlight on "Joint Play"

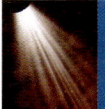

In addition to active and passive range of motion, one other type of motion occurs at a joint; it is called joint play. Joint play is the small amount of motion that is permissible at a joint at the end of a joint's passive range of motion. Two types of manipulations are possible within the realm of joint play. One type is a low-velocity stretching of the joint and is usually called joint play or **Grade IV joint mobilization**[11] (see left photo). The other type is a high-velocity manipulation that is called a **Grade V joint mobilization** or an adjustment[11] and is usually used by chiropractic and osteopathic physicians. Although Grade IV and V joint mobilizations may be directed toward increasing axial motions at the joint, most often they are focused on increasing the non-axial component motion at the joint. Depending on the scope of license, manual therapists may be permitted to do Grade IV joint mobilization. However, Grade V joint mobilizations are usually performed only by physicians (see right photo).

When a chiropractic/osteopathic adjustment is performed, a popping sound often occurs. During an adjustment, the bones of the joint are not "cracked" together as is commonly thought. What occurs is that the bones of the joint are distracted away from each other. This causes an increase in the space within the joint capsule, resulting in a lower pressure within the joint. This causes the gases that are dissolved within the synovial fluid to come out of solution and become gaseous. This change in the state of the gases of the joint fluid causes the characteristic popping sound that is associated with osseous adjustments. An analogy can be made to the popping sound that occurs when a champagne bottle is opened. When a champagne cork is first removed from the bottle, a popping sound occurs; if the cork is then immediately placed back in the bottle and immediately removed again, no popping sound occurs the second time it is removed. However, if the cork is placed back in the bottle, left there for 20 minutes or so, and then removed again, the popping sound will occur once again because the gases had sufficient time to go back into solution. Similarly, if a joint is adjusted two times in a row quickly, there will be no popping sound the second time because the gases within the joint cavity, like the gases within the champagne bottle, did not have sufficient time to go back into solution. Keep in mind that the point of an adjustment is not to make the popping sound, but rather to increase the range of motion of the joint by stretching the capsule/ligaments of the joint. The popping sound is often just a good indicator that this objective was successfully achieved.

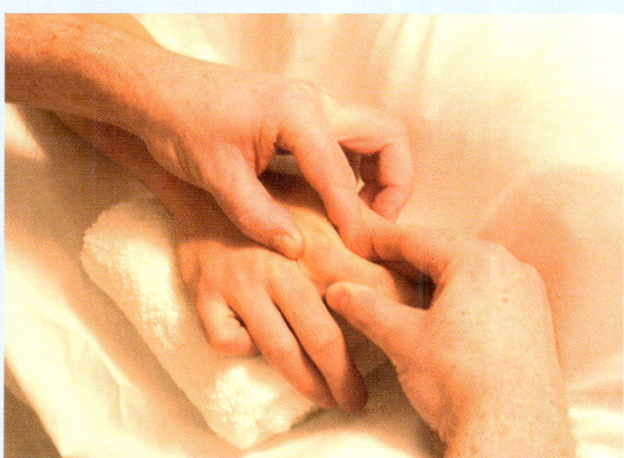

From Dixon M: *Joint play the right way for the peripheral skeleton: the training manual*, ed 2, Port Moody, British Columbia, 2003, Arthrokinetic Publishing.

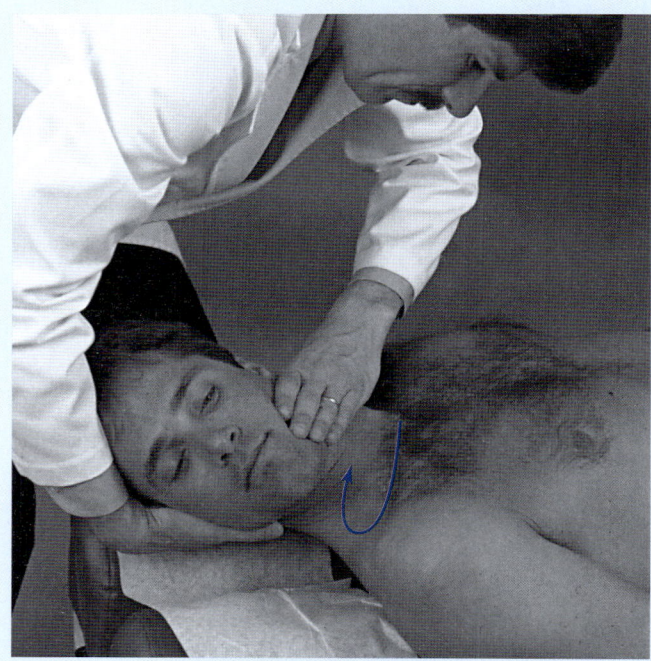

From Bergmann TF, Peterson DH: *Chiropractic technique: principles and procedures*, ed 3, St Louis, 2010, Mosby.

- **Muscle spasm end-feel** occurs when the end of motion is caused by a muscle spasm; this end-feel is abrupt and sudden. Muscle spasm end-feel is always pathologic.
- **Springy-block end-feel** occurs when the end range of joint motion is blocked and the joint springs back as a result of the presence of a loose body of tissue that becomes jammed between the two bones of the joint. An example is a torn meniscus between the femur and tibia at the knee joint. Another example is a small piece of bone that has broken off one of the bones of the joint (this fragment of bone is often called a **joint mouse**). Springy-block end-feel is always indicative of a pathologic joint.
- **Empty end-feel** is so named because there is no mechanical obstruction to joint motion, but the client stops motion because of pain or the fear that pain will occur if motion were to continue. If empty end-feel occurs because of the presence of actual pain, it is indicative of a pathologic condition. If it occurs because a client preemptively stops the motion because of the fear that pain will occur, it certainly is likely that a pathologic condition is present. It is also often present in a client who once had a painful pathologic condition and has now become patterned to stop motion because of the fear that the condition is still present or that it will return.

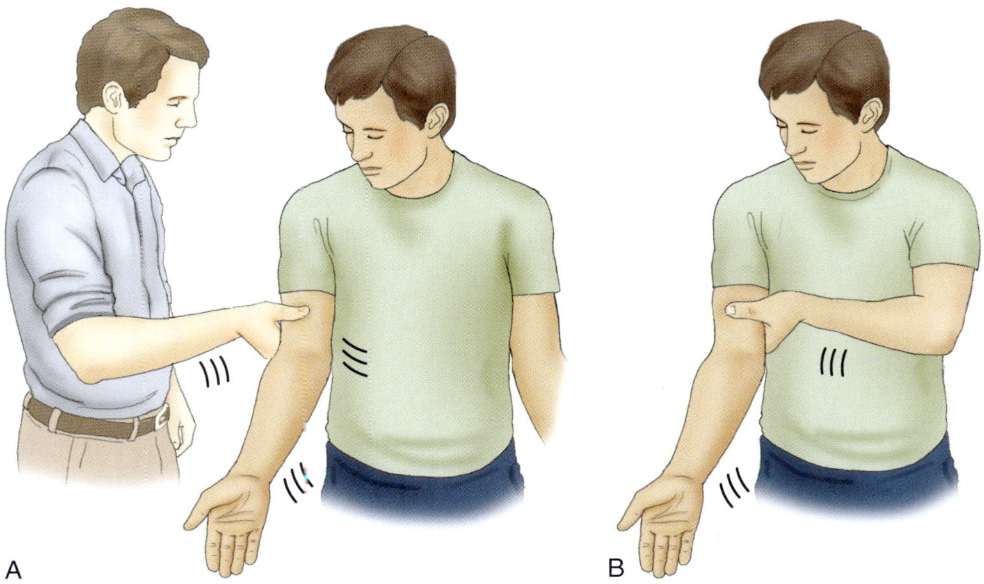

CHAPTER 16 Types of Joint Motion and Musculoskeletal Assessment

FIGURE 16-3 Two examples of passive joint motion. **A**, A therapist is flexing the client's right arm at the GH joint. **B**, Client is using the left upper extremity to flex the right arm at the GH joint. Both cases illustrate passive motion because the mover muscles of flexion of the right arm at the GH joint are relaxed and another force is creating the motion.

SECTION 16.2 RESISTED MOTION/MANUAL RESISTANCE

- **Resisted motion** occurs when a resistance force stops the contraction of the muscles of the joint from being able to create motion at that joint.[5]
  - Therefore resisted motion results in an isometric contraction of the muscles of the joint with no actual joint motion occurring.
- This force of resistance that stops motion from occurring can be provided by a therapist or trainer, an object, or even the client himself/herself. Figure 16-4 illustrates examples of resisted motion.
- Resisted motion is often called **manual resistance**.[5]

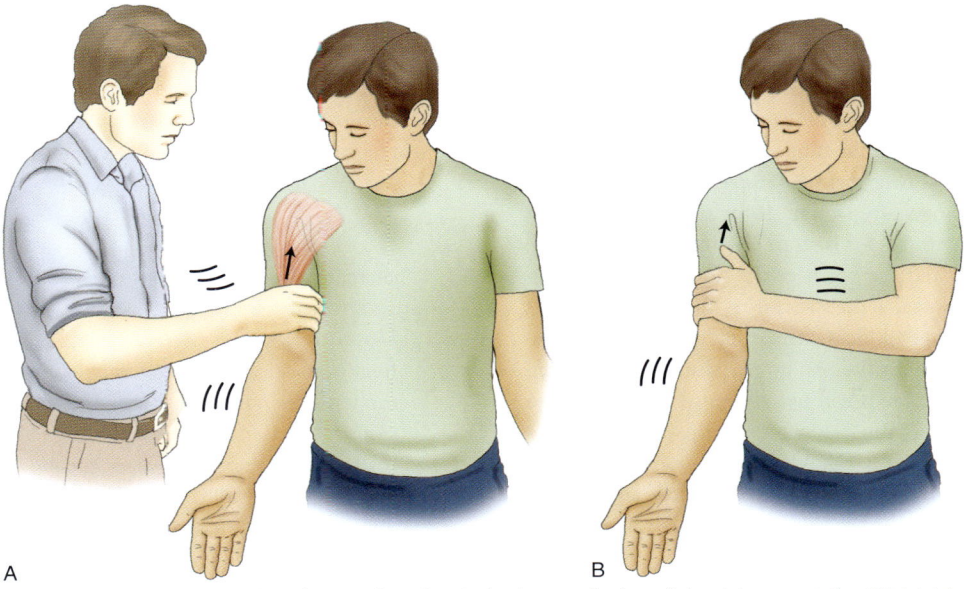

FIGURE 16-4 Two examples of resisted motion. In both cases flexion of the right arm at the GH joint is being resisted from occurring by another force. In **A**, the force resisting and stopping motion is coming from a therapist. In **B**, the client is using the left upper extremity to provide resistance to the motion.

SECTION 16.3 MUSCULOSKELETAL ASSESSMENT: MUSCLE OR JOINT?

- Most musculoskeletal conditions are either injury to the musculature (and the associated tendons) of a joint or to the ligament/joint capsule complex of a joint (Box 16-2).

BOX 16-2

If a muscle is injured and torn, it is defined as a **strain**[4]; an injured tendon that is inflamed is defined as **tendinitis**[4] (also spelled tendonitis). If a ligament or joint capsule is injured and torn, it is defined as a **sprain**.[4] Musculoskeletal injuries are often classified as either muscular in origin (i.e., muscle strain, tendinitis) or joint in origin (i.e., ligamentous/joint capsule in origin).

- Knowledge of active range of motion, passive range of motion, and resisted motion (manual resistance) can be valuable in assessing these musculoskeletal conditions (Box 16-3).

BOX 16-3

There can be a fine line between diagnosis and assessment. A **diagnosis** may be defined as the assigning of a name or label to a group of signs and/or symptoms by a qualified health care professional, whereas an **assessment** may be defined as a systematic method of gathering information to make informed decisions about treatment.[4] The information provided in this section is to assist manual and movement therapists, trainers, and other bodyworkers in assessing their clients' musculoskeletal conditions, not making diagnoses. An excellent text written for the world of massage and bodywork that deals with the assessment of musculoskeletal conditions is *Orthopedic Assessment in Massage Therapy* (2006) by Whitney Lowe, published by David Scott.

- Assessment requires critical thinking, and critical thinking requires a fundamental understanding of how the various parts of the musculoskeletal system function.
- The basis of an assessment **test procedure** is that it challenges a structure by placing a stress on it.[4] If the structure is healthy, then it will be able to meet this stress in a symptom-free (e.g., pain-free) manner and the result of the test procedure is declared negative. However, if the structure is injured in some way, symptoms (e.g., pain) will most likely result and the test procedure result is declared positive. An injured muscle that is asked to contract (or is stretched) will usually cause pain, as will an injured ligament or joint capsule that is stretched or compressed in some manner.
- Active range of motion, passive range of motion, and manual resistance are valuable test procedures that can be used for assessing musculoskeletal soft tissue conditions.
- When assessing musculoskeletal soft tissue injuries, it is helpful to divide the soft tissues of the body into two major categories: (1) mover muscles and (2) the ligament/joint capsule complex.

We can then look at the stresses placed on these soft tissues with active range of motion, passive range of motion, and resisted motion.
- If these procedures are performed on a client with musculoskeletal pain, the origin of the pain can usually be determined.
- Note: Two other important categories of musculoskeletal assessment exist and should not be ignored. These are antagonist musculature and bony/cartilage articular surface (Box 16-4).

ACTIVE RANGE OF MOTION:

- When active range of motion is performed, both mover muscles and the ligament/joint capsule complex are stressed.
  - Mover muscles are stressed because they are asked to contract concentrically to create the joint motion that is occurring. If the mover muscles and/or their tendons are injured in some way, this will likely result in pain.
  - The ligament/joint capsule complex is stressed because the joint is moved, causing stretching and/or compression to various parts of the capsule and ligaments of the joint. If these structures are injured, pain will likely result.
- Therefore active range of motion would be expected to generate pain in almost any musculoskeletal injury of mover musculature or ligament/joint capsule tissue. For this reason, active range of motion is useful as an initial screening procedure to determine if any type of soft tissue injury or dysfunction is present.[4]

PASSIVE RANGE OF MOTION:

- When passive range of motion is done, only the ligament/joint capsule complex is stressed.
  - The ligament/joint capsule complex is stressed because the joint is being moved, causing stretching and/or compression to various parts of the capsule and ligaments of the joint. If these structures are injured, pain will likely result.
- However, mover muscles are not stressed because they are passive (i.e., relaxed as another force creates the joint action).

MANUAL RESISTANCE:

- When manual resistance is performed, only the mover musculature is stressed.
  - Mover muscles are stressed because they are asked to contract isometrically in an attempt to create joint motion. This motion does not actually occur because the resistance force stops the mover muscle from being able to shorten and actually move the joint; however, the mover muscle still works by isometrically contracting. Therefore if it or its tendons are injured in some way, pain will likely result.
  - The ligaments and joint capsule are not stressed because the joint does not actually move in any way. Therefore no force is placed on them; they are neither stretched nor compressed in any way.

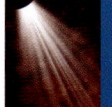

BOX 16-4 — Spotlight on Orthopedic Assessment and Antagonist Musculature and Articular Surface Tissue

Active range of motion, passive range of motion, and manual resistance testing are usually looked at from the perspective of their effect upon active mover musculature and passive ligamentous tissue. However, two other tissues/structures can be assessed using these assessment test procedures. These two tissues are the antagonist musculature at the joint, and the articular surface tissue (articular cartilage and the underlying subchondral bone).

Antagonist Musculature:
Antagonist musculature, if injured or spasmed, could cause pain with active and passive range of motion.

- Active range of motion and passive range of motion would both cause pain if the antagonist musculature were injured and/or tight, because any motion of the joint requires the antagonist muscles to lengthen and stretch, and an injured or tight antagonist muscle will be resistant to stretch, most likely resulting in pain.
- Manual resistance would not cause pain in the antagonist musculature that is on the other side of the joint from where the mover musculature that is isometrically contracting and attempting to shorten is located. (In reality, the terms mover musculature and antagonist musculature do not even apply here, because no joint motion actually occurs and movers and antagonists are defined by their role relative to an actual joint motion.) Because no motion occurs, the muscles on the other side of the joint (i.e., antagonist musculature) are not lengthened and stretched and are therefore not stressed.
   Understanding this, we realize that painful passive range of motion can indeed indicate muscular injury, but only of the antagonist muscles on the other side of the joint. If this is the case the client can usually localize the pain to the other side of the joint; localization of pain there indicates to the therapist that the pain is in antagonist musculature. To confirm this, manual resistance can be done to these muscles. If they are unhealthy, then causing them to isometrically contract by resisting their contraction should elicit pain.

Articular Surface Tissue:
- Active and passive range of motion and manual resistance are also valuable toward assessing the health of the articular surface tissues. Because motion to one side, whether it is active or passive, results in compression upon the joint surfaces on the side to which motion occurs, clients with inflammation/injury to the articular cartilage and/or the underlying subchondral bone may experience pain during these motions. Unlike the stretching tensile forces experienced by ligamentous/capsular tissue and antagonist musculature, this pain would be experienced on the side to which motion occurs, not the side that is stretched. Pain may also result from joint motion restriction due to intrinsic fascial tissue adhesions within the capsule and/or ligaments. Obstruction of the proper kinematic movement pattern of the joint can minimize the proper glide of the articular surfaces, resulting in excessive compression force upon the joint surfaces.
  - Unlike active and passive range of motion, in which motion results in compression force being applied to one side of the articular surfaces of the bones at the joint, pain due to joint surface pathology does not usually occur with manual resistance because no motion occurs. However, if manual resistance is performed assertively, the strong isometric muscle contraction that occurs can result in compression of the articular surfaces due to the stabilization aspect of the mover musculature's contraction force being directed toward the joint. This should be considered when performing differential assessment testing.

- Note: Every test procedure has a certain degree of sensitivity and accuracy. Sometimes a **false-negative result** occurs wherein the client has a negative test result (i.e., the client does not report pain [or does not exhibit whatever sign or symptom is indicative for that test procedure]) on performing the procedure, yet he or she actually does have the musculoskeletal condition.[6] In other words, the negative result is incorrect (in other words, false). A **false-positive result** would be defined as a test result wherein the client does report pain (or whatever sign or symptom is indicative for the condition being tested for) on performance of the procedure but does not actually have the musculoskeletal condition. In other words, the positive result is incorrect (in other words, false).[6] These physical test procedures that deal with the musculoskeletal system are usually called **orthopedic test procedures**. It should always be kept in mind that test procedures such as these are not 100% accurate.

ORDER OF ASSESSMENT PROCEDURES:

- Following is the order of steps to be followed when assessing a client with musculoskeletal soft tissue pain[4]:
  1. Begin with active range of motion. A client who experiences pain with active range of motion is confirmed as having either mover muscular *and/or* ligament/joint capsule complex injury.
  2. Next assess passive range of motion. If passive range of motion results in pain, the client's ligament/joint capsule complex is injured.
  3. Then assess resisted motion. If resisted motion results in pain, then the mover musculature is injured.
- It is important to remember that a client may have injury to more than one type of tissue (e.g., mover muscles and the ligament/joint capsule complex can be injured). If you find that one type of tissue is injured, continue to assess the other tissue.
- In fact, given the concept of compensation, whenever one tissue of the body is dysfunctional, other tissues try to compensate for the functional weakness. Therefore the presence of one condition usually, in time, creates the presence of other conditions (Box 16-5).
- Figure 16-5 demonstrates a flow chart for using these test procedures for musculoskeletal assessment.

BOX 16-5

Too often we look to pigeonhole a client's condition into a neat little box, either assessing the client as having a strain to muscular tissue or a sprain to ligamentous/joint capsular tissue. In reality, clients who have had a traumatic accident of some sort rarely have a pure strain or a pure sprain because any traumatic injury that causes damage to one of these tissues often causes damage to the other. Of course, the extent of damage to each tissue is not necessarily the same. Although a strain and sprain may both be present, the relative proportion of each one may vary. Determining the proportion of each one can be done with the same active, passive, and manual resistance test procedures, but it usually requires more experience and judgment to make finer distinctions. This is because it is important not only to note whether the client feels pain or not but also to note at what point pain begins and what degree of pain exists during the procedures. Although manual and movement therapists, trainers, and other bodyworkers can address ligamentous/joint capsule problems with joint range of motion and other test procedures, muscular problems are usually the primary concern. For that reason, particular attention should be paid to the muscular elements of injury.

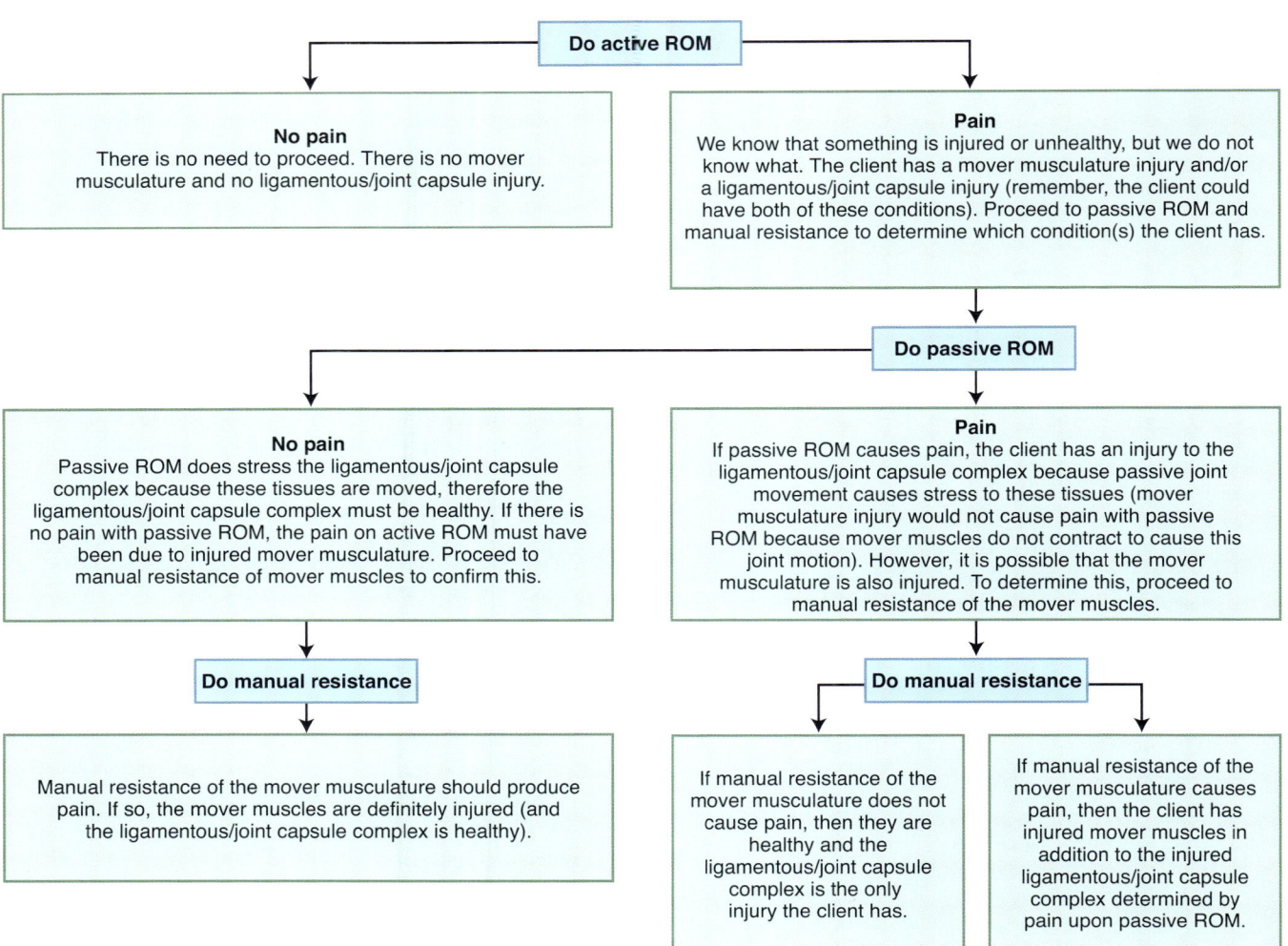

FIGURE 16-5 Flow chart demonstrates the proper sequence to follow for the orthopedic test procedures of active range of motion, passive range of motion, and manual resistance to assess a musculoskeletal soft tissue injury. *ROM*, Range of motion.

SECTION 16.4   MUSCLE PALPATION

- Regarding musculoskeletal assessment, perhaps no skill is more important or more valuable than assessment of resting muscle tone by muscle palpation. For this reason, it is extremely important for manual therapists to have a solid foundation in how to palpate the skeletal muscles of the body.
- Most textbooks on muscles offer a method to palpate each skeletal muscle of the human body. Although providing these palpation directions can be helpful, memorization of them on the part of the student should not be necessary. If a student knows the attachments and actions of the muscles, palpation can be figured out. The best way to become a better palpator is to spend more time palpating. Beyond that, if the student has extra time, that time should be spent reinforcing the knowledge of the attachments and actions of a muscle, not spent trying to memorize palpation directions.
- The student does not need to memorize the actions of a muscle—only the attachments need to be memorized. With use of the five-step approach to learning muscles presented in Section 13.3, once the attachments are known, the line of pull of the muscle relative to the joint is known. Knowledge of this allows the actions to be figured out. Less memorization and more understanding eases the stress of being a student and allows for better critical thought and clinical application!

FIVE-STEP MUSCLE PALPATION GUIDELINE:

- Following are the five basic guidelines to follow when looking to palpate the **target muscle** (i.e., the muscle that you desire to palpate) (Figure 16-6):
  1. Know the attachments of the target muscle so that you know where to place your palpating fingers.
  2. Know the actions of the target muscle so that you can ask the client to contract it. A contracted muscle is palpably firmer and easier to feel and discern from the adjacent soft

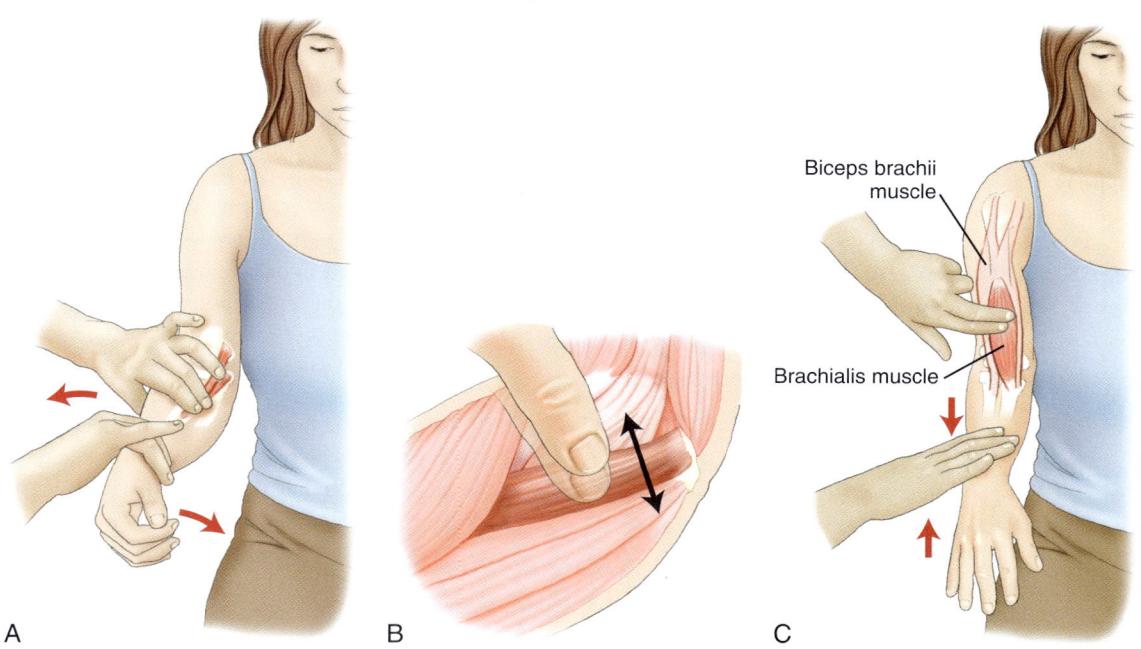

FIGURE 16-6 Five basic guidelines for palpating a muscle. **A,** Person palpating the pronator teres muscle while the client attempts to pronate the forearm at the radioulnar (RU) joints against resistance. **B,** Close-up of the palpating fingers strumming perpendicular to the fiber direction of the pronator teres. **C,** Palpation of the brachialis muscle through the biceps brachii using the neurologic reflex, reciprocal inhibition, to relax the biceps brachii. The client is flexing her forearm (against gentle resistance by the therapist) to bring out the brachialis so it can be more easily palpated.

BOX 16-6

Assessment of a muscle is usually performed to determine the resting tone of the muscle. Asking a client to contract a muscle is done only to help us find and locate the muscle. Once the muscle has been located, it is important to then ask the client to relax the muscle so that we can assess its resting tone.

tissues (Box 16-6). In effect, when contracted, the target muscle becomes a hard, soft tissue amongst a sea of soft, soft tissues. When asking the client to contract the target muscle, given that most target muscles have a number of joint actions they can perform, it is important to find the best joint action of the target muscle to ask the client to engage. The best joint action is usually the one that is most different from the joint actions of the adjacent muscles of the region. This way, as best as possible, we isolate the contraction of the target muscle so that the other nearby muscles remain relaxed and soft.

3. Add resistance. Especially for a target muscle that is deep and more difficult to discern from adjacent musculature, it is often helpful to resist the client's contraction of the target muscle. Adding resistance causes the client to generate a forceful isometric contraction of the target muscle, making it even more palpable and discernable from adjacent muscles. When adding resistance, it is important that you do not place your hand that gives resistance beyond any joint other than the joint where the muscle is contracting. Otherwise, other muscles may contract that will cloud your ability to discern the target muscle. For example, when resisting the client from pronating the forearm at the radioulnar joints, do not contact the client distal to the wrist joint (see Figure 16-6, *A*).

4. Strum across the muscle. Once a muscle is contracted and taut, it can more easily be felt by strumming across the muscle. Whatever the direction of the fibers is, palpate (i.e., strum) the muscle perpendicular to that direction (see Figure 16-6, *B*).

5. Use reciprocal inhibition. The idea of making a target muscle contract is to make it stand out from adjacent muscles. Therefore we ask the client to perform an action of the target muscle that is different from the actions of the nearby muscles. However, sometimes the action (or actions) of the target muscle is the same as the action (or actions) of the adjacent muscles. In these instances, if we ask the client to perform the action of the target muscle, then the adjacent muscle will also contract and it will be difficult to discern and feel the target muscle. This is especially true when the target muscle is deep to the adjacent muscle and contraction of this adjacent muscle would completely block our ability to palpate the deeper target muscle. In these instances, knowledge of the neurologic principle of reciprocal inhibition can be extremely valuable. (Note: For more information on the principle of reciprocal inhibition, see

Section 19.3.) Reciprocal inhibition can be used by asking the client to do an action that is antagonistic to another action of the adjacent muscle that we want to relax. Doing this will cause this adjacent muscle to relax[1] so that we can better palpate the target muscle. For example, when palpating the brachialis through the biceps brachii, have the client in a position of forearm pronation. Because the biceps brachii is a supinator, it will be reciprocally inhibited (relaxed), allowing palpation of the brachialis through it (see Figure 16-6, C; Box 16-7).

BOX 16-7

Using reciprocal inhibition can be extremely valuable when trying to relax an adjacent or superficial muscle that blocks our ability to palpate the target muscle. However, even though reciprocal inhibition tends to relax this other muscle, if the client contracts the target muscle too forcefully, the nervous system will override the neurologic reflex of reciprocal inhibition and direct the muscle (that we wanted to relax) to contract. In this situation, reciprocal inhibition is overridden because the nervous system feels that it is more important to contract all muscles that can add to the strength of the joint action that the client is being asked to do, including contracting the muscle that was otherwise being reciprocally inhibited. For this reason, whenever using the principle of reciprocal inhibition, the client should not be asked to contract the target muscle too forcefully. In other words, only gentle resistance should be given to the contraction of the target muscle!

- Following are additional palpation guidelines that may prove useful:
  1. Begin by palpating the target muscle in the easiest place possible. Once the target muscle has been palpated, it is usually easier to continue following it, even if it is deep to other muscles. For this reason, you must begin by finding and palpating the target muscle in the easiest location possible; then follow it to its attachments.
  2. It is usually best to palpate with the pads of the fingers because they are the most sensitive.
  3. Use appropriate pressure! Less can be more regarding palpatory pressure. Deeper pressure can be uncomfortable for the client and lessen your palpatory sensitivity.[7] Having said that, many therapists press too lightly to feel deeper structures. Ideal palpatory pressure is *gentle but firm* and will also vary based on the depth of the muscle that is being palpated.
  4. When you ask the client to actively contract a muscle so that you can palpate it (whether you resist the contraction or not), do not have the client sustain the isometric contraction for too long, because it may cause fatigue or injury to the client.
  5. It is often helpful to ask the client to alternately contract and relax the target muscle. By doing this, you can better feel the changes in tissue texture when the muscle contracts and relaxes.
  6. If a client is ticklish, have the client place his or her hand over your palpating hand. This will often lessen or eliminate the ticklishness. Being ticklish is oversensitivity as a result of a sense of intrusion on one's space (you cannot tickle yourself). By having the client's hand over your hand, that sense of intrusion is eliminated or diminished.

SECTION 16.5 DO WE TREAT MOVERS OR ANTAGONISTS?

- When it comes to musculoskeletal treatment, treatment of muscles is usually the primary focus for most manual and movement therapists, trainers, and other bodyworkers. However, a question arises: Which muscles do we treat?
- We have learned that muscles may act in many roles. Muscles may contract as movers, antagonists, fixators (i.e., stabilizers), neutralizers, and support muscles.[8]
- When a client comes to the office and states that he or she has tightness/pain when turning the head to the right (i.e., right rotation of the head and neck at the spinal joints), what muscles come to mind to be assessed and treated?
  - When this question is asked of beginning students of kinesiology, 80% to 90% of the answers are muscles such as left upper trapezius, left sternocleidomastoid, right splenius capitis or cervicis, and so forth. In other words, most students immediately focus on the movers of the action of right rotation. Given that *mover actions* is the vehicle that we use to teach and learn muscles, this reaction should probably be expected. However, on further thought, why would we look to assess and treat movers of the action? Are the movers injured and not able to create their mover actions without pain? Perhaps this is the case; however, when motion is restricted and/or painful, the most likely culprits are the antagonists.
- The most common problem causing restricted range of motion in clients is tight muscles. Which muscles, if they are tight, would cause pain with right rotation? Right rotators? No. The left rotators that must lengthen and stretch when right rotation occurs are the muscles that will generate pain if they are tight. In other words, it will usually be tight antagonists that will be generating pain when a client performs a joint motion that is restricted and painful.
- This does not mean that we will not treat many clients with muscles that create pain when they perform their mover actions or muscles that are painful when they act as fixators, neutralizers, or support muscles. Any muscle of a muscle group can be involved in a pain and dysfunction. But when restricted range of motion is present, it simply means that more often it will be tight antagonists on the other side of the joint that will create pain when they are lengthened and stretched by a joint action. Mover muscles will usually generate pain during stronger contractions against resistance.
- Tight musculature is not the only tissue that can restrict motion. Any soft tissue on the "other side" of the joint must lengthen for joint motion to occur. For this reason, the concept of antagonist musculature should be expanded to be **antagonist soft tissue**. This includes all fascial tissue as well: ligaments, joint capsules, and other fascial planes of tissue (it can even be expanded to include skin and subcutaneous fascial tissue). Seen in this light, the musculoskeletal system would be better viewed as the **myo-fascio-skeletal system** (Box 16-8).

BOX 16-8

Although there are many factors that are involved in maintaining a healthy musculoskeletal system, perhaps three can be singled out as the most important. These are flexibility of soft tissues, strength of musculature, and proper neural control. As discussed in this chapter, flexibility of soft tissues is important to allow full range of motion. Strength of musculature is important to both create this motion as well as stabilize the joints during motion. And proper neural (motor) control is important to co-order the musculature in temporal and spatial sequence to allow for healthy posture and movement patterns. Given the inclusion of the nervous system control, perhaps our term myo-fascio-skeletal should be expanded even more broadly to be **neuro-myo-fascio-skeletal system**. It is only when all of these factors are assessed and treated that the client's "musculoskeletal" health can be optimized.

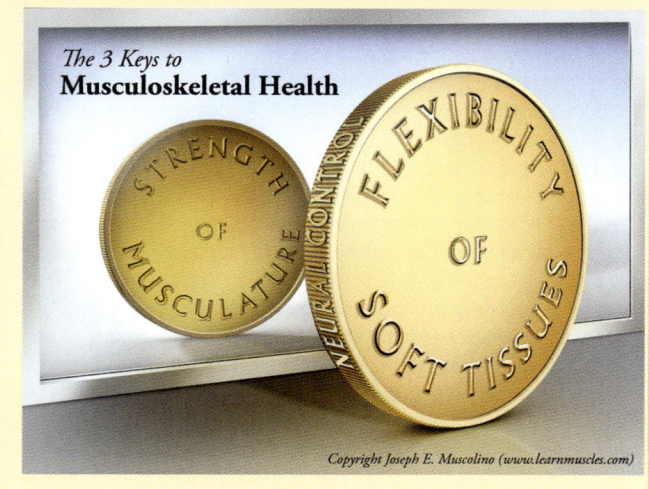

Courtesy Giovanni Rimasti

SECTION 16.6 DO WE TREAT SIGNS OR SYMPTOMS?

○ When assessing a client's musculoskeletal condition, it is important to distinguish between signs and symptoms.
○ **Signs** are objective (i.e., they are observable and measurable by someone other than the client).[6] An example is a person's temperature. The client does not need to tell us that he or she has a fever; it is observable by palpation and measurable with a thermometer. Another example is the tone/tension level of a client's muscle. We do not need a client to tell us that he or she has a tight muscle; it can be objectively felt by the therapist.
○ **Symptoms** are subjective (i.e., only the client can report them).[6] An example is a client *feeling* feverish. No one but the client can report if the client feels feverish; that is a subjective statement only the client can report. Another example is a client's pain as a result of tight musculature. Only the client can experience and report the client's pain; no other person can tell a client what his or her pain level is (Box 16-9).
○ It is crucially important to consider *both* the subjective symptoms that a client reports and the objective signs that we as therapists can determine. If a therapist bases all treatment on a client's subjective report of pain, the ability to accurately assess and effectively treat the cause of a client's condition is greatly diminished.
○ Furthermore, relying solely on a client's subjective pain to determine when treatment is appropriate and necessary can be dangerous for the health of the client. The experience of subjective symptoms usually lags far behind the presence of objective signs.
   ○ A mildly or moderately tight muscle is usually not felt by a client; the muscle usually has to get markedly tight before the client even experiences pain because of the tight muscle. Unfortunately, by that time the problem is larger, more chronically patterned into the client's body, and more difficult to improve with treatment.
○ An analogy often made to clients to help them understand this concept is to explain that a cavity in a tooth begins forming long before the toothache appears. Waiting for muscle pain to appear before having soft tissue manipulation, undergoing other bodywork, or beginning a program of stretching and strengthening exercise is similar to waiting for a toothache to appear before deciding to brush one's teeth (Box 16-10).
○ It is in the clients' best interest to encourage them to proactively approach their health. As therapists and trainers it is our job to educate clients about their musculoskeletal health and to treat signs, not just symptoms (Box 16-11).
○ Another analogy used when explaining the value of manual and movement therapy, exercise, and other bodywork to a client who is focusing only on the level of his or her pain and other symptoms, is to liken a person's condition and symptoms to a glass of water (Figure 16-7). In this analogy, water in the glass represents an accumulation of bad health on the part of the client (it would be a measure of the objective degree of the problem). The more water in the glass, the unhealthier the client.

BOX 16-9

Perhaps the best definition of pain comes from Margo McCaffery, a nurse in private practice. Her definition of pain is "whatever the experiencing person says it is, existing whenever he says it does."* The beauty of this definition is that it squarely recognizes that pain is a subjective symptom and must be defined by the client; it is not within the realm of a therapist or physician to define the client's pain! Therapists and physicians define signs, not symptoms. Symptoms must be reported by the client.

*From Porth CM: *Pathophysiology, concepts of altered health states*, ed 3, Philadelphia, 1990, JB Lippincott.

BOX 16-10

When evaluating the client's signs and symptoms, it is important to not rely only on subjective symptoms such as pain. As critically thinking therapists, we do not want to chase the client's pain because often the underlying mechanism or one of the underlying perpetuating factors for the client's condition lies elsewhere in the body, and may be asymptomatic. For this reason, it is important to thoroughly evaluate the client to determine all underlying mechanisms and perpetuating factors. Having said this, it is also important to keep in mind that there is often a fairly large lag between objective pathology and subjective symptomology. The body has a redundancy built into its design that allows for a good amount of structural dysfunction before pain or other symptoms are necessarily experienced by the client. For example, the accompanying radiograph demonstrates a fairly severe scoliosis in a middle-aged, white-collar worker client. Upon first glance, it would be tempting to assign this client with all sorts of symptoms, chief amongst them pain. Yet this person has no chronic pain pattern to her lower back, middle back, or neck at all (perhaps because she engages in a 20-minute stretching and strengthening routine every morning). Although this may be an extreme case, most people with an advanced scoliosis would probably experience some pain or at least discomfort, it illustrates the point that we need not obsess on every structural deviation that we find with our clients. Each pathological finding should be considered as one puzzle piece of the picture of the person's overall structural and functional health and must be considered along with each other physical examination piece, as well as the person's clinical history and report of presenting complaints.

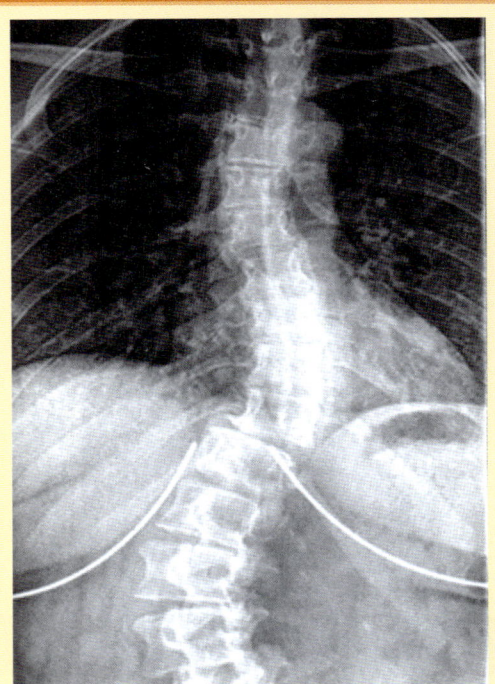

Courtesy Joseph E. Muscolino

However, as long as the water is contained in the glass, the client experiences no symptoms because of the condition. However, once the glass is unable to contain the water and some of it spills out onto the counter, the client feels pain. In this analogy, the amount of water on the counter is equivalent to the degree of subjective pain experienced by the client. However, the total of the water on the counter *and* the water that fills the glass is a more accurate representation of the objective degree of the client's actual condition. If we treat the client only long enough to eliminate the water that has spilled onto the counter, then even though the person now feels fine, the glass is full to the top and the slightest additional stress to the system will cause water to spill over again and create pain once again. At this point it is likely that an uneducated client will say that massage, exercise, and bodywork are nice, but their effects do not last. This type of approach does not help the health of the client and does not

BOX 16-11

Although it is often in the best interest of the client to have manual and movement therapy, receive other bodywork, or begin a physical exercise regimen of stretching and strengthening even when he or she is not experiencing pain or other symptoms, we must be careful that we always keep the client's best interest at heart when recommending a plan of care. It is highly unethical to recommend care to our clients that we know is unnecessary or inappropriate. Furthermore, it is also unethical to push our clients into having care that they do not want to have, whether we feel it is in their best interest or not. Our role is to educate and encourage the client about his or her musculoskeletal health and offer options for care; it is up to the client to accept or decline that advice and care.

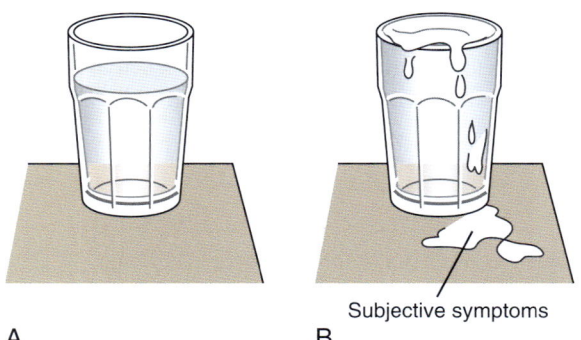

FIGURE 16-7 Analogy to a glass of water and a client's objective and subjective ill health/dysfunction. Amount of water in glass **A** represents the degree of objective ill health of the client. However, as long as the glass contains the water, no subjective symptoms exist (i.e., the client feels fine). As soon as the level of dysfunction increases to the point that water spills out of the glass **(B)**, the water that spills out represents the subjective symptoms of the client (i.e., the client now feels the problem and knows that it is present).

help the reputation of our work. Although we cannot fully empty the client's glass and return the client back to the health he or she had as a child or teenager, we should at least endeavor to do more than just stop the glass from spilling over. Instead we should try to somewhat lessen the water level below the top of the glass. By doing this, the client will have some leeway to encounter stress without every little stressor recreating the pain pattern. A reasonable approach like this is what is ultimately in the best interest of the client.

◯ Treating symptoms is analogous to only mopping up the water that has spilled on the counter. Treating signs is equivalent to treating the client to lessen the level of water in the glass and improve the client's condition now and into the future. What do you treat? Symptoms or signs?

SECTION 16.7 UNDERSTANDING RESEARCH

IMPORTANCE OF RESEARCH:

◯ As manual and movement therapies enter their place among the professions of what is known as integrative or complementary alternative medicine (CAM), the need for research becomes clear. We may know many wonderful things that these therapies and training can do for our clients, but others do not, and our word is not always enough. Conducting research studies shows to the world that the beneficial effects are many and are reproducible. Reproducibility means that it doesn't just work for our clients; it will also work for their clients. It is the basis for *evidence-based care*. For this reason, manual and movement therapies are stepping to the plate, and an increasing amount of research is being done.

◯ The first step toward research literacy is having a familiarity and comfort level with reading and critically thinking through research articles. Yet for those of us who are not familiar with reading and making sense of these articles ourselves, it may be a daunting task when we are asked to read the first few articles. The good news is that most research articles are organized in a similar manner and if we are familiar with its structure, it is easier to read, understand, and navigate the article. To facilitate the process of becoming familiar with the structure of a research article, it is helpful to break down a typical research article into its basic elements. The main purposes of each section, and the definitions of some of the key terms that tend to appear in a research article, are also stated.

◯ However, as valuable as research and evidence-based care are, it should be recognized that there are limitations to this approach.
  ◯ Not all research studies are carried out in a competent manner. As the following section will demonstrate, there are a great number of factors inherent in a quality research study.
  ◯ There are times when the authors of the research study draw conclusions that may not be valid given the framework and findings of the study.
  ◯ A broader limitation is that the very essence of a research study is to isolate one parameter and measure its effect. Yet, the health of body functioning can never rely on any one factor. By virtue of the complexity of our anatomy and physiology, it can be challenging, difficult, or impossible to effectively study the effect of any one aspect of someone's health or any one clinical treatment modality.
  ◯ The world of manual therapy has one particular challenge when it comes to research. The members of the treatment group (that receives the therapeutic treatment) and control group (that receives no treatment or a sham treatment) are supposed to be blind to the fact that they did or did not receive the therapeutic treatment. This is easy to accomplish when both treatment and control groups are given a little white pill, one being the effective treatment and the other being a "sugar pill." However, with manual therapy, it is challenging if not impossible for each of the groups to not know (be blind to) the fact that manual therapy was or was not administered. The work-around for this challenge is often to compare manual therapy to another therapy that already has an established record of results. For example, massage/soft tissue manipulation therapy might be compared to acupuncture.
  ◯ And finally, not all research is in. In fact, all research will never be in. But in the world of manual therapy, there is an especially large gap in evidence-based research. While this gap is gradually being filled in, there is the need to treat now the clients that we have now.

So, in the face of all these challenges, where possible, we try to provide the justification of our care by relying on a solid research study, and/or on the review of a body of studies on one topic, called a *metastudy*.[9] But when research is not available so solid evidence-based work is not possible, we should endeavor to critically think through the mechanisms of the client's condition and choose the most effective treatment techniques based on treating the mechanism(s) of the underlying condition. By critically thinking, we are empowered to creatively apply our care.

ANATOMY OF A RESEARCH ARTICLE:

◯ A research article is usually arranged into six sections with the following headers[9]:
  1. Abstract
  2. Introduction
  3. Methods
  4. Results
  5. Discussion
  6. References

◯ Sometimes, the header for one or some of these sections is slightly different. For example, *methods* might be called *materials and methods* or *methodology*; or *results* might be called *findings*. When present, these alternate names are usually close enough to the listed names that the reader will not be confused.

PURPOSE OF EACH SECTION:

- Abstract: The main purpose of the **abstract** is to summarize the entire research article. The value of the abstract is that when you are doing a literature search and trying to find all articles dealing with a particular topic, reading the abstract can help you decide if that particular article will be useful to you. In other words, the abstract can potentially save you from reading the entire paper only to find out that the article does not address the topic you are investigating.[9]
- Introduction: The **introduction section** is just that; it introduces you to the topic of the research study of the article. Often the introduction lays out the history of the research studies done in the past for this particular topic, stating what was found in them. It then continues to explain why this particular study is valuable or needed. It will usually also state what the specific objective of this research study is.[9]
- Methods: The **methods section** explains the nuts and bolts of how the research study was conducted. It states how many participants were in the various groups, how they were chosen, what the exact procedure was for the treatment group and the control group, and so on. One can look at the methods section as being like a recipe that was followed.[9]
- Results: As the name implies, the **results section** states the results of the study. This section refrains from drawing any subjective conclusions as to the meaning of the results; it merely objectively states what the findings were.[9]
- Discussion: The **discussion section** now discusses the results that were stated in the results section. This is where the meaning of the results is interpreted and conclusions are drawn. This section will, it is hoped, also state whatever limitations the study was found to have. It will usually also state what the implications of the findings of the research study are—that is, what the implications might be for the manual therapist practicing massage (if the research study involved massage) or the therapist or trainer doing stretching or strengthening exercise (if the research study involved these therapies), as well as what the implications are for future research studies involving this topic.[9]
- References: The **references section** is valuable for two reasons. It tells the reader how thorough and current the people conducting the research project were in reading the literature before choosing to conduct their study. The references section also gives the reader a list of other articles that cover the same topic; for anyone doing a literature search, this is extremely valuable because it points to other research articles that may be of value.[9]

SOME KEY TERMS DEFINED:

- There are certain terms that are often used in a research article. Following are the meanings of some of the more common terms that you are likely to encounter.
- Hypothesis: A **hypothesis** is the premise/idea that the research study is attempting to prove or disprove.[9] In effect, it is the theme or purpose of the study. An example of a hypothesis might be "Massage therapy decreases the pain level in people with low back pain." The study would then be designed to try to find the answer that either proves this to be true or proves this to be not true.
- Population: The term **population** is used to describe the population of people that can participate in the study.[9] For example, the population for a particular study might be adults aged 25 to 60 years who have low back pain. (Note: The population is defined by inclusion and exclusion criteria; see next paragraphs.)
- Criterion/parameter: A **criterion** or **parameter** is one aspect, characteristic, or standard of something. For example, a participant's height, weight, or age, whether she or he has a certain medical condition, or whether or not she or he receives treatment are all examples of criteria/parameters. It is usually desirable to have all parameters of the treatment and control groups identical except for one. This way, any difference in results found between these groups can be confidently attributed to the one parameter that was different. This one different parameter is usually the treatment being studied, in our example, low back massage. Note: The word *criterion* is singular; the word *criteria* is plural.
- Inclusion criteria: The **inclusion criteria** are the criteria or parameters that a participant must have to be included within the study.[9] For example, following the example in the previous paragraph, a criterion is that the participant must have low back pain; another criterion is that the person must be 25 to 60 years old.
- Exclusion criteria: The **exclusion criteria** are the criteria or parameters that a participant is not allowed to have to participate in the study.[9] Continuing with our example, an exclusion criterion is that the person cannot be younger than 25 or older than 60. Exclusion criteria often become much more specific: another exclusion criterion might be that the participant cannot have a herniated lumbar disc.
- **Random sample**: It is not feasible for a research study to be done on the entire population because it is usually too large. In our example, there might be tens of millions of people aged 25 to 60 who have low back pain; it is simply too difficult and expensive to do a study on that many people. Therefore, to do this study, it is necessary to take a *sample* of those people. Hence a sample is a smaller subgroup of the entire population being studied. The term *random* refers to the sample of people from the population being chosen at random. In other words, no bias was used in choosing the participants who will be in the study; this means that everyone within the population that you want to study has an equal chance of being a participant in the study. Having a random sample increases the likelihood that the sample group is representative of the larger population and is therefore valid.[9] This means that whatever results are obtained for the sample group will also be true for the entire population.
- Treatment group and control group: The random sample of people (of the population) that is involved in the study is divided into two groups of participants: the treatment group and the control group. The **treatment group** is the group of participants who receive the treatment; in our example, they receive massage therapy to the low back. The **control group** is the group of participants who do not receive the treatment[9]—that is, they do not receive massage therapy to the low back. The idea is that there should be only one parameter that is different between the treatment and control groups; that parameter is the treatment (low back massage therapy) whose efficacy/value the research study is trying to determine. Note: Just as the sample group is supposed to be chosen at random from the population, the treatment and

control groups should essentially be chosen at random from the sample group.

- Placebo: The term **placebo** refers to a *sham treatment* that has no effect that is of interest on the outcome of the study. The placebo treatment is given to the participants in the control group; its purpose is to keep the participants in the control group from knowing that they are not in the treatment group.[9] For example, when a research study is done to test the efficacy of a drug, the placebo given to the control group is usually a sugar pill that looks identical to the real drug. Placebo sham treatments keep the participants *blind* to which group they are in—in other words, not knowing which group they are in.
- Double blind: The term **double blind** refers to both the participants and the examiners (i.e., the people conducting the study) not knowing which group, treatment or control, the participants are in. In effect, both participants and examiners are *blind* to this knowledge.[9] Having a double blind study is considered to be the *gold standard* in research. Note: A problem for the massage world is that it is virtually impossible to have a double blind study with massage therapy because it is difficult to have a placebo sham treatment. The participants in the treatment and control groups pretty much know whether or not they received massage.

A FEW STATISTICS TERMS:

- Standard deviation: When conducting a research study, a **standard deviation** measures how similar the results are for the members of the treatment group relative to the average result for the entire treatment group when measuring a particular value[9] (such as pain or range of motion).

  By definition, one standard deviation in each direction captures 68% of all the participants in the treatment group.[10] To understand this, let's look at an example where the value we are measuring is the client's pain, using a pain scale that ranges from 0 to 10 (where 0 is no pain at all and 10 is the worst pain imaginable). In our example, the average participant in the treatment group reported a decrease in low back pain from a level of 7 to a level of 3; therefore the average pain decrease is measured as $7 - 3 = 4$ degrees of improvement.

  Given that one standard deviation in each direction includes 68% of all the participants in the treatment group. If the treatment group has a standard deviation of one, then that standard deviation would include all people who improved to be within 1 degree of the average pain level at the end of the study. Given that the average pain level is 3, one standard deviation in this case would include all people whose pain level falls between 2 and 4. This shows that 68% of participants improved to be between 2 and 4. In this case, having a small standard deviation of 1 in each direction shows that the improvement of the group is very consistent (i.e., the results are very similar to the average).

  If, instead, the treatment group has a standard deviation of 3, this would include all participants who improved to be within three degrees of the average pain level at the end of the study. Given that the average pain level is 3, one standard deviation would include all people whose pain level falls between 0 and 6. In this case, 68% of the participants improved to be between 0 and 6, which is a larger and more diverse span. In this case, having a larger standard deviation shows that the improvement of the group is much less consistent (i.e., the results are not very similar to the average).

  Note: By definition, 1 standard deviation in each direction is defined as consisting of 68% of the group; 2 standard deviations in each direction is defined as consisting of 95% of the group; and 3 standard deviations in each direction is defined as consisting of 99.7% of the group.[10]

- Mean: The term **mean** is synonymous with the term *average*.[9]
- Median: The term **median** is not the same as mean/average. The median of a group of numbers is the middle score.[9] Let's look at example 1 with the following group of five numbers: 2, 4, 6, 8, and 10. These numbers add up to 30. The mean of this group is computed as 30 divided by 5 = 6; and the median is the middle of the five numbers, which is also 6. In this example, the mean and the median happen to be the same. Now let's look at example 2, also with five numbers that add up to 30: 1, 1, 1, 12, and 15. Now, the mean is still computed as 30 divided by 5 = 6. However, the median number is now 1, which is quite different than the mean number of 6. When interpreting results, usually either the mean or the median is used to describe the results. When the scores are very similar (i.e., homogeneous), the mean is usually used because it well represents the results of the group. When the scores are quite dissimilar (i.e., heterogeneous), the median is usually used because it better represents the results of the group.

REVIEW QUESTIONS

evolve *Answers to the following review questions appear on the Evolve website accompanying this book at:* http://evolve.elsevier.com/Muscolino/kinesiology/.

1. What is the difference between active and passive range of motion?

2. Give an example of active range of motion; give an example of passive range of motion.

3. What type of joint motion is possible at the end of passive joint motion?

4. What is the difference between joint play and an osseous adjustment?

5. Give an example of a ballistic motion.

6. What are the six types of joint end-feel?

7. Resisted motion results in what type of muscular contraction?

8. What is an orthopedic test procedure?

9. Describe how active range of motion, passive range of motion, and resisted motion can be used to assess musculoskeletal soft tissue injuries.

10. What is the difference between a sprain and a strain?

11. What is the difference between an assessment and a diagnosis?

12. What are the five major guidelines to palpating a muscle?

13. Describe and give an example of reciprocal inhibition when palpating a muscle.

14. Explain why tight/injured antagonists are more likely the cause of a problem than tight/injured mover muscles.

15. If a client were to arrive at your office with decreased flexion of the right thigh at the hip joint, what musculature would most likely need to be treated (i.e., what musculature would you first look to assess and treat)?

16. What is the difference between signs and symptoms?

17. Describe how signs and symptoms are used in assessing a client's condition.

18. What are the six major sections of a research paper?

REFERENCES

1. Hamill J, Knutzen KM: Biomechanical basis of human movement, ed 12, Baltimore, 2003, Lippincott Williams & Wilkins.
2. Magee DJ: Orthopedic physical assessment, ed 5, St Louis, 2008, Saunders.
3. Hamilton N, Weimar W, Luttgens K: Kinesiology: Scientific basis of human motion, ed 12, New York, 2012, McGraw Hill.
4. Lowe W: Orthopedic assessment in massage therapy, Sisters, OR, 2006, Daviau-Scott.
5. Neumann DA: Kinesiology of the musculoskeletal system: Foundations for physical rehabilitation, ed 3, St Louis, 2017, Elsevier.
6. Stedman's medical dictionary, ed 27, Baltimore, 2000, Lippincott Williams & Wilkins.
7. Chaitow L, Delaney JW: Clinical application of neuromuscular techniques: Volume 1: The upper body, Edinburgh, 2000, Churchill Livingstone.
8. Hall SJ: Basic biomechanics, ed 6, New York, 2012, McGraw Hill.
9. Baumgartner TA, Hensley LD: Conducting & reading research in health & human performance, ed 4, New York, 2006, McGraw Hill.
10. Kazmier LJ: Schaum's outline of business statistics, ed 4, New York, 2004, McGraw Hill.
11. Slater H, de las Penas CF: Joint mobilization and manipulation of the elbow. In de las Penas CF, Cleland JA, Dommerholt J, editors: Manual therapy for musculoskeletal pain syndromes: An evidence- and clinical-informed approach, Oxford, 2015, Elsevier, pp 458–466.

CHAPTER 17

Determining the Force of a Muscle Contraction

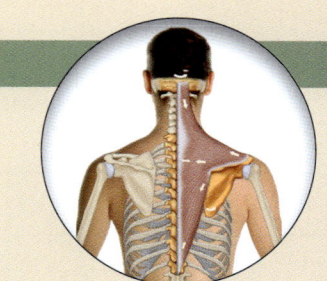

CHAPTER OUTLINE

Section 17.1	Partial Contraction of a Muscle	Section 17.6	Leverage of a Muscle
Section 17.2	Muscle Fiber Architecture	Section 17.7	Leverage of a Muscle—More Detail
Section 17.3	Active Tension versus Passive Tension	Section 17.8	Classes of Levers
Section 17.4	Active Insufficiency	Section 17.9	Leverage of Resistance Forces
Section 17.5	Length-Tension and Force-Velocity Relationship Curves		

CHAPTER OBJECTIVES

After completing this chapter, the student should be able to perform the following:

1. Define the key terms of this chapter and state the meanings of the word origins of this chapter.
2. Do the following related to partial contractions of a muscle:
   - Describe how a muscle can have a partial contraction
   - Explain the meaning of the Henneman size principle.
   - Explain the difference between the intrinsic strength of a muscle and the extrinsic strength of a muscle.
3. Describe the various types of muscle fiber architecture, and explain the advantages and disadvantages of longitudinal versus pennate muscles.
4. Describe active tension and passive tension of a muscle
5. Do the following related to active insufficiency:
   - Explain the relationship between the sliding filament mechanism and shortened active insufficiency and lengthened active insufficiency.
   - Give an example of shortened active insufficiency and lengthened active insufficiency.
6. Do the following related to length-tension and force-velocity relationship curves:
   - Explain the meaning of the active, passive, and total tension curves of the length-tension relationship curve.
   - Describe the relationship between the concepts of the sliding filament mechanism, active length-tension relationship curve, and active insufficiency.
7. Explain the relationship between leverage and the extrinsic strength of a muscle.
8. Do the following related to leverage of a muscle:
   - Describe the advantage and disadvantage of a muscle with greater leverage.
   - Define the terms *internal force* and *external force*, and give an example of each.
   - Explain why a muscle with an attachment that has a less than optimal angle of pull loses extrinsic strength.
   - Explain how to determine the lever arm of a muscle.
9. List the three classes of levers, and give a mechanical object and muscular example of each one.
10. Do the following related to leverage of resistance forces:
    - Define the resistance force to a muscle's contraction, and give two examples of a resistance force.
    - Sketch the region of the body where a muscle is contracting, and draw the arrows that represent the force of the muscle contraction and the resistance force that opposes the muscle contraction.

OVERVIEW

The all-or-none–response law states that a muscle fiber either contracts all the way or not at all. Therefore a muscle fiber cannot have a partial contraction. The all-or-none–response law also applies to motor units, because if any one muscle fiber of the motor unit is instructed to contract, then every muscle fiber of that motor unit will contract. Therefore a motor unit cannot have a partial contraction either. However, the all-or-none–response law does not apply to an entire muscle. A muscle is an organ made up of many motor units, some of which may be ordered to contract and others not. Therefore a muscle can have a partial contraction. How strong a muscle's contraction will be is dependent on many factors. It is the focus of this chapter to examine the factors that affect the strength of a muscle's contraction, whether it is a partial or full contraction. Some of these factors are intrinsic to the muscle, such as the active tension and passive tension of the muscle. A number of factors are extrinsic to the muscle, such as the leverage of the muscle's pulling force, including the angle at which the muscle pulls on its bony attachment. Gravity must also be considered in evaluation of the ability of a muscle contraction to create movement of the body. This chapter explores these intrinsic and extrinsic factors that determine the pulling force (i.e., the strength) of a muscle's contraction.

KEY TERMS

Active insufficiency
Active tension
Axis of motion (AK-sis)
Bipennate muscle (buy-PEN-nate)
Effort arm
External forces
Extrinsic strength (ek-STRINS-ik)
Fan-shaped muscle
First (1st)-class lever
Force-velocity relationship curve
Fusiform-shaped muscle (FUSE-i-form)
Henneman size principle (HEN-i-man)
Internal forces
Intrinsic strength (in-TRINS-ik)
Lengthened active insufficiency
Length-tension relationship curve
Lever
Lever arm
Leverage
Longitudinal muscle
Mechanical advantage
Mechanical disadvantage

Moment arm
Multipennate muscle (MUL-tee-PEN-nate)
Muscle fiber architecture
Optimal angle of pull
Passive tension
Pennate muscle (PEN-nate)
Pennation angle (pen-NAY-shun)
Rectangular-shaped muscle
Resistance to movement
Rhomboidal-shaped muscle (rom-BOYD-al)
Second (2nd)-class lever
Shortened active insufficiency
Sphincter muscle (SFINGK-ter)
Spindle-shaped muscle
Spiral muscle
Squat bend
Stoop bend
Strap muscle
Third (3rd)-class lever
Triangular-shaped muscle
Unipennate muscle (YOU-nee-PEN-nate)

WORD ORIGINS

- Active—From Latin *activus*, meaning *doing, driving*
- Bi—From Latin *bis*, meaning *two, twice*
- Extrinsic—From Latin *extrinsecus*, meaning *from without, outside*
- Intrinsic—From Latin *intrinsecus*, meaning *on the inside*
- Lever/leverage—From Latin *levis*, meaning *light, not heavy*
- Longitudinal—From Latin *longitudo*, meaning *length*
- Motor—From Latin *moveo*, meaning *a mover*
- Multi—From Latin *multus*, meaning *many, much*
- Passive—From Latin *passives*, meaning *permit, endures*
- Pennate—From Latin *penna*, meaning *feather*
- Tension—From Latin *tensio*, meaning *to stretch*
- Uni—From Latin *unis*, meaning *one*

SECTION 17.1 PARTIAL CONTRACTION OF A MUSCLE

- A muscle is an organ composed of many muscle fibers that are grouped into motor units. According to the all-or-none–response law, a muscle fiber contracts either all the way or not at all. Because whatever instruction is given to one muscle fiber is given to all muscle fibers of a motor unit, the all-or-none law also applies to a motor unit (i.e., either all muscle fibers of a motor unit contract all the way or they do not contract at all). (Note: For more information on motor units and the all-or-none–response law, see Sections 12.9 and 12.10.)
- Physiologists who study muscle function often like to say that when it comes to ordering musculature of the body to contract, the brain thinks in motor units, not muscles. Although this might be a strong statement, a certain truth to it exists. Neurons do not control muscles per se; they control the contraction of motor units. In that sense, it is the coordination of motor units of the body, not muscles, that creates the movement patterns of the body!
- When one looks at the contraction of motor units, a hierarchy of motor unit recruitment exists.[1]
  - Generally, when a muscle needs a weak contraction, a smaller motor unit is recruited to contract.
  - If the muscle then needs a stronger contraction, the muscle recruits a larger motor unit *in addition to* the smaller one that is already contracting.
  - Starting with small motor units and then incrementally adding increasingly larger motor units causes a smooth transition to occur as a muscle begins its contraction and then increases the strength of its contraction.
  - This hierarchy of how motor units are recruited to contract is called the Henneman size principle.[1]
  - A relationship exists between the size of a motor neuron, the size of a motor unit, and the type of muscle fibers that are within that motor unit. Generally, smaller motor units are innervated by smaller motor neurons and contain red, slow-twitch muscle fibers, which are more adapted toward creating joint stabilization, whereas larger motor units are innervated by larger motor neurons and contain white, fast-twitch muscle fibers, which are more adapted toward creating joint movement. Therefore when a joint action is ordered by the central nervous system (CNS), the smaller motor units that initially contract are meant to create stabilization of the joint before larger motor units are recruited to create the larger motion at that joint. (For more on joint stabilization, see Sections 15.5 and 15.6.)
- Although muscle fibers and motor units obey the all-or-none–response law, muscles can have partial contractions.
- A number of factors should be considered in examining the intrinsic strength of a muscle's contraction. The most obvious factor regarding the strength or degree of a muscle's contraction is simply how many motor units are ordered to contract by the nervous system.
- If every motor unit of a muscle contracts, then the muscle will contract at 100% of its maximum strength (i.e., the muscle will have a full contraction).
- If only some motor units are ordered to contract, then the muscle will have a partial contraction.
- The degree of this partial contraction is determined not only by the number of motor units that contract but also by the number of muscle fibers in these motor units.
- If, for example, a muscle has a total of 1000 fibers and three of its motor units contract, and if these three motor units each have 50, 100, and 250 muscle fibers in them respectively, then a total of 400 muscle fibers out of 1000 muscle fibers are contracting, yielding a 40% contraction of the muscle.
- If instead, a muscle with a total of 1000 fibers has three motor units contract with 100, 200, and 300 fibers each, then that muscle has 600 muscle fibers contract out of 1000 muscle fibers and has a 60% contraction of the muscle.
- In both cases three motor units contracted, but the degree of strength of the contraction was determined by the number of muscle fibers that contracted, not the number of motor units.
- Therefore a better determination of the strength of a muscle's contraction would be to count the number of muscle fibers that contract (Box 17-1).

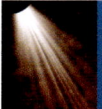

BOX 17-1 Spotlight on Intrinsic versus Extrinsic Strength of a Muscle

The strength of a muscle can be defined as the strength of its pulling force on its bony attachment(s). The overall strength of a muscle is a combination of two aspects: (1) the muscle's intrinsic strength and (2) the muscle's extrinsic strength.[5] The **intrinsic strength** of a muscle is defined as the strength that the muscle generates within itself (i.e., intrinsically). It is a result of the strength that the muscle generates internally because of the sliding filament mechanism (i.e., active tension) and the elastic recoil property of the tissues of the muscle (i.e., passive tension). The intrinsic strength of a muscle is independent of the external surroundings. However, the intrinsic strength of a muscle is not the totality of the strength that a muscle displays when it contracts and pulls on its attachments. To complete the picture, the extrinsic strength of the muscle must also be taken into account. The **extrinsic strength** of a muscle takes into account all the factors outside of the muscle itself. These factors include such things as the leverage that the muscle has on its attachments, as well as the angle of the muscle's pull relative to the joint where the movement is occurring. Only when considering intrinsic and extrinsic factors can the sum total of a muscle's effect on its attachments (i.e., its strength) be understood. (Factors that affect the intrinsic strength of a muscle are covered in Sections 17.1 through 17.5; extrinsic factors that affect the muscle's strength are covered in Sections 17.6 through 17.9.)

- However, not all muscle fibers are the same. For example, when a person does strengthening exercises and builds up the muscles, the number of muscle fibers does not change; what changes is the size of each fiber. With exercise, the number of sarcomeres and the number of contractile proteins (i.e., actin, myosin) increases. As a result, some muscle fibers are larger and stronger than others.

- Therefore a better determinant of the strength of a muscle's contraction is the number of cross-bridges that are made between myosin and actin. A muscle is really nothing more than a great number of sarcomeres with cross-bridges that create a pulling force!
- Note: Even the simple number of myosin-actin cross-bridges is not the final determinant. Another factor must be considered (i.e., the orientation of the pull of the cross-bridges relative to the line of pull of the muscle itself). The orientation of the pull of the cross-bridges is determined by the orientation of the pull of the muscle fibers (i.e., the architecture of the muscle fibers relative to the muscle). For more on the architecture of muscle fibers, see the following section, Section 17.2.

SECTION 17.2   MUSCLE FIBER ARCHITECTURE

- The orientation—in other words, the arrangement of muscle fibers within a muscle—is called **muscle fiber architecture**.
- Muscles have two general architectural types in which their fibers are arranged: (1) longitudinal and (2) pennate.[2]

LONGITUDINAL MUSCLES:

- A **longitudinal muscle** has its fibers running longitudinally (i.e., along the length of the muscle).[3] Most fibers of a longitudinal muscle run along the length of the muscle from attachment to attachment. (For more information on how muscle fibers are arranged within a muscle, see Section 12.3.)
  - Therefore the force of the contraction of the fibers is in the same direction as the length of the muscle.
- Longitudinal muscles can be divided into various categories based on the shape. The following are the most common types of longitudinal muscles[3] (Figure 17-1):
  - **Fusiform** (also known as **spindle**)
  - **Strap**
  - **Rectangular**
  - **Rhomboidal**
  - **Triangular** (also known as **fan-shaped**)
- Note: Other types of muscles such as a **sphincter muscle** (circular muscle—e.g., the orbicularis oculi) and a **spiral muscle** (muscle with a twist—e.g., the latissimus dorsi) may also be placed into the category of longitudinal muscles.[3]

PENNATE MUSCLES:

- A **pennate muscle** has its fibers arranged in a featherlike manner.[4]
- The word *pennate* means *featherlike*. The word *pen* has the same origin, because pens were originally made from quills (i.e., feathers).
- Like a feather, the fibers are not arranged along the length of the muscle; rather, a central fibrous tendon runs along the length of the muscle. The muscle fibers themselves are arranged obliquely (i.e., at an angle) to the central tendon of the muscle.[3]
  - Therefore the force of the contraction of the fibers is not in the same direction as length of the muscle[2]!
- Pennate muscles are divided into three types: (1) unipennate, (2) bipennate, and (3) multipennate[3] (Figure 17-2).
  - A **unipennate muscle** has a central tendon within the muscle, and the fibers are oriented diagonally off one side of the tendon. An example of a unipennate muscle is the vastus lateralis muscle of the quadriceps femoris group.[4]
  - A **bipennate muscle** has a central tendon within the muscle, and the fibers are oriented diagonally off both sides of the tendon. An example of a bipennate muscle is the rectus femoris muscle of the quadriceps femoris group.[4]
  - A **multipennate muscle** has more than one central tendon with fibers oriented diagonally either to one and/or both sides. In effect, a multipennate muscle has combinations of unipennate and bipennate arrangements. An example of a multipennate muscle is the deltoid muscle.[4]

LONGITUDINAL AND PENNATE MUSCLES COMPARED:

- In comparison, a longitudinal muscle has long muscle fibers; a pennate muscle has short muscle fibers.
  - However, a pennate muscle has more muscle fibers than a longitudinal muscle.[3]
- Furthermore, the fibers of a longitudinal muscle are oriented along the length of the muscle, whereas the fibers of a pennate muscle are oriented at an oblique angle to the length of the muscle.
  - However, if a longitudinal muscle and a pennate muscle of the same overall size are compared, they will both contain the same mass of muscle tissue. Hence they will both contain the same number of sarcomeres and therefore the same number of myosin-actin cross-bridges.
- Because a muscle fiber can shorten to approximately ½ of its resting length when it maximally concentrically contracts, longitudinal muscles, having longer fibers, shorten more than pennate muscles.[5]
  - Therefore a longitudinal muscle is ideally suited to create a large range of motion of a body part at a joint.
- Pennate muscles have shorter fibers but have a greater number of them than longitudinal muscles.
  - Given that a pennate muscle has the same number of sarcomeres generating strength as a same-sized longitudinal muscle, but that same strength is concentrated over a shorter range of motion (because of the shorter fibers arranged at an oblique angle to the direction of the muscle [Box 17-2]), a pennate muscle exhibits greater strength over a shorter range of motion.[4]
  - Therefore a longitudinal muscle is generally better suited for a greater range of motion contraction but with less force, whereas a pennate muscle is generally better suited for greater strength contraction over a shorter range of motion.[5]

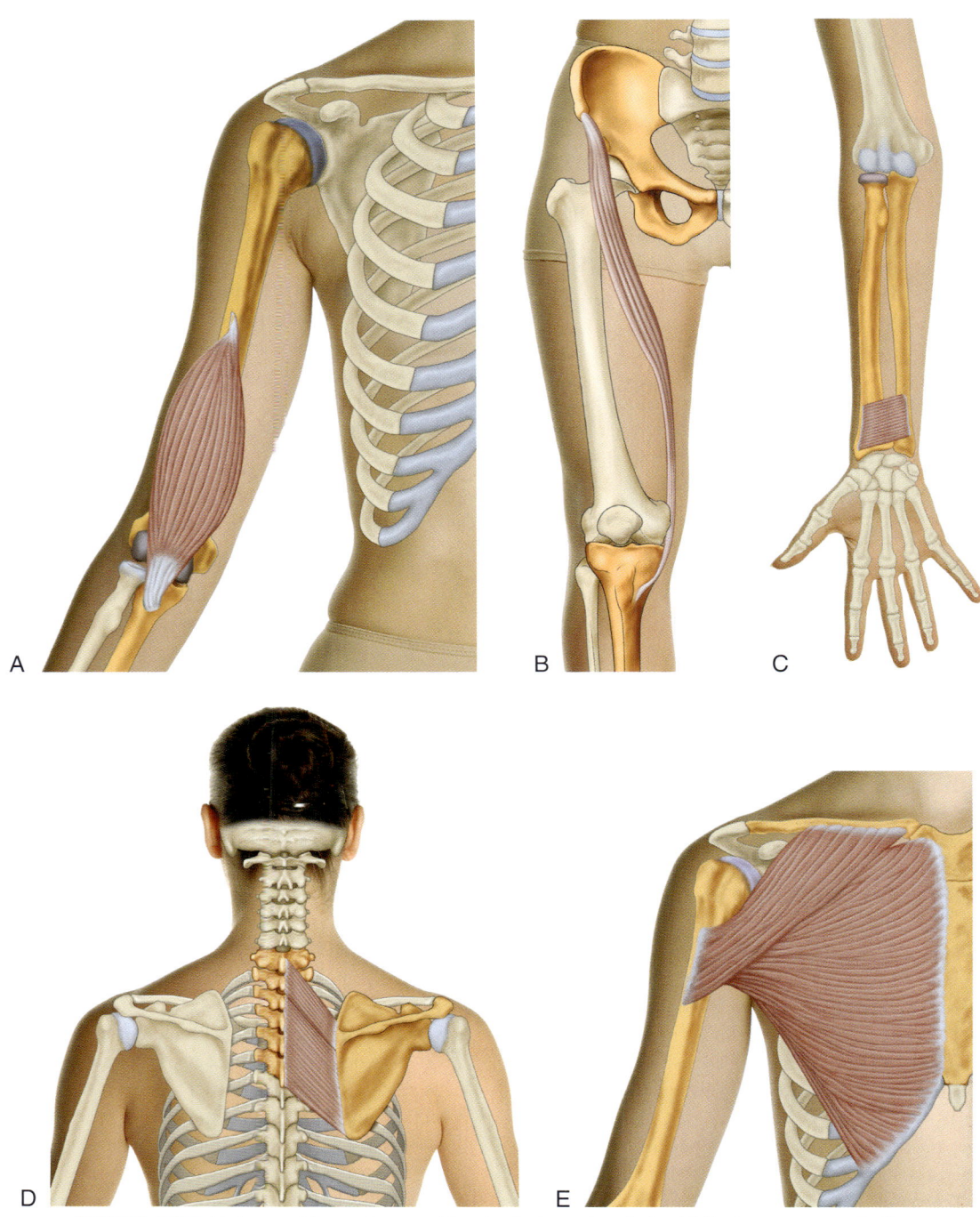

FIGURE 17-1 Various architectural types of longitudinal muscles. **A,** Brachialis demonstrates a fusiform-shaped (also known as spindle-shaped) muscle. **B,** Sartorius demonstrates a strap muscle. **C,** Pronator quadratus demonstrates a rectangular-shaped muscle. **D,** Rhomboid muscles demonstrate rhomboidal-shaped muscles. **E,** Pectoralis major demonstrates a triangular-shaped (also known as fan-shaped) muscle. *(From Muscolino JE: The muscular system manual: the skeletal muscles of the human body, ed 4, St Louis, 2017, Mosby.)*

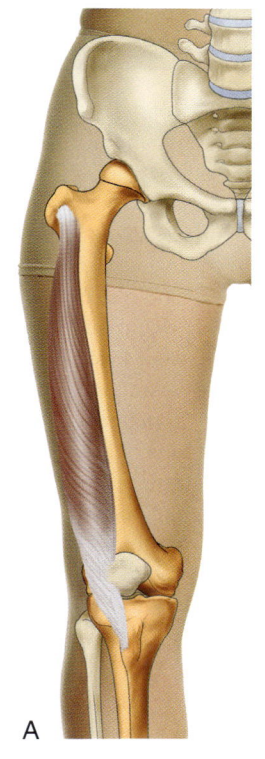
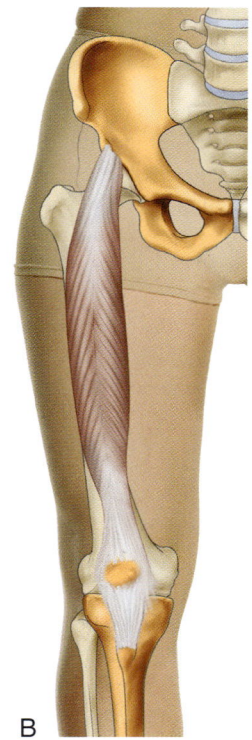
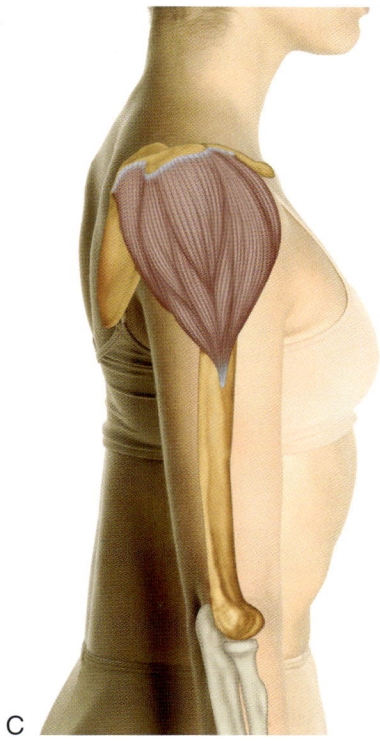

FIGURE 17-2 The three architectural types of pennate muscles. Pennate muscles have one or more central tendons running along the length of the muscle from which the muscle fibers come off at an oblique angle. **A,** Vastus lateralis is a unipennate muscle. (Note: Central tendon is not visible in the anterior view.) **B,** Rectus femoris is a bipennate muscle. **C,** Deltoid is a multipennate muscle. *(From Muscolino JE: The muscular system manual: the skeletal muscles of the human body, ed 4, St Louis, 2017, Mosby.)*

A   B   C

BOX 17-2 Spotlight on the Pennation Angle

In determining the strength of a muscle, especially pennate muscles, one other factor needs to be taken into consideration—that is, the **pennation angle**. The pennation angle is the angle of the muscle fiber relative to the central tendon of the muscle. If a muscle fiber is parallel to its tendon (i.e., running along the length of the muscle as in longitudinal muscles), then its pennation angle is zero degrees and all of its pulling force pulls along the length of the tendon, pulling the attachments of the muscle toward the center of the muscle. However, as the angle of the muscle fiber becomes more oblique (as in pennate muscles), the pennation angle increases, the pull of the fiber is less in line with the tendon, and less of its contraction force contributes to the pull on the attachments. For this reason, as much as pennate muscles are designed to generate a greater force over a relatively small range of motion, some of the strength is lost because of the greater pennation angle (see figures).

In other words, the greater the pennation angle, the more fibers can be fit in the same mass and the greater relative strength over a shorter range of motion; however, some of the intrinsic strength of the muscle fibers is lost because they are not pulling along the length of the muscle! To determine the effect of the pennation angle on the strength of the muscle, trigonometry is used. A trigonometric formula can be used to determine what percentage of a pennate fiber's contraction contributes to the pulling force that occurs along the length of the muscle, because it is this force that effectively pulls the muscle's attachments toward the center of the muscle. For example, a fiber with a pennation angle of 30 degrees contributes 86% of its force to pulling the attachments toward the center, and a fiber with a pennation angle of 60 degrees contributes 50% of its force to pulling the attachments toward the center.[6]

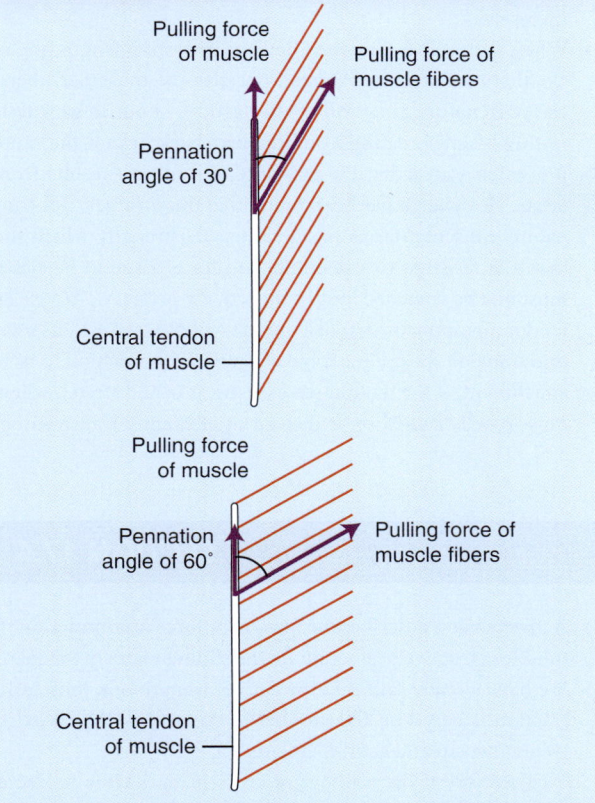

SECTION 17.3   ACTIVE TENSION VERSUS PASSIVE TENSION

- When we talk about a muscle generating a forceful contraction, it is important to remember that a muscle can generate two types of forces: (1) an active force and (2) a passive force.
- The term *tension* is used to describe the pulling force that a muscle generates.
- Interestingly, the word *tension*, which is used to describe pulling forces and therefore the degree of a muscle's contraction (i.e., its pulling force), actually means *stretch*. Perhaps the derivation of its use is that when something is being pulled on, it is stretched.
  - Therefore a muscle may pull on its attachments with active tension and with passive tension.

ACTIVE TENSION:

- **Active tension** of a muscle is generated by the sliding filament mechanism (i.e., its contraction). This tension is termed *active* because the muscle is actively creating this force (i.e., the muscle is expending energy in the form of adenosine triphosphate [ATP] to generate a contraction via actins being pulled toward the center of the sarcomere by the cross-bridges of myosin).[6]
  - Hence this aspect of a muscle's pulling force is called *active tension*.

PASSIVE TENSION:

- A muscle can also generate a **passive tension** force that can contribute to its tension pulling force.[6]
- This passive force is created primarily by the muscle fibers themselves.
- When a muscle is stretched beyond its resting length, the muscle fibers are stretched longer. Because the muscular fibers are elastic in nature, they will try to elastically bounce back to their resting length, creating a pulling force back toward the center.[6]
- It is often stated that the elasticity of a muscle results from its fascia. However, it has been found that this is largely not true. By nature, muscular fascia has great tensile strength, which means that it is resistant to stretching; and for a tissue to be elastic, it must first be stretched longer. Indeed, the primary purpose of the tendon (or aponeurosis) of a muscle—in other words, its fascia—is to transmit the pulling force of a muscle contraction to its bony attachment. If the tendon were elastic, it would stretch when the muscle belly pulled on it instead of efficiently transmitting the force of the muscle contraction to the attachment. Instead, it has been found that the elasticity of muscle tissue resides primarily within the muscle fibers themselves. Specifically, it results from the elasticity of the large titin proteins that are found within the muscle fibers[6] (for more on titin, see Section 12.11).
- An analogy can be made to a rubber/elastic band. When an elastic band is stretched, its natural elasticity creates a pulling force that would pull on whatever is holding the elastic band in this stretched position. In a similar manner, all soft tissue, including muscular tissue, is elastic.
  - Therefore a stretched muscle would have an elastic pulling force that would pull the muscle's attachments toward the center of the muscle.
- This pulling force adds to the tension that a muscle generates on its attachments[6] (Box 17-3).
- This elastic tension force is termed *passive tension* because a muscle does not actively generate it (i.e., the muscle expends no energy to create it; it is inherent in the natural elasticity of the tissue).

BOX 17-3

Most sports have a backswing before the actual stroke is performed; examples include the backswing in tennis, golf, or baseball. One reason for a backswing is that it first stretches the muscle that will be performing the stroke. This adds the passive elastic recoil force to the active contraction force of the muscle when it performs the stroke. The net result is a more powerful pulling force by the muscle!

TOTAL TENSION:

- Hence the active tension of a muscle is generated by its contractile actin and myosin filaments, and the passive tension of a muscle results from its natural elasticity.
- Therefore the total tension of a muscle, both its active and passive tension, must be measured for determination of the force of a muscle's contraction.[7]

SECTION 17.4   ACTIVE INSUFFICIENCY

- Active tension describes the tension or force of contraction that a muscle can actively generate via the sliding filament mechanism.
- We have already said that the active strength of a muscle's contraction is based on the number of cross-bridges that exist between myosin and actin filaments.
  - Therefore if the number of cross-bridges were to decrease, the strength of the muscle's contraction would decrease.[6]
- If the strength of a muscle's contraction decreases sufficiently, the muscle could be said to be insufficient in strength.
  - Hence an actively insufficient muscle is a muscle that cannot generate sufficient strength actively via the sliding filament mechanism.[2]
  - Therefore **active insufficiency** is the term used to describe a muscle that is weak because of a decrease in the number

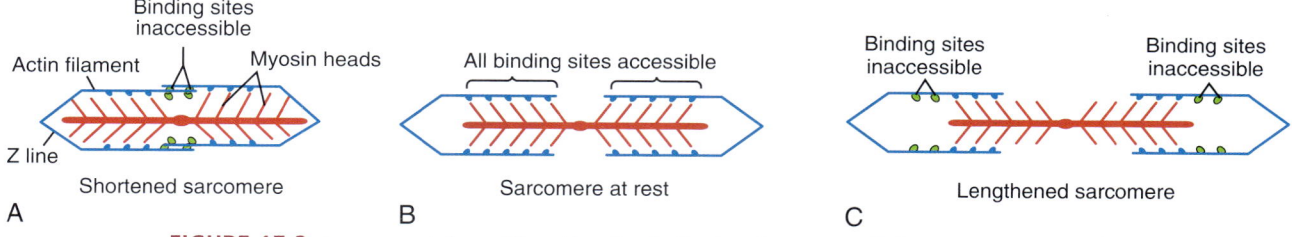

FIGURE 17-3 Sarcomere at three different lengths. **A,** Shortened sarcomere. **B,** Same sarcomere at resting length. **C,** Same sarcomere lengthened. (Note: The sarcomere at resting length can produce the greatest number of myosin-actin cross-bridges and therefore can produce the strongest contraction.) Fewer possible cross-bridges formed when the sarcomere is shorter or longer results in weakness of the muscle, called active insufficiency (i.e., shortened active insufficiency in **A**; lengthened active insufficiency in **C**).

of myosin-actin cross-bridges during the sliding filament mechanism.
○ Two states of active insufficiency exist: (1) shortened active insufficiency and (2) lengthened active insufficiency.

SHORTENED ACTIVE INSUFFICIENCY:

○ **Shortened active insufficiency** of a muscle occurs when a muscle is shorter than its resting length and weak because of a decrease in myosin-actin cross-bridges.[2]
○ To understand why this situation occurs, we will compare a sarcomere at resting length with a sarcomere that is shortened (Figure 17-3).
○ Figure 17-3, *B* shows a sarcomere at rest. At rest, we see that every myosin head is able to form a cross-bridge by binding to the adjacent actin filament. Given this maximal number of cross-bridge formation, the sarcomere at rest can generate maximal pulling force and is therefore strong.
○ In Figure 17-3, *A* we see a sarcomere that is shortened. In a shortened sarcomere, the actin filaments overlap one another in such a way that some of the binding (active) sites on one of the actin filaments are blocked by the other actin filament (and some of the binding sites of the actin filament that is overlapping the other are too close toward the center and also not accessible by the myosin heads). Therefore the myosin heads that would normally form cross-bridges by attaching to those binding sites are unable to do so. This results in fewer cross-bridges. A sarcomere that forms fewer cross-bridges cannot generate as much pulling force, and its strength is diminished. Because a shortened muscle is composed of shortened sarcomeres, a shortened muscle exhibits shortened active insufficiency and is weaker because it forms fewer myosin-actin cross-bridges!

LENGTHENED ACTIVE INSUFFICIENCY:

○ **Lengthened active insufficiency** of a muscle occurs when a muscle is longer than its resting length and weak because of a decrease in myosin-actin cross-bridges.[2]
○ To understand why this situation occurs, compare a sarcomere at resting length with a sarcomere that is lengthened (see Figure 17-3).

○ Again, Figure 17-3, *B* shows a sarcomere at rest in which every myosin head is able to form a cross-bridge by binding to the adjacent actin filament. Given this maximal number of cross-bridge formation, the sarcomere at rest can generate maximal pulling force and is therefore strong.
○ In Figure 17-3, *C* we see a sarcomere that is lengthened. In a lengthened sarcomere, the actin filaments are pulled so far from the center of the sarcomere that many of the myosin heads cannot reach the actin filaments to form cross-bridges. Therefore many of the myosin heads that would normally form cross-bridges are unable to do so. This results in fewer cross-bridges. A sarcomere that forms fewer cross-bridges cannot generate as much pulling force, and its strength is diminished. Because a lengthened muscle is composed of lengthened sarcomeres, a lengthened muscle exhibits lengthened active insufficiency and is weaker because it forms fewer myosin-actin cross-bridges!
○ Excellent examples of both shortened active insufficiency and lengthened active insufficiency are shown in Figure 17-4. When a person makes a fist, the muscles that make the fist are the flexors of the fingers and thumb, and the specific muscles responsible for this action are primarily the extrinsic flexors that attach proximally in the arm/forearm (flexor digitorum superficialis, flexor digitorum profundus, flexor pollicis longus). These extrinsic flexors cross the wrist joint anteriorly to enter the hand; then they cross the metacarpophalangeal (MCP) and interphalangeal (IP) joints to enter the fingers.
○ If the wrist joint is flexed as in Figure 17-4, *A,* these extrinsic muscles would shorten across the wrist joint, and because of shortened active insufficiency, would be unable to generate sufficient strength to move the fingers and make a strong fist (Box 17-4).
○ If the wrist joint is extended instead (as in Figure 17-4, *C*), these muscles would be stretched longer across the wrist joint and, because of lengthened active insufficiency, would be unable to generate sufficient strength to move the fingers and make a strong fist. Compare your ability to make a fist when your wrist joint is flexed or extended with your ability to make a fist when your wrist joint is in a neutral position (see Figure 17-4, *B*).

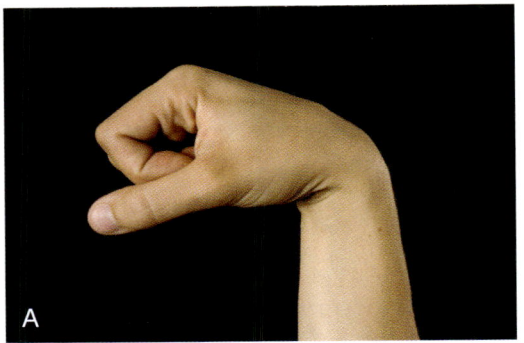
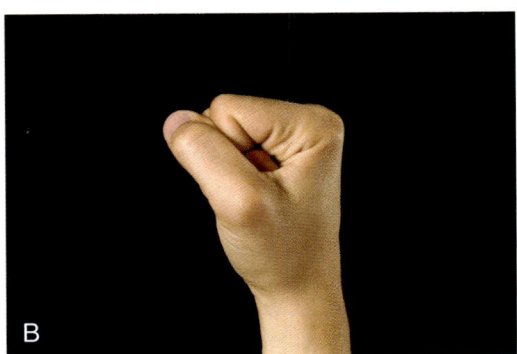
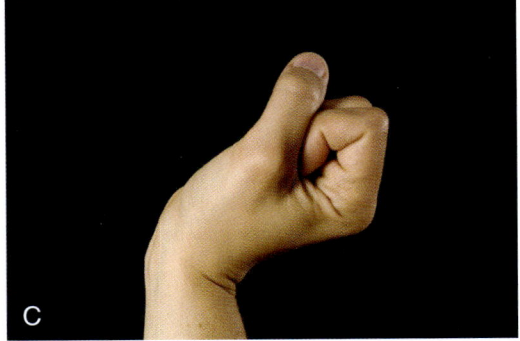

FIGURE 17-4 Concept of active insufficiency of the extrinsic finger flexor muscles that attach proximally in the arm/forearm. When these muscles contract to make a fist with the hand flexed at the wrist joint, these muscles become shortened and actively insufficient, resulting in a fist that is weak **(A)**. When these muscles contract to make a fist with the hand extended at the wrist joint, these muscles become lengthened and actively insufficient, also resulting in a fist that is weak **(C)**. However, when a fist is made with the hand in neutral position at the wrist joint, the strength of the fist is optimal **(B)**. *(Courtesy Joseph E. Muscolino.)*

BOX 17-4

Another classic example that demonstrates shortened active insufficiency is abdominal curl-ups (i.e., crunches). A number of years ago, when people did sit-ups, they were done with the hip and knee joints straight. However, that style sit-up was found to excessively strengthen and most likely tighten the iliopsoas muscle, which could then have deleterious effects on the posture of and compression upon the spine. Now it is routinely taught to bend the hip and knee joints when doing a sit-up (now termed a curl-up or crunch). The reason for bending the hip joint is to shorten the iliopsoas by bringing its attachments closer together (flexing the thigh at the hip joint brings the lesser trochanter closer to the pelvis and spine). By doing this, the iliopsoas becomes shortened and actively insufficient; therefore it is not as readily recruited during the curl-up and is not strengthened as much. It should be noted that it is often recommended to not go past 30 degrees with a curl-up because at that point the iliopsoas will more likely be recruited despite being actively insufficient.

SECTION 17.5 LENGTH-TENSION AND FORCE-VELOCITY RELATIONSHIP CURVES

- Given the concepts of passive tension and shortened and lengthened active insufficiency, it is clear that the length of a muscle has an effect on the tension that it can generate[5] (i.e., the strength of its pulling force).
- The relationship between the length of a muscle and the active tension that a muscle can generate is related to the length of the sarcomeres and the tension that the sarcomeres can generate, as has been explained in earlier sections of this chapter. This relationship can be depicted on a graph called the **length-tension relationship curve**[8] (Figure 17-5).
- The length-tension relationship curve is a graph that compares the length of a sarcomere with the percentage of maximal contraction that the sarcomere can generate. Because a muscle is effectively composed of many sarcomeres, the relationship between the length and tension of a sarcomere can be extrapolated to the relationship between the length and tension of

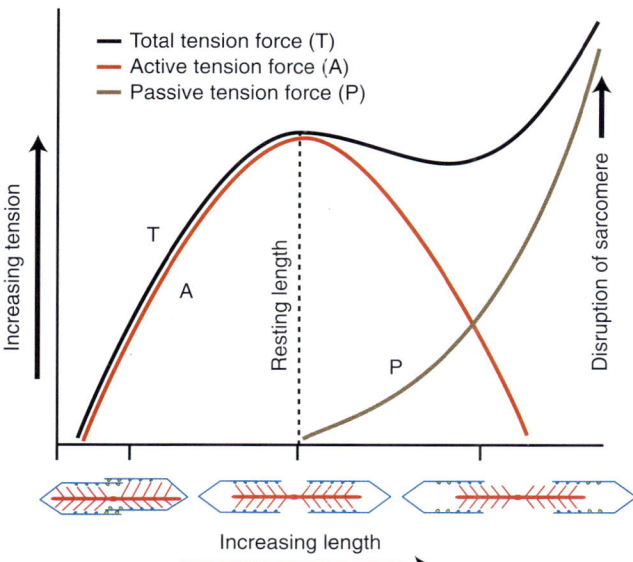

FIGURE 17-5 Three sarcomere length-tension relationship curves. These curves depict the relationship between the length of a sarcomere and the tension that it generates (i.e., its pulling force) at that length. The *red line* represents the active tension force that a sarcomere can generate when it contracts via the sliding filament mechanism. The *brown line* represents the passive tension force that the sarcomere generates when it is stretched. The *black line* represents the sum total of the active tension curve and the passive tension curve; therefore it represents the total pulling force of the sarcomere.

an entire muscle. (Note: The active length-tension relationship curve depicted in Figure 17-5 was created by measuring the contractile force of an isometric contraction for the continuum of lengths displayed. Some researchers caution that the values derived may not be 100% accurately correlated to concentric and eccentric contractions.)

Extrapolating these values for an entire muscle, we see the following:
- The red line in Figure 17-5 considers only the active tension as the length of a muscle changes. The shape of this curve is a bell curve wherein the greatest tension is clearly when the muscle is at resting length. When the length of the muscle changes in either direction (i.e., gets longer or shorter), the active tension that the muscle can generate decreases.
  - Lessened active tension when a muscle is shortened is called *shortened active insufficiency*.
  - Lessened active tension when a muscle is lengthened is called *lengthened active insufficiency*.
- The brown line in Figure 17-5 considers only the passive tension as the length of the muscle changes. We see that passive tension is nonexistent when the muscle is shortened. However, as the muscle lengthens beyond resting length, the passive tension of the muscle increases.
  - This increased passive tension of a muscle as it lengthens is called *passive tension* and results from the natural elasticity of the tissue.
- The black line in Figure 17-5 considers both the active tension and the passive tension of a muscle as its length changes.
  - We see that the overall tension (i.e., pulling force of the muscle) increases from a shortened length to resting length. The tension force in this range of the muscle's length is caused by increasing active tension.
  - The pulling force then stays fairly high beyond resting length for quite some time. Most of the tension in this range of the muscle's length results from increasing passive tension.
  - It is important to note that (as the graph shows) even though the total tension/pulling force of a muscle is greatest when it is longest, working a muscle at a much lengthened state is very dangerous, because at the end of this curve is tearing/disruption of the muscle tissue!
  - The length-tension relationship curve expresses the tension force of a muscle relative to its length. At each length of the muscle, the tension that it can generate can be located on the curve. However, this relationship is technically for an isometrically contracting muscle. That is, each point along the curve displays the isometric strength of the muscle at that static length. There is another curve that is used to express the tension force of a muscle but better expresses the muscle's tension force when the muscle is moving.[6]
  - This curve is called the **force-velocity relationship curve** (Figure 17-6). Regarding concentric contractions (shown on the right side of the curve), the force-velocity relationship curve essentially states that the tension force of a muscle is greatest when the muscle is contracting slowly. As the velocity of the muscle contraction increases, its tension force decreases. In other words, the faster a muscle contracts, the weaker its contraction force becomes; the slower a muscle contracts, the stronger its contraction force becomes.[6]

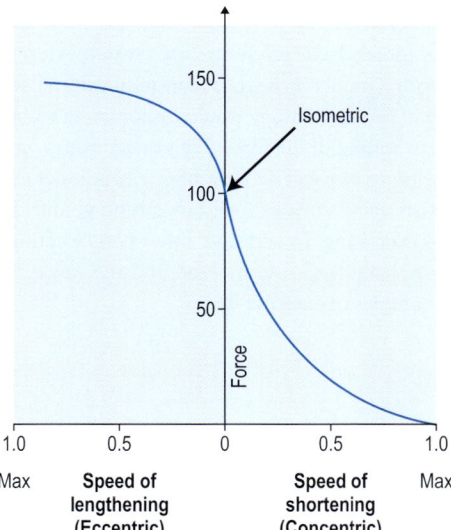

FIGURE 17-6 Illustration of the force-velocity relationship curve. This curve correlates the tension force that a muscle can develop relative to its velocity (i.e., speed) of contraction. Concentric contraction is shown on the right; eccentric contraction on the left. Regarding concentric contraction, the slower a muscle contracts, the stronger its contraction force; the faster a muscle contracts, the weaker its contraction force. *(Modified from Watkins, J: Pocket podiatry: functional anatomy, ed 1, Edinburgh, 2010, Churchill Livingstone.)*

- The reasoning behind this concentric contraction force-velocity relationship can be explained by the cross-bridge formation of the sliding filament mechanism. As the speed of a muscle contraction increases, there is less time for cross-bridges to form. With fewer cross-bridges formed, the force of the muscle's contraction decreases.[4]
- Eccentric contraction force-velocity relationship is shown on the left side of the curve. The force of eccentric contractions is less dependent on the velocity of the muscle contraction and stays fairly constant. The force of an eccentric contraction can also be seen to be consistently high. Much of this force results from the addition of passive tension as the myofascial tissue resists stretching (Box 17-5).

BOX 17-5

Muscles are strengthened by placing a demand for contraction force on them. The force-velocity relationship curve demonstrates that a muscle produces the greatest force when it is eccentrically contracting and when it is slowly concentrically contracting. Therefore it stands to reason that a muscle will be most powerfully strengthened during the eccentric contraction phase of an exercise and when it is slowly concentrically contracting. When working with clients whose goal is to strengthen their musculature, having them perform the exercise slowly and making sure that they properly execute the eccentric contraction phase are important.

SECTION 17.6   LEVERAGE OF A MUSCLE

- Up until now we have been discussing factors that affect the intrinsic strength of a muscle. However, extrinsic factors also affect the strength with which the muscle can move a body part.
- A major extrinsic factor is the leverage of the muscle.[6]
  - Leverage affects the force that a muscle can generate when moving a body part.
  - **Leverage** is a term that describes the mechanical advantage that a force can have when moving an object.[9]
  - Note: When we study motion of the body, it is useful to realize that any movement that occurs will always be the sum total of all forces that act on that body part. Therefore it is important to have a sense of every force that is at work in a given situation. All forces can be divided into two categories[6]: (1) internal forces and (2) external forces. **Internal forces** are generated internally, inside the body; muscles create internal forces. **External forces** are created externally, outside the body. Gravity is the most common external force, and no study of the kinesiology would be complete without a strong understanding of the force that gravity exerts on the motion of the body. However, many other examples of external forces exist: using springs, resistance tubing, and Thera-Bands when exercising. In addition, other people acting on us provide external forces; even wind and the waves of the ocean are examples of external forces.

LEVERS:

To understand the idea of the mechanical advantage of leverage, one should consider the concept of levers.[6]
- A **lever** is a rigid bar that can move (Figure 17-7).
- Movement of a lever occurs at a point that can be called the **axis of motion**.
- This movement occurs because of a force that acts on the lever.
- The distance from the axis of motion to the point of application of force on the lever is defined as the **lever arm**. (Note: Technically, the definition of a lever arm is the distance from the axis of motion to the point of application of force on the lever, only if the application of the force is perpendicular to the lever.

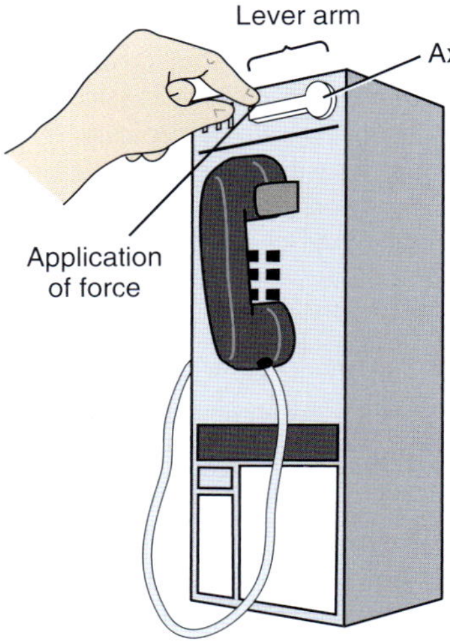

FIGURE 17-7 Illustration of a simple lever (i.e., a coin return on a pay phone). The lever is the rigid bar that someone pushes on to have the coins returned; the movement of the lever is created when someone pushes on it. The distance from the axis of motion of the lever to where the person pushes on the lever is called the lever arm.

When the application of force is not perpendicular, the definition of a lever arm is slightly different.) (See Section 17.7 for more information.)
- A lever arm is also referred to as a **moment arm** or an **effort arm**.

LEVERAGE:

- The longer the lever arm is, the less effort it takes to move the lever. This less effortful movement of a longer lever is called *leverage*. Thus the longer the lever arm is, the greater is the leverage.
- Leverage can be used to move a weight. When we want to move a weight that is otherwise too heavy to move, or we simply want to move a weight with less effort, we can use the concept of leverage to our advantage. In fact, the term **mechanical advantage** is

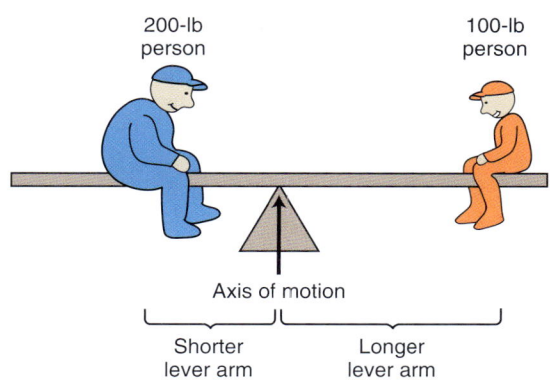

FIGURE 17-8 Illustration of the mechanical advantage of leverage. Two people are sitting on opposite sides of a seesaw. The lighter person on the right side is able to create a force that balances the heavier person on the left by the increased leverage of sitting farther away from the center of the seesaw.

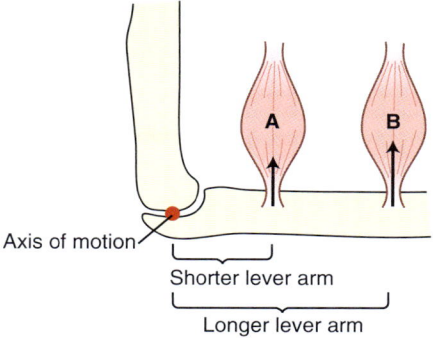

FIGURE 17-9 Illustration of the increased force that a muscle can generate by attaching farther from the joint. Two muscles of the same size and intrinsic strength are crossing the same joint and attaching to the same bone. However, muscle B attaches onto the bone twice as far from the joint as muscle A. This gives muscle B greater leverage and therefore greater force to move the bone at the joint crossed. The axis of motion is located at the joint.

- used to describe the advantage of being able to move heavy objects with less effort.[9]
- However, nothing is free; even the mechanical advantage of a longer lever arm comes with a price. Although a longer lever arm makes it easier to move an object that might otherwise be too difficult to move, the disadvantage is that the lever arm must be moved a great distance to move the object a short distance. No work or effort is actually saved. In effect, increased leverage simply spreads what would be a large effort into a smaller effort over a greater distance!
- A seesaw is as an example of the mechanical advantage of leverage. A seesaw is a lever. On a seesaw, the further from the axis of motion that a person sits, the more force the person exerts on the seesaw due to increased leverage. If two people sit on opposite sides of a seesaw and one person weighs ½ the weight of the other person, the lighter person would be able to balance the heavier person by sitting farther (twice as far) from the axis of motion of the seesaw. In this example, the lighter person gains the mechanical advantage of greater leverage by increasing the lever arm on his side of the seesaw by sitting farther from the center of the seesaw (i.e., the axis of motion) (Figure 17-8).
- Another everyday example of the concept of leverage is the location of a doorknob on a door. A doorknob is nearly always located as far from the hinges (i.e., the axis of motion) as possible. This increased leverage (i.e., having a longer lever arm) provides increased mechanical leverage for opening or closing of the door. In the same manner, when a muscle attaches farther from a joint, it gains mechanical advantage or leverage because the lever arm is longer.

LEVERAGE IN THE HUMAN BODY:

- Leverage is an important concept when it comes to the biomechanics of the musculoskeletal system.
- In the human body, bones are levers, muscles create the forces that move these levers, and the axis of motion is located at the joint.[5]
- The mechanical advantage or leverage of a muscle increases as its attachment site on the bone is located farther from the joint.[8]

- As an example, consider two muscles that are the same size and therefore have the same intrinsic strength. Both of these muscles attach to the same bone and move it at the same joint. If muscle B were to attach twice as far from the joint as muscle A, muscle B would generate twice the force for movement on its attachment as muscle A, even though both muscles have the same intrinsic strength.
  - Therefore the location of the attachment of a muscle, although not changing the muscle's intrinsic strength, does change the force for movement that the muscle exerts on its attachment—in other words, its strength (Figure 17-9). Leverage is an example of an extrinsic factor that affects the force that a muscle exerts on its attachment(s).
- The disadvantage to the greater leverage of muscle B is that muscle B must contract a greater distance to move the bone the same amount that muscle A can move it with a shorter distance of contraction. Thus although muscle B can double the strength of its force by being twice as far from the joint as muscle A, muscle B must contract twice as far to move the bone the same amount that muscle A does. The consequence of having to contract a greater distance is that it is difficult to generate great speed of the body part that is being moved, because the muscle must contract a great amount in exchange for a small amount of movement[6] (Box 17-6).

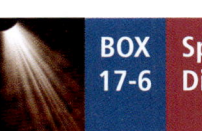

BOX 17-6 Spotlight on Advantage and Disadvantage of Leverage

Regarding the advantages and disadvantages of the leverage of muscle attachments, the following two rules can be stated:
1. Muscles with good leverage can generate greater extrinsic strength of contraction compared with muscles with poor leverage.
2. Muscles with poor leverage can generate greater speed of movement of the body part compared with muscles with good leverage.

SECTION 17.7 LEVERAGE OF A MUSCLE—MORE DETAIL

- Another factor must be considered when evaluating the strength of a muscle based on its leverage—the angle of pull of the muscle at its bony attachment.
- Technically, a lever arm is defined based on the application of force to move the lever as being perpendicular to the lever (i.e., the pull of the muscle on its attachment should be perpendicular to the bone to which it attaches). However, the pull of a muscle on a bone is rarely ever perfectly perpendicular. Therefore to evaluate the leverage of a muscle, we must consider the angle of the pull of the muscle on the bone.

ANGLE OF PULL OF THE MUSCLE:

- The angle of pull that a muscle has relative to the bone to which it attaches is quite important. The effective strength of a muscle to move a body part at a joint is based on its ability to move the bone in the direction of the motion that is to occur. If the angle of pull is directly in line with that motion, then all of the force of the muscle's contraction will contribute to moving the bone in that direction.[5]
- The term **optimal angle of pull** is used to describe the optimal angle of pull that a muscle has on the bone to which it attaches. As a rule, the optimal angle of pull is perpendicular to the long axis of the bone[10] (Figure 17-10).
- If instead the muscle's line of pull is at an oblique angle to the bone, not all the force of the muscle will go toward moving the bone in the direction of the motion. (Note: This is similar to the discussion of the pennation angle of muscle fibers of pennate muscles; see Section 17.2.) The greater the obliquity of the muscle's attachment, the less of the force of the muscle contraction contributes to the motion at the joint[10] (see muscle B in Figure 17-10). Simple trigonometry is used to figure out what percentage of a muscle's pulling force contributes to the motion that is occurring.
- Generally, the optimal angle of pull is the angle that most efficiently moves the bone at the joint crossed, and any obliquity in the angle of the muscle's pull will result in a decrease in efficiency of movement when the muscle contracts. However, the advantage of an increased obliquity (i.e., a less-than-optimal angle of pull) is that a greater portion of the force of the muscle's contraction goes into stabilizing the joint.

Joint Stability:

- As stated, increased obliquity of a muscle's pull decreases the muscle's ability to move the joint but increases its stability of the joint. This is because any deviation from perpendicular increases the angle of pull of the muscle along the long axis of the bone toward the joint. This results in a portion of the muscle's contraction pulling the bone in toward the joint. This compression force of the bone in toward the joint increases the stability of the joint. Inherent in the term *optimal angle of pull* is a bias toward joint movement and a bias against joint stabilization. A muscle with an optimal angle of pull contributes 100% of its pulling force to motion, but nothing to joint stabilization. However, joint stabilization is extremely important toward protecting a joint against injury. Therefore it is the role of a muscle not only to move a bone at a joint, but to also contribute toward stability of the joint (Figure 17-11).

LEVER ARM DEFINITION REFINED:

- In Section 17.6 it was stated that the definition of a lever arm is the distance along a lever from the axis of motion for the lever to the point of application of force on the lever. Applying this definition to the musculoskeletal system, a lever arm would be defined as the distance from the center of the joint

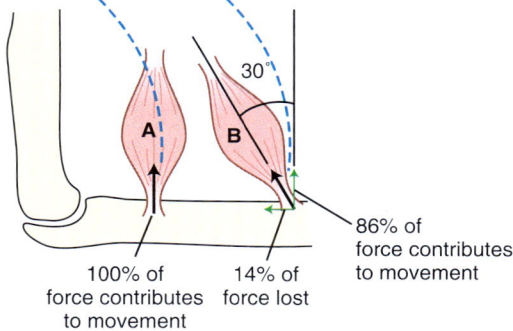

FIGURE 17-10 Illustration of the effect of the angle of pull of a muscle on its bony attachment. The efficiency of the pulling force toward creating movement of the bone at the joint crossed is best when the muscle's angle of pull is perpendicular to the bone. Any change from that angle will result in a weaker force placed on the bone. Muscle *A* has an optimal angle of pull; it attaches into the bone at exactly 90 degrees (i.e., perpendicularly); therefore 100% of the strength of its contraction force goes toward moving the bone. Muscle *B* attaches into the bone at an oblique angle of 30 degrees. Through use of trigonometry, the percentage of its contraction force that contributes to motion at the joint can be calculated to be 86%; therefore with regard to creating movement, 14% of its contraction force is lost.

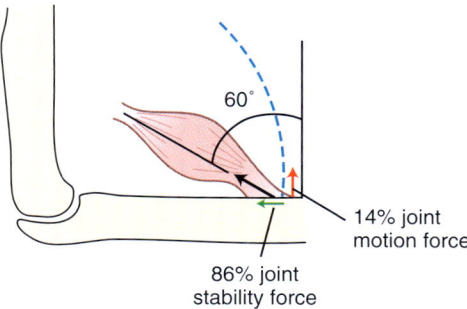

FIGURE 17-11 Whatever portion of a muscle's line of pull does not contribute to motion at the joint instead contributes to stability of the joint by pulling the bone along its long axis into the joint. In this figure, the 86% of the muscle's pulling force that is lost to motion is valuable because it adds to the stability of the joint, protecting the joint from injury.

(i.e., the axis of motion) to the point of attachment of the muscle (i.e., the point of application of force) onto the bone. However, this definition of a lever arm does not take into account the angle of the muscle's pull. To account for the change in leverage force of a muscle when its angle of pull is other than perpendicular to the bone, the definition of a lever arm must be slightly refined.
  ○ A more accurate definition of a musculoskeletal lever arm is the measurement of the line that begins at the center of the joint and meets the line of pull of the muscle at a perpendicular angle.
○ Figure 17-12, A illustrates the precise definition of a lever arm. We see a line drawn that is the shortest distance from the center of the joint to the line of pull of the muscle. Note that this lever arm is less than what it would be if it were measured from the center of the joint to the point of attachment of the muscle. Therefore using the line of pull of the muscle as the defining distance for the definition of leverage changes the determination of leverage force. By amendment of the definition of a lever arm in this manner, the angle of the muscle's attachment into the bone is taken into consideration (and trigonometric formulas can be avoided).
○ Figure 17-12, B shows the same muscle when the joint is in a different position. Note that the lever arm has changed. Therefore the leverage of the muscle changes from one joint position to the other. It must be noted and emphasized that as a bone moves through its range of motion at a joint, although the attachments of a muscle remain constant, the angle of pull of the muscle relative to the bone constantly changes. This means that the lever arm and therefore the leverage of the muscle's force change.
  ○ Therefore the effective extrinsic strength of the muscle's contraction constantly changes as the joint position changes during a muscle's contraction!

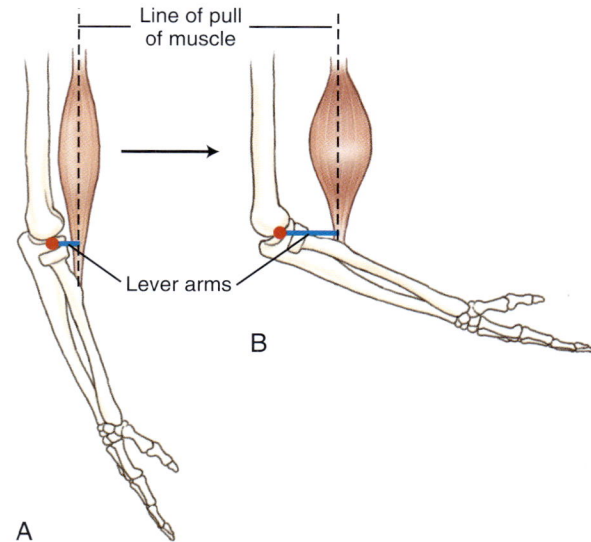

FIGURE 17-12 The precise definition of a musculoskeletal lever arm is the shortest distance from the center of the joint (i.e., the axis of motion) to the line of pull of the muscle. **A** and **B** illustrate the lever arms of the same muscle when the joint is in two different positions. (Note: The lever arm is greater in **B** than in **A**.)

SECTION 17.8   CLASSES OF LEVERS

○ Levers are divided into three classes.
  ○ These classes are first-class, second-class, and third-class levers.[6]
  ○ The difference among the three classes of levers is the relative location of the application of force to cause movement *(F)* and the force of **resistance to movement** *(R)* relative to the axis of motion *(A)*[9] (Figure 17-13).
○ Relating this to the musculoskeletal system, it can be said that the difference among the three classes of levers is the relative location of the line of pull of the muscle *(F)* and the weight of the body part *(R)* relative to the center of the joint *(A)*.
  ○ The resistance to movement would be whatever force resists the motion from occurring. In the musculoskeletal system, apart from additional forces that might enter the picture, the resistance to motion would be the weight of the body part that has to be moved (or the body parts that have to be moved). For example, if a muscle attaches onto the hand and moves the hand at the wrist joint, the resistance to movement is the weight of the hand. However, if the muscle attaches onto the forearm and moves the forearm at the elbow joint, the resistance to movement is the weight of the forearm, as well as the weight of the hand (which must also be moved along with the forearm).

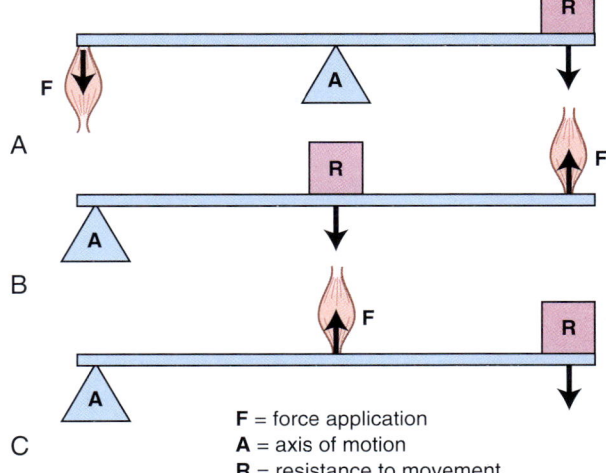

F = force application
A = axis of motion
R = resistance to movement

FIGURE 17-13 Illustration of the concept of the three classes of levers. These classes are based on the relative positions along the lever of the application of force, the resistance to movement, and the axis of motion. **A** is a first-class lever, **B** is a second-class lever, and **C** is a third-class lever.

PART 4 Myology: Study of the Muscular System

- We usually think of the resistance to movement as being the weight of whatever body part(s) must be moved. However, it is possible for other forces to come into play. For example, if a muscle must contract and move the upper extremity, the resistance force increases if the hand is holding a weight. Another example is if an exercise is being done in which springs or Thera-Bands are used to increase the resistance of the exercise.

FIRST-, SECOND-, AND THIRD-CLASS LEVERS:

- A **first-class lever** has the force that causes motion and the force of resistance to motion on opposite sides of the axis of motion.[11]
- A **second-class lever** has the force that causes motion and the force of resistance to motion on the same side of the axis of motion, and the force that causes motion is farther from the axis than the force of resistance.[11]
  - Therefore second-class levers inherently have greater leverage for strength of pulling force.
- A **third-class lever** has the force that causes motion and the force of resistance to motion on the same side of the axis of motion, and the force that causes motion is closer to the axis than the force of resistance.[11]
  - Therefore third-class levers inherently have less leverage for strength of pulling force.

First-Class Levers:

- The typical example of a first-class lever is a seesaw (Figure 17-14, A).
- With a seesaw, the axis of motion is located between the force for motion and the resistance to motion.
- An example of musculature in the human body that is a first-class lever is the extensor musculature that attaches to the back of the head[6] (Figure 17-14, B).
- Note: The definition of a first-class lever is that the force creating movement (F) and the force resisting movement (R) are on opposite sides of the axis of motion (A). However, which force is farther from the axis of motion, and hence which force has greater leverage and therefore mechanical advantage for power, is not specified (whereas second- and third-class levers are defined based on which force [F or R] is greater). Therefore knowing that a muscle is a first-class lever does not immediately tell us about its relative leverage force compared with the leverage force of the resistance (i.e., it does not tell us if the muscle has a relative leverage advantage or leverage disadvantage). Each first-class lever muscle must be individually looked at to determine its relative leverage advantage/disadvantage. (Note: Leverage of the resistance force is covered in Section 17.9.)

Second-Class Levers:

- The typical example of a second-class lever is a wheelbarrow (Figure 17-15, A).
- With a wheelbarrow, both the force that causes motion and the force of resistance to the motion are on the same side of the axis of motion, and the force that causes the motion (i.e., the person lifting up on the handles) is farther from the axis than the

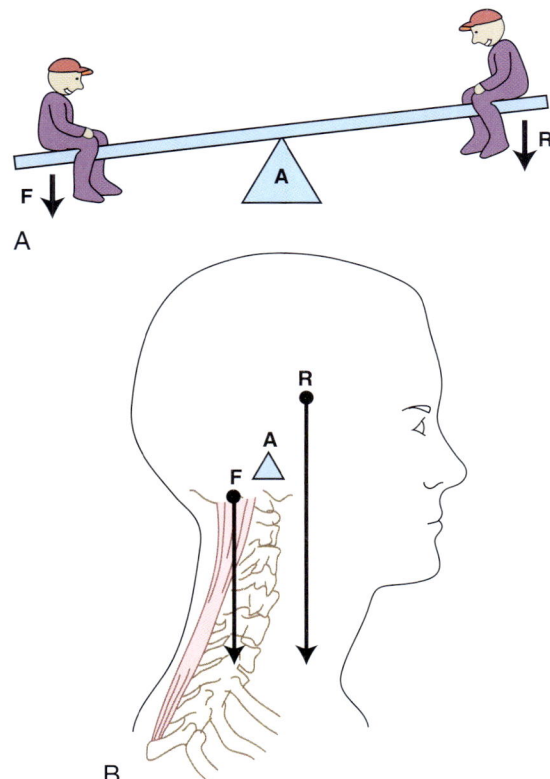

FIGURE 17-14 Two examples of a first-class lever. A first-class lever is one in which the force applied to the lever *(F)* and the resistance to movement of the lever *(R)* are on opposite sides of the axis of motion of lever *(A)*. **A** is a seesaw; **B** is the extensor musculature acting on the head.

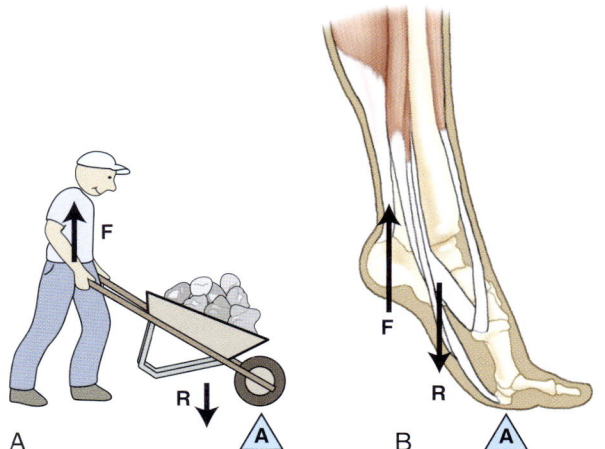

FIGURE 17-15 Two examples of a second-class lever. A second-class lever is one in which both the force applied to the lever *(F)* and the resistance to movement of the lever *(R)* are on the same side of the axis of motion of the lever *(A)*; however, the force causing motion *(F)* is farther from the axis than is the resistance *(R)*. **A,** Wheelbarrow. (The mechanical advantage of a wheelbarrow should be noted; by virtue of being a second-class lever, it allows us to lift and move objects that might otherwise be too heavy for us.) **B,** Plantarflexor musculature of the lower extremity acting on the foot. Its mechanical advantage allows it to lift the entire body (i.e., a heavy weight) relative to the toes at the metatarsophalangeal joints!

resistance force (i.e., weight of the loaded wheelbarrow). Because the force that causes motion is farther from the axis of motion than the resistance force, wheelbarrows have a great amount of leverage and therefore allow us to lift and move heavy loads with relative ease.
- An example of musculature in the human body that is a second-class lever is the plantarflexor musculature of the lower extremity, which attaches into the calcaneus. When the plantarflexor musculature contracts with the foot on the ground, its contraction lifts the entire body relative to the toes at the metatarsophalangeal joints of the foot[6] (Figure 17-15, B).
- Attaching farther from the axis of motion on the foot than the location of the force of resistance to contraction (i.e., the point of center of weight of the body) affords the plantarflexor musculature a great deal of leverage force to lift the entire weight of the body.
- Note: The disadvantage of this muscle (as well as every second-class lever muscle) is that it must concentrically contract a great distance to create a small range of motion; therefore its ability to move the body quickly is less.

Third-Class Levers:
- A typical example of a third-class lever is a pair of tweezers (Figure 17-16, A).
- With a pair of tweezers, both the force that causes motion and the force of resistance to the motion are on the same side of the axis of motion, and the force that causes the resistance (i.e., the resistance of the object being held) is farther from the axis than the force that causes motion (i.e., the person squeezing the tweezers).
- An example of a muscle in the human body that is a third-class lever is the brachialis, which attaches to the proximal end of the forearm (Figure 17-16, B).
- Attaching so far proximally on the forearm does not give the brachialis much leverage for strength of contraction, but as with all muscles that are third-class levers, it means that a small amount of brachialis contraction will move the forearm through a large range of motion. Therefore the mechanical advantage the brachialis gives up in leverage for lifting heavy weights, it gains in speed of motion of the forearm.

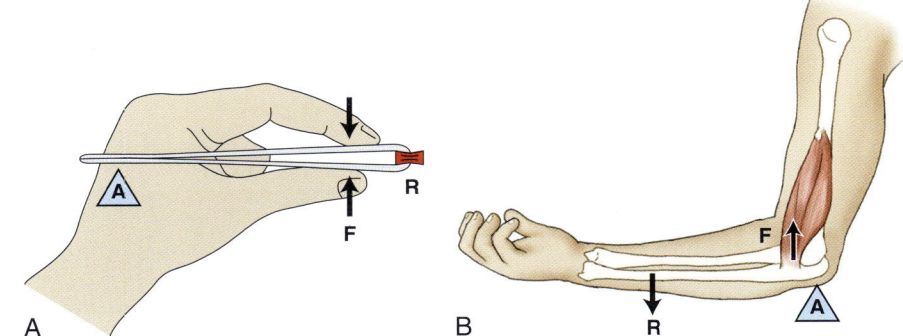

FIGURE 17-16 Two examples of a third-class lever. A third-class lever is one in which both the force applied to the lever (F) and the resistance to movement of the lever (R) are on the same side of the axis of motion of the lever (A). **A,** Pair of tweezers. **B,** Medial view of the brachialis muscle of the upper extremity. As a third-class lever, the brachialis loses leverage for strength of contraction, but by virtue of being a third-class lever, it gains the ability to quickly move the forearm through its range of motion!

SECTION 17.9 LEVERAGE OF RESISTANCE FORCES

- Up until now we have spoken about leverage only from the point of view of the leverage of a muscle that is creating a force to move or stabilize the body. However, the force of resistance to our muscle's force may have greater leverage than our muscle does. When this occurs, whether our muscle's role is to move the body part against the resistance force or to hold the body part stable against the resistance force, our muscle is often at a **mechanical disadvantage** when working against a force with greater leverage.[12] For this reason, it is just as important to know the leverage of the resistance force that our muscle must work against as it is to know the leverage of our muscle's force. In effect, the mechanical disadvantage (or advantage) of a muscle is the difference between these two leverage forces.
- *Mechanical disadvantage* occurs with third-class levers, because third-class levers are defined as having the resistance force farther from the joint than the muscular attachment. It may also occur with first-class levers if the resistance force is located farther from the joint than the muscular attachment. When the role of the muscle is to isometrically contract and stabilize the joint (to prevent movement), the muscle needs to contract forcefully enough to meet the strength of the resistance force; when the role of the muscle is to concentrically contract and move

the joint, the muscle needs to contract more forcefully than the strength of the resistance force. Needing to generate contraction strength when the muscle is at a mechanical disadvantage increases the risk of a muscular strain.

- Figure 17-17, *A* depicts a muscle that is flexing the forearm at the elbow joint. When the forearm is in a position of 90 degrees of flexion, the resistance force (i.e., the weight of the forearm and hand) has a large lever arm that increases the resistance force that our forearm flexor muscle must overcome to be able to move the forearm. Figure 17-17, *B* depicts the same scenario after our muscle has succeeded in flexing the forearm at the elbow joint to a position that is near full flexion. In this position, the lever arm of the resistance force of the weight of the forearm and hand has greatly decreased. This decreased lever arm means that the resistance force of the weight of the forearm and hand has greatly decreased. Therefore the forearm flexor muscle does not need as powerful a contraction to move the forearm further into flexion. However, it should be noted that the lever arm (and therefore the leverage) of the muscle has also decreased in the position in Figure 17-17, *B* as compared with the position in Figure 17-17, *A*.
- Understanding the mechanical advantage and disadvantage of a muscle or muscle group is critically important when clinically evaluating the physical stress that a client's musculature is experiencing during postures and activities (Boxes 17-7 and 17-8).

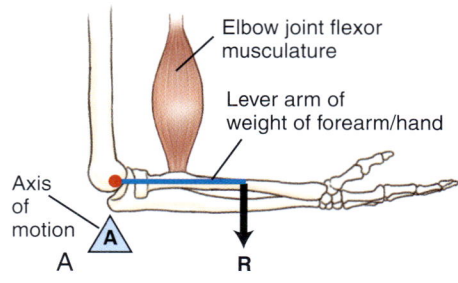

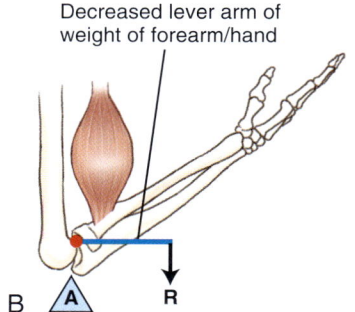

FIGURE 17-17 Illustration of the changing leverage of the force of gravity as a result of the weight of the forearm and hand when the angle of the elbow joint changes. **A,** The weight of the forearm and hand creates a resistance force *(R)* to flexor musculature of the elbow joint. **B,** Lesser leverage of this resistance force than **A** because of the decreased lever arm when the elbow joint is in a position of greater flexion.

BOX 17-7 Spotlight on Leverage and Holding an Object

If a person is carrying a weight in the hand and the weight is being held in front of the body, the extra weight in front of the body would tend to make the trunk fall forward into flexion (at the spinal joints). If this weight is held farther away from the body, the lever arm of the weight of the object increases and its force on our body increases. To keep the trunk from falling forward into flexion, the back extensors must contract to equal the force that the weight of the object is creating on the body. The farther the weight is held away from the body, the greater the force on the body, and the greater the back extensors must contract. For example, a 10-lb weight that is held against the front of the body magnifies its force approximately seven times to 70 lb if it is held away from the body at arm's length. For this reason, holding a heavy object far away from us is extremely stressful to our back muscles. To feel this, hold this book close to your body with one hand and palpate your erector spinae musculature with your other hand. Continue palpating your erector spinae musculature as you take the book farther away from your body. You should clearly feel the erector spinae's increased contraction as the book is moved farther from the body. Knowledge of this principle allows us to better understand and examine the habits and work practices of our clients and better advise them regarding how to lift and carry in a manner that is less stressful and healthier. The application of this concept is also extremely important when evaluating the physical stress on the body of a client when performing exercises with weights.

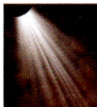

BOX 17-8 Spotlight on Leverage and Bending Over

It is very common for a client to report that he or she bent over to pick up something and the back "went out." Often what occurs in these scenarios is that the extensor musculature in the back is strained and/or spasms. The client often cannot understand why this occurred, because whatever object was being picked up was not that heavy. Many times nothing was even being picked up; perhaps the client was just bending over to tie a shoelace. What is often not understood is that bending over in and of itself is stressful, because the back extensor musculature must eccentrically contract to slow down the descent of the trunk into flexion. If the client then comes back up from the bent over position, extensor muscles of the trunk must concentrically contract to lift the weight of the upper body (i.e., trunk, neck, head, and both upper extremities) back into extension.

When these actions occur, the muscles of the back are actually lifting quite a heavy weight. Even if nothing was picked up in the hands, the muscles are lifting the weight of the body! Figure 1 depicts a typical **stoop bend** in which the back bends (i.e., the spine flexes); Figure 2 depicts a straight back **squat bend** in which the back has stayed straight and more vertical. Notice the large lever arm (LA) for the center of weight (CW) of the upper body of the person with the stoop bend; the extensor muscles of the back must contract forcefully to counter this force. It is no wonder that so many people strain and injure their backs when stooping over, regardless of whether a heavy object was being picked up or not. Compare the stoop bend with the decreased lever arm of the upper body weight when the person does a squat bend. For this reason, squat bending in which the knees and hips are bent is the safer way to bend over (see Note 1). If a heavy object is being lifted in the hands, it only magnifies the importance of this concept.

It should also be noted that many people are aware that the safe way to bend is to bend the knees and hips and keep the back straight. However, they do not realize that it is also important to keep the back not only straight, but as vertical as possible. If the back is straight, but inclined forward (i.e., the pelvis is anteriorly tilted at the hip joints) as in Figure 2, then the lever arm for the weight of the upper body still increases. Although healthier than the stoop lift, this inclined squat lift is not as healthy as the vertical back squat lift depicted in Figure 3 (see Note 2).

Note 1. Squat bending in which the spinal joints are extended (i.e., the back is straight) is healthier than stoop bending in which the spinal joints are flexed (i.e., the back is hunched forward) for two reasons:
A. The squat bend tends to decrease the leverage of the body weight by keeping the trunk more vertical. If the leverage of the body weight is less, then the extensor muscles of the trunk do not need to contract as forcefully and the likelihood of a strain of the extensor musculature is low.
B. In the squat bend, the spinal joints are extended and therefore in the more stable closed-packed position. Therefore it is less likely that the spinal joints will be sprained with a squat bend.

Note 2. For all the cautioning that is done to encourage people to bend (and/or lift) in a healthy manner with a vertical back squat lift, it is amazing how few people actually bend in this manner on a regular basis. It turns out that many people resist this healthier method of bending for two good reasons:
A. Squat lifting places more pressure on the knee joints.
B. It actually takes more energy to squat bend than it does to stoop bend; so to save a few calories of energy, many people keep stoop bending and putting their backs in peril.

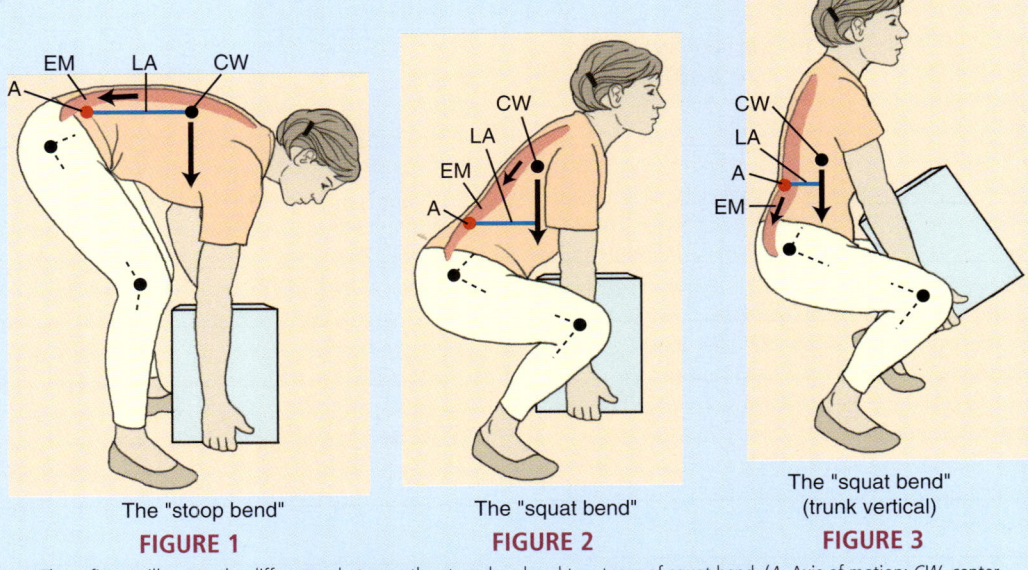

FIGURE 1 The "stoop bend"
FIGURE 2 The "squat bend"
FIGURE 3 The "squat bend" (trunk vertical)

These figures illustrate the differences between the stoop bend and two types of squat bend. (*A*, Axis of motion; *CW*, center of weight of the trunk and upper body; *EM*, extensor musculature of the spine; *LA*, lever arm.) (Note: The spine has multiple joints; therefore multiple axes of motion exist. To simplify this, the lumbosacral joint has been used in all cases as the axis of motion to determine the relative lever arms.)

REVIEW QUESTIONS

Answers to the following review questions appear on the Evolve website accompanying this book at: http://evolve.elsevier.com/Muscolino/kinesiology/.

1. How can a muscle have a partial contraction?

2. What is the Henneman size principle?

3. What factor determines the intrinsic strength of a muscular contraction?

4. What factors determine the extrinsic strength of a muscular contraction?

5. Name two types of longitudinal muscle fiber architecture and three types of pennate muscle fiber architecture.

6. What is a pennation angle?

7. What is the difference between active tension and passive tension of a muscle?

8. What is the term used to describe the fact that a muscle's contraction is weakened when it is lengthened beyond resting length?

9. Why is the strength of a muscular contraction weakened when it is shortened beyond resting length?

10. What do the three length-tension relationship curves describe?

11. What is a lever? What is a lever arm?

12. What is the definition of *leverage?*

13. What advantage does a muscle gain by having greater leverage?

   _____

   _____

14. What disadvantage does a muscle have if it has greater leverage?

   _____

   _____

15. What is the optimal angle of pull for a muscle?

   _____

16. What is the definition of a first-class lever?

   _____

   _____

17. What is the similarity between a second-class lever and a third-class lever?

   _____

   _____

18. Name a muscle that acts as part of a third-class lever system.

   _____

19. What is the importance of the resistance force to movement?

   _____

   _____

   _____

20. What is the resistance force to a person's anterior hip joint musculature flexing the thigh at the hip joint from anatomic position?

   _____

   _____

REFERENCES

1. Enoka RM: Neuromechanics of human movement, ed 3, Champaign, IL, 2002, Human Kinetics.
2. Lieber RL: Skeletal muscle, structure, function, & plasticity: The physiological basis of rehabilitation, ed 2, Baltimore, 2002, Lippincott Williams & Wilkins.
3. Watkins J: Structure and function of the musculoskeletal system, Champaign, IL, 1999, Human Kinetics.
4. Hamilton N, Weimar W, Luttgens K: Kinesiology: Scientific basis of human motion, ed 12, New York, 2012, McGraw Hill.
5. Hall SJ: Basic biomechanics, ed 6, New York, 2012, McGraw Hill.
6. Neumann DA: Kinesiology of the musculoskeletal system: Foundations for physical rehabilitation, ed 3, St Louis, 2017, Elsevier.
7. Nordin M, Frankel VH: Basic biomechanics of the musculoskeletal system, ed 3, Baltimore, 2001, Lippincott Williams & Wilkins.
8. Oatis CA: Kinesiology: The mechanics and pathomechanics of human movement, Philadelphia, 2004, Lippincott Williams & Wilkins.
9. Levangie PK, Norkin CC: Joint structure and function: A comprehensive analysis, ed 5, Philadelphia, 2011, FA Davis.
10. Patton KT, Thibodeau GA: Anatomy & physiology, ed 9, St Louis, 2015, Elsevier.
11. Smith LK, Weiss EL, Lehmkuhl LO: Brunstrom's clinical kinesiology, ed 5, Philadelphia, 1996, FA Davis.
12. McLester J, St. Pierre P: Applied biomechanics: Concepts and connections, Belmont, 2008, Thomson Wadsworth.

CHAPTER 18
Biomechanics

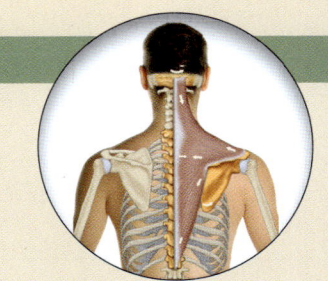

Co-authored by Scott Gaines and Joseph E. Muscolino

CHAPTER OUTLINE

Section 18.1 Introduction to Biomechanics
Section 18.2 A Brief Introduction to Forces
Section 18.3 Basic Principles in Mechanics
Section 18.4 Describing Human Movement—Analyzing Kinematics
Section 18.5 Describing the Forces of Human Movement—Analyzing Kinetics

CHAPTER OBJECTIVES

After completing this chapter, the student should be able to perform the following:

1. Define the key terms of this chapter.
2. Discuss the basis of biomechanics, including why it is important, and its two primary goals.
3. Do the following related to forces:
   - Discuss the two ways forces can affect a body.
   - Give examples how the human body adapts to forces, including traction, compression, shear, twist, and bending.
   - Discuss the stress/strain relationship curve.
4. Do the following related to basic principles in mechanics:
   - Discuss the three fundamental units in mechanics.
   - Explain the difference between a scalar and vector.
   - Describe resultant vectors.
5. Do the following related to describing human movement and analyzing kinematics:
   - Describe position and direction in 3D space.
   - Describe how motion can be categorized as linear or rotary.
   - Describe linear motion (distance versus displacement).
   - Describe rotary motion (angular distance versus angular displacement).
   - Define and explain the difference between speed and velocity, as well as angular speed and angular velocity.
   - Compare linear and angular acceleration.
6. Do the following related to describing the forces of human movement and analyzing kinetics:
   - Describe the concepts of mass, inertia, and momentum.
   - Discuss Newton's three laws of motion.
   - Describe the concepts of statics and dynamics.
   - Discuss the vertical and horizontal components of ground reaction forces.
   - Explain the components of torque and why it is important to human movement analysis.
   - Analyze the human body by creating a basic free-body diagram.

OVERVIEW

Biomechanics is the study of how forces affect living systems. For the purposes of this book, we will be focusing primarily on human musculoskeletal biomechanics. In other words, we will be looking at how the body (primarily though muscles) generates forces to create (or inhibit) movement. We will also be looking at how external forces on the body, such as those due to gravity, affect the body. The primary goal of this chapter is to empower you with the knowledge to be able to critically use biomechanical and physiological principles to analyze an individual's needs in order to optimize their movement so as to maximize performance and minimize injury.

KEY TERMS

- Acceleration
- Active forces
- Angular acceleration
- Angular displacement
- Angular distance
- Angular speed
- Angular velocity
- Anthropometry
- Balance
- Bending
- Biomechanics
- Center of gravity (COG)
- Center of mass (COM)
- Compression
- Degrees
- Displacement
- Distance
- Distraction
- Dynamics
- Elastic region
- Equilibrium
- Eustress
- External forces
- Force
- Gravity
- Ground reaction force (GRF)
- Inertia
- Internal forces
- Kinematics
- Kinetics
- Linear motion
- Mass
- Mechanical strain
- Mechanical stress
- Momentum
- Newton's First Law of Motion: Law of Inertia
- Newton's Second Law of Motion: Law of Acceleration
- Newton's Third Law of Motion: Law of Action-Reaction
- Passive forces
- Plastic region
- Qualitative analysis
- Quantitative analysis
- Radians
- Resultant vector
- Rotary motion
- Scalar
- Shear
- SI
- Speed
- Statics
- Torque
- Traction
- Twist
- Ultimate strength
- Vector
- Velocity
- Weight
- Yield strength

TABLE 18-1 Reference Table for Mechanical Terms and Their Symbols Utilized in This Chapter

Mechanical Term	Symbol	SI (System International) Units	SI Unit Symbol
Time	t	seconds	s
Mass	m	kilograms	kg
Linear Displacement/Position	x	meters	m
Angular Displacement/Position	theta (θ)	radians or degrees	rad
Linear Velocity	v	meters per second	$\frac{m}{s}$
Angular Velocity	omega (ω)	radians per second	$\frac{rad}{s}$
Linear Acceleration	a	velocity per second	$\frac{m}{s^2}$
Angular Acceleration	Alpha (α)	angular velocity per second	$\frac{rad}{s^2}$
Momentum	p	mass times velocity	$kg \frac{m}{s}$
Force	F	mass times acceleration	$\frac{kg \, m}{s^2}$ = Newton (N)
Torque	Tau (τ)	force times moment arm	N m
Stress and Pressure	Pascal (P)	Force per unit area	$\frac{N}{m^2}$

SECTION 18.1   INTRODUCTION TO BIOMECHANICS

WHAT IS BIOMECHANICS AND WHY IS IT IMPORTANT?

- Biomechanics is an incredibly broad field. In order to properly define biomechanics, it is best to break it down into its root word origins.
  - Bio—*life*
  - Mechanics—*branch of physics that analyzes forces on a body and their effects*
  - Therefore biomechanics can be seen as *the science which evaluates the motion of a living organism and the action of forces on it.*[9]
- Because this is a kinesiology text, the study of forces and how they affect human musculoskeletal motion will be the focus of this chapter. It is essential for all manual and movement professionals to have a fundamental understanding of biomechanics, as forces not only create all human movement, but also stimulate various adaptions of all bodily tissues. These adaptions can have positive or negative effects on one's performance and quality of life. Amazing feats of athleticism can be performed with proper biomechanics. Likewise, the vast majority of musculoskeletal injuries are caused by forces improperly applied to the body's tissues.[3,13]

ANATOMY, PHYSIOLOGY AND KINESIOLOGY— WHERE DOES BIOMECHANICS FIT IN?

- As kinesiology is the study of human movement, biomechanics is often seen as a subdiscipline of kinesiology that specifically uses the principles of mechanics to analyze and solve problems related to the structure (anatomy) and function (physiology) of the human body.[7]
- Another perspective is that biomechanics is analogous to physiology in that it, as a discipline, analyzes how an organism "functions" (from a mechanical standpoint). In an ideal scenario, optimizing "function" (both mechanics and physiology) will optimize performance for an individual.[6]

(Note: The use of the word *performance* in this chapter does not solely refer to athletic performance, but how the body performs mechanically [i.e., how well one moves]. With this in mind, remember that *life is a performance*) (Figure 18-1).

THE RELATIONSHIPS BETWEEN STRUCTURE (ANATOMY) AND FUNCTION (BIOMECHANICS AND PHYSIOLOGY), MOBILITY AND STABILITY

- Musculoskeletal anatomy is also directly related to its biomechanical function. This is especially evident in the structure of joints. As Levangie and Norkin (1992) point out:
  - *The design of a joint is determined by its function and the nature of its components.*

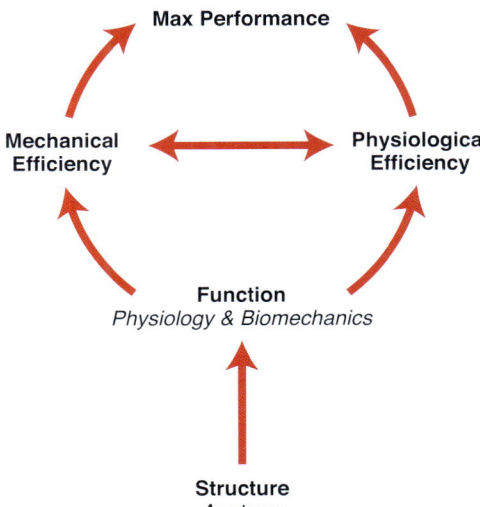

FIGURE 18-1 The relationship between structure, function, and performance. (©Scott Gaines, 2016)

- *Once a joint is constructed, the structure of the joint will determine its function.*
- *Joints that serve a single function are less complex than joints that serve multiple functions.*
- In this way the human body is mechanically analogous to other joints and levers found in the world. For example, let's imagine a large family gathering. Two tables will be used in order to seat the large number of family members—a large dining room table and a portable folding table. The legs of a folding table pivot at their hinge so that the table may be moved easily. While this table is mobile, it is not nearly as stable as the big, wooden dining room table. The dining room table, on the other hand, is very stable but is very hard to move. Note that mechanically, mobility and stability are inversely related. Furthermore, if one tried to fold the leg of the big dining room table, as if it had a hinge like the portable table, with enough force, the leg would break. Its structure would not allow that function and rupture/injury would occur (Figure 18-2).
- The same will be found in the human body. Joints that are very mobile, such as the glenohumeral (shoulder), which has three degrees of freedom, will not be as stable as the elbow joint, which has one degree of freedom (Figure 18-3).[5,10,11]
- The point being that structure and function are directly related. Hence it is vital that in order to be safe and effective, the manual and movement professional must understand the basic sciences of both structure (anatomy) and function (physiology and biomechanics) of the human body.

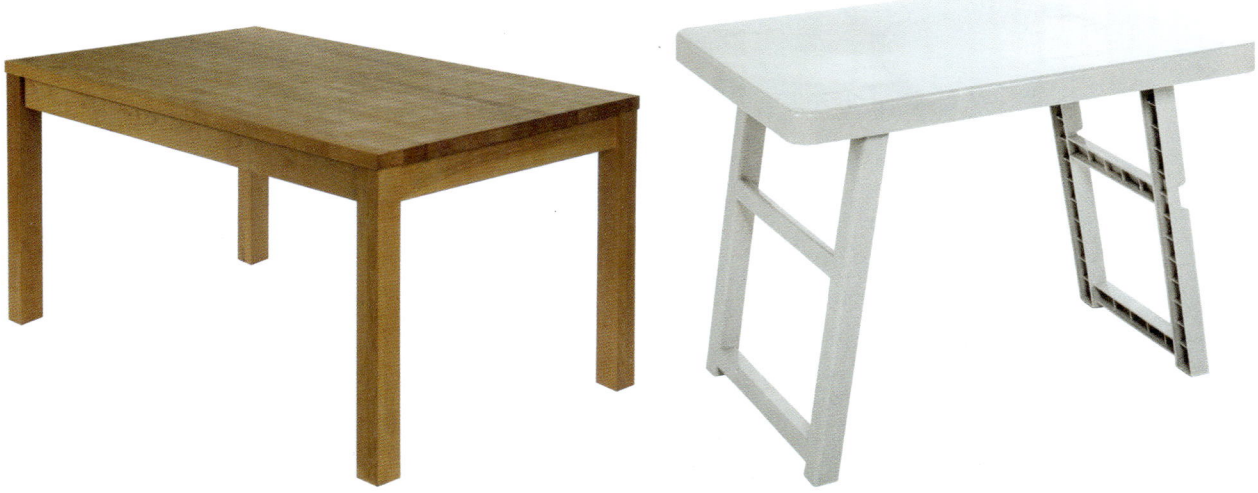

FIGURE 18-2 Example of stability versus mobility in the world (©istock.com).

THE TWO PRIMARY GOALS OF BIOMECHANICS

- The study of human musculoskeletal biomechanics has two primary emphases:
  1. Performance/movement enhancement
     - This is done primarily by using a biomechanical analysis to improve movement, technique, equipment, or training.
  2. Injury prevention and rehabilitation
     - This is done by reducing injury by using a biomechanical analysis to improve techniques and develop new equipment designs.[9]

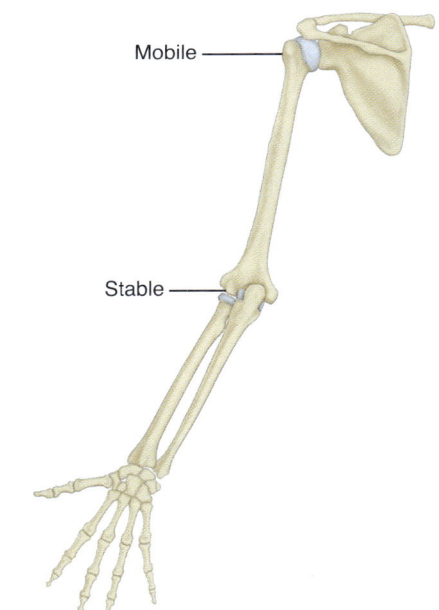

FIGURE 18-3 Example of stability versus mobility in the body.

- Biomechanics allows us to answer the question *"What's happening in this _____ (e.g., postural pattern/movement pattern/exercise/sport/drill), and how can we make it better?"* One example is the overhead squat assessment (Figure 18-4).

OPTIMIZING HUMAN POSTURE AND MOVEMENT THROUGH A QUALITATIVE BIOMECHANICAL ANALYSIS

- As stated above, the primary goal of this chapter is to empower you with the knowledge to be able to critically use biomechanical and physiological principles to *analyze* an individual's biomechanical needs. This is necessary to *optimize* their posture and movement so as to *maximize* performance and *minimize* injury.[9] This chapter will give you the knowledge to perform a basic analysis, while the remainder of this text will give you the information needed to optimize an individual's posture and movement. This begs the question, "How do we analyze human posture and movement?" This can be done quantitatively (a **quantitative analysis** using numbers) or qualitatively (a **qualitative analysis** using non-numerical descriptions).[4,7,9] While we will be reviewing some mathematical formulas in mechanics to understand the relationships between different concepts, this chapter will primarily focus on a *qualitative* approach to biomechanical analysis:
  - Step 1: Analyze the posture/motion (**kinematics** is the study of motion with NO regard to the forces that cause the motion)
  - Step 2: Analyze the forces (**kinetics** is the study of forces acting on a body)
  - Step 3: Compare to the "ideal" for the individual[6,7,9]
- The remainder of this chapter will focus on steps 1 and 2, while the remainder of the text will give you insight on determining the "ideal" posture and movement for an individual (Figure 18-5).

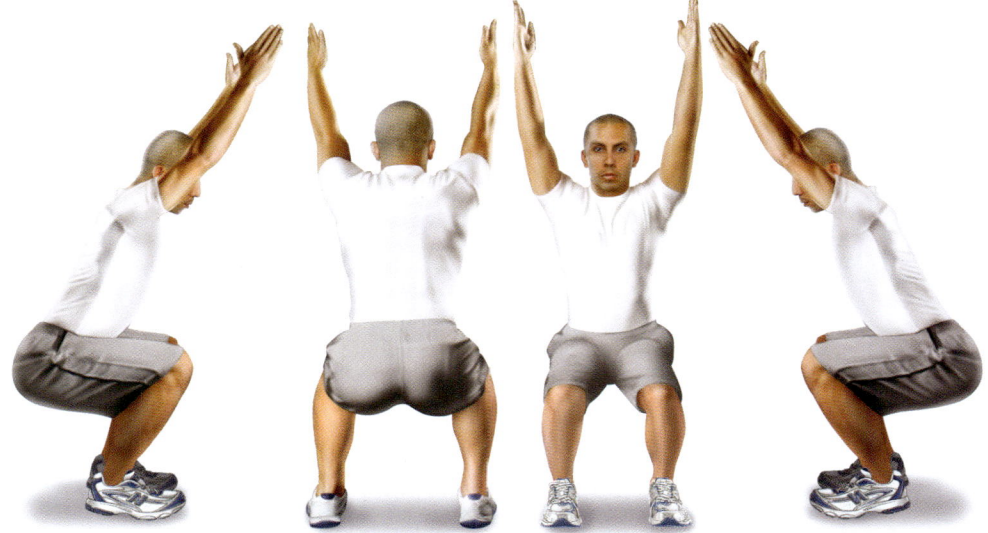

FIGURE 18-4 The overhead squat assessment.

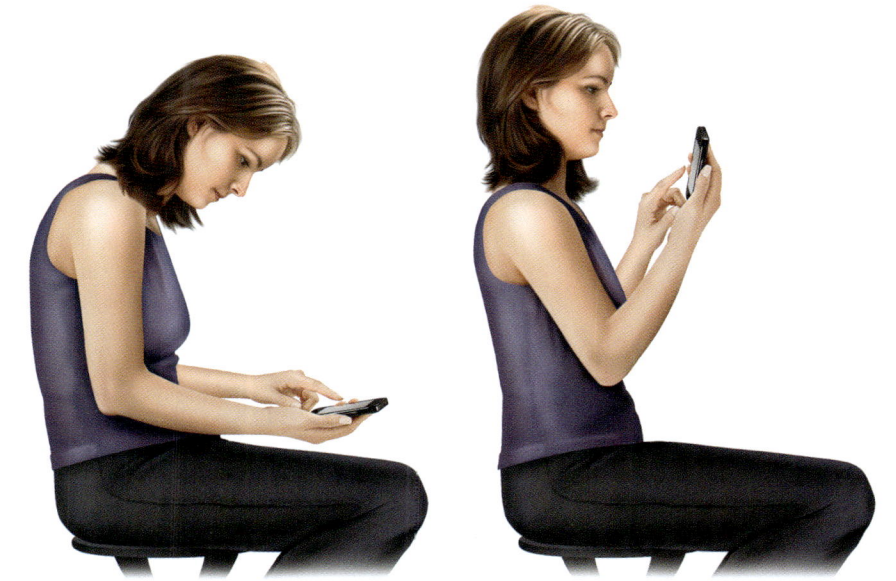

FIGURE 18-5 Being able to biomechanically analyze an individual's posture and movement is essential for the manual and movement professional. (From Muscolino JE: *Body mechanics: The price of smart phones*, Massage Therapy Journal, Springer, 2015. Art by Giovanni Rimasti.)

SECTION 18.2 A BRIEF INTRODUCTION TO FORCES

WHAT ARE FORCES?

- Forces will be defined with great detail later in this chapter. To get started, think of forces as simply a *push or a pull* of one body on another (please note, the word "body" in this case just means a physical object, not necessarily a human body).[2,3,7,9]
  - In most cases a force will be a push or a pull of two bodies *in contact*. However, there are exceptions to this; the most important example of a force with no contact is that of bodyweight.

Weight is the force due to **gravity** acting upon an object's mass, always pulling the object *down* (toward the center of the earth). Being that gravity is causing the force and there is no direct contact between two objects, it is an exception to the rule above.

- Forces can affect a body in two ways:
  1. Forces can move the body through space and/or
  2. Deform the body (i.e., create changes in its shape—see below)[11]

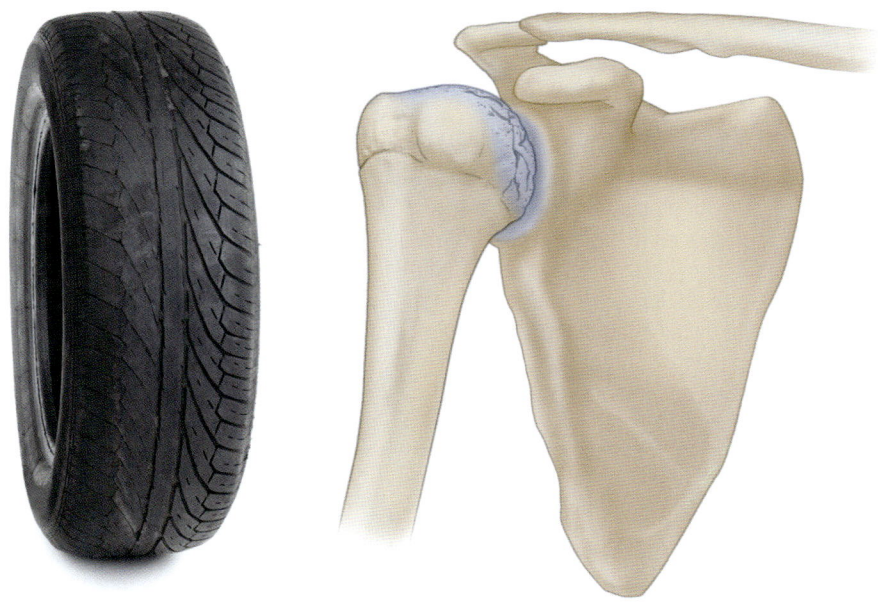

FIGURE 18-6 Forces can create deformations in solid materials such as a worn tire or arthritic shoulder (Tire ©istock.com).

- For the purposes of studying human musculoskeletal biomechanics, forces can be divided into two groups: external forces and internal forces.
  - **External Forces**—as the name implies, external forces arise from outside the body. The most common external force is weight. So a dumbbell in the hand is an external force. What is not so obvious is that one's own bodyweight is an external force (the primary one acting on us at all times). Other external forces include drag, friction, springs, and elastomers (e.g., elastic tubing or bands).
  - **Internal Forces**—these forces arise from within the body. These forces can be further classified as active or passive forces.
    - **Active forces**—produced by the skeletal muscles.
    - **Passive forces**—produced by the connective tissues (e.g., fascia, ligaments, tendons, etc.) These forces typically assist the muscles in producing motion and protect the integrity of a joint by restricting unwanted motion. (Note: Under certain circumstances, fascia can transition to allow for the creation of active forces. See Chapter 4, Section 4.3).[10]
- For proper joint movement (arthrokinematics) to occur, internal forces must be generated via proper activation of the musculoskeletal system by the nervous system (providing there are no structural abnormalities preventing proper movement).[10] However, if there is improper activation of the skeletal muscles, improper joint movement may result, ultimately leading to wear and tear on the joint.
  - Again, this is perhaps best seen with a nonhuman analogy. Imagine you are driving your car and the wheels are out of alignment (just as improper joint motion is "out of alignment"). What would happen to one's tires if driven repeatedly out of alignment? They would wear down sooner on one side of the tire. The same happens in joints.
- Likewise, if external forces are not applied to the body in accordance to the body's structure, injury can result (Figures 18-6 and 18-7 and Table 18-2).

HOW DOES THE BODY ADAPT TO MECHANICAL STRESS? TRACTION, COMPRESSION, SHEARING, TWISTING, AND BENDING

- The term *stress* often holds a negative connotation in people's minds (e.g., "I'm stressed out!"). However, depending on the type of stress we are referring to, it can be good (**eustress**) or

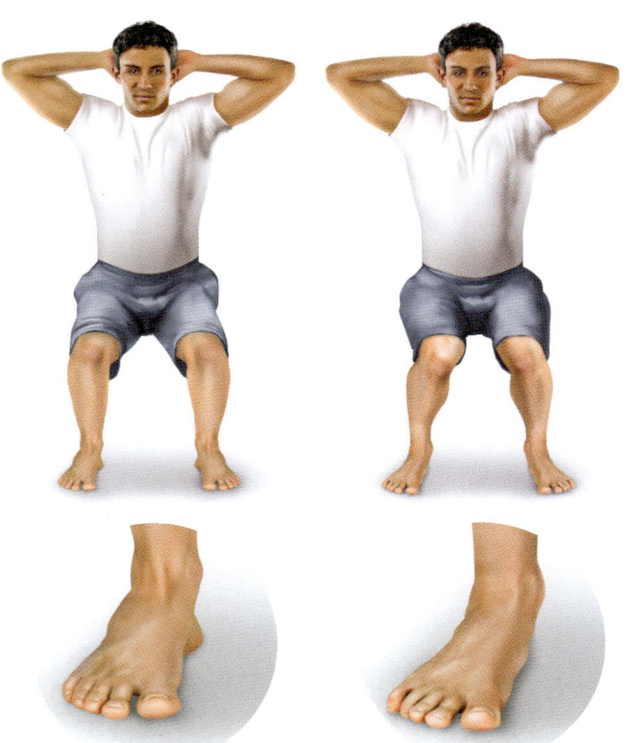

FIGURE 18-7 Overpronation of the foot can ultimately damage the knee joint.

Table 18-2

	Positive ("Good") Forces	Negative ("Bad") Forces
Internal Forces	Proper activation of muscles (muscles are activated in the proper order, at the proper intensity, at the proper time) for proper joint movement	Improper activation of muscles leading to improper joint movement
External Forces	The body is positioned to properly accept forces from outside the body (e.g., weight, friction, drag) in accordance with the body's structure	Forces enter the body not in accordance with the structure and function of the body
Result	The work input by the internal forces is efficiently transferred to work output (e.g., propulsive forces) Positive structural adaptations (Growth) Increased velocity	Not as efficient Higher risk of connective tissue damage (negative structural adaptations) Decreased velocity

bad (distress). **Mechanical stress** is specific to the forces within a body. This is described as the amount of "**force**" within a body, divided by the "area" over which the force is applied (Stress = F/A). It is these forces within the body that will affect body tissues. A particular mechanical stress can cause damage (i.e., injury) to tissues, while another may stimulate hypertrophy (cause growth) of other tissues. On the other hand, the lack of stress can stimulate tissue atrophy (wasting).[13]

- "*The same forces that move and stabilize the body also have the potential to deform and injure the body.*"[10]

- Common forces on bodily tissues (Figure 18-8):
  - **Traction** (**distraction**, stretch)—Forces upon the structure are directed away from the contact surfaces.
  - **Compression** (squash)—Forces upon the structure are directed toward the contact surfaces.
  - **Shear** (friction)—Forces that lie parallel to the contact surfaces of the structures. Two forces are present and are in opposite directions. Think of friction or a rubbing force.
  - **Twist** (torsion)—Opposing forces rotate in opposite directions around the body's longitudinal axis.

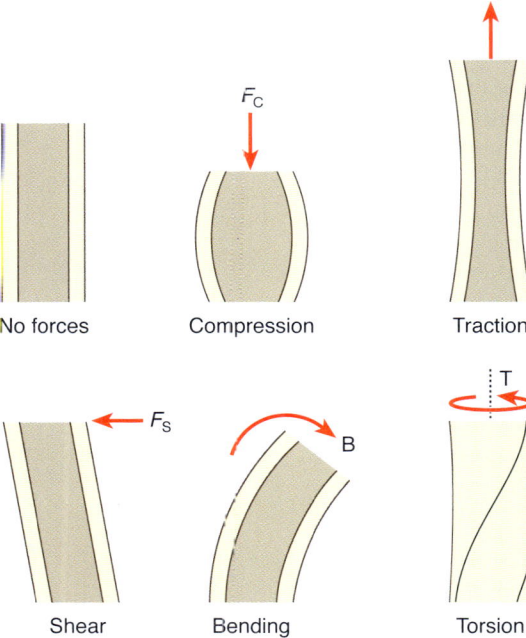

FIGURE 18-8 Common forces on tissues of the body. *(Modified from Adams M, Bogduk N, Burton K, and Dolan, P: Biomechanics of Back Pain, ed 3, London, 2013, Churchill Livingstone.)*

- **Bending**—Forces working together in the same direction cause compression on one side of the body and traction on the other.

STRESS/STRAIN RELATIONSHIP CURVE

- When forces (mechanical stress) are placed upon a solid object, it can create physical changes in the object. Mechanical strain is the change in length of an object (i.e., the deformation) divided by its original length. In other words, **Mechanical Strain** = $\Delta L/L$, where "Δ" is delta, meaning change. Therefore, $\Delta L = L - L_0$ (where "L" is the final length and "L_0" is the initial length). Depending on the nature of the object, if the force of the stress is low, then when it is removed, the object reverts back to its original length (i.e., shape). This level of stress is known as the **elastic region**. **Yield strength** is the point beyond which a material will not return to its original dimensions once the force is removed. This level of stress for a material is known as the **plastic region**. If more stress is applied, eventually the **ultimate strength** of the tissue/structure is reached; beyond this, rupture occurs. Graphing these points yields the stress/strain relationship curve (Figure 18-9). Please note, every solid will have a different stress/strain curve (e.g., a rubber band will have a large elastic region, but a pencil would have a relatively small one).[10,13]
- *The quick take-away: "Stress" can be "good" or "bad"; it depends on the magnitude of stress on the various parts of the body and if those areas (e.g., joints) biomechanically are able to accept the stress.*[6]
- Example: Bones are subjected to forces all the time. In fact, forces are required for normal bone growth (see Wolff's law in Chapter 3). However, if forces are applied in such a manner that they are beyond physiological range of the tissue, rupture can occur (Figure 18-10, Box 18-1)

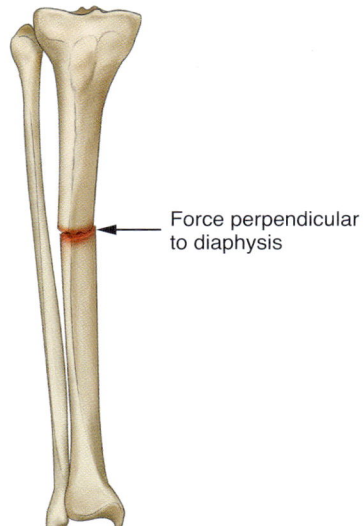

FIGURE 18-10 Stress upon a bone exceeding its plastic region.

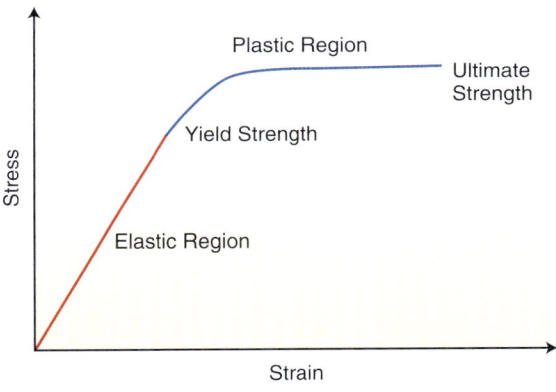

FIGURE 18-9 Stress/strain relationship curve.

BOX 18-1 Think about it . . .

Whiting and Zernicke (2008) describe a way of looking at mechanisms for musculoskeletal injuries as variations of "overload" (load being an external force). While the body is under various loads at all times (many of them required for normal body function), only when the loads are said to exceed *physiological range* does the probability of injury increase. In other words, the load exceeds the tissue's maximum tolerance, and injury results.[13]

SECTION 18.3 BASIC PRINCIPLES IN MECHANICS

THE THREE FUNDAMENTAL UNITS IN MECHANICS (MEASURING SPACE, TIME, AND MATTER)

- As mechanics is the study of how physical bodies react to forces and move through space over time, we must have ways of measuring these variables. The **SI** (SI is from the French, *Système International d'Unités*; i.e., the metric system) is typically used.[6,9] The three fundamental units in mechanics are the following:
  1. Physical bodies (i.e., mass) = kilogram (kg)
  2. Space (i.e., distance) = meter (m)
  3. Time = seconds (s)
- Note: All formulas in classical mechanics can be simplified into these three units.

596 PART 4 Myology: Study of the Muscular System

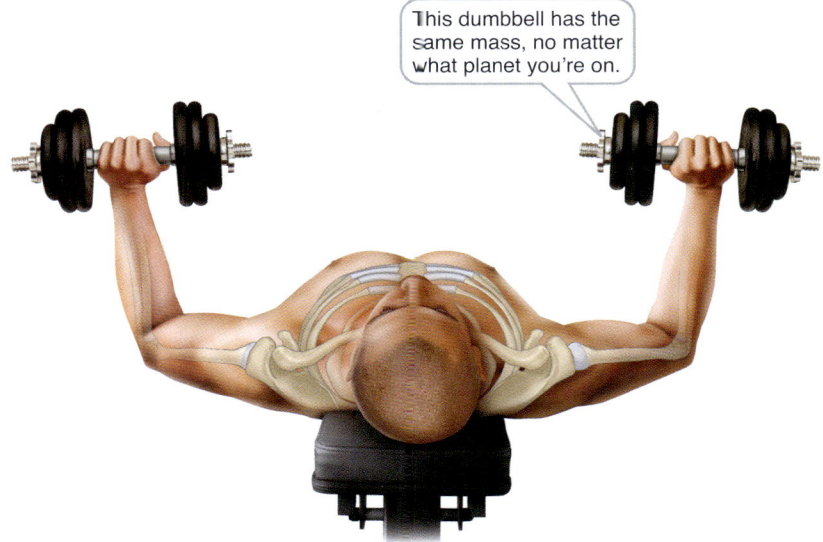

FIGURE 18-11 The mass of a dumbbell is constant.

SCALARS AND VECTORS

- As mechanics can be used to quantitatively describe the world around us, it uses two types of quantities to represent concepts like mass, time, and distance: scalars and vectors.[1]
  - **Scalars**—A term describing distance, speed, or mass, which has magnitude but no direction. In other words, it is a quantity that can be *fully described* by its magnitude (i.e., a number).[1,2,7,9]
    - For example: mass (m) is a scalar quantity measuring the amount of physical matter that comprises an object. The mass of the dumbbells seen in Figure 18-11 would be the same on the moon as it would be on earth (even though its weight would be very different) (Figure 18-11).
  - **Vectors**—A term describing something that has both magnitude and direction (e.g., displacement, velocity, force).
  - Graphically, vectors are represented by an *arrow*. The direction and length of the arrow demonstrate the equivalent of a force and how it is applied to an object (see also Chapter 6, Section 6.30). When represented in mathematical notation, vectors are represented by either boldface type or with a small right arrow above the names (e.g., **v** or $\vec{v}$).[1,2,7,9]
  - Examples: Force and velocity. Weight is a force vector due to gravity (**w** = mg). Given that gravity acting on the scalar mass of the dumbbells now creates the force of weight, the weight of the dumbbells is now shown as a vector (Figure 18-12).

Vectors Have Several Characteristics

- Point of application
- Direction
- Magnitude

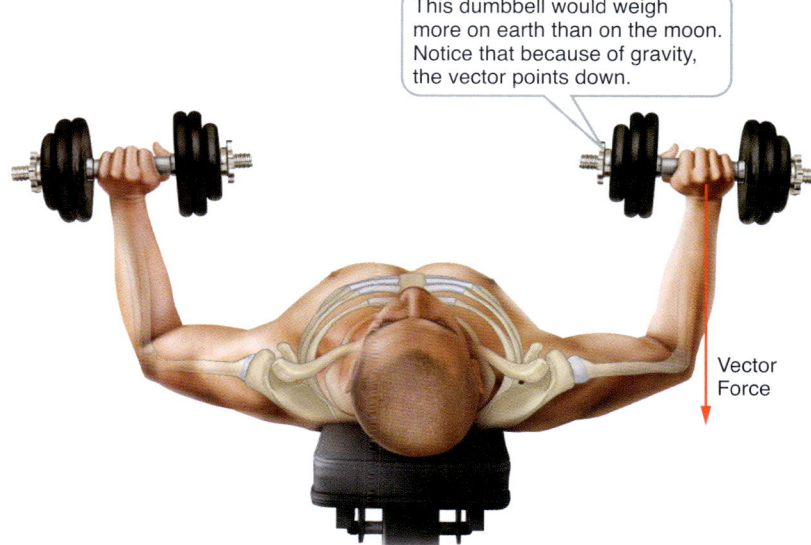

FIGURE 18-12 The weight of the dumbbells is represented by a vector force.

CHAPTER 18 Biomechanics

RESULTANT VECTORS

- As forces are the cornerstone to mechanics and forces are vectors, it is important to be able to visualize all forces as arrows. The start (head) of the arrow is placed where the force is being applied (i.e., the point of application, which in the case of weight would be the object's geometric center—its center of mass). The direction of the arrow corresponds to the direction of force's push or pull. Last, the length of the arrow corresponds to the magnitude of the force.[7,14]
- When multiple forces are acting upon an object, the net force on the object can be found by "resolving the vectors," in other words, by finding the resultant of the vectors in question. A resultant is simply the sum of two or more vectors (i.e., we are adding all the force vectors together to find the net vector force). **Resultant vectors** can be found graphically using the methods below.
  - Tip-to-tail method
    - Put the tip (head) of the first vector (A) on the tail of the second vector (B) and then draw the resultant vector from the tail of A to the tip of B (Figure 18-13).
  - Parallelogram method
    - Connect the tails of the vectors to be added and then create a parallelogram (Figure 18-14, Figure 18-15).

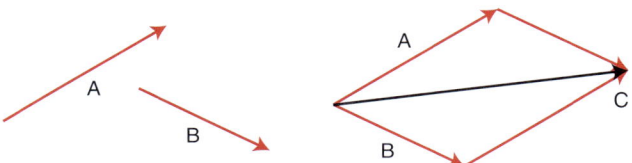

FIGURE 18-14 Parallelogram method for resolving vectors.

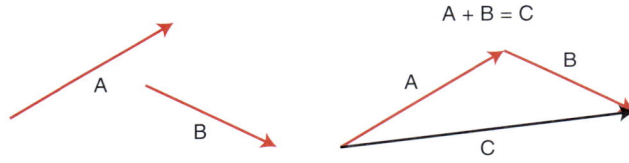

FIGURE 18-13 Tip to tail method for resolving vectors.

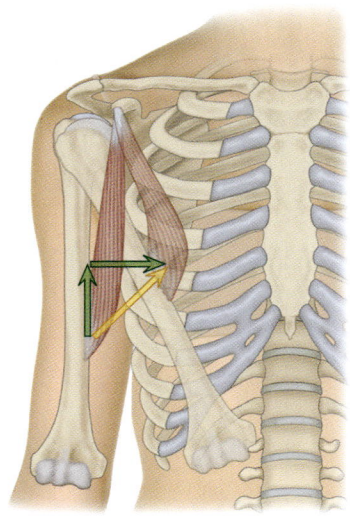

FIGURE 18-15 An internal force vector due to the action of the coracobrachialis. Note the resultant force vector represented in yellow and its component cardinal plane vectors in green.

SECTION 18.4 DESCRIBING HUMAN MOVEMENT—ANALYZING KINEMATICS

- The first step in analyzing human movement is to analyze an individual's kinematics. Kinematics is the study of motion with no regard to the forces that cause the motion.[9,14] Kinematics takes into account an object's:
  1. *Position* in space
  2. How *far* it moves (if at all)
  3. How *fast* it moves
  4. How *quickly* it changes its movement

Please note, as we describe an object's motion using kinematics, we will not be considering the nature of the object itself (i.e., its mass). We will only be examining movement. (The nature of the object being moved will be analyzed in the next step as we examine kinetics).

Note: When thinking "Kinematics," think "Movement"

DESCRIBING POSITION AND DIRECTION IN 3D SPACE

- Because we live in three-dimensional space, we must have a way to describe an object's location in space. In mechanics we use Cartesian coordinates (Figure 18-16).[7,9,14]

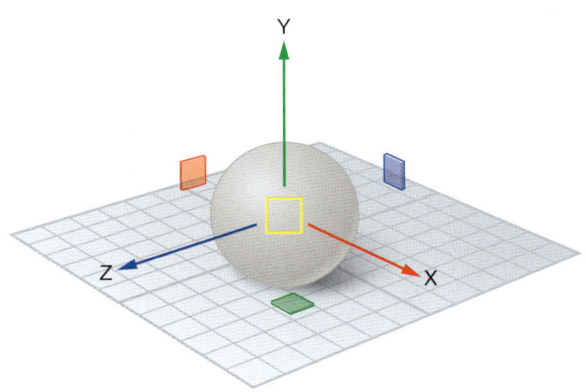

FIGURE 18-16 Plotting points using Cartesian coordinates.

- Plotting points using Cartesian coordinates along X, Y, and Z planes is analogous to plotting points along the sagittal, frontal, and transverse cardinal planes in kinesiology. For a qualitative biomechanical analysis we utilize the reference planes and axes of motion discussed in Chapter 2 to describe human movement (Figure 18-17).

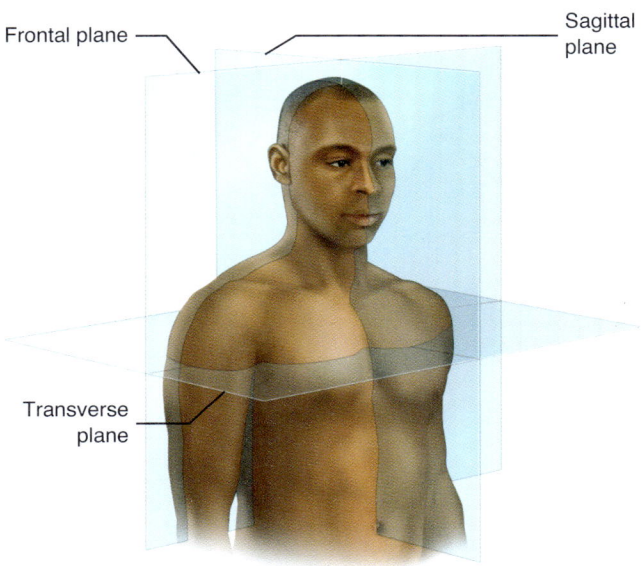

FIGURE 18-17 Sagittal, frontal, and transverse cardinal planes.

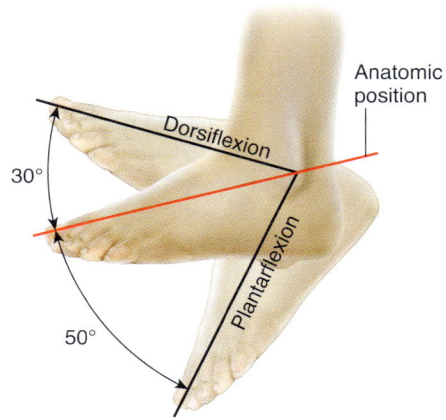

FIGURE 18-19 The foot rotates about the ankle joint (a hinge joint) in a near rotary/axial manner.

DESCRIBING MOTION

- Motion can be categorized as linear or rotary.
    a. **Linear motion** (i.e., nonaxial, glide, slide, translational motion) is when all components of an object move together as one unit.
        i. Rectilinear motion is when a body moves along a perfectly straight line (Figure 18-18, *A*).
        ii. Curvilinear motion is when a body moves along a curved line (Figure 18-18, *B*).
    b. **Rotary motion** (i.e., axial, angular, circular motion) is the movement of an object or segment around a fixed axis in a curved path. Each point on the object/structure moves through the same angle, at the same time. An example would be a door with the hinge as the axis around which the door rotates. There are few, if any, joints in the human body which move around a truly fixed axis. However, for simplicity's sake, joint motions are often described as being rotary/axial movements (Figure 18-19).
    c. **General plane motion** is a special case of curvilinear motion where the object is segmented and free to move rather than rigid or fixed. In this case, an object rotates about an axis, while the axis itself is translated in space by motion of an adjacent segment. In a sense, it is a combination of rotary and translational movements. As the body can be seen as a linked series of joints, this is very common in the human body. For example, if one were to bring a cup to one's mouth by flexing at both the shoulder and the elbow joints, the path of the hand would be curvilinear within a plane (general plane motion). (Figure 18-20)[7,9,14]

DESCRIBING LINEAR MOTION—LINEAR KINEMATICS (DISTANCE VERSUS DISPLACEMENT)

- Linear motion can be measured either by using a scalar (distance) or by a vector (displacement). While in everyday conversation these two terms are often used interchangeably, they are actually very different.
    a. **Distance**
        1. A *scalar* quantity and refers to the sum of all movements in whatever directions these movement occurred

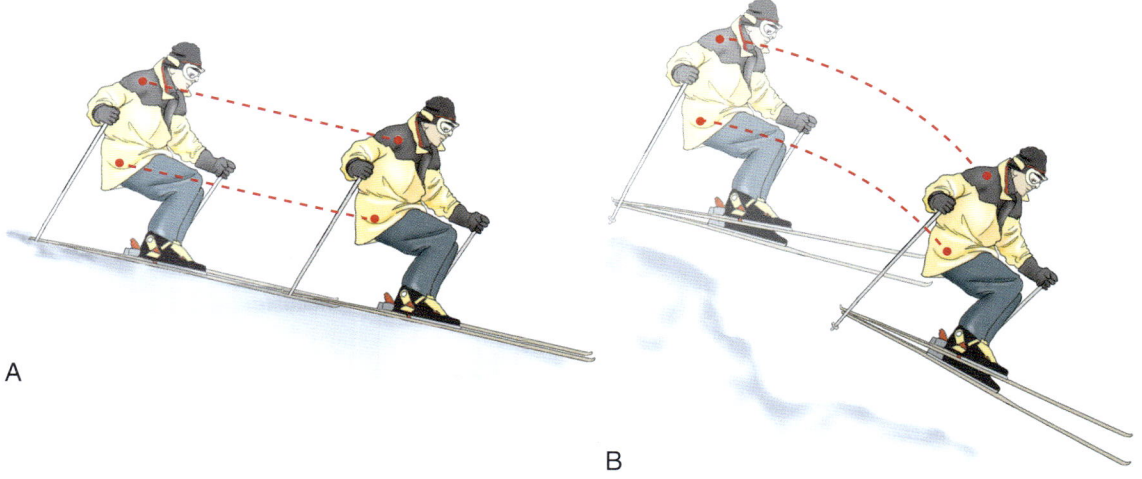

FIGURE 18-18 Linear motion **A**, Rectilinear motion. **B**, Curvilinear motion.

CHAPTER 18 Biomechanics

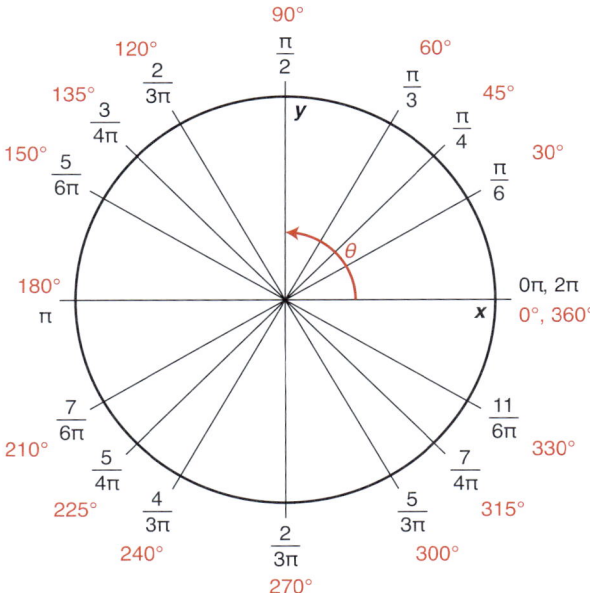

FIGURE 18-21 Various angles of a circle represented in both degrees and radians.

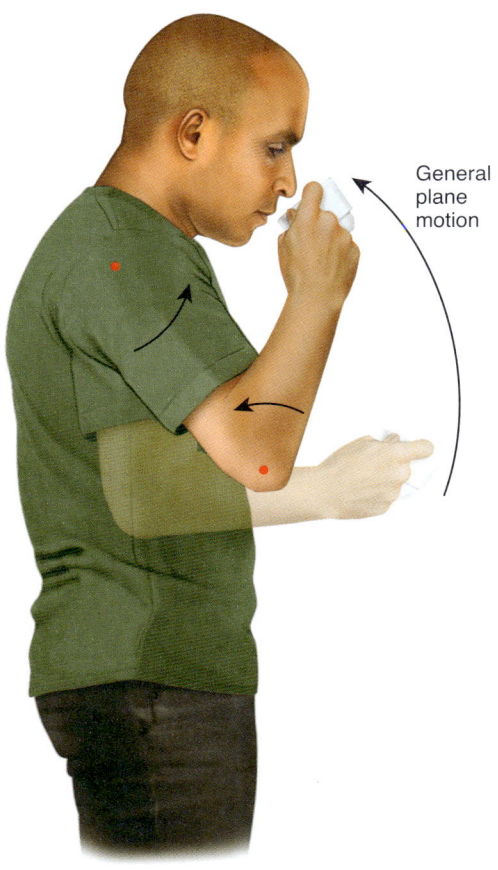

FIGURE 18-20 An example of general plane motion.

b. **Displacement**
   2. A *vector* quantity describing a change in position, measured by a straight line that connects the beginning and end points of motion.
○ Probably the best way to understand the difference is with an example. If one were to compete in the Kona Ironman competition, the last leg of the race is a run. The run starts and ends at the same location. If one were to measure the *distance* from the start of the run to the end, it would be 26.2 miles (a marathon). However, the displacement from the start of the run to the end is zero—it's at the same location.
○ In this case, displacement may not seem to be very useful. In reality, in a quantitative biomechanical analysis, it is preferred. Because displacement is a vector, it not only gives us a magnitude, it also gives us a direction (distance can be looked at as the magnitude of the displacement vector). Ultimately, the direction of the displacement vector will be essential in determining the direction of the net force which caused the movement because it will indicate what musculature is engaging during the movement pattern.[1,3,7,9]

DESCRIBING ROTARY MOTION—ANGULAR KINEMATICS (ANGULAR DISTANCE VERSUS ANGULAR DISPLACEMENT)

○ Rotary/angular motion is measured either in **degrees** or **radians**.
   ○ Degrees: There are 360° in a circle.

Radian: distance travelled/radius. Put simply, a radian is the relationship of the radius of a circle and its circumference. If one were to take the radius of any circle and place it on the circumference of the circle, the corresponding arc would be 1 radian (1 radian = 57.3°). Furthermore, it would require exactly pi (π = 3.14159...) radians to transverse half a circle (180° = π).

○ Typically, radians are better for most quantitative biomechanical calculations. It is essential when equations are being used where the angle is not within a trigonomic function. However, degrees tend to be better for a qualitative analysis, which, as previously noted, is the primary focus of this chapter (Figure 18-21).[9]
○ **Angular distance** (φ) is when a rotating body moves from one position to another, the angular distance through which it moves is equal to the length of the angular path.
○ **Angular displacement** (θ) is analogous to linear displacement, in that it is equal in magnitude to the angle between the initial and final position of the body.[7,9]
○ Note: The difference between angular distance and angular displacement is similar conceptually to the difference between distance and displacement discussed above.
○ For example, if a person were to maximally flex the thigh at the hip joint to 120 degrees, both the angular displacement and the angular distance would be 120 degrees. But when the thigh has returned to the starting position by extending at the hip joint, the thigh would have traveled a total of 240 degrees of angular distance, but 0 degrees of angular displacement (Figure 18-22).

DESCRIBING HOW FAST AN OBJECT MOVES—LINEAR KINEMATICS (SPEED VERSUS VELOCITY)

○ We will now examine the rate of change of an object's position as a function of time. Again, we have both a scalar and a vector to represent this rate of change. **Speed** is a scalar, describing how

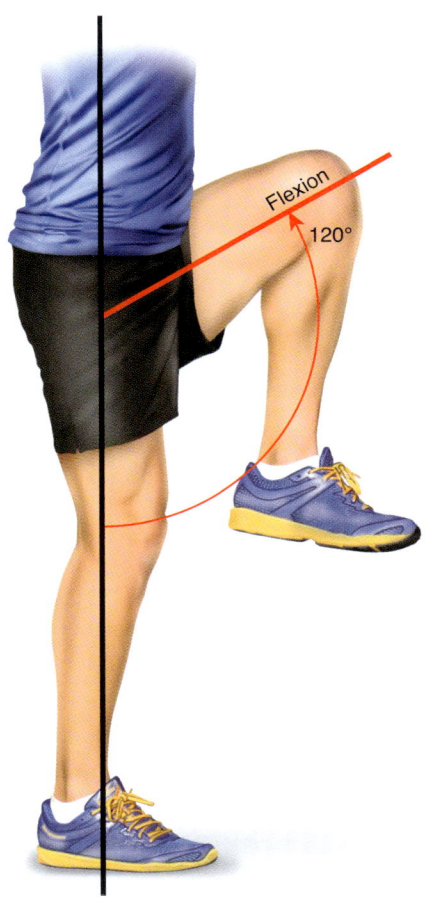

FIGURE 18-22 Angular displacement versus angular distance.

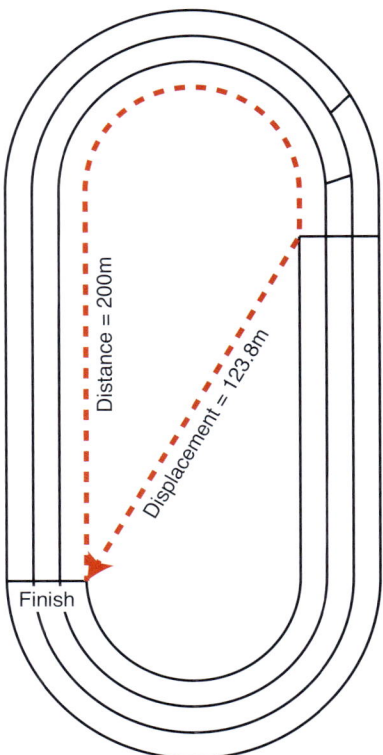

FIGURE 18-23 Distance versus displacement during a race on a track. *(Modified from Blazevich, A.J.: Sports biomechanics. The basics: optimising human performance. ed 2, London, 2012, A&C Black Publishers an imprint of Bloomsbury Publishing PLC.)*

fast an object is moving. **Velocity** is a vector, describing both how fast an object is moving, as well as the direction in which it is moving (an object's speed can be looked upon as the magnitude of its velocity vector).[4,7,9,14]

- **Speed** (v) = change in distance divided by the change in time
- **Velocity** (**v** or $\vec{v}$) = change in displacement divided by the change in time

$$\vec{v} = \frac{dx}{dt}$$

(Note: "d" means "change in" so dx = change in distance and dt = change in time.)

- Let's take an example of a track athlete running the 200 m. If she ran the event in 22.5 seconds, then her average speed would be 200m/22.5s = 8.89ms^{-1}. However, because velocity looks at a straight line from start to finish (and it is a curved track), her average velocity would be 123.8m/22.5s = 5.50ms^{-1} (Figure 18-23). Again, speed would seem to be the more useful number in this situation. However, the velocity vector becomes very important as we start to look at a concept known as instantaneous velocity.
- Average versus Instantaneous Velocity
  - Let's examine another sprinter. This time let's have a sprinter who runs the 100-m dash in 10 seconds (Figure 18-24). He would like to improve his technique. If we know his time is 10 seconds to complete the 100m, and we know he wants to be faster than this speed, but we don't know much else, where does he need to improve?[3]
  - Now let's imagine we can collect data of where the athlete is at every second of the event. We can now determine his average velocity of not just the entire event, but also from second to second. Using the chart below we could determine the athlete's velocity from the 3rd second of the race to the 4th second (Figure 18-25).
  - If we are able to get more precise data, we can determine the *instantaneous velocity* (Figure 18-26).

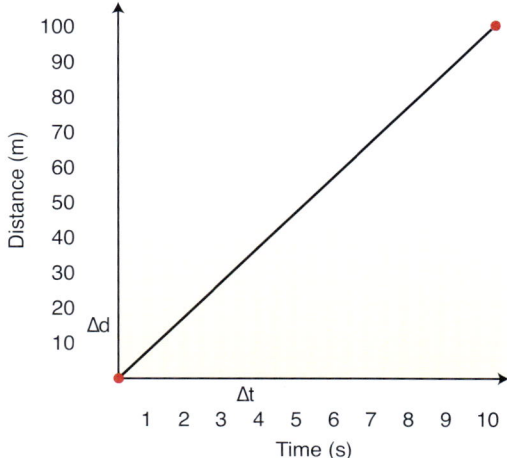

FIGURE 18-24 Average velocity of sprinter completing 100-m dash.

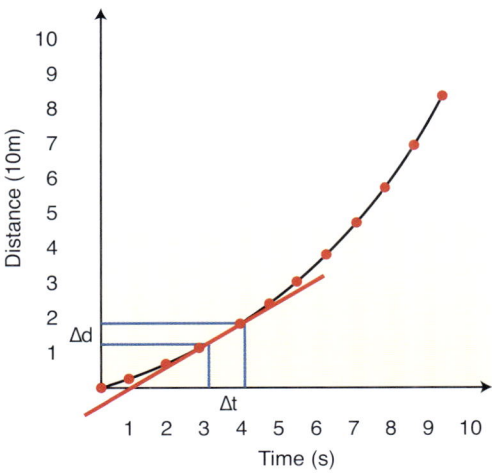

FIGURE 18-25 The average velocity of a sprinter from 3 seconds in the race to 4 seconds. (©Scott Gaines, 2016)

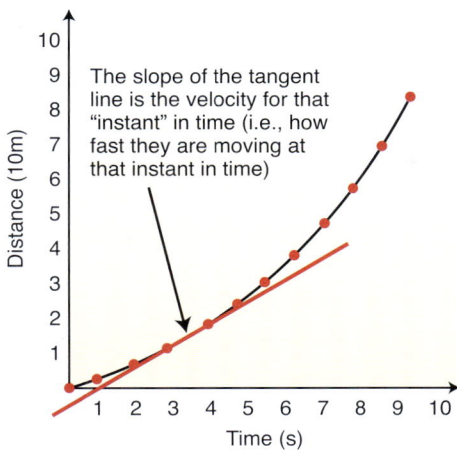

FIGURE 18-26 Graph of the instantaneous velocity of a sprinter at a moment in time between 3 and 4 seconds in the race. (©Scott Gaines, 2016)

DESCRIBING HOW FAST AN OBJECT MOVES AROUND AN AXIS—ANGULAR KINEMATICS (ANGULAR SPEED VERSUS ANGULAR VELOCITY)

- Again, we see there are corresponding rotary components to linear speed and velocity. It is important that manual and movement professionals appreciate and understand the rotational component to movement, as the body tends to work as a series of levers (e.g., the long bones) that rotate about specific axes (i.e., joints).[7,9,14]
  - **Angular speed** (σ = "*sigma*") = angular distance/change in time:
    - $\sigma = \dfrac{d\varphi}{dt}$
  - **Angular velocity** (ω = "*omega*") = angular displacement/change in time (Figure 18-27):
    - $\omega = \dfrac{d\theta}{dt}$
  - Because angular velocity is a vector, it has not only a magnitude but also a direction. As it is rotational, counter-clockwise is considered positive (+) while clockwise is considered negative (−).

For example, if a person moves the arm at the glenohumeral joint from anatomic position to full flexion (180 degrees) in one second, the angular velocity would be $\omega = \dfrac{\pi\ rad}{s}$ or $\dfrac{180°}{s}$ (Figure 18-27).

DESCRIBING HOW FAST AN OBJECT CHANGES SPEED—LINEAR AND ANGULAR ACCELERATION

- **Acceleration** is a vector quantity demonstrating the rate of change of an object's velocity (change in velocity/change in time). In other words, it is how quickly something "speeds up" or "slows down."[7,9]

  a = change in velocity (dv) divided by the change in time (dt):

  $$a = \dfrac{dv}{dt}$$

- Note: "Deceleration" is actually negative acceleration.

Angular acceleration (α) = angular velocity (dω) divided by the change in time (dt):

$$\alpha = \dfrac{d\omega}{dt}$$

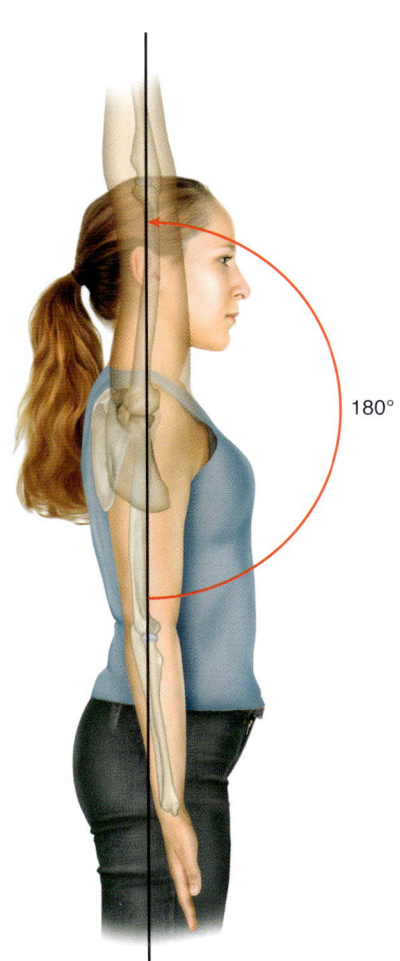

FIGURE 18-27 Example of angular velocity of the arm at the glenohumeral joint.

Acceleration: The Link Between Kinematics and Kinetics

○ As previously stated, kinematics is the study of motion without regard to the forces that cause motion. Kinetics on the other hand, is the study of forces acting on a body. So where does acceleration fit in? As we will discuss in the next section, forces change an object's velocity. In other words, *forces are the reason that objects accelerate* (Table 18-3).[6]

Table 18-3 Kinematics Summary

	Linear	Angular
Position	Measured in meters in 3D space using Cartesian coordinates	Measured in degrees or radians
Change in position	Scalar = Distance Vector = Displacement	Scalar = Angular Distance Vector = Angular Displacement
Rate of change in position	Scalar = Speed Vector = Velocity	Scalar = Angular Speed Vector = Angular Velocity
Rate of change of the rate of change in position	Acceleration	Angular Acceleration

SECTION 18.5 DESCRIBING THE FORCES OF HUMAN MOVEMENT—ANALYZING KINETICS

MASS MATTERS

○ As we begin our conversation about kinetics, it is important to note that we are now taking into account the nature of the object we're observing. In other words, we are taking into account the object's **mass** (m). Note that up until this point while analyzing kinematics, mass was never taken into account. Mass is defined as the amount of physical matter that comprises the object.[1,4,7,9]

  ○ Another way to look at mass is the product of density (concentration of physical matter) and volume (amount of space the mass occupies).

  $$\text{Mass} = \text{Density} (\rho) \times \text{Volume} (V):$$
  $$m = \rho V$$

  ○ Therefore, if one object has greater concentration of mass relative to another object, it would have a higher density (for example, bone is more dense than muscle which itself is more dense than fat).

○ **Inertia** is the property of an object to resist its current state of motion (which could be zero motion). In other words, inertia resists change...

Note: The amount of inertia is proportional to its mass.

  ○ In other words, the greater the mass, the greater the inertia, [...] state of motion.

MOMENTUM

○ If we want [...] (momentum) of a particular [...] more than just the object's [...] the object's mass.

  Momentum — [...] object's motion

  $$\text{Momentum (p)} = \text{mass times velocity:}$$
  $$p = mv$$

(Note: We use "p" for momentum because m was already taken for mass.)[7,9]

○ As an example, imagine on the ground in front of you are two balls, a bowling ball and a soccer ball. Both balls are the same size in diameter; however, the bowling ball has much greater mass than the soccer ball. Hence the bowling ball would have greater inertia, and it would be harder to get it moving. However, if we were able to roll both balls at the same velocity, the bowling ball would have greater momentum and would be harder to stop.

NEWTON'S THREE LAWS OF MOTION

○ Sir Isaac Newton, a 17th- to 18th-century English physicist and mathematician created three laws that describe both statics and dynamics of objects. Statics studies the forces on an object at rest or at constant velocity and dynamics studies how forces affect the motion of an object.[7,9]

Newton's First Law of Motion: Law of Inertia

○ An object continues in its state of rest or of uniform speed in a straight line unless it is compelled to change that state by forces acting on it.

If $\vec{F}_{NET} = 0$, then $\vec{v}$ = constant or zero.

  ○ What this means is that . . .
    ○ An object at rest stays at rest or an object moving at a certain speed in a certain direction maintains its trajectory unless another force acts upon it, causing it to change. Inertia is simply an object's ability to resist change to its position or motion. It requires more energy to get an object moving or to change its direction than to keep it moving at a constant speed in a constant direction.
    ○ A good example of this is throwing a ball. Once the ball is thrown, it will keep on going at the same velocity (speed and direction) unless another force changes the ball's trajectory (path). On earth there is air friction that

pushes against the ball. Gravity also changes its direction by making it fall down toward the earth. Finally, the ball stops when it hits the ground. Therefore air friction, gravity, and the resistance of the ground are forces acting on the ball.
- Likewise, the larger, more massive the individual, the more the individual's body will resist change. A large 300-lb (136.1-kg) football lineman will need to exert a greater amount of muscular force than a 175-lb (79.4-kg) wide receiver to change his motion.

Newton's Second Law of Motion: Law of Acceleration

- The acceleration of an object is directly proportional to the net force acting on it and is inversely proportional to its mass. The direction of the acceleration is in the direction of the applied net force. Note: This is where we get our definition of force!

$$\text{Force} = \text{Mass} \times \text{Acceleration:}$$
$$F = ma$$

- What this means is . . .
  - An object's acceleration is directly related to the force acting on it. The object will move in the direction of that force acting upon it.
  - If you push a bike, it will accelerate in the direction you are pushing it. It will also accelerate faster if you push it harder (greater force).
  - This concept is important in technique analysis in order to appreciate the how, what, and why something is happening.
  - Another way to look at this law is that a force is something that, when applied to an object, will change that object's motion (i.e., momentum).

Therefore a force can be seen as a push or a pull that will change an object's current motion (i.e., will start something in motion, stop its motion, speed it up, or slow it down).

Newton's Third Law of Motion: Law of Action-Reaction

- Whenever one object exerts a force on a second object, the second exerts an equal and opposite force on the first object.
  - During an action such as a foot-strike while running, there is a **ground reaction force (GRF)** (a fundamental force in the world of biomechanics). The force generated against the earth is the same as the force the earth is generating back. The difference is that the body's mass is insignificant in comparison to the Earth's. Therefore the body will move upward against gravity rather than the Earth moving away from the body.
  - Another example can be appreciated by looking at the forces that are applied to a manual therapist's body when doing soft tissue manipulation (massage) to the client's body. When the therapist presses into the client's body, the client's body presses back with an equal force into the therapist's body. This equal and opposite force into the therapist's body can be quite appreciable, especially when the therapist is employing deep pressure and using a smaller contact, such as the thumb.[7,9]

STATICS AND DYNAMICS REVISITED

- As mentioned above, **statics** is the study of systems in constant motion (including zero motion). In other words, the body in question is under *constant* momentum. In order for this to be true, there must be no net forces on the object (note: it does not mean there are no forces; it's just that the forces on the object cancel each other out). Therefore a book sitting on the table is static because it has constant (zero in this case) motion. However, there are forces on the book. Specifically, the force due to gravity (its weight) and the equal and opposite reaction of the table pressing on the book.[9]
  - Here's another example of statics. Imagine standing upright, perfectly still. Of course, one would still have some movement (breathing, heart beating, blood pumping, etc.); however, let's focus on the musculoskeletal movement. In this example, there is no gross musculoskeletal movement; however in order to remain upright, postural muscles must contract to create forces to maintain the position of the joints (see equilibrium section below). So forces are occurring within the system, but there are no *net* forces and hence it is a static position.
- **Dynamics** on the other hand is the study of systems in which acceleration is present. This means that there are *net* forces on the body, changing its momentum (motion). Whenever an object is moving and it changes speed or direction, forces are not constant and hence there is a net acceleration.[9]
  - Now imagine moving from the static standing position to a seated position. Gravity would be pulling down, primarily pulling trunk, hips, and knees into flexion and the ankles into dorsiflexion. Extensor muscles of the trunk, hip, and knee, and plantarflexors of the ankle would eccentrically decelerate to control/restrain the action of gravity. Forces are involved just as before, but now there is acceleration present (i.e., it is dynamic).

Note: While a dynamic biomechanical analysis is ideal, analyzing statics is much simpler and usually sufficient.

REVISITING FORCES ON THE HUMAN BODY

- Center of mass/center of gravity
  - Every physical body has a point about which its mass is evenly distributed (i.e., **center of mass [COM]**). When subjected to gravity, it can be considered the point in the body at which gravity acts and can be described as the body's **center of gravity (COG)**. A body behaves as if its entire mass acts or is acted upon at its center of gravity. For our purposes, COM and COG can be used interchangeably.[7]
  - For the average person standing in anatomic position, the body's COG will be just anterior to the second sacral vertebra (S2) (Figure 18-28).
  - The human body can also be seen as a series of segments linked together by joints. Each segment has its own weight and hence its own COG that contributes to the body's total body weight (Figure 18-29).[7]
    - If the body is not in anatomic position, the COG will shift. The COG may actually be located outside the body (Figure 18-30).

604   PART 4   Myology: Study of the Muscular System

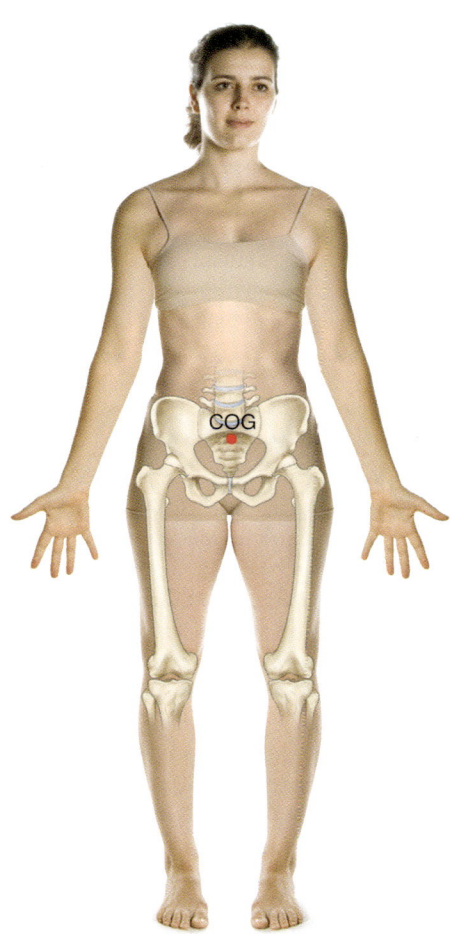

FIGURE 18-28 Representation of anatomic position with center of gravity (COG) highlighted.

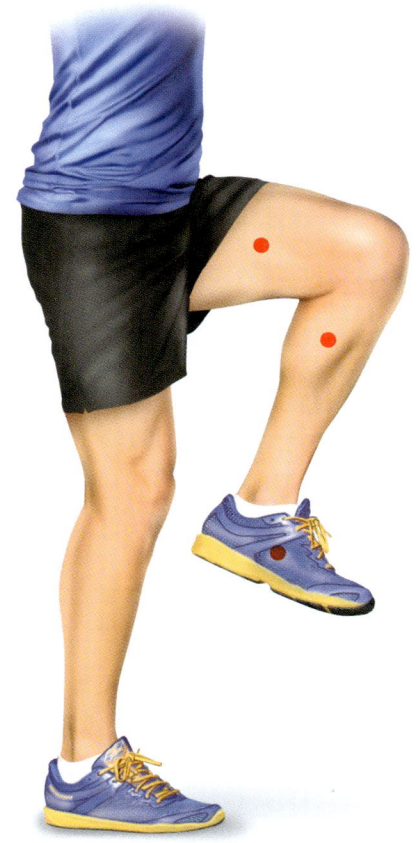

FIGURE 18-29 Each segment in the left lower extremity (thigh, leg, and foot) has its own center of gravity (COG), represented by a red dot.

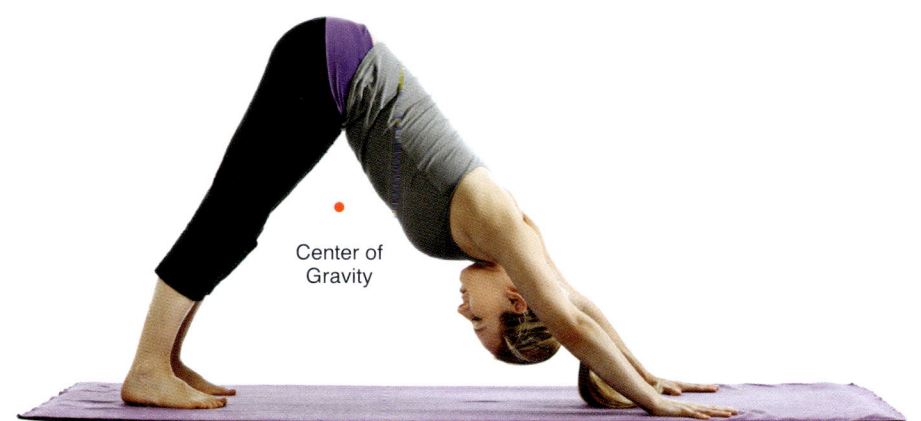

FIGURE 18-30 When not in anatomic position, the center of gravity (COG) of the human body can actually shift to be located outside of the body (©istock.com).

GROUND REACTION FORCES

- Force vectors (remember, when you think vectors, think arrows) can be broken down into x, y, and z components. For the purposes of understanding ground reaction forces, we will examine basic running gait. Let's take a look at two of the components that make up the GRF at foot-strike. These components are the vertical component force (F_y) and the horizontal component force (F_x) (Figure 18-31).

The Vertical Component—F_Y

- Ground reaction force at each foot-strike is studied extensively for performance enhancement and in the investigation of running-related injuries. The vertical component of the GRF during running is two to three times bodyweight depending on running style. Runners are typically classified as rearfoot, midfoot, or forefoot strikers (depending on the portion of the shoe/foot that tends to contact the ground first) (Figure 18-32).[3]
  - Figure 18-32 shows the vertical component of the GRF for a rearfoot striker and a midfoot striker. Note: There is a larger impact peak (point a) for the rearfoot striker, followed by a slight decrease (b) then a propulsive peak (c).

The Horizontal Component—F_x

- Runners generally increase stride length as running speed increases. Longer strides tend to generate GRFs with a larger "braking" horizontal component. This is one reason why longer strides (over-striding) can be counterproductive. Research has shown that a braking horizontal component force of 6% of bodyweight can increase the metabolic cost of running by up to 30%. This is wasted effort (Figure 18-33).[3]
  - The graph in Figure 18-33 represents the horizontal GRF (F_x) over time of an over-strider. Notice that the initial horizontal force over time (or impulse) is pressing forward into the ground so the ground reaction force (F_x) is backward. It's a braking force that slows performance! Only later in the stance phase (the phases of gait will be covered in Chapter 20) do the forces switch directions. The body creates a backward force against the ground and the GRF creates a propulsive force to accelerate the runner forward (remember Newton's Third Law: For every action, there is an equal and opposite reaction). To increase efficiency during running, braking forces must be reduced and propulsive forces increased.[3]

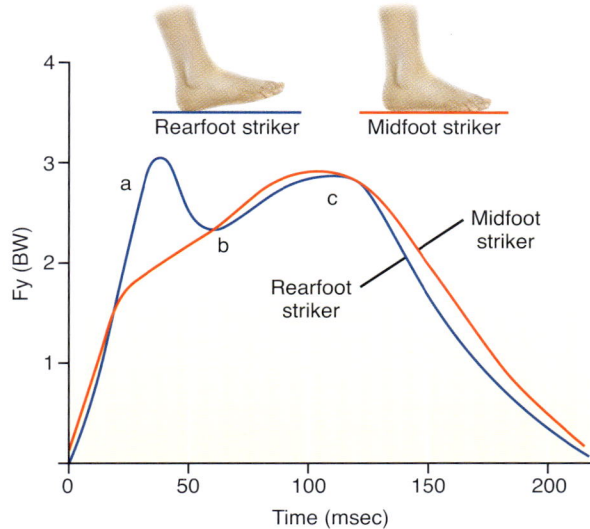

FIGURE 18-32 Vertical ground reaction force (GRF) for both rearfoot strikers and midfoot strikers.

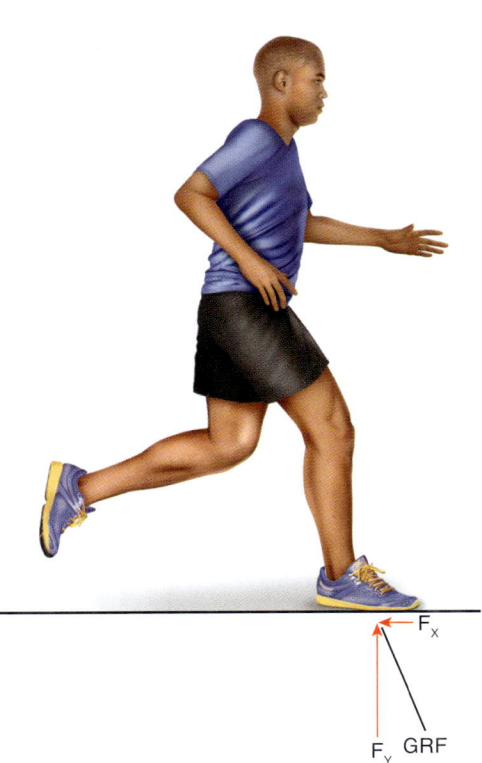

FIGURE 18-31 The resultant force vector from the ground reaction force (GRF) during footstrike.

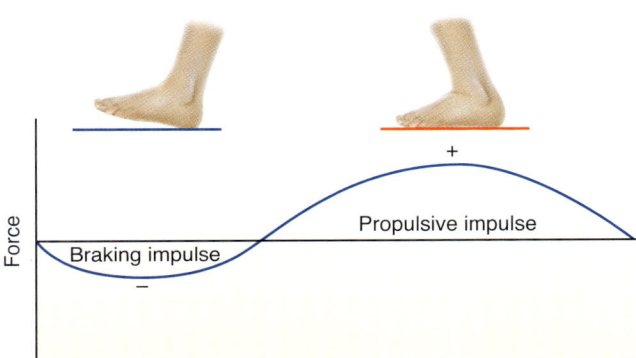

FIGURE 18-33 The horizontal component of the ground reaction force (GRF) for a rearfoot striker.

THE IMPORTANCE OF THE ROTATIONAL ANALOG TO FORCE—TORQUE ("FORCES THAT CAUSE ROTATION")

- What is torque (a.k.a. "moment of force")?
  - A **torque** is rotational force and is represented by the Greek letter tau (τ).

  $$\text{Torque} = \tau = F\, r\, \sin\theta$$

- Note: It has three components:
  1. F = the force applied to the lever
  2. r = the distance of the application of force to the axis (lever arm)
  3. $\sin\theta$ = the angle of application (force angle)
- It is also written:

  $$\tau = F\,(MA)$$

- MA = moment arm
  - MA is the shortest distance between the axis and line of force (always perpendicular)
  - MA is simply the force angle ($\sin\theta$) × the lever arm (r)
- Why is torque so important?
  - While muscles will work together to create a linear resultant force, in order for joints to move, the linear force will move a bone around its axis of rotation (i.e., the joint).[5,9]

In order to create typical axial joint movement, the force generated by muscles must create torque around a joint.[6]

TORQUE AND LEVERS

- As mentioned above in the angular kinematics section, the human body can be seen as a series of levers (bones) that move around an axis. Rotation occurs when a force (known as an effort force) is applied to the lever and creates a torque to overcome an opposing force at some other point in the opposite direction, known as the resistance force (for example, the concentric contraction force of a muscle upon a bone/body part opposes the resistance force of gravity upon that bone/body part).
- A lever system allows the effort force to perform one of two tasks:
  - The effort force is able to create a greater torque than a larger resistance force due to a longer lever arm (in this case the effort force has "mechanical advantage"). For example, lifting a heavy object with a crowbar.
    - Note: The "mechanical advantage" (MA) of a lever is the ratio of its output force to its input force.
  - The effort force is able to move the body part against the resistance force farther and/or faster than the effort arm is moved (in this case the resistance force is smaller and has the "mechanical advantage"). An example of this is throwing a baseball or rowing a boat.
  - The vast majority of the time, our muscles will work at a mechanical disadvantage, having to produce a relatively large force to overcome a smaller resistance. This allows our bodies to have greater speed and range of motion.[12]
  - Note: Levers and lever systems are covered in more detail in Chapter 17.

EQUILIBRIUM, STABILITY, BALANCE, AND BASE OF SUPPORT

- **Equilibrium** is often equated with the concept of "balance."
- Perhaps better defined, the term **balance** could be defined as an individual's ability to control equilibrium.
- There are two types of equilibrium: static equilibrium and dynamic equilibrium.
  - *Static equilibrium* is a motionless state, where there are no net forces or torques on a body (notice again that this does not mean there are no forces or torques, just that the forces and torques that do exist cancel each other out). For example, when one is standing perfectly still.
  - Similarly, the concept of *dynamic equilibrium* is used to describe the balance of the body, but in motion. In this case, the forces and torques on the body are working to opposed directed inertial (movement forces).
- *Stability* is the resistance to a change or a resistance to a disruption in equilibrium (i.e., resistance to linear and angular acceleration that would move the body). Factors that affect stability include:
  - The mass of the object. The greater the mass, the more inertia and the more it will resist movement; hence the greater the stability.
  - The amount of friction between a body and the surface it is in contact with. The greater the friction, the greater the force needed for movement and the greater the stability.
  - The size of the object's *base of support* (the area beneath an object or person that is bound by the outermost regions of contact between a body and its support surface). The larger the base of support, the more stable the object.
  - The height of the object's COG. The lower the COG, the greater the stability.[7]

ANALYZING THE HUMAN BODY VIA A FREE-BODY DIAGRAM

- In Section 18.1, a three-step process was introduced to qualitatively analyze human posture:
  - Step 1: Analyze the posture/motion (kinematics is the study of motion with no regard to the forces that cause the motion)
  - Step 2: Analyze the forces (kinetics is the study of forces acting on a body)
  - Step 3: Compare to the "ideal" for the individual[9]
- Now that we have covered the foundational mechanics, we can put the steps into action with a free body diagram. A free body diagram is an essential tool for movement analysis. In a free body diagram, all the forces on an object at an instant in time are shown with arrows representing their relative magnitude and direction. For manual and movement professionals, certain assumptions can be made to make the process easier for analyzing posture.
  - No tissue deformation
  - No friction in the system
  - The action of all the muscle fibers in a muscle can be summarized in a single resultant force vector
  - No acceleration present (a static system)[11]

- Step 1: Analyze the kinematics
  - Draw a basic image of the body or body segments in question
  - Make special note of joint relationship to anatomic position
    - **Anthropometry** is the science of measurements and proportions of the human body. As each person is unique, the manual and movement professional must be able to take into account anthropometric differences (e.g., limb length differences) into their analysis.
- Step 2: Analyze the kinetics
  - Draw force vectors for all external forces
    - COG of whole body
    - COG of body segments (if necessary)
    - Any other external load/forces entering the body
  - Determine the direction of internal forces needed for equilibrium
  - Draw representative force vectors for all internal forces based on equilibrium
- Step 3: Compare to the "ideal"
  - Using the information from the remainder of this text, one should be able to determine where biomechanical deficiency may lie and how to best address it.[9]

REVIEW QUESTIONS

Answers to the following review questions appear on the Evolve website accompanying this book at: http://evolve.elsevier.com/Muscolino/kinesiology/.

1. What is Biomechanics?

2. How is biomechanics analogous to physiology?

3. How are mobility and stability mechanically related?

4. What are the two primary emphases in the study of biomechanics?

5. What are the two forms of biomechanical analysis?

6. How are weight and force related?

7. Is bodyweight considered an internal force or an external force?

8. What are the primary producers of active forces within the body?

9. When a force is placed on a solid object and the material changes and will not return to its original shape, this level of stress is known as the _____.

10. What's the difference between a scalar and a vector?

11. What is kinematics?

12. What is the difference between rectilinear motion and curvilinear motion?

13. What the difference between linear distance and displacement?

14. How is speed related to velocity?

15. What will cause an object to accelerate?

16. Momentum can be seen as a measurement of an object's _____.

17. According to Newton's Second Law of Motion, Force = _____.

18. Will an individual's COM always be in the same place?

19. What is "torque" also known as?

20. In a concentric muscle action, what produces the effort force?

21. What are the four factors that affect stability?

22. In the Analyze-Optimize-Maximize-Minimize process, what is analyzed first? Second?

REFERENCES

1. Abernethy B: The biophysical foundations of human movement, Champaign, IL, 2005, Human Kinetics.
2. Ackland TR: Applied anatomy and biomechanics in sport, Champaign, IL, 2009, Human Kinetics.
3. Blazevich AJ: Sports biomechanics, The basics: Optimising human performance, ed 2, London: 2012, A&C Black Publishers.
4. Burkett BA: Sport mechanics for coaches, Champaign, IL, 2010, Human Kinetics.
5. Floyd RT: Manual of structural kinesiology, New York, NY 2011, McGraw-Hill.
6. Gaines SE: NESTA personal fitness trainer manual, Rancho Santa Margarita, CA, NESTA.
7. Hall SJ: Basic biomechanics, ed 6, New York, NY, 2011, McGraw-Hill.
8. Levangie P: Joint structure and function: A comprehensive analysis, ed 4, Philadelphia, PA, 2005, F.A. Davis.
9. McGinnis PM: Biomechanics of sport and exercise, Champaign, IL, 2005, Human Kinetics.
10. Neumann DA: Kinesiology of the musculoskeletal system: Foundations for physical rehabilitation, ed 3, St. Louis, MO, 2017, Elsevier.
11. Oatis CA: Kinesiology: The mechanics and pathomechanics of human movement, Philadelphia, PA, 2004, Lippincott Williams & Wilkins.
12. Saladin K: Anatomy & physiology: The unity of form and function, ed 7, New York, NY, 2014, McGraw-Hill.
13. Whiting WC: Biomechanics of musculoskeletal injury, ed 2, Champaign, IL, 2008, Human Kinetics.
14. Zatsiorsky VM: Kinematics of human motion, Champaign, IL, 1998, Human Kinetics.

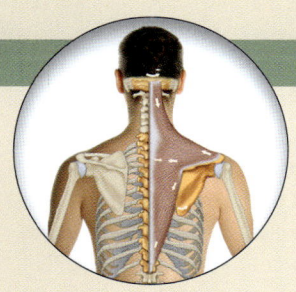

CHAPTER 19
The Neuromuscular System

CHAPTER OUTLINE

Section 19.1	Overview of the Nervous System	Section 19.6	Muscle Spindles
Section 19.2	Voluntary Movement versus Reflex Movement	Section 19.7	Golgi Tendon Organs
		Section 19.8	Inner Ear Proprioceptors
Section 19.3	Reciprocal Inhibition	Section 19.9	Other Musculoskeletal Reflexes
Section 19.4	Overview of Proprioception	Section 19.10	Pain-Spasm-Pain Cycle
Section 19.5	Fascial/Joint Proprioceptors	Section 19.11	Gate Theory

CHAPTER OBJECTIVES

After completing this chapter, the student should be able to perform the following:

1. Define the key terms of this chapter and state the word origins of this chapter.
2. Compare and contrast sensory, integrative, and motor neurons.
3. Describe the structural and functional classifications of the nervous system.
4. Do the following related to voluntary movement versus reflex movement:
   - Compare and contrast the neuronal pathways for the initiation of voluntary movement and a spinal cord reflex.
   - Describe the difference between true reflexive behavior and learned/patterned behavior.
   - Describe the relationship between neural facilitation and resting muscle tone.
5. Describe the neuronal pathways for and the purpose of reciprocal inhibition, as well as describe how reciprocal inhibition can be used to aid muscle palpation and muscle stretching.
6. Do the following related to proprioception:
   - Define and discuss proprioception.
   - List the three major categories of proprioceptors and the specific proprioceptors found in each major category.
   - Compare and contrast the function of Pacini's corpuscles and Ruffini's endings.
7. Do the following related to muscle spindles and Golgi tendon organs:
   - Compare and contrast the neuronal pathway mechanism and the function of muscle spindles and Golgi tendon organs.
   - Discuss the relationship between muscle spindles, Golgi tendon organs, and muscle stretching.
   - Discuss the concept of muscle facilitation and muscle inhibition.
   - Discuss the differences (including implications for treatment) between trigger points and global tightening of a muscle.
8. Do the following related to inner ear proprioceptors:
   - Describe the mechanisms and functions of inner ear proprioceptors.
   - Compare and contrast dynamic and static proprioception.
   - Describe the relationship between inner ear proprioceptors and neck proprioceptors and the implications for bodywork and/or exercise.
9. Describe the mechanism and purpose of the flexor withdrawal, crossed extensor, tonic neck, cervico-ocular, righting, and cutaneous reflexes.
10. Do the following related to the pain-spasm-pain cycle:
    - Discuss the mechanism and importance of manual and movement therapy to the pain-spasm-pain cycle.
    - Describe the function of muscle splinting and body armoring.
11. Describe the mechanism of the gate theory, including the implications for manual and movement therapy.

OVERVIEW

We have now studied the bones and joints of the skeletal system and the muscles of the muscular system. Bones provide rigid levers and come together to form the joints of the body; muscles attach to the bones and create movement at the joints. In this manner, the bones, joints, and muscles function together as the musculoskeletal system. However, this system cannot function in a harmonious fashion on its own. Indeed, its elements can be likened to the members of a symphony orchestra who are missing their conductor. Just as a conductor is needed to direct and coordinate the musicians of an orchestra, a conductor is needed to direct and coordinate the muscles of the musculoskeletal system. The conductor of the musculoskeletal system is the nervous system. It is the purpose of this chapter to examine the role that the nervous system plays in directing movement of the body. Indeed, a fine appreciation of the biomechanical functioning of the human body cannot exist without an understanding of the integrated role of the nervous system. In short, this chapter explores the functioning of the neuromusculoskeletal system.

KEY TERMS

Active isolated stretching (AIS)
Agonist contract (AC) stretching
Afferent neuron (A-fair-ent NUR-on)
Alpha motor neurons (AL-fa NUR-onz)
Ampulla (am-POOL-a, am-PYUL-a)
Ascending pathways
Body armoring
Central nervous system
Cerebral motor cortex (se-REE-bral, KOR-tex)
Cervico-ocular reflex
CNS
Co-contraction
Contract relax (CR) stretching
Counter irritant theory
Crista ampullaris (KRIS-ta AM-pyul-AR-is)
Crossed extensor reflex
Cutaneous reflex (cue-TANE-ee-us)
Descending pathways
Dermatome
Dizziness
Efferent neuron (E-fair-ent NUR-on)
Electrical muscle stimulation
Endogenous morphine (en-DAHJ-en-us)
Endorphins (en-DOOR-fins)
Equilibrium
Extrafusal fibers (EX-tra-FUSE-al)
Fascial/joint proprioceptors (PRO-pree-o-SEP-torz)
Feldenkrais technique (FEL-den-krise)
Flexor withdrawal reflex
Free nerve endings
Gamma motor neurons (GAM-ma, NUR-onz)
Gamma motor system
Gate theory
Global tightening
Golgi end organs (GOAL-gee)
Golgi tendon organ reflex
Golgi tendon organs
Homunculus
Hypnic jerk (HIP-nik)
Inner ear proprioceptors (PRO-pree-o-SEP-torz)
Integrative neuron (NUR-on)
Interstitial myofascial receptors (IN-ter-STISH-al MY-o-fash-al)
Intrafusal fibers (IN-tra-FUSE-al)
Inverse myotatic reflex (MY-o-TAT-ik)
Joint proprioceptors (PRO-pree-o-SEP-torz)
Krause's end bulbs (KRAUS-es)
Labyrinthine proprioceptors (LAB-i-rinth-EEN PRO-pree-o-SEP-torz)
Labyrinthine righting reflex
Learned behavior
Learned reflex
Locked long
Locked short
Lower crossed syndrome
Lower motor neuron (LMN) (NUR-on)
Macula (MACK-you-la)
Mechanoreceptors (mi-KAN-o-ree-SEP-torz)
Meissner's corpuscles (MIZE-nerz CORE-pus-als)
Merkel's discs (MERK-elz)
Motor homunculus
Motor neuron (NUR-on)
Muscle facilitation
Muscle inhibition
Muscle memory
Muscle proprioceptors (PRO-pree-o-SEP-torz)
Muscle spindle reflex
Muscle spindles
Muscle splinting
Myotatic reflex (MY-o-TAT-ik)
Nerve impulse
Neural facilitation (NUR-al)
Neuron (NUR-on)
Otoliths (O-to-liths)
Pacini's corpuscles (pa-SEEN-eez CORE-pus-als)
Pain-spasm-pain cycle
Patterned behavior
Peripheral nervous system (PNS)
Plyometric training (ply-o-MET-rik)
Post-isometric relaxation (PIR) stretching
Primary motor cortex
Primary sensory cortex
Proprioception (PRO-pree-o-SEP-shun)

Proprioceptive neuromuscular facilitation (PNF)
  (PRO-pree-o-SEP-tiv) stretching
Reciprocal inhibition
Reflex arc
Resting tone
Righting reflex
Ruffini's endings (ru-FEEN-eez)
Semicircular canals
Sensory homunculus

Sensory neuron
Stretch reflex
Target muscle
Tendon reflex
Tonic neck reflex (TON-ik)
Trigger points
Upper crossed syndrome
Upper motor neuron (UMN)
Vestibule (VEST-i-byul)

WORD ORIGINS

- Ampullaris—From Latin *ampulla,* meaning *a two-handed bottle*
- Cortex—From Latin *cortex,* meaning *outer portion of an organ, bark of a tree*
- Crista—From Latin *crista,* meaning *crest*
- Endogenous—From Greek *endon,* meaning *within,* and *gen,* meaning *production*
- Equilibrium—From Latin *aequus,* meaning *equal,* and *libra,* meaning *a balance*
- Exogenous—From Greek *exo,* meaning *outside,* and *gen,* meaning *production*
- Facilitation—From Latin *facilitas,* meaning *easy*
- Inhibition—From Latin *inhibeo,* meaning *to keep back* (from Latin *habeo,* meaning *to have*)
- Interstitial—From Latin *inter,* meaning *between,* and *sisto,* meaning *to stand* (*Interstitial* means to stand between or to be located between.)
- Macula—From Latin *macula,* meaning *a spot*
- Proprioception—From Latin *proprius,* meaning *one's own,* and *capio,* meaning *to take*

SECTION 19.1   OVERVIEW OF THE NERVOUS SYSTEM

- The following overview of the nervous system is not meant to be comprehensive; it is meant to overview only the aspects of the nervous system pertinent to muscle contraction.
- The nervous system is made up of nerve cells, also known as neurons (Figure 19-1).
- A **neuron** is specialized to carry an electrical signal known as a **nerve impulse**.[1]
- The typical neuron is composed of dendrites, a cell body, and an axon.
  - The dendrites carry the nerve impulse toward the cell body; the axon carries the nerve impulse away from the cell body.[1]
- Functionally, a neuron can be sensory, integrative, or motor.[2]
- A **sensory neuron** carries a sensory stimulus.
  - Sensory neurons are also known as **afferent neurons**.

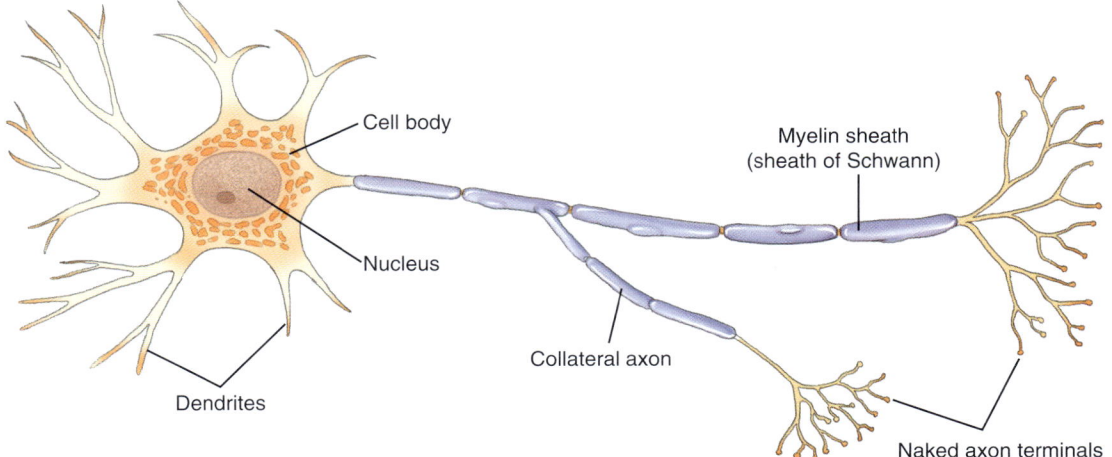

FIGURE 19-1 A nerve cell (also known as a neuron). A neuron is a type of cell that is specialized to carry a nerve impulse. The typical neuron has dendrites that carry the nerve impulse toward the cell body and an axon that carries the nerve impulse away from the cell body.

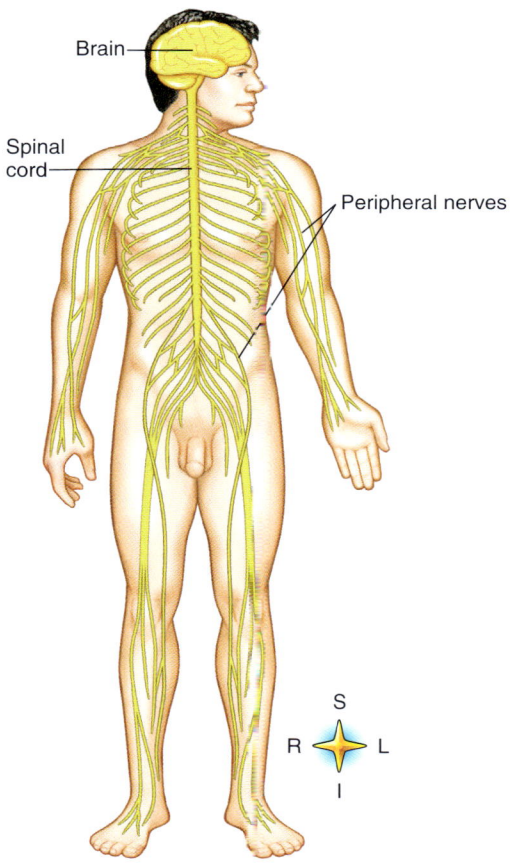

FIGURE 19-2 The two major structural divisions of the nervous system: (1) the central nervous system (CNS) and (2) the peripheral nervous system (PNS). The CNS is located in the center of the body and is composed of the brain and spinal cord. The PNS is located peripheral to the CNS and is composed of 31 pairs of spinal nerves and 12 pairs of cranial nerves. (Note: The cranial nerves are not shown.) *(Modified from Patton KT, Thibodeau GA: Anatomy and physiology, ed 7, St Louis, 2010, Mosby.)*

- An **integrative neuron** integrates/processes the sensory stimuli received from the sensory neurons.
- A **motor neuron** carries a message that directs a muscle to contract.
  - Motor neurons are also known as **efferent neurons**.
- On a large scale, the nervous system can be structurally organized into the **central nervous system (CNS)** and the **peripheral nervous system (PNS)** (Figure 19-2).

CENTRAL NERVOUS SYSTEM STRUCTURE:

- The central nervous system (CNS) is located in the center of the body (hence the name *central*) and is composed of the brain and spinal cord.
- The brain and spinal cord contain sensory, integrative, and motor neurons.[3]

Brain:

- The brain is composed of three major parts: (1) the cerebrum, (2) brainstem, and (3) cerebellum.[4]
  - The cerebrum is the largest part of the brain. The outer aspect of the cerebrum is called the *cortex* and is composed of gray matter. The inner aspect of the cerebrum is primarily made up of white matter, with some isolated clusters of gray matter called *nuclei* or *ganglia*.
  - White matter of the nervous system is white because of the presence of myelin. When myelin is present, it wraps around neuronal axons, insulating them and helping to speed the conduction of nerve impulses (see Figure 19-1). Gray matter is made up of dendrites, cell bodies, and unmyelinated axons of neurons. It is in the gray matter regions that connections and processing occur. Decisions made in these gray matter regions are then carried via white myelinated neurons to distant sites within the body. Gray matter regions may be likened to think tanks where questions are pondered and answered; white matter tracts are then analogous to the highways that carry these answers to other locations.

Spinal Cord:

- The spinal cord is composed of an outer area of white matter and an inner area of gray matter.[4]
- The gray matter is where the connections occur.

- The outer white matter region of the spinal cord is made up of white matter tracts.
  - These white matter tracts are composed of ascending and descending pathways of information. The **ascending pathways** carry sensory information. The **descending pathways** carry motor information.
  - The ascending white matter tracts carry sensory information up from lower levels of the spinal cord to higher levels of the spinal cord and/or the brain. The descending tracts carry motor information down from the brain to the spinal cord or from higher levels of the spinal cord to lower levels of the spinal cord.

PERIPHERAL NERVOUS SYSTEM STRUCTURE:

- The peripheral nervous system (PNS) is located peripherally and is composed of peripheral spinal and cranial nerves.[5]
  - Entering and exiting the CNS are 31 pairs of spinal nerves and 12 pairs of cranial nerves.[6]
  - Note: A nerve of the peripheral nervous system (PNS) is technically an organ because it contains two different tissues organized for a common purpose, transmission of information via nerve impulses. It is also similar in organization to a muscle. A muscle is composed of bundles of muscle cells and is separated and enveloped by connective tissue coverings that surround each individual muscle cell (i.e., endomysium), each bundle of muscle cells (i.e., perimysium), and the entire muscle (i.e., epimysium). A nerve is composed of bundles of neurons (i.e., nerve cells) and is separated and enveloped by connective tissue coverings; each neuron is covered by endoneurium; each bundle of neurons is covered by perineurium; and the entire nerve is covered by epineurium.
  - The PNS contains sensory and motor neurons.[7]
  - A peripheral nerve can contain all sensory neurons, in which case it is said to be a *sensory nerve*, or it can contain all motor neurons, in which case it is said to be a *motor nerve*. It can also contain both sensory and motor neurons, in which case it is said to be a *mixed nerve*.

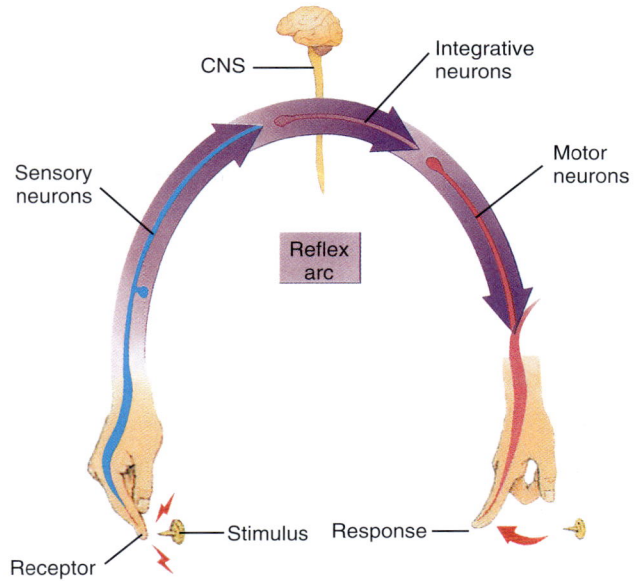

FIGURE 19-3 Illustration of the functional flow of information within the nervous system. *(Modified from Patton KT, Thibodeau GA:* Anatomy and physiology, *ed 7, St Louis, 2010, Mosby.)*

FUNCTION OF THE NERVOUS SYSTEM:

Generally, the flow of information within the nervous system proceeds in the following order (Figure 19-3):
- Sensory neurons located within peripheral nerves of the PNS carry sensory information (i.e., stimuli) from the periphery of the body into the CNS (Box 19-1).
- The CNS then processes that sensory input via its integrative neurons.
- A motor response is carried back out from the CNS to the periphery within motor neurons of a peripheral nerve of the PNS. This motor response directs contraction of musculature.
  - How much integration occurs with the CNS varies tremendously, depending on whether the movement being directed is a voluntary movement or a reflex movement.[7]

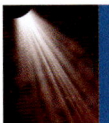 **BOX 19-1** **Spotlight on Dermatomes**

Somatic sensory touch sensation from the skin is illustrated by what is called a dermatomal map. The word "dermatome" literally means "cut skin" ("derm" means "skin" and "tome" means "cut") because the skin can be looked at as being divided or *cut up* by the sensory nerve roots. So each **dermatome** is the area of skin that is innervated by a single peripheral nerve root. These sensory nerve roots come from the spinal cord (spinal nerves C1-C8, T1-T12, L1-L5, and S1-S5) with two exceptions. First, C1 spinal nerve has no sensory component, hence no dermatome. Second, the face receives sensory innervation from a cranial nerve, not a spinal nerve. Specifically, it receives innervation from Cranial Nerve V (the trigeminal nerve, named for having three branches), hence three dermatomes known as *V1*, *V2*, and *V3* exist in the face.

The clinical significance of dermatomes is that if the client presents with paresthesia (abnormal sensation) such as numbness, tingling, or pain, then knowing the dermatome of the paresthesia can point to the level of a possible condition of nerve compression (often caused by a bulging or herniated spinal disc, or perhaps a bone spur). For example, tingling in the thumb might be traced back to a herniated disc pressing on the sensory nerve root of C6; or pain in the plantar foot might be found to be caused by a bone spur pressing on the sensory nerve root of L5.

Continued

BOX 19-1 Spotlight on Dermatomes—Cont'd

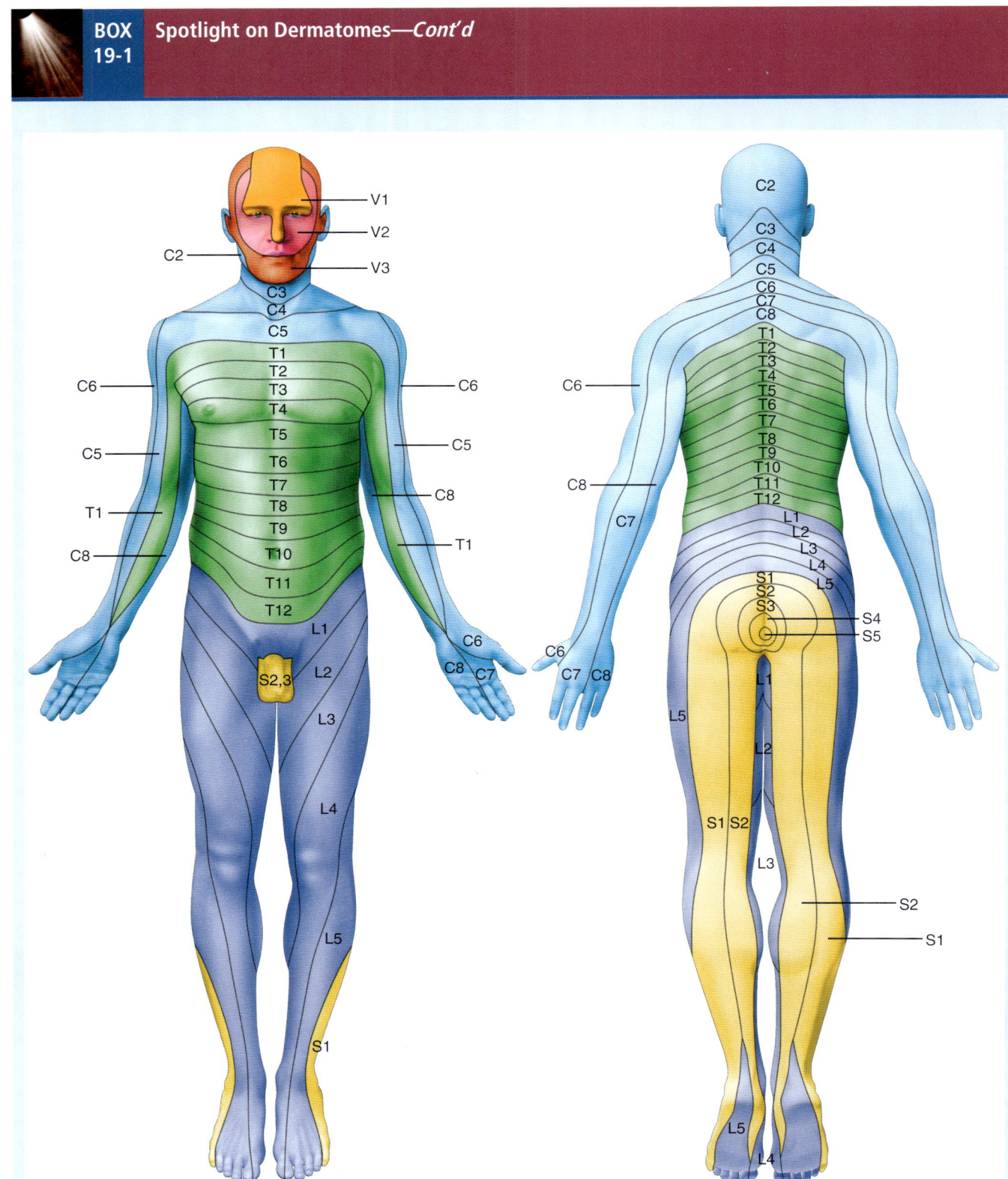

SECTION 19.2 VOLUNTARY MOVEMENT VERSUS REFLEX MOVEMENT

The nervous system can direct two types of movement: (1) voluntary movement and (2) reflex movement.

INITIATION OF VOLUNTARY MOVEMENT:

- All voluntary motor control of movement originates in the outer portion of the cerebrum called the *cerebral cortex*[7] (Figure 19-4, *A*).
- When the integration and processing of sensory stimuli within the brain result in the determination that a joint action will be made, this decision is passed along to the **cerebral motor cortex** of the brain. The cerebral motor cortex then sends a directive down through the spinal cord within descending white matter tract pathways (Box 19-2).[7]
- Most but not all voluntary movements are directed by the brain via the spinal cord to peripheral spinal nerves. The directions for some movements leave the brain directly via peripheral cranial nerves.[8]

BOX 19-2

There are two regions of the brain that are largely responsible for processing somatic touch sensation and voluntary movement. Somatic touch is received by and processed in the *somatic sensory cortex*, also known as the ***primary sensory cortex***, which is located on the postcentral gyrus of the parietal lobe (directly posterior to the central sulcus that divides the frontal and parietal lobes). Voluntary movement is processed in and directed by the *motor cortex*, also known as the ***primary motor cortex***, which is located in the precentral gyrus of the frontal lobe (directly anterior to the central sulcus). The representation of our body in each case is called a **homunculus** (literally means "little person"); hence there is a **sensory homunculus** and a **motor homunculus**. Note that the proportions of the body parts for each homunculus is not proportional to the actual size of these body parts, but rather is proportional to the sensory or motor representation of those body parts in the brain.

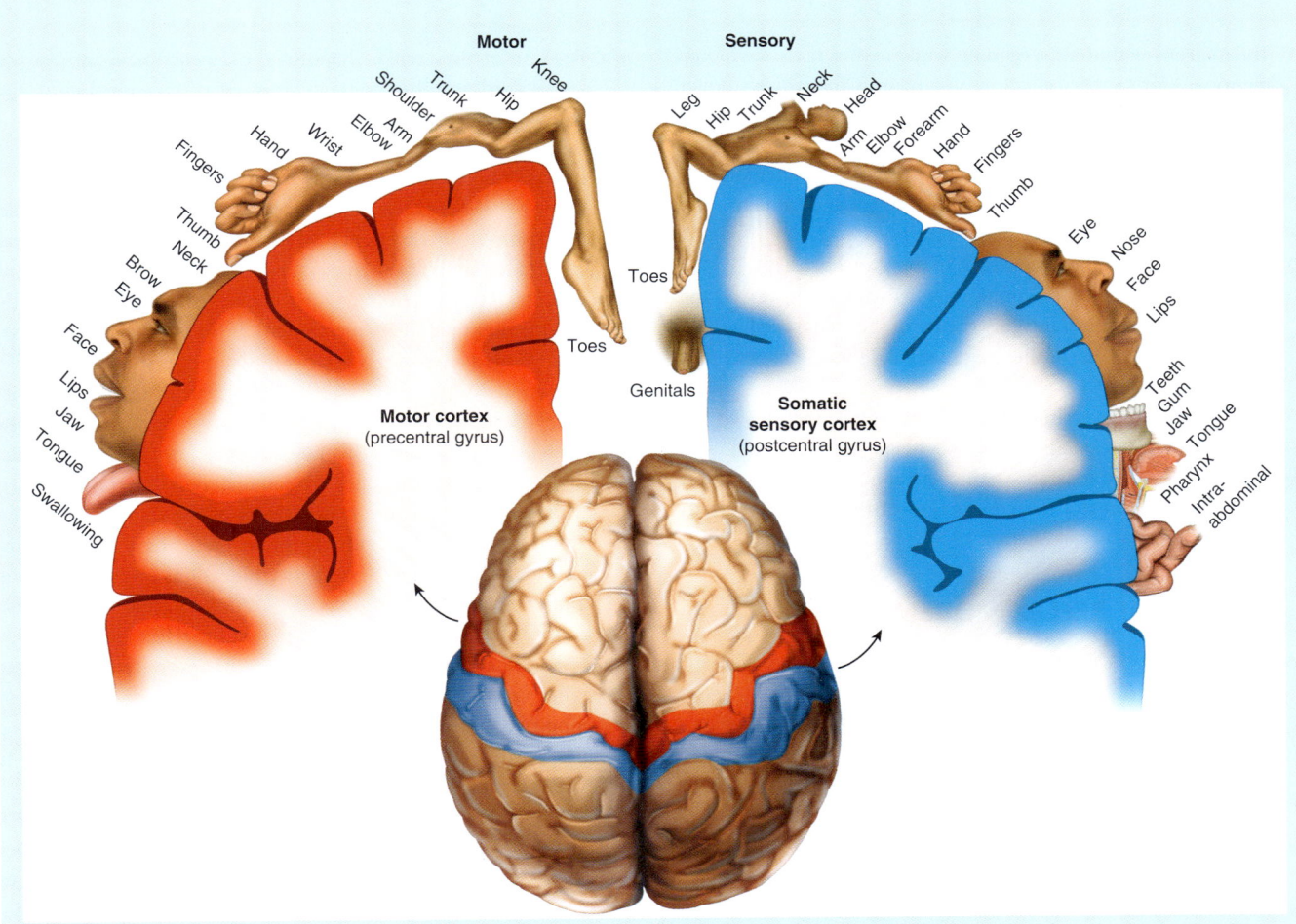

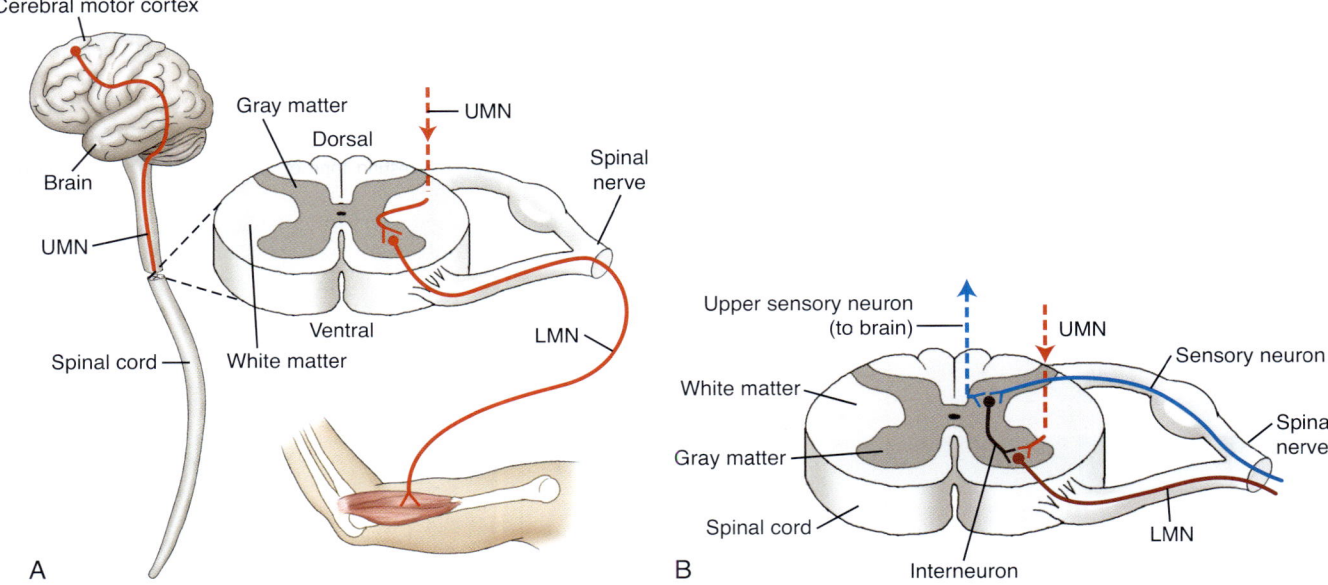

FIGURE 19-4 **A,** Pathways within the nervous system for initiation of voluntary movement. An upper motor neuron (UMN) originates within the motor cortex of the cerebrum and travels down through a descending white matter tract of the spinal cord where it then enters the gray matter of the spinal cord and synapses with a lower motor neuron (LMN). The LMN then exits the spinal cord and travels within a peripheral spinal nerve to connect with a muscle. **B,** Simple reflex arc that consists of a sensory neuron, interneuron, and LMN. Awareness of a reflex occurs via connections that travel up to the brain to alert the brain to what has just happened. The brain can influence a spinal cord reflex via UMNs that travel down through descending white matter tracts of the spinal cord.

- The neurons within a descending white matter tract are motor neurons. More specifically, a motor neuron that travels down in a descending white matter tract is called an **upper motor neuron (UMN)**.[9]
  - Lower areas of the brain, such as the basal ganglia and the cerebellum, also feed into these pathways and influence the production of the movement of the body.
- The UMN ends in the gray matter of the spinal cord.
- The UMN synapses (i.e., connects with) with the **lower motor neuron (LMN)** within the gray matter of the spinal cord.[5]
- The LMN travels out of the gray matter of the spinal cord in a peripheral nerve.
- These LMNs then end at the neuromuscular junctions of the fibers of a muscle, where the muscle fibers are directed to contract. (Note: For the details of the neuromuscular junction and how the LMN creates the contraction of the muscle fibers to which it is attached, see Section 12.8.)

INITIATION OF REFLEX MOVEMENT:

- Reflex movement is much simpler than voluntary movement (see Figure 19-4, *B*).[10]
- A sensory stimulus enters the spinal cord via a sensory neuron.
- The sensory neuron either synapses directly with an LMN within the spinal cord, or it synapses with a short interneuron that then synapses with an LMN within the spinal cord.
- This LMN is the same LMN involved in voluntary movement (mentioned previously).
- The LMN then travels out of the spinal cord to end at the neuromuscular junctions of the fibers of a muscle, where the muscle fibers are directed to contract.

- Because of the arclike shape of the sensory neuron into the spinal cord and the motor neuron out of the spinal cord, the pathway of a reflex is often called a **reflex arc**.
- Reflexes are "hardwired" in the body—in other words, they are innate (inborn) (Box 19-3).
- These reflexes are meant to be protective in nature. Before a child can know from experience which circumstances are safe and which are not, reflexes give automatic responses that are meant to protect the child from possible danger. For example, the startle reflex causes the child to turn toward the source of any loud noise. This brings attention to a potentially dangerous stimulus.
- Conscious awareness of a reflex is not part of the reflex arc itself.[11] However, we do know that we have performed a reflex after it has happened. This knowledge occurs because of connections between the reflex arc and the brain that travel upward within ascending white matter tracts of the spinal cord to the brain; connections within the brain then bring the information to the cerebral cortex. These connections give us conscious awareness of what reflex has just occurred. (Note: Again, these connections are technically not part of the reflex arc itself.)
- In addition, descending connections exist from the brain to the reflex arc via the UMNs. These connections have the ability to modify the action of the reflex. This modification may increase the response of a reflex or it may inhibit it. If the inhibition is strong enough, the reflex may be entirely overridden.
- Using the example of the loud noise that caused the startle reflex mentioned earlier, as we age, we may find that certain loud noises are not a threat. Therefore experience teaches us when it is safe to override the startle reflex with descending influence from the brain. As we get older, we depend more and more on this descending influence to determine our actions instead of pure reflexive behavior.

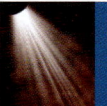

BOX 19-3 Spotlight on Learned Behavior and Neural Facilitation

Sometimes the term **learned reflex** is used. Technically, this term is incorrect because reflexes are not learned; all reflexes are innate. The correct term that should be used is **learned behavior** or **patterned behavior**. A learned/patterned behavior describes an activity that is learned and so well patterned that it is carried out in what appears to be a "reflexive" manner. However, this learned/patterned behavior does not involve a reflex arc. The patterning of a learned behavior initially involves association within the brain between a certain stimulus and a certain response. After many repetitions, the association becomes so well patterned that our response becomes automatic without the necessity of conscious thought. A classic example of learned behavior is Pavlov's dog salivating after hearing a bell because the dog learned to associate the sound of the bell with being fed. Many if not most of our daily activities are learned behavior patterns. We rarely think of the muscles that we need to contract to walk across the room, tie our shoes, speak, or drive a car along a route that we have taken many times before. In fact, it is likely that we may be driving our car while drinking a café latte and having a conversation at the same time, and we may realize halfway home that we have not even thought about which turns we have taken. If asked, we may not even know which road we are on; the body has been carrying out a series of learned behaviors as if it were operating on autopilot, with little or no conscious awareness!

The explanation that is given for how all associations are made, as well as why learned behaviors become so rooted in our nervous system, is the process of **neural facilitation**. Functionally, neural facilitation patterning that is made between a certain stimulus and a certain response becomes easier and easier to make as the association becomes reinforced through intensity or repetition.[20] Structurally, neural facilitation results from actual physical changes in the pathways of neurons that lower their threshold to form a certain pattern of connections (see figure). The result is a pattern of thinking and a pattern of behaving that becomes learned. The more this pattern is reinforced, the more entrenched this pattern becomes.

Some crucially important applications of the concept of learned behavior (i.e., neural facilitation) are found in the health field. Application can be made to the fields of manual and movement therapy and fitness training. Just as certain tasks and movement patterns are learned and patterned, the **resting tone** of our musculature can be learned and patterned. Normally, the resting tone of all our musculature should be relaxed. However, for many reasons the resting tone of a client's muscle may increase when certain stressful circumstances occur. If the relationship of this muscle tightening is not addressed, the pattern of this muscle tightening because of certain stimuli such as being stressed psychologically can become entrenched. As a result, each time in the future when the client becomes psychologically stressed, it will be a triggering stimulus that will more easily cause the muscle to tighten up. In time, the stimulus/tight muscle response can become a learned behavior that occurs without us having any realization of the link between the two. As therapists working on the musculoskeletal system, changing this pattern of muscle tightness involves more than just working on the muscle itself; it involves working with the nervous system to retrain its responses. In effect, we have to help the client's nervous system unlearn a certain pattern of response and relearn a new and healthier pattern of response.

An equally important application of neural facilitation to exercise exists. The pattern of co-ordering muscles (i.e., coordination) is also a learned/patterned behavior. When working with a client who exhibits poor technique when doing an exercise, this poor technique pattern is most likely entrenched via neural facilitation. To correct this faulty technique pattern, the client must create a new pattern that is healthy and proper to replace the old unhealthy pattern. In this regard, repetition is essential toward creating a new healthy neural facilitation pattern.

The concept of learned behavior/neural facilitation can also be applied to movement patterns and movement therapies. Often our movements are learned patterns that have become ingrained without conscious realization. As a result, poor movement patterns may be adopted that are inefficient, unhealthy, and functionally limiting. It is important to realize that these patterns exist within the nervous system, not within the musculoskeletal system. Therefore correction of these faulty patterns may be most efficiently accomplished by addressing the nervous system directly. **Feldenkrais technique** is a movement therapy that seeks to create client awareness of their movements including their faulty patterns of movement. Once aware, if the client desires to change his or her movement patterns, new patterns that are healthier and functionally freer may be learned.

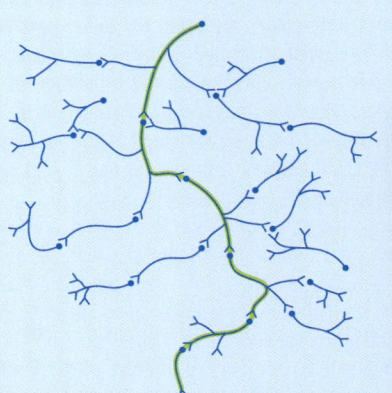
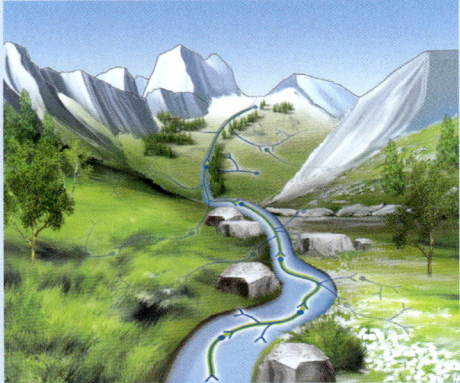

A pattern of neuronal synaptic connections being made via neural facilitation is analogous to water etching a deeper and deeper pathway into the side of a mountain over a period of time. *(Courtesy of Giovanni Rimasti)*

SECTION 19.3 RECIPROCAL INHIBITION

- **Reciprocal inhibition** is the name given to the neurologic reflex that causes the antagonist to a joint action to relax when the mover of that joint action is directed to contract.[9]
- Muscles that are on the opposite sides of a joint have opposite actions at that joint (i.e., their actions are antagonistic to each other).
- If one of these muscles contracts to move the joint, it is termed the *mover;* the muscle on the opposite side is then termed the *antagonist*. (Note: For more information on movers and antagonists, see Sections 15.1 and 15.2.)
- If the mover contracts and shortens, the antagonist on the opposite side of the joint must relax and lengthen to allow that joint action to occur; otherwise, the mover will not be able to efficiently move the joint.
- When the mover and antagonist both contract at the same time, it is called **co-contraction**.
- Co-contraction is by definition unwanted if a joint action is to occur, because the antagonist will fight the mover and lessen or stop the joint action from occurring.
- For this reason, whenever the nervous system desires a joint action to occur, it not only sends facilitatory impulses to the LMNs that control the mover(s) of that action but also sends inhibitory impulses to LMNs that control the antagonist(s) of that action.
- Note: Generally, all nerve impulses can be considered to be either facilitatory or inhibitory. Facilitatory impulses facilitate the muscle contraction's occurrence (i.e., they send a signal to the muscle asking it to contract); inhibitory impulses inhibit the muscle contraction's occurrence (i.e., they send a signal to relax the muscle so that it does not contract).
- These inhibitory impulses cause the antagonist muscles of that joint action to relax so that they cannot contract and fight the mover muscles.
- This neurologic reflex that sends inhibitory impulses to the antagonists is called *reciprocal inhibition*.
- Therefore, reciprocal inhibition helps to create joint actions that are strong and efficient (Box 19-4). Figure 19-5 demonstrates an example of reciprocal inhibition.

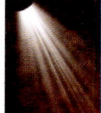

BOX 19-4 Spotlight on Reciprocal Inhibition

Reciprocal Inhibition and Muscle Palpation
The neurologic reflex of reciprocal inhibition can be very usefully applied to muscle palpation. When trying to palpate and locate a **target muscle** (i.e., the particular muscle that you want to palpate), it is helpful to make the target muscle contract so that it stands out and can be easily felt and discerned from adjacent muscles. To do this, we need to have the client perform a joint action of the target muscle that the adjacent muscles cannot perform. However, sometimes it is not possible to find a joint action that only the target muscle performs (i.e., the other muscles that are adjacent to it all perform the same action and will contract when the target muscle contracts). This makes it extremely hard to discern the target muscle. In these cases reciprocal inhibition can be used to stop the other, adjacent muscles from contracting so that only the target muscle contracts; this allows for easier identification and palpation of the target muscle.

For example, if we want to palpate the brachialis, we ask the client to flex the forearm at the elbow joint so that the brachialis contracts and is more palpable. However, flexion of the forearm at the elbow joint also causes the biceps brachii to contract. Because the biceps brachii is superficial to most of the brachialis, its contraction blocks our ability to palpate the majority of the brachialis. In this case we need the brachialis to contract but the biceps brachii to stay relaxed. This can be accomplished by using reciprocal inhibition. Ask the client to flex the forearm at the elbow joint while the forearm is fully pronated at the radioulnar (RU) joints. The biceps brachii is a supinator of the forearm; having the client pronate the forearm reciprocally inhibits all supinators, including the biceps brachii.

This allows us not only to better discern the brachialis lateral and medial to the biceps brachii where it is superficial but also to palpate the brachialis through the biceps brachii (see Figure 16-6, C).

One cautionary note to keep in mind when using reciprocal inhibition to aid muscle palpation: any reflex can be overridden, including reciprocal inhibition. If the client forcefully contracts, most or all movers of that joint action will be recruited to contract, including ones that are otherwise being reciprocally inhibited. Generally, when using the principle of reciprocal inhibition, do not allow the client to contract forcefully.

Reciprocal Inhibition and Stretching
Reciprocal inhibition can also be used to increase the effectiveness of a stretch. Stretches are often done in a passive manner. That is, the joint that is being stretched is moved passively in one direction, causing a stretch of the muscles on the other side of the joint (i.e., the antagonists). However, reciprocal inhibition can be used to increase the effectiveness of this stretch. Instead of having the client stretch passively, have the client actively contract the mover (i.e., agonist) muscles during the stretching maneuver. Actively contracting the movers will reflexively create a reciprocal inhibition to the antagonist muscles on the other side of the joint (which are the muscles that we are trying to stretch), causing them to relax, thus increasing the effectiveness of the stretch. This type of stretching is sometimes called **agonist contract (AC) stretching** and is the basis for Aaron Mattes's method of **active isolated stretching (AIS)**[21] (for more on the use of reciprocal inhibition and stretching, see Section 22.4). Note: Agonist contract stretching is also sometimes referred to as proprioceptive neuromuscular facilitation (PNF) stretching.

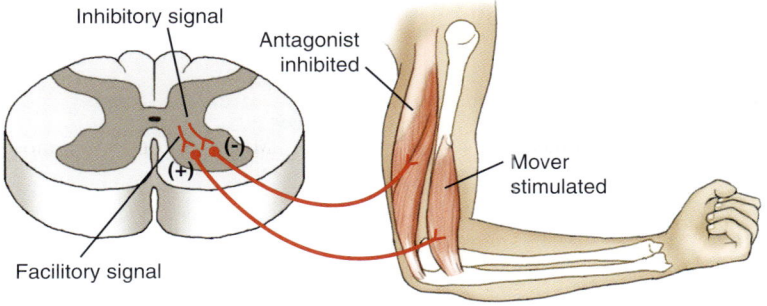

FIGURE 19-5 Neurologic reflex of reciprocal inhibition. When the lower motor neurons (LMNs) that control a mover muscle are facilitated to direct the mover to contract, the LMNs that control the antagonist muscle of that joint action are inhibited from sending an impulse to contract to the antagonist muscle. The result is that the antagonist muscles are inhibited from contracting and therefore relax. This relaxation allows the antagonist muscles to lengthen and stretch, thereby allowing the mover muscles to create their joint action without opposition.

SECTION 19.4 OVERVIEW OF PROPRIOCEPTION

- The word *proprioception* literally means the body's sense of itself.
- **Proprioception** is the ability of the nervous system to know the body's position in space and the body's movement through space.[4]
- When we are young, we are usually taught that five senses exist: (1) sight, (2) hearing, (3) taste, (4) smell, and (5) touch. Another sense is called *proprioception*. As important as proprioception is, most people take this vital sense for granted.
- The sense of proprioception gives us awareness of the body's position in space and the body's movement through space.
- A proprioceptor is a receptor cell that is sensitive to a stimulus. When this stimulus occurs, the proprioceptor is stimulated, causing an impulse to travel through the sensory neuron to which it is attached. This sensory neuron then carries that impulse into the CNS.[4]
  - Note: Each sensory receptor cell of the body is sensitive to a particular type of stimulus. For example, visual receptors (i.e., rods and cones) in the retina of the eye are sensitive to light; taste bud receptors on the tongue are sensitive to dissolved chemicals in the saliva. Most proprioceptor receptors are called **mechanoreceptors** because they are sensitive to mechanical pressure stimuli.
- Many types of proprioceptors are found in the human body (Box 19-5). Generally they can be divided into three major categories[10]:
  1. **Fascial/joint proprioceptor**
  2. **Muscle proprioceptors**
  3. **Inner ear proprioceptors**

- Fascial/joint proprioceptors are located in and around the capsules of joints and provide information about the joint's static position and its dynamic movement. This information is used to give us conscious awareness of the positions and movements of the parts of the body.
  - They are also located in all other types of deep fibrous fascia of the body.
  - The two major types of fascial/joint proprioceptors are **Pacini's corpuscles** and **Ruffini's endings**.[10]
- Muscle proprioceptors are located within the muscles of the body and not only provide proprioceptive awareness about the position and movement of the body but also function to create proprioceptive reflexes that protect muscles and tendons from injury.
  - Two major types of muscle proprioceptors exist: (1) **muscle spindles** and (2) **Golgi tendon organs**.[10]
- Inner ear proprioceptors provide information about the static position and dynamic movement of the head.[10]
  - Proprioceptive sensation from the inner ear (both static and dynamic) is often referred to as the sense of **equilibrium**.
  - The inner ear static proprioceptors for head position are located in the vestibule of the inner ear.[5]
  - The inner ear dynamic proprioceptors for movement are located in the semicircular canals of the inner ear.[5]

BOX 19-5 Spotlight on Other Proprioceptors

Although three major categories of receptors are considered to be proprioceptors, any receptor that aids in the awareness of the body's position and movement can be considered to be proprioceptive in nature, even if its primary function is to provide us with another sense. Examples of these receptors that also have a proprioceptive function are vision, pain, and touch.

The sense of sight, although crucially important toward allowing us to know the objects in our surroundings, is also important toward giving us our own body's orientation in space. If a person is suspected of driving under the influence of alcohol, the police will often administer a sobriety test in which the person is asked to touch a finger to the nose. The ability to do this requires the proprioceptive awareness of the positions of the finger and nose, as well as the proprioceptive awareness of the movement of the upper extremity as the finger is moved toward the nose. Because alcohol particularly impairs centers of proprioception in the brain, this is a valuable test to determine a person's sobriety. However, when this test is administered, the person is instructed to close the eyes because vision would otherwise help guide the finger to the nose, destroying the test's accuracy. Although not technically considered to be proprioceptive by some sources, vision certainly aids in our proprioceptive awareness.

The sense of pain can also aid our ability to sense the position and/or movement of the body. Using the sobriety test again as an example; try the sobriety test on yourself in two ways: (1) do it as described previously and (2) try it after squeezing your nose hard enough to be painful. The presence of pain impulses coming from the nose will help someone to locate the nose with a finger. Although the primary function of pain is to alert our nervous system to possible tissue damage in the body, it should come as no surprise that pain in a body part also increases our awareness of that body part.

Touch receptors may also be proprioceptive in nature. Although touch is usually considered important toward alerting us to the physical presence of objects that are close to the body, touch that is sensed in a body part, similar to pain, also increases the nervous system's awareness of that body part. Interestingly, two major mechanoreceptors of touch located fairly deeply in the skin are Pacini's corpuscles and Ruffini's endings. These are the same receptors that are located within joint capsules and considered to be joint proprioceptors (see Section 19.5). Other touch mechanoreceptors located more superficially in the skin are **Meissner's corpuscles**[3], **Merkel's discs**[3], **Krause's end bulbs**[22], and **free nerve endings**[3] (see figure).

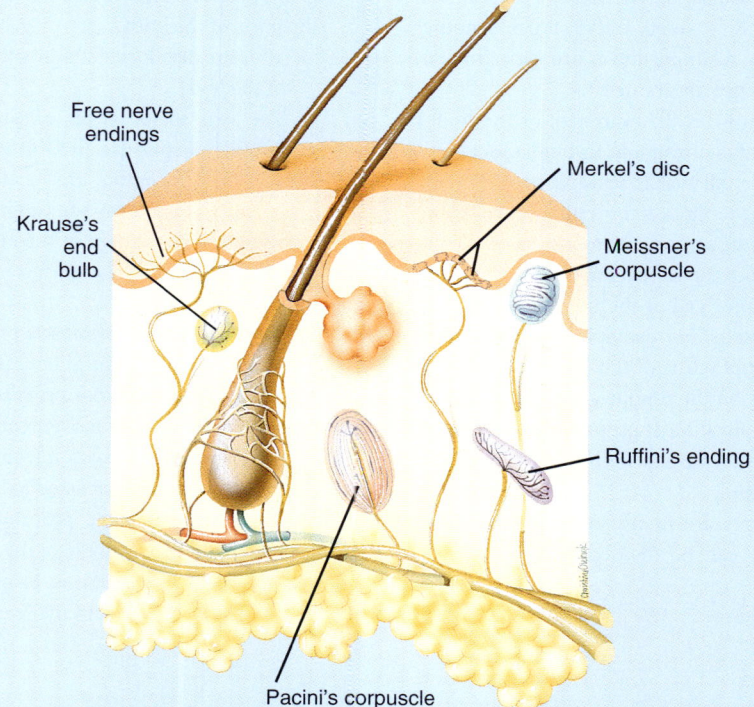

(Modified from Patton KT, Thibodeau GA: *Anatomy and physiology,* ed 7, St Louis, 2010, Mosby.)

SECTION 19.5 FASCIAL/JOINT PROPRIOCEPTORS

- Fascial/joint proprioceptors are located deeper in the body within dense fascia, both in and around joint capsules, as well as within deep muscular fascia. They are often referred to simply as *joint proprioceptors*.

JOINT PROPRIOCEPTORS:

- **Joint proprioceptors** are mechanoreceptors located in and around the capsules of joints.
- When the position of a joint changes, the soft tissues around the joint are compressed on one side of the joint and stretched on the other side of the joint.
- When this compression and stretching occurs, it creates a mechanical force on the joint proprioceptors that deforms them. Because they are mechanoreceptors, they are sensitive to this mechanical deformation, and this stimulus causes the joint proprioceptors to fire, sending their signal into the central nervous system (CNS) (Figure 19-6).
- Based on which side(s) of the joint has proprioceptors stimulated and in what pattern this stimulation occurs, the CNS is able to determine the position that the joint is in.
- For example, if the hip joint flexes (whether the thigh flexes toward the pelvis or the pelvis anteriorly tilts toward the thigh), the joint proprioceptors located on the anterior and posterior sides of the hip joint are deformed and stimulated, causing signals to be sent into the CNS. Knowing that it is the anterior and posterior proprioceptors that fired, and knowing the pattern of how this firing occurred, the CNS knows that the joint is flexed. If the joint action had been extension instead, the pattern of anterior and posterior receptors would have been different and the CNS would have interpreted the position as extension. Similarly, impulses from lateral and medial proprioceptors would signal abduction/adduction movements. Medial and lateral rotations would be indicated by the characteristic pattern of compression that they would create. This concept can be applied to any joint of the body.

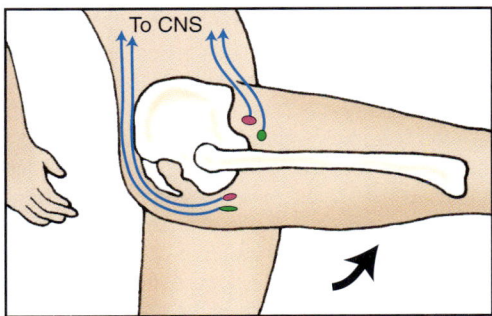

FIGURE 19-6 Flexion of the hip joint, which deforms the proprioceptors (i.e., Pacini's corpuscles, Ruffini's endings) located around the joint by compressing those located anteriorly and stretching those located posteriorly. Deformation of the proprioceptors stimulates them, which causes nerve impulses to travel to the central nervous system (CNS). The pattern of proprioceptive signals sent to the CNS is interpreted by the brain and informs us of the position and movement of the hip joint.

- Two types of joint proprioceptors exist[10]: (1) **Pacini's corpuscles** and (2) **Ruffini's endings** (see the figure in Box 19-5).
  - Pacini's corpuscles, often called Pacinian corpuscles, are named for Italian anatomist Filippo Pacini (1812-1883).
  - Ruffini's endings, often called Ruffini's corpuscles, are named for Italian anatomist Angelo Ruffini (1864-1929).
- Note: A third group of mechanoreceptors (i.e., proprioceptors) is found within joint capsules; they are known as **interstitial myofascial receptors**. Interstitial receptors are actually the most numerous receptors found within deep dense fascia. They are small receptors that are believed to be involved in pain reception and proprioception. Some are fast adapting and some are slow adapting.[12]
- Both Pacini's corpuscles and Ruffini's endings are sensitive to mechanical force as described previously. The difference between them lies in how quickly they adapt to the application of the mechanical force.
- Pacini's corpuscles adapt quickly to mechanical force. This means that as they are being deformed, they send impulses into the CNS, apprising it of the movement that is causing the deformation. However, as soon as the movement ceases, the corpuscles adapt to this new level of deformation and stop sending impulses into the CNS. As a result, Pacini's corpuscles are sensitive to and stimulated only by changes in position (i.e., movement).[10]
- Ruffini's endings are slow to adapt. This means that as they are being deformed, they send impulses into the CNS, apprising it of the movement that is causing the deformation. However, when the movement ceases and the change in deformation stops, Ruffini's endings continue to send impulses into the CNS. As a result, Ruffini's endings are sensitive to and stimulated by a change in position (i.e., movement) and the static position of the joint[10] (Box 19-6).

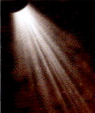 **BOX 19-6** Spotlight on Ruffini's Endings

Even Ruffini's endings have a limit to how long they will continue to be stimulated before adapting to the new position of the joint. If you have ever stayed very still in one position for an extended period of time (perhaps 15 to 20 minutes), you may have experienced a loss of Ruffini's ending proprioception from a joint; this results in an inability to feel the position of the body part(s) of that joint. If you cannot see the body part, it literally feels as if the body part is missing. The proprioceptive feel of the region can be immediately regained if you move the joint even a slight amount because this movement stimulates Pacini's corpuscles and Ruffini's endings in the joint once again.

(Note: This phenomenon is not the same as when a body part "falls asleep," which occurs when the blood supply to a body part such as the foot is lost, resulting in the nerves of the foot losing their blood supply. Having lost their blood supply, the nerves are no longer able to send any signals, including proprioceptive signals, into the central nervous system [CNS]. When this occurs, loss of sensation may also occur, but the return of sensation takes much longer and usually feels like "pins and needles" as the blood supply gradually returns and the nerves "reawaken.")

ESSENTIAL FACTS:

- Pacini's corpuscles give us proprioceptive information only about the movement of our joints.
- Ruffini's endings give us proprioceptive information about the movement of our joints and the static position of our joints.[10]

OTHER FASCIAL PROPRIOCEPTOR LOCATIONS:

- Aside from their location within joint capsules, all types of proprioceptors that are located within joint capsules are also located in all other types of deep fibrous fascia (i.e., ligaments, muscular fascia, tendons, aponeuroses, and intermuscular septa).
- Pressure applied to these fascial/joint proprioceptors has been found to have direct reflex effects, causing an increase in circulation of blood to the local area, a decrease in the tone of the muscles in the local area, and a decrease in sympathetic nervous system output. This pressure reflex has been found to occur during the application of manual and movement therapies, as well as exercise.

SECTION 19.6   MUSCLE SPINDLES

- A **muscle spindle** is a type of muscle proprioceptor that is located within a muscle and is sensitive to a stretch (i.e., lengthening of the muscle).[4]
- Muscle spindle cells are located within the belly of a muscle and lie parallel to the fibers of the muscle.
- The number of muscle spindles that a muscle contains varies from one muscle to another in the body. The muscles with the greatest proportion of muscle spindles are the muscles of the suboccipital group of the neck. Other muscles with a very high concentration of muscle spindles are the intertransversarii and the rotatores of the spine. Some sources state that because small deep muscles such as these contain such a high number of muscle spindles, their primary importance is to act as proprioceptive organs, not to contract and move or to contract and stabilize body parts.[13]
- Muscle spindle cells contain fibers that are known as **intrafusal fibers**. In contrast, regular muscle fibers are known as **extrafusal fibers**.[2]
- These intrafusal fibers of the muscle spindle are contractile like extrafusal fibers (i.e., they are able to contract and shorten).
- A muscle spindle is sensitive to the stretch (i.e., the lengthening) of the muscle within which it is located. More specifically, it is sensitive to two aspects of the stretch[2]:
  1. The amount of stretch of the muscle
  2. The rate (i.e., speed) of the stretch of the muscle
- When the muscle is stretched sufficiently, the muscle spindle is also stretched and becomes stimulated, creating an impulse in a sensory neuron that enters the spinal cord to alert the CNS that the muscle has just been stretched.
- Because a stretched muscle may be overly stretched and torn, this impulse in the spinal cord causes a reflex contraction of the muscle (Figure 19-7). By contracting and shortening, the muscle stops any excessive stretching that might tear the muscle (Box 19-7).
- This reflex is called the **muscle spindle reflex** or the **stretch reflex**.[11]
  - The muscle spindle reflex is also known as the **myotatic reflex**.
- Therefore a muscle spindle and its stretch reflex are protective in nature. They prevent a muscle from being overly stretched and torn (Box 19-8).
- Because muscles are less likely to be torn when they are relaxed and more likely to be torn when they are tight, muscle spindles

BOX 19-7

Because of the presence of the muscle spindle stretch reflex, stretches must be done slowly and in a fairly gentle manner; they cannot be forced. Heavy-handed and/or excessively fast stretches will by definition result in tightening of the muscles involved. Furthermore, although it was done for many years, it is now known that fast bouncing when you stretch is unhealthy. The reason for this is that fast bouncing quickly lengthens the muscle that is being stretched. Unfortunately, a quick lengthening of the muscle activates the muscle spindle reflex, which results in a contraction and tightening of the muscle. Although the purpose for the bouncing stretch is to relax and lengthen the muscle, this purpose is defeated if the muscle ends up being tighter.

Having said this, there is evidence that a gentle controlled bounce added to a stretch can be beneficial because it has been found to stimulate the fascial tissue that is stretched. Given that muscle spindle activity is controlled by the gamma motor system, the muscle spindle reflex threshold for engagement can be trained. The key is to slowly add in the bounce component to the stretch over a period of time, perhaps weeks, months, or longer.

BOX 19-8

Although muscle spindle stretch reflexes are protective in nature, they also serve another purpose (i.e., to increase the strength of a muscle contraction immediately after it has been quickly stretched). If you observe any sport that involves throwing, kicking, or swinging, you will notice that the athlete uses a backswing before the actual throw, kick, or swing. For example, before serving a tennis ball, the tennis player quickly brings the racquet back. The purpose of this fast backswing immediately before the forward swing to actually hit the ball is to trigger the stretch reflex so that the power of the forward swing will be augmented by the reflex contraction of the stretch reflex. **Plyometric training** uses this concept and involves exercises that rapidly stretch a muscle and then immediately follows the stretch with contraction of the same muscle.[23] (Note: The addition of the passive force of elastic recoil created by stretching the muscle during the backswing is a further benefit gained by preceding a stroke with a backswing. This phenomenon is called productive antagonism and is covered in Section 15.2.)

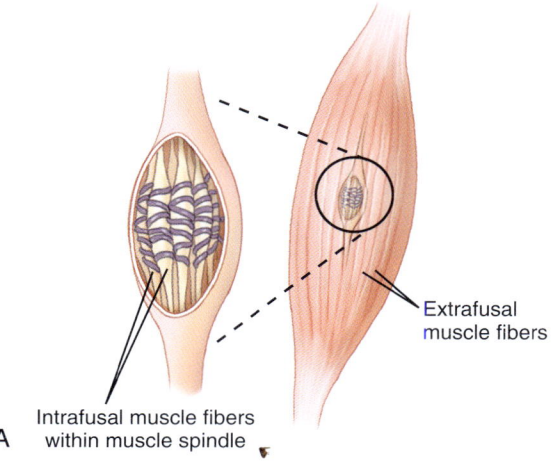
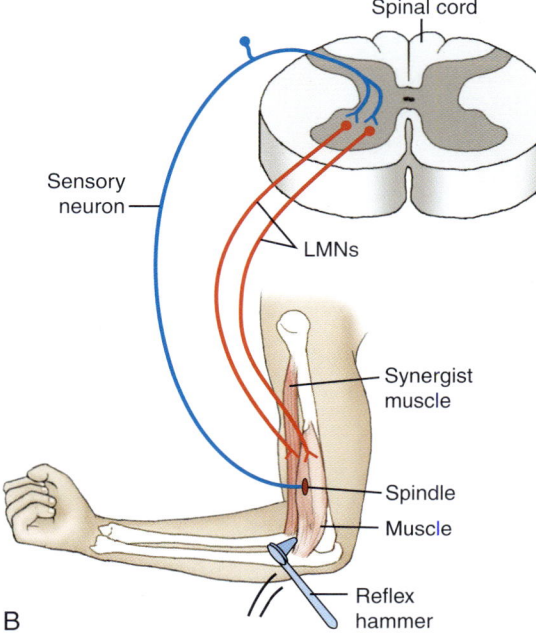

FIGURE 19-7 A, Illustration of how a muscle spindle is located within the belly of a muscle and runs parallel to the extrafusal muscle fibers of the muscle. **B,** Muscle spindle reflex. When the tendon of the muscle is tapped with the reflex hammer, the tendon elongates and creates a pulling force on the muscle belly. This in turn stretches the muscle spindles located within the belly, triggering a stretch reflex. The stretch reflex occurs when a sensory neuron from the muscle spindle carries a nerve impulse into the spinal cord, where it synapses with the lower motor neuron (LMN) that returns to the muscle and causes it to contract (as well as causing synergistic muscles that perform the same action to contract as shown). Any strong or fast stretch of a muscle may result in the stretch reflex, causing the muscle to contract.

need to be able to adapt to these different circumstances. Therefore it is important that the sensitivity of a muscle spindle to the stretch of the muscle be regulated.

- The sensitivity of a muscle spindle is set by the **gamma motor system**.[3]
  - The gamma motor system has upper motor neurons (UMNs) and lower motor neurons (LMNs). Gamma UMNs travel from the brain down to the spinal cord, where they synapse with gamma LMNs in the gray matter of the spinal cord. Gamma LMNs then travel from the spinal cord out to the muscle spindle.[3]
- Motor neurons that are directly concerned with controlling muscle contraction are called *alpha motor neurons*. This is done to differentiate them from the **gamma motor neurons** of the gamma motor system. Therefore alpha upper motor neurons (UMNs) and alpha lower motor neurons (LMNs), as well as gamma UMNs and gamma LMNs, exist. The alpha system directs muscle contraction by directing the regular extrafusal fibers of the muscle to contract. The gamma motor system directs muscle spindle contraction by contracting the intrafusal fibers of the muscle spindle to contract.
- The gamma LMN is responsible for directly setting the sensitivity of the muscle spindle (Figure 19-8). It does this by contracting and shortening the intrafusal fibers of the muscle spindle so that they are tauter. The shorter and tauter a muscle spindle is, the more sensitive it is to a stretch of the muscle.[3]
  - A muscle spindle has a spindle-like or fusiform shape. The two ends of the muscle spindle are contractile (i.e., they can contract and shorten when stimulated by the gamma LMN). The central section houses the sensitive receptor portion of the spindle and is noncontractile. The sensitivity of a muscle spindle to stretch is caused by the gamma LMN causing a contraction at both ends of the spindle cell. This in turn stretches the noncontractile central portion from both ends, making it tauter and more sensitive, and therefore it is more likely that a stretch of the muscle will cause the muscle spindle to trigger its stretch reflex.[14]
- However, the ultimate control of the gamma LMN rests with the UMNs of the gamma motor system. These gamma UMNs reside in the brain. The degree of sensitivity that these UMNs exert on the LMNs is based on subconscious processing of many factors within the brain. Some of these factors include previous and present physical traumas to the region of the body where the muscle is located, the need for stability in the region, and general emotional and physical stress levels (Box 19-9).
  - The regions of the brain that primarily influence and control gamma UMNs are brainstem nuclei, the hypothalamus and amygdala (limbic system structures), and the cerebellum.

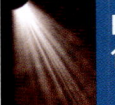

BOX 19-9 Spotlight on Muscle Spindles and Muscle Facilitation

For manual and movement therapists and trainers, a major concern (likely a major concern for other bodyworkers as well) is working on our clients' tight muscles. A muscle that is tight when it is being directed to contract and work to move the body is not a concern. We are concerned with the muscles of our clients that are tight when they should be relaxed (i.e., when they are at rest). In other words, our concern is when the resting tone of a muscle is too tight. At rest, muscles are rarely totally relaxed. Some degree of contraction is usually present to maintain the proper posture of the joints of the body. This resting tone of our muscles is set by the gamma motor system that resides in the brainstem and works without our conscious control. However, the resting tone of muscles often gets too tight. Whether this is a result of injury to the area, chronically bad posture, or any other reason, the gamma upper motor neurons (UMNs) of the brain order the gamma lower motor neurons (LMNs) to tighten the muscle spindles within the musculature. When the muscle spindles are tauter, they more readily trigger the stretch reflex, resulting in alpha LMNs that direct the muscle fibers of the muscle to tighten. Therefore it is actually the gamma motor system's control of the muscle spindle that sets the resting tone of a muscle (indirectly by setting the sensitivity of the muscle spindles to the stretch reflex). Whatever tone the gamma motor system sets for the spindles will shortly thereafter become the tone for the muscle itself. In this manner, the gamma motor system may create **muscle facilitation** or **muscle inhibition**. If the tone of the muscle's spindles (and therefore the tone of the muscle itself) is set high, the muscle is said to be facilitated. If the tone of the muscle's spindles (and therefore the tone of the muscle itself) is set low, the muscle is said to be inhibited.

When a muscle is facilitated, it is poised to be able to respond to any stimulus and contract more quickly than if it were not facilitated. The downside of muscle facilitation is that the muscle may tighten more easily; manual and movement therapists are very sensitive to this condition of their clients. However, the upside of muscle facilitation is that the muscle is more responsive to the surrounding environment and can react more quickly and efficiently. This is extremely important during sporting events and exercise in general; trainers are very sensitive to this aspect of their clients' muscle tone. On the other hand, when a muscle's spindles are lax and therefore not set as sensitive, the muscle is said to be inhibited. An inhibited muscle is most likely more relaxed (i.e., less tight); however, it is also less able to respond to stimuli and tighten quickly and efficiently when the need arises. The balance between facilitation and inhibition of a muscle is important. In a healthy individual the relative proportion of this balance should be flexible and able to shift between greater or lesser facilitation or greater or lesser inhibition as the circumstances change and the need arises.

Interestingly, it seems that there are certain patterns of resting tone dysfunction within the body. Sources have divided most muscles of the body into two groups: those that tend toward becoming facilitated/tight, and those that tend toward becoming inhibited/weak. While this division should not be taken as absolute, these patterns do seem generally to be true. Examples of muscles that tend toward being overly facilitated are neck extensors, pectoralis major and minor, subscapularis, lumbar erector spinae, hip flexors and adductors, hamstrings, and foot plantarflexors. Examples of muscles that tend toward being overly inhibited are longus colli and capitis (deep neck flexors), lower trapezius and rhomboids, infraspinatus and teres minor, thoracic erector spinae, rectus abdominis, gluteus maximus, vastus lateralis and medialis, and foot dorsiflexors. As a general rule, it seems that flexors and medial rotators needed to achieve fetal position tend to be overly facilitated, whereas extensors and lateral rotators tend to be overly inhibited! An application of the asymmetry of this facilitation/inhibition pattern is that it predisposes the human body to two well-known postural distortion patterns known as the **upper crossed syndrome** and the **lower crossed syndrome**[24] (see accompanying illustration). In the two crossed syndromes, the facilitated muscles shorten and tighten, often described as **locked short**. The inhibited muscles are lengthened out by the locked short muscles, and they often tighten as a result and are described as **locked long**. Hence both muscle groups end up being locked—in other words, tight.

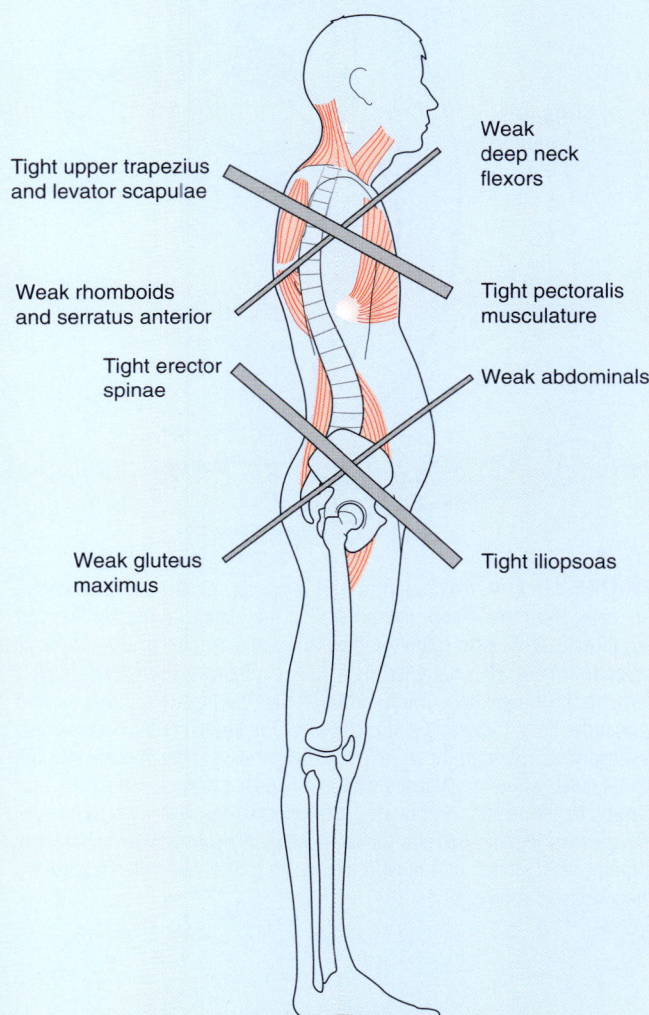

Modified from Chaitow L, DeLany JW: Clinical application of neuromuscular techniques, Vol 2: The lower body, Edinburgh, 2002, Churchill Livingstone.

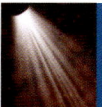

BOX 19-9 Spotlight on Muscle Spindles and Muscle Facilitation—*Cont'd*

For manual and movement therapists, it is important to make a distinction between the two general types of muscle tightness that may be encountered: (1) local small areas of hypertonicity (i.e., **trigger points**) and (2) **global tightening** of the entire muscle. Although trigger points are created locally and require specific local work to remedy, a muscle that is globally tight is not really a local problem. The true cause is the sensitivity setting of the spindles by the gamma motor system of the brain (i.e., the muscle is overly facilitated). Therefore even though we may address this problem locally by treatment to the muscle itself, we must be aware that the root cause lies within the central nervous system (CNS). Whatever attention can be given to encourage the gamma motor portion of the nervous system to relax its activity (i.e., its facilitation of the muscle) may ultimately prove to be the most valuable aspect of our treatment. While being careful to not overstep the boundaries of our professions, when looking at gamma motor system facilitation, we must consider many parameters of the client's health. These parameters include both physical and emotional/psychological factors. The subconsciously perceived fragility and vulnerability of the region of the body where the muscle is located are particularly important. Also of importance is the chronicity of neural facilitation patterning of how the client's body responds to stressors of all types—or put more simply, where he or she tends to "hold stress."

- Note: The term **muscle memory** is often used to describe the postural tone of the muscular system. It is common to ascribe muscle memory to the muscular system itself; however, as the foregoing discussion has explained, aside from trigger points, the contractile tone of a muscle is set by the gamma motor system's control of the muscle spindle reflex. Hence, muscle memory resides in the nervous system, not the muscular system.

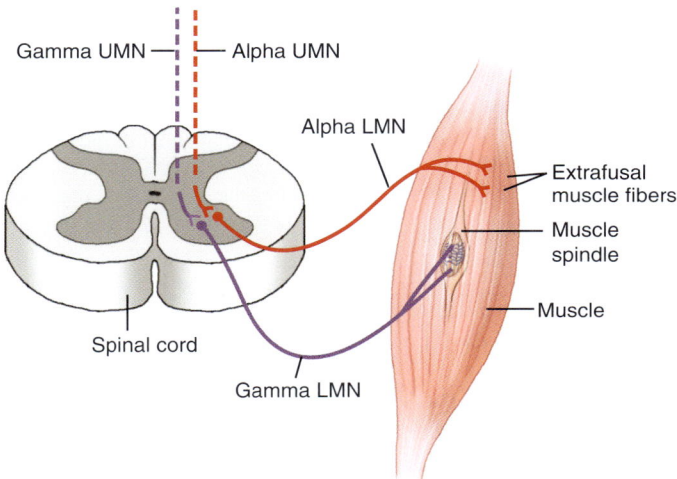

FIGURE 19-8 Innervation of a muscle spindle by the gamma motor system. A gamma lower motor neuron (LMN) travels from the spinal cord and synapses with the intrafusal fibers of a muscle spindle. The gamma LMN can contract the muscle spindle, making it tauter and therefore more sensitive to stretch. The more sensitive a muscle spindle is, the more likely it is to trigger a stretch reflex when it is stretched. (Note: The LMN that travels from the spinal cord and synapses with the regular extrafusal fibers of the muscle is called an alpha LMN to distinguish it from the gamma LMN. Just as alpha LMNs are controlled by alpha UMNs, gamma LMNs are controlled by gamma UMNs.)

SECTION 19.7 GOLGI TENDON ORGANS

- A **Golgi tendon organ** is a type of muscle proprioceptor that is located within a tendon of a muscle and is sensitive to a pulling force that is placed on the tendon.[10]
- Pulling forces on a tendon primarily occur when the tendon's muscle belly contracts; therefore Golgi tendon organs sense contraction of the muscle belly.
- Golgi tendon organs are located within the tendon of a muscle near the musculotendinous junction.[10]
- Golgi receptors are also located within joint capsules and ligaments; they are referred to as **Golgi end organs**.
- Golgi tendon organs are attached in series (end to end) to a number of muscle fibers. When these muscle fibers contract and

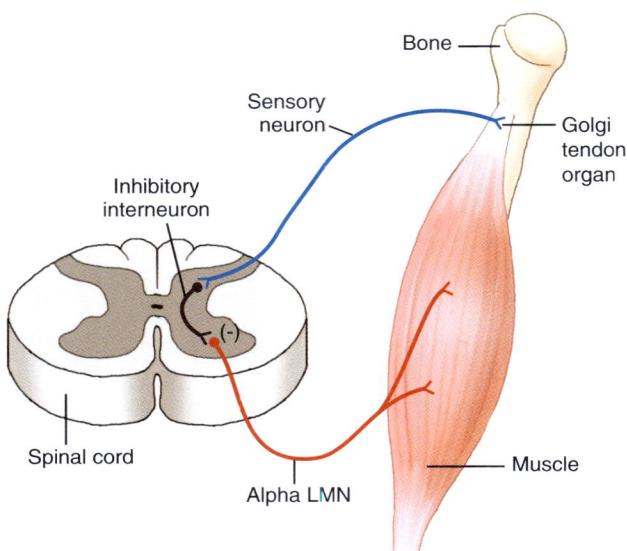

FIGURE 19-9 Illustration of the neural pathways of the Golgi tendon organ reflex. A Golgi tendon organ is located within a muscle's tendon and is sensitive to a stretch placed on the tendon. When a Golgi tendon organ is stimulated by a stretch on the tendon of the muscle in which it is located, it causes a relaxation of the muscle, thereby eliminating the excessive stretch from being placed on the tendon. This reflex is accomplished by the sensory neuron from the Golgi tendon organ synapsing with and stimulating an interneuron, which in turn inhibits the alpha lower motor neurons (LMNs) that control the muscle fibers. Inhibition of a muscle's alpha LMNs results in a relaxation of the muscle.

- ○ This reflex is called the **Golgi tendon organ reflex** or simply the **tendon reflex**.[11]
  - ○ Because the Golgi tendon organ reflex has the opposite effect of the *myotatic reflex* of the muscle spindle, it is also referred to as the **inverse myotatic reflex**.
- ○ The relaxation of the muscle is accomplished by the sensory neuron from the Golgi tendon organ synapsing with an interneuron that inhibits the alpha LMN to the muscle. If the alpha motor neuron to the muscle is inhibited from carrying an impulse, the muscle will be inhibited from contracting and will therefore relax.[14]
  - ○ Therefore a Golgi tendon organ and its tendon reflex are protective in nature. They prevent a tendon from being overly stretched and torn by a muscle that otherwise might contract too forcefully (Box 19-10).

 BOX 19-10

The Golgi tendon organ reflex is often used as a part of the physical therapy treatment called **electrical muscle stimulation** (EMS) (also referred to as E-stim). An EMS machine puts an electrical current into the client's muscle that is similar to the electrical current that would come from the alpha lower motor neuron (LMN); this causes the muscle to contract. The treatment is applied for 5 to 10 minutes, keeping the muscle in a sustained isometric contraction. In response to this contraction, the Golgi tendon organ reflex is triggered, resulting in relaxation of the muscle.

shorten, they create a pulling force on the Golgi tendon organ. A Golgi tendon organ is sensitive to the pulling force of the muscle fibers to which it is attached.[10]
- ○ When the muscle contracts and shortens sufficiently, the Golgi tendon organ is stretched, becomes stimulated, and creates an impulse in a sensory neuron that enters the spinal cord to alert the CNS that the muscle has just contracted and shortened, pulling on its tendon(s).
- ○ Because a pulling force on a tendon may stretch and tear it, this impulse in the spinal cord causes a reflex relaxation of the muscle (Figure 19-9). By relaxing the muscle, the muscle no longer creates a pulling force that might tear the tendon.[10]

ESSENTIAL FACTS:

- ○ Muscle spindles and Golgi tendon organs are similar in that they are both protective in nature.
- ○ They differ regarding which structure they each protect and the result of their reflexes.
  - ○ The muscle spindle reflex results in contraction of a muscle and acts to prevent a muscle from being overly stretched and torn.
  - ○ The Golgi tendon organ reflex results in relaxation of a muscle and acts to prevent the tendon from being overly stretched and torn (by an overly contracting muscle) (Box 19-11).

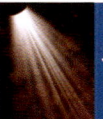

BOX 19-11 Spotlight on the Golgi Tendon Organ Reflex and Stretching

Using the Golgi tendon organ reflex can be a powerful tool to increase the effectiveness of a stretch with your client. When doing a stretch in this manner, have the client actively isometrically contract the muscle that you want to stretch against your resistance. After the isometric contraction, ask the client to relax the muscle; you can then stretch the muscle further than you would have been able to otherwise because of the reflex inhibition of the muscle by the Golgi tendon organ reflex.

This type of stretching is known as **CR stretching** or **PIR stretching**. CR stands for **contract relax stretching** because the client contracts and then relaxes; PIR stands for **post-isometric relaxation stretching** because the client isometrically contracts and then relaxes. It is also commonly referred to as **PNF stretching**; PNF stands for **proprioceptive neuromuscular facilitation** because a proprioceptive neuromuscular reflex (the Golgi tendon organ reflex) is used to facilitate the stretch.[25] Note: There is some controversy as to the role of the Golgi tendon organ reflex with CR stretching

Although the exact manner in which this type of stretching is carried out varies from therapist to therapist, it is customary to have the client hold the isometric contraction for approximately 5 to 8 seconds each time before the relaxation/stretch is performed; this can be repeated

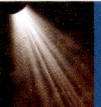

> **BOX 19-11** Spotlight on the Golgi Tendon Organ Reflex and Stretching—*Cont'd*

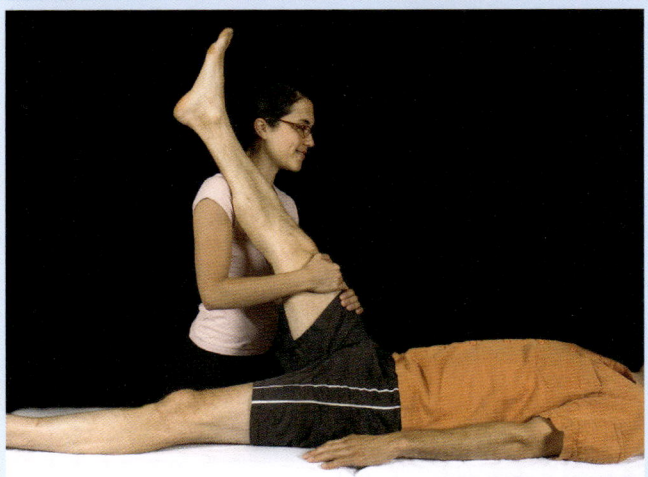

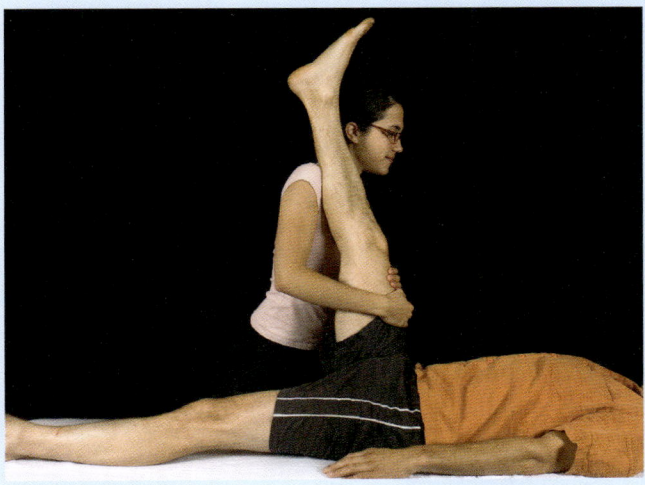

approximately three to four times, usually with a stronger isometric contraction each time. Although the hamstrings are usually the muscles used when demonstrating CR stretching (and are shown here in the accompanying figure), this type of stretching is extremely effective and can be used for any muscle of the body.

An interesting footnote to CR stretching is that when performed on one side of the body, it can help the same muscles on the other side of the body relax, even though the muscles on that side were not directly touched and stretched. To try this using the hamstrings as an example again, evaluate the maximum passive range of motion of the client's hamstring muscles bilaterally. Then do the CR stretch technique three to four times as described here on only one side of the body. After completing the stretch on one side, check the range of motion of the untouched side; its passive range of motion should have increased! The reason for this is that the effect of stretching one side of the body affects the sensitivity of the gamma motor system in the brain. Therefore the upper motor neurons (UMNs) of the gamma motor system relax the muscle spindles bilaterally for that muscle group (i.e., the hamstrings on both sides of the body will have the sensitivity of the muscle spindles relaxed, resulting in a greater passive range of motion on both sides).

Contract-relax (CR) stretching is demonstrated in these two photos. The first photo illustrates the first step of CR stretching, in which the therapist asks the client to take a deep breath and either let it out or hold it in while isometrically contracting the hamstrings against resistance for 5 to 8 seconds. The second photo illustrates the second step, in which the client relaxes and exhales while the therapist gently stretches the client's hamstrings. This two-step process should be repeated approximately three to four times. Each time, the client can gradually increase the force of the isometric contraction, and the therapist should be able to gently increase the range of motion of the stretch. *(Courtesy Joseph E. Muscolino.)*

SECTION 19.8   INNER EAR PROPRIOCEPTORS

- Inner ear proprioceptors provide information as to the static position and dynamic movement of the head.
- Inner ear proprioception is often referred to as the *sense of equilibrium*.
- Note: The term *equilibrium* is used to describe our ability to maintain our balance both during statically held positions and during dynamic movements. Although the inner ear is usually credited with giving us the sensory information to have this ability, all proprioceptors are involved in maintaining equilibrium.[5]
- Two types of proprioceptive organs are located in the inner ear (Figure 19-10):
  1. The **macula** (plural maculae), which provides static proprioception informing the brain of the static position of the head[5] (Figure 19-11)
  2. The **crista ampullaris**, which provides dynamic proprioception informing the brain of the movement of the head[5] (Figure 19-12)
- Note: The inner ear is often called the *labyrinth*. For this reason, the inner ear proprioceptors are often referred to as the **labyrinthine proprioceptors**.[10] Information from the labyrinthine proprioceptors of the inner ear, as well as the sense of hearing from the cochlea of the inner ear, travels in cranial nerve (CN) VIII, which is named the *vestibulocochlear nerve*.

STATIC PROPRIOCEPTION:

- Two maculae are located within the **vestibule** of the inner ear.[5]
- A macula consists primarily of a mass of gelatinous substance. Within the gelatinous substance are hair cells that are attached

FIGURE 19-10 Structure of the inner ear, which includes the three semicircular canals, the vestibule, and the cochlea. The vestibule houses the maculae, which detect static equilibrium. Each semicircular canal contains an ampulla (housing a crista ampullaris—not shown in this Figure; see Figure 19-12), which detects dynamic equilibrium. (Note: The cochlea is the part of the inner ear that is involved with the sense of hearing.)

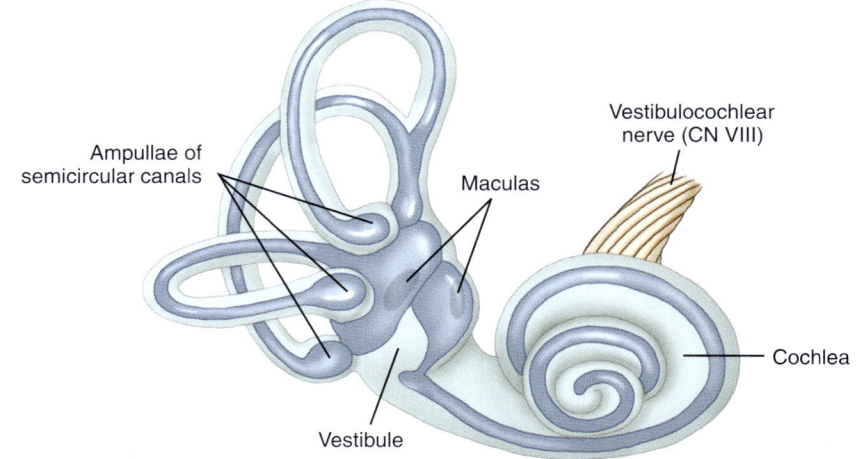

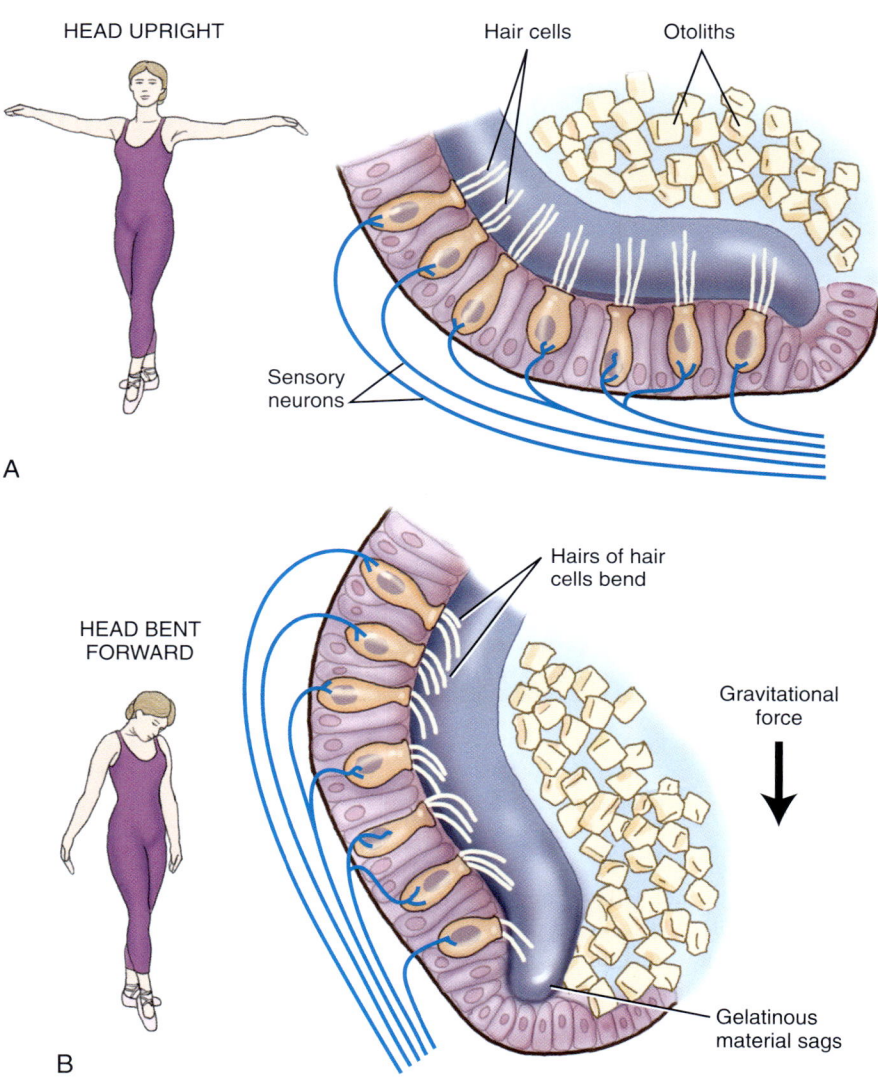

FIGURE 19-11 Maculae of the inner ear. A macula is composed of a gelatinous substance that has crystals called otoliths embedded within it. Also located within the gelatinous substance are hair cells attached to sensory neurons. **A,** Macula when the head is held up straight. **B,** When the head is bent forward, the gelatinous material sags because of the weight of the otoliths being pulled by gravity. This causes the hair cells to bend, triggering nerve impulses to travel to the brain, alerting the brain of the changed position of the head. In this manner, the macula detects static positions of the head.

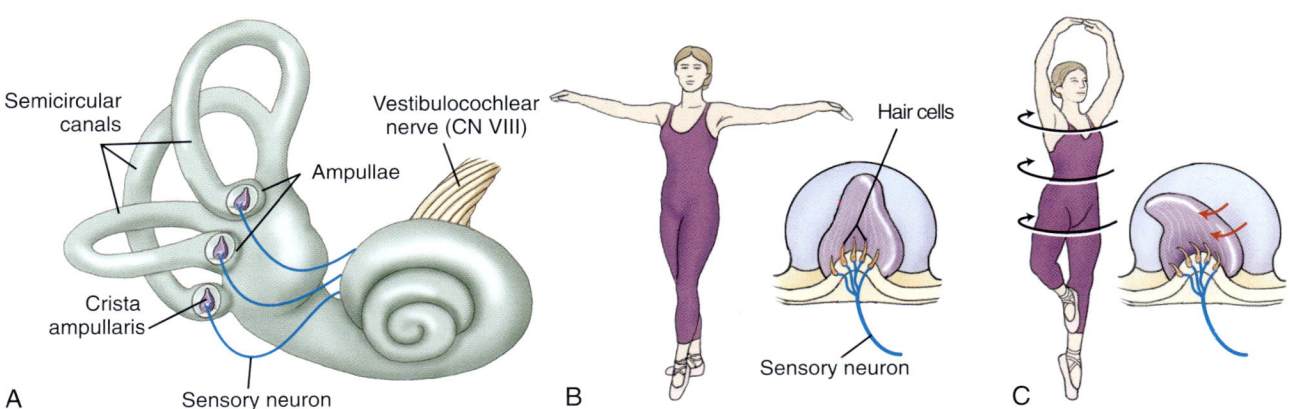

FIGURE 19-12 A, Crista ampullaris of the semicircular canals of the inner ear. Three semicircular canals exist, one in each of the three cardinal planes (sagittal, frontal, and transverse). **B,** A crista ampullaris is composed of hair cells and is located within the ampulla of a semicircular canal. **C,** When a person moves the head within a cardinal plane, the fluid within the canal that is oriented within that cardinal plane is set in motion, causing the hair cells of the crista ampullaris to be bent (in this figure, the ballerina spins within the transverse plane). This triggers the neurons attached to the hair cells to send this information to the brain, alerting the brain to the movement of the head.

○ to sensory neurons, and crystals called **otoliths**. The purpose of the otoliths is to increase the weight of the gelatinous substance, making it more responsive to changes in position (see Figure 19-11, *A*).
○ When the position of the head changes, such as when the head tilts (i.e., flexes) forward, the otoliths fall with gravity, dragging the gelatinous substance with them. The movement of the gelatinous substance causes the hairs to bend, resulting in impulses being sent through sensory neurons that travel to the brain (see Figure 19-11, *B*).
○ Based on which hair cells are bent and how they are bent (i.e., based on the pattern of nerve impulses received from the maculae), the brain can determine the position of the head relative to gravity.
○ It is important to emphasize that the maculae can only detect the static position of the head itself, not the position of the trunk or any other body part.

DYNAMIC PROPRIOCEPTION:

○ Three crista ampullaris structures are located within the **semicircular canals** of the inner ear (one is located in each of the three semicircular canals) (see Figure 19-12, *A*).[5]
○ One semicircular canal is located in each of the three cardinal planes; sagittal, frontal, and transverse.
○ A semicircular canal is a fluid-filled canal that is semicircular in shape. It has an expanded end that is called the **ampulla**, where the crista ampullaris is located.
○ A crista ampullaris is a structure that has hair cells attached to sensory neurons (see Figure 19-12, *B*).

○ When the head moves, depending on the direction of movement, fluid is set in motion within one or more of the semicircular canals (see Figure 19-12, *C*).
  ○ For example, if the motion of the head is forward or backward (i.e., within the sagittal plane), the fluid within the sagittally oriented semicircular canal is set in motion, and impulses from the sensory neurons from that semicircular canal are sent to the brain.
  ○ If the motion of the head is sideways (i.e., within the frontal plane), impulses are sent to the brain from the frontally oriented semicircular canal.
  ○ If the motion of the head is rotary (i.e., within the transverse plane), impulses are sent to the brain from the transversely oriented semicircular canal.
○ Any oblique plane movement of the head results in a pattern of impulses from two or three semicircular canals that the brain can decipher and interpret as that particular oblique direction of motion.
○ It is important to emphasize that the crista ampullaris structures of the semicircular canals can only detect motion of the head itself; they cannot detect motion of the trunk or any other body part.

ESSENTIAL FACTS:

○ The macula of the inner ear provides the brain with proprioception about the static position of the head.
○ The crista ampullaris of the inner ear provides the brain with proprioception about the dynamic movement of the head.

Righting Reflex:

○ Proper proprioceptive information from the inner ears and the eyes is crucially important for the sense of proprioception (i.e., for interpreting position and movement). This proprioceptive input is best interpreted when the head is level. (Note: To prove this, try maintaining a position of lateral flexion of the head and neck for an extended period of time. It will quickly be felt to be uncomfortable to sense proprioception in this position.) Hence a reflex called the righting reflex acts to keep the head level.[5] (Note: For more on the righting reflex, see Section 19.9.) Whenever the head becomes unlevel, the righting reflex directs the muscles of the body to alter the position of the joints to bring the head back to a level position. The righting reflex can be very important posturally. One example of this is the effect of the righting reflex caused by a collapsed arch in the foot. A collapsed arch in the foot creates one lower extremity that is shorter than the other; the result of this is that the body would lean toward the lower side, resulting in the head being unlevel. The righting reflex will create a compensation so that the head returns to being level. In this instance, the righting reflex will cause the spine to curve scoliotically so that the head is level (see Figure 20-5).

Equilibrium and Dizziness:

○ As we have seen, proprioceptive information regarding the position and movement of the body is provided by many sources. Whenever a disagreement exists between what the various proprioceptors of the body report regarding the position and/or movement of the head (perhaps as a result of injury or malfunction of certain proprioceptors), the brain experiences proprioceptive confusion. We feel and describe proprioceptive confusion as dizziness[5] (Box 19-12).

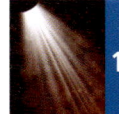

BOX 19-12 Spotlight on the Inner Ear and Neck Proprioceptors

The inner ear proprioceptors are located within the head. Consequently, they can report to the brain the position and movement of only the head. They cannot know the position or movement of the trunk (or of any other body part). However, it is imperative for the brain to know what the position and movement of the trunk are as well, because the trunk is the heaviest body part, and maintaining proper static and dynamic posture of the trunk is important so that we do not fall. How then does the brain know about trunk posture? The critical link to know trunk posture is provided by the joint and muscular proprioceptors of the neck. These proprioceptors report the posture of the neck (i.e., whether it is straight or bent). If the brain knows the position of the head from the inner ear receptors, and it then knows whether the neck is straight or bent (and if it is bent, in what position it is bent), then the brain can determine the position of the trunk.

For example, if the inner ear proprioceptors report that the head is inclined forward, the brain needs to know whether or not the trunk is also inclined forward. If the neck proprioceptors report that the neck is straight, then the brain knows that the trunk must also be inclined forward; therefore the brain would have to order back extensor muscles to contract to keep the trunk from falling into flexion. However, if the neck proprioceptors instead report that the neck is flexed, then the brain can determine that the trunk is vertical and no postural muscles would have to be activated to keep the trunk from falling.

This role of the neck proprioceptors is critically important and has an important clinical application to manual and movement therapy. If the neck has been injured (e.g., as the result of a whiplash accident or an asymmetric muscle spasm in the neck), incorrect proprioceptive signals may be sent from the neck proprioceptors to the brain. Because these incorrect proprioceptive signals will contradict other proprioceptive signals (e.g., signals from the eyes), proprioceptive confusion will most likely result. Because proprioceptive confusion is experienced as dizziness, the client may become dizzy. In other words, not all dizziness comes from inner ear infections as is often believed. When dizziness does result from a neck that is unhealthy musculoskeletally, manual and movement therapists are empowered to work on the necks of these clients and may possibly relieve them of the dizziness that they are experiencing!

SECTION 19.9   OTHER MUSCULOSKELETAL REFLEXES

Other than reciprocal inhibition, muscle spindle, and Golgi tendon organ reflexes, a number of other musculoskeletal reflexes occur in the human body. Following are some such reflexes that are applicable to movement, in other words, to the study of kinesiology.

FLEXOR WITHDRAWAL REFLEX:

○ The flexor withdrawal reflex involves a flexion withdrawal movement of a body part when that body part experiences pain.[3] Like most reflexes, the flexor withdrawal reflex is mediated by the spinal cord. Any conscious knowledge that we have flexed and withdrawn a body part in response to pain occurs after the reflex has occurred (by information that goes up through ascending white matter tracts of the spinal cord to the brain). Figure 19-13 illustrates the flexor withdrawal reflex.

○ The flexor withdrawal reflex is a protective reflex meant to prevent injury to the body by removing the body part from possible injury.

○ Note that reciprocal inhibition is a necessary component of the flexor reflex. As the flexor muscles are ordered to contract, the extensor muscles on the same side of the body are inhibited from contracting (i.e., ordered to relax), otherwise flexion away from the pain-causing object would not be efficiently possible. (Note: The reciprocal inhibition component of the flexor withdrawal reflex has not been shown in Figure 19-13.)

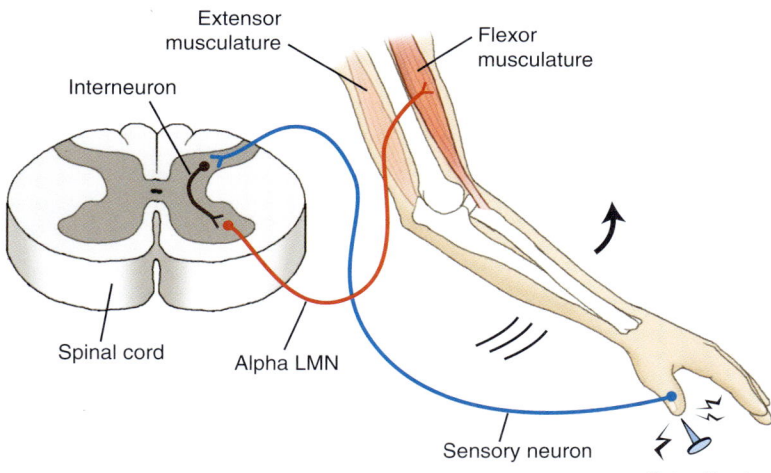

FIGURE 19-13 Illustration of the flexor withdrawal reflex, which is reflex mediated by the spinal cord. When a painful stimulus has occurred, it travels via a sensory neuron into the spinal cord, where it synapses with an interneuron, which then synapses with an alpha lower motor neuron (LMN). The alpha LMN then directs the flexor musculature in that region of the body to contract so that the body part is flexed and withdrawn from the cause of the painful stimulus.

CROSSED EXTENSOR REFLEX:

- The **crossed extensor reflex** is a reflex that works in conjunction with the flexor withdrawal reflex.[3] As the body part that experiences pain flexes and withdraws, the extensor muscles of the contralateral (i.e., opposite side) extremity contract to move that extremity into extension. Figure 19-14 illustrates the crossed extensor reflex.
  - The crossed extensor reflex is so named because this reflex crosses to the other side of the spinal cord to create a contraction in the contralateral extensor muscles.
  - The purpose of the crossed extensor reflex is to create a balanced posture of the body when one side flexes and withdraws. For example, if one lower extremity flexes and withdraws, the contralateral lower extremity must go into extension to support the body from falling; if one upper extremity flexes and withdraws, then extension of the contralateral upper extremity helps to create a more balanced posture.
  - Note that reciprocal inhibition is a part of the crossed extensor reflex. As the extensor muscles are ordered to contract, the flexor muscles on that side of the body are inhibited from contracting (i.e., ordered to relax); otherwise, extension of the contralateral extremity would not be efficiently possible. (Note: The reciprocal inhibition component of the crossed extensor reflex is not shown in Figure 19-14.)

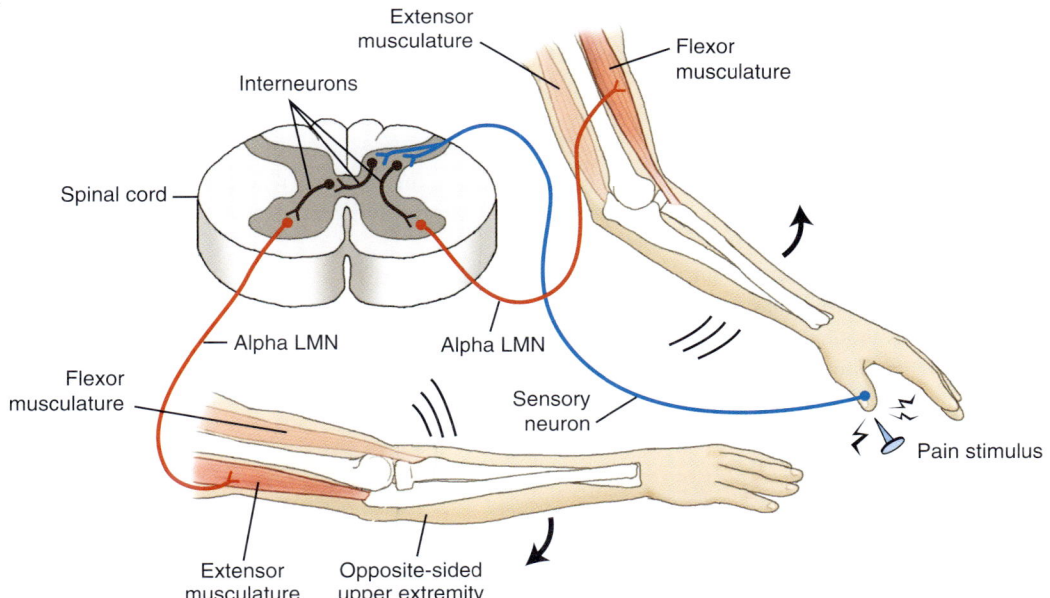

FIGURE 19-14 Illustration of the crossed extensor reflex and the flexor withdrawal reflex. When the flexor withdrawal reflex causes flexion and withdrawal of the extremity on the same side as the painful stimulus, the information that enters the spinal cord also crosses over to the other side of the cord and synapses with alpha lower motor neurons (LMNs), which direct the extensor musculature of the opposite-sided extremity to contract. This additional reflex component that crosses to the other side of the cord and directs extensor contraction is called the crossed extensor reflex.

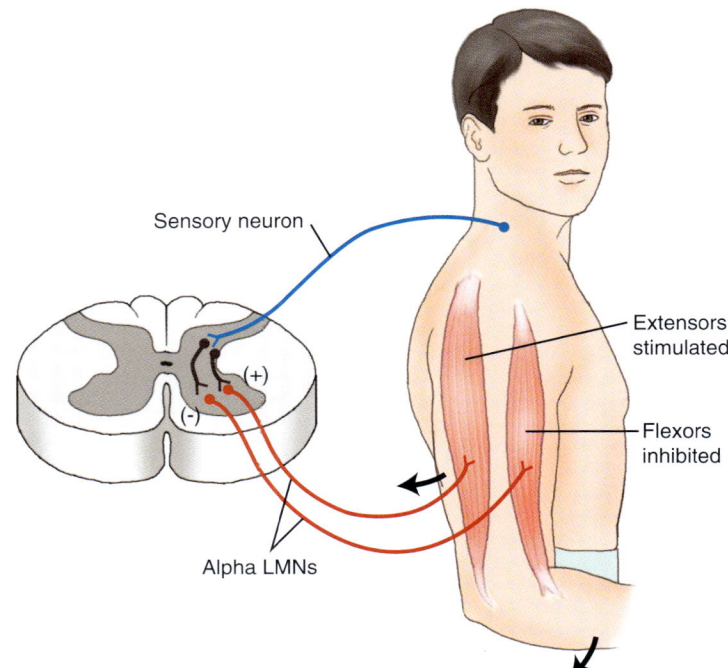

FIGURE 19-15 Illustration of the tonic neck reflex, which orders contraction of extremity muscles when the neck moves. In this illustration, when the neck rotates to the right, the extensors of the right upper extremity are reflexively ordered to contract (and via reciprocal inhibition, the flexors are inhibited and therefore relax). The flexors of the left upper extremity would also be ordered to contract (and via reciprocal inhibition, the extensors of the left upper extremity would be inhibited and relax). (Note: The left upper extremity component of the tonic neck reflex is not shown in this figure.)

TONIC NECK REFLEX:

- The **tonic neck reflex** orders contraction of the muscles of the arms based on the change in position of the neck.[10] For example, if the neck rotates to the right, extensor muscles of the right arm are ordered to contract and flexor muscles of the left arm are ordered to contract (of course, reciprocal inhibition inhibits the flexors on the right and the extensors on the left). Figure 19-15 demonstrates the tonic neck reflex.
  - The purpose of the tonic neck reflex is to help orient the body in the direction to which the head is oriented (i.e., where we are facing and looking).

CERVICO-OCULAR REFLEX:

- The **cervico-ocular reflex** is meant to coordinate eye movement with cervical spinal movement.[15] For example, if we look to the right with our eyes, the central nervous system will interpret this to mean that we will be orienting our head and neck to the right, so it will facilitate this motion, both by facilitating right rotator musculature and inhibiting left rotation musculature (Box 19-13).

RIGHTING REFLEX:

- The **righting reflex** is meant to keep us upright in a balanced position. If the inner ear perceives that our posture is such that we might fall, then that information is sent into the brain, which then sends signals down through the spinal cord to many levels, ordering muscle contractions to try to keep us upright.[16] One example of the righting reflex is when a person attempts to do a back dive into a pool. As soon as the head inclines backward, reflex contraction of the flexor musculature of the trunk and arms occurs to try to bring the person back into an upright posture (Figure 19-16; Box 19-14). Allowing this reflex to occur would result in a failed back dive and most likely a painful entry into the water. Having to override this reflex is one reason why a back dive seems so difficult for a beginner.
  - The righting reflex is also known as the **labyrinthine righting reflex**.

CUTANEOUS REFLEX:

- The **cutaneous reflex** causes relaxation in musculature after either soft tissue manipulation and/or an application of heat (Figure 19-17).

BOX 19-13

The cervico-ocular reflex can be used to advantage by manual and movement therapists and trainers for their clients with restricted cervical spinal motion. First ask the client to look with the eyes a number of times, perhaps three to five repetitions, toward the side whose motion is restricted. Then have the client actively, or the therapist could passively, move the neck to that side. On re-assessment, the restricted range of motion will likely be found to be increased.

BOX 19-14

Many people often experience a sudden and strong muscular twitch when falling asleep. This is called a **hypnic jerk**. Although the cause is not known for sure, it is believed that when we start to fall asleep, our muscles relax, causing a small but sudden change in joint position. This is sensed by our proprioceptors and sent to our central nervous system, where it is interpreted as if we have lost our balance and are falling. In response, the central nervous system orders muscular contraction to stop the perceived fall.

CHAPTER 19 The Neuromuscular System

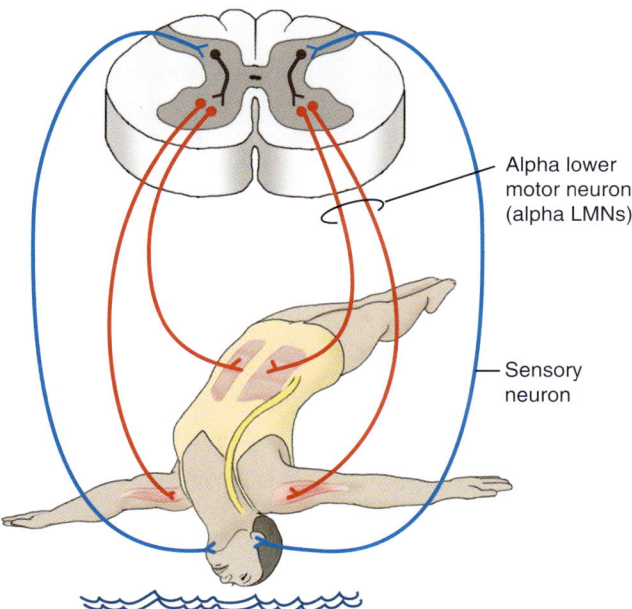

FIGURE 19-16 Illustration of the righting reflex. In this illustration, when a person attempts a back dive into a swimming pool, the head is no longer vertical. As a result, the righting reflex orders flexor musculature of the trunk and upper extremities to contract in an attempt to "right" the orientation of the head, bringing it back to a vertical orientation. A successful back dive requires the righting reflex to be overridden.

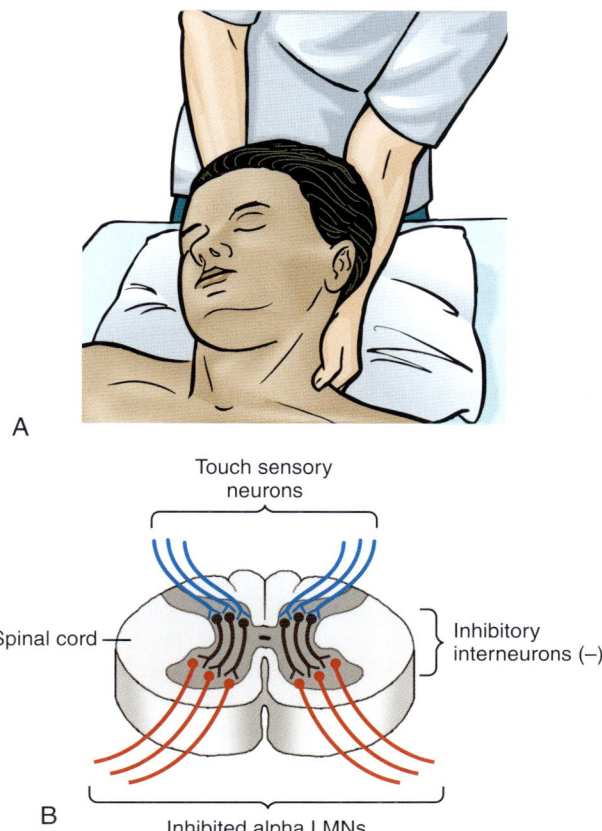

FIGURE 19-17 Illustration of the cutaneous reflex, which results in relaxation of musculature in response to touch and/or heat applied to the skin. Stimulation from touch travels into the spinal cord within sensory neurons. Within the cord, these sensory neurons synapse with inhibitory interneurons that inhibit alpha lower motor neurons (LMNs) from carrying nerve impulses. When alpha LMNs are inhibited, the musculature controlled by them relaxes. *(A, From Fritz S: Mosby's fundamentals of therapeutic massage, ed 4, St Louis, 2009, Mosby.)*

SECTION 19.10 PAIN-SPASM-PAIN CYCLE

○ The **pain-spasm-pain cycle** describes the vicious cycle of pain causing muscular spasm, which causes further pain, which causes further spasming, and so forth.

PAIN CAUSES SPASM:

○ From an evolutionary standpoint, pain in the body was often caused by physical trauma such as a broken bone and/or a bleeding wound. If movement of a physically damaged body part such as this were to occur, the broken bone and bleeding wound would never have the opportunity to heal. For this reason, **muscle splinting** often occurs in the region of the injury. Muscle splinting is caused by the nervous system directing the musculature of the region to contract (i.e., spasm). In effect, by spasming the surrounding muscles, the area is splinted and cannot move, affording the injury a chance to heal[17] (Box 19-15).

 BOX 19-15

Body armoring is a term used to describe when a person armors the body by splinting/spasming muscles in a region of the body for emotional or psychologic reasons. An example often given is if a person has a "broken heart," he or she may tighten the muscles of the pectoral region to "armor" the heart. Whether the root cause of muscle splinting/spasming is physical or emotional/psychological, once long-standing isometric tightening of musculature occurs, it is likely to lead into the pain-spasm-pain cycle.

SPASM DOES NOT GO AWAY:

○ The presence of muscular spasm (caused by the pain) affords the damaged body part a chance to heal. However, with the physical lifestyle that people generally had before modern civilized society, some physicality of the body was required to survive. Perhaps water had to be gotten from the stream or well, or food had to be gathered from the woods or picked from the garden. There was no indoor plumbing, and it was not possible to call in sick to work or have meals delivered. As much as it seemed that the body was telling us to not use the body part, it simply was not possible to stop all physical activity. As a result of gradually having to use the body in a physical manner, the muscle spasms that were initially created to splint the injured body part and give it chance to heal were gradually worked free, and the area was gradually coaxed into loosening up. However, in our modern nonphysical lifestyle, physicality is often not required of us and, as a result, these muscle spasms, once begun, tend to continue.

CONTINUED SPASM CAUSES FURTHER PAIN:

- As muscle spasming continues, pain increases because of two factors:
  1. The spasmed muscle itself. Because of the strong pull of its own contraction, the spasmed muscle causes pain by pulling on its attachments. In addition, most any movement that asks the spasmed muscle to stretch creates further pain because it is spasmed and resistant to stretch.
  2. Compromised blood flow. Continued muscle spasm closes off venous return of blood back to the heart. As venous return is blocked, waste products of metabolism build up in the body tissues distal to the site of the spasming. These waste products of metabolism contain acidic substances that irritate the nerves of the region, causing pain. If the spasming is sufficiently strong, even arterial supply can be closed off, resulting in **ischemia**, depriving body cells of needed nutrients, and further irritating nerves. All of this further irritation of nerves creates further pain. Thus the pain-spasm-pain cycle is complete and will continue to viciously cycle and worsen[13] (Box 19-16).

- With the pain-spasm-pain cycle, pain and spasming are root causes that perpetuate each other.
- The role of the manual or movement therapist or trainer/instructor in this scenario is to try to break this cycle. Addressing either of these factors (i.e., the pain or the spasm) directly or indirectly can help to achieve this. By working on these factors, manual and movement therapists and trainers can be a powerful part of the healing process for the client experiencing the pain-spasm-pain cycle.
  - The trainer has the tools to guide the client through exercises that will gradually stretch and loosen the musculature and also facilitate venous return of blood. Furthermore, exercise has been shown to increase the release of **endorphins**, which help to block pain.[18]
  - The term *endorphin* comes from **endogenous morphine**, which literally means morphine produced within the body (*endogenous* means *formed within*). Morphine is a powerful pain-killing substance that is produced from plants and therefore comes from outside the body; therefore it is exogenous (*exogenous* literally means *formed outside*). When scientists saw that the human body already had receptors to this *exogenous* morphine from plants, they reasoned that there must be an internal chemical of the body for which these receptors were present. Based on this, they went searching for a substance produced within the body that would bind to these receptors and alleviate pain as morphine does. When they found this substance, they named it *endogenous morphine* or *endorphin* for short.
- The manual or movement therapist may work directly on the spasmed muscles by using soft tissue techniques such as soft tissue manipulation and stretching to relax the musculature. Manual and movement therapists can also do soft tissue manipulation and joint range of motion techniques that are focused directly on increasing venous circulation.

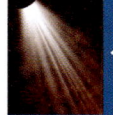

BOX 19-16 Spotlight on Isometric Muscle Spasm and Venous Circulation

The heart creates sufficient blood pressure to push the blood through the arteries to the level of the capillaries. For blood to return to the heart within the venous system, veins with unidirectional valves and thin walls depend on skeletal muscular contractions to collapse the walls of the veins and push the blood back in the direction of the heart. Each muscle contraction collapses and pushes blood located in the vein; each subsequent relaxation of the muscle then allows the vein to fill up again with intercellular tissue fluid containing waste products of metabolism. The next contraction then recollapses the vein and pushes this blood toward the heart. Thus the venous system relies on alternating contractions and relaxations of the adjacent skeletal musculature. However, long-standing (i.e., isometric) muscle spasming causes a collapse and blockage of the veins that compromises or entirely stops local venous circulation for the duration of the muscle spasm. As a result, waste products of metabolism are allowed to build up. Many of these waste products are acidic and irritate the local tissues, resulting in further pain thereby perpetuating the pain-spasm pain cycle.

SECTION 19.11 GATE THEORY

- The **gate theory** proposes that a "gating mechanism" is present in the nervous system that blocks the perception of pain when faster signals of movement or pressure occur at the same time.[13]
  - Note: Neurons do not all carry their impulses at the same speed. Larger and/or myelinated neurons conduct their impulses faster than smaller and/or nonmyelinated neurons. The sense of pain is carried in slow neurons; the senses of movement and pressure are carried in fast neurons.
- It is believed that this gating mechanism exists in the spinal cord.[13]
- The name of this mechanism and how it works can be explained by making an analogy to a horse race in which a gate at the end of the race only allows the winner (i.e., the fastest horse) to enter. Once the fastest horse enters, the gate closes and blocks the entrance of the other, slower horses.
- Relating this analogy to our nervous system, a similar gating mechanism is believed to exist in the spinal cord. When a number of sensory signals from the periphery enter the spinal cord at the same time, this gate allows the passage of impulses from the neurons that conduct their impulses the fastest, and it blocks transmission of the impulses of the slower neurons. Because pain is carried in slower neurons, the transmission of pain signals can be blocked by movement and/or pressure impulses carried in faster neurons. In effect, the sensation of pressure and/or movement can close the gate and block transmission of pain signals[19] (Figure 19-18; Box 19-17). Everyday examples that illustrate the gate theory are abundant. Two examples follow (Box 19-18).

BOX 19-17

From an evolutionary point of view, the effects described by the gate theory can be seen to be very valuable and protective in nature. Hundreds/thousands of years ago, physical encounters often involved fighting or taking flight from a dangerous, potentially life-threatening situation (e.g., battle with a wild animal or another person). During the actual battle, it was imperative that we could efficiently fight or take flight (a sympathetic nervous system–mediated response), or we would die; being distracted by pain caused by our wounds would have only hampered our ability to fight or take flight in that circumstance. After the activity was completed and we were no longer in a potentially dangerous circumstance, then we could safely experience our pain and "lick our wounds." In present times we are less often placed in actual life-threatening physical situations where the effects described by the gate theory are necessary to save our lives. However, the effects described by the gate theory still occur within the body and help protect us in any situation in which a danger is perceived by our more primitive nervous system.

- Example 1: If a person burns or cuts the finger and pain is felt, it is common to see the person shake the injured hand or squeeze the hand near the wound. While either of these activities is being done, the pain is blocked because the shaking causes movement signals to enter the spinal cord and/or the squeezing causes pressure signals to enter the spinal cord at the same time as the pain. Because movement and pressure signals both travel faster than pain signals, either one would help to block the sensation of the pain via the gate theory.
- Example 2: When a person exercises more than usual while working out or playing a sport, very often no pain is felt during the actual exercise. To some degree, this is because of the gate theory. During exercise, the constant input of movement and pressure sensory signals helps to block the pain signals at the gate. It is only later that evening or perhaps the next morning that the person realizes that he or she overdid it and was hurt.

BOX 19-18

Another interesting clinical application of the gate theory to bodywork and training is the use of pain relief topical balms containing such substances as menthol, oil of wintergreen, and eucalyptus. Almost all of these balms work on the principle of the gate theory; they irritate the skin and distract the body from the pain. The term **counterirritant theory** is often used to describe the mechanism by which these balms function to relieve pain. Because their true function is to indirectly relieve pain by the counterirritant theory, in effect, they all have the same intrinsic value (apart from the strength of the formula and therefore the intensity of the irritation that they cause). Therefore using the one that the client finds the most pleasing is recommended!

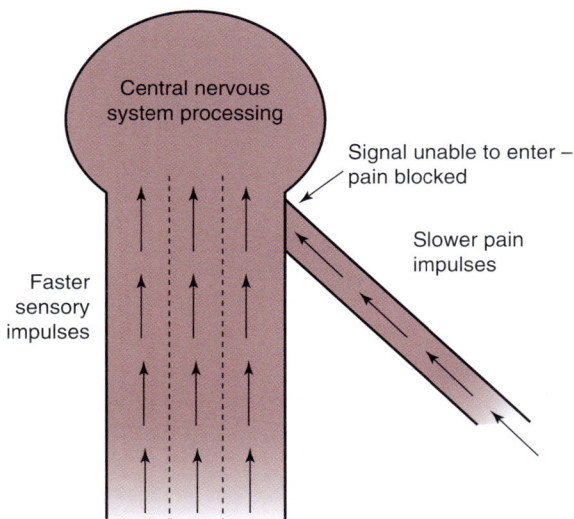

FIGURE 19-18 Illustration of the concept of the gate theory using an analogy to roads. Because of the presence of traffic in the faster lanes of the expressway, traffic from the smaller local road is blocked from entering the expressway and reaching its destination. In this analogy, the expressway carries the faster sensations of pressure and/or movement, and the local road carries the slower sensation of pain. Thus via the gate theory, the sensation of pain in the CNS can be blocked from reaching the brain because of the simultaneous presence of pressure and/or movement. *(Modified from Fritz S: Mosby's essential sciences for therapeutic massage: anatomy, physiology, biomechanics, and pathology, ed 3, St Louis, 2009, Mosby.)*

- Understanding the gate theory leads us to two very important clinical applications:
  1. Clinical application 1: It is an age-old maxim in the world of alternative health that we should be in touch with the body and listen to what it tells us. However, understanding the gate theory, we realize that we are not always able to perceive all that is happening in the body. When we are very physically active, we may be causing physical damage yet not know it because our pain signals are being blocked as the gate theory describes. In cases like these, when giving advice to clients as to what they may safely do regarding physical exercise/exertion, it is important to caution them that they may not know that they are overdoing it during the actual physical activity and should judge more by how they feel after the exercise (anywhere from the remainder of that day until when they wake up the next morning).
  2. Clinical application 2: We go to school and continuing education seminars to learn how best to apply treatment techniques, and we know that properly applied techniques are more beneficial than improperly applied ones. However, to some degree, no matter what touch, exercise, or movement therapy we apply to the client (as long as it is not injurious), the client's pain will tend to be blocked as described by the gate theory. In addition, of course, any blockage of pain may help to break the pain-spasm-pain cycle. (Note: For information on the pain-spasm-pain cycle, see Section 19.10.)

REVIEW QUESTIONS

evolve Answers to the following review questions appear on the Evolve website accompanying this book at: http://evolve.elsevier.com/Muscolino/kinesiology/.

1. What is the function of a sensory neuron, and what is the function of a motor neuron?

2. List the neurons involved in a spinal cord reflex arc.

3. List the neurons involved in initiation of voluntary movement.

4. What is the difference between patterned behavior and true reflexive behavior?

5. Give an example of an application of neural facilitation to manual and movement therapy and/or exercise.

6. What is the definition of reciprocal inhibition?

7. How can reciprocal inhibition be used to aid muscle stretching?

8. What is the definition of *proprioception?*

9. List the three major categories of proprioceptors.

10. Which fascial/joint proprioceptor detects static joint position?

11. What is the effect of a muscle spindle reflex?

12. What is the effect of a Golgi tendon organ reflex?

13. Bouncing when stretching activates which proprioceptive reflex?

14. Contract relax (CR) stretching uses which proprioceptive reflex?

15. Which inner ear proprioceptor detects motion of the head?

16. Which proprioceptor (along with inner ear proprioceptors) is particularly important for determining the posture of the trunk?

17. Which reflex is responsible for pulling the left foot away if it steps on a tack?

18. Which reflex is responsible for tightening the quadriceps femoris muscles of the right lower extremity in question 17?

19. Why does the pain-spasm-pain cycle perpetuate itself?

20. According to the gate theory, what sensations can help block pain?

REFERENCES

1. Watkins J: Structure and function of the musculoskeletal system, Champaign, IL, 1999, Human Kinetics.
2. Leonard CT: The neuroscience of human movement, St. Louis, 1998, Mosby.
3. Enoka RM: Neuromechanics of human movement, ed 3, Champaign, IL, 2002, Human Kinetics.
4. Magill RA: Motor learning and control: Concepts and applications, ed 9, New York, 2007, McGraw Hill.
5. Thibodeau GA, Paton KT: Anatomy & physiology, ed 5, St Louis, 2003, Mosby.
6. Palastanga N, Field D, Soames R: Anatomy and human movement, ed 4, Oxford, 2002, Butterworth-Heinemann.
7. Shumway-Cook A, Woolacott MH: Motor control: Translating research into clinical practice, ed 4, Baltimore, 2012, Lippincott Williams & Wilkins.
8. Kandel ER, Schwartz JH, Hessell TM: Principles of neural science, ed 4, New York, 2000, McGraw Hill.
9. Neumann DA: Kinesiology of the musculoskeletal system: Foundations for physical rehabilitation, ed 3, St Louis, 2017, Elsevier.
10. Hamilton N, Weimar W, Luttgens K: Kinesiology: Scientific basis of human motion, ed 12, New York, 2012, McGraw Hill.
11. Smith LK, Weiss EL, Lehmkuhl LO: Brunstrom's clinical kinesiology, ed 5, Philadelphia, 1996, FA Davis.
12. Archer P, Nelson LA: Applied anatomy & physiology for manual therapists, Philadelphia, 2012, Lippincott Williams & Wilkins.
13. Chaitow L, Delaney JW: Clinical application of neuromuscular techniques: Volume 1: The upper body, Edinburgh, 2000, Churchill Livingstone.
14. MacIntosh BR, Gardiner PF, McComas AJ: Skeletal muscle: Form and function, ed 2, Champaign, IL, 2006, Human Kinetics.
15. Baloh RW, Honrubia V: Clinical neurophysiology of the vestibular system, ed 3, Oxford, 2001, Oxford University Press.

16. McGinnis PM: Biomechanics of sport and exercise, ed 3, Champaign, IL, 2013, Human Kinetics.
17. Scrivani SJ, Mehta NR, Keith DA, et al: Facial pain. In Fishman SM, Ballantyne JC, Rathmell JP, editors: Bonica's management of pain, ed 4, Baltimore, 2010, Lippincott Williams & Wilkins.
18. Kenney WL, Wilmore JH, Castill DL: Physiology of sport and exercise, ed 5, Champaign, IL, 2012, Human Kinetics.
19. Marcus DA: Chronic pain: A primary care guide to practical management, ed 2, New York, 2009, Humana Press.
20. Hamill J, Knutzen KM: Biomechanical basis of human movement, ed 12, Baltimore, 2003, Lippincott Williams & Wilkins.
21. Mattes AL: Active isolated stretching: The Mattes method, Sarasota, 2000, Aaron Mattes.
22. Stedman's medical dictionary, ed 27, Baltimore, 2000, Lippincott Williams & Wilkins.
23. Potach DH, Chu DA: Plyometric training. In Baechle TR, Earle RE, editors: Essentials of strength training and conditioning, ed 3, Champaign, IL, 2008, Human Kinetics.
24. Page P, Frank CC, Lardner R: Assessment and treatment of muscle imbalance: The Janda approach, Champaign, IL, 2010, Human Kinetics.
25. Jeffreys I: Warm-up and stretching. In Baechle TR, Earle RE, editors: Essentials of strength training and conditioning, ed 3, Champaign, IL, 2008, Human Kinetics.

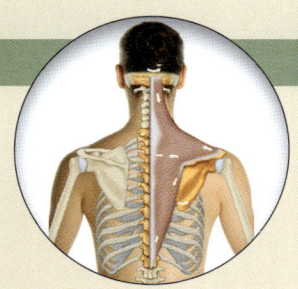

CHAPTER 20
Posture and the Gait Cycle

CHAPTER OUTLINE

Section 20.1	Importance of "Good Posture"	Section 20.5	General Principles of Compensation within the Body
Section 20.2	Ideal Standing Plumb Line Posture	Section 20.6	Limitations of Standing Ideal Plumb Line Posture
Section 20.3	Analyzing Plumb Line Postural Distortions	Section 20.7	Gait Cycle
Section 20.4	Secondary Postural Distortions and Postural Distortion Patterns	Section 20.8	Muscular Activity during the Gait Cycle

CHAPTER OBJECTIVES

After completing this chapter, the student should be able to perform the following:

1. Define the key terms of this chapter and state the meanings of the word origins of this chapter.
2. Do the following related to posture:
   - Describe good and bad posture, and give examples of the effects of bad posture.
   - Define *stress*, and discuss the positive and negative effects of stress on the body.
3. Discuss the value of plumb line postural assessment, and list the landmarks for posterior and lateral plumb line assessments.
4. Do the following related to plumb line postural distortions:
   - Give and discuss an example of a postural distortion in each of the three cardinal planes (sagittal, frontal, and transverse).
   - Explain the concept of center of weight, and discuss its application to postural analysis.
5. Do the following related to secondary postural distortions and postural distortion patterns:
   - Explain the relationship between a primary postural distortion, a secondary postural distortion, and a postural distortion pattern.
   - Compare and contrast consequential secondary postural distortions and compensatory secondary postural distortions.
   - Give an example of a consequential secondary postural distortion, a compensatory secondary postural distortion, and a postural distortion pattern.
6. Discuss and give examples of three general principles of compensation within the body.
7. Discuss the limitations of using a plumb line for postural analysis.
8. Do the following related to gait cycle:
   - Describe the major phases and landmarks of the gait cycle.
   - Describe the relative rigidity/flexibility of the foot and its relation to the gait cycle.
9. State when each of the major muscles of the lower extremity contract during the gait cycle (i.e., relate the timing of its contraction to the landmarks of the gait cycle).

OVERVIEW

This chapter covers the two topics of posture and gait. The word *posture* means *position*. Because the human body can be placed in an infinite number of possible positions, it can assume an infinite number of postures. When we examine a client's posture, we look to see how balanced and efficient it is. Based on balance and efficiency, we often describe the client as having **"good posture"** or **"bad posture."** Common bad postures, in other words, postural distortion patterns, of the human body are covered in the next chapter (Chapter 21).

In addition to assessing a client's static postures, it is also important to consider the balance and efficiency of the human body in movement. In contrast to the term *posture,* which describes the static position of the body, the term **"acture"** is sometimes used to describe the balance and efficiency of the body during movement. We then explain and discuss the dynamic movement pattern of walking, called the *gait cycle*. Included in this discussion is an analysis of the timing of engagement of the major muscles of the lower extremity during the gait cycle.

KEY TERMS

- "Acture" (AK-cher)
- Agonist/antagonist pair (AG-o-nist/an-TAG-o-nist)
- Anterior shin splints
- "Bad posture"
- Center of weight
- Compensatory secondary postural distortion
- Consequential secondary postural distortion
- Counterbalance (COUNT-er-BAL-ans)
- Double-limb support
- Dynamic posture
- Early swing
- Electromyography (EMG) (e-LEK-tro-my-OG-ra-fee)
- Foot-flat
- Foot slap
- Gait (GATE)
- Gait cycle
- "Good posture"
- Heel-off
- Heel-strike
- Late swing
- Midstance
- Midswing
- Planting and cutting
- Plumb line (PLUM)
- Posterior shin splints
- Postural distortion pattern
- Posture
- Primary postural distortion
- Protracted head
- Secondary postural distortion
- Shin splints
- Stance phase
- Step
- Step angulation
- Step length
- Step width
- Stress
- Stressors
- Stride
- Swing phase
- Toe-off

WORD ORIGINS

- Acture—From Latin *actus,* meaning *to act*
- Counterbalance—From Latin *contra,* meaning *against; bi,* meaning *two;* and *lanx,* meaning *dish*
- Dynamic—From Greek *dynamis,* meaning *power*
- Dysfunction—From Greek *dys,* meaning *bad,* and Latin *functio,* meaning *to perform*
- Electromyography—From Greek *electron,* meaning *amber* (origin: static electricity can be generated by friction against amber); *mys,* meaning *muscle;* and *grapho,* meaning *to write*
- Plumb—From Latin *plumbum,* meaning *lead*
- Posture—From Latin *positura,* meaning *to place*
- Primary—From Latin *primarius,* meaning *of the first rank*
- Secondary—From Latin *secundus,* meaning *second in order of rank*
- Stress—From Latin *stringere,* meaning *to draw tight*

SECTION 20.1 IMPORTANCE OF "GOOD POSTURE"

- **Posture** means *position.*
- The position that a person's body is in is important because holding the body statically in a position places stresses on the tissues of the body.[1]
  - Muscles may have to work, causing them to be stressed.
  - Ligaments, joint capsules, and other soft tissues of the body may have pulling forces placed on them, causing stress to these tissues.
  - Articular surfaces of bones may be compressed, causing stress to them.
- It is impossible to entirely eliminate muscles from working, soft tissues from being pulled, and compression forces from existing in the body. However, when these stresses become excessive, injury and damage to tissues of the body may occur (Box 20-1).
- When we examine a client's posture to see if it is "good" or "bad," we are looking to see how the position of the client's body may create stresses to the tissues of the body.
- "Good posture" is healthy because it is balanced and efficient; therefore it does not place excessive stresses on the tissues of the body.[2]
- "Bad posture" is unhealthy because it is not balanced and not efficient; therefore it does place excessive stresses on the tissues of the body.[2]
  - Bad, unhealthy postures place excessive stresses on the tissues of the body. Most commonly, muscles, ligaments, and/or bones are stressed by unhealthy postures.

CHAPTER 20 Posture and the Gait Cycle 641

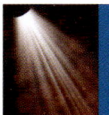

BOX 20-1 Spotlight on Stress

The term stress is often misused and misunderstood. **Stress** is caused by stressors, and a **stressor** is defined simply as anything that requires the body to change. Stressors may be physical or psychological/emotional. Because any change is potentially dangerous, stressors are viewed by the body as alarming and generally handled by the sympathetic branch of the autonomic nervous system. Having excessive stress is deleterious to the body, because the body is constantly keying up for possible dangers. However, to have no stress is not only equally unhealthy but also essentially impossible. Being alive implies change and growth, and it is the presence of stressors that challenges us to change and grow. An absence of all stress means a total absence of growth. Having a healthy amount of stress gives us the challenges we need to grow. In short, it is not stress that should be avoided; it is excessive stress that should be avoided.

SECTION 20.2 IDEAL STANDING PLUMB LINE POSTURE

○ When posture is analyzed, most often it is standing posture that is examined.
○ Although standing posture does yield some important information, its value can be limited. The analysis of any posture is valuable only if the client spends time in that posture. Therefore if a client spends the bulk of the day sitting at a desk or computer, it would be much more valuable to assess the healthiness of that posture. Furthermore, most people sleep at least 6 to 8 hours a night; that translates to literally ¼ to ⅓ of our lives! If sleeping posture is unhealthy, that will also have a great influence on the health of the client, most likely a greater influence than standing posture does. Although this textbook does not examine each of these other postures, the fundamental principles addressed for standing posture can be extrapolated to apply to most other postures. In short, for every posture of the client, look for the stresses that would result to the tissues of the body.
○ Standing posture is usually analyzed by comparing the symmetry of the body against a perfectly vertical line that is created by a plumb line.[3]
○ The word *plumb* of "plumb line" comes from the Latin word for lead. A **plumb line** is created by attaching a small heavy weight (originally made of lead) to a string. The weight pulls the string down, creating a straight vertical line that one can use to analyze the symmetry of the body in standing posture. Although one can buy fancy plumb line devices made for postural analysis, a string and a weight bought very inexpensively from a hardware store and attached to the ceiling create a perfectly good postural plumb line.
○ When looking at the body in plumb line posterior and lateral views, we look for symmetry and balance of the parts of the body (Figure 20-1).
○ Note: For transverse plane postural distortions, see Section 20.6.

FRONTAL PLANE POSTURAL EXAMINATION (POSTERIOR PLUMB LINE):

○ A posterior postural examination yields information about postural distortions that exist in the frontal plane (see Figure 20-1, A).
○ When looking at the posterior view plumb line posture, are the left and right sides of the body symmetric and balanced in the frontal plane? The ideal posterior plumb line posture is to have

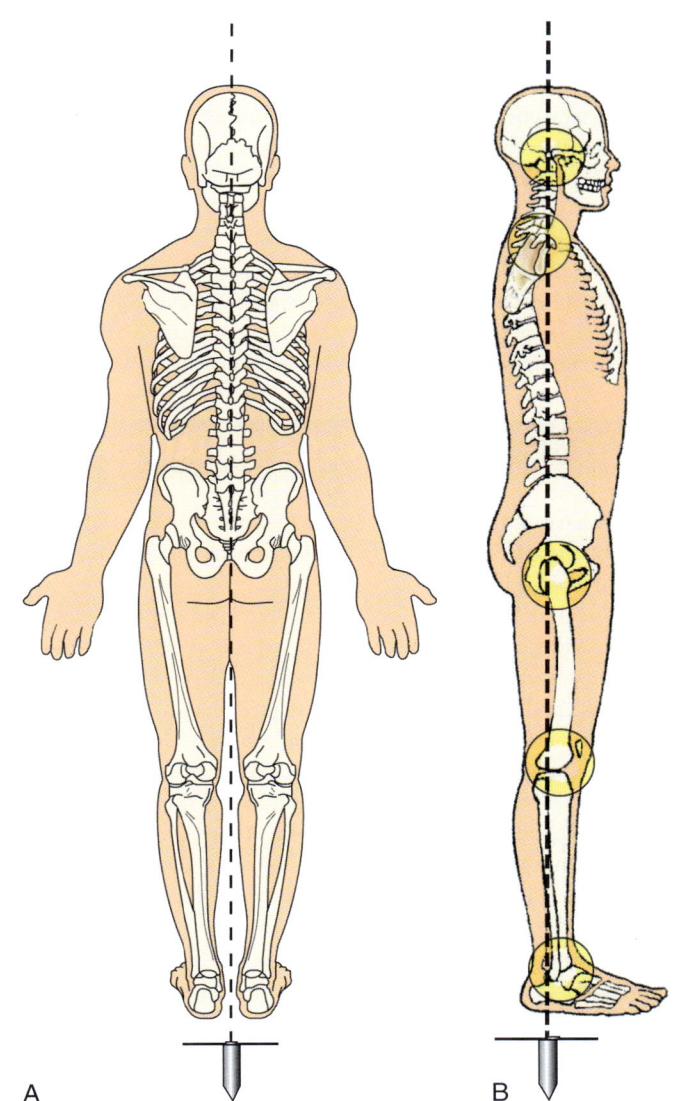

FIGURE 20-1 Plumb line postural assessments. **A,** Posterior view. **B,** Lateral view. With ideal posture from the posterior view, the plumb line should bisect the body into equal right and left halves. With ideal posture from the lateral view, the plumb line should descend through the ear (i.e., external auditory meatus), acromion process of the scapula, greater trochanter of the femur, knee joint, and lateral malleolus of the fibula.

the line travel straight down the center of the body, evenly dividing the body into two equal left and right halves. Look to see if left and right sides are equal in position.
- During a posterior postural exam, the following are fundamental things to check[4]:
  - Are the shoulder heights equal, or is one side higher than the other?
  - Are the iliac crest heights equal, or is one side higher than the other?
  - Are the knee joints straight, or does the client have genu valgum or genu varum? (Note: Genu valgum and genu varum are covered in Section 9.15.)
  - Does the client collapse over one or both of the arches (excessive pronation of the foot at the subtalar joint), resulting in an iliac crest height that is lower than the other?

SAGITTAL PLANE POSTURAL EXAMINATION (LATERAL PLUMB LINE):

- A lateral postural examination yields information about postural distortions that exist in the sagittal plane (see Figure 20-1, *B*).
- When looking at the lateral view plumb line posture, are the anterior and posterior sides of the body symmetric and balanced in the sagittal plane?
- The ideal lateral plumb line posture is to have the line travel straight down through the ear (i.e., external auditory meatus), the acromion process of the scapula, the greater trochanter of the femur, the knee joint, and the lateral malleolus of the fibula.[4]
- Look to see if each body part is balanced over the body part that is below it. Are joints excessively flexed or extended? Are the curves of the spine normal?
- During a lateral postural exam, the following are fundamental things to check[4]:
  - Are the spinal curves increased or decreased?
  - Is the head balanced over the trunk, or is it anteriorly held?
  - Is the trunk balanced over the pelvis?
  - Does the pelvis have excessive anterior or posterior tilt?
  - Are the knee or hip joints hyperextended?

TRANSVERSE PLANE POSTURAL EXAMINATION:

- Postural distortions that exist in the transverse plane are rotational distortions and are perhaps the most challenging to see and assess. (Note: Some common examples of transverse plane rotational postural distortions include scoliosis, medially rotated arms at the glenohumeral joints, and medially or laterally rotated thighs at the hip joints.) This is because a vertical plumb line cannot be used to assess a transverse plane distortion, because the transverse plane is horizontal.
- Ideally, the best view from which to see a transverse plane postural distortion is superior. From above, any transverse plane rotation distortion would show as an asymmetry. However, short of positioning yourself above a client by standing on a ladder, this is logistically difficult. For this reason, special attention must be paid when looking for transverse plane rotation distortions from the front, back, or sides!

SECTION 20.3 ANALYZING PLUMB LINE POSTURAL DISTORTIONS

- We have said that when we look at the body in plumb line posterior and lateral views, we look for symmetry and balance of the parts of the body.
- When the body is not posturally symmetric and balanced, we can say that one or more postural distortions exist. As we have stated, each postural distortion places excessive stress on tissues of the body and may lead to injury and damage.
- When analyzing posture, two things should be determined[5]:
  - What stressful effects will the client's postural distortion place on the tissues of the body? Knowing the stressful effects will allow us to relate the posture of the client to the symptoms that the client is experiencing.
  - What is causing this postural distortion (i.e., what activities and habit patterns of the client are causing the postural distortion[s])? Knowing the activities and habit patterns that the client engages in allows us to understand how this postural distortion occurred in the first place. This allows us to give postural lifestyle advice to help prevent these postural distortions from occurring or worsening in the future.

POSTURAL ASSESSMENT:

- When assessing the cause of a client's postural problem, it is easy to try to blame the problem on just one factor. Although this does sometimes happen, it is rare for a person's condition to be caused by just one thing. The cause for most conditions is multifactorial, meaning that many factors contribute to the condition. When you have found one cause for a problem, do not stop searching for others. It is in the client's interest for you to be thorough so that you can give better advice as to how to change all the pertinent habit patterns that contribute to the problem; this will help the client to be healthier in the future. Usually, many *straws weigh down the camel's back;* all blame should not be placed on one straw that is found. Look to find all or at least most of the straws that contribute to the problem!

FRONTAL AND SAGITTAL PLANE DISTORTIONS:

- Any deviation from ideal posture in the posterior view means that the client has a postural distortion within the frontal plane.
- Any deviation from ideal posture in the lateral view means that the client has a postural distortion within the sagittal plane.

EXAMPLES OF POSTURAL DISTORTIONS:

Two common postural distortions, one in the frontal plane and one in the sagittal plane, are shown in Figures 20-2 and 20-3.
- Figure 20-2 is a posterior view that illustrates the frontal plane postural distortion of a person with the right shoulder higher

CHAPTER 20   Posture and the Gait Cycle   643

muscles. To then understand why the client has this postural distortion, it is important to do a thorough history to look for the activities and habit patterns the client has that might create it. It might be determined that the client habitually carries a purse on the right side. In this case constant elevation of the right shoulder girdle to hold a purse from falling off the shoulder has led over the years to this frontal plane postural distortion (Box 20-2).

❍ Figure 20-3 is a lateral view that illustrates the sagittal plane postural distortion of a person with a protracted (i.e., anteriorly held) head. We begin by looking at the stresses this posture places on the tissues of the body. To hold the head anteriorly means that the center of weight of the head is no longer over the trunk; it is over thin air. Therefore the head and neck should fall into flexion, resulting in the chin landing against the chest. The only reason this does not occur is that musculature of the posterior neck (that performs extension of the neck and head) must be isometrically contracting, creating a counterforce to gravity, preventing the head and neck from falling into flexion. Long-standing isometric contraction of the muscles of the posterior neck such as the upper trapezius and semispinalis capitis can lead to trigger points and pain in these muscles. To then understand why the client has this postural distortion, it is important to obtain a thorough history to look for the activities and habit patterns the client has that might create this. It might be determined that the client habitually reads with a book in the lap. In this case a constant habit of reading with a book in the lap has led over the years to this sagittal plane postural distortion (Boxes 20-3 and 20-4).

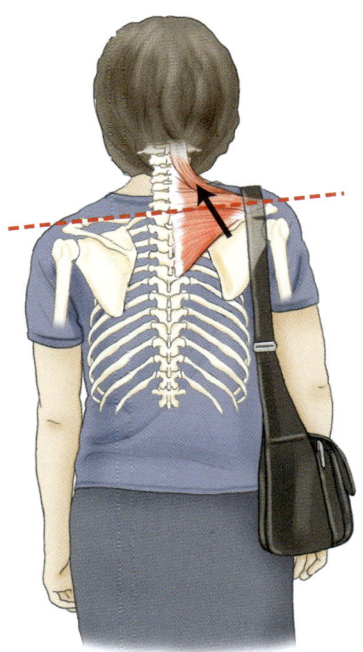

FIGURE 20-2 Person who on postural assessment is found to have a frontal plane postural distortion; her right shoulder girdle is higher than the left. Long-term carrying of a purse on the right side has led to chronic hypertonicity of her right-sided scapular elevator musculature to prevent the purse from falling off.

than the left. We begin by looking at the stresses this posture places on the tissues of the body. To hold the right shoulder high means that the baseline resting tone of the musculature of elevation of the right shoulder girdle (i.e., elevators of the right scapula at the scapulocostal [ScC] joint) must be tighter on the right than on the left. Long-standing isometric contraction of elevators of the right scapula such as the upper trapezius and levator scapulae can lead to trigger points and pain in these

BOX 20-2   Spotlight on Carrying a Shoulder Bag

Carrying a purse or any type of shoulder bag is an extremely common habit that can lead to postural distortion. Although the weight of the bag is important because that weight bears down through the strap into the musculature of the shoulder girdle, the weight is not the most important aspect. Even carrying an empty shoulder bag will create the postural distortion of spasmed muscles that perform elevation of the shoulder girdle. The reason is that the natural slope of the shoulder is such that a bag would fall off. To prevent that from occurring, the person isometrically contracts musculature to elevate the scapula to prevent this. This long-standing isometric contraction eventually leads to the chronic postural problem, regardless of the weight of the bag (although greater weight means that the muscles will have to contract more forcefully). Wearing a bag that has a strap that goes over the opposite shoulder and across the body is healthier, because it eliminates the necessity of having to isometrically contract musculature to change the slope of the shoulder.

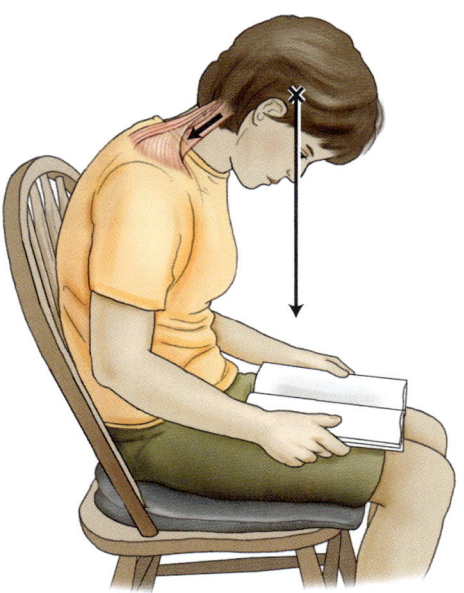

FIGURE 20-3 Person with a sagittal plane postural distortion; her head is held anteriorly. This results in the center of weight of the head no longer being balanced over the trunk. Long-term reading with a book down in her lap has led to chronic hypertonicity of her posterior extensor head/neck musculature. (Note: The *X* indicates the center of weight of the head, which falls anterior to the trunk.)

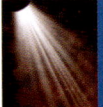

BOX 20-3 Spotlight on Center of Weight

The concept of the **center of weight** is critical to the idea of a balanced posture. The center of weight of an object is an imaginary point where all the weight of the object could be considered to be located. If the center of weight of an object is over the object below, then the object on top will be balanced on the object below it. If instead the center of weight of the upper object is not over the object below, then the upper object is not balanced and would fall unless some force holds it in place (see accompanying illustration). This concept applies to the major parts of the human body. The head should be balanced by having its center of weight over the trunk, the trunk should be balanced by having its center of weight over the pelvis, and so forth. If the head's center of weight is not over the trunk (e.g., it is protracted and anterior to the trunk), then extensor muscles must be in a constant isometric contraction to hold the head (and neck) in position so that it does not fall into flexion.

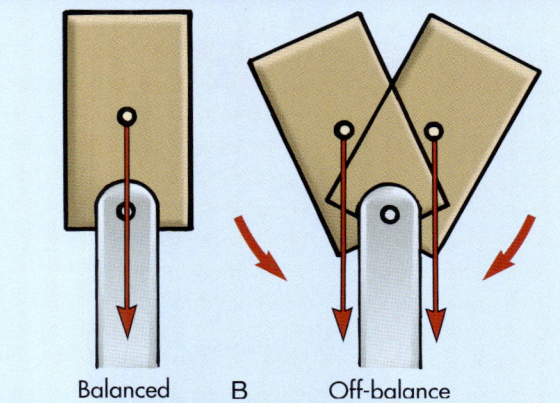

A Balanced   B Off-balance

(Modified from Fritz S: Mosby's fundamentals of therapeutic massage, ed 5, St Louis, 2013, Mosby.)

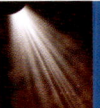

BOX 20-4 Spotlight on Protracted Head Posture

A **protracted head** (i.e., anteriorly held head) is one of the most common postural distortion patterns. Almost every activity that we do is down and in front of us. From the day that a child is given crayons and a coloring book, through the years of sitting at a desk to read and write in elementary, middle, and high school and college, we tend to hold the head anteriorly to read, write, and study. Furthermore, activities such as desk jobs, crafts such as sewing or needlepoint done in the lap, caring for children who are being held in parents' arms, preparing and cutting food while cooking, holding a smart phone or PDA (personal digital assistant) down low in front of us, and working at a computer with a monitor that is too low all tend to place the head in an anteriorly held posture. It is no wonder that so many people have an anteriorly held head posture and the muscles of their posterior necks are so commonly tight. Use of a bookstand or an inclined desk, such as those used by architects and engineers, are easy ways to prevent this problem! (See Section 21.3 for more on the posture of a protracted head.)

SECTION 20.4 SECONDARY POSTURAL DISTORTIONS AND POSTURAL DISTORTION PATTERNS

- A **primary postural distortion** of the body is a postural distortion that is caused by a problem in that area of the body.[6]
- A **secondary postural distortion** is a postural distortion that is caused by a problem in another area of the body, in other words, it occurs secondary to this other problem.[6]
- A **postural distortion pattern** is a set of interrelated postural distortions located in the body, including both the primary postural distortion and the secondary postural distortion(s).
- Not every postural distortion is primary. Sometimes a postural distortion pattern is created secondary to another postural distortion that already exists.
- Understanding when a postural distortion is primary versus secondary is important for manual and movement therapists, because massage, bodywork, or exercise of the muscles of a secondary postural distortion, no matter how good it feels to the client, will never eliminate the problem. This is because the cause of the problem lies elsewhere.
- A secondary postural distortion may exist as a consequence of the primary postural distortion, in which case it is called a **consequential secondary postural distortion**. Alternatively, it may be specifically created by the body as a compensation for the primary postural distortion, in which case it is called a **compensatory secondary postural distortion**.

CONSEQUENTIAL SECONDARY POSTURAL DISTORTIONS:

- Figure 20-4 is a posterior view of a person with a high right shoulder similar to the person in Figure 20-2. However, in this case the high right shoulder is not a primary postural distortion caused by tight musculature of the right shoulder girdle; rather it is caused by the person's collapsed left arch, which has dropped the entire left side of the client. Because the left side is lower, the right shoulder is seen as higher. In this case the person's

CHAPTER 20 Posture and the Gait Cycle 645

- Figure 20-5 illustrates a person with a collapsed arch of the left foot, which is a primary postural distortion. We have seen that an uncompensated dropped left arch would cause the entire left side of the person's body to drop (as shown in Figure 20-4), resulting in a low left shoulder girdle and a relatively high right shoulder girdle. However, in this person's case the spine has developed a scoliotic curve to compensate for the low left side. Through curving of the spine, the shoulder heights have been brought to level. Therefore this scoliosis is a compensatory secondary postural distortion that has been created as a compensation for the dropped left arch. Although work done on the scoliosis may feel good and be beneficial, it will never correct the scoliotic curve, because the cause is elsewhere. Correction of the dropped left arch is necessary to correct the scoliosis.
- When analyzing posture, although a primary postural distortion at one level may travel inferiorly and create secondary postural

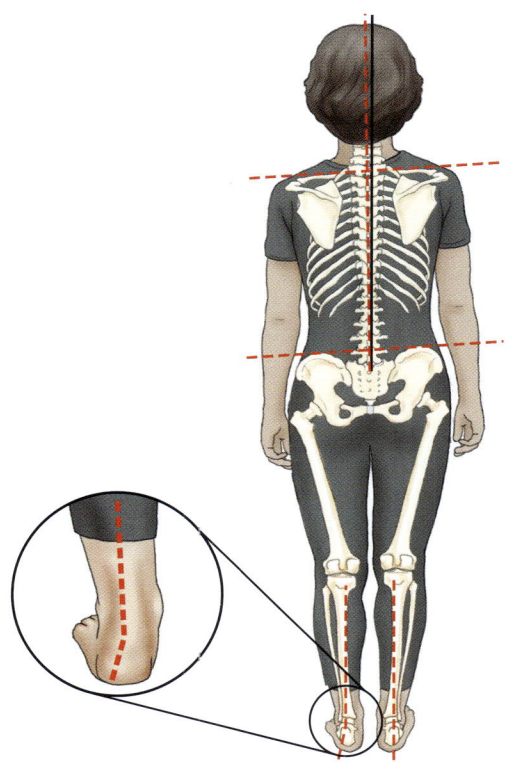

FIGURE 20-4 Person who on postural assessment is found to have a frontal plane postural distortion seemingly identical to what was found in Figure 20-2 (i.e., her right shoulder girdle is higher than the left). In this case, it is caused by a collapsed arch in her left foot that has caused her entire left side to drop, making the right shoulder girdle relatively higher. Her low left shoulder is a consequential secondary postural distortion.

right-sided musculature of scapular elevation is not the reason for the elevated right shoulder girdle. Even if bodywork into these muscles feels good, the postural distortion of the high right shoulder will never be changed by working this region, because it is not the cause of the problem. The high right shoulder is a consequential secondary postural distortion, in other words, it is simply the consequence of another (primary) postural distortion that has not been compensated for, the collapsed left arch. In this case, correcting the collapsed left arch of the person's foot must be addressed to correct the high right shoulder.
- As Figure 20-4 illustrates, sometimes a secondary postural distortion is merely the consequence of another postural distortion that is primary. However, sometimes a secondary postural distortion is purposely created by the body as a compensation for a primary postural distortion.

COMPENSATORY SECONDARY POSTURAL DISTORTIONS:

- Sometimes the body creates a secondary postural distortion as a compensation mechanism for another primary postural distortion. These compensatory secondary postural distortions are meant to correct or prevent consequential secondary postural distortions that might otherwise occur.[7]

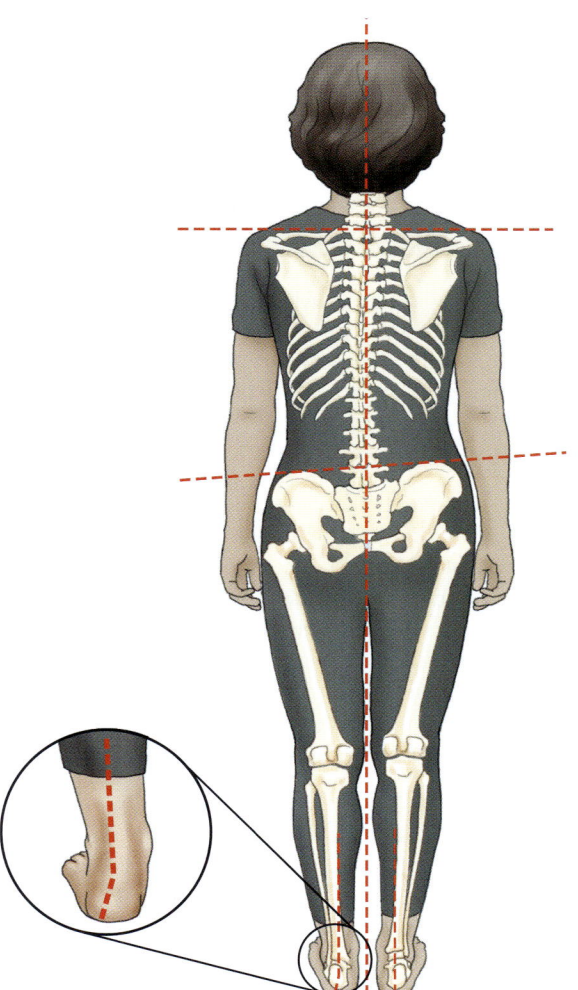

FIGURE 20-5 Same person as in Figure 20-4 with a collapsed left arch, which is a primary postural distortion. The only difference is that now the person's spine has compensated for the dropped arch by having a (left thoracolumbar) scoliotic curve. This scoliosis is a compensatory secondary postural distortion that brings the left shoulder girdle back to being the same height as the right shoulder girdle.

distortions lower down in the body, it is more common for a lower primary postural distortion to create secondary postural distortions higher up in the body. To draw an analogy to the structure of a building, it is more likely that a building with a foundation that is improper will develop cracks in the plaster on the third floor than it is that a problem on the third floor will create a problem with the building's foundation. Generally when putting together the various clues that one sees when analyzing a client's posture, it is best to think from the bottom up.

POSTURAL DISTORTION PATTERNS:

○ Whether a person's secondary postural distortion is simply a consequence of an uncompensated primary postural distortion as in Figure 20-4 or is a compensation for a primary postural distortion as in Figure 20-5, we still see that once a primary postural distortion exists in the body, secondary postural distortions are likely to develop. In other words, a local primary postural distortion tends to create a larger postural distortion pattern that may spread throughout the body.[5]

○ These larger global distortion patterns mean that many local distortions will be present when a client's posture is examined.

By possessing a fundamental understanding of the musculoskeletal structure and function of the body and by critically thinking, the examiner usually can determine which postural distortion is the causative primary distortion. Although work on all postural distortions, including secondary distortions, feels good and may be beneficial, it is only through the correction of the primary postural distortion that a client's entire postural distortion pattern can be corrected.

○ Although it is true that a secondary postural distortion is functionally caused by another "primary" postural distortion and that the secondary postural distortion cannot be corrected unless the primary one is first eliminated, unfortunately, not every secondary postural distortion will automatically disappear when the primary distortion is eliminated. If a secondary postural distortion has been present long enough, the soft tissues of the body will have most likely structurally changed to adapt to this postural distortion.[7] To correct these structural changes, it may be necessary to work directly on them. In effect, the functional secondary postural distortion in time becomes its own structural primary postural distortion. This is one reason why the longer a client waits to address a problem, the more difficult it becomes to resolve it.

SECTION 20.5 GENERAL PRINCIPLES OF COMPENSATION WITHIN THE BODY

○ Understanding and being able to apply the principle of postural compensation throughout the body is an important skill for any therapist or trainer who works clinically. Following are some of the general principles of how postural compensation occurs in the body.

COUNTERBALANCING BODY PARTS:

○ When a body part is deviated to one side, the body part above it will usually be deviated to the opposite side to **counterbalance** the weight of the body.
  ○ One example of this is when a person is very heavy and has a large abdomen. The weight of the abdomen throws the center of weight of the lower trunk anteriorly. To compensate for this, the upper trunk will usually be deviated posteriorly to counterbalance the anteriorly deviated lower trunk. As a result, the center of weight of the trunk as a whole is centered and balanced.

HYPOMOBILITY/HYPERMOBILITY OF JOINTS:

○ When a joint of the body becomes hypomobile (i.e., its movement becomes restricted), other joints often compensate by becoming hypermobile[8] (Box 20-5).
  ○ An example of this is a spinal joint that has lost mobility (i.e., is hypomobile). For full range of motion of that region of the spine to occur, an adjacent spinal joint must compensate by increasing its mobility (i.e., becoming hypermobile).
  ○ Another example is that if one shoulder joint is painful and cannot be moved (thus hypomobile), the other shoulder joint will be used more and in time will likely become hypermobile.

 BOX 20-5

An interesting addendum exists to a joint hypermobility that is caused as a compensation for a hypomobility. In time, the excessive motion and use of the hypermobile joint will often result in overuse and pain. The consequence of this will likely be muscle spasm to prevent the painful use. This muscle spasm will then decrease movement of that joint, resulting in another hypomobile joint. Now two hypomobile joints exist, which will then create another hypermobility, which by the same process will likely result in a third hypomobile joint. Like dominoes falling, once one hypomobile joint exists, it sets a compensation pattern in motion that tends to spread throughout the body!

TIGHTENED ANTAGONIST MUSCLES:

○ Opposing muscles on opposite sides of a joint usually need to balance their pull on the bone to which they attach. Indeed, the proper posture of the body part involved depends on a balanced pull of these muscles. If the tone of one of these muscles changes, it will usually cause a compensatory change in the tone of the muscles on the other side of the joint. For example, if a muscle on one side of a joint becomes tighter and therefore shortens, the opposing muscle on the other side of the joint will often become tighter in an attempt to even out the pulling force on their common attachment. Otherwise, the attachment would be unevenly pulled in one direction and a postural distortion would result.

- Opposing muscles located on opposite sides of a joint are often called an **agonist/antagonist pair**. The muscles of an agonist/antagonist pair should usually be balanced in tone.[9] If an agonist becomes excessively shortened and tightened (i.e., facilitated), two things may happen to the antagonist:
  1. It can become lengthened and weakened (i.e., inhibited), allowing the tight agonist to excessively pull on the common attachment and resulting in a postural distortion of the body part involved.[1]
  2. It can tighten as a compensation to try to even out the pull of the agonist to prevent the postural distortion[7]; this results in tight muscles on both sides of the joint! The musculature on each side may be the same length, in which case bony posture remains symmetrical. Or one side may be longer or shorter, in which case bony posture is asymmetrical (and the two groups of musculature may be described as "locked short" and "locked long").
- One common example of compensations between opposing muscles is tightness of the muscles of the neck. For example, if the musculature of the left side of the neck becomes tight, the musculature of the right side of the neck will often become tight in an attempt to prevent the head and neck from being pulled to the left.

SECTION 20.6 LIMITATIONS OF STANDING IDEAL PLUMB LINE POSTURE

- Although use of a plumb line can be very helpful when analyzing a client's posture, plumb line postural analysis has certain limitations, discussed in the following sections.

TRANSVERSE PLANE POSTURAL DISTORTIONS:

- As mentioned in Section 20.2, plumb line postural analyses give us a way to look for postural distortions within the frontal and sagittal planes. The plumb line is effective in these cases because it is vertically oriented and the sagittal and frontal planes are vertically oriented. However, a vertical plumb line cannot be effectively used to check for rotational distortions that occur within the transverse plane because the transverse plane is horizontal in orientation. Because a plumb line is not effective for evaluating and assessing transverse plane postural distortions, they are easy to miss and must be more carefully looked for than frontal and sagittal plane distortions.
  - To see a rotation of a body part, a superior view is best (see Figure 20-6, *A*). Unfortunately, viewing a client from above is logistically difficult. For this reason, transverse plane postural distortions must usually be seen and assessed from anterior, posterior, and/or lateral views, but the plumb line is not very helpful in this examination (see Figure 20-6, *B*).

STANDING POSTURE ONLY:

- Plumb line posture is generally useful for examining only our client's standing posture. If the client does not spend much of the day standing, analyzing standing posture may be largely irrelevant to his or her health. In this case it would be better to analyze the postures that the client more frequently assumes.[1]

QUESTIONABLE IMPORTANCE OF STATIC POSTURAL ANALYSIS:

- Static posture is just one piece of the puzzle in assessing a client's health. Many other pieces exist. Static postural analysis is an analysis of structure. Although structure does certainly affect function, the relationship is not always direct and immediate. The human body has a great deal of ability to deal with deviations from "ideal" posture, and deviations from ideal are not necessarily reflected in signs and symptoms on the part of the client. Certainly poor posture creates stresses on tissues of the body that predispose us to problems; however, these problems may not manifest for a very long time, or they may never manifest. Be careful to not make too strong of a relationship between every little postural distortion and the client's presenting problem(s). Keep in mind that ideal posture is just that—ideal. Not everyone must have the same exact ideal posture; the human body comes in many shapes and forms, and it is important to not try to force every body into one standardized ideal!
- What may be of much greater importance is not someone's static posture but what might be called his or her **dynamic posture**,[10] or "acture." **Acture** is a term used to describe the fluidity of someone's movement patterns. Some people when standing still may have a static posture that is less than desirable, but when they move, their movements may be clean, efficient, graceful, and healthy. In this regard, the dynamic aspect of acture may be as important as, if not more important than, the static aspect of posture.

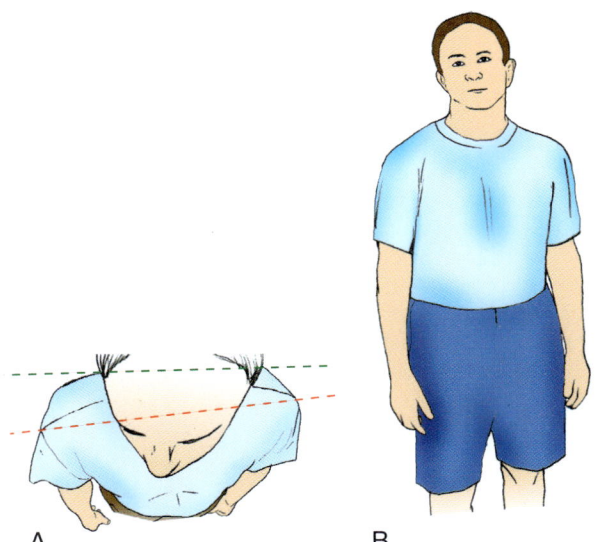

FIGURE 20-6 Individual with a mild/moderate scoliosis. A scoliosis has a rotational postural distortion in the transverse plane. The best view for any transverse plane postural assessment is superior. **A,** Superior view. Reader should note how clearly the asymmetry of the posture of the upper trunk can be seen. **B,** Anterior view, which is the more common view that we have when trying to assess transverse plane postural distortions. This perspective is not as ideal, but subtle visual clues are present. The orientation of the trunk should be noted; it is not facing perfectly anterior. In addition, the asymmetry of the arms by the sides of the body should be noted; the right hand is held farther from the body than is the left hand.

SECTION 20.7 GAIT CYCLE

- Gait is defined as the manner of walking.[12]
- The gait cycle is defined as the cyclic pattern of engagement of muscles and joints of the body when walking.[1]
- Walking requires a very complex coordination of muscle contractions. Although most adults take the ability to walk for granted, children need years to learn how to walk in a coordinated fashion. With advancing years, people are often challenged once again by the demands of walking.
- It is estimated that an individual does not develop a mature gait pattern until approximately the age of 7 years.[11]
- Whether our clients are children, adults, or senior citizens, athletes or nonathletes, understanding the demands of gait can be extremely valuable for therapists and trainers, given the effects that gait can have on musculoskeletal health.

GAIT CYCLE SPECIFICS:

- When we walk, our gait has a repetitive or cyclic pattern. We step forward with our right foot, then our left foot, then our right foot again, then our left foot again, and so forth. Whether we walk 50 feet or 50 miles, this cyclic pattern is the same. The term *gait cycle* is used to describe this cyclic pattern of gait.
- Figure 20-7 illustrates the gait cycle. We see that it begins when one heel strikes the ground and ends when the same-side heel strikes the ground again.
- The term stride is used to define one cycle of the gait cycle.
  - One stride consists of two steps: (1) a left step and (2) a right step.
  - Technically the step of one foot begins when the heel of the other foot strikes the ground and ends when its heel strikes the ground. Each step makes up 50% of the gait cycle (or stride). In other words, two steps occur in one stride (Box 20-6).

GAIT CYCLE PHASES AND LANDMARKS:

- The gait cycle has two main phases (Figure 20-7): (1) the stance phase and (2) the swing phase. These phases are correlated with the major landmarks of the gait cycle.
  - Stance phase begins at heel-strike and ends at toe-off.
  - Swing phase begins at toe-off and ends at heel-strike.

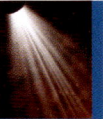

BOX 20-6   Spotlight on Foot Facts

A number of additional terms are often used when describing a step of the gait cycle:
- Step length is defined as the length between two consecutive heel strikes (i.e., the length of a step). Average step length of an adult is approximately 28 inches (72 cm).
- Step width is the width (i.e., lateral distance) between the centers of two consecutive heel strikes. Average step width of an adult is approximately 3 inches (7 to 9 cm).
- Step angulation is the angle created between the direction in which one is moving and the long axis of the foot. A step angulation of approximately 7 to 10 degrees is considered normal.

In addition, the normal pace of walking is approximately 100 steps per minute (approximately 2½ miles per hour [4 kilometers per hour]); and on average, each foot strikes the ground 2000 to 10,000 times daily!

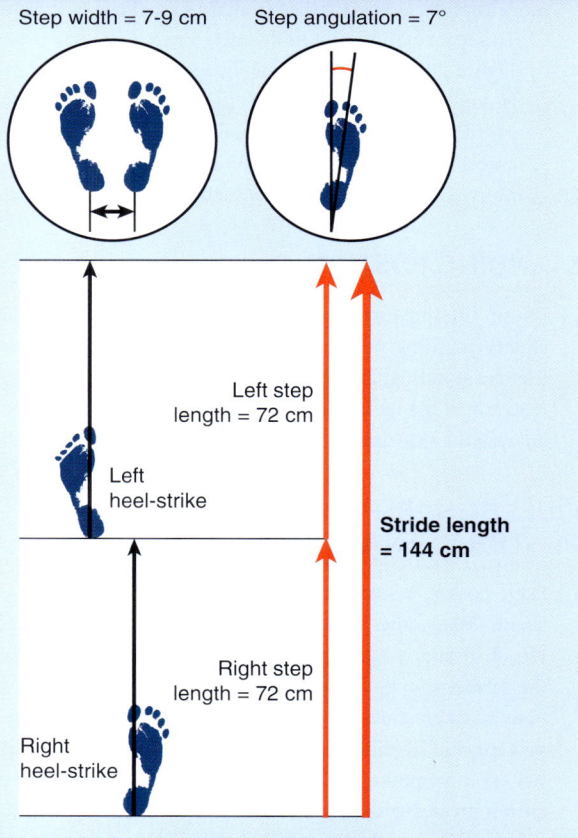

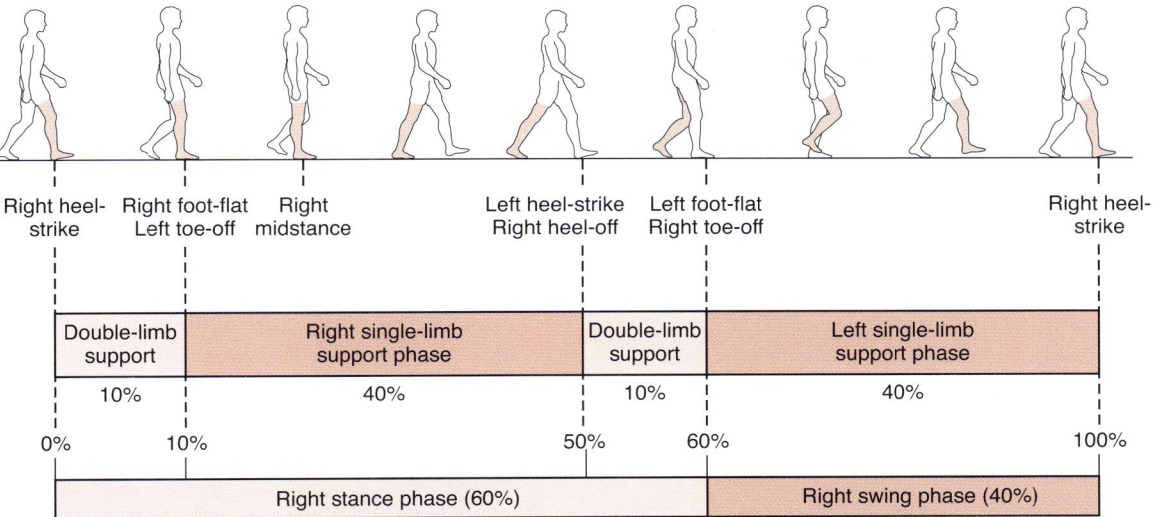

FIGURE 20-7 Gait cycle. The gait cycle begins with one heel-strike and ends with the same-side heel-strike. One gait cycle is composed of one stride, which in turn is composed of two steps. Phases and landmarks of the gait cycle. The gait cycle can be divided into two main phases: (1) the stance phase and (2) the swing phase. The stance phase is defined as when the foot is on the ground and accounts for 60% of the gait cycle for each foot; the swing phase is defined as when the foot is swinging in the air and accounts for 40% of the gait cycle for each foot. The period of double-limb support in which both feet are on the ground should be noted; walking is defined by the presence of double-limb support. The major landmarks of stance phase are heel-strike, foot-flat, midstance, heel-off, and toe-off. The swing phase is often divided into an early swing, midswing, and late swing. *(Modified from Cameron M, Monroe L: Physical rehabilitation: evidence-based examination, evaluation, and intervention, ed. 1, St. Louis, 2007, Saunders.)*

Stance Phase:

❍ Stance phase contains the following five landmarks of the gait cycle (Box 20-7).[1]
1. **Heel-strike** is defined as the moment that a person's heel strikes (i.e., makes contact with) the ground.
   Heel-strike is the landmark that begins stance phase (and ends swing phase).
2. **Foot-flat** is defined as the moment that the entire plantar surface of the foot comes into contact with the ground (i.e., the foot is flat).
3. **Midstance** is the midpoint of stance phase and occurs when the weight of the body is directly over the lower extremity. Midstance occurs when the greater trochanter is directly above the middle of the foot.
4. **Heel-off** is defined as the moment that the heel leaves the ground.
5. **Toe-off** is defined as the moment that a person's toes push off and leave the ground. Toe-off is the landmark that ends stance phase (and begins swing phase).

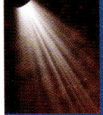

| BOX 20-7 | Spotlight on the Function of the Foot during the Gait Cycle |

When walking, the foot must be supple and flexible during the early stages of the stance cycle to adapt to the uneven surfaces of the ground. This requires the foot to be in its open-packed position, which is pronation (primarily composed of eversion). Pronation allows the arch structure to collapse, thus allowing the foot to adapt to the contour of the ground. However, during the later stages of the stance cycle when toeing-off (i.e., pushing off) the ground, the foot must be stiff and stable to propel the body forward. This requires the foot to be in its closed-packed position, which is supination (primarily composed of inversion). Supination holds the arches high and creates a more rigid, stable foot for propulsion. The ability of the foot to change from being supple (able to pronate) to rigid (held in supination) is largely created by the laxity/tautness of the plantar fascia of the foot. When the plantar fascia is taut, the arch structure is supported and the foot becomes somewhat rigid; when the plantar fascia is lax, the arch structure is more mobile and the foot becomes supple. The ability of the plantar fascia to change from being lax to being taut is created by the windlass mechanism (see Section 9.17). During the early stages of the stance cycle when the foot is in anatomic position, the plantar fascia is lax, resulting in a supple foot. However, during the later stages of the stance cycle when extension occurs at the metatarsophalangeal (MTP) joints, because of the windlass mechanism, the plantar fascia is pulled taut around these joints. The resulting tension in the plantar fascia is then transferred to the arch structure of the foot, causing it to rise, creating a rigid foot for propulsion. Thus the foot shifts between being supple and flexible during the early stance cycle to adapt to the ground, and being stable and rigid during the late stance cycle for propulsion.[7]

- Note: Although the order of landmarks of the stance phase of the gait cycle is classically considered to be heel-strike, foot-flat, midstance, heel-off, and toe-off, in that order, not all people walk in this pattern. Instead, some people reach out and begin stance phase with their toes contacting the ground before their heels.

Swing Phase:

- Swing phase begins with toe-off and ends with heel-strike.[1]
- Swing phase is often subdivided into three approximately equal sections: (1) **early swing**, (2) **midswing**, and (3) **late swing**.
- When analyzing gait, our first assumption might be that stance phase and swing phase each account for 50% of the gait cycle; however, this is not true. Stance phase of each foot actually accounts for 60% of the gait cycle, with the swing phase of that foot accounting for the other 40%. The reason for this is that a period of **double-limb support** exists in which both feet are in contact with the ground[1] (see Figure 20-7; Box 20-8).
- For therapists and trainers, knowledge of the gait cycle is important because it allows us to understand the demands placed on the musculature, joints, and other soft tissues of the lower extremity when walking.
- Lower extremity muscle contraction can generally be stated to occur during the gait cycle for three conceptual reasons: (1) muscles concentrically contract to create the motion needed during the gait cycle; (2) muscles eccentrically contract to decelerate the momentum motion of the gait cycle; and (3) muscles isometrically contract to stabilize and prevent motion of a body part.[12]
- During the early to middle stages of the stance phase, muscles of the lower extremity are primarily eccentrically contracting to slow the momentum of the body's movement. Furthermore, during the early to middle stages, joints of the foot must be sufficiently supple to both adapt to the uneven surfaces of the ground and to absorb the stresses of the foot striking the ground.
- During the middle to late stages of the stance phase, muscles of the lower extremity are primarily concentrically contracting to create the propulsion force of the body's movement. Furthermore, during the middle to late stages, the joints of the foot must be sufficiently rigid to be able to allow the foot to act as a rigid lever for propulsion of the body forward.

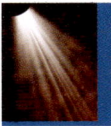

BOX 20-8 Spotlight on Walking versus Running

It is not the speed of movement that distinguishes walking from running, but the presence of double-limb support. By definition, walking has double-limb support and running does not. Interestingly, as a person speeds the pace of walking, the period of double-limb support grows increasingly smaller and smaller. At the moment that double-limb support disappears, by definition we are running.

SECTION 20.8   MUSCULAR ACTIVITY DURING THE GAIT CYCLE

- The patterns of muscular coordination that occur during the gait cycle can be quite complex. Although the entire body is involved in the gait cycle, we will limit our discussion to the functional muscle groups of the lower extremity.
- Understanding these conceptual roles can be very important when working with clients who are experiencing lower extremity problems, because improper mechanics during the gait cycle often lead to functional problems throughout the body. The best way to understand and assess the cause of these improper mechanics is to have a clear understanding of the proper mechanics of gait. Once a clear assessment has been made, appropriate treatment can be given.

Following are the three major conceptual roles of the musculature of the lower extremity during the gait cycle:

1. Muscles can contract concentrically to create (i.e., accelerate) a movement of the lower extremity.
2. Muscles can contract eccentrically to slow down (i.e., decelerate) a movement of the lower extremity.
3. Muscles can contract isometrically to stabilize (stop movement of) a body part.

Following is a survey of the major role(s) of the individual functional muscle groups of the lower extremity during the gait cycle. The role of the contraction of each of the major muscles of the lower extremity within the gait cycle has been determined by electromyography (EMG) (Box 20-9). (For each of these functional groups, please refer to Figure 20-8.)

BOX 20-9

Electromyography (EMG) is an assessment tool used to determine when a muscle is contracting. Because the contraction of a muscle involves a depolarization of the muscle's membrane, electricity is generated whenever a muscle contracts. That electricity can be measured by EMG. Two methods of EMG exist: one is to place surface electrodes on the skin that measure the electrical signal created by the muscles beneath them; for superficial muscles this method works fine. However, for deeper muscles, needle electrodes must be inserted into the musculature to elicit accurate results. With either method, the protocol of EMG is to put electrodes in place and then ask the person to carry out a specific movement pattern; based on the results of the EMG, it can be determined not only which muscles contracted during the movement pattern but also exactly when and how strongly each of the muscles contracted. Although analysis of a muscle's potential actions is possible based on an understanding of a muscle's line of pull relative to the joint it crosses, it does not tell us exactly which one of a number of possible muscles that have a particular joint action is recruited by the nervous system to contract during specific movement patterns. That information can be provided by EMG. For this reason, EMG is considered to be the most accurate means to determine the roles of muscles in movement patterns.

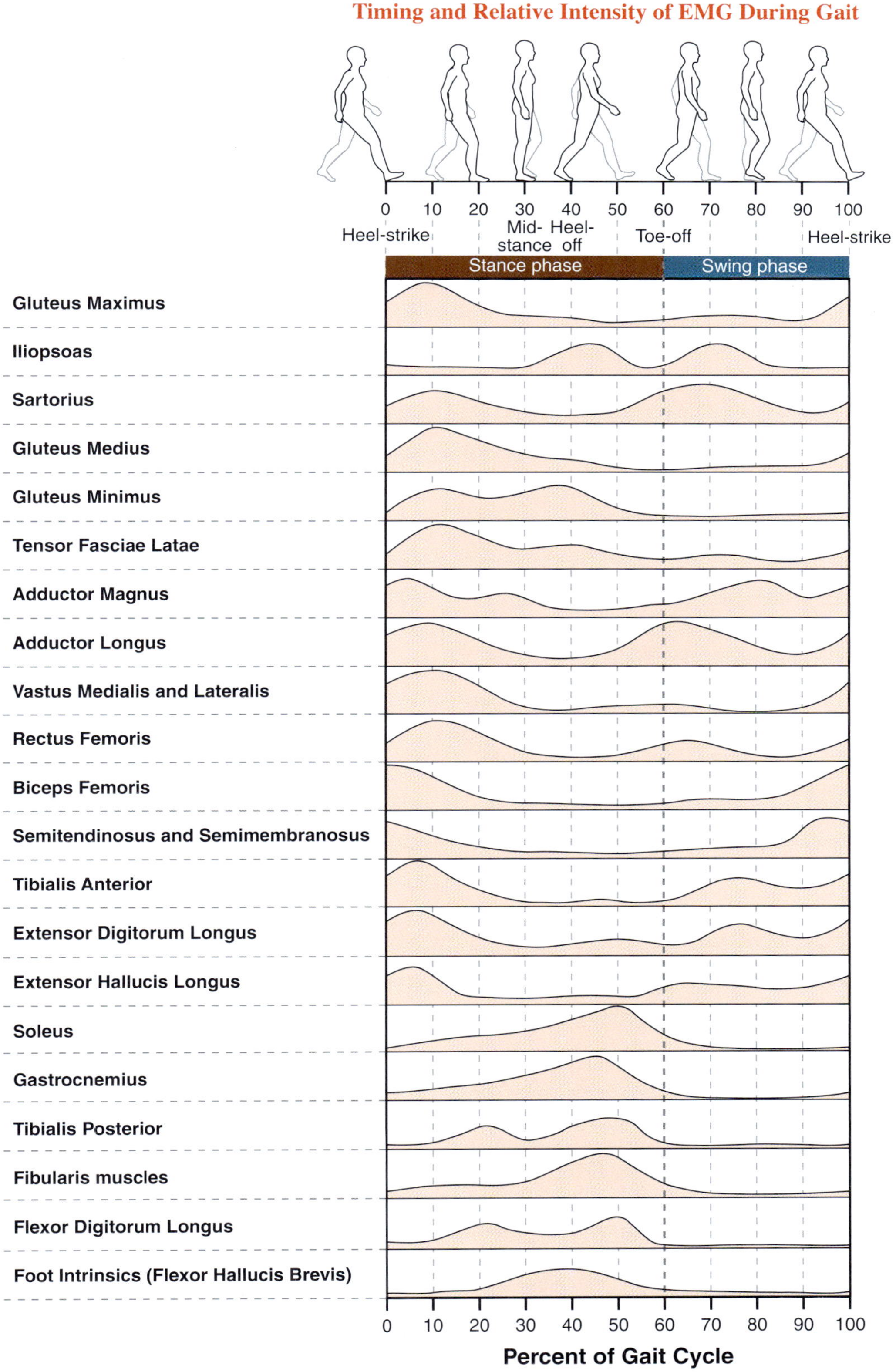

Timing and Relative Intensity of EMG During Gait

FIGURE 20-8 Intensity of the contractions of the major muscles of the lower extremity correlated with the phases and landmarks of the gait cycle, determined by electromyography (EMG). (Note: All references are for the right side.) *(Modified from Neumann DA:* Kinesiology of the musculoskeletal system: foundations for physical rehabilitation, *ed 2, St Louis, 2010, Mosby.)*

HIP JOINT FLEXOR MUSCLES:

○ Hip joint flexors have two roles during the gait cycle[7]:
  1. The primary role of hip joint flexors is to contract concentrically to create the forward swing of the lower extremity (i.e., flexion of the thigh at the hip joint) during the early aspect of the swing phase. Interestingly, contraction of the hip flexor muscle group is necessary only during the first half of the swing phase. This is because the second half of the swing phase is completed by momentum—in other words, swing phase is a ballistic motion.
  2. Hip joint flexors contract eccentrically to decelerate the extension of the thigh at the hip joint that is occurring between midstance and toe-off of the stance phase.
○ Major hip joint flexors are the iliopsoas, sartorius, and rectus femoris.

HIP JOINT EXTENSOR MUSCLES:

○ Hip joint extensors have two roles during the gait cycle[7]:
  1. Hip joint extensors contract eccentrically to decelerate the forward-swinging limb at the late aspect of the swing phase (i.e., their force of extension on the thigh at the hip joint slows down flexion of the thigh at the hip joint, which occurs during the swing phase).
  2. Hip joint extensors isometrically contract forcefully on heel-strike of the stance phase to stabilize the pelvis from anteriorly tilting at the hip joint (hip extensors are posterior tilters of the pelvis). This contraction is necessary to help prevent the pelvis and upper body from being thrown forward because of momentum when the lower extremity's forward movement is stopped by striking the ground.
○ Major hip joint extensors are the hamstrings (i.e., biceps femoris, semitendinosus, and semimembranosus) and the gluteus maximus.

HIP JOINT ABDUCTOR MUSCLES:

○ The role of the hip joint abductors during the gait cycle is primarily important with regard to their action on the pelvis, not the thigh.[7]
○ The major function of the hip joint abductors is to contract, creating a force of depression on the same-side pelvis during the stance phase of gait. They are particularly active during the first half of the stance phase, from heel-strike to midstance. By creating a force of depression on the pelvis on the stance (i.e., support) limb side, they stabilize the pelvis (and upper body), stopping it from depressing to the other side (i.e., the swing-limb side). Without this stabilization, the pelvis would fall toward the swing-limb side, because when the body is in single-limb support, the center of weight of the body is not balanced over the support limb but rather located over thin air, toward the swing-limb side.
○ Major hip joint abductors are the gluteus medius and gluteus minimus. The tensor fasciae latae, sartorius, and upper fibers of the gluteus maximus are also active as hip joint abductors.
○ Depression of the pelvis at the hip joint is the reverse action of abduction of the thigh at the hip joint. In other words, all thigh abductor musculature can either abduct the thigh or depress the same-side pelvis at the hip joint. This scenario illustrates the importance of understanding the concept of reverse actions. During the gait cycle, we are in stance phase (i.e., closed-chain with the distal attachments of muscles fixed) 60% of the time. Therefore lower limb reverse actions actually occur more frequently than what are considered to be lower limb standard actions. (For more details on the concept of reverse actions, see Section 6.29.)
○ As stabilizers (i.e., fixators) of the pelvis, the hip abductors are usually considered to contract isometrically. Actually, the pelvis is permitted to drop slightly toward the swing-limb side; therefore the hip abductor musculature's contraction is slightly eccentric.

HIP JOINT ADDUCTOR MUSCLES:

○ Hip joint adductors have two roles during the gait cycle[7]:
  1. Hip joint adductors contract at heel-strike. It is believed that this contraction aids the hip joint extensors' stabilization of the hip joint as the force of hitting the ground travels up through the lower extremity.
  2. Hip joint adductors contract again just after toe-off. This contraction most likely aids in flexion of the thigh at the hip joint.
○ Note: Generally the adductor muscle group has the ability to extend the thigh when it is flexed and flex the thigh when it is extended. Many muscles change their actions when their line of pull relative to the joint changes with a change in joint position. This is an example of why muscles' *anatomic actions* should not be memorized. (See Section 13.10 for an explanation of *anatomic actions*.) A muscle's action should be understood to be a function of its line of pull relative to the joint it crosses; if the joint position changes, the action of the muscle can change (see Section 13.10)!
○ Major hip joint adductors are the adductors longus, brevis, and magnus, as well as the pectineus and gracilis.

HIP JOINT MEDIAL ROTATOR MUSCLES:

○ Hip joint medial rotators are active during the stance phase of gait.[7]
○ During stance phase, the thigh is relatively fixed (because the foot is fixed to the floor) and the pelvis is mobile. Therefore the medial rotators of the hip joint perform their reverse action of ipsilateral rotation of the pelvis at the hip joint, pulling the entire pelvis forward. (Note: For the relationship between medial rotators of the thigh at the hip joint and ipsilateral rotators of the pelvis at the hip joint, see Section 9.7.) Ipsilateral rotation of the pelvis helps to advance the swing-limb forward.
○ Major hip joint medial rotators are the tensor fasciae latae and the anterior fibers of the gluteus medius and minimus.

HIP JOINT LATERAL ROTATOR MUSCLES:

○ Hip joint lateral rotators are primarily active during the stance phase of gait.[7]
○ Hip joint lateral rotators are believed to be important toward controlling the hip joint medial rotators' action on the pelvis (i.e., the hip joint lateral rotator muscles' action of contralateral rotation of the pelvis controls the ipsilateral rotation of the pelvis of the medial rotator muscles).

- Another function of the lateral rotators is to prevent excessive medial rotation of the thigh at the hip joint. This can occur if the client excessively pronates the foot at the subtalar joint on that side. With excessive pronation in stance phase, the calcaneus is somewhat fixed, requiring the talus to medially rotate. Because the ankle joint and extended knee joint do not allow rotation, this medial rotation of the talus carries the leg and thigh along with it, thereby transferring the medial rotation force all the way to the hip joint.
- The reverse action of lateral rotation of the thigh at the hip joint is contralateral rotation of the pelvis at the hip joint, which can be an important joint action in the stance phase (Box 20-10).
- Major hip joint lateral rotators are the gluteus maximus, the posterior fibers of the gluteus medius and minimus, and the deep lateral rotators of the thigh (piriformis, superior and inferior gemelli, obturators internus and externus, and quadratus femoris).

KNEE JOINT EXTENSOR MUSCLES:

- Knee joint extensors have two roles during the gait cycle[7]:
  1. Knee joint extensors contract concentrically at the end of swing phase to extend the leg at the knee joint and reach out with the leg in preparation for heel-strike.
  2. Knee joint extensors contract even more powerfully during the first half of the stance phase from heel-strike to midstance, to eccentrically contract and decelerate the knee joint flexion that occurs early in stance phase just after heel-strike (due to body weight moving forward on a fixed foot) and to then concentrically contract to create extension of the knee joint as we approach midstance.
- Major knee joint extensors are the quadriceps femoris group (i.e., vastus lateralis, vastus medialis, vastus intermedius, and rectus femoris [which is also a hip joint flexor]).

KNEE JOINT FLEXOR MUSCLES:

- Knee joint flexors have three roles during the gait cycle[7]:
  1. Knee joint flexors contract eccentrically to decelerate knee joint extension just before heel-strike.
  2. Knee joint flexors contract just after heel-strike. This may occur to stabilize the knee joint in the early stage of the stance phase.
  3. Knee joint flexors contract during the swing phase to keep the foot from dragging on the ground as the swing limb is brought forward.
- Major knee joint flexors are the hamstring muscles (i.e., biceps femoris, semitendinosus, and semimembranosus) and the gastrocnemius.

BOX 20-10

The reverse action of the lateral rotator muscles of the hip joint is contralateral rotation of the pelvis at the hip joint (see Section 9.7). Contralateral rotation of the pelvis is extremely important when **planting and cutting** in sports. Planting and cutting are done when a person plants a foot on the ground and then cuts (i.e., changes the direction in which he or she is running by turning the body to orient to the opposite side). For example, you plant your right foot and then turn to the left (see figure).

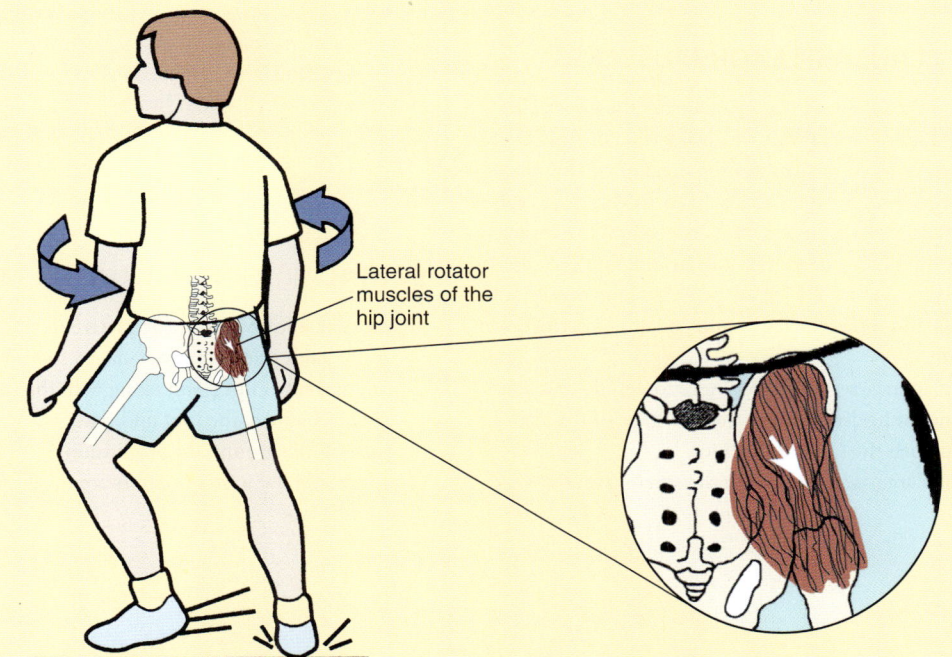

(Modified from Neumann DA: Kinesiology of the musculoskeletal system: foundations for physical rehabilitation, ed 2, St Louis, 2010, Mosby.)

- Note: Interpreting the role of the knee joint flexor musculature in the gait cycle can be difficult, because the hamstrings are also hip joint extensors.

ANKLE JOINT DORSIFLEXOR MUSCLES:

- Ankle joint dorsiflexors have two roles during the gait cycle[7]:
  1. Ankle joint dorsiflexors eccentrically contract to decelerate plantarflexion of the foot at the ankle joint during early stance phase between heel-strike and foot-flat. This allows the foot to be lowered to the ground in a controlled and graceful manner as the body weight transfers over the stance limb (Box 20-11).
  2. Ankle joint dorsiflexors contract concentrically during the swing phase of the gait cycle. This is necessary to create dorsiflexion of the foot at the ankle joint to keep the toes from scraping on the ground as the swing limb is brought forward.
- Major ankle joint dorsiflexors are the muscles of the anterior compartment of the leg (i.e., tibialis anterior, extensor digitorum longus, extensor hallucis longus, fibularis tertius).

BOX 20-11

If the foot is not brought to the ground in a controlled and graceful manner at the beginning of the stance phase, it is called **foot slap**, named for the characteristic slapping noise that the foot makes as it impacts the ground. Foot slap is usually caused by nerve compression on the nerve segments of the deep fibular nerve (a branch of the sciatic nerve) that provides motor innervation to the muscles of the anterior compartment of the leg, in other words, the dorsiflexors of the foot at the ankle joint.[7]

ANKLE JOINT PLANTARFLEXOR MUSCLES:

- Ankle joint plantarflexors have two roles during the gait cycle[7]:
  1. Ankle joint plantarflexors eccentrically contract during most of the stance phase to decelerate dorsiflexion of the ankle joint. However, because the foot is fixed to the floor, this force of plantarflexion is necessary to decelerate the reverse action of the leg moving anteriorly toward the foot (i.e., dorsiflexion or extension of the leg at the ankle joint). Without this plantarflexion force, the leg would collapse anteriorly at the ankle joint.
  2. Ankle joint plantarflexors contract more forcefully in a concentric manner at heel-off during the late stage of the stance phase to help push the foot off the floor.
- Major ankle joint plantarflexors are the gastrocnemius and soleus.

SUBTALAR JOINT SUPINATOR MUSCLES:

- Subtalar joint supinators have two roles during the gait cycle[7]:
  1. Subtalar joint supinators contract eccentrically during the stance phase from heel-strike to foot-flat to decelerate pronation of the foot at the subtalar joint. Note: During this phase of the gait cycle, pronation of the foot at the subtalar joint is a passive process caused by the body weight moving over the arch of the foot and is necessary to collapse the arch and allow it to adapt to the uneven contour of the ground.
  2. Subtalar joint supinators then concentrically contract between foot-flat and toe-off to supinate the foot at the subtalar joint.
- Major subtalar joint supinators are the tibialis posterior, tibialis anterior, flexor digitorum longus, flexor hallucis longus, and intrinsic muscles of the foot (Box 20-12).
- Note: As a group, intrinsic muscles of the foot are credited with supporting the arch structure of the foot. Because excessive pronation involves a collapse of the medial longitudinal arch of the foot, intrinsic muscles of the foot are considered to be supinators and active in preventing excessive pronation of the foot. However, when shoes are worn all day, much of the need for intrinsic foot muscles to contract is lost, and these muscles often weaken. Weakness of the intrinsic muscles of the foot may add to the propensity of a person to develop the postural distortion pattern of a collapsed arch, in other words excessive pronation.

BOX 20-12

A person with an excessively pronated foot will often overwork the foot supinators, trying to counter the tendency to overly pronate when weight bearing. As a result, pain may develop in the supinator muscles, especially the tibialis posterior and/or tibialis anterior. This condition is often called **shin splints**. The term **anterior shin splints** is often applied when the tibialis anterior is involved, and the term **posterior shin splints** is often used when the tibialis posterior is involved.[13]

SUBTALAR JOINT PRONATOR MUSCLES:

- Subtalar joint pronators are active during the later stance phase of the gait cycle, from foot-flat to toe-off.[7] They are believed to co-contract at this point along with the subtalar joint supinators to help stabilize the foot and make it more rigid as it readies to push off the ground for propulsion.
- Major subtalar joint pronators are the fibularis longus and brevis.

REVIEW QUESTIONS

Answers to the following review questions appear on the Evolve website accompanying this book at: http://evolve.elsevier.com/Muscolino/kinesiology/.

1. Define "good posture" and "bad posture."

2. What is the definition of a *stressor*?

3. A posterior view plumb line analysis is best for assessing a postural distortion in what plane?

4. List the landmarks used for doing a lateral view plumb line analysis of posture.

5. Give an example of a frontal plane postural distortion and a sagittal plane postural distortion.

6. Explain how the concept of center of weight is important to posture.

7. Define the term *secondary postural distortion*, and give an example of a secondary postural distortion.

8. Give two examples of why a client might have a high right shoulder.

9. List three general principles of compensation within the body.

10. Give one example of an agonist/antagonist pair.

11. Explain how the spine might compensate for a low iliac crest height.

12. Why is it that use of a plumb line is not effective when assessing transverse plane postural distortions?

13. What are the two main phases of the gait cycle?

14. What are the five main landmarks of the gait cycle?

15. Define and describe *double-limb support*.

16. What is the role of foot pronation when the foot is on the ground during the gait cycle?

17. How are the lateral rotators of the thigh at the hip joint involved in planting and cutting?

18. What is the major role of the hip joint abductors during the gait cycle?

REFERENCES

1. Oatis CA: Kinesiology: The mechanics and pathomechanics of human movement, Philadelphia, 2004, Lippincott Williams & Wilkins.
2. Spirduso WW, Francis KL, MacRae PG: Physical dimensions of aging, ed 3, Champaign, IL, 2005, Human Kinetics.
3. Loudon JK, Manske RC, Reiman MP: Clinical mechanics and kinesiology, Champaign, IL, 2013, Human Kinetics.
4. Shultz SJ, Houglum PA, Perrin DH: Examination of musculoskeletal injuries, ed 4, Champaign, IL, 2015, Human Kinetics.
5. Page P, Frank CC, Lardner R: Assessment and treatment of muscle imbalance: The Janda approach, Champaign, IL, 2010, Human Kinetics.
6. Simancek J: Deep tissue massage treatment, ed 2, St Louis, 2013, Elsevier.
7. Neumann DA: Kinesiology of the musculoskeletal system: Foundations for physical rehabilitation, ed 3, St Louis, 2017, Elsevier.
8. King MA: Static postural assessment. In Clark MA, Lucette SC, editors: NASM essentials of corrective exercise training, Baltimore, 2011, Lippincott Williams & Wilkins, pp 92-104.
9. Baechle TR, Earle RW, Wathen D: Resistance training. In Baechle TR, Earle RE, editors: Essentials of strength training and conditioning, ed 3, Champaign, IL, 2008, Human Kinetics.
10. Hamilton N, Weimar W, Luttgens K: Kinesiology: Scientific basis of human motion, ed 12, New York, 2012, McGraw Hill.
11. Froehle AW, Nahhas RW, Sherwood RH, et al: Age-related changes in spatiotemporal characteristics of gait accompanying ongoing lower limb linear growth in late childhood and early adolescence. Gait Posture 38(1):14-19, 2012.
12. Shumway-Cook A, Woolacott MH: Motor control: Translating research into clinical practice, ed 4, Baltimore, 2012, Lippincott Williams & Wilkins.
13. Werner R: A massage therapist's guide to pathology, ed 4, Philadelphia, 2004, Lippincott Williams & Wilkins.

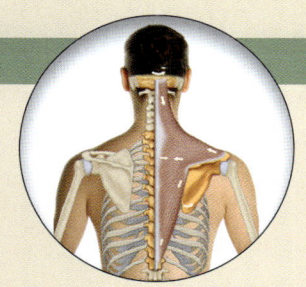

CHAPTER 21
Common Postural Distortion Patterns

CHAPTER OUTLINE

Section 21.1	Lower Crossed Syndrome		Section 21.10	Rigid High Arch
Section 21.2	Rounded Low Back/Pelvis		Section 21.11	Hallux Valgus
Section 21.3	Upper Crossed Syndrome		Section 21.12	Hammertoes
Section 21.4	Flat Back		Section 21.13	Morton's Foot
Section 21.5	Elevated/Depressed Pelvis		Section 21.14	Genu Valgum/Genu Varum
Section 21.6	Scoliosis		Section 21.15	Genu Recurvatum
Section 21.7	Elevated Shoulder Girdle		Section 21.16	Pigeon-toe/Toe-in
Section 21.8	Pelvic/Spinal Rotational Distortion		Section 21.17	Cubitus Valgus
Section 21.9	Overpronation			

CHAPTER OBJECTIVES

After completing this chapter, the student should be able to perform the following:

1. Define the key terms of this chapter and state the meanings of the word origins of this chapter.
2. Discuss the definition, etiology, effects, and treatment approach for lower crossed syndrome.
3. Discuss the definition, etiology, effects, and treatment approach for rounded low back/pelvis.
4. Discuss the definition, etiology, effects, and treatment approach for upper crossed syndrome.
5. Discuss the definition, etiology, effects, and treatment approach for flat back.
6. Discuss the definition, etiology, effects, and treatment approach for elevated/depressed pelvis.
7. Discuss the definition, etiology, effects, and treatment approach for scoliosis.
8. Discuss the definition, etiology, effects, and treatment approach for elevated shoulder girdle.
9. Discuss the definition, etiology, effects, and treatment approach for pelvic/spinal rotational distortion.
10. Discuss the definition, etiology, effects, and treatment approach for overpronation.
11. Discuss the definition, etiology, effects, and treatment approach for rigid high arch, hallux valgus, hammertoes, Morton's foot, genu valgus/genu varum, genu recurvatum, pigeon-toe/toe-in, and cubitus valgus.

OVERVIEW

Chapter 20 covered the topic of posture, addressing the concepts of postural distortion patterns, including postural compensations patterns in the body. This chapter now covers the more common postural distortion patterns found in the human body. We begin with the major dysfunctional patterns of the pelvis and spine, then focus on the lower extremity, and conclude with the upper extremity. For each condition, the definition, etiology (in other words the cause[s]), effects, and treatment approach for manual/movement therapy are discussed.

Although each postural distortion pattern is covered separately in its own section, it is important to keep in mind that each dysfunctional pattern has close- and far-reaching effects throughout the body; indeed, one dysfunctional pattern often predisposes or causes the body to experience other dysfunctional distortion patterns. For this reason, understanding the inter-relationships between these patterns is extremely important.

KEY TERMS

Adaptive shortening
Bowleg
Bunion
C curve
Carrying angle
Clubfoot
Collapsed arch
Cubitus valgus (CUE-bi-tus VAL-gus)
Cubitus varum (CUE-bi-tus VAR-um)
Depressed pelvis
Double S curve
Dropped arch
Elevated pelvis
Elevated shoulder girdle
Excessive anterior tilt of the pelvis
Femoral torsion
Flat back
Flat foot
Forefoot varus (VAR-us)
Forward head carriage
Genu recurvatum (JEN-you REE-ker-VAT-um)
Genu valgum (JEN-you VAL-gum)
Genu valgus (JEN-you VAL-gus)
Genu varum (JEN-you VAR-um)
Genu varus (JEN-you VAR-us)
Greek foot
Hallux valgus (HAL-uks VAL-gus)
Hammertoes
High arch
Hiking of the hip
Hyperkyphotic thoracic spine (HI-per-ki-FOT-ik thor-AS-ik)
Hyperlordotic lumbar spine (HI-per-lor-DOT-ik LUM-bar)
Hyperlordotic upper cervical spine (HI-per-lor-DOT-ik, SERV-i-kul)
Hypolordotic cervical spine (HI-po-lor-DOT-ik, SERV-i-kul)
Hypolordotic lower cervical spine (HI-po-lor-DOT-ik, SERV-i-kul)
Hypolordotic lumbar spine (HI-po-lor-DOT-ik, LUM-bar)
Hypokyphotic thoracic spine (HI-po-ki-FOT-ik, thor-AS-ik)
Idiopathic scoliosis (ID-ee-o-PATH-ik SKO-lee-os-is)
Interdigital neuroma (noor-O-ma)
Knock-knees
Kyphotic lumbar spine (ki-FOT-ik LUM-bar)
Lower crossed syndrome
Metatarsus adductus (MET-a-TARS-us ad-DUK-tus)
Metatarsus varus (MET-a-TARS-us VAR-us)
Military neck
Morton's foot
Morton's toe
Morton's metatarsalgia (MET-a-tars-AL-ja)
Morton's neuroma (noor-O-ma)
Overpronation (OV-er-pro-NAY-shun)
Oversupination (OV-er-SUE-pin-A-shun)
Pelvic/spinal rotational distortion
Pes cavus (PEZ CAVE-us)
Pes planus (PEZ PLANE-us)
Pigeon-toe
Posteriorly tilted pelvis
Protracted head (PRO-tract-ed)
Protracted shoulder girdles (PRO-tract-ed)
Rib hump
Rigid flat foot
Rigid high arch
Rounded low back/pelvis
Rounded shoulders
S curve
Scoliosis (SKO-lee-os-is)
Short leg
Supple flat foot
Swayback
Tibial torsion
Toe-in
Upper crossed syndrome

WORD ORIGINS

- Cubitus—From Latin *cubitus,* meaning *forearm, elbow*
- Genu—From Latin *genu,* meaning *knee*
- Hallux—From Latin *hallex,* meaning *big toe*
- Hyper—From Greek *hyper,* meaning *above, over*
- Hypo—From Greek *hupo,* meaning *under*
- Idiopathic—From Greek *idios,* meaning *private,* denoting *unknown;* and *pathos,* meaning *feeling, suffering*
- Kyphotic—From Greek *kyphosis,* meaning *bent, humpback*
- Lordotic—From Greek *lordosis,* meaning *a bending backward*
- Recurvatum—From Latin *recurvare,* meaning *to bend back*
- Scoliosis—From Greek *scoliosis,* meaning *curvature, crooked*
- Valgus—From Latin *valgus,* meaning *twisted, bent outward, bowlegged*
- Varum—From Latin *varum,* meaning *crooked, bent inward, knock-kneed*

CHAPTER 21 Common Postural Distortion Patterns

SECTION 21.1 LOWER CROSSED SYNDROME

DEFINITION

○ **Lower crossed syndrome** (LCS) refers to the characteristic sagittal plane postural dysfunction of the lumbopelvic region in which the client exhibits **excessive anterior tilt of the pelvis** and a **hyperlordotic lumbar spine**.[1] This term was coined by Vladimir Janda, a respected Czech neurologist and rehabilitation therapist. LCS is so named because an "X" (in other words a cross) can be placed against the lower body (lumbar spine and pelvis). One arm of the cross represents the two overly facilitated ("tight") groups of anterior pelvic tilt musculature (the hip flexors and low back extensors) and the other arm of the cross represents the two overly inhibited ("weak") groups of posterior pelvic tilt musculature (hip extensors and trunk flexors) (Figure 21-1). The resultant imbalance of anterior/posterior tilt musculature results in the postural dysfunctional pattern of excessive anterior pelvic tilt, which then results in compensatory hyperlordosis of the lumbar spine. Note: Excessive anterior tilt of the pelvis accompanied by hyperlordosis of the lumbar spine is sometimes described as *swayback*.[2] However, the use of this term can be misleading because it is also sometimes used to describe a rounded low back/pelvis (excessive posterior tilt of the pelvis accompanied by kyphosis of the lumbar spine).

ETIOLOGY

○ As stated, the major cause of LCS is an imbalance of sagittal plane anterior tilt and posterior tilt musculature of the pelvis, such that the anterior pelvic tilt musculature is tighter, creating a greater pulling force at baseline tone than the posterior tilt musculature. The anterior tilters are described as being overly facilitated[1] and are locked short.[3] But even the lengthened weaker posterior tilt muscles may tighten in an attempt to oppose the locked short muscles. For this reason, they may be described as being locked long.[3] The net result of these pulling forces is excessive anterior tilt of the pelvis. There are two major groups that create pelvic anterior tilt: hip flexors and low back extensors[2]; and there are two major groups that create pelvic posterior tilt: hip extensors and anterior abdominal wall musculature[2] (Box 21-1). It should be noted that both locked short and locked

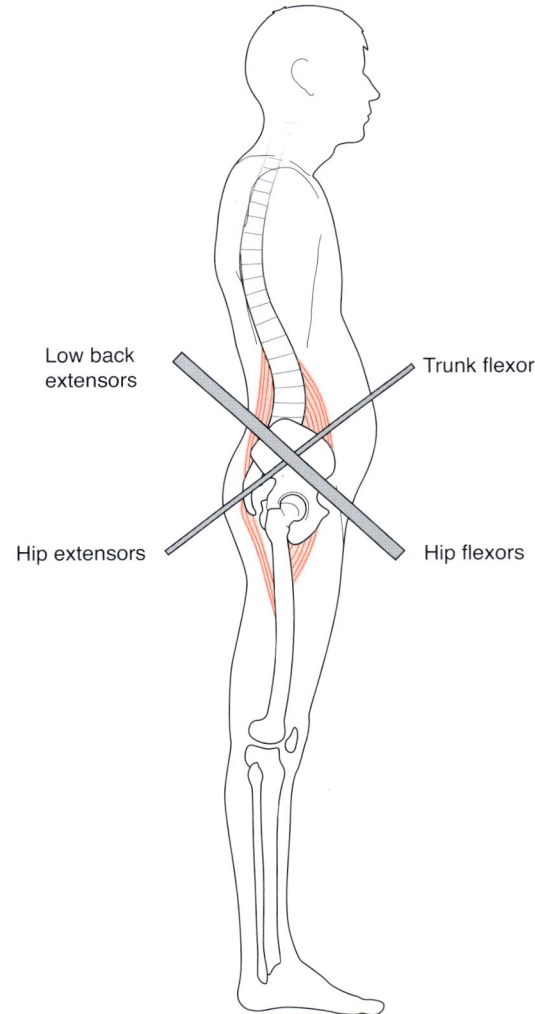

Figure 21-1 Lower crossed syndrome is a sagittal plane postural distortion pattern of the pelvis and lumbar spine that usually has repercussions into the upper body. *Adapted from Chaitow L:* Muscle energy techniques, *ed 4, Edinburgh, 2013, Elsevier, Ltd.*

BOX 21-1 Sagittal plane tilters of the pelvis[4]

Anterior Tilters (Overly Facilitated/Locked Short)
Hip flexors:
○ Gluteus minimus (anterior fibers)
○ Gluteus medius (anterior fibers)
○ Tensor fasciae latae
○ Rectus femoris
○ Sartorius
○ Iliacus
○ Psoas major
○ Pectineus
○ Adductor longus
○ Gracilis
○ Adductor brevis
○ Adductor magnus (anterior head)

Low back (trunk) extensors:
○ Quadratus lumborum
○ Iliocostalis
○ Longissimus
○ Multifidus

Posterior Tilters (Overly Inhibited/Locked Long)
Hip extensors:
○ Gluteus maximus
○ Gluteus medius (posterior fibers)
○ Gluteus minimus (posterior fibers)
○ Semitendinosus
○ Semimembranosus
○ Biceps femoris (long head)
○ Adductor magnus (posterior head)

Anterior abdominal wall (trunk flexors):
○ Rectus abdominis
○ External abdominal oblique
○ Internal abdominal oblique

long muscles end up being both overly tight and being weakened with regard to their ability to contract with force.[3]

- Hip flexor musculature tends to become tight because of the excessive amount of time that we spend seated. Seated position shortens and slackens hip flexor musculature, which then adaptively shortens and becomes locked short (Box 21-2). When hip flexor musculature becomes tight, it does not result in flexion of the thigh at the hip joint. Rather, its tension plays out upon the pelvis, pulling the pelvis into anterior tilt.[2] Similarly, low back extensor musculature tends to become tight because it must eccentrically contract whenever we bend our trunk forward, isometrically contract when we hold forward bent positions, and concentrically contract when returning from forward bent posture. Excessive use of the low back extensors both pulls the lumbar spine into extension and anteriorly tilts the pelvis.

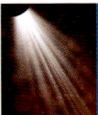

BOX 21-2   Spotlight on Adaptive Shortening

Adaptive shortening is the term that describes the concept that when a soft tissue is kept in a shortened position for a long period of time, it adapts to that shortened position by increasing its tension/tautness.[5] Applying this concept to musculature, if a muscle is kept in a shortened state for an extended period of time, even if it is relaxed and slackened in this shortened state, it will increase its baseline contractile tension (tone) and become less flexible. This change in tension occurs due to the central nervous system so that the muscle will be responsive if ordered to contract by the nervous system. This is important because if the muscle is slackened, then when the nervous system orders it to contract, the slack will have to be taken out before its contraction will result in a pulling force on its attachment and therefore movement of the body part. This delay in movement can mean the difference between life and death in physically threatening circumstances. For this reason, a shortened slackened muscle will become a shortened tightened muscle, in other words, a locked-short muscle. One very common example of this in the human body is the hip joint flexor musculature; spending prolonged periods of time sitting with the hip joints in a position of flexion often results in adaptive shortening of the hip flexor musculature. If musculature or any soft tissue is left shortened for long periods of time, fascial adhesions will also accumulate, resulting in further adaptive shortening.

- This can be contrasted with hip extensors, largely composed of gluteal musculature, which is commonly weak,[6] and anterior abdominal wall musculature, which is also commonly weak. The sum total of tight anterior tilt musculature with weak posterior tilt musculature is an excessively anteriorly tilted pelvis. (Note: an ideal "neutral" pelvis is generally described as having a sacral base angle of approximately 30 degrees; an excessively anteriorly tilted pelvis would have a sacral base angle of greater than 30 degrees[2]—see Section 9.8.)
- Because the pelvis is the base upon which the spine sits, if the pelvis is excessively anteriorly tilted, the lumbar spine must compensate by increasing its lordotic curve of extension to bring the upper body back to level; it is important for the eyes and inner ears to be level for proprioception.
- Other contributory causes of lower crossed syndrome are excessive body weight carried in the abdominal area[7] (for example, pregnancy or increased abdominal fat), which pulls the lumbar lordotic curve forward and down, hyperextension of the knee joint[1] (when the knee joint hyperextends, the femoral heads are pushed anteriorly, thereby pushing the pelvis anteriorly, predisposing anterior tilt), and postural compensation when wearing high-heeled shoes[8] (Box 21-3).

EFFECTS

- The effects of lower crossed syndrome are many. Excessive anterior tilt posture of the pelvis perpetuates locked-short hip flexors and low back extensors as well as locked-long hip extensors and trunk flexors of the anterior abdominal wall. Locked muscles, especially locked short muscles, often experience pain. If the psoas major becomes tight and painful, it can also increase compression upon the lumbar spinal joints. Locked musculature, both short and long, usually becomes weak[1] (as per the length-tension relationship curve—see Section 17.5). Weak muscles tend to be less effective at being able to respond to the demands placed upon them. As a result, they may become overworked and strained, often developing myofascial trigger points.
- It is interesting to note that not only does knee joint hyperextension (a postural distortion pattern known as genu recurvatum; see Section 21.15) create excessive anterior tilt of the pelvis, but excessive pelvic anterior tilt also predisposes the knee joint to fall into hyperextension. In closed chain kinematics, when the pelvis falls into anterior tilt, it pushes posteriorly on the femoral heads, pushing the femurs posteriorly, thereby pushing the knee joint into hyperextension.
- Further, given that a strong anterior abdominal wall assists in stabilizing the lumbar spine,[8] weakened anterior abdominal wall musculature would be less able to stabilize the spine, possibly resulting in long-term low back injury or dysfunction. The hyperlordotic lumbar curve characteristic of lower crossed syndrome also shifts weight bearing in the spine posteriorly onto the facet joints. This can result in excessive compression upon the lumbar facet joints, which can lead to facet syndrome and perhaps early onset of degenerative osteoarthritic changes.[2] Of course, if weight bearing is shifted onto the facet joints, it is commensurately decreased upon the disc joints; this could be considered to be a somewhat positive effect of a hyperlordotic lumbar spine. Increased extension of the lumbar spine also decreases the size of the intervertebral foramina, possibly causing compression of a spinal nerve. And finally, when the lumbar spine is hyperlordotic, the thoracic spine begins is curvature oriented excessively posterior, requiring an excessive kyphotic curve of flexion to return the center of weight of the upper trunk back to neutral. Thoracic hyperkyphosis then often results in hypolordosis of the lower cervical spine, hyperlordosis of the upper cervical spine, and forward (protracted) head carriage, along with the sequelae of these conditions (see Section 21.3 on upper crossed syndrome).

TREATMENT APPROACH

- The manual and movement therapy treatment approach for LCS is primarily to stretch and relax anterior pelvic tilt musculature and strengthen posterior pelvic tilt musculature.[1]

BOX 21-3 — High-Heeled Shoes

- Wearing high-heeled shoes creates many sagittal plane distortions and is perhaps one of the worst offenders to posture, because high-heeled shoes begin their effects at the very foundation of the body; the sequelae then occur all the way up the body

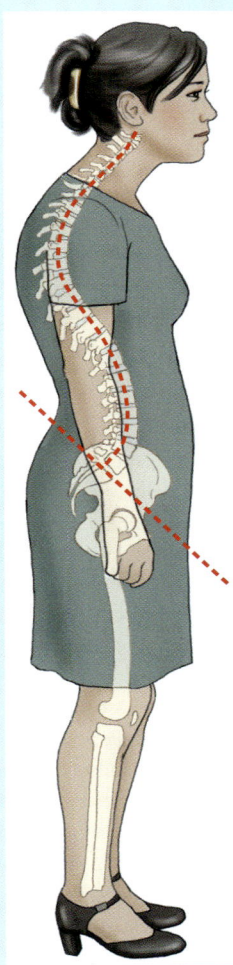

- High-heeled shoes place the foot into plantarflexion, which is an unstable position for the ankle and subtalar joints, increasing the chance of sprain.[8]
- With elevation of the heels, more body weight is shifted anteriorly on the foot. The ability of the transverse arch of the foot to absorb this weight bearing is overcome, and the arch weakens and splays out, resulting in a widening of the forefoot. If the shoe is too tight, this then pushes the proximal phalanx of the big toe laterally, resulting in hallux valgus.
- Loss of the transverse arch of the foot is usually accompanied by loss of both longitudinal arches of the foot. This then leads to increased tension forces placed on the plantar fascia, increasing the likelihood of plantar fasciitis and a calcaneal heel spur.
- Furthermore, because of the position of plantarflexion, the plantarflexor musculature becomes shortened and tightened, and the dorsiflexor musculature becomes lengthened and weakened. This often results in spasms in the gastrocnemius and soleus muscles. Ironically, because of the plantarflexor shortening, women who wear high-heeled shoes often complain of pain when they do wear flat shoes because the plantarflexors are so tight that they cannot stretch sufficiently when the person is in flats. As a result, many of these people continue to wear high-heeled shoes, erroneously believing that high-heeled shoes are better for the body than flats because the flats cause immediate pain! The remedy is to gradually switch the client from wearing higher-heeled shoes to lower high-heeled shoes, and eventually to flats over a period of months, if not a year or more.
- Moving up the body, when high-heeled shoes are worn, the body weight is thrown forward because wearing high-heeled shoes is effectively like standing on a surface that is a steep downgrade. As a result, the trunk will fall into flexion if the body weight is not brought back to be balanced over the lower extremities. This is often accomplished by increasing the anterior tilt of the pelvis, which results in an increased lordotic curve of the low back (lower crossed syndrome) and the compensatory patterns that ensue due to that (often upper crossed syndrome with its resultant effects). Thus wearing high-heeled shoes often results in foot problems, lower crossed syndrome and upper crossed syndrome.
- Note: If a client feels that high-heeled shoes must be worn, then a healthier way to compensate for high-heeled shoes is to bring the body weight backward by posteriorly tilting the pelvis, which avoids the increased lumbar lordosis with all of the unhealthy effects that would follow. However, depending upon the height of the heels, this may lead to an unhealthy posterior tilt of the pelvis with the effects of that postural distortion pattern (rounded low back). However, regardless of the compensation for the spine, all the unhealthy effects to the lower extremity from wearing high-heeled shoes remain.

SECTION 21.2 ROUNDED LOW BACK/PELVIS

DEFINITION

○ A **rounded low back/pelvis** is marked by a **posteriorly tilted pelvis** with a **kyphotic lumbar spine**[2] (Figure 21-2). This postural dysfunction is extremely important because it is occurring more and more frequently in recent years. Note: Rounded low back/pelvis is sometimes described as "swayback." However, the use of this term can be misleading because swayback is also sometimes used to describe the posture of an excessively anteriorly tilted pelvis with a hyperlordotic lumbar spine (in other words, the posture involved in lower crossed syndrome).

ETIOLOGY

○ The most common cause of a kyphotic lumbar spine is a collapsing of the low back and pelvis into flexion to round forward when working down in front of oneself. This condition is becoming extremely common in recent years due to the increased use of digital devices such as laptop computers, tablets, and smart phones (see Figure 21-2). A rounded low back/pelvis can also be caused by excessively tight hamstrings.[6] Hamstrings are posterior tilt musculature of the pelvis. If they are tight, they can pull the pelvis into posterior tilt, which then results in lumbar kyphosis, hence rounded low back.

EFFECTS

○ Rounded low back/pelvis shifts the weight bearing of the lumbar spine anteriorly, which increases compression upon the intervertebral discs.[2] This drives the nucleus pulposus posteriorly into the posterior annular fibers as they are being pulled taut and subjected to increased tension due to the position of flexion. These factors increase the likelihood of pathologic disc changes, resulting in disc bulging and/or herniation. Of course, if weight is shifted anteriorly, it is shifted off of the facet joints, resulting in an unloading of the facet joints. This could be considered to be a positive effect. But this posture places the facet joints into a position of flexion, which is an open-packed unstable position for the joints.[2] Decreased stability may predispose toward increased aberrant motions of these joints with resultant degenerative osteoarthritic changes. Another effect is that lumbar spine flexion results in increased size of the lumbar intervertebral foramina, which could help to decrease pressure upon a nerve in the intervertebral foramina.

TREATMENT APPROACH

○ The manual and movement therapy treatment approach for rounded low back/pelvis should be two-pronged. First, the client must be counseled to change their postural patterns so that they do not collapse into the dysfunctional posture.[8] Using lumbar support pillows and avoiding use of digital devices down in front of them is key. Second, strengthening the low back extensor musculature is important to prevent the collapse of the lumbar spine into flexion and pelvis into posterior tilt; and, if needed, stretching/loosening the hamstring musculature is important.[2]

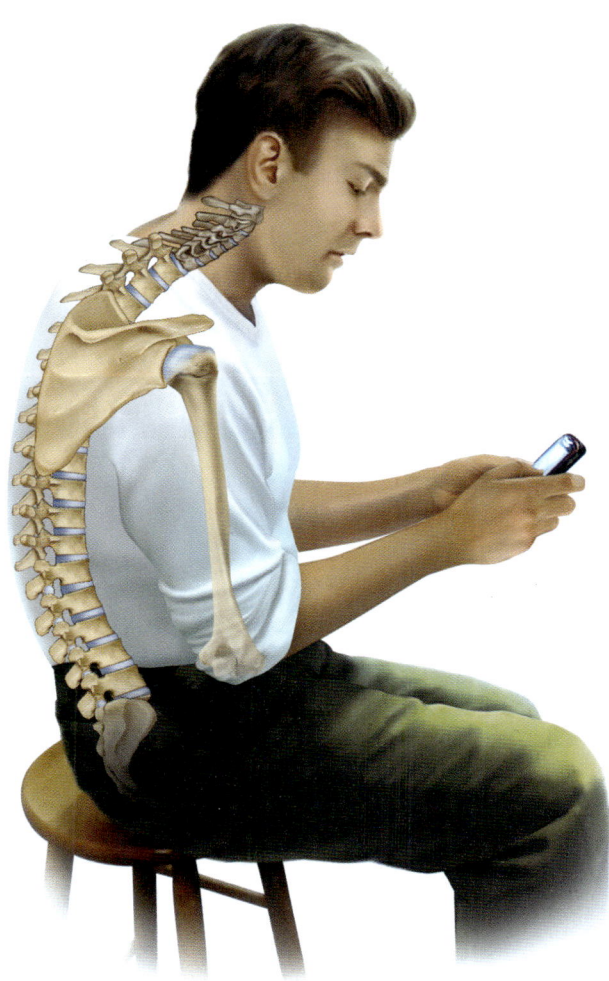

Figure 21-2 Rounded low back/pelvis is a sagittal plane distortion pattern of the thoracolumbar spine that involves kyphosis of the lumbar spine and hyperkyphosis of the thoracic spine. *(From Muscolino JE: The Price of Smart Phones, Massage Ther J Winter 2015:17–24. Illustration by Giovanni Rimasti.)*

SECTION 21.3 UPPER CROSSED SYNDROME

DEFINITION

- **Upper crossed syndrome** (UCS), like lower crossed syndrome, is a postural dysfunctional pattern that was named by Vladimir Janda, the Czech neurologist and rehabilitation therapist. Upper crossed syndrome involves a **hyperkyphotic thoracic spine** (at the spinal joints) with **protracted shoulder girdles** (scapulae and clavicles protracted at the scapulocostal and sternoclavicular joints; also known as **rounded shoulders**) and medial rotation of the arms[1] (humeri at the glenohumeral joints). As a result of the thoracic hyperkyphosis, UCS also involves a **hypolordotic lower cervical spine** with **hyperlordotic upper cervical spine** and a **protracted head**[1] (**forward head carriage**). UCS is so named because an "X" (in other words a cross) can be placed against the upper body (upper trunk, neck, and head). One arm of the cross represents the two overly facilitated ("tight") groups of trunk flexor/shoulder girdle protractor/glenohumeral medial rotation musculature and cervicocranial extensor musculature; and the other arm of the cross represents the two overly inhibited ("weak") groups of trunk extensor/shoulder girdle retractor/glenohumeral joint lateral rotator musculature and deep neck flexors (Figure 21-3). The resultant imbalance of musculature results in the postural dysfunctional pattern found in this condition. UCS is an extremely prevalent condition, and only becoming more so with the increased use of handheld digital devices such as smart phones.[9]

ETIOLOGY

- Similar to rounded low back, UCS is primarily caused by poor posture, especially postures that involve working down in front of ourselves, whether it is reading and writing involved with deskwork, computer work, working with a digital device, or any task that involves working down in front. UCS can also be caused by both lower crossed syndrome and rounded low back/pelvis postural distortion patterns[1] (see Sections 21-1 and 21-2).
- Once the thoracic spine begins to round forward into hyperkyphosis, and the shoulder girdles and arms collapse forward and medially, gravity further aggravates the problem (Box 21-4). Then as the posture is assumed for longer periods of time, the anterior chest musculature becomes overly facilitated and locked short, and the posterior upper back and scapular musculature becomes overly inhibited and locked long (Box 21-5).

EFFECTS

- The effects of UCS are many. The locked short and locked long muscles become tight at baseline tone and may become symptomatic as a result of the internal tension created by excessive contraction. The hyperkyphotic thoracic spine causes excessive compression upon the anterior aspects of the discs and vertebral bodies, increasing the likelihood of disc pathology and degenerative osteoarthritic changes along the vertebral bodies.[2]

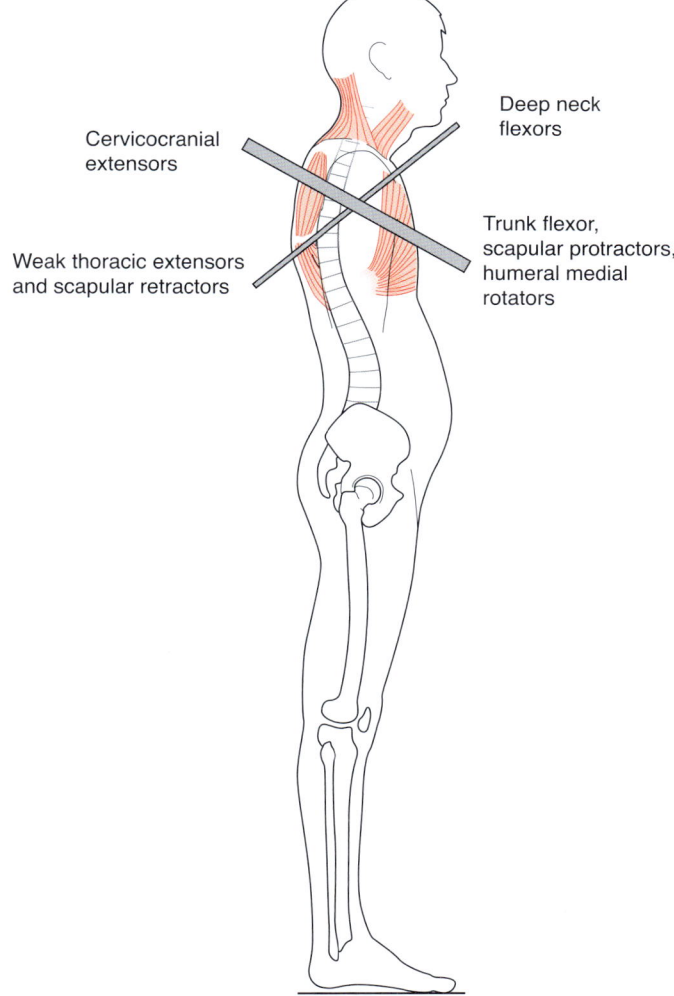

Figure 21-3 Upper crossed syndrome is a sagittal plane postural distortion pattern that involves the upper trunk, shoulder girdles and arms. It also has repercussions upon the posture of the neck and head. *Adapted from Chaitow L: Muscle energy techniques, ed 4, Edinburgh, 2013, Elsevier, Ltd.*

BOX 21-4

It should be noted that most postural distortions are a factor of letting the posture of a region of the body fall with gravity. It can almost be likened to a war that the body wages with gravity through the years. The problem is that gravity never tires and usually wins out in the long run. Look at the posture of senior citizens, and it can be seen that most exhibit postures in which a part of the body or many parts of the body have given in to gravity and are slumped forward. Much of the answer to winning the war with gravity is to keep the muscles that oppose gravity strong and healthy. Of course, keeping the antagonists to these muscles loose is also important so that these antagonists do not help gravity pull us down.

BOX 21-5	Musculature of Upper Crossed Syndrome
Overly Facilitated (Locked Short)	**Overly Inhibited (Locked Long)**
Pectoralis minor	Thoracic paraspinal musculature
Pectoralis major	Rhomboids
Sternocleidomastoid	Middle and lower trapezius
Subscapularis	Infraspinatus
	Teres minor
	Longus musculature of the neck

The posture of the lower cervical spine is projected anterior to the body due to the vertical orientation of the base of T1 upon which C7 sits. This results in a hypolordotic lower cervical spine, which is then compensated for by a hyperlordotic upper cervical spine with forward head carriage.[2] Beyond the increased anterior compression in the lower cervical spine and increased posterior compression in the upper cervical spine, this cervicocranial posture results in the center of weight of the head being held anterior to the trunk. This forward imbalance should cause the head and neck to fall into flexion, however, this is prevented by constant isometric contraction of the posterior cervicocranial musculature.[10] This often leads to neck pain as well as tension headaches. The forward posture into flexion also chronically stretches out the posterior ligament complex of the cervical spine, lengthening and weakening these structures. As posterior cervical ligamentous fascial tissues weaken, they are less able to assist the posterior cervicocranial musculature in preventing the head and neck from falling into flexion. Thus, even greater stress is placed upon the posterior cervicocranial musculature. And as the cervical musculature becomes chronically tight, joint mobility is decreased, resulting in loss of cervical range of motion. Further, due to the loss of the cervical curve, shock absorption in the cervical spine decreases, increasing the likelihood of the development of degenerative osteoarthritic changes. The posture of the neck may even create a constant pull on the anterior hyoid musculature that may transmit its tension into the mandible, possibly resulting in temporomandibular joint syndrome.[11] And the locked short posture of the scalenes can result in anterior scalene syndrome, a version of thoracic outlet syndrome in which the brachial plexus of nerves and the subclavian artery can become impinged between the anterior and middle scalene muscles.[12] Beyond all this, because the thoracic spine becomes locked/rigid into flexion, a greater demand is placed on the adjacent regions of the spine, cervical and lumbar, to move (especially into extension), causing use/overuse of these regions, increasing physical stresses and pathologic changes to these regions.

○ The protracted posture of the shoulder girdles can cause a decrease in the costoclavicular space between the clavicle and first rib, and/or a compression of the pectoralis minor against the underlying rib cage. These postural changes can result in compression upon the brachial plexus of nerves and/or the subclavian artery and vein. Compression of these neurovascular structures between the clavicle and first rib is called costoclavicular syndrome, another version of thoracic outlet syndrome. And compression of these neurovascular structures between the pectoralis minor and rib cage is called pectoralis minor syndrome, a third version of thoracic outlet syndrome.[13] Further, the over dominance of the pectoralis musculature often leads to flaring (lateral tilt/medial rotation) of the scapula, which creates an unstable base from which upper extremity muscular contraction must work, thereby weakening and overstraining upper extremity musculature. Further, when the humerus becomes locked in medial rotation, the greater tubercle of the head of the humerus becomes aligned with the acromion process of the scapula, thereby decreasing the space for the supraspinatus distal tendon and the subacromial bursa when the arm is lifted into abduction in the frontal plane.[2] The result is shoulder impingement syndrome of the supraspinatus tendon and subacromial bursa. Dysfunction of the trapezius can also lead to an inability of the trapezius (upper and lower parts) to adequately stabilize the scapula from downwardly rotating when the arm is raised into abduction or flexion, which can further lead to shoulder impingement syndrome. And a posture of protraction of the scapulae with medial rotation of the humeri close in on the chest, making it difficult for the thorax to expand, thereby making it difficult to take in a deep breath. Therefore, UCS can even inhibit the ability to oxygenate the cells of the body.

TREATMENT APPROACH

○ Like rounded low back/pelvis condition, correcting UCS requires a two-pronged approach of counseling the client regarding their postural tendency toward rounding, and strengthening and stretching the appropriate musculature. Although it is valuable to strengthen and stretch and work with manual therapy upon all "locked" musculature, both front and back, the major emphasis should be upon strengthening the posterior trunk extensor/shoulder girdle retractor/arm lateral rotation musculature, and to stretch and perform manual therapy on the anterior pectoral region (pectoralis minor and major) and arm medial rotators.

SECTION 21.4 FLAT BACK

DEFINITION

- A **flat back** is a postural distortion pattern in which, as the name implies, the curves of the spine are decreased. The lumbar lordosis is decreased, the thoracic kyphosis is decreased, and the cervical lordosis is decreased[14] (a decreased cervical lordosis is often described as a **military neck**). Therefore the client has a **hypolordotic lumbar spine**, a **hypokyphotic thoracic spine**, and a **hypolordotic cervical spine** (Figure 21-4).

ETIOLOGY

- The cause of a flat back usually begins with the sagittal plane posture of the pelvis. If the anterior tilt of the pelvis is decreased, the sacral base becomes more horizontal, resulting in a flattening (hypolordosis) of the lumbar spine, with a concomitant flattening of the thoracic and cervical spine (Box 21-6).

EFFECTS

- One effect of the postural condition of flat back is that the lumbar and cervical spines shift their weight anterior (because the lordotic curves of extension decrease), thereby shifting their weight onto the discs (and off the facets); and the thoracic curve shifts its weight posteriorly (because the kyphotic curve of flexion decreases), thereby shifting its weight onto the facets and off of the discs.[2] Another effect of a flat back is that shock absorption in the spine decreases. The curves are part of what allows the spine to absorb the compression forces of body weight down the spine and ground reaction forces (when walking or running) up the spine. Decreased shock absorption results in greater physical stress to the spinal joints; this then results in an increased chance of earlier degenerative osteoarthritic changes to the spine.[10]

TREATMENT APPROACH

- Although strengthening, stretching, and manual therapy is generally beneficial for all musculature, the treatment approach for a flat back is to correct the posture of the pelvis by focusing on strengthening the anterior tilters of the pelvis and stretching and performing manual therapy on the posterior tilters[14] (likely the hamstrings). Depending on how chronic the postural pattern is, joint mobilization might be necessary to loosen fascial restrictions.

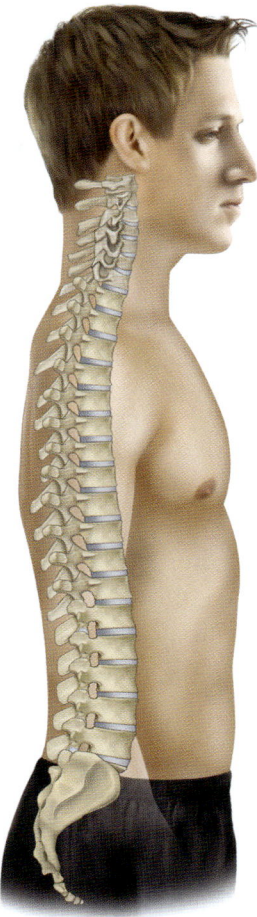

Figure 21-4 Flat back is a sagittal plane postural distortion pattern in which all the curves of the spine are decreased.

BOX 21-6

The sagittal plane tilt of the pelvis is the primary factor responsible for determining the degree of sagittal plane curvature of the spine. The relationship between the pelvis and spine is that as the pelvis changes its sagittal plane tilt, the base of the sacrum, which is the pedestal upon which the spine sits, changes its angulation. The ideal "neutral" pelvis is usually said to be one in which the sacral base angle is approximately 30 degrees (see Figure A). In other words, the neutral pelvis is anteriorly tilted 30 degrees.[2] Because of this tilt, the lumbar spine begins its posture on a sacral base that is oriented somewhat vertically forward. As a result, for the center of weight of the body to be balanced over the pelvis, the lumbar spine must compensate by having a curve of lordosis, in other words a curve of extension, to bring the center of weight back posteriorly over the pelvis. The greater the anterior tilt of the pelvis, the greater the vertical orientation of the sacral base and the greater the lumbar lordotic curve necessary. This is the posture of lower crossed syndrome (see Figure B). If the pelvic anterior tilt is decreased, the orientation of the sacral base is less vertical, in other words, more horizontal; therefore, the lumbar compensation necessary decreases and the lumbar curve decreases commensurately becoming hypolordotic. If the sacral base angle were to be zero, the sacral base would be perfectly horizontal and there would be no need at all for a lordotic curve of extension to bring the body weight back posteriorly. Figure C demonstrates what is described as flat back. If the pelvic anterior tilt is not just decreased, but actually reversed into posterior tilt, then the sacral base will be oriented somewhat vertically in the posterior direction and the lumbar compensation necessary would actually be a kyphotic curve of flexion to bring the center of weight of the body anteriorly over the pelvis; this posture is termed rounded back (see Figure D).

Similar to how the tilt of the pelvis affects the lumbar curve, the lumbar curve affects the thoracic curve. The thoracic curve effectively starts its curve on the superior surface of L1. Therefore the orientation of the body of L1 creates the pedestal upon which the thoracic spine begins. So when the lumbar curve changes, it impacts the curve of the thoracic spine. A hyperlordotic lumbar curve usually results in a hyperkyphotic thoracic spine; and a hypolordotic lumbar spine usually results in a hypokyphotic thoracic spine. Thus, the greater the curve of the pelvis, the greater the lumbar and thoracic curves; the less the curves of the pelvis, the less the lumbar and thoracic curves. Ironically, a kyphotic lumbar spine (rounded back) also usually results in a hyperkyphotic thoracic spine because it is part of the slumped posture involved with rounding the entire body forward to work in front of oneself.

And of course, the curve of the cervical spine begins on the superior surface of the body of T1, and is therefore determined by the curve of the thoracic spine. The impact of the posture of the thoracic spine upon the cervical spine is quite interesting. When the thoracic spine is hyperkyphotic, the lower cervical spine is projected anteriorly and is usually hypolordotic in the lower neck, but then the upper cervical spine must become hyperlordotic to compensate so that the eyes and inner ears are level for proprioception. This results in the typical forward head carriage that is so common. If the thoracic spine is hypokyphotic, then the entire cervical spine is usually hypolordotic, and the posture of the head is usually centered over the trunk.

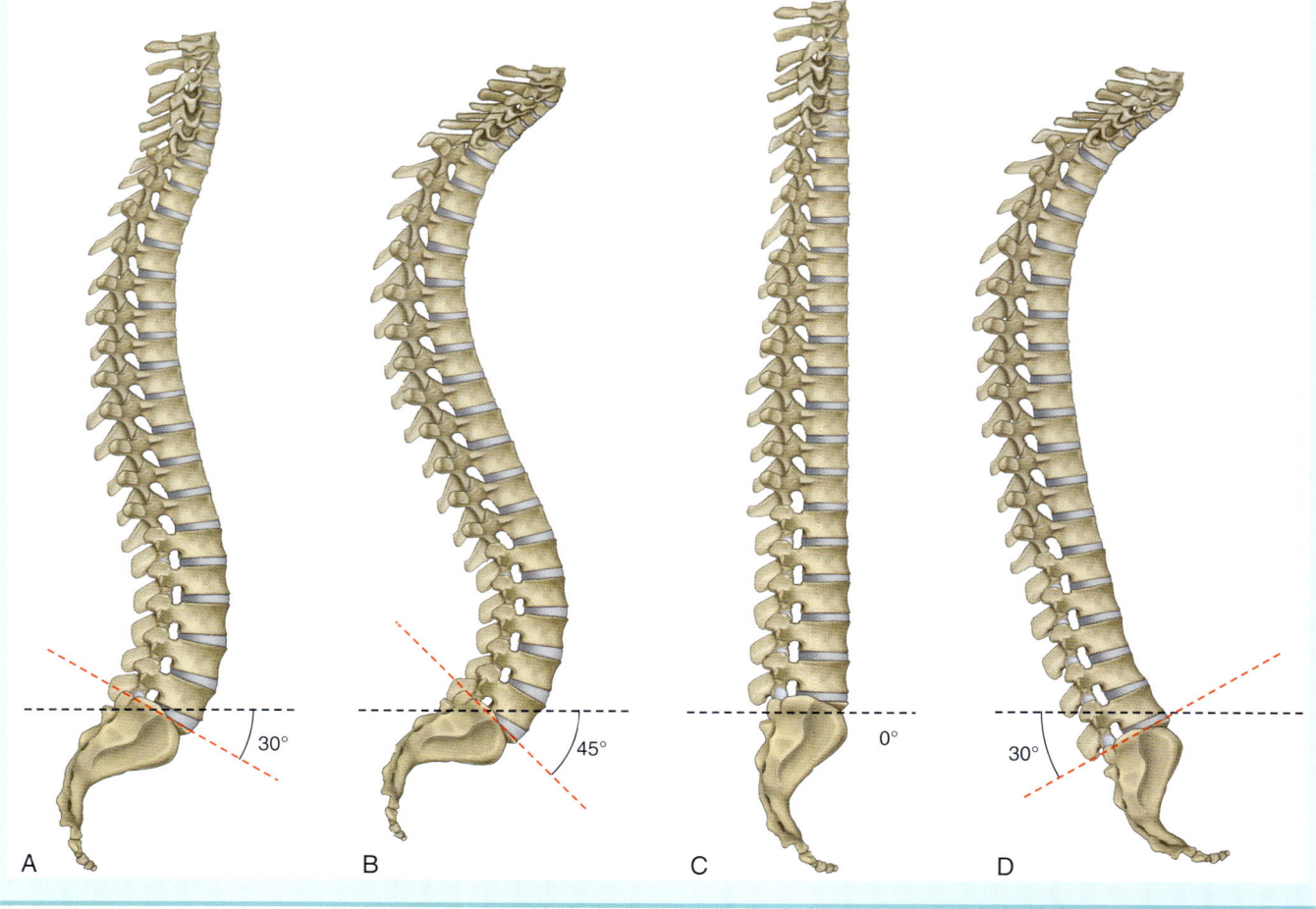

A B C D

SECTION 21.5 ELEVATED/DEPRESSED PELVIS

DEFINITION

○ An **elevated pelvis** or **depressed pelvis** is a frontal plane postural distortion pattern of the pelvis in which the pelvis is elevated on one side and depressed on the other side; in other words, the iliac crest heights are not level. The side on which the pelvis is elevated is often described as *hiking of the hip*.

ETIOLOGY

○ An elevated pelvis is usually caused by overly facilitated (tight) same-side lateral flexion musculature of the trunk that crosses the lumbosacral joint to attach onto the pelvis; most often the quadratus lumborum is involved.[15] Tight adductor musculature can also result in an elevated pelvis on that side. A depressed pelvis can result from tight hip joint abductor musculature on that side, for example the gluteus medius; and of course, depressing the pelvis on one side causes the other side to elevate (and vice versa), so a tight gluteus medius would result in the pelvis elevating on the opposite side (Figure 21-5). The challenge when the client presents with an unlevel pelvis in the frontal plane is to determine which musculature is responsible. Note: Although tight musculature is usually described as the cause, it is really an asymmetry of pull that causes the change in height of the pelvis in the frontal plane. For this reason, weak musculature could also be the cause or part of the cause of this frontal plane postural distortion.[15]

○ Another cause of an elevated/depressed pelvis is a "short limb" on one side. This could be a structural short limb due to a femur or tibia that is literally shorter on one side than the other. Or it could be a functional short limb that is due to a soft tissue asymmetry such as a dropped arch on one side, which would drop the height of the limb on that side.[15] A condition such as genu valgus (see Section 21.14) could also result in a short limb. Genu valgus is usually described as a structural deformity, but it usually begins as an imbalance of soft tissue forces, so it could also be considered to be a functional postural distortion pattern.

EFFECTS

○ The first effect of an elevated/depressed pelvis is that some musculature becomes locked short and other musculature becomes locked long, with all the usual sequelae that accompany tight musculature. Another effect of an unlevel pelvis is that the spine will likely compensate with a scoliotic curve to bring the eyes and inner ears back to level for proprioception.[2]

TREATMENT APPROACH

○ The manual and movement therapy treatment approach for an elevated/depressed pelvis is to determine what is causing the frontal plane asymmetry in iliac crest height. If musculature is determined to be the cause, the overly facilitated/tight

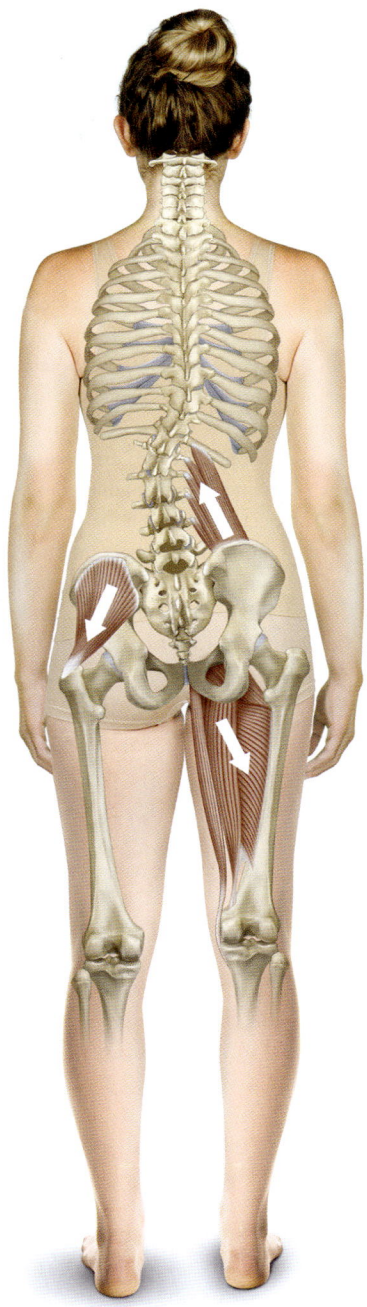

Figure 21-5 An elevated/depressed pelvis is a frontal plane postural distortion pattern.

musculature should be stretched and have manual therapy performed on them. Weak antagonist musculature should be strengthened. Any joint dysfunction hypomobilities should be mobilized. If the cause lies in the lower extremity, then this needs to be assessed and treated.

SECTION 21.6 SCOLIOSIS

DEFINITION

○ A **scoliosis** is a frontal plane postural distortion of the spine in which the spine has curves when viewed from posterior to anterior (or anterior to posterior).[8] Because of the coupling of lateral flexion with rotation, a scoliosis also has a transverse plane component.[10] Generally, a lumbar scoliosis couples lateral flexion with contralateral rotation; for example, left lateral flexion couples with right rotation; this results in the spinous processes turning into the concavity of the curve, making the degree of scoliotic curve visually appear to be less than what it is. A cervical scoliosis couples lateral flexion with ipsilateral rotation; for example, left lateral flexion couples with left rotation. The lower thoracic spine usually follows the pattern of the lumbar region and the upper thoracic spine usually follows the pattern of the cervical spine. A scoliosis can be described as being either a "**C curve**," an "**S curve**," or a "**double S curve**"[5]; and each scoliotic curve is named for its side of convexity (Figure 21-6).[2] The degree of a scoliotic curve can be measured by the angle formed from the intersecting lines drawn along the superior bodies of the highest and lowest vertebrae of the curve[2] (see Figure 21-6, C). Like most postural distortions of the body, a scoliosis can be a primary problem or a secondary problem.

ETIOLOGY

○ One type of scoliosis is known as **idiopathic scoliosis** because its cause is not known (idiopathic means of unknown cause). This is a primary form of scoliosis that can be quite severe and usually affects adolescent/teenage girls.[12] However, a scoliosis can be mild or moderate in severity and be secondary to a simple mechanical asymmetry of musculature of posture. For example, if a muscle such as the quadratus lumborum is excessively tight on one side, it can pull the lumbar spine into lateral flexion on that side (and/or pull the pelvis up into elevation on that side, which would also result in lateral flexion of the lumbar spine to that side). Posturally, any condition that creates a short lower extremity, often referred to as a **short leg**, on one side (such as asymmetrical muscular pull upon the pelvis in the frontal plane or overpronation/dropped arch) would result in an unlevel iliac crest height,[15] which would then create a scoliosis as a compensation to bring the eyes and inner ears back to level for proprioception.[2] A scoliosis could even develop secondary to an asymmetrical postural habit in which the client leans into lateral flexion on one side; perhaps due to a habit of sitting in a desk chair and leaning to one side.

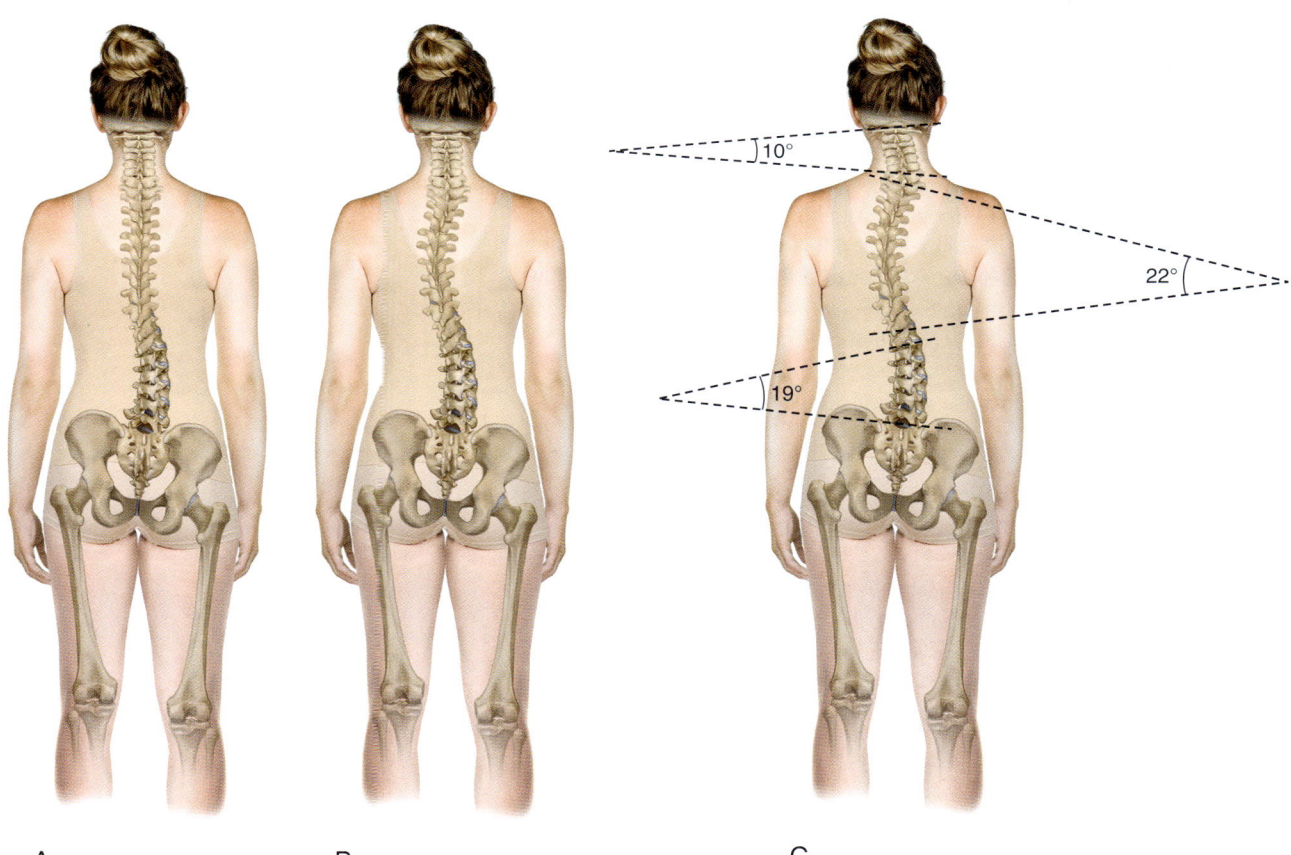

Figure 21-6 Scoliosis. **A,** A right lumbar "C scoliosis." Note the rotation that couples with the lateral flexion. **B,** A right lumbar left thoracic "S scoliosis." **C,** A right lumbar, left lower thoracic, right cervicothoracic "double S scoliosis." Each scoliotic curve has been measured in **C**.

EFFECTS

- Regardless of whether a scoliosis is a primary or secondary problem, it causes locked-short musculature in the concavity of the curve and locked-long musculature on the convex side of the curve. Because of the nature of the scoliotic curve, there are asymmetrical forces placed upon the vertebrae themselves. Compression forces upon the vertebrae are increased in the concavity and tension forces are increased on the side of convexity. These forces can add stress to the ligament/joint capsules as well as the joint surfaces, possibly resulting in degenerative osteoarthritic changes. Furthermore, scoliotic curves usually lead to a loss of range of motion in the direction opposite to the posture of the scoliotic curve; for example, a right lumbar scoliosis would likely exhibit decreased right lateral flexion and decreased left rotation. Scolioses in the thoracic region also cause postural distortion to the rib cage as well; this distortion is termed a **rib hump**,[10] and when severe enough, is usually visible. A thoracic scoliosis will usually have similar effects on the associated soft tissues of the rib cage. Although rare, if a scoliotic curve were to become severe, it could impact on the ability of the heart to beat and the lungs to fill with air.[16]

TREATMENT APPROACH

- Generally, the manual and movement therapy approach for a scoliotic curve is to perform manual therapy and stretch to the concave side,[17] and to strengthen the musculature on the side of convexity. However, manual therapy is beneficial for all dysfunctional soft tissue, whether it is locked short or locked long.[12]
- If the scoliosis is secondary to another condition that is causing a short lower extremity, this condition must be addressed and alleviated or the scoliosis will persist.[12]
- Note: Idiopathic scoliosis in adolescent/teenage girls can be severe and should be referred to a chiropractic or orthopedic physician for consultation.

SECTION 21.7 ELEVATED SHOULDER GIRDLE

DEFINITION

- An **elevated shoulder girdle** is a frontal plane postural distortion in which, as the name of the condition implies, the shoulder girdle is posturally held in elevation (Figure 21-7). This problem may be a primary problem because of tight musculature of the area or it may be secondary to another postural distortion pattern.

ETIOLOGY

- When an elevated shoulder girdle is a primary problem, there are many possible causes, including carrying a bag or purse on the shoulder (regardless of the weight of the bag), crimping a phone between the shoulder and head, and improper desk

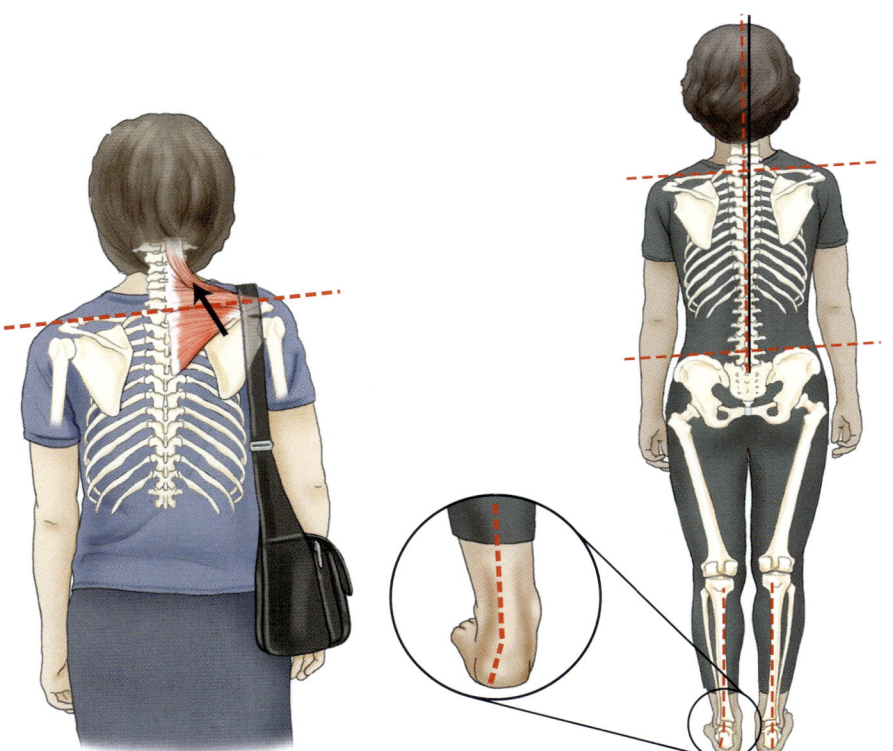

Figure 21-7 An elevated right shoulder girdle. **A,** The right shoulder is high due to tight musculature of elevation of the right scapula due to carrying a bag on the right shoulder. **B,** The right shoulder is high due to an uncompensated right high iliac crest (due to overpronation of the arch-structure of the left foot).

height that requires the shoulders to be raised when working and typing.[17] The upper shoulder girdle region is also a common region in which people hold psychological stress.[17] When an elevated shoulder girdle is secondary to another postural condition, it is usually secondary to a scoliotic curve or to an elevated iliac crest height on that side that is not compensated for.[2]

EFFECTS

- When a high shoulder girdle is a primary muscular problem, the major effects are local tightness of the musculature. Because these muscles have their other attachments in the neck, pain will usually spread into the neck. If the neck muscles stay tight long enough, cervical spinal joint dysfunction and headaches may also occur.[17] When a high shoulder girdle is secondary to another postural distortion, the muscles of the shoulder region may not be tight. However, any postural distortion that is allowed to exist long enough will gradually cause adaptive shortening (and therefore tightening) of the muscles that are held in the shortened posture.

TREATMENT APPROACH

- The manual and movement therapy approach for treatment of an elevated shoulder girdle is determining the cause of the condition. If it is a primary problem, then counseling the client regarding postural habits that perpetuate the problem is important, as well as manual therapy and stretching to the associated musculature.[17] If the elevation is occurring secondary to another condition, then finding and treating the cause is necessary. However, if this condition is chronic, beyond finding and taking care of the primary cause, manual therapy and stretching the musculature of the high shoulder girdle may also be necessary.

SECTION 21.8 PELVIC/SPINAL ROTATIONAL DISTORTION

DEFINITION

- **Pelvic/spinal rotational distortion** pattern is, as the name indicates, a rotational postural distortion pattern of the pelvis and spine. Most often if the pelvis is rotated to one side, the spine compensates for it by rotating to the opposite side (Figure 21-8).

ETIOLOGY

- One cause for a rotated spine and/or pelvis is scoliosis. Although a scoliotic curve is defined by its frontal plane lateral flexion deformity, lateral flexion in the frontal plane couples with rotation in the transverse plane, so scoliosis involves rotation as well.[2]
- More often, a rotated pelvis and spine is due to an imbalance in the transverse plane rotational musculature at the hip joint. If, for example, the lateral rotation musculature is overly facilitated/tight, instead of pulling the thigh into lateral rotation, it may pull the pelvis into rotation to the opposite side of the body (contralateral rotation). Similarly, tight medial rotation musculature may pull the pelvis into rotation to the same side of the body (ipsilateral rotation). Once the pelvis is rotated right or left, the spine will usually rotate in the opposite direction to compensate for the pelvic rotation, bringing the face back to orient forward.[2]

EFFECTS

- The effects of pelvic/spinal rotational distortional pattern are two-fold. First, there will usually be tight musculature of both the pelvis at the hip joint and the spine at the spinal joints, with locked-short and locked-long muscles, with all the signs and symptoms that follow from tight musculature. Second, there will be greater physical stress upon the joint surfaces due to

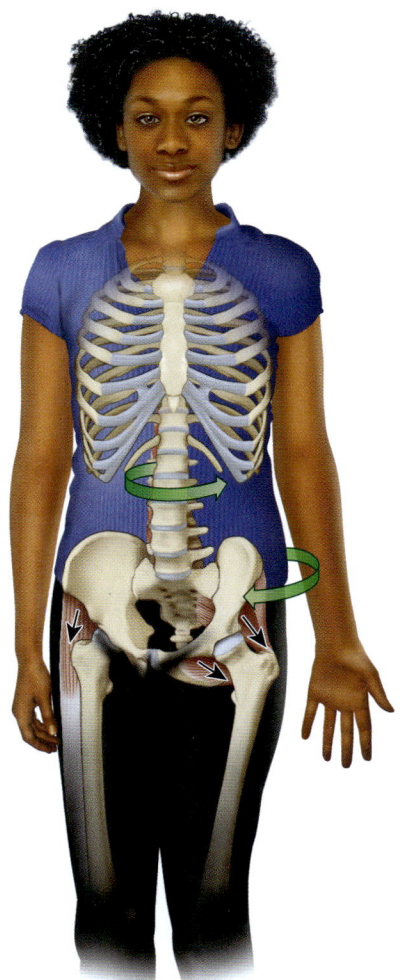

Figure 21-8 Pelvic/spinal rotational distortion pattern with right rotation of the pelvis and left rotation of the spine.

the rotational malpositioning of the joints, which can result in compression and possible consequent inflammation and pain. This is especially true in the lumbar spine because each segmental lumbar vertebral joint level allows only one degree of rotation in each direction.[2] Any greater rotation tends to approximate and jam the facets, increasing the likelihood of facet syndrome. Rotation also increases stress upon the annular disc fibers, predisposing the disc joints to weakening, and therefore possible bulging and herniation.

TREATMENT APPROACH

○ The manual and movement therapy treatment approach depends upon the cause of the condition. Most often, this postural distortion pattern is caused by imbalance in the baseline tone of the transverse plane musculature of the hip joint. Therefore this musculature should be assessed and treated appropriately with manual therapy, stretching, and strengthening. These treatment modalities should also be applied to any myofascial imbalance in the spine. With chronic cases, joint mobilization is very useful toward increasing motion in the affected joints.

SECTION 21.9   OVERPRONATION

DEFINITION

○ **Overpronation** is a frontal plane postural distortion of the foot in which the foot excessively pronates; in other words, the arch structure of the foot overly collapses. A **collapsed arch/dropped arch** is known as a *flatfoot*. Some people have a **rigid flatfoot** in which the arch is never present (Figure 21-9, *A*). Other people have a **supple flatfoot** in which the arch is lost only on weight bearing (Figure 21-9, *B* and *C*). Supple flat foot is the more common type of flat foot. A flat foot is also known as **pes planus**.[2]

ETIOLOGY

○ A rigid flat foot is usually caused by a structural configuration of the bones of the foot, or by the long-term accumulation of fibrous adhesions in a chronic supple flat foot, gradually creating rigidity. A supple flat foot is usually caused by a combination of lax (weak) ligaments and weak musculature. The primary ligaments that when weak can cause overpronation are the spring ligament, long plantar ligament, short plantar ligament, and the plantar fascia. Because many muscles assist in maintaining the arch structure of the foot, there are many muscles, that when weak, can contribute to overpronation[2] (Box 21-7).
○ These muscles can be divided into the following groups: subtalar joint supinators (plus the fibularis as a "stirrup muscle"), plantar intrinsics, and hip joint lateral rotators/abductors.
○ Supination musculature opposes pronation. Therefore if the supinators are weak, overpronation is possible. Because the

BOX 21-7	Principal Muscles That Need to Be Strengthened in a Client with Overpronation

Subtalar Joint	Plantar Intrinsics	Hip Joint
Tibialis posterior	Abductor hallucis	Gluteus maximus
Flexor digitorum longus	Abductor digiti minimi pedis	Deep lateral rotator group
Flexor hallucis longus	Flexor digitorum brevis	Gluteus medius
Tibialis anterior		Gluteus minimus
Extensor hallucis longus		
Gastrocnemius		
Soleus		
Fibularis ("stirrup muscle")		

principal component of supination is inversion of the foot, then all invertors are supinators. The fibularis longus muscle also tends to increase the arch structure of the foot because it, along with the tibialis anterior, forms a "stirrup" that supports the arch of the foot.

○ Plantar intrinsic muscles in Plantar Layer I attach into the plantar fascia.[4] Therefore, these muscles help to maintain the tone of

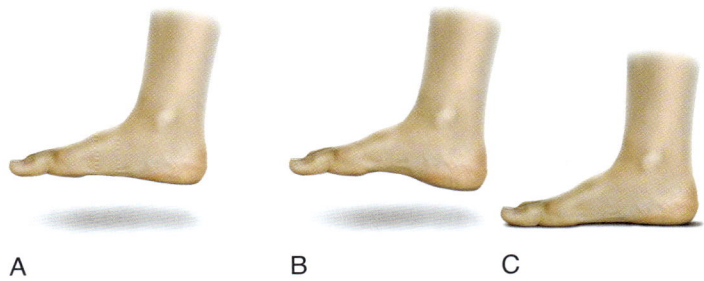

Figure 21-9 Overpronation/flat foot. **A,** Rigid flat foot. **B,** Supple flat foot, non–weight-bearing. **C,** Supple flat foot, weight-bearing.

the plantar fascia so that it can better support the arch structure of the foot. Unfortunately, because we place our feet into shoes, movement of our toes is largely irrelevant when walking and standing. For this reason, plantar intrinsic musculature is underutilized and therefore weakens, causing the concomitant weakness of the plantar fascia, and therefore the arch (Box 21-8).

BOX 21-8   Barefoot and Minimalist Shoes

An understanding that shoes remove the need for our musculature to support our arch structure and therefore results in a weakening of these muscles, with a resultant predisposition toward collapsing the arch, is the reason that going barefoot or wearing "minimalist shoes" is becoming so popular. And this logic makes sense. It seems silly that we place our feet into shoes from before we can even stand or walk. And the more rigid the shoes, the less the need for our lower extremity musculature to engage to support the foot. However, it should be pointed out that if a person has been wearing shoes for his or her entire life, and then suddenly decides to throw them away and either go barefoot or switch to minimalist shoes, the deconditioned musculature will likely be overwhelmed with the sudden demand placed upon them. This may result in a greater collapsing of the arch structure, which will place a greater load on the ligamentous fascial tissue of the foot, likely overstretching it, thereby permanently weakening it and making the job of the musculature to prevent overpronation even greater. This greater demand is also likely to overwhelm and injure the ligaments and other soft tissues of the foot and the rest of the lower extremity. Any change in demand upon muscles and other soft tissues of the body must always be done gradually and prudently. The decision to switch to minimalist shoes may be a wise one, but should be transitioned toward over many months or more.

BOX 21-9   Pronation and Hip Joint Rotation

The open chain transverse plane component of pronation is lateral rotation (abduction) of the calcaneus relative to the talus at the subtalar joint. However, in closed chain kinematics with the foot weight bearing on the ground, the transverse plane component of pronation involves medial rotation of the talus.[2] However, the ankle joint does not allow rotation so when the talus medially rotates, the tibia must medially rotate with it. And because when the knee joint is in extension it does not allow rotation, when the tibia medially rotates, the femur must medially rotate with it. The result is that pronation causes the entire lower extremity to medially rotate. The hip joint is the first joint that allows rotation and can therefore either manifest and/or counter this medial rotation. This is one of the reasons that hip joint lateral rotation musculature is so massive: to prevent the arch structure of the foot from collapsing and causing the lower extremity to fall into medial rotation. Therefore strengthening lateral rotation musculature of the hip joint can help to maintain the arch structure of the foot. This can be easily seen and demonstrated. While standing up, contract your gluteal musculature (pinch your butt cheeks together), and notice that your arches rise. The reasoning is the mechanism explained here, but in the opposite direction. Because the extended knee joint does not allow rotation, laterally rotating the thigh causes the tibia to laterally rotate with it; and because the ankle joint does not allow rotation, laterally rotating the tibia causes the talus to laterally rotate with it; and lateral rotation of the talus causes the talus to supinate at the subtalar joint. Hence, the lateral rotation force caused by musculature at the hip joint is transferred distally to the subtalar joint, causing it to supinate, thereby raising the arch.

- And because overpronation causes the entire lower extremity to fall into medial rotation, hip joint lateral rotation musculature helps to prevent the lower extremity from medially rotating and therefore helps to prevent the foot from overpronating (Box 21-9). And because medial rotation of the lower extremity (specifically the thigh) tends to couple with adduction, the medially rotated thigh that accompanies the overpronated foot also usually falls into adduction. Therefore hip joint abduction musculature, if weak, can cause or contribute to overpronation.
- And of course, if the aforementioned muscles being weak can cause overpronation, then their antagonists (subtalar joint evertors and hip joint medial rotators/adductors), if tight, could cause or contribute to overpronation.
- There are other factors that can cause or contribute to an overly pronated foot. Being overweight increases the chance that the foot will overpronate. Our weight bears through the arch structure of the foot when standing. If the weight increases, a greater demand us placed upon the soft tissues that must maintain the arch, likely overwhelming them, with the resultant arch collapse. Walking on hard surfaces (e.g., asphalt and concrete roads and sidewalk, marble and hard wood floors) also increases the forces that are transmitted into our feet and lower extremities, increasing the demand on the soft tissues whose job it is to support the arch. Another factor is the transverse plane posture of the hip joint. Excessively tight hip joint lateral rotation musculature at baseline tone can cause the thigh to be excessively laterally rotated, which causes the foot to turn outward. The result is that when walking, instead of the weight of the body traveling through the foot from heel-strike to toe-off, it passes directly over the medial longitudinal arch, tending to collapse it.

EFFECTS

- The effects of overpronation are many. Each time that the foot overpronates, the plantar fascia is stretched/overstretched[13]; and via Wolff's law, chronic repetitive overstretching of the plantar fascia often leads to heel spur formation (calcium deposition) upon the underside of the calcaneus where the plantar fascia attaches. Also, overpronation, by definition, involves a loss of the arch-structure of the foot. When the transverse arch overly collapses, adjacent metatarsal bones collapse into each other, increasing the likelihood that the plantar digital nerve between them is compressed. This condition is known as

Morton's neuroma; it is also known as *Morton's metatarsalgia* or *interdigital neuroma* (although technically it is not a neuroma). Compression of the plantar digital nerve between the third and fourth metatarsals or second and third metatarsals is most common.[13] And overpronation also predisposes the client toward developing hallux valgus[13] (see Section 21.11).

❍ The loss of the fluid movement pattern of supination to pronation is important toward shock absorption during the gait cycle. Therefore overpronation can lead to increased physical stress into all weight-bearing joints of the body. Overpronation also causes the entire lower extremity to fall into medial rotation, which places increased demand on the lateral rotation musculature of the hip joint, often leading to pain and dysfunction. Increased medial rotation of the lower extremity is also usually accompanied by increased adduction of the thigh at the hip joint, which predisposed the client toward genu valgus, which then increases stress forces on both the medial side (tension stress) and lateral side (compression stress) of the knee joint.[13] And increased medial rotation of the lower extremity is often accompanied by excessive anterior tilt of the pelvic bone on that side, leading to increased stress at the sacroiliac joints as well as increased lordosis of the lumbar spine.

❍ Further, if only one foot overpronates, the arch dropping causes a decrease in the length of that lower extremity, which drops the iliac crest height creating an unlevel pelvis. This often leads to a compensatory scoliosis to bring the head back to level.[2] Hence muscular and joint imbalances can occur throughout the entire body.

TREATMENT APPROACH

❍ The manual and movement therapy approach for treatment of the client with overpronation is to determine and address the cause(s). Rigid flat foot is addressed primarily by manual therapy, stretching, and joint mobilization to increase the flexibility of the tissues to allow for the arch to be regained. Supple flat foot can be addressed by strengthening the musculature that would support the arch and/or wearing an orthotic that supports the arch. Any aggravating factors would certainly need to be reduced or eliminated.

SECTION 21.10   RIGID HIGH ARCH

DEFINITION

❍ A healthy functioning arch should have the ability to raise (supinate) and lower (pronate). However, some people have a **rigid high arch** that does not adequately lower/pronate when necessary; as a result, it is stuck in supination. A rigid high arch is also known as **pes cavus** and sometimes referred to as a **high arch** or **oversupination**.[13]

ETIOLOGY

❍ The usual cause of a rigid high arch is congenitally taut ligaments and fascial tissue in the foot.[13] As a result, the bones of the foot cannot drop into pronation (Figure 21-10). (Note: Other, more severe causes of a rigid high arch include cerebral palsy and poliomyelitis.[2])

EFFECTS

❍ The major effect of a rigid high arch is the loss of the ability of the foot to absorb shock, especially when walking or running. As a result, greater stress is placed on the foot as well as the rest of the weight-bearing joints of the body. Because a high arch results in less of the foot meeting the ground, physical stress to the foot is magnified at the areas of the foot that do meet the ground, the heel (calcaneus) and ball (metatarsal heads) of the foot. Consequently, foot pain is common in people with rigid high arches. Joint pain in the other joints of the lower extremity

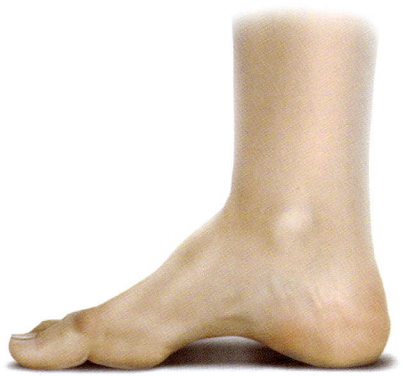

Figure 21-10 Rigid high arch of the foot.

and spine is also common. And, because pronation of the foot tends to increase genu valgum force at the knee, a rigid high arch may predispose toward genu varum at the knee joint.[2]

TREATMENT APPROACH

❍ The manual and movement therapy treatment approach for a rigid high arch is moist heat, manual therapy, stretching, and joint mobilization aimed at loosening the taut soft tissues. Orthotics are also often recommended to support and cushion the high arch.[2]

SECTION 21.11 HALLUX VALGUS

DEFINITION

- **Hallux valgus** is a condition in which the proximal phalanx of the big toe deviates laterally (adducts toward the second toe) at the metatarsophalangeal (MTP) joint, and the metatarsal of the big toe deviates medially[2] (Figure 21-11). This condition is known in lay terms as a **bunion** because of the characteristic bony protuberance of the big toe on the inside of the foot. However, it should be emphasized that bunion and hallux valgus are not synonymous; rather, a bunion is a common aspect of hallux valgus.[13]

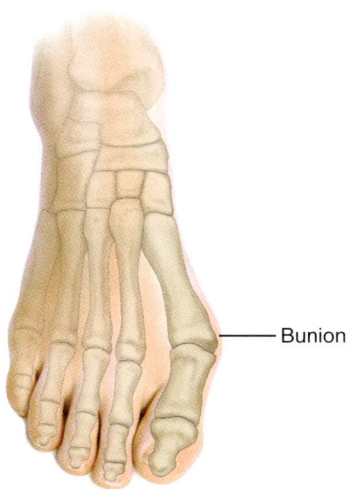

Figure 21-11 Hallux valgus. The proximal phalanx of the big toe deviates laterally; the metatarsal of the big toe deviates medially.

ETIOLOGY

- The principal cause of hallux valgus is improper shoe wear.[2] Most problematic is a shoe that is too narrow at the toe box, especially shoes that have a pointed toe box.[13] This places pressure on the proximal phalanx of the big toe, pushing it laterally at the MTP joint. High-heeled shoes are also problematic because they increase the weight-bearing force at the MTP joints, increasing the deviation and instability of the joints. Overpronation also seems to be an aggravating factor because it involves lateral rotation (abduction) of the foot at the subtalar joint, splaying it outwards; this results in the body's weight passing over the medial side of the MTP joint of the big toe, further pushing it laterally, increasing the valgus deformity.[13] Additionally, individuals with hypermobile ligaments/fascial tissue are more prone to this condition because their ligaments are less able to resist the deviation of the big toe. There is controversy regarding whether there is a genetic component, but there does seem to be a genetic predisposition for certain individuals to acquire this condition.[13]
- Once the proximal phalanx of the big toe begins to deviate laterally, pressure is also placed on the metatarsal of the big toe at the MTP joint, pushing/deviating it medially away from the second metatarsal bone. This pushes the head of the metatarsal medially, creating the characteristic bony protuberance/bunion, which is a visible marker for this condition.[2]

EFFECTS

- The most noticeable effect of hallux valgus is the protuberance of the first metatarsal head on the medial side of the foot. Pressure of the metatarsal head against the shoe then results in irritation and inflammation of the bony tissue of the metatarsal head, leading to inflammation and hyperostosis (calcium deposition/osteoarthritis).[2] The associated soft tissues also become irritated and inflamed, leading to pain. Because the deviation of the first metatarsal is not just medial but also somewhat dorsal away from the ground, greater pressure is placed on the metatarsal heads of the other toes to meet the ground and weight bear, leading to irritation/inflammation, and often increased skin build up (keratosis) and pain there as well. This shift of weight bearing away from the big toe is augmented by the client's desire to avoid the pain of weight bearing through the affected joint, thereby further shifting/increasing weight-bearing stress to the other toes.[2] It should be noted that the proximal phalanx of the big toe not only deviates laterally, but also everts (rotating around its long axis so that the plantar surface comes to face laterally). This alters the line of pull of the abductor hallucis muscle so that it now passes on the plantar side of the MTP joint instead of the medial side. This results in this muscle losing its ability to abduct the big toe, which leaves the adductor hallucis unopposed to further deviate the big toe into valgus/adduction.[2]
- Further, because the big toe deviates laterally against the second toe, sores in the skin often develop where these two toes meet and the skin abrades. Finally, because pain is common upon weight bearing and especially when walking, an antalgic gait (changing the pattern of the gait to avoid pain) often leads to asymmetric forces throughout the foot, the rest of the lower extremity, and even the spine, possibly leading to dysfunction and pain far throughout the body.

TREATMENT APPROACH

- The manual and movement therapy treatment approach to hallux valgus depends on the severity of the condition. The first approach should be conservative and comprises counseling the client regarding a change in footwear. Further, because lateral deviation of the proximal phalanx of the big toe is adduction of the proximal phalanx at the MTP joint, it would follow that increasing the strength of the abductor hallucis muscle (assuming that it still has a line of pull to create abduction), along with manual therapy and stretching to loosen the adductor hallucis muscle, would be beneficial.[13] Joint mobilization of the metatarsal and proximal phalanx of the big toe at the MTP joint (especially inversion of the metatarsal and axial abduction and traction with medial nonaxial glide of the proximal phalanx) is also beneficial. Any other aggravating factors should also be addressed. If conservative care is not successful, then surgery is often performed,[2] usually to shave down the bunion and realign the metatarsal and proximal phalanx.

SECTION 21.12 HAMMERTOES

DEFINITION

- **Hammertoes** are a postural distortion pattern that usually affects toes two through four. The characteristic pattern is for the metatarsophalangeal (MTP) joint of the toe to be extended, the proximal interphalangeal (PIP) joint to be flexed, and the distal interphalangeal (DIP) joint to be extended[13] (Figure 21-12). The name is given because the bend at the MTP, PIP, and DIP joints makes the toe appear to be a hammer.

ETIOLOGY

- The cause of hammertoes is improper footwear, specifically shoes that are too short. This causes the length of the toes to shorten by extending at the MTP joint and flexing at the PIP joint, and extending at the DIP joint. High-heeled shoes aggravate this condition because body weight is shifted forward, further jamming and shortening the toes (Box 21-10).

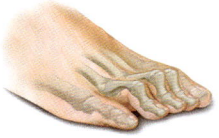

Figure 21-12 Hammertoes of the second, third, and fourth toes. The MTP joint is extended, the PIP joint is flexed, and the DIP joint is extended.

pain.[13] Further, the shortening of the toes results in concomitant shortening of the soft tissues that cross the joints. Fascial ligaments and joint capsules shorten on one side of the joint and are lengthened on the other side. Similarly, muscles and their tendons shorten/lengthen across the joints (Box 21-11). In time, these changes become rigid due to adaptive shortening and due to the accumulation of fascial adhesions. In very chronic cases, bony changes may even occur.

BOX 21-10 Hammertoes

Looking at the mechanics of hammertoes elucidates how this postural distortion pattern occurs. To accommodate the shortened shoe, the overall length of the toe must decrease. It accomplishes this by bending in opposite directions are the various joints, extending at one joint, flexing at the next, and then extending at the last one. Exactly why the characteristic pattern at each joint occurs is as follows: The proximal phalanx cannot flex at the MTP joint because the ground obstructs this movement from occurring, so the MTP joint must extend. Extension at the MTP joint requires compensatory flexion at one of the interphalangeal joints. This cannot occur at the DIP joint because that would require the proximal and middle phalanges to be extended/straight, which would cause the toe to be overly extended up into the air, which the dorsal surface of the shoe would not allow to occur. Further, if the toe were that far up into the air, flexion at the DIP alone would be insufficient to bring the distal end of the toe back to the ground for stability and weight bearing. Consequently, the compensatory flexion occurs at the PIP joint. For the toe to now be grounded for balance, the distal phalanx must meet the ground; this requires the DIP to extend. Therefore a hammertoe accommodates a shorter shoe length by shortening the toe with extension at the MTP joint, flexion at the PIP joint, and extension at the DIP joint.

BOX 21-11

It is often said that hammertoes result in muscle imbalances. It is interesting to examine the effects upon the various muscles across these joints. The extensor digitorum longus would be shortened across the MTP and DIP joints, but stretched longer across the PIP joint; the net effect would be shortening of this muscle. The extensor digitorum brevis would be similarly shortened. The flexor digitorum longus would be shortened across the PIP joint, but stretched longer across the MTP and DIP joints; the net effect would likely be lengthening of this muscle. The flexor digitorum brevis would be stretched across the MTP joint but stretched longer across the PIP joint, so this muscle's length would likely not change a great deal.

TREATMENT APPROACH

- The first manual and movement therapy approach when working with a client who has hammertoes is to counsel them regarding healthy footwear. Manually, the aim of treatment is to try to mobilize the tissues that have become locked short or locked long. This can be done with manual therapy (soft tissue manipulation) as well as stretching. Joint mobilization is also very beneficial.[13] Given the usual chronic nature of this condition when a client comes in for care, it is important to also instruct the client how to do their own manual therapy and stretching for the toes; instructing the client to perform these home-care exercises after soaking the foot in a warm bath is helpful. Strengthening the toes may also be helpful. Exercises like picking up marbles with the toes and/or scrunching up with the toes a towel placed on the floor are often recommended.

EFFECTS

- There are a number of effects of hammertoes. The bend in the toes causes the skin around the PIP joint to rub up against the shoe, resulting in inflammation, callus buildup, and often

SECTION 21.13   MORTON'S FOOT

DEFINITION

❍ **Morton's foot** is a congenital condition in which the first metatarsal is shorter than the second metatarsal. This is a fairly common structural variant, occurring in approximately 10% of the population. As a result of the second metatarsal being longer than the first metatarsal, the second toe is usually longer, protruding farther anteriorly than the first (Figure 21-13). However, it is possible for the second toe to be longer than the big toe due to longer phalanges; technically, this is not Morton's foot. By definition, Morton's foot is determined by the relative lengths of the first and second metatarsals, not the overall lengths of the first two toes. Morton's foot is also know as *Morton's toe* or *Greek foot*[13] (classical Greek and Roman art idealized the second toe being longer).

ETIOLOGY

The cause of Morton's foot is genetic.[13] The first metatarsal is shorter than the second metatarsal.

EFFECTS

❍ The principal effect of Morton's foot is that it alters the normal biomechanics of the foot as the foot moves through the gait cycle.[13] At toe-off during the gait cycle, body weight should be pushing off the big toe (primarily at the metatarsophalangeal [MTP] joint). However, with Morton's foot, because the second metatarsal is longer with its head protruding farther anteriorly, the propulsion for toe-off shifts there. However, the second toe is not as large and therefore not as well adapted to deal with this increased stress, leading to increased callusing, as well as pain at the second toe. Also, toward the end of toe-off during the gait cycle, with the pivot point located at the second MTP joint, the foot often collapses inward onto the first MTP joint, resulting in increased pronation of the foot. For this reason, Morton's foot is thought to predispose the foot toward overpronation, with all the effects associated with this condition.

TREATMENT APPROACH

❍ Assuming that Morton's toe is associated with altered biomechanics and/or pain, treatment is usually aimed at altering the mechanics of the foot during the gait cycle by means of either a pad under the first metatarsal head or an orthotic. In occasional cases, surgery is performed. Manual and movement therapy should be oriented at the possible altered biomechanical effects due to Morton's foot.[13]

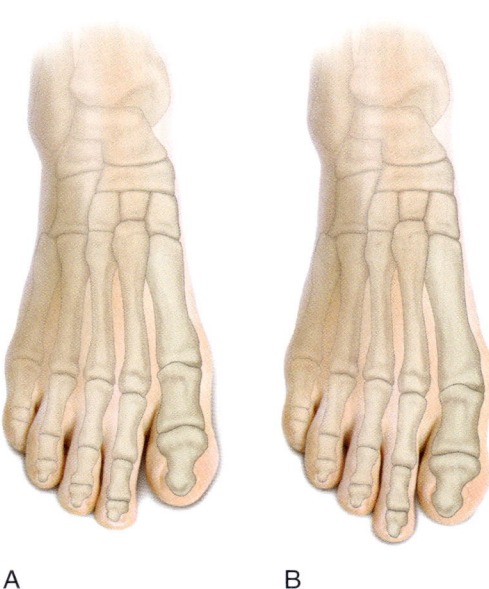

Figure 21-13 Morton's foot. **A,** True Morton's foot: the first metatarsal is shorter than the second metatarsal. **B,** A longer toe caused by longer phalanges of the second toe; this is not Morton's foot.

SECTION 21.14   GENU VALGUM/GENU VARUM

DEFINITION

❍ Genu valgum and genu varum are frontal plane angulations measured between the shaft of the femur and the shaft of the tibia. **Genu valgum** (also known as **genu valgus**) refers to a lateral deviation of the tibia, in effect abduction of the leg at the knee joint; **genu varum** (also known as **genu varus**) refers to a medial deviation, in effect, adduction of the leg at the knee joint. In ideal healthy posture, there should be an approximate 5- to 10-degree genu valgus angle because the femur slants in medially and the tibia is vertical.[5] Any angulation greater than 10 degrees would be considered excessive genu valgum and is known in lay terms as *knock-knees* (Figure 21-14, *A*). If the tibia deviates medially at the knee joint, it is measured as a genu varum angle and known in lay terms as *bowleg* (Figure 21-14, *B*).

❍ Because women have a wider pelvis than men, their femurs tend to have a greater medial slant; therefore, the incidence of genu valgum in women is much greater than in men.

❍ It is interesting to note that in Western cultures, excessive genu valgus occurs more often than genu varum; but genu varum occurs more frequently than genu valgum in Eastern cultures. A couple of factors may account for this. In Eastern cultures, babies are often held and carried against the mother's body with the baby's hip joints in abduction and lateral rotation, thereby predisposing toward genu varum posture. Also, the characteristic squat position that many Easterners assume also tends to increase lateral rotation and abduction at the hip joints.

CHAPTER 21 Common Postural Distortion Patterns

culature across the knee joint, known as the Q-angle (see Section 9.15). The Q-angle tends to pull the patella laterally. As the genu valgus angle increases, the Q-angle increases. The problem with this is that it allows the lateral retinacular fibers of the vastus lateralis to shorten and tighten, thereby increasing tension laterally at the knee joint. Similarly, an increased Q-angle tends to stretch and weaken the vastus medialis, thereby weakening its retinacular fibers across the medial side of the knee joint.[13]

EFFECTS

- At the knee joint, an increased genu valgum angle increases tension forces medially and increases compression forces laterally. As a result, the medial collateral ligament is often overstretched and injured, resulting in pain as well as further genu valgum weakness. Because the medial collateral ligament has fascial attachments into the medial meniscus, the medial meniscus may also be injured. Compression forces laterally may damage the lateral meniscus and/or cause bone compression leading to osteoarthritic degeneration. Genu varum increases tension forces laterally and increases compression forces medially.[13] This can cause damage and injury to the lateral collateral ligament as well to the meniscus on either side of the joint.

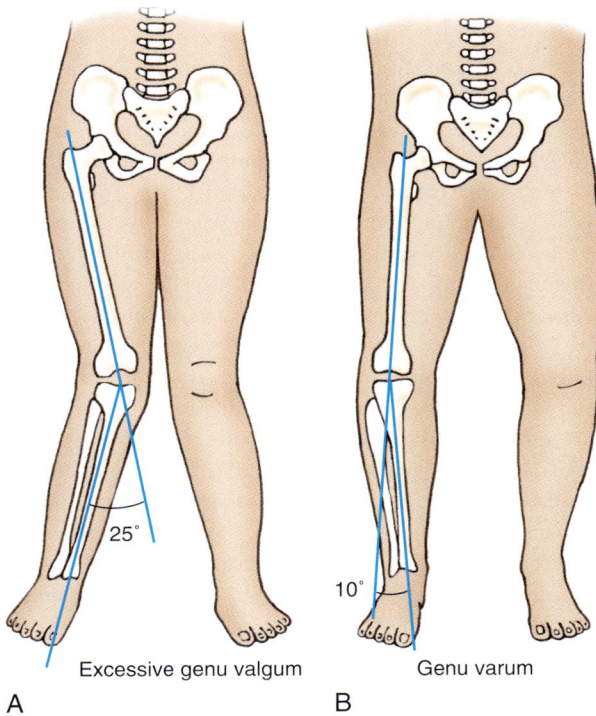

Figure 21-14 Frontal plane postural distortion patterns at the knee joint. **A,** An excessive genu valgum angulation of 25 degrees. **B,** A genu varum angulation of 10 degrees.

TREATMENT APPROACH

- The manual and movement therapy treatment approach for excessive genu valgum is to strengthen the medial tissues across the knee joint, principally the muscles of the pes anserine group, and loosen the tissues that cross the knee joint laterally, principally the lateral collateral ligament, lateral retinacular fibers, and the iliotibial band. It is also to remove any factors that would tend to exacerbate genu valgum, such as overpronation of the foot that causes the hip joint to fall into adduction and medial rotation[6]; in other words, strengthen foot supination musculature and hip joint abduction and lateral rotation musculature; and loosen foot pronation and hip joint adduction and medial rotation musculature.
- The treatment approach for genu varum is to strengthen the lateral tissues across the knee joint,[6] principally the biceps femoris of the hamstring group, and loosen the tissues that cross the knee joint medially, principally the medial collateral ligament, medial retinacular fibers, and the pes anserine group. It is also to remove any factors that would tend to exacerbate genu varum, such as a rigid high arch and a hip joint that is deviated toward abduction and lateral rotation. Adduction musculature should be strengthened, and hip joint abductors and lateral rotators should be loosened.

ETIOLOGY

- The cause of genu valgum is an imbalance of soft tissue forces across the medial and lateral sides of the knee joint. The medially oriented tissues, principally the medial collateral ligament, pes anserine muscles, and medially oriented retinacular fibers of the quadriceps femoris musculature, resist genu valgum. The laterally oriented structures, principally the lateral collateral ligament, biceps femoris, iliotibial band, and laterally oriented retinacular fibers, pull toward genu valgum. If the medial structures are weaker than the lateral structures, the knee joint will fall into genu valgum.
- Other postural distortion patterns can predispose toward genu valgum. Overpronation drops the lower extremity in medially, creating a genu valgus torque. At the hip joint, weak abductor musculature and/or tight adductor musculature tends to create increased adduction of the thigh at the hip joint.[1] This increases the medial slant of the femur, thereby increasing genu valgum. Another factor that can increase genu valgum is the pull of the quadriceps mus-

SECTION 21.15 GENU RECURVATUM

DEFINITION

- **Genu recurvatum** is a sagittal plane deformity at the knee joint in which the knee falls into hyperextension. The angle for extension at the knee can be measured by the intersection of two lines: one running through the center of the shaft of the femur and the other running through the center of the shaft of the tibia (Figure 21-15). Typically, full knee joint extension creates an angle of approximately 5-10 degrees of extension beyond neutral posture.[5] This occurs for two reasons. The tibial plateau slopes slightly posteriorly; and when standing, the center of body weight falls slightly anterior to the knee joint, tending to push the knee joint into extension. The knee joint is considered to have genu recurvatum when the angle of extension measures greater than 10 degrees.[5]

PART 4 Myology: Study of the Muscular System

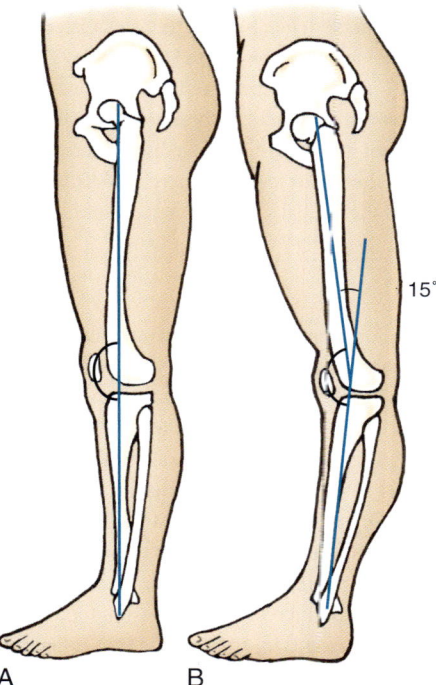

Figure 21-15 Genu recurvatum. **A,** An extension angle across the knee joint of zero degrees. **B,** a genu recurvatum angle of 15 degrees.

ETIOLOGY

- The cause of genu recurvatum is an imbalance in sagittal plane soft tissue tension across the knee joint. Given that posterior soft tissues are flexors at the knee joint, they resist knee joint extension. Therefore laxness/weakness of the posterior soft tissues of the knee joint allow the knee joint to fall into hyperextension.[13] These tissues are principally the muscles of the hamstring group (as well as the popliteus and gastrocnemius) and the posterior joint capsule and ligaments. On the opposite side of the joint, anterior soft tissues create knee joint extension. Therefore excessive tightness of the anteriorly located quadriceps musculature increases the likelihood of genu recurvatum. An excessively anteriorly tilted pelvis also tends to push the knee joint into genu recurvatum by pushing the femoral head anteriorly, thereby slanting the femur posteriorly from proximal to distal.[13]

EFFECTS

- As the knee joint falls into genu recurvatum, the force of body weight increasingly moves anterior to the center of the joint, thereby further increasing the force toward genu recurvatum. The effect of this is that the posterior soft tissues are increasingly stretched out and weakened, making their task to restrain genu recurvatum even more challenging.[18] This can result in excessive stress and strain on these tissues, possibly leading to dysfunction and pain. On the anterior side, the quadriceps musculature tends to become locked short and can similarly become dysfunctional and painful. The hyperextended position of the knee joint also causes increased compression force at the anterior margins of the femur and tibia, increasing the likelihood of anterior meniscus compression and knee joint osteoarthritic degeneration.[2] Hyperextension also forces the patella posteriorly against the femur, increasing compression force upon the joint surfaces of the patellofemoral joint, likely causing dysfunction and osteoarthritic degeneration (patellofemoral syndrome).
- The effects of genu recurvatum upon the pelvis and spine can vary. The posture of genu recurvatum is such that the proximal end of the tibia leans posteriorly and the proximal end of the femur leans anteriorly (see Figure 21-15, B). The body is now leaning forward (like the Leaning Tower of Pisa) and must get its weight back posteriorly to counterbalance its center of gravity. So where and how does this posterior shift occur? If the hip flexor musculature and the anterior hip joint capsular fibers are loose, the pelvis can posteriorly tilt to bring body weight posteriorly. This flattens the lumbar spine and/or causes a kyphotic rounded low back. However, if the hip flexor musculature and anterior hip joint capsular fibers are tight/taut, then the pelvis must follow the femur and will be excessively anteriorly tilted; and the compensation to bring body weight back posteriorly will have to occur in the lumbar spine by an increase in the lordosis/extension of the lumbar curve (hence increased anterior pelvic tilt and lower crossed syndrome).

TREATMENT APPROACH

- The treatment approach for manual and movement therapists/trainers is to improve the soft tissue balance across the knee joint in the sagittal plane. This is accomplished by strengthening the hamstrings and loosening/relaxing the quadriceps femoris.[13]

SECTION 21.16 PIGEON-TOE/TOE-IN

DEFINITION

- The term **pigeon-toe** is a lay term that refers to any posture that causes the foot to **toe-in** toward the midline of the body (Figure 21-16). As such there are many causes of this postural distortion pattern. Note: Toe-in posture is common in young children under the age of three.[19] Usually, this posture is outgrown by approximately age six.

Following are five postural distortions that can cause pigeon-toe (toe-in) posture:

1. **Tibial torsion**. Tibial torsion is a twisting of the tibia that results in a toe-in posture.[6] This condition is usually outgrown during childhood development.
2. **Forefoot varus**. Forefoot varus (also known as **metatarsus adductus** or **metatarsus varus**) is an excessive adduction (inversion/supination) of the forefoot. Forefoot varus can simply

CHAPTER 21 Common Postural Distortion Patterns 679

adults is a simple imbalance between medial and lateral rotation soft tissues at the hip joint. This is the form of toe-in posture that will be discussed here.

ETIOLOGY

- An imbalance of medial rotation compared with lateral rotation soft tissues may be due to an imbalance in the musculature or in the fascial ligament/joint capsule complex. Baseline tone imbalance of the musculature could be due to medial rotator muscles that are tighter than lateral rotator muscles at the hip joint. Baseline tone/tautness imbalance of the ligamentous/capsular tissue commonly occurs when the more posterior ischiofemoral ligament fibers are excessively taut.
- There are a number of reasons that these soft tissue imbalances might be present. One reason is that they are leftover from childhood when medial rotation in-toeing was the postural pattern. Thus neural plasticity (muscle memory) tone has become entrenched and/or fascial adhesions have formed. Another reason for the soft tissue imbalance is overly facilitated/tight baseline tone of the adductor group of muscles (which are also medial rotators) or tensor fasciae latae, or overly inhibited/weak lateral rotator musculature, especially the deep lateral rotator group, due to postural and/or movement patterns as adults. People who overly pronate also tend to have an overly medially rotated lower extremity; specifically the thigh is overly medially rotated at the hip joint[13] (see Section 21.9). And increased tone of medial rotation musculature can also be due to habitual facilitation of this musculature, perhaps due to an antalgic gait. For example, a client with an injured medial meniscus might medially rotate the thigh at the hip joint to avoid the pain associated with bearing weight over the medial meniscus when walking.

EFFECTS

- A toe-in posture due to a transverse plane imbalance of soft tissue tension across the hip joint results in locked-short (medial rotation) and locked-long (lateral rotation) musculature, with the concomitant dysfunction and pain that often accompanies these conditions: increased global muscle tension, weakness, myofascial trigger points, and pain. Medially rotating the thigh at the hip joint can also create asymmetrical forces across the knee, hip, sacroiliac, and spinal joints, with dysfunction, structural injury, and pain possible with the associated musculature, fascial ligamentous/joint capsular tissue, and articular surfaces.

TREATMENT APPROACH

- If the cause of toe-in posture is a simple transverse plane soft tissue imbalance, then the manual and movement therapy approach is to relax and loosen the soft tissues that pull toward medial rotation and strengthen the soft tissues that pull toward lateral rotation.

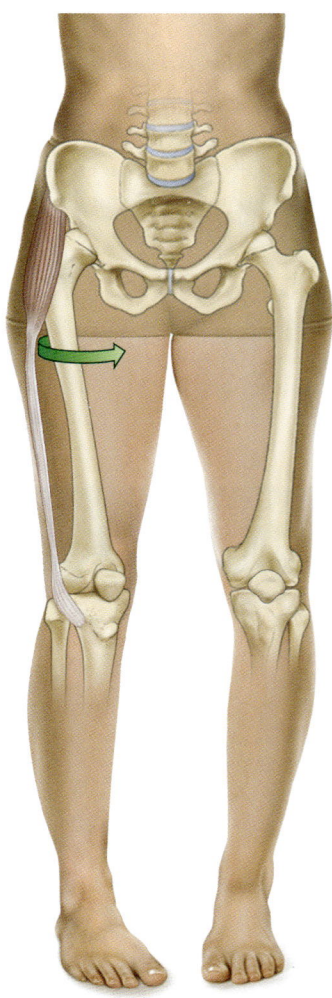

Figure 21-16 Pigeon-toe (toe-in) posture resulting from medial rotation of the thigh at the hip joint.

be part of an overly supinated foot. Or, ironically, it can present with a rearfoot valgus, in other words, rearfoot pronation, which is necessary to compensate and bring the foot flat to the ground during midstance. Forefoot varus should be grown out of during childhood.[19]

3. **Femoral torsion**. There is a femoral torsion angle (also known as an angle of anteversion; see Section 9.10) that measures the angle between the orientation of the head/neck of the femur and the shaft of the femur. The greater the angle of anteversion, the more that the hip joint needs to compensate by medially rotating the femur/thigh at the hip joint. Young children have an increased angle of anteversion that should decrease as the child grows.[20]
4. **Clubfoot**. More serious cases of the foot toe-in posture can be classified as clubfoot. This usually involves a major structural deformity that requires immediate treatment beginning at birth.[21]
5. Transverse plane soft tissue imbalance at the hip joint. Likely the simplest and most straightforward reason for a toe-in posture in

SECTION 21.17 CUBITUS VALGUS

DEFINITION

- The ulna of the forearm deviates laterally in the frontal plane compared with the humerus of the arm. The term **cubitus valgus** (*valgus* describes a lateral deviation) is used to describe this angulation (Figure 21-17). Cubitus valgus at the elbow joint is also known as the **carrying angle** because it allows objects carried in the hand to be held in the frontal plane away from the body. The usual cubitus valgus angle in a man is approximately 5-10 degrees; in a woman, it is approximately 10-15 degrees.[22] It is typically greater in a woman because the female pelvis is wider.[5] Interestingly, in both males and females, the cubitus valgus angle has been found to be slightly greater in the dominant arm, possibly related to increased use and stress upon the elbow joint.[5] A cubitus valgus angle approximately 20 degrees or greater is described as excessive cubitus valgus.[2] If the forearm actually deviates medially at the elbow joint, it is described as **cubitus varum**.[2]

ETIOLOGY

- The cause of an excessive cubitus valgus angle may be genetic or may be due to an injury (likely fracture) at the growth plate of the distal humerus.[13] An excessive cubitus valgus angle might also be aggravated/increased due to laterally directed forces place upon the medial side of the forearm, pushing the forearm laterally in the frontal plane. These forces may occur due to a macrotrauma, such as a fall on an outstretched hand; they may also occur due to repeated microtrauma, such as pushing with the hand forcefully outward on an object, with the elbow positioned excessively toward the midline of the body. These forces are especially likely to increase the cubitus valgus angle if the soft tissues on the medial side of the elbow joint (medial ligamentous/capsular fibers and the muscles and tendons of the common flexor belly/tendon [Box 21-12]) are weak/lax; and/or if the soft tissues on the lateral side of the elbow joint (lateral ligamentous/capsular fibers and the muscles and tendons of the common extensor belly/tendon) are tight/taut.

BOX 21-12	Muscles of the Common Flexor Belly/Tendon

Pronator teres
Flexor carpi radialis
Palmaris longus
Flexor carpi ulnaris
Flexor digitorum superficialis

EFFECTS

- An excessive cubitus valgus angle places tensional stress across the soft tissues on the medial side of the elbow joint, with resultant dysfunction, structural damage, and pain. These tissues include the medial collateral ligament, medial fibers of the elbow joint capsule, the ulnar nerve, and the myofascial tissues of the common flexor belly/tendon. Increased cubitus valgus may also create instability at the elbow joint and place increased stress upon the articular surfaces of the humerus and ulna. Because of the stable interlocking bony shapes of the humerus and ulna at the elbow joint, increased cubitus valgus instability is relatively rare, but this postural distortion pattern can occur.

TREATMENT APPROACH

- The manual and movement therapy approach to treatment is focused on counseling the client to avoid postures that would aggravate this condition and offering exercises to strengthen the muscles of the common flexor belly/tendon. Loosening any taut laterally oriented tissues that cross the elbow joint might also be beneficial. Manual therapy and stretching would be directed toward any dysfunctional soft tissues in the region, most likely the myofascial tissue of the common flexor belly/tendon.[13]

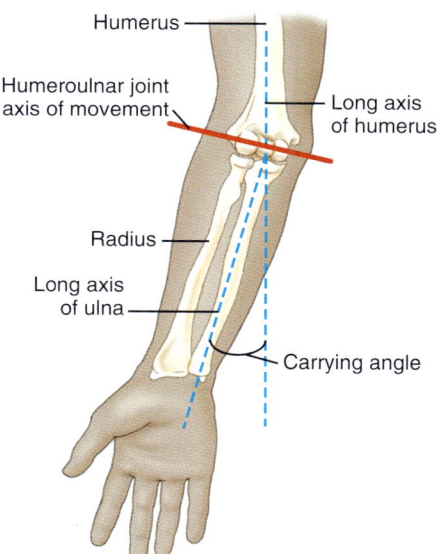

Figure 21-17 Cubitus valgus (carrying) angle.

REVIEW QUESTIONS

Answers to the following review questions appear on the Evolve website accompanying this book at: http://evolve.elsevier.com/Muscolino/kinesiology/.

1. Compare and contrast lower and upper crossed syndromes.

2. What is the definition of a scoliotic curve?

3. What is the principal cause of rounded low back/pelvis?

4. What is the relationship between the tilt of the pelvis and the curves of the spine?

5. Describe overpronation of the foot.

6. What muscles should be strengthened in a client with genu valgus?

7. What causes hammertoes?

8. What are the effects of a protracted head on the neck musculature?

9. Explain how the spine might compensate for a low iliac crest height.

10. Define *adaptive shortening*, and give an example.

REFERENCES

1. Page P, Frank CC, Lardner R: Assessment and treatment of muscle imbalance: The Janda approach, Champaign, IL, 2010, Human Kinetics.
2. Neumann DA: Kinesiology of the musculoskeletal system: Foundations for physical rehabilitation, ed 3, St Louis, 2017, Elsevier.
3. Myers TW: Anatomy trains: Myofascial meridians for manual & movement therapists, ed 3, Italy, 2014, Churchill Livingstone Elsevier.
4. Muscolino JE: The muscular system manual: The skeletal muscles of the human body, ed 4, St Louis, 2017, Elsevier.
5. Levangie PK, Norkin CC: Joint structure and function: A comprehensive analysis, ed 5, Philadelphia, 2001, FA Davis.
6. Sahrmann SA: Diagnosis and treatment of movement impairment syndromes, St Louis, 2002, Mosby.
7. Bompa T, Buzzichelli C: Periodization training for sports, ed 3, Champaign, IL, 2015, Human Kinetics.
8. Hamilton N, Weimar W, Luttgens K: Kinesiology: Scientific basis of human motion, ed 12, New York, 2012, McGraw Hill.
9. Muscolino JE: The price of smart phones. Massage Therapy Journal, 54(2):17-24, 2015.

10. Oatis CA: Kinesiology: The mechanics and pathomechanics of human movement, Philadelphia, 2004, Lippincott Williams & Wilkins.
11. Chaitow L: Cranial manipulation theory and practice: Osseus and soft tissue approaches, ed 2, Edinburgh, 2005, Elsevier Churchill Livingstone.
12. Werner R: A massage therapist's guide to pathology, ed 4, Philadelphia, 2004, Lippincott Williams & Wilkins.
13. Lowe W: Orthopedic assessment in massage therapy, Sisters, 2006, Daviau Scott.
14. Solberg G: Postural disorders and musculoskeletal dysfunction: Diagnosis, prevention, and treatment, Edinburgh, 2007, Churchill Livingstone.
15. Kendall FP, McCreary EK, Provance PG, et al.: Muscles: Testing and function, ed 5, Baltimore, 2005, Lippincott Williams & Wilkins.
16. Cramer GD, Darby SA: Basic and clinical anatomy of the spine, spinal cord, and ANS, St Louis, 1995, Mosby.
17. Lowe W: Functional assessment in massage therapy, ed 3, Bend, 1997, OMERI.
18. Palastanga N, Field D, Soames R: Anatomy and human movement, ed 4, Oxford, 2002, Butterworth-Heinemann.
19. Staheli LT: Fundamentals of pediatric orthopedics, ed 4, Philadelphia, 2008, Lippincott Williams & Wilkins.
20. Hamill J, Knutzen KM: Biomechanical basis of human movement, ed 12, Baltimore, 2003, Lippincott Williams & Wilkins.
21. Jenkins DB: Hollinshead's functional anatomy of the limbs and back, ed 8, Philadelphia, 2002, WB Saunders Company.
22. Smith LK, Weiss EL, Lehmkuhl LO: Brunstrom's clinical kinesiology, ed 5, Philadelphia, 1996, FA Davis.

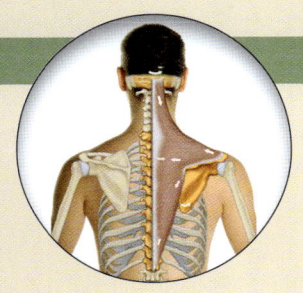

CHAPTER 22

Stretching

CHAPTER OUTLINE

Section 22.1 Introduction
Section 22.2 Basic Stretching Techniques: Static Stretching versus Dynamic Stretching
Section 22.3 Advanced Stretching Techniques: Pin and Stretch Technique
Section 22.4 Advanced Stretching Techniques: Contract Relax and Agonist Contract Stretching Techniques

CHAPTER OBJECTIVES

After completing this chapter, the student should be able to perform the following:

1. Define the key terms of this chapter and state the meanings of the word origins of this chapter.
2. Do the following related to stretching:
   - Describe the relationship between a line of tension and stretching.
   - Discuss the purpose and benefit of stretching and describe why stretching is done.
   - Explain how stretches can be reasoned out instead of memorized.
   - Describe the relationship of the pain-spasm-pain cycle and the muscle spindle reflex to the force exerted during a stretch.
   - Discuss when stretching should be done, especially with respect to an exercise workout routine.
3. Compare and contrast static stretching with dynamic stretching.
4. Discuss how and why the pin and stretch technique is done.
5. Do the following related to contract relax and agonist contract stretching techniques:
   - Describe how to perform the contract relax, agonist contract, and contract relax agonist contract stretching techniques.
   - Discuss the similarities and differences between contract relax stretching and agonist contract stretching.

OVERVIEW

This chapter discusses the therapeutic tool of stretching. It begins with an explanation of some of the choices that are available to the therapist and trainer when stretching a client. Basic questions pertaining to stretching are then posed and answered so that the therapist and trainer can better understand how to incorporate stretching into therapeutic practice. The two basic stretching techniques, static stretching and dynamic stretching, are then described and contrasted, with an explanation of when each method is best applied. The chapter concludes with a discussion of the advanced stretching techniques: pin and stretch, contract relax (CR) stretching (often known as *PNF stretching*), and agonist contract (AC) stretching. A brief description is then given of contract relax agonist contract (CRAC) stretching.

KEY TERMS

Active tension
Agonist contract (AC) stretching (AH-go-nist)
Antagonist contract stretching
Contract relax agonist contract (CRAC) stretching
Contract relax (CR) stretching
Dynamic stretching
Golgi tendon organ (GTO) reflex (GOAL-gee)
Good pain
Line of tension
Mobilization
Multiplane stretching
Muscle spindle reflex
Myofibroblast (MY-o-FI-bro-blast)

Neural inhibition stretching
Passive tension
Pin and stretch
Post-isometric relaxation (PIR) stretching
Proprioceptive neuromuscular facilitation (PNF) stretching (PRO-pree-o-SEP-iv noor-o-MUS-kyu-lar)
Reciprocal inhibition
Static stretching
Stretching
Target muscle
Target tissue
Tension

WORD ORIGINS

- Active—From Latin *activus,* meaning *doing, driving*
- Agonist—From Greek *agon,* meaning *a fight, a contest*
- Antagonist—From Greek *anti,* meaning *against, opposite,* and *agon,* meaning *a fight, a contest*
- Dynamic—From Greek *dynamis,* meaning *power*
- Facilitation—From Latin *facilitas,* meaning *easy*
- Golgi—Named for *Camillo Golgi,* Italian pathologist
- Inhibition—From Latin *inhibeo,* meaning *to keep back* (from Latin *habeo,* meaning *to have*)
- Myofibroblast—From Greek *mys,* meaning *muscle,* and Latin *fibra,* meaning *fiber,* and from Greek *blastos,* meaning *to bud, to build, to grow*
- Passive—From Latin *passivus,* meaning *permits, endures*
- Postisometric—From Latin *post,* meaning *behind, after,* and Greek *isos,* meaning *equal,* and Greek *metrikos,* meaning *measure, length*
- Proprioceptive—From Latin *proprius,* meaning *one's own,* and *capio,* meaning *to take*
- Reciprocal—From Latin *reciprocus,* meaning *alternate*
- Stretch—From Old English *streccan,* meaning *to extend, lengthen*
- Tension—From Latin *tensio,* meaning *to stretch*

SECTION 22.1 INTRODUCTION

- Stretching is a powerful therapeutic tool that is available to manual therapists and athletic trainers to improve the health of their clients. Very few people disagree about the benefits of stretching; multiple studies have shown that regular stretching is successful toward lengthening and loosening tight/taut myofascial tissue.[1] However, there is a great deal of disagreement about how stretching should be done. There are many possible choices. For example, stretching can be performed statically or dynamically. Three repetitions (reps) can be done, each one held approximately 10 to 20 seconds, or 10 reps can be performed, each one held for approximately 2 to 3 seconds. A technique called *pin and stretching* can be done, or stretches that use neurologic reflexes to facilitate the stretch, such as contract relax (CR) and agonist contract (AC) stretching, can be performed. There are also choices regarding when stretching is best done: stretching can be done before or after strengthening exercise.
- To best understand stretching so that we can apply it clinically for the optimal health of our clients, let's first look at the fundamental basis of stretching by posing and answering the following five questions: What is stretching? Why is stretching done? How do we figure out how to stretch muscles? How forcefully should we stretch? When should stretching be done? Then we can examine the types of stretching techniques that are available to the client and therapist/trainer.

1. WHAT IS STRETCHING?

- Simply defined, **stretching** is a method of physical bodywork that lengthens and elongates soft tissues. These soft tissues may be muscles and their tendons (collectively called *myofascial units*), ligaments, joint capsules, and/or other fascial planes. When performing a stretch on our client, we use the term **target tissue** to describe the tissue that we intend to stretch, or **target muscle** when we specifically want to stretch a muscle or muscle group. To create a stretch, the client's body is moved into a position that creates a **line of tension** that pulls on the target tissues, placing a stretch on them (Figure 22-1). If the stretch is effective, the tissues will be lengthened.

CHAPTER 22 Stretching

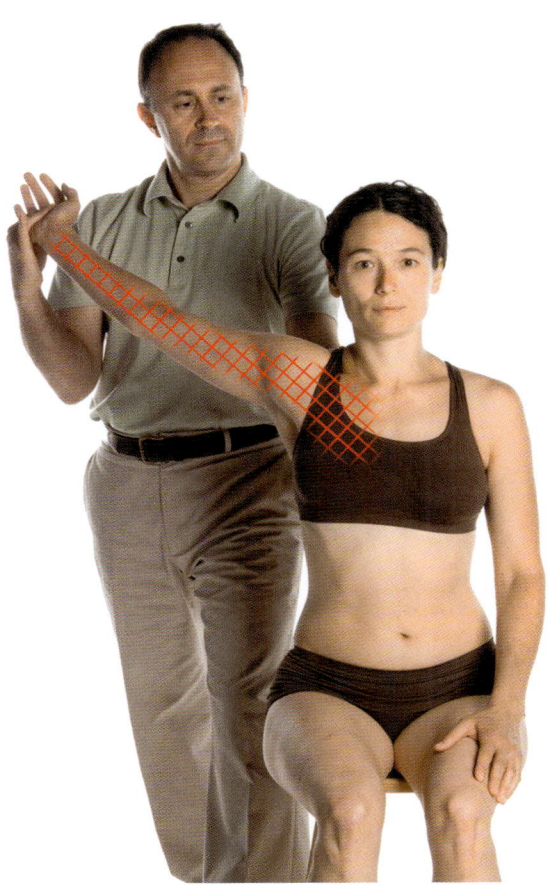

FIGURE 22-1 A client's right upper extremity is stretched. The line of tension created by this stretch is indicated by hatch marks and extends from the client's anterior forearm to the pectoral region. A stretch is exerted on all tissues along the line of tension of the stretch.

2. WHY IS STRETCHING DONE?

- Stretching is done because soft tissues may increase in tension and become shortened and contracted. Shortened and contracted soft tissues resist lengthening and limit mobility of the joint that they cross.[2] The tension of a tissue can be described as its resistance to stretch. The specific joint motion that is limited will be the motion of a body part (at the joint) that is in the opposite direction from the location of the tight tissues. For example, if the tight tissue is located on the posterior side of the joint, anterior motion of a body part at that joint will be limited, and if the tight tissue is located on the anterior side of the joint, posterior motion of a body part at that joint will be limited. Figure 22-2, *A* shows a decreased flexion of the thigh at the hip joint because of taut tissues, tight hamstrings, at the posterior side of the hip joint. Similarly, tight hamstrings would also limit anterior tilt of the pelvis at the hip joint because anterior pelvic tilt is the reverse action of flexion of the thigh at the hip joint. If anterior hip joint tissues, especially hip joint flexor muscles, such as the tensor fasciae latae seen in Figure 22-2, *B* are tight, a decrease in range of motion of extension of the thigh at the hip joint will occur. Similarly, tight anterior hip joint tissues also limit posterior tilt of the pelvis at the hip joint (posterior pelvic tilt is the reverse action of extension of the thigh at the hip joint).

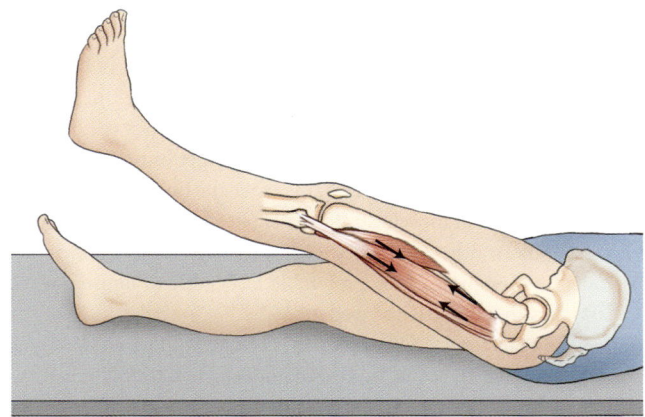

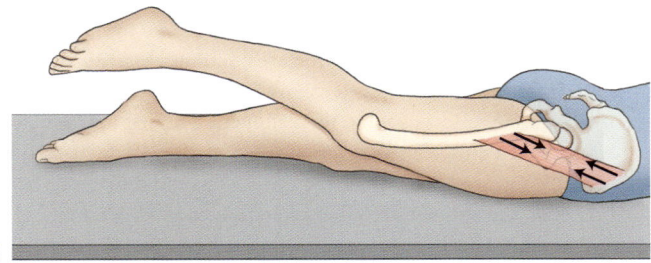

FIGURE 22-2 A, Tight hip extensors (hamstrings shown here) limit flexion of the thigh at the hip joint. **B,** Tight hip flexors (tensor fasciae latae shown here) limit extension of the thigh at the hip joint.

- As stated, a shortened and contracted tissue can be described as having greater **tension**. Two types of tissue tension exist, passive tension and active tension. All soft tissues can exhibit increased passive tension. **Passive tension** results from the natural elasticity of a tissue. In muscle tissue, it is proposed that passive tension results from the presence of the protein titin within the sarcomere[3] (for more on titin, see Section 12.11). Passive tension can also be increased because of fascial adhesions that build up over time in soft tissues.
- In addition, muscles may exhibit increased active tension. **Active tension** results when a muscle's contractile elements (actin and myosin filaments) contract via the sliding filament mechanism, creating a pulling force toward the center of the muscle. Whether a soft tissue has increased passive or active tension, this increased tension makes the tissue more resistant to lengthening. Therefore stretching is done to lengthen and elongate these tissues, hopefully restoring full range of motion and flexibility of the body.[3]
- Muscles have classically been considered to be the only tissue that can exhibit active tension. However, recent research has shown that fibrous connective tissues often contain cells called **myofibroblasts**, which evolve from fibroblasts normally found in them. Myofibroblasts contain contractile proteins that can actively contract. Although not present in the same numbers as in muscle tissue, connective tissue myofibroblasts may be present in sufficient numbers to be biomechanically significant, which must be considered in assessment of the active tension of that connective tissue[4] (for more on myofibroblasts, see Section 4.3).

3. HOW DO WE FIGURE OUT HOW TO STRETCH MUSCLES?

○ If our target tissue to be stretched is a muscle, the question is: How do we figure out what position the client's body must be put in to achieve an effective stretch of that target muscle or muscle group? Certainly, there are many excellent books available for learning specific muscle stretches. However, better than relying on a book or other authority to give us stretching routines that must be memorized, it is preferable to be able to figure out the stretches that our clients need.

○ Figuring out a stretch for a muscle is actually quite easy. Our goal is to lengthen the muscle. To accomplish this, simply recall the joint actions that were learned for the target muscle, and then do the opposite of one or more of its actions. Because the actions of a muscle are what the muscle does when it shortens, then stretching and lengthening the muscle would be achieved by having the client do the opposite of the muscle's actions. Essentially, if a muscle flexes a joint, then extension of that joint would stretch it; if the muscle abducts a joint, then adduction of that joint would stretch it; if a muscle medially rotates a joint, then lateral rotation of that joint would stretch it. If a muscle has more than one action, then the optimal stretch would consider all its actions.[2]

○ For example, if the target muscle that is being stretched is the right upper trapezius, given that its actions are extension, right lateral flexion, and left rotation of the neck and head at the spinal joints, then stretching the right upper trapezius would require either flexion, left lateral flexion, and/or right rotation of the head and neck at the spinal joints.

○ When a muscle has many actions, it is not always necessary to do the opposite of all of them; however, at times it might be desired or needed. If the right upper trapezius is tight enough, simply doing flexion in the sagittal plane might be sufficient to stretch it. However, if further stretch is needed, then left lateral flexion in the frontal plane and/or right rotation in the transverse plane could be added as shown in Figure 22-3.

○ Even if not every plane of action is used for the stretch, it is still important to be aware of all the muscle's actions or a mistake might be made with the stretch. For example, if the right upper trapezius is being stretched by flexing and left laterally flexing the client's head and neck, it is important to not let the client's head and neck rotate to the left, because this will allow the right upper trapezius to be slackened and the tension of the stretch will be lost. Furthermore, given that the right upper trapezius also elevates the right scapula at the scapulocostal joint, it is important to make sure that the right scapula is depressed or at least not allowed to elevate during the stretch, or the tension of the stretch will also be lost.

○ It can be very difficult to isolate a stretch so that only one target muscle is stretched. When a stretch is performed, usually an entire functional group of muscles is stretched at the same time (Box 22-1).

○ For example, if a client's thigh is stretched into extension at the hip joint in the sagittal plane, the entire functional group of sagittal plane hip joint flexors will be stretched (the functional group of flexors of the hip joint includes the tensor fasciae latae [TFL], anterior fibers of the gluteus medius and minimus, sartorius, rectus femoris, iliopsoas, pectineus, adductor longus, gracilis, and adductor brevis). To isolate one of the hip joint flexors usually

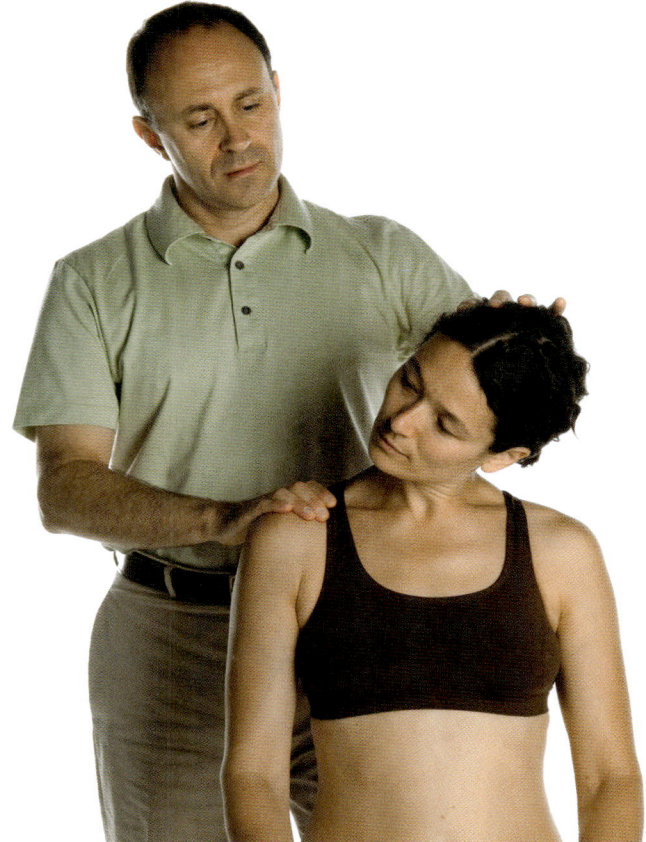

FIGURE 22-3 The right upper trapezius is stretched in all three planes. The movements of a stretch of a target muscle are always antagonistic to the joint actions of that muscle. In this case, the right upper trapezius is an extensor in the sagittal plane, right lateral flexor in the frontal plane, and left rotator in the transverse plane of the head and neck at the spinal joints. Therefore, to stretch the right upper trapezius, the client's head and neck are flexed in the sagittal plane, left laterally flexed in the frontal plane, and right rotated in the transverse plane.

requires fine-tuning the stretch to achieve the desired result. If the stretch is done into extension in the sagittal plane and adduction in the frontal plane, then all hip joint flexor muscles that are also frontal plane adductors will be slackened and relaxed by the adduction, but the stretch on those hip flexor muscles that are also abductors (such as the TFL, the sartorius, and the anterior fibers of the gluteus medius and minimus) will be increased.

○ If medial rotation of the thigh at the hip joint in the transverse plane is also added to the stretch so that the thigh is now being

 BOX 22-1

Whenever a stretch affects a functional group of muscles, in other words, a number of muscles, the tightest muscle within the line of tension of the stretch will usually be the limiting factor of how forcefully the stretch can be done. The problem with this is that if a different muscle is the therapist/trainer's target muscle to be stretched, it will not be successfully stretched because the stretch was limited by the tighter muscle.

extended in the sagittal plane, adducted in the frontal plane, and medially rotated in the transverse plane, then all hip joint flexors and abductors that are also transverse plane medial rotators will be slackened and relaxed by medial rotation, but the stretch on muscles that perform flexion, abduction, and lateral rotation of the thigh at the hip joint will be increased. In this case, the sartorius will be the principal target muscle to be stretched because it is the only hip joint flexor and abductor muscle that also laterally rotates the thigh at the hip joint (the iliopsoas will also be stretched because it is a flexor and lateral rotator at the hip joint, and some sources state that it can also abduct[5]). Of course, given that the sartorius is also a flexor of the leg at the knee joint, it is imperative that the knee joint be extended during the stretch, or the sartorius would be slackened by a flexed knee joint and the effectiveness of the stretch for the sartorius would be lost.

- Had lateral rotation of the thigh at the hip joint been added as the third transverse plane component instead of medial rotation, then the sartorius, being a lateral rotator, would have been slackened and the TFL and anterior fibers of the gluteus medius and minimus, being medial rotators, would have been preferentially stretched instead. To then isolate the stretch to just the TFL or just the anterior fibers of the gluteus medius or minimus is difficult if not impossible, because these muscles all share the same actions in all three planes and therefore are stretched by the same joint position.
- Stretching a muscle across more than one cardinal plane is called **multiplane stretching**.
- Therefore whenever a client's body part is moved into a stretch in one direction—in other words, in one plane—the entire functional group of muscles located on the other side of the joint is stretched. To then fine-tune and isolate the stretch to one or only a few of the muscles of this functional group requires adding other components to the stretch. These other components might involve adding other planes to the stretch, or they may involve adding a stretch to another joint if the target muscle crosses more than one joint—in other words, is a multijoint muscle.
- Figuring out exactly how to fine-tune a stretch to isolate a target muscle depends on a solid foundation of knowledge of the joint actions of the muscles involved. Once this knowledge is attained, applying it can eliminate the need for memorizing tens or hundreds of stretches. In the place of memorization comes an ability to critically reason through the steps necessary to figure out whatever stretches are needed for the proper treatment of our clients!
- Note: If the target tissue to be stretched is not a muscle but rather a ligament, a region of a joint capsule, or some other fascial plane of tissue, its stretch can still be reasoned out instead of memorized. One way to do this is to think of this fascial tissue as though it were a muscle; figure out what its action would be if it were a muscle, and then perform the action that is antagonistic to that action. Even simpler, move the client's body part at the joint that this tissue crosses in the direction that is away from the side of the joint where it is located. For example, if the target tissue is a ligament located anteriorly at the hip joint, then simply move the client's thigh posteriorly at the hip joint (or posteriorly tilt the pelvis at the hip joint) to stretch it. Doing this will work for most anteriorly located fascial tissues at the hip joint, except for the ones that are arranged horizontally in the transverse plane. To stretch these, a transverse plane rotation motion is needed.

4. HOW FORCEFULLY SHOULD WE STRETCH?

- Stretching should never hurt. If stretching causes pain, it is likely that the target muscles or muscles in the vicinity of the target tissues will tighten in response to the pain via the pain-spasm-pain cycle (for more on the pain-spasm-pain cycle, see Section 19.10).[6] Furthermore, if the target muscle is stretched either too quickly or too forcefully, the **muscle spindle reflex** may be engaged, resulting in a tightening of the target muscle.[3] Given that a stretch should relax and lengthen tissue, stretching that causes musculature to tighten defeats the purpose of the stretch.
- For this reason, a stretch should never be done too quickly; stretching should always be done slowly and rhythmically.[2] If a bounce is to be added, it should be a gentle bounce and should be gradually introduced into the stretching protocol over the course of many weeks or months. Furthermore, the therapist/trainer should be prudent and judicious regarding how far a client is stretched. And a stretch should never cause pain; theoretically, a stretch can be done as hard as possible, but always without pain. When in doubt, it is best to be conservative regarding the speed and forcefulness of a stretch. It is wiser to gently and slowly stretch a client over a number of sessions to safely achieve the goal of loosening the target tissues. It may take more sessions, but a positive outcome is essentially guaranteed. Imprudent stretching not only may set back the progress of the client's treatment program but may also cause damage that is difficult to reverse (Box 22-2).

BOX 22-2

Clients often describe a stretch as being painful but go on to say that the pain feels good. For this reason, a distinction should be made between what is often described by the client as **good pain** and true pain (or what might be called bad pain). Good pain is often the way that a client describes the sensation of the stretch; therefore causing good pain as a result of a stretch is fine. However, if a stretch causes true pain—in other words, the client winces and resists or fights the stretch—then the intensity of the stretch must be lessened. Otherwise, not only will the stretch not be effective, but the client is likely to be injured. A stretch should never be forced.

5. WHEN SHOULD STRETCHING BE DONE?

- Stretching should be done when the target tissues are most receptive to being stretched. Target tissues are most receptive when they are already warmed up.[7]
- Warming/heating the soft tissues of the body facilitates stretching them in two ways: first, heat is a central nervous depressant helping the musculature relax[8]; second, myofascial tissue is more easily stretched when warm.[8]
- Not only do cold tissues resist stretching, resulting in little benefit, they are also more likely to be injured when stretched.[9] For this reason, if stretching is linked to a physical exercise workout, the stretching should be done after the workout when the tissues are warmed up, not before the workout when the tissues are cold. This general principle is true if the type of stretching is the classic form, called *static stretching*. If dynamic stretching is done instead, then

- it is safe and appropriate to stretch before an exercise regimen when the tissues are cold, because dynamic stretching is a method of warming the tissues in addition to stretching them. For more on static versus dynamic stretching, see the next section.
- If the client wants to stretch but does not have the opportunity to first engage in physical exercise to warm the target tissues, then the client may warm them by applying moist heat. There are a number of ways to do this. Taking a hot shower or bath, using a whirlpool, and placing a moist heating pad or hydrocollator pack on the target tissues are all effective ways to warm target tissues before stretching them. Of all these choices, perhaps the most effective one is taking a hot shower, because not only does it warm the tissues, but the pressure of the water hitting the skin also physically creates a massage that can help to relax the musculature of the region.

SECTION 22.2 BASIC STRETCHING TECHNIQUES: STATIC STRETCHING VERSUS DYNAMIC STRETCHING

- Classically, stretching has been what is called **static stretching**, meaning that the position of the stretch is attained and then held statically for a period of time (Figure 22-4). The length of time recommended to statically hold a stretch has traditionally been 10 to 30 seconds, and three reps have usually been recommended.[2] However, the wisdom of this "classic" technique of stretching has recently been questioned[2] (Box 22-3). Regardless of controversy, based upon the characteristic property of soft tissue called creep (see Section 4.6), static stretching must have efficacy. Creep states that a sustained force placed upon a soft tissue will gradually deform it (i.e., change its form).[3] The word *deform* usually has a negative connotation, but in this case the connotation is positive. The form is changed from being tight and short to being long and loose, in other words, stretched.

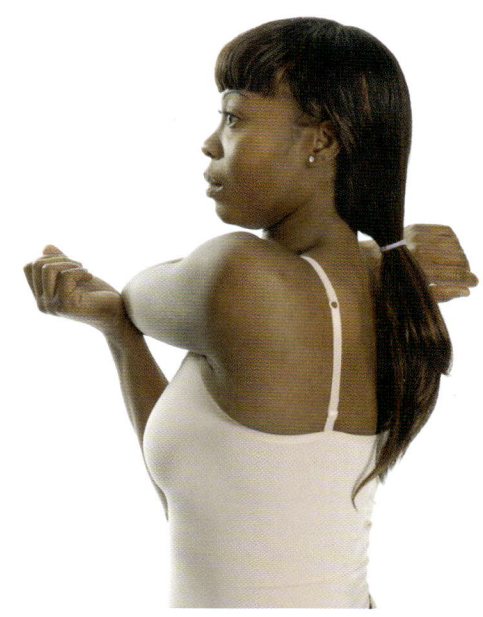

FIGURE 22-4 A client is performing a static stretch of her left arm and scapular region. Static stretches are done by bringing the body part to a position of stretch and then statically holding that position for a period of time. (From Muscolino JE: Stretch your way to better health, *Massage Ther J* 45:167, 2006. Photo by Yanik Chauvin.)

BOX 22-3

Some sources state that static stretching done before strengthening exercise is actually deleterious to the performance of the exercise. Their reasoning is that when muscles are stretched, they are neurologically inhibited from contracting and consequently less able to contract quickly when needed to protect a joint from a possible sprain or strain during strenuous exercise.[1] What is most important before engaging in any type of strengthening exercise is to warm up the body.

- The alternative to static stretching is called **dynamic stretching**, also known as **mobilization stretching**. Dynamic stretching is done by moving the joints of the body through ranges of motion instead of holding the body in a static position of stretch. The idea is that whenever a joint is moved in a certain direction, the tissues on the other side of the joint are lengthened and stretched.[2] Following the example of Figure 22-2, if the hip joint is flexed (whether by the usual action of flexion of the thigh at the hip joint or the reverse action of anterior tilt of the pelvis at the hip joint), then the tissues on the other side of the joint, the hip joint extensor muscles and other posterior soft tissues, will be stretched. Similarly, if the hip joint is extended (whether by extending the thigh at the hip joint or posteriorly tilting the pelvis at the hip joint), the hip joint flexor muscles and other anterior tissues will be stretched.
- By this concept, any joint motion of the body stretches some of the tissues of that joint. Of course, it is important when doing dynamic stretching that the joint motions are performed in a careful, prudent, and graded manner, gradually increasing the intensity of the motions. For this reason, dynamic stretching begins with small ranges of motion carried out with little or no resistance. It then gradually builds up to full ranges of motion. If dynamic stretching is done before a physical workout, then the ranges of motion that are performed should be the same ranges of motion that will be asked of the body during the physical workout.[10] And if the exercise entails some form of added resistance, then the added resistance of the exercise should gradually be added to the dynamic stretching after the full ranges of motion of the joints are accomplished.
- For example, before playing tennis, one would go through the motions of forehand, backhand, and serving strokes without a racquet in hand, beginning with small swings and building up to full range of motion swings. Then the same order of motions would be repeated, but this time with the added resistance of having the tennis racquet in hand (but not actually hitting a ball), starting with small swings and gradually working up to full range of motion swings. Finally, the person adds the full resistance of hitting the tennis ball while playing on the court, again, starting with gentle, short swings and gradually building up to full range of motion and powerful swings (Figure 22-5).

- The advantage of dynamic stretching is that not only is it a stretch, it is also an effective exercise warm-up. Arterial, venous, and lymph circulation is increased, synovial fluid movement is increased, the joints are brought through their ranges of motion, and the neural pathways that will be used during the exercise routine engaged.[10] Even though dynamic stretching is the ideal method to employ before engaging in physical exercise, it can certainly be done at any time.

- Given the benefits of dynamic stretching, is there still a place for classic static stretching? Yes. As explained earlier, static stretching is beneficial if the tissues are first warmed up. This means that static stretching can be very effective after an exercise routine is done (or if the tissues are first warmed up by applying moist heat).

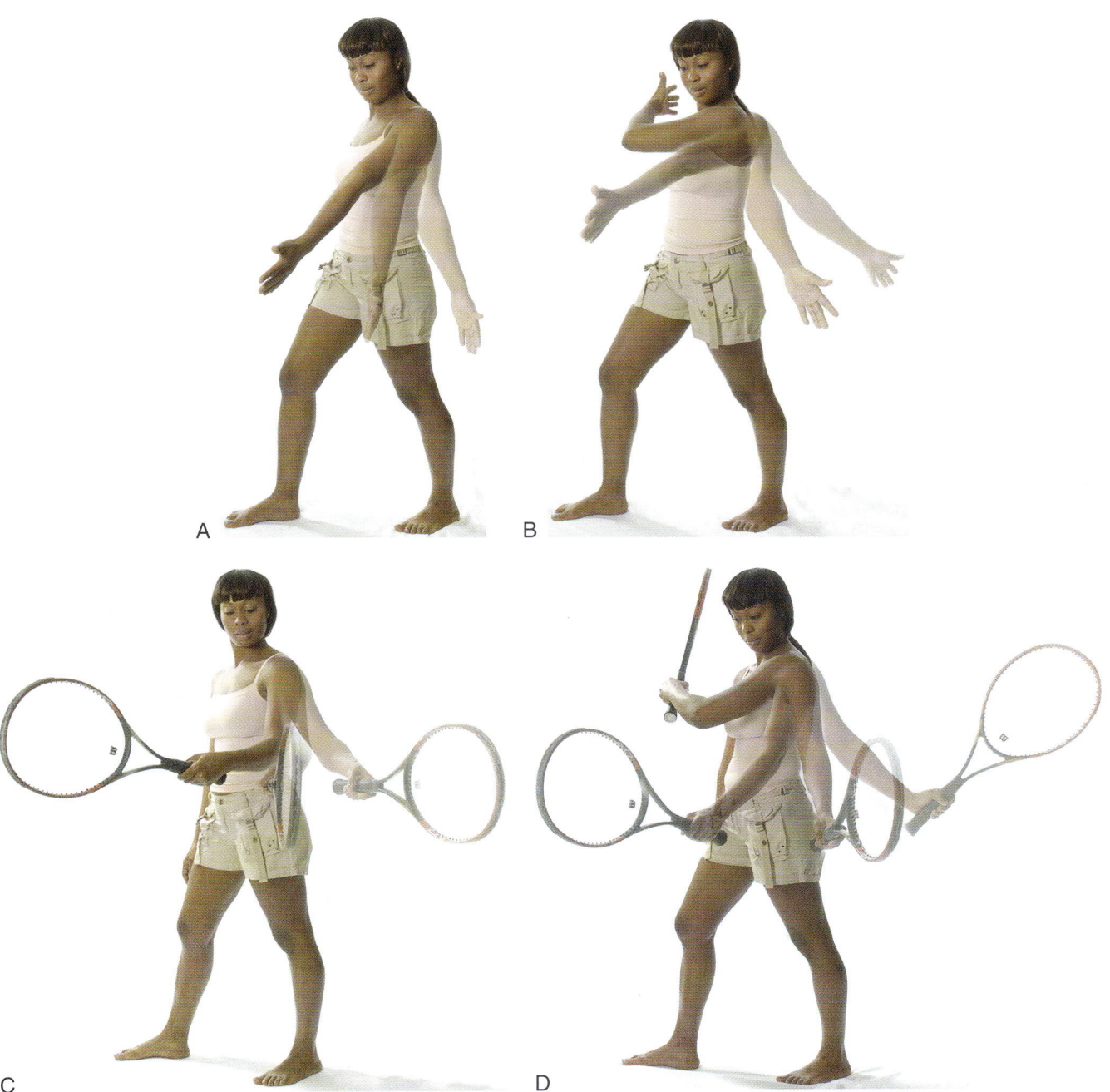

FIGURE 22-5 Illustration showing the beginning stages of dynamic stretching for a forehand stroke in tennis. In **A,** a short forehand swing is done without holding a racquet. In **B,** a full range of motion swing is done without the racquet. The person then progresses to holding a racquet to provide greater resistance, first with a short swing as seen in **C,** and then with a full range of motion swing as seen in **D.** After this, the person is ready to progress to the added resistance of playing tennis and hitting the ball. Note that with dynamic stretching, when the arm is brought posteriorly for the backswing, the muscles in front of the shoulder joint are stretched, and when the person swings forward with the forehand stroke, the muscles in back of the shoulder joint are stretched. *(From Muscolino JE: Stretch your way to better health,* Massage Ther J *45:167, 2006. Photos by Yanik Chauvin.)*

SECTION 22.3 ADVANCED STRETCHING TECHNIQUES: PIN AND STRETCH TECHNIQUE

- Beyond the choice of performing a stretch statically or dynamically, there are other, more advanced stretching options. One of these advanced options is pin and stretch technique. **Pin and stretch** technique is a stretching technique in which the therapist/trainer pins (stabilizes) one part of the client's body and then stretches the tissues up to that pinned spot.
- The purpose of the pin and stretch is to direct a stretch to a more specific region of the client's body. As stated previously, when a body part is moved to create a stretch, a line of tension is created. Everything along the line of tension will be stretched. However, if we want only a certain region of the soft tissues along that line of tension to be stretched, then we can specifically direct the stretch to that region by using the pin and stretch technique.[11]
- For example, if a side-lying stretch is done on a client as demonstrated in Figure 22-6, *A,* the entire lateral side of the client's body from the therapist/trainer's right hand on the client's distal thigh to the therapist/trainer's left hand on the client's upper trunk will be stretched. The problem with allowing the line of tension of a stretch to spread over such a large region of the client's body is that the intensity of the stretch is diluted over this large expanse, and if one region of soft tissue of the client's body within that line of tension is very tight, it might stop the stretch

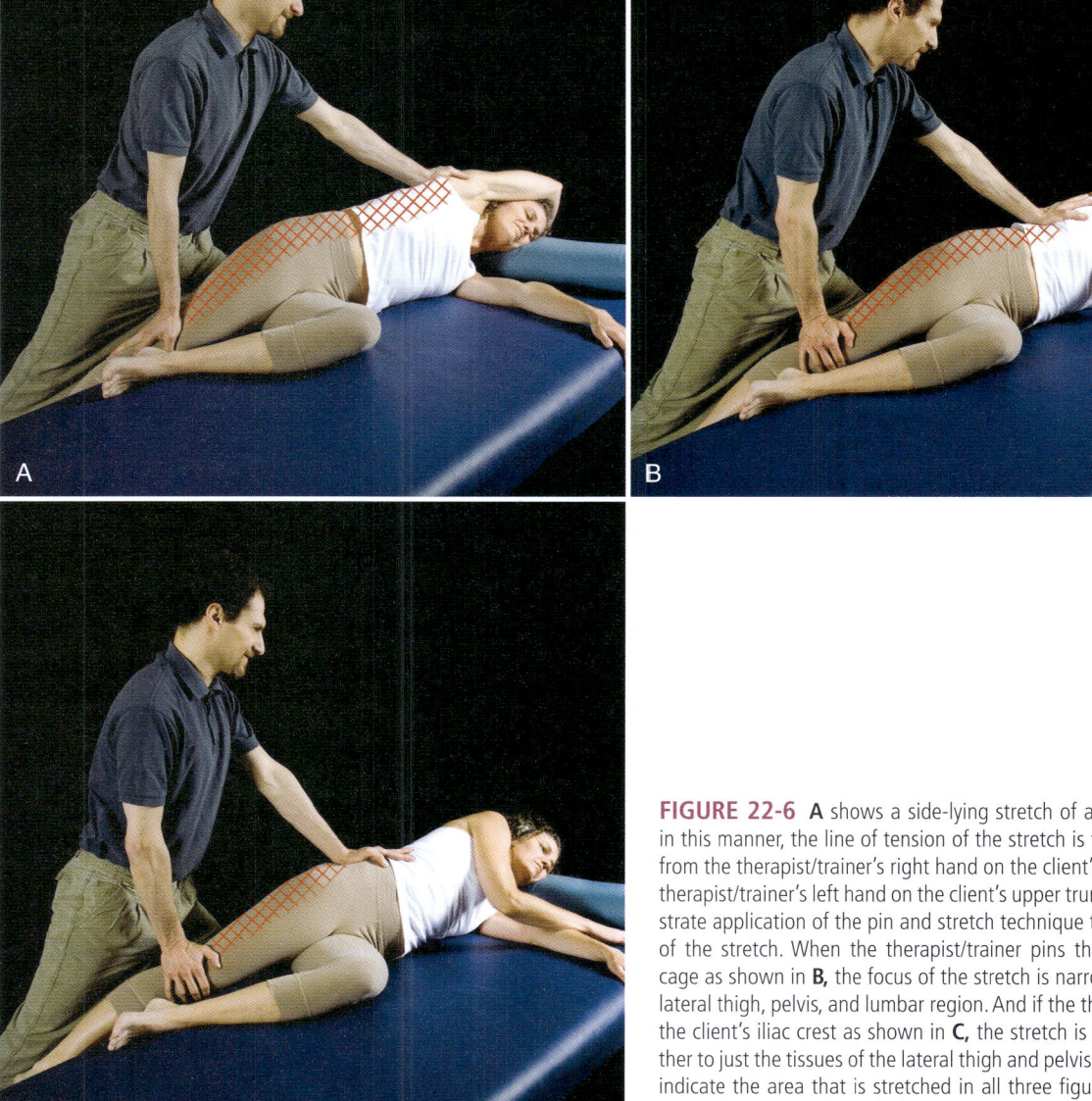

FIGURE 22-6 **A** shows a side-lying stretch of a client. When done in this manner, the line of tension of the stretch is very broad, ranging from the therapist/trainer's right hand on the client's distal thigh to the therapist/trainer's left hand on the client's upper trunk. **B** and **C** demonstrate application of the pin and stretch technique to narrow the focus of the stretch. When the therapist/trainer pins the client's lower rib cage as shown in **B,** the focus of the stretch is narrowed to the client's lateral thigh, pelvis, and lumbar region. And if the therapist/trainer pins the client's iliac crest as shown in **C,** the stretch is narrowed even further to just the tissues of the lateral thigh and pelvis. Note: Hatch marks indicate the area that is stretched in all three figures. *(Modified from Muscolino JE:* Stretching the hip, *Massage Ther J 46:167, 2007. Photos by Yanik Chauvin.)*

- from being felt in another area of the line of tension that we are specifically targeting to stretch.
- To focus the line of tension and direct the stretch to our target tissues, we can use the pin and stretch technique. If the therapist/trainer pins the client's lower rib cage, as seen in Figure 22-6, *B*, the stretch will no longer be felt in the client's lateral thoracic region; instead it will be specifically directed to the client's lateral thigh, pelvis, and lumbar region. If the therapist/trainer instead pins the client's iliac crest, as seen in Figure 22-6, *C*, the stretch will no longer be felt in the client's lateral lumbar region and will now be directed to only the lateral musculature and other soft tissues of the client's thigh and pelvis. In effect, the pin and stretch technique pins and stabilizes a part of the client's body, thereby focusing and directing the force of the line of tension of the stretch to the specific target tissue(s).
- Continuing with this example, if the target tissues are the gluteus medius and quadratus lumborum (as well as other muscles of the lateral pelvis and lateral lumbar region), pinning the client at the lower rib cage, as seen in Figure 22-6, *B*, would be the ideal approach. If the target tissue is limited to the gluteus medius (and other muscles/soft tissues of the lateral pelvis), the ideal location to pin the client during this side-lying stretch is at the iliac crest, as seen in Figure 22-6, *C*. As can be seen here, pin and stretch is a powerful technique that allows for much greater specificity when stretching a client.
- This concept of pin and stretch can also be applied to one specific muscle. This allows the focus of the stretch to be applied to one end of the muscle instead of being applied across the entire length of the entire muscle. This is extremely helpful when there is a tight area at one end of the muscle, but when the entire muscle is stretched, the other end of the muscle gives with the stretch, preventing the effect of the stretch from lengthening the region of tightness. In effect, we have a "hypermobile" region of the muscle compensating for the tight "hypomobile" region. By pinning the muscle and then stretching it, the stretch is focused on the area of the muscle that is between the pinned point and the attachment that is moved. For this reason, pin and stretch technique applied to a muscle is effective when the region of the muscle that requires the stretch is toward the distal end of the muscle, in other words, the attachment that can be easily moved.

SECTION 22.4 ADVANCED STRETCHING TECHNIQUES: CONTRACT RELAX AND AGONIST CONTRACT STRETCHING TECHNIQUES

- Two other advanced stretching techniques that are extremely effective are the **contract relax (CR) stretching** technique and the **agonist contract (AC) stretching** technique. Both of these advanced stretching techniques are similar in that they employ a neurologic reflex to inhibit, in other words relax, the target muscle from contracting, thereby facilitating the stretch. For this reason, these techniques are termed **neural inhibition stretches**. The CR technique has classically been described as utilizing the neurologic reflex called the *Golgi tendon organ (GTO) reflex* (although there is some controversy regarding this). The AC technique uses the neurologic reflex called *reciprocal inhibition*.[7]

CONTRACT RELAX STRETCHING:

- Contract relax (CR) stretching is perhaps better known as **proprioceptive neuromuscular facilitation (PNF) stretching**; it is also known as **post-isometric relaxation (PIR) stretching**.
- The name *contract relax* is used because the target muscle is first *contracted*, and then it is *relaxed*. The name *proprioceptive neuromuscular facilitation* is used because a *proprioceptive neurologic reflex (GTO reflex)* is used to *facilitate* the stretch of the target muscle. The name *post-isometric relaxation* is used because after (i.e., *post*) an *isometric* contraction, the target muscle is *relaxed* (because of the GTO reflex). In each case the name describes how the stretch is done.
- CR stretching is done by first having the client isometrically contract the target muscle with mild to moderate force against resistance provided by the therapist/trainer, then the therapist/trainer stretches the target muscle by lengthening it immediately afterward. The isometric contraction is usually held for approximately 5 to 10 seconds (although some sources recommend holding the isometric contraction for as long as 30 seconds),[10] and this procedure is usually repeated three to four times.[7]
- It is customary for each rep of a CR stretch to begin where the previous rep ended. However, it is possible and sometimes desirable (for client comfort) to take the client off stretch to some degree before beginning the next rep. Given that the mechanism of CR stretching is the GTO reflex, what is most important is that the client be able to generate a forceful enough contraction to stimulate this reflex. Sometimes this is not possible if the client is trying to contract when the target muscle is stretched extremely long.
- Even though the contraction of a CR stretch is usually isometric, it can be done concentrically. In other words, when the client contracts against the resistance of the therapist/trainer, the client can be allowed to slightly shorten the muscle and move the joint. Whether the contraction is isometric or concentric, what is important is that tension is developed in the muscle belly that pulls on the muscle's tendon, initiating the GTO reflex to increase effectiveness of the stretch.
- A number of different breathing protocols can be employed. The client can be asked to exhale while isometrically contracting against resistance, and then relax and complete the exhalation while the therapist performs the stretch. Or the client can exhale while isometrically contracting against resistance, then relax and take another breath in, and then remain relaxed and exhale again while the therapist performs the stretch. Or the client can be asked to hold in the breath while isometrically

> **BOX 22-4**
>
> If CR stretching will be combined with AC stretching to perform CRAC stretching, then it is usually necessary for the client to hold in the breath while isometrically contracting the target muscle.

contracting against resistance, and then relax and exhale while the target muscle is being stretched (Box 22-4). What is most important regarding the breathing protocol during CR stretching, and in fact during any stretch, is that the client relaxes and exhales while the stretch is being performed by the therapist/trainer.[7]

- The muscle group that is usually used to demonstrate CR stretching is the hamstring group; however, this method of stretching can be used for any muscle of the body (Figure 22-7).
- The basis for CR stretching is the **Golgi tendon organ (GTO) reflex**, as follows: if the target muscle is forcefully contracted, the GTO reflex is engaged and results in inhibition of the target muscle (i.e., the muscle is inhibited, in other words stopped from contracting). This is a protective reflex that prevents the forceful contraction from tearing the muscle and/or its tendon.[3] As therapists/trainers, we can use this protective reflex to facilitate stretching our client's musculature, because muscles that are neurologically inhibited are more easily stretched. (For more on the GTO reflex, see Section 19.7.)

AGONIST CONTRACT (AC) STRETCHING:

- Like CR stretching, agonist contract (AC) stretching also uses a neurologic reflex to neurally inhibit/relax the target muscle and "facilitate" its stretch; however, instead of the GTO reflex, AC stretching uses reciprocal inhibition (Box 22-5).
- Sometimes the term *PNF stretching* is used to describe AC stretching as well as CR stretching.
- **Reciprocal inhibition** is a neurologic reflex that creates a more efficient joint action by preventing two muscles that have antagonistic actions from contracting at the same time.[3] When a muscle is contracted, muscles that have antagonistic actions to the contracted muscle are inhibited from contracting and relaxed so they can be lengthened, in other words, stretched. For example, if the brachialis contracts to flex the forearm at the elbow joint, reciprocal inhibition would inhibit the triceps brachii from contracting and creating a force of elbow joint extension, which if allowed to occur would oppose the action of elbow joint flexion by the brachialis. (For more on the reciprocal inhibition reflex, see Section 19.3.)

> **BOX 22-5**
>
> Agonist contract (AC) stretching that uses the neurologic reflex of reciprocal inhibition is the basis for Aaron Mattes's active isolated stretching (AIS) technique.

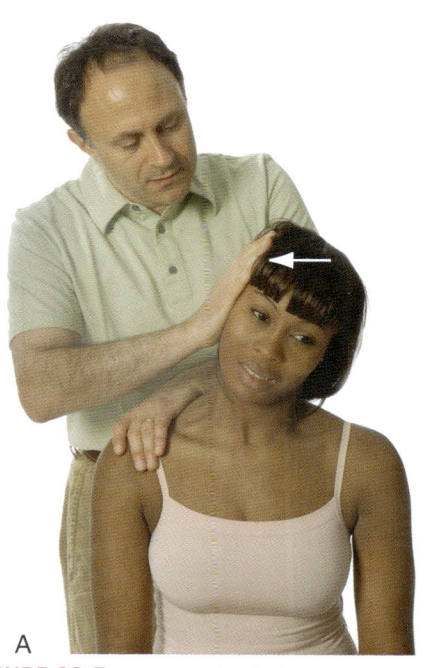
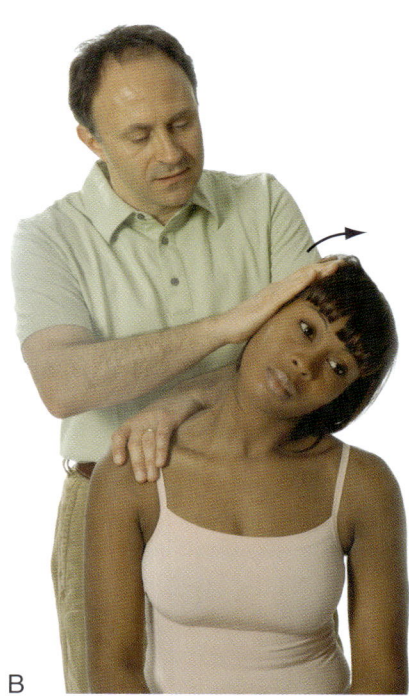

FIGURE 22-7 Contract relax (CR) stretching of the right lateral flexor musculature of the neck and head is shown. In **A,** the client is isometrically contracting the right lateral flexor musculature against resistance provided by the therapist/trainer. In **B,** the therapist/trainer is now stretching the right lateral flexor musculature by moving the client's neck and head into left lateral flexion. This procedure is usually repeated three to four times. *(From Muscolino JE:* Stretch your way to better health, *Massage Ther J 45:167, 2006. Photos by Yanik Chauvin.)*

- Regarding the agonist contract (AC) stretching technique, the name *agonist contract* is used because the *agonist* (mover) of a joint action is *contracted,* causing the antagonist (the target muscle that is to be stretched) on the other side of the joint to be relaxed (by reciprocal inhibition). Some sources describe this technique as **antagonist contract stretching** because they look at it from the point of view that the client contracts the antagonist to the target muscle that is to be stretched.[11]
- To use reciprocal inhibition when stretching a client, have the client perform a joint action that is antagonistic to the joint action of the target muscle. This will inhibit the target muscle, allowing for a greater stretch to be done at the end of this active movement (Figure 22-8). Generally, the position of stretch is held for only 1 to 3 seconds; this procedure is repeated approximately 10 times.[12]
- Regarding the breathing protocol, the client is usually asked to breathe in before the movement, exhale during the concentric contraction movement, and then relax and complete the exhalation while the therapist/trainer augments the stretch. An alternative would be to add in another breath cycle. This would be done by having the client breathe out during the concentric contraction movement, but then take in another breath and then breathe out while the therapist/trainer augments the stretch.

CONTRACT RELAX AND AGONIST CONTRACT STRETCHING COMPARED AND COMBINED:

- The two methods of CR and AC stretching can be powerful additions to your repertoire of stretching techniques and may greatly benefit your clients.
- To simplify the difference between CR and AC stretching, consider this: with CR stretching, the client actively isometrically contracts the target muscle, and then the therapist/trainer stretches it immediately afterward. With AC stretching, the client actively moves his or her body into the stretch of the target muscle, and then the therapist/trainer augments/further stretches the target muscle immediately afterward.
- Put another way, with CR stretching, the client contracts the target muscle to stimulate the GTO reflex to relax it, whereas with AC stretching, the client moves their body in such a way that the target muscle is an antagonist to the movement and is reciprocally inhibited and relaxed.
- CR and AC stretching can be combined and performed sequentially on the client, beginning with CR stretching followed by AC stretching; this protocol is called **contract relax agonist contract (CRAC) stretching** (Figure 22-9). CRAC stretching begins with the client isometrically contracting the target muscle against the therapist/trainer's resistance for approximately 5 to 8 seconds while holding in the breath (Figure 22-9, *A*); this is the CR aspect of the stretch. Next, the client actively contracts the antagonist muscles of the target muscle by moving the joint toward a stretch of the target muscle while breathing out (Figure 22-9, *B*); this is the AC aspect of the stretch. Then the client relaxes and the therapist/trainer moves the client into a further stretch of the target muscle while the client continues to breathe out (Figure 22-9, *C*). Combining CR with AC stretching can create an even greater stretch for the client's target musculature.[10]

CONCLUSION:

- Stretching can be a very powerful treatment option. There are many choices when it comes to choosing the most effective stretching technique. Basic stretching techniques involve the choice between static and dynamic stretching. Current

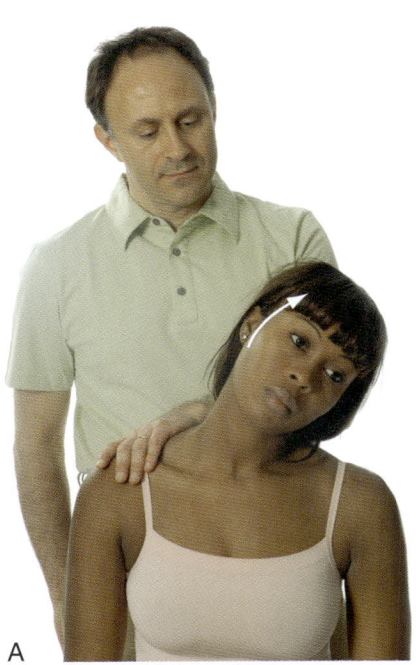 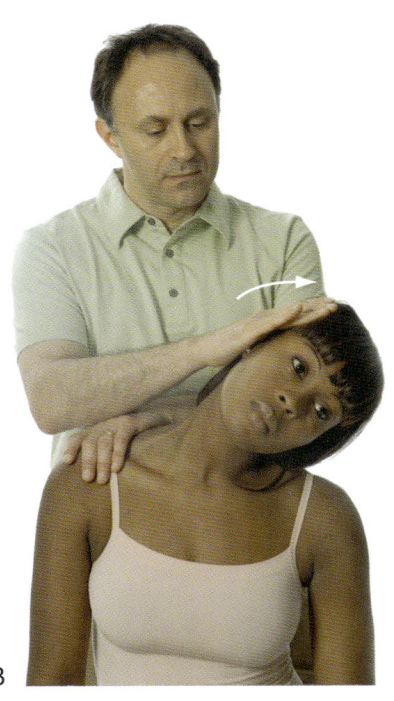

FIGURE 22-8 Agonist contract (AC) stretching for the right lateral flexor musculature of the neck is shown. **A** shows the client actively performing left lateral flexion of the neck, which both mechanically stretches the right lateral flexor musculature of the neck and results in reciprocal inhibition of the right lateral flexors. **B** shows that at the end of range of motion of left lateral flexion, the therapist/trainer then stretches the client's neck farther into left lateral flexion, thereby further stretching the right lateral flexor musculature of the neck. This procedure is usually repeated 8 to 10 times. *(Modified from Muscolino JE:* Stretch your way to better health, Massage Ther J *45:167, 2006. Photos by Yanik Chauvin.)*

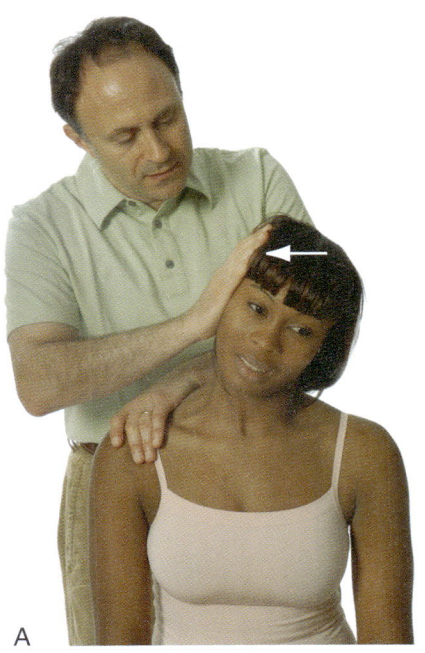 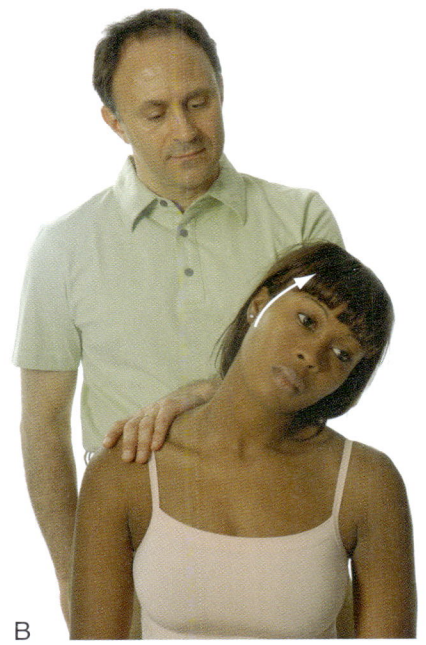 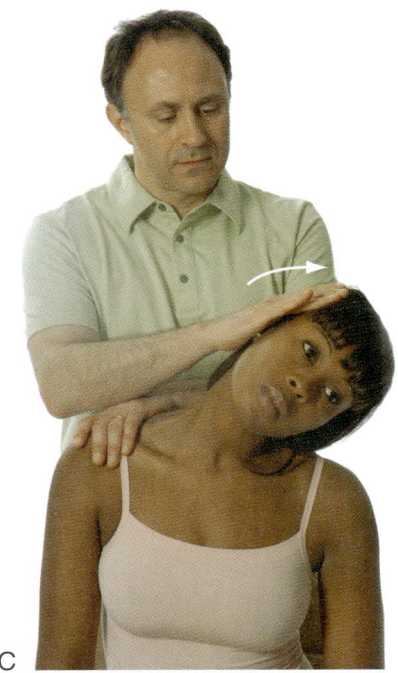

FIGURE 22-9 Contract relax agonist contract (CRAC) stretching is demonstrated for the right lateral flexion musculature of the neck. **A** shows CR stretching technique with the client isometrically contracting the right lateral flexion musculature of her neck against the resistance of the therapist/trainer. At the end of this isometric contraction, the client actively moves her neck into left lateral flexion as shown in **B**. This active motion is part of the AC stretching technique. In **C**, the therapist/trainer now stretches the client's neck farther into left lateral flexion. *(Modified from Muscolino JE: Stretch your way to better health,* Massage Ther J *45:167, 2006. Photos by Yanik Chauvin.)*

research seems to favor dynamic stretching as the preferred protocol before a physical activity is to be performed; and static stretching as optimally performed after the physical activity.[1] Of course, it is possible to combine these two methods and perform a hybrid stretching protocol: Perhaps 30–40 seconds of dynamic stretching repetitions followed by one long-held static stretch of 20 seconds. The best choice likely depends on the unique circumstances of each client. Beyond the choice of static versus dynamic stretching, advanced stretching techniques, such as pin and stretch, CR, AC, and CRAC stretching techniques, are extremely effective therapeutic tools when working clinically.

REVIEW QUESTIONS

evolve Answers to the following review questions appear on the Evolve website accompanying this book at: http://evolve.elsevier.com/Muscolino/kinesiology/.

1. What is stretching?

2. What is the name given to the muscle or other soft tissue that the therapist/trainer intends to stretch?

3. Why is stretching done?

4. What is passive tension?

5. What is active tension?

6. What are myofibroblasts, and what is their importance?

7. How can a stretch for a muscle be figured out instead of memorized?

8. What reflex might be triggered if a muscle is stretched either too far or too fast? And what would be the result of that reflex?

9. What joint actions would best stretch the right upper trapezius?

10. What name is given to the fact that we consider the actions in all the cardinal planes when stretching a target muscle?

11. When should stretching be done?

12. Contrast static and dynamic stretching.

13. Describe pin and stretch technique.

14. What is the neurologic basis for contract relax (CR) stretching?

15. What is the neurologic basis for agonist contract (AC) stretching?

16. What are two other names for contract relax (CR) stretching?

17. What is the neurologic basis for active isolated stretching (AIS) technique?

18. What muscle is contracted during the contract relax (CR) stretching technique? What muscle is contracted during the agonist contract (AC) stretching technique?

19. Approximately how many reps should be done with contract relax (CR) stretching and with agonist contract (AC) stretching?

20. When contract relax (CR) and agonist contract (AC) stretching are combined, which one is usually done first?

REFERENCES

1. Ylinen J: Stretching therapy for sport and manual therapies, China, 2008, Churchill Livingstone.
2. Armiger P, Martyn MA: Stretching for functional flexibility, Baltimore, 2010, Lippincott Williams & Wilkins.
3. Neumann DA: Kinesiology of the musculoskeletal system: Foundations for physical rehabilitation, ed 3, St Louis, 2017, Elsevier.
4. Myers TW: Anatomy trains: Myofascial meridians for manual & movement therapists, ed 3, Edinburgh, 2014, Churchill Livingstone.
5. Kendall FP, McCreary EK, Provance PG: Muscles: Testing and function, ed 4, Baltimore, 1993, Williams & Wilkins.
6. Scrivani SJ, Mehta NR, Keith DA, et al: Facial pain. In Fishman SM, Ballantyne JC, Rathmell JP, editors: Bonica's management of pain, ed 4, Baltimore, 2010, Lippincott Williams & Wilkins.
7. McAtee RE, Charland J: Facilitated stretching, ed 2, Champaign, IL, 1999, Human Kinetics.
8. Fritz S: Mosby's essential sciences for therapeutic massage: Anatomy, physiology, biomechanics, and pathology, ed 4, St. Louis, 2014, Elsevier.
9. McArdle WD, Katch FI, Katch VL: Essentials of exercise physiology, Media, 1994, Williams & Wilkins.
10. Jeffreys I: Warm-up and stretching. In Baechle TR, Earle RE, editors: Essentials of strength training and conditioning, ed 3, Champaign, IL, 2008, Human Kinetics.
11. Fritz S: Sports & exercise massage, ed 2, St Louis, 2013, Elsevier.
12. Mattes AL: Active isolated stretching: The Mattes method, Sarasota, FL, 2000, Aaron Mattes.

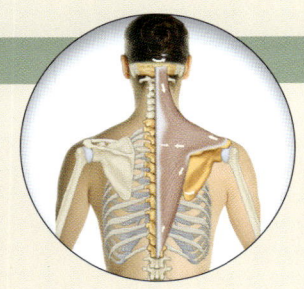

CHAPTER 23
Principles of Strengthening Exercise

Alexander Charmoz and Joseph E. Muscolino

CHAPTER OUTLINE

Section 23.1	Reasons for Exercise	Section 23.4	Execution of Exercise
Section 23.2	Types of Exercise	Section 23.5	Exercise Technique
Section 23.3	Types of Resistance	Section 23.6	Program Design

CHAPTER OBJECTIVES

After completing this chapter, the student should be able to perform the following:

1. Define the key terms of this chapter and state the meanings of the word origins of this chapter.
2. Define exercise, and explain the different motivations that a client might have for beginning an exercise program.
3. Do the following related to types of exercise:
   - Compare isolation exercise and compound exercise.
   - Define *functional strength,* and apply it to an individual's goal by means of exercise.
   - Understand the relationship between muscles that stabilize and muscles that mobilize, and know how to apply this knowledge in a gym setting.
   - Identify open and closed kinetic chain movements for any given exercise.
4. Do the following related to types of resistance:
   - Discuss bodyweight resistance, including plyometrics, speed training, agility training, balance training, and unilateral training.
   - Discuss external resistance, including free weights.
   - Compare and contrast the different types of external resistance including static, variable, progressive, nonprogressive, linear, and nonlinear.
   - Explain the benefits of aqua therapy.
   - Describe a cambered pulley and how it differs from a regular pulley.
   - Discuss what the benefits and hazards of a Smith machine are, and give examples of alternate methods that could accomplish a similar task.
5. Do the following related to the execution of exercise:
   - Define *volume, sets,* and *repetitions*.
   - Discuss rep ranges, including comparing and contrasting myofibrillar and sarcoplasmic hypertrophy.
   - Compare and contrast aerobic versus anaerobic exercises.
   - Define *time under tension (TUT)* and describe how tempo affects an exercise routine.
   - Explain why it can be important to identify a client's repetition (rep) max.
   - Discuss rest intervals and define *workload*.
   - Identify some of the recovery factors that will have an impact on how much rest a client might need between workouts.
6. Do the following related to exercise technique:
   - List the different ways a workout can be split up, and explain the advantages/disadvantages of each one.
   - Explain why changing the angle of a joint relative to the resistance curve can alter the outcome of an exercise.
   - Discuss range of motion as applied to exercise and how it might be manipulated to help a client reach his or her goals.
   - Discuss how form is important during exercise, and explain the various factors that will determine proper form.
   - Define the SAID principle and how it applies to the body via exercise.
7. Do the following related to exercise program design:
   - List the specific exercise programs that are discussed in this chapter and identify how a client might benefit by participating in them.
   - Identify the special equipment discussed in this chapter and explain what its purpose is.

OVERVIEW

This chapter covers strengthening exercise and is designed to help a trainer or perhaps manual or movement therapist better serve clients in a gym environment. By breaking down exercise into several subcategories, decisions can be made that can influence the training program of clients to better help them reach their goals safely and effectively. Strengthening exercise is a complex subject but can be defined simply: it involves placing the body under physical stress by asking musculature to contract against some kind of resistance. As tissues become stressed and broken down, our bodies undergo a physiologic repair process that results in increased myofascial strength, neurologic coordination, and cardiovascular health. Resistance variables are discussed and applied to help the trainer/therapist identify the benefits of various types of equipment. These variables are chosen based on the desired outcome of the client's program, which can be determined by the client's motivations. By combining the right equipment with the right exercise, and its proper execution, the client's time in the gym can be maximized and the risk of injury can be reduced. Exercise technique and program design are broken down and discussed so that the right decisions can be made and applied to any and every client. Finally, a list of specific programs and special gym equipment is provided to help the trainer/therapist be more familiar with current techniques and applications. Note: If the Evolve icon (evolve) is placed after a reference to a specific exercise, an illustration or photograph of that exercise is shown on the Evolve website for reference.

KEY TERMS

1 rep max (1 RM)
Active recovery
Activities of daily living
Aerobic exercise
Agility drill
Ammonia/smelling salts (a-MONE-ya)
Anaerobic exercise (AN-a-ROW-bik)
Anaerobic glycolysis (gly-KO-li-sis)
Aqua therapy
Assistance lifts
Bench shirts/squat suits
Cable machines
Cambered pulley
Chalk
Cheating
Closed kinetic chain exercise
Compensation
Compound exercise
Compressive force
Constant resistance
Critical point acceleration
Crossfit
Cross-education
Delayed onset muscle soreness (DOMS)
Dip belts
Drop sets
Dynamic balance
Endurance training
Exercise
External resistance
Form
Functional exercise
Gloves
Hybrid fibers (HI-brid)
Isolation exercise
Isometric exercise
Karvonen formula (kar-VO-nin)
Kettlebell
Kickboxing
Knee wraps
Kreb's cycle
Leverage machines
Mind-body connection
Mind-to-muscle connection
Mobility muscles
Muscle activation technique (MAT)
Multijoint muscle
Myofibrillar hyperplasia (MY-o-FIB-ri-lar HI-per-PLA-zha)
Myofibrillar hypertrophy (hi-PER-tro-fee)
Open kinetic chain exercise
Partial rep
Phosphate system (FOSS-fate)
Pilates
Plyometric exercise (ply-o-MET-rik)
Postural muscles
Power
Pre-exhaust
Progressive resistance
Range of motion
Regressive resistance
Repetition
Repetition (Rep) max
Rest interval
Rest/Pause
Resting metabolic rate (RMR)
Rippetoe's starting strength
SAID principle
Sarcoplasmic hypertrophy (sar-ko-PLAZ-mik hi-PER-tro-fee)
Set
Shearing force
Shoes
Single-joint muscle
Speed training
Stabilization exercise

Static balance
Static resistance
Strength endurance
Strengthening exercise
Stretch-shorten cycle
Stretching exercise
Supersets
Tempo
Time under tension
Tone

Unilateral training
Variable resistance
Vibration training
Volume
Weightlifting belt
Westside barbell
Workload
Wrist straps
Yoga

WORD ORIGINS

- Acceleration—From Latin *accelerare*, meaning *to quicken*
- Aerobic—From Latin *aer*, meaning *air*, and Greek *bios*, meaning *life*
- Ammonia—From Greek *ammoniakon*, meaning *belonging to Ammon*
- Anaerobic—From Latin *a*, meaning *not, without*; and *aer*, meaning *air*; and Greek *bios*, meaning *life*
- Aqua—From Latin *aqua*, meaning *water*
- Cambered—From Latin *camur*, meaning *crooked, arched*
- Compensation—From Latin *compensatus*, meaning *to counterbalance*
- Exercise—From Latin *exercitare*, meaning *to train, to drill*
- Fiber—From Latin *fibra*, meaning *fiber*
- Fibrillar—From Latin *fibra*, meaning *fiber*
- Glycolysis—From Greek *glykeros*, meaning *sweet*, and *lysis*, meaning *loosening*
- Hybrid—From Latin *hybrida*, meaning *mongrel*
- Hyperplasia—From Greek *hyper*, meaning *above, over*; and *plasis*, meaning *formation*
- Hypertrophy—From Greek *hyper*, meaning *above, over*; and *trophe*, meaning *nourishment*
- Isolation—From Latin *insula*, meaning *island*
- Isometric—From Greek *isos*, meaning *equal*, and *metron* meaning *measure*
- Kinetic—From Greek *kinesis*, meaning *motion*
- Metrics—From Greek *metrikos*, meaning *measure*
- Mobility—From Latin *mobilis*, meaning *movable*
- Muscle—From Latin *musculus*, meaning *little mouse*
- Myo—From Greek *mys*, meaning *muscle*
- Plasm—From Latin *plasma*, meaning *to mold*
- Plyo—From Greek *pleion*, meaning *more*
- Posture—From Latin *positura*, meaning *position*
- Repetition—From Latin *repetere*, meaning *to do again*
- Resistance—From Latin *re*, meaning *against*, and *sistere*, meaning *to take a stand*
- Sarco—From Greek *sarcoma*, meaning *fleshy substance*
- Stabilization—From Latin *stabilitas*, meaning *firmness*
- Tempo—From Latin *tempus*, meaning *time*
- Tone—From Latin *tonus*, meaning *sound*
- Variable—From Latin *variare*, meaning *to change*

SECTION 23.1 REASONS FOR EXERCISE

DEFINING EXERCISE:

- **Exercise** can be defined as performing active or passive movements for the purpose of restoring, maintaining, or improving health of the body.[1] Two general types of exercise exist: strengthening exercise and stretching exercise.
  - **Strengthening exercises** are designed to increase the force that a muscle can generate when it contracts.
  - **Stretching exercises** are designed to increase the ability of soft tissues of the body to lengthen/stretch.
- To optimize musculoskeletal health, it is important to balance our exercise regimen with strengthening and stretching exercises. By strengthening the muscles in our body, we increase our ability to create movement, as well as our ability to stabilize our joints, potentially decreasing the risk of injury. By stretching our muscles (and other soft tissues) to become more flexible, we allow for more mobility within our joints, which can also prevent injury[2] (Box 23-1).
- A client may have one or several goals regarding how he or she would like to use exercise to benefit his or her health.

 BOX 23-1

There is an inverse relationship between joint stability and mobility, meaning that the more flexible a joint is, the less stable it is. An unstable joint can be more easily subluxated (dislocated) than a stable one. On the other hand, the more stable a joint is, the less mobile it is, and the easier it might be to strain a muscle or sprain a ligament of that joint.

Assessing the motivations that a client has for beginning an exercise program is important for helping that person reach those goals quickly, as well as keeping the client interested in the program. See the Evolve site for a sample client evaluation form.

REASONS FOR EXERCISE:

- The following are some generic reasons why one might wish to begin an exercise program.
  - **Wellness and overall health:** One of the most common reasons why someone might choose exercise is to improve the way he or she feels throughout the day. This can include reducing stress, improving energy levels, preventing injury, and/or improving the ability to perform day-to-day activities.
  - Benefits of exercise can also include lowering the risk of many diseases, including cardiovascular disease, diabetes, hypertension, stroke, osteoporosis, arthritis, obesity, depression, and even certain forms of cancer.[1] Fortunately, those who choose to exercise for reasons other than health will enjoy these lowered risks as well!
- **Rehabilitation:** When the body undergoes any form of trauma, a healing cycle must take place in order to restore the proper function of the affected area. Trauma that occurs to connective tissue such as ligament or tendon, as well as trauma that occurs to bone or cartilage, can be better healed by combining various stretching and strengthening exercises into an exercise program. Rehabilitation is also common after surgical procedures to help speed the healing process. Physical therapists specialize in treating clients who have the specific goal of restoring function to an injured part of the body.[3]
- **Improving at a sport or activity:** Many clients are either recreational or competitive athletes who are looking to improve their ability at a certain sport through exercise. By analyzing the strengths and weaknesses of the client as well as the specific repetitive movements that are in the sport, an exercise program can be developed that will increase the athlete's performance.[4]
- **Increasing strength:** The desire to become stronger at certain tasks or activities can be very appealing to a client. Strength can be defined and applied in many different ways, and there may be a variety of reasons and motivations behind a client's desire to increase strength. For some, strength can build confidence and improve the sense of overall well-being. Those who perform manual labor (for work or otherwise) will also benefit from an increase in strength. At the competitive level, powerlifters, Olympic weightlifters, and strongmen all rely on their relative strength. Because of the specific weight classes that separate the competitors in these activities, it is desirable to become stronger without increasing weight.[5]
- **Improving physical appearance:** Many clients have goals that pertain to either increasing muscle mass or decreasing body fat. Often these goals will go hand in hand. The sport of bodybuilding capitalizes on this concept of having large, clearly defined muscles and a low percentage of body fat. Although most clients will never aspire to compete in a bodybuilding show, they may have smaller, more modest goals of changing their physical appearance to a level of personal satisfaction (Box 23-2).

BOX 23-2

The word *tone* is often used when a client is describing fitness goals. In the world of exercise, the term **tone** is used to describe the ability to distinctly see the superficial muscles of the body. (Not to be confused with the kinesiology term *tone*, which refers to the state of contraction/pulling force of the muscle). This word can be the source of much confusion, which is perpetuated largely by the media. Many exercises are described as toning exercises, which implies that they will reduce body fat and increase the definition of the musculature to a specific area. It is incorrect and unfair to say that only certain exercises are toning exercises. All strengthening exercises burn calories, which may cause a reduction in body fat, and all strengthening exercises can cause hypertrophy of musculature. In this context, every strengthening exercise is a toning exercise.

- Our bodies are constantly in a state of energy consumption, meaning that a certain number of calories is being burned at any given moment. This process is known as the **resting metabolic rate (RMR)**. RMR accounts for approximately 60% to 75% of our total calorie expenditure throughout the day (with the other 25% to 40% coming from physical activity and digestion of food).[6] It has been shown that an increase in muscle mass will increase RMR, resulting in a greater number of calories burned at rest,[6] which can aid in fat loss. Just how much it increases RMR is still a subject of debate, because of the complexity of calculating and measuring the number of variables that exist. On average, studies show that 1 lb of muscle can burn 5 to 15 calories a day.[7] It might not sound like much, but when you take into consideration that skeletal muscle can account for up to 40% of total body weight, we can see that the calories burned from muscle mass can appreciably add to RMR. In fact, it would take approximately 4 lb of fat to equal the calorie expenditure of 1 lb of muscle mass. This is not to say that nutrition, cardiovascular exercise, and certain lifestyle choices can be neglected, but it does show that resting metabolism can be altered and that it is not simply genetics that determine it.

SECTION 23.2 TYPES OF EXERCISE

- When beginning any strengthening exercise program, it is important to take into consideration the multitude of factors that can influence the outcome, as well as the desired result of the training program. Earlier we mentioned many of the reasons why one might choose to exercise; now we will explore the specific ways in which the trainer or therapist can structure the client's workouts appropriately.

ISOLATION VERSUS COMPOUND EXERCISES:

- Strengthening exercises can be split into two distinct movement categories: an isolation exercise and a compound exercise.
  - **Isolation exercise** is defined as a single joint in motion under resistance with the purpose of targeting a specific muscle or muscle group.[5] The surrounding joints, although possibly stimulated, will remain motionless in order to stabilize the body so that one specific motion may occur. An example is the standing dumbbell biceps curl. Although elbow joint flexion is the only motion occurring, muscles that stabilize the shoulder, spinal, and hip joints contract to keep the body still during the exercise.
  - **Compound exercise** is defined as more than one joint in motion under resistance with the purpose of targeting a certain number of muscles or muscle groups. These exercises are sometimes referred to as *movement patterns* because they can mimic certain day-to-day motions.[5] The muscle groups tend to work synergistically (together) in order to create a relatively more powerful movement when compared with an isolation exercise. An example is the push-press, an exercise that involves a simultaneous squatting and overhead pressing motion evolve. Because several joints are being used for one common task (pressing a weight overhead), a heavier load can be used when compared with a single-joint exercise.
- It is commonly thought that an isolation exercise will stimulate a certain muscle or muscle group more than a compound exercise does. Although this may be true in some cases, it is by no means a universal rule. A good example is comparing the barbell bench press (also known as a barbell chest press, a compound exercise [see Figure 23-2]) with the seated chest fly machine (an isolation exercise evolve). The pectoralis major and anterior deltoid are prime movers in both of these exercises and are equally stimulated during each activity. This is contrary to the belief that an exercise designed to isolate the pectoralis major and anterior deltoid provides superior stimulation. The decision to choose between an isolation exercise and a compound exercise should be based on the goals of the client, and ultimately, variety in exercise selection is going to produce the best results.

FUNCTIONAL EXERCISES:

- An exercise that translates to an improvement in an activity or sport is commonly referred to as a **functional exercise**. When a client has goals that include *functional strength*, it is important

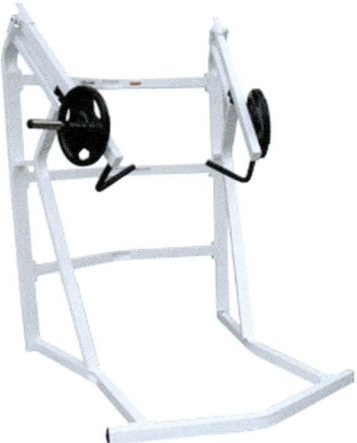

FIGURE 23-1 The jammer press is one example of how an exercise machine can increase the performance of an athlete in a sport. By mimicking a movement pattern that is similar to pushing or tackling, this machine is functional in that it translates to strengthening the athlete in those specific areas. (© Maxim Strength Fitness Equipment Pty Ltd., www.maximfitness.net).

to assess what types of activities the client participates in during the day as well as in his or her line of work.[8]
- Somebody who works for a moving company, for example, may want to work on strengthening the low back and lower extremities by training various *movement patterns* that mimic the day-to-day motions of the job.
  - Athletes also use movement patterns that pertain to their particular sport. Certain sport-specific gyms are equipped with special machines to help the athlete, such as the *jammer press* (Figure 23-1), used in rugby to mimic a simultaneous squatting and pushing motion.

STABILIZATION EXERCISES:

- Although movement of one or more joints is common in exercise, it does not have to occur in order to be effective. At any point in time, a muscle can be responsible for one of three tasks: to create movement, to slow down movement, or to prevent movement. Exercises that prevent movement are known as *stabilization exercises*.
  - A **stabilization exercise** is defined as a stress being applied to the body while the body attempts to remain motionless, in order to preserve the structural integrity of the tissues and thus make them stronger.[9] A stabilization exercise can also be called an **isometric exercise**.
  - Certain muscles are sometimes classified as *stabilization muscles,* or more commonly **postural muscles**, and are often neglected or underworked. These muscles tend to be relatively deep, short, and thick in comparison with the more superficial muscles that many classify as **mobility muscles**.[10] An example of a postural muscle group is the transversospinalis group in the low back, which contributes to the

alignment and stabilization of the spine. Although these muscles have actions and reverse actions, they are typically trained in a fashion that reinforces little or no movement. By contrast, the erector spinae group is generally looked on as a mobility muscle because it pulls the spine into extension, among its other actions.

- It is important to realize that all muscles in the body can create movement, slow down movement, and/or prevent movement. Whatever movement the client chooses to perform should be based on the needs and goals (as well as the limitations) of that person. There is no rule regarding a muscle's role, but there certainly are many common movements that occur that can dictate what role might be necessary in a given situation. For this reason, the terms *origin* and *insertion*, which describe the attachment sites of a muscle, are being phased out because of their implication that the insertion is always the mobile attachment.

OPEN VERSUS CLOSED KINETIC CHAIN EXERCISES:

- Once the exercise has been selected as either an isolated or compound movement, it can be analyzed further to determine which type of movement is occurring in space. The body is capable of producing either open kinetic chain exercises or closed kinetic chain exercises.
- An **open kinetic chain exercise (OKCE)** is defined as any movement occurring in the body in which the distal attachment (usually the hand or foot) is free to move, and the resistance applied to the proximal body is greater than the resistance applied to the distal attachment.[3] An example of an OKCE is the barbell bench press (a compound movement), in which the client lies down on a bench and slowly lowers a weighted bar to the chest; then the client applies force away from the body and the bar is pushed upward away from the body. During this time, the trunk remains still (Figure 23-2, *A*). As a rule, with OKCEs, the distal attachments of muscles move.
- A **closed kinetic chain exercise (CKCE)** is defined as any movement occurring in the body in which the distal attachment is fixed and the body must overcome the resistance applied to it in order to move.[3] An example of a CKCE is the push-up (also a compound movement). It is very similar in design to the barbell bench press, but the client's hands are fixed to the floor. When the client applies force downward, the trunk and pelvis rise away from the floor (see Figure 23-2, *B*). As a rule, with CKCEs the proximal attachments of muscles move.
- An OKCE often involves movement of the elbow or knee joint and usually results in a **shearing force**. A shearing force causes sliding of one bone along another at a joint. Although this is what usually occurs, an OKCE can also create compressive force as well. A **compression force** causes an approximation (squeezing together) of the joint surfaces of the bones. Inversely, a CKCE typically results in one or more compressive joint forces but can also produce a shearing force.[1] The easiest way to determine what kind of exercise is being performed is to look at the core (trunk and pelvis) and determine if it is in motion or not.
- For example, when a seated cable pull-down is performed, the arms will bring the handle down toward the body while the body remains seated. If too much resistance is on the bar, however, the body will rise up to the machine, resulting in a pull-up (Figure 23-3).
- As stated, CKCEs commonly result in movement of the proximal attachment of a muscle instead of the distal attachment; this is termed a *reverse action*. In Figure 23-3, it is a reverse action because the trunk/pelvic attachment moves toward the arm instead of the arm moving toward the trunk/pelvis (Box 23-3).

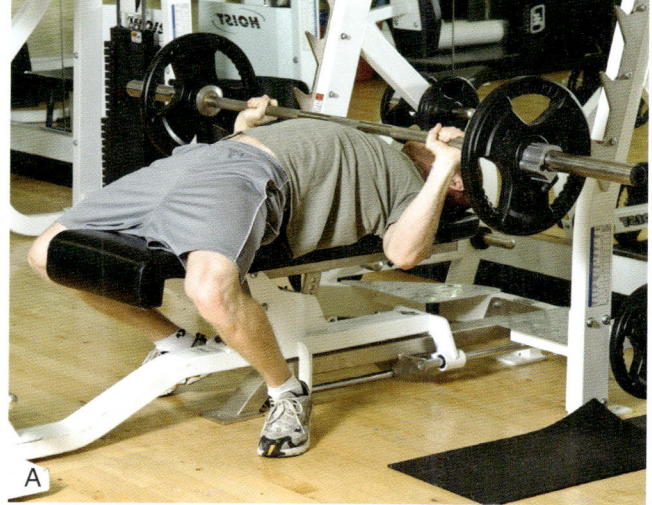

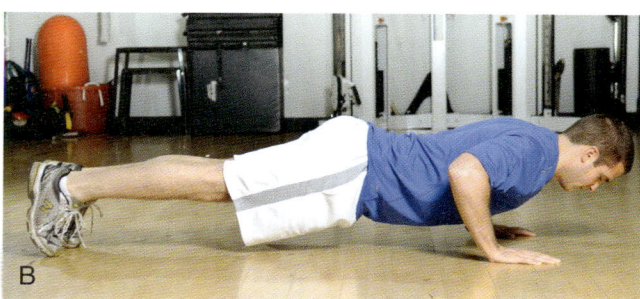

FIGURE 23-2 A, During a barbell bench press, the core of the body remains still and the distal end of the upper extremities move as they push the bar up and away from the chest. The barbell bench press is an open kinetic chain exercise. **B,** In contrast, during a push-up, the hands are fixed to the floor and remain still, so the core of the body moves instead, rising away from the floor. A push-up is a closed kinetic chain exercise.

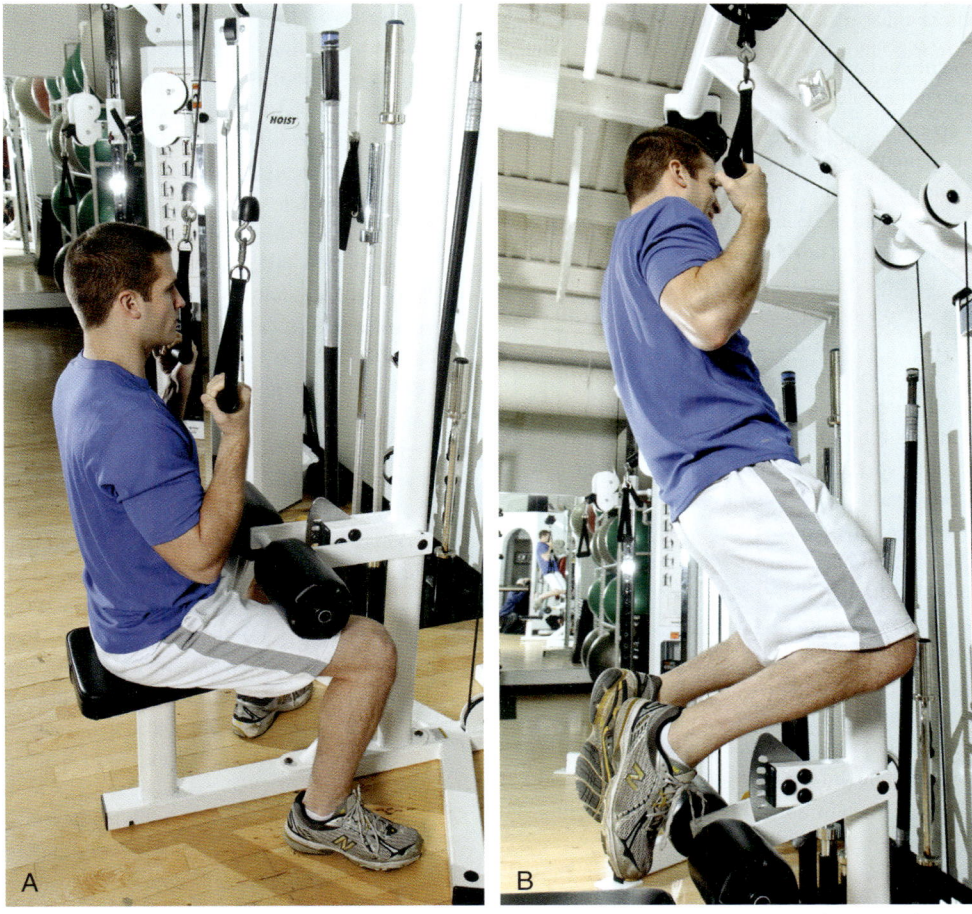

FIGURE 23-3 A, The client is performing a seated lat pull-down, which is an example of an open kinetic chain exercise. **B,** If the same exercise is performed with too much weight, the client will not be able to pull the distal attachment toward the more proximal body; instead, the proximal body will be pulled up toward the machine. This exercise has now become a closed kinetic chain exercise.

 BOX 23-3

It is possible to perform both open and closed kinetic chain movements in the same exercise. A simple example is walking. During the gait cycle, the foot of the support limb is on the ground and is therefore closed chain while the foot of the swing limb is moving in free space and is therefore open chain. It is also possible to create a scenario in which one movement is both open and closed—in other words, it is a partially closed chain movement. An example of this is cycling. If the resistance of the gear is minimal, the activity is an open chain exercise because the pedal moves freely. If the resistance increases (such as when going uphill), the activity is both open and closed chain because when the cyclist pushes down on the pedal, the pedal will somewhat yield and move downward (open chain), but the cyclist's body will also be pushed upward (closed chain).

In fact, a motion as simple as a boxer's punch combines open kinetic chain and closed kinetic chain movement as well as stabilization and mobility within the same joints in a matter of a single second!

SECTION 23.3   TYPES OF RESISTANCE

○ Once an exercise has been selected, the decision must be made as to which type of resistance will be applied to the body. Resistance can come in many shapes and forms, and each method can help in its own unique way. Types of resistance can be divided into two broad categories: bodyweight resistance and external resistance.

BODYWEIGHT RESISTANCE:

○ The simplest form of resistance is the kind that involves no equipment at all; instead, the client uses his or her own body weight to apply force to the targeted muscles. An example of this is a squat evolve. During the concentric portion of the movement, the client must overpower the force of gravity applied to the body in order to move from a squatted position to a standing position. The muscles in action are not only overcoming gravitational force but are also stabilizing the trunk in order to direct the movement in the proper direction. The overall weight of the body determines the amount of resistance that the muscles involved need to overcome (Box 23-4).

> **BOX 23-4**
>
> Something fun you can try is to perform a push-up on a typical bathroom weight scale to see how much resistance is being applied through your arms. Then, by elevating your legs onto a chair, you can see how the resistance increases depending on the angle of the body. Of course, a handstand push-up would be equivalent to the whole weight of your body, as well as requiring the greatest amount of stabilization when compared with a regular push-up.

- It is important to note that the body is always under a state of resistance: the resistance of gravity. By simply lifting an upper extremity into the air, its weight (approximately 5% of total body weight) is providing resistance that the mover muscles must overcome. This is why astronauts must use special training methods when in space, because without the resistance of gravity, their muscles would quickly atrophy and weaken! (See Figure 23-4.)
- Bodyweight exercises are common among athletes and those wishing to improve their day-to-day functional strength. When certain exercises such as the squat are mastered and can no longer provide enough desired resistance, the movement can be manipulated in many different ways. Various methods of bodyweight resistance exercises include plyometrics, speed, endurance, agility, balance, and unilateral training.

Plyometrics:

- A **plyometric exercise** is typically defined as a movement in which a muscle or muscle group is quickly stretched and then immediately thereafter contracts with a maximal concentric force, usually resulting in the feet (or hands) leaving the ground. By rapidly stretching the muscles involved and then contracting them, a ballistic movement is created that allows for a very high level of force output[12] (see Section 19.6 for the relationship of plyometric exercise to the muscle spindle reflex). This technique of training eccentric-concentric sequence movements is also known as the **stretch-shorten cycle**.
  - An example of a plyometric exercise is the squat jump (Figure 23-5). In this exercise, the client quickly drops down into a squatting position and then applies maximal force during the concentric contraction to jump into the air. As the amount of force applied to the muscles overcomes the force of gravity, the client becomes momentarily airborne. The client is then instructed to land softly using the legs to absorb the impact as the body returns to the ground.
  - External resistance, such as from elastic bands or weights, can be added for additional challenge to a plyometric exercise. These movements tend to be closed kinetic chain exercises, but there are some that are open chain as well. For example, medicine balls are commonly used to challenge the upper extremities (Figure 23-6). Available in several different sizes, weights, and compositions, medicine balls can help the client develop power, coordination, and aerobic capacity. Many athletes incorporate this type of training into their program because of these benefits.

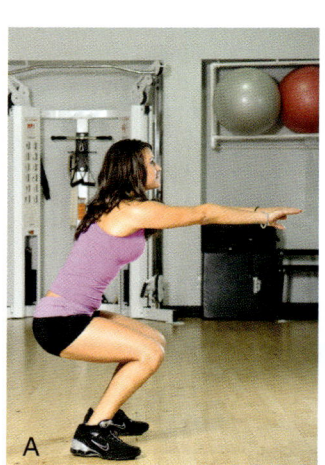

FIGURE 23-4 In order to create artificial gravity, the Space Cycle, a machine designed for astronauts, uses the principles of centrifugal force by rotating in circles around the central vertical axis (like a merry-go-round) at a speed that increases as the cyclist pedals with the feet (there is also a hand pedal attachment for an upper body workout). The faster the apparatus rotates, the more artificial gravity is created, with as much as seven times the Earth's gravity having been recorded. While the machine is in motion, the user inside the cage can perform various exercises against the resistance of the gravity that the client creates with the centrifugal force. (Photo courtesy VJ Caiozzo, University of California, Irvine.)

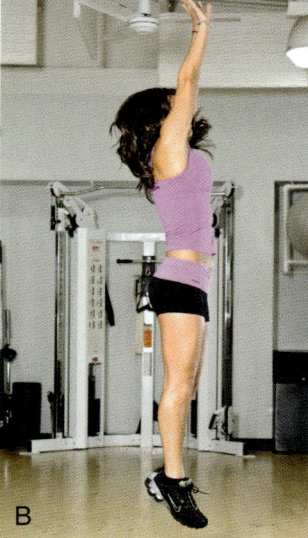

FIGURE 23-5 The squat jump is one of the most common plyometric exercises. Many sports involve some form of jumping, and this exercise is designed to help train the body to achieve an optimal movement pattern for this action, as well as strengthen the muscles and connective tissues during the impact phase of the landing.

CHAPTER 23 Principles of Strengthening Exercise

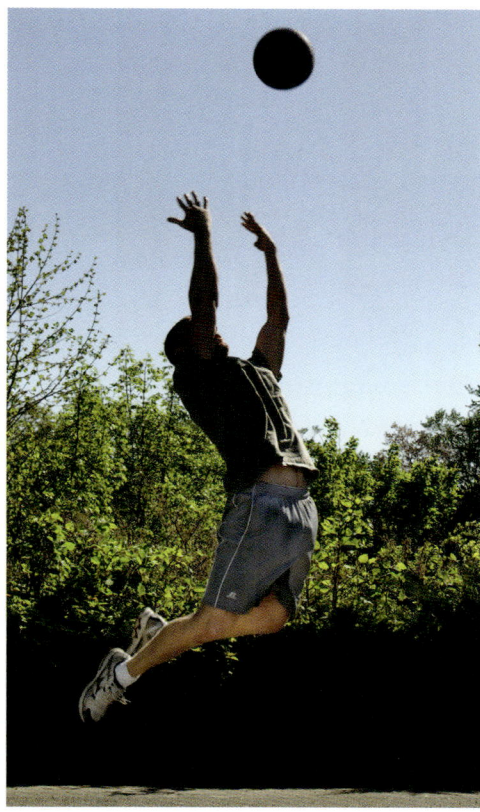

FIGURE 23-6 A full-body plyometric exercise. The client squats down with the medicine ball held at waist level, then jumps into the air and releases the ball overhead and behind with maximal force. Exercises such as these can provide a fun alternative for your clients if you have the proper space and resources.

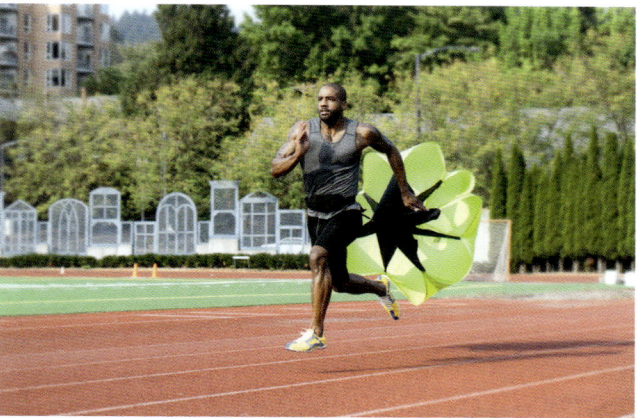

FIGURE 23-7 An athlete performing sprints with a sprinting parachute. In this exercise, the parachute creates air resistance, which increases the drag coefficient and forces the athlete to work harder to achieve a certain speed. The benefit of this type of training is that the athlete's muscles will adapt to a heavier drag, and when the parachute is removed, the athlete will become faster under normal conditions. The degree of specific carry-over of this type of training relating to improved acceleration is still debated by fitness professionals. (© istock.com)

Speed Training:

- **Speed training** is designed to increase maximal speed of a client who participates in sports that require short bursts of energy, such as track and field, baseball, and football. Sprinting relies on the ability to create fast, powerful, and coordinated muscle contractions. Note: Sprint training may be performed with special tools, such as a sprinting parachute, that provide additional resistance[13] (Figure 23-7; Box 23-5).

Endurance Training:

- **Endurance training** is a type of training used to increase the aerobic capacity of the body to allow for repetitive movements that are sustained for a long period of time. It is a popular way of training for specific sports, long distance races, or recreational activities. Specific events, such as marathons, triathlons, and bicycle road races, are designed specifically for this purpose. Sports such as soccer and tennis may incorporate endurance training because of their prolonged physical requirements.[14]

Agility Training:

- Agility drills are often used to train athletes, as well as anyone who wishes to improve coordination, proprioception, and dynamic balance. An **agility drill** is defined as an exercise that requires quick movement combined with changes of direction from the whole body. The client is also trained mentally, as he or she is forced to think and react quickly, training the reflexes. This type of training can simulate the chaotic environment of sports and other daily activities[15] (Figure 23-8).

Balance Training:

- **Dynamic balance** is defined as the ability of the body to balance while in motion. Examples of dynamic balance include agility drills in which the client must land on one leg and transfer force to change direction while keeping the center of gravity in line with the body. Dynamic balance can also be seen in plyometric exercises, such as alternating lunge jumps, in which the client performs a jumping lunge, switching leg positions in the air with each jump.[16]
- If balance is trained while the body is not in motion, it is referred to as **static balance** training. Static balance training can be achieved in a number of ways, but the simplest example would

BOX 23-5

It is commonly thought that the lower extremities provide acceleration and speed to the body. However, it is the location of the center of mass—in other words, the weight of the body's heaviest parts—that more directly influences acceleration and speed. The trunk and the head account for approximately 50% of a runner's acceleration, whereas each lower extremity contributes approximately 17% and each upper extremity 5%. What this means is that the proper technique of body position is one of the keys to developing and maintaining speed.

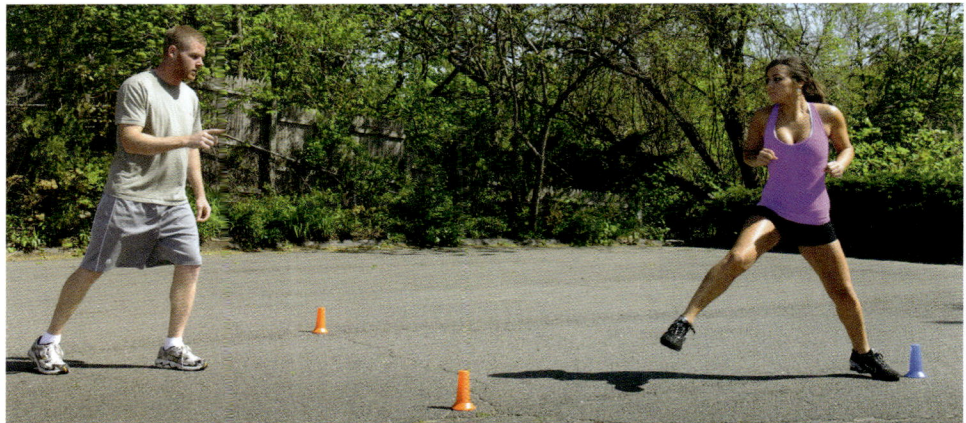

FIGURE 23-8 An example of an agility drill, using cones. The client is instructed to run to the cones in either a predetermined order or a random order that is decided by the trainer and shouted out to the client during the exercise. Such exercises can be performed on a variety of surfaces and in an unlimited number of ways.

be to attempt to stand on one leg for a period of time.[16] There is a variety of tools that are designed to challenge static balance; they are covered in Section 23.6.

Unilateral Training:

○ If further challenge to a bodyweight exercise is desired, **unilateral training** can be incorporated into an exercise by performing it on one leg. An example of this is the one-legged squat, or *pistol squat* (Figure 23-9). In this movement the client performs the squat exercise with one leg in the air, resulting in a much heavier load on the fixed leg as well as a much greater requirement for core stabilization (Box 23-6).

 BOX 23-6

Did you know that training only one limb can produce strength gains in the other limb? This phenomenon is known as **cross-education**. It can be used clinically in rehabilitation to help strengthen an area that is recovering from a traumatic injury or surgery. Average strength gains from cross-education account for approximately 60% translation to the untrained limb.[19]

EXTERNAL RESISTANCE:

○ If a bodyweight exercise is not desired, then the client must turn to some form of external resistance in order to achieve the desired goal.
○ **External resistance** is defined simply as any force that is placed on the body that is not part of the body. External resistance can be combined with the force of gravity to create a far greater force than gravity alone would provide.[17]

Free Weights—Dumbbells and Barbells:

○ Dumbbells and barbells are among the most popular of the available options. Both barbells and dumbbells have a bar with weights attached to both ends. By definition, a barbell has a

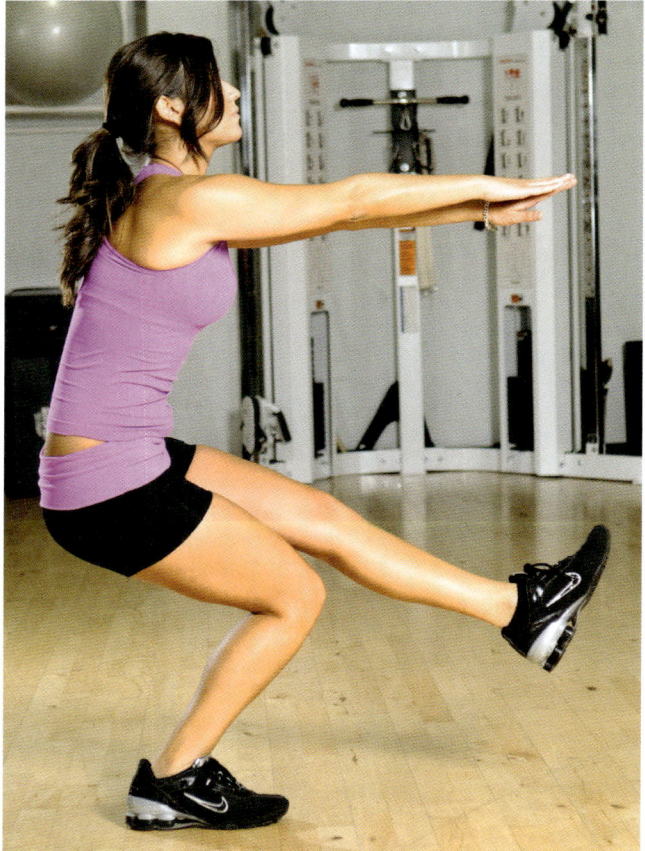

FIGURE 23-9 The pistol squat is a more advanced version of the bodyweight squat. It requires a high level of balance, flexibility, stabilization, and strength. If the client wishes to perform this exercise but is unable to, there are progressive steps that can be taken, including holding onto a band with both hands (with the band placed horizontally in front of the client to act as a counter-balance evolve), shortening the range of motion of the squat, and/or using a bench to sit on at the bottom of each repetition.

longer bar and is typically held with both hands; a dumbbell is usually held with one hand. Dumbbells and barbells are a type of resistance known as *free weight* or *dead weight*.

- Dumbbells require a great degree of stabilization because they demand 360 degrees of control while in motion. During a dumbbell bench press, the client will hold one dumbbell in each hand (usually of equal weight) and perform the movement with both arms simultaneously, trying to direct all the energy in the correct path. The smaller the amount of energy wasted attempting to keep the weights stable, the greater the energy that can be directed toward performing the movement (Figure 23-10; Box 23-7).
- Barbells, on the other hand, require a slightly smaller demand for stabilization than dumbbells. Because the arms are fixed on one single attachment (the barbell), they should move together in synchronization during the exercise. Therefore, the advantage of a barbell over a dumbbell is that the weight will require less neural control and coordination by the central nervous system to keep it steady, which can result in the ability to use a heavier load compared with a set of dumbbells. This advantage is dependent on the amount of time spent on training with either apparatus. Although it is true that a dumbbell requires overall greater neural control, the brain must spend time learning each and every new movement, and training with a barbell will require new movement pattern learning before its advantages can be employed.
- If stabilization strengthening is not desired, then a machine might be used in place of free weights. One such example is known as the *Smith machine*, which guides the bar along a fixed track that can move only up and down. This results in a similar movement pattern as the dumbbell bench press but requires no stabilization of the weight (Figure 23-11). The disadvantage to undertraining stabilization muscles is that it can lead to strength imbalances and possible eventual joint injury.[10]

Constant versus Variable Resistance:

- Free weight is dependent on gravity to provide the resistance for an exercise. Twenty pounds will always weigh 20 lb; this principle is referred to as **constant resistance** (or **static resistance**). The advantages of constant resistance are that it is simple to set up

> **BOX 23-7**
>
> Exercises with dumbbells do not always have to be performed with both arms in simultaneous motion. For example, to add additional stabilization demands to a dumbbell bench press, the client can perform alternating unilateral movement by pushing one arm up at a time. One dumbbell can also be placed on the floor, and the client can perform the movement one arm at a time, which would require the torso to remain in position with resistance being applied to only one side of the body.

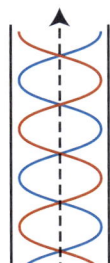
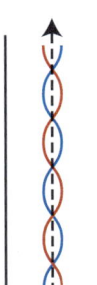

FIGURE 23-10 The dashed black arrow represents the desired direction of movement, with the black lines being boundaries of which the weight must be balanced in order to continue on its path. The red and blue lines in the example on the left demonstrate wasted energy, which is being used to stabilize the weight and is thus lost from contributing toward upward motion. The red and blue lines on the right demonstrate energy that is creating a much better direction of upward force, which would allow for heavier weight to be used than that used in the first example.

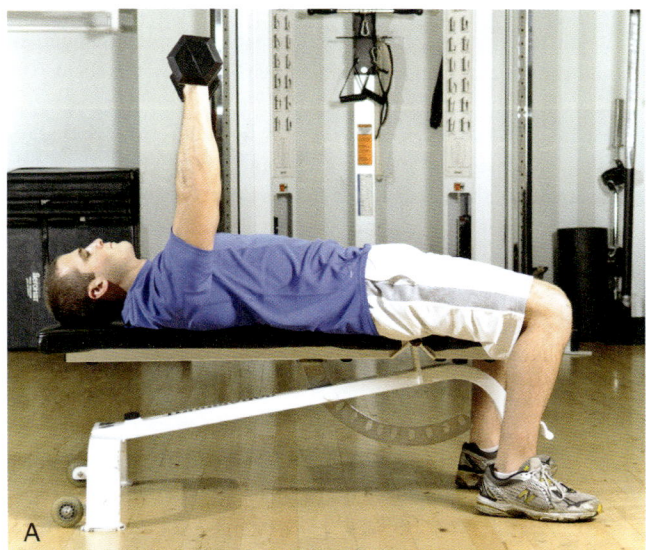
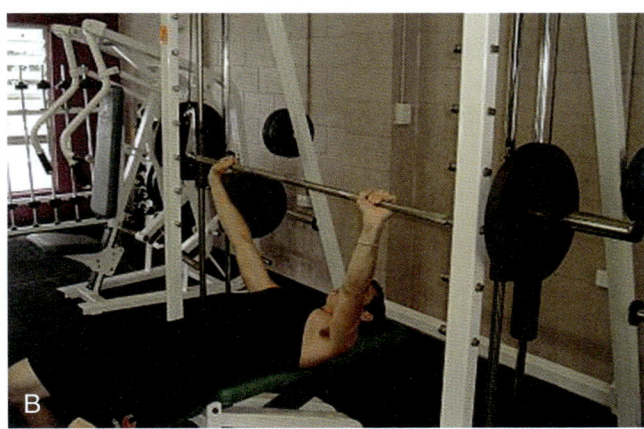

FIGURE 23-11 Here we see two different exercises with similar movement patterns. In **A**, the client is performing a dumbbell bench press; in **B**, the client is performing a bench press on a Smith machine. The stabilization demands involved with the dumbbell bench press are much higher than in the same exercise performed on a Smith machine, because the Smith machine guides the resistance along a vertical track. *(B, Courtesy Paul Rogers)*.

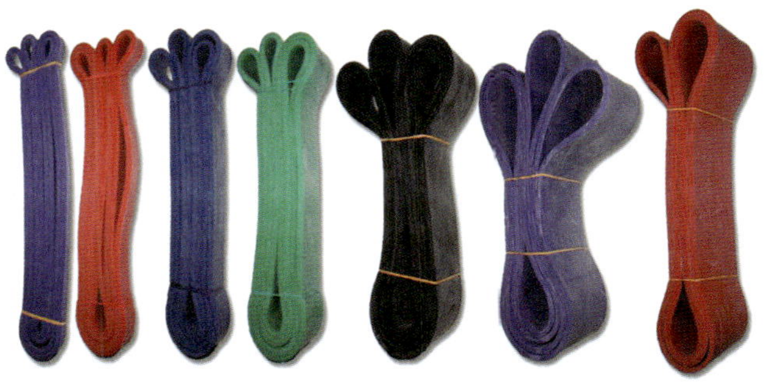

FIGURE 23-12 Exercise bands come in a wide variety of lengths, thicknesses, and design. It is important to match the appropriate band with the appropriate exercise, which may involve some trial and error. It is a good idea to have several types of bands available for a variety of situations. *(Courtesy Iron Woody Fitness Bands.)*

Progressive Resistance—Bands, Tubing, and Chains:

- **Progressive resistance** is defined as any form of variable resistance that increases its load (resistance) throughout the range of motion of the exercise. The use of bands and tubing allows for progressive resistance.
- Bands are affordable, and offer a simple setup that allows for infinite possibilities of angles and tension curves. Typically constructed out of rubber, they may be referred to as *exercise tubing* or *resistance bands*. They come in a wide selection of lengths and thicknesses, which ultimately determine for which exercise they are best suited. They are also often color coded with each color denoting a different degree of resistance (Figure 23-12).
- Bands are useful for any training program but have become especially popular in the world of physical therapy (PT). Progressive tension has been shown to be useful in working a weak or recovering muscle. At the beginning concentric range of motion for the chosen exercise, the muscle does not have as much strength as it does in the middle or the end of the range of motion. Band tension caters to this by progressively increasing resistance as it is stretched longer during the movement so that the muscle can work harder where it is strongest. By simply moving closer to or farther away from the origin of the band, the client can alter the tension to suit his or her level of strength. A technique that is sometimes applied is to have the client start at a challenging distance and then take small steps toward the origin of the tubing as the muscle fatigues. This ensures that the client can maintain good form and perform additional repetitions (Figure 23-13).

and use and that the *line of pull* will always be directly downward, with gravity. Many training programs use a combination of bodyweight and free weight exercises that require no special equipment and can be easily understood and performed by the client. The alternative to constant resistance is known as variable resistance.

- **Variable resistance** is defined as any form of resistance that results in a change of load (i.e., resistance) throughout the range of motion of the exercise. The change can come in either a linear or a nonlinear form, and the load can either increase or decrease depending on how it is set up.[18] Although a decreasing load can have benefits, the most common form of variable resistance involves an increasing load and is known as *progressive resistance*.

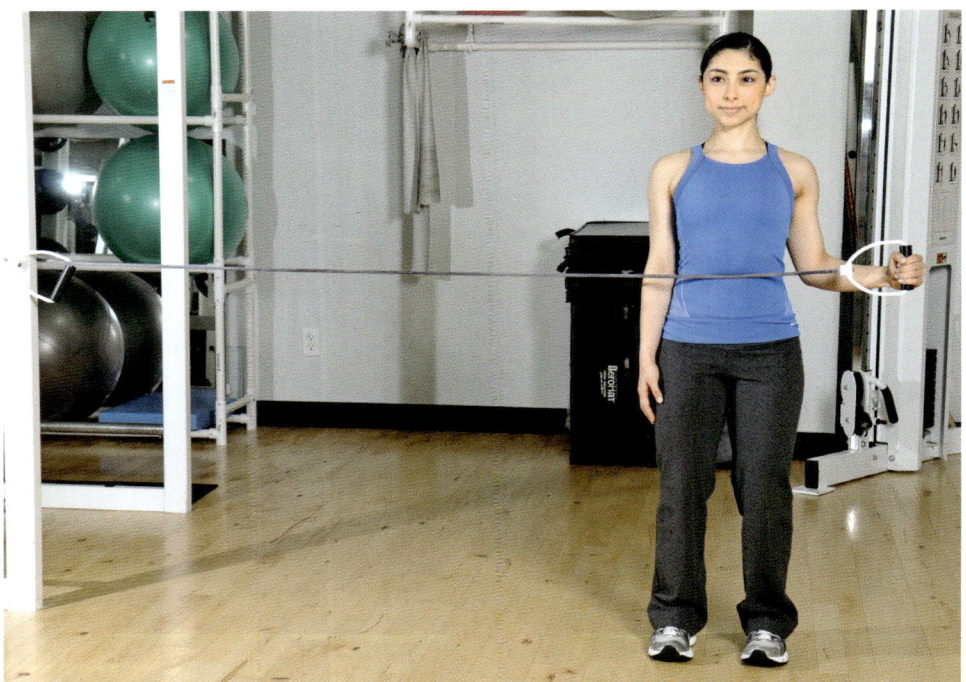

FIGURE 23-13 The client is performing humeral lateral rotation against the tension of the exercise tube. Depending on the resistance of the tube, the client will want to adjust his or her location so that a proper strength curve is created.

- Bands can also be attached to free weight to provide a combination of constant and variable resistance. For example, in the sport of competitive power lifting, many athletes train the bench press exercise by attaching one or more bands to a loaded bar and then securing them to the floor or the bottom of the bench (Figure 23-14). When the bar is pushed off the chest, the bands provide an increase in tension as the arms extend. The contrast to this exercise is also used by powerlifters and is known as *reverse band tension*. In this setup the athlete will secure the bands around a loaded bar but will secure them to a point above the athlete (usually a power rack) instead of the floor. This provides a decrease in tension as the lifter lowers the bar to the chest and is an example of **regressive resistance**.
- Variable resistance can also come in the form of linear progression. An example of linear variable resistance is the use of chains. Commonly used in the sport of competitive powerlifting, chains can be attached to a loaded barbell or dumbbell, or used independently to provide a further challenge to an exercise. An example of their use is during the bench press, when the chains are attached on each end of the bar and curled into a pile on the floor (Figure 23-15). As the athlete lifts the bar off the chest, the links begin to leave the floor, offering extra poundage as well as increased stability demands as the arms extend to finish the movement. Chains can be used in various thickness and lengths depending on the goals of the individual.

Progressive Resistance—Machines:

- Similar in characteristics to bands are spring-loaded machines. A spring behaves identically to a band in that it provides variable, progressive, nonlinear resistance throughout the range of motion of the exercise. The most commonly used machine that employs springs is used in Pilates and is known as the *reformer* (Figure 23-16). This machine uses a series of closed kinetic chain exercises under the resistance of springs, which the client or instructor can add to or subtract from the sliding base.

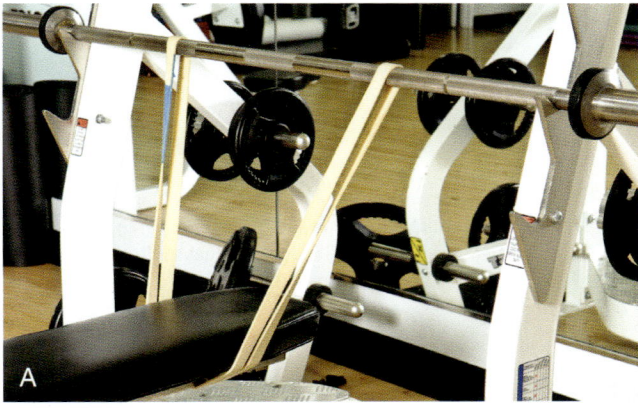
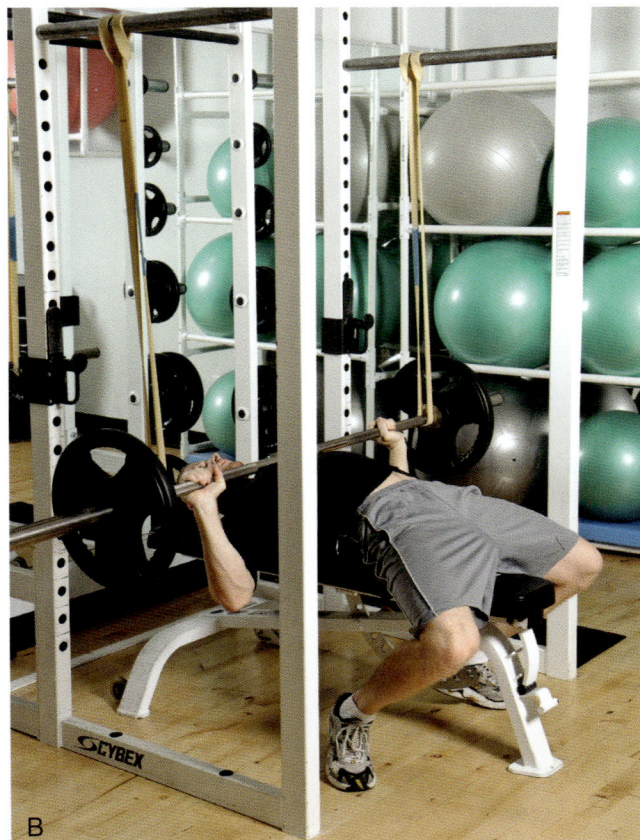

FIGURE 23-14 A, One possible setup for applying band tension to a barbell exercise. The band is looped underneath the bench and secured to the bar at equidistant points from the center. When the bar is pushed up and away from the body, the band tension increases. In **B,** we see an example of the opposite form of tension, called regressive tension. With the bands secured from a point higher than the barbell, and looped around each end, the bands are stretched and decrease the load as the bar is lowered to the chest. When the bar is pushed back up, the bands slacken and the client will be handling a higher percentage of the actual loaded barbell.

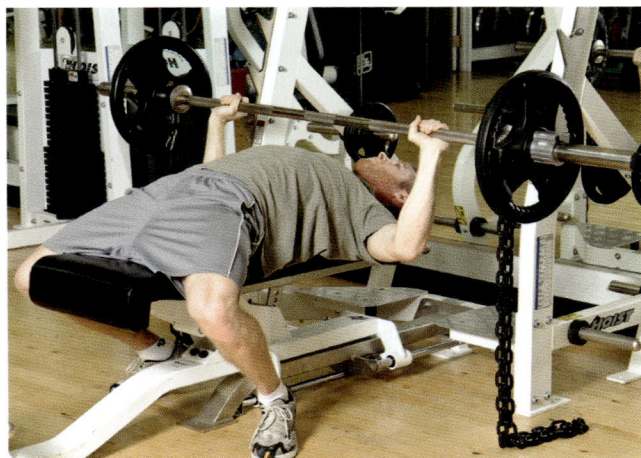

FIGURE 23-15 Setup of a barbell bench press using chains attached to either side of the bar. Depending on the thickness of the chains as well as how many times they are looped around the bar, the amount of resistance can vary. The difference between tension created by a band and tension created by a chain is that the chain provides a linear resistance curve, in that each link that is raised off the floor weighs the same amount (assuming you are using the same size links throughout). The tension created by a band, however, becomes exponentially greater as the band is stretched out farther.

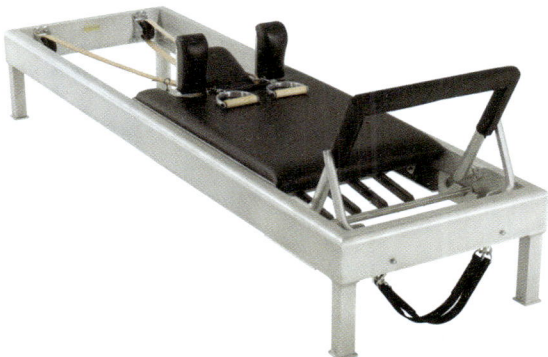

FIGURE 23-16 Gratz Pilates Classic Universal Reformer. *(Photo courtesy of Gratz Industries.)*

- Some other forms of progressive resistance include rod tension, hydraulic tension, and electronic tension.
  - Rod tension uses a series of bendable rods, which are typically controlled by a cable and pulley system. They are not common in commercial gyms but are popular in home equipment such as the Bowflex line (Figure 23-17).
  - Hydraulic and/or pneumatic tension employs the use of compressed liquid or air to provide resistance. It is a rather expensive option and is also quite rare. Typically, the user will control the degree of pressurization using a gauge with manual controls (Figure 23-18).
  - Electronic tension uses a computer to provide electrically assisted resistance, which can be manually set by the client. It is most commonly used in the field of physical therapy (Figure 23-19).
  - Another form of electronic tension is known as **vibration training**. Vibration training has been gaining popularity in the world of physical therapy and is also now available to consumers. Studies have shown that performing an exercise while the engaged muscles are vibrated by an external apparatus can lead to increased strength and power gains compared with regular exercise.[19] Although this equipment is available to the general public, it is recommended that the parameters be set and monitored by a professional in order for the full benefit of this type of training to be attained (Figure 23-20).

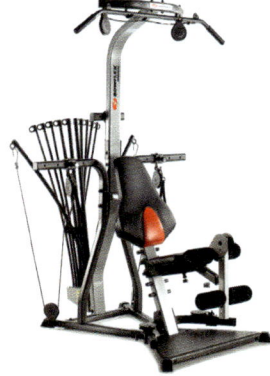

FIGURE 23-17 Commonly found in home gyms, the Bowflex line has become very popular because of its compact, lightweight design. By attachment of multiple rods to the cables, resistance can be increased to provide further challenge. As the rod bends, the tension increases; this is similar to the variable tension created by a band. *(Courtesy Nautilus [Bowflex], Inc.)*

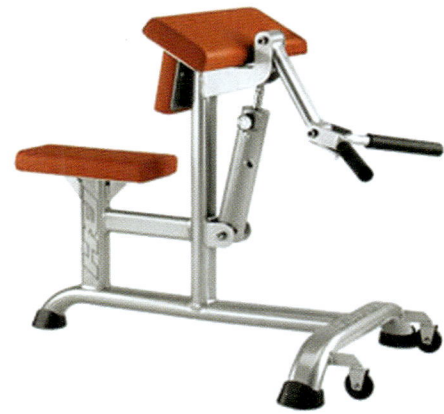

FIGURE 23-18 Here we see an example of a machine that provides progressive resistance through hydraulic tension. The degree of resistance is set in pounds per square inch (PSI) using a manual control. This machine is used to perform a preacher biceps curl. *(Courtesy BH North America Corporation, 2010.)*

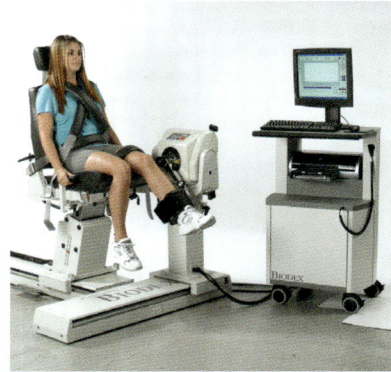

FIGURE 23-19 The client is using an isokinetic machine, which uses a computer to provide electrically assisted resistance to flexion of the left leg at the knee joint. The machine is designed to keep the speed of the joint at a constant rate, so that the client can apply maximal contraction throughout the range of motion. The machine is programmed to match its resistance to the resistance being applied by the client. *(Photo courtesy Biodex Medical Systems, Inc.)*

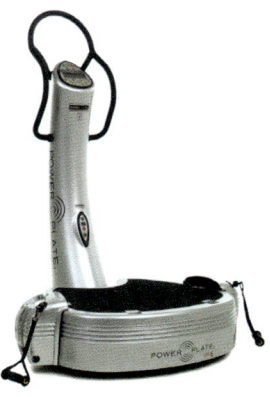

FIGURE 23-20 A vibration machine. The client performs various exercises under a determined frequency and amplitude on the platform. *(Courtesy Power Plate, Irvine, CA.)*

Aqua Therapy:

○ One unique way of providing resistance is by performing exercise in water, known as **aqua therapy**. The resistance of the water is considered progressive and nonlinear because it increases relative to the speed of the exercise being performed. Often used in the field of rehabilitation, aqua therapy offers a low-impact environment that is easy on recovering joints and connective tissues. In the world of sports, aqua therapy is also useful in enhancing power in the athlete. Plyometrics performed in the water require powerful concentric contractions and provide resistance in every direction. This provides a unique stimulation to the body and reduces the delayed onset muscle soreness caused by eccentric contractions[20] (Figure 23-21).

Cable and Leverage Machines:

○ Exercise machines are the most common sight in almost every gym, and there are many different styles of machines made by many different manufacturers. The two most common types of machines can be categorized as cable machines and leverage machines.

○ **Cable machines** use a series of cables and pulleys that typically attach to a weight stack and are manipulated by an interchangeable attachment that allows the user to do a variety of exercises. The cable is made of either a thick wire or a belt, and the pulleys are typically round in design and can vary in number from one to several. The resistance is considered to be nonvariable and linear because the weight stack is working with gravity to provide a fixed weight.

○ The benefit of a cable machine over free weights is that the client can manipulate the line of pull for many different exercises, allowing for an unlimited combination of angles to work with.[21] By analyzing a movement such as the dumbbell chest fly, we see that the client is lying supine on a bench with a dumbbell in each hand and the arms abducted out to the side (Figure 23-22). As the arms horizontally flex (adduct) toward the midline of the body, we see that the resistance from gravity decreases as the moment arm of the resistance decreases (as the arms approach the top of the arc). This decreases the challenge to the target muscle, which

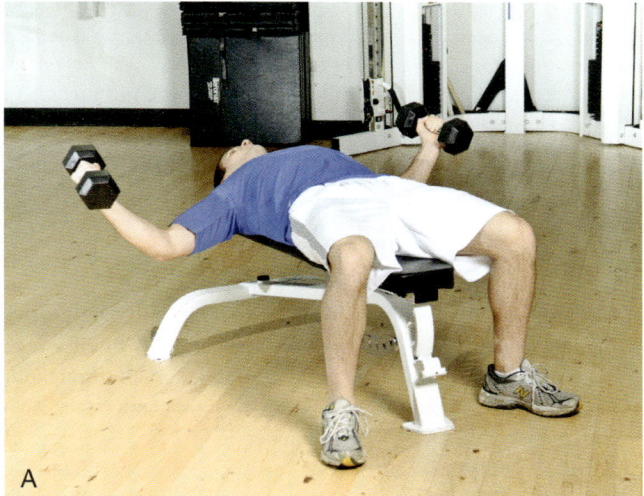

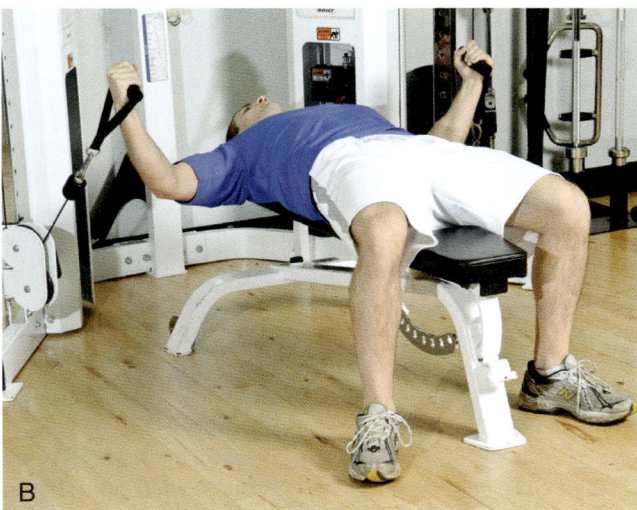

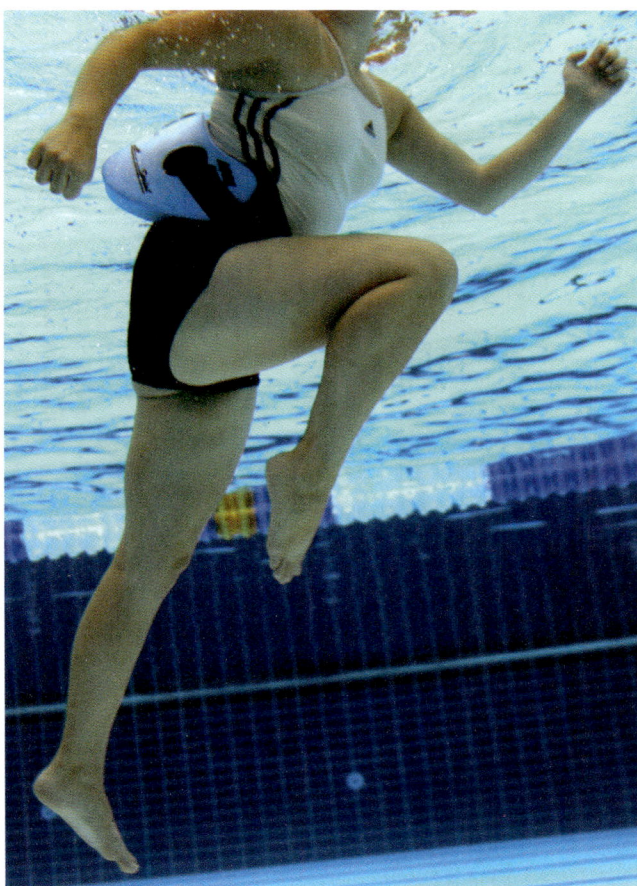

FIGURE 23-21 Aqua therapy. Here we see a sprinting drill being performed in a pool. Note that the water is at neck level. This provides a high level of support on impact. If the same exercise were to be performed in water that was at waist level, the support would be significantly less. (© Nigel Farrow, Loughborough University.)

FIGURE 23-22 Dumbbell chest fly and cable chest fly. Here we see two similar exercises being performed, with dumbbells in **A** and with cables in **B**. In the dumbbell chest fly it is apparent that the desired path of the dumbbell does not match well with the resistance created by gravity. When cables are used, we can see that the client is following a better trajectory for the desired movement, as the line of pull is now more congruent with the direction of the exercise.

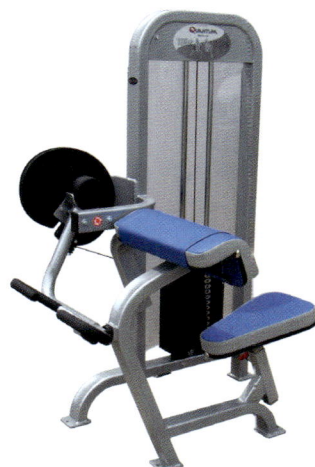

FIGURE 23-23 An example of a cambered pulley machine. Pulleys can vary in design but must be asymmetrical in order to manipulate the line of pull. They are commonly used on single-joint machines, such as the ones used to perform open kinetic chain movements for the biceps curl and leg extension. *(Courtesy Quantum Fitness.)*

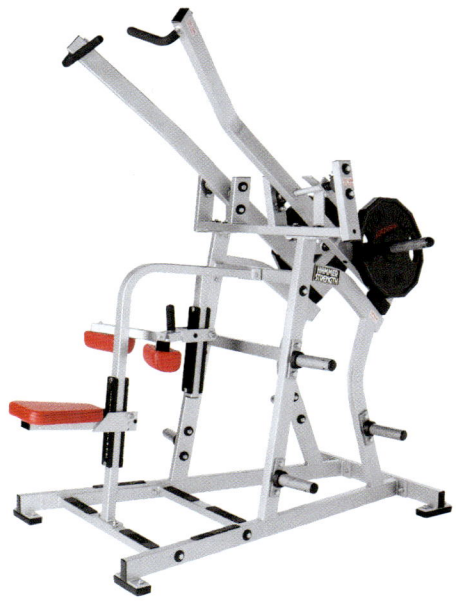

FIGURE 23-24 Leverage machine employing a first-class lever. To use this machine, the client sits on the pad, securing his or her legs under the two pads above. Then, grasping the two handles, the client pulls them downward, raising the weight attached to the opposite end. Much like a playground seesaw, the resistance applied by the client must be enough to overpower the weight attached to the opposite side in order for it to move. *(Courtesy Life Fitness, Schiller Park, IL.)*

is not optimally exercised in this phase of the range of motion. Similarly, when the moment arm is greatest (the arms are the farthest out to the side), the challenge to the target muscle is greatest; unfortunately, this is when the muscle is stretched and is longer and weaker. Hence the ability of the muscle to carry out this exercise in a healthy manner while protecting the shoulder joint is tenuous. By using cables set at an angle for this exercise, we can maintain a constant tension on the muscles throughout the range of motion, and by angling the pulleys out to the side, we can decrease stress on the shoulder and elbow joints.

- Cable machines can also provide variable resistance through the use of **cambered pulleys** (Figure 23-23). Pulleys are typically designed to be round. If a pulley is not round, it is described as a *cambered pulley*. Because of its asymmetrical shape, the leverage force varies and can be manipulated to a greater or lesser degree as the exercise is performed. Cambered pulleys provide a greater moment arm and therefore a greater resistance force when the moment arm and strength of the muscle are greatest, and a lesser moment arm, and therefore smaller resistance force, when the moment arm and strength of the muscle are weakest. This allows the client to work harder where he or she is strongest and gain a relative leverage advantage in a weaker range of motion.
- **Leverage machines** are defined as any piece of equipment that employs a weight attached to the end of a lever, which moves around a central pivot point. Because leverage changes depending on its relationship with gravity, this form of resistance is considered to be variable. As discussed in Section 17.8, there are three classes of levers: first class, second class, and third class. These various types of setups can be seen on the different machines found in a gym (Figure 23-24).
  - Leverage resistance does not always require a bulky, expensive machine. A neat piece of equipment known as the Landmine (Figure 23-25) can provide a client with several options and is easily set up. Rowing and pressing can be combined with core stabilization for a challenging full body workout.

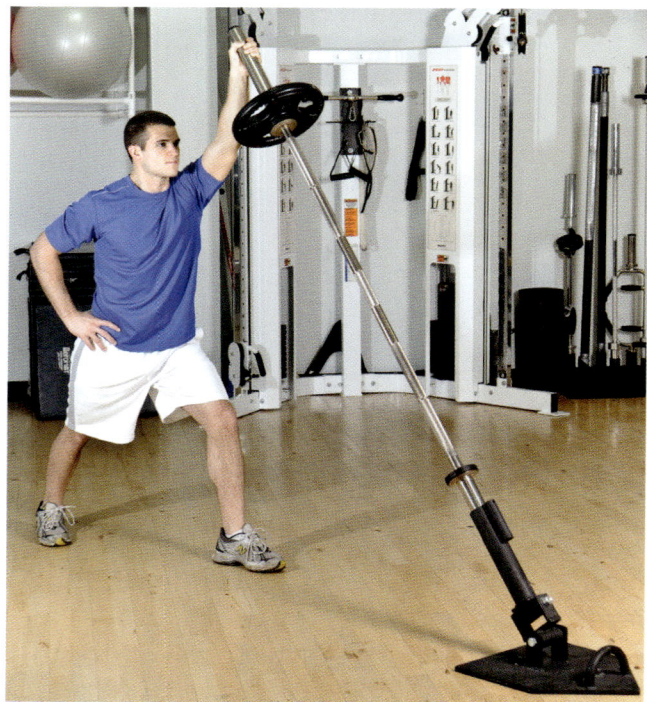

FIGURE 23-25 The Landmine in action. A barbell is placed inside the tube, which is secured to the floor by the metal plate. Additional resistance can be added by putting plates onto the free end of the barbell. Here the client is standing in the center while twisting the bar from side to side using his arms and torso. This is just one of many exercises that can be performed with this piece of equipment.

A Note of Caution:
- With regard to using machines to exercise, it must be noted that the body will not always respond positively to an artificially created environment. By forcing the joints into a rigid range of motion, stabilizer muscles may become weak over time and underdeveloped relative to the mover musculature.[22]
- In the previous example regarding the Smith machine (see Figure 23-11, *B*), we see that the bar is fixed to a vertical track. When performing an exercise such as a bench press, we see that the bar is only free to move directly up and down. When this exercise is performed with a free weight barbell, the trajectory of the bar is not strictly up and down. As a matter of fact, no single free weight barbell bench press is identical to another. The brain will alter the path of the bar ever so slightly in order to distribute the stress of the load differently.
- Furthermore, some machines have limited adjustment settings, and the client may find that he or she does not fit properly when seated. For these reasons, choosing a machine for some exercises may not be optimal.

SECTION 23.4 EXECUTION OF EXERCISE

- Throughout the fitness world, there is a universal consensus of terminology that is used to identify different variables of an exercise program. This section covers these variables and explains the reasons why they might be manipulated to help clients achieve their goals. These variables are volume, rep ranges, aerobic/anaerobic, time under tension, tempo, rep max, rest interval, workload, and recovery.

VOLUME:

- **Volume** is defined as the total amount of an exercise that is performed. Total volume is determined by the number of sets and repetitions performed of that exercise.
    - A **set** is the number of times a certain exercise is performed before one moves on to a different exercise.
    - A **rep** (or **repetition**) is the number of times that movement occurs without rest during the set.
- When combined, the number of sets and reps of a particular exercise determines the total volume of that exercise. For example, three sets of 10 reps would equal a total volume of 30 reps; 10 sets of three reps would produce the same total volume as three sets of 10 reps. Mathematically, the result is equal, but physiologically the two examples would yield different results. The best way to determine how many sets and reps are appropriate or necessary for an individual is based on several factors. The goals of the client should first be analyzed to figure out what the best approach should be.

REP RANGES:

- Typically, someone who is training to increase strength will attempt to lift a relatively heavy weight. This is commonly associated with low rep ranges (usually one to five).[5] An athlete who competes in power lifting, Olympic weightlifting, strength competitions, or sports requiring a lot of explosive power will employ these lower rep ranges in their routines. Because this type of exercise requires short bursts of energy, the muscles do not undergo a significant amount of stimulation before hypertrophy begins. Maximal strength is heavily reliant on the ability of the brain to send signals to as many motor units as it can in the muscle groups involved so that it can use as many muscle fibers as possible on command. Of course, once the brain has been trained to maximize these motor units, the muscle must become bigger in order to handle a heavier load. Muscles with a high ratio of fast twitch fibers tend to respond the best to this type of training.[23] Once muscular hypertrophy begins, it can be accomplished in three ways:
    - **Myofibrillar hypertrophy** is the physiological process in which the muscle increases in (cross-sectional) size because of an increase of contractile proteins (actins and myosins).[23] Myofibrillar hypertrophy of a muscle tends to occur best in a repetition range of 8 to 14 but can be seen anywhere in 5 to 20 reps.[5] (Remember that tempo and ability to stimulate the muscle will play a role in how effective a rep is.)
    - **Sarcoplasmic hypertrophy** is the physiological process in which the sarcoplasmic fluid increases in volume, which creates a larger muscle without an increase of strength.[24] Sarcoplasmic hypertrophy of a muscle tends to occur most predominantly in higher repetition ranges (usually 10 to 20). Myofibrillar hypertrophy and sarcoplasmic hypertrophy occur simultaneously, but the degree to which they occur depends on the repetition ranges and total volume.
    - **Myofibrillar hyperplasia** is a physiological adaptation that results in an increase in the number of muscle fibers within a muscle.[23] Although it is not yet entirely understood, this phenomenon is thought to occur as a result of the action of growth hormones such as IGF-1 and human growth hormone.[23] Stretching and inflammation can also cause a similar effect. In some cases the cause of hyperplasia is unknown.
- If the goal of the client is to increase strength endurance, then a different strategy should be employed. **Strength endurance** is defined as the ability of the muscle or muscle groups to repeat a certain motion for an extended period of time, whether it is for one minute or several hours. Repetitions can range from 15 to as many as the body can handle.[4] Running, for example, requires strength endurance of many muscles in the body, even though it is often called *cardiovascular exercise* and is associated with only the heart and lungs. Muscles that are composed of a high ratio of slow twitch muscle fibers tend to respond best to this type of training.[25] By teaching the brain to signal only the minimum number of motor units needed to complete each stride, we let the others recover so that the muscle can continue to be supplied with constant energy (Box 23-8).

BOX 23-8

There is strong evidence that to some degree the fiber type within a muscle can be altered through physical training. Within the classes of fast and slow twitch fibers, there is a class of intermediate fibers that display characteristics of one or both of these fiber types. Slow twitch intermediate fibers, which have a relatively large number of capillaries to supply oxygen to a muscle, when properly exercised, can be hypertrophied, resulting in a larger diameter of the muscle fiber. If the muscle fiber itself hypertrophies and its capillary supply does not increase, then its relative proportion of muscle mass to capillary increases and it is altered to behave more like a fast twitch fiber. By contrast, a fast twitch intermediate fiber has a relatively low concentration of capillaries. If exercise results in an increase in the capillary supply and the muscle fiber mass does not increase, then its proportion changes in the opposite direction and it behaves more like a slow twitch fiber. In other words, the type of exercise performed can be suited to preferentially increase either the muscle fiber size (anaerobic exercise) or the capillary supply (aerobic exercise).[31] These fibers are sometimes referred to as **hybrid fibers** because of their transitional qualities.

○ It is important to note that although there are commonly accepted repetition ranges for a desired result, there is a large gray area that must be accounted for when designing a program—that is, it is very hard to isolate one desired result of resistance training from another. Training to increase the maximal strength of a muscle may also result in an increase of its endurance capability. Similarly, training to increase the endurance of a muscle may also result in an increase in its maximal strength. Hypertrophy of a muscle can occur from several combinations of sets and reps and will ultimately be determined by hormonal and nutritional factors that occur post-workout. Using a combination of sets, reps, and exercises is typically the best option for maintaining health in many aspects as well as for preventing burning out with one single method of training.

AEROBIC VERSUS ANAEROBIC EXERCISES:

○ By altering repetition ranges, it is possible to manipulate the source of energy that is used by our bodies to fuel our muscles. In discussion of these energy systems, exercise can be categorized into aerobic exercise and anaerobic exercise (see Section 12.7 for more information).
  ○ **Aerobic exercise** is an exercise that is performed for a sustained period of time. After the body has exhausted its resources of free adenosine triphosphate (ATP), creatine phosphate (CP), and glycogen to fuel the muscles, it must use oxygen to convert glucose and glucose derivatives created from fats, proteins, and other carbohydrates into usable ATP. The exercise is described as *aerobic* because of the dependence of the muscles on oxygen.[4]
  ○ **Anaerobic exercise** is an exercise that is performed for a short period of time. The muscles are fueled by free ATP, CP, or glycogen. The exercise is described as *anaerobic* because of the ability of the muscles to function without the presence of oxygen.[4]
○ Our muscles have an immediate supply of ATP, which is ready to be used at any given moment. This stored supply of ATP is responsible for approximately the initial 2 to 3 seconds of muscle contraction.[26] Because the storage supply of ATP in the muscle is limited, the body must be able to regenerate ATP quickly in order to sustain an exercise. ATP regeneration can occur in three ways. The first method, known as the **phosphate system**, occurs via a transfer of energy from stored CP molecules. This process occurs for approximately 30 seconds.[26] The second method involves the process of breaking down glucose (a simple sugar carbohydrate) in the sarcoplasm and is termed **anaerobic glycolysis**. This can help supply energy to a muscle for approximately 30 to 120 seconds.[26] The third method, known as the **Kreb's cycle**, involves the system of breaking down glucose into ATP in the presence of oxygen in the mitochondria. This method is prevalent in aerobic exercise. This process of oxidizing sugars into energy yields a large number of ATP molecules and is predominately responsible for fueling a muscle for periods longer than 2 minutes[26] (Figure 23-26; Box 23-9).

BOX 23-9

By using a heart rate monitor during exercise, it is possible (to a degree) to keep track of which energy system you are working in. The **Karvonen formula**, developed by Dr. M. Karvonen, offers a semiaccurate way of determining percentages of your maximum heart rate. By knowing these numbers, it is possible to monitor how hard you are exercising and which source of energy you are using during exercise. The formula is as follows: Subtract your age from 220; this number is termed the maximum heart rate. Now subtract your resting heart rate from the maximum heart rate, which will give you your heart rate reserve. Now, to find 80% of your maximum training heart rate, multiply your heart rate reserve by 0.80 and then add your resting heart rate again. This number is generally considered to be the peak exercise level that is safe for an individual. Some sources advocate a different percentage, ranging from 65% to 85% instead of a rigid 80%. The level of conditioning of the athlete will affect what this percentage is. As a general rule of thumb, elite athletes can train at a higher percentage of their maximal heart rate than can individuals who are unconditioned. The following is an example of calculating a client's training heart rate.

Brian is 26 years old and has a resting heart rate of 72. The formula for Brian would look like this:

$$220 - 26 = 194 \text{ (maximum heart rate)}$$
$$194 - 72 = 122 \text{ (heart rate reserve)}$$
$$122 \times 0.80 = 98 + 72 = 170 \text{ (80\% of maximum training heart rate)}$$

Therefore 170 would be roughly 80% of Brian's maximal training heart rate. To find a different percentage, simply replace the 0.80 with a different number.

It is important to note that this formula is meant as a general guideline and should be treated with caution. For high-performing athletes, people taking certain prescription medications, and special populations including children and the elderly, this formula may not produce accurate parameters.

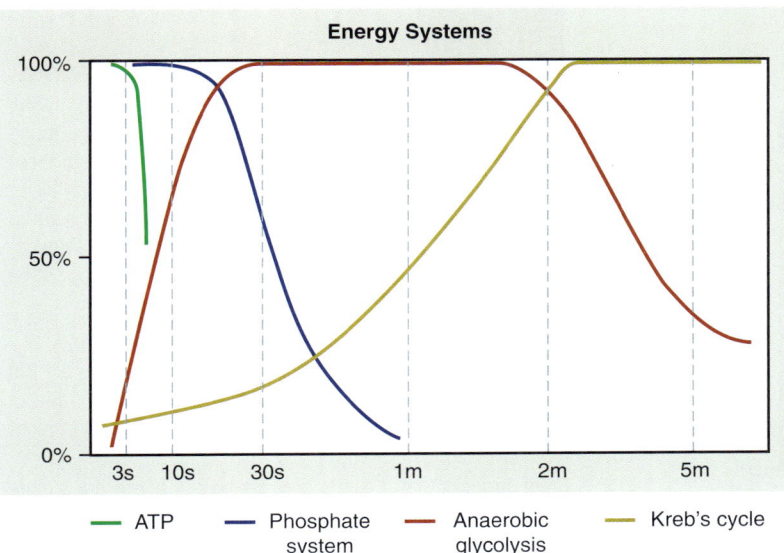

FIGURE 23-26 Adenosine triphosphate (ATP) is a source of energy that is stored in our muscle cells and is immediately available to fuel a muscle. Because we can store only a limited amount, our bodies must be able to regenerate it. ATP regeneration can be accomplished via the phosphate system, anaerobic glycolysis, and the Kreb's cycle. S, Seconds; m, minutes.

TIME UNDER TENSION AND TEMPO:

- When performing a chosen number of repetitions in a given set, the muscles involved are under tension for a certain amount of time. This is commonly referred to as **time under tension (TUT)**. The ability of a muscle to contract relies on its ability to create binding sites on the actin for the myosin heads to attach onto, creating cross-bridges. When the muscle can no longer create these cross-bridges, it becomes fatigued, and nociceptors begin to send pain signals to the brain.[27] This is imperative to injury prevention because it is a sign of temporary damage to the muscle fibers, which need a short amount of rest in order to function properly again. Through adequate training, rest, and nutrition, clients can be conditioned to increase the amount of time under tension their muscles can experience before total fatigue sets in. Time under tension is reliant on both the number of reps in the set and the tempo at which the reps are performed. Those who train to increase the size of their muscles tend to pay attention to this training variable, although no concrete studies have been able to conclude an optimum time under tension.
- **Tempo** is the speed at which an exercise is performed. It is typically categorized into three separate parts: eccentric tempo, isometric tempo, and concentric tempo. In most exercise programs it will be listed in the order of eccentric, isometric, and concentric; 3-2-1, for example, would refer to a 3-second eccentric count, a 2-second isometric count, and a 1-second concentric count. A set of 10 repetitions using this 3-2-1 tempo would result in a total time under tension of 60 seconds. If the tempo signature were altered to 2-1-1, the total time under tension would be only 40 seconds, and the number of reps would need to increase to 15 in order to match the previous example.
- Tempo is a subject of debate among some fitness experts. Although a variety of tempos can be used for an exercise and produce good results, there is a general consensus that during the concentric portion of the movement, the client should contract his or her muscles as quickly as possible in order to maximize stimulation. Although this might result in a fast movement, it is important to control the speed enough to properly stabilize the weights, as well as to prevent hyperextension of the joints. The tempo of the eccentric contraction is important because if the muscles do not slow the movement of the weight to its original position, they do not receive as much stimulation. For example, allowing gravity to bring a dumbbell down from a standing biceps curl does not have the same benefit as using the muscles involved to slowly lower the weight. Not only does it increase the total time under tension of the muscles, but it also helps prevent injury by allowing the load to transfer slowly onto the closed elbow joint as the arm straightens.
- Olympic weightlifters rarely use eccentric contractions in their training because the two lifts in which they compete—the *snatch* and *clean and jerk*—rely on concentric-only movements. The plates are covered in rubber coating, and the lifter will either dump the weights onto a platform or rack them on a stand (Figure 23-27). Spending energy on lowering the bars is wasted energy and is better used on the explosive concentric movements involved in their lifts. This helps by allowing the athlete to handle a much higher-volume workout and preserve cellular energy for a longer period of time.
- The isometric tempo is important because it controls what is known as critical point acceleration.
- **Critical point acceleration** is defined as the transitional point at which the muscle is stretched to its safe limit and transitions back into a state of shortening. This involves both the stretch reflex and elastic energy (recoil) of the myofascial tissue.[17] An athlete training for a sport uses this to advantage by transmitting power from the stretched state of the muscle to its concentric contraction. Examples include the backswing in tennis, golf, or baseball. It is important to move immediately from the backswing to the concentric contraction to take advantage of the stretch reflex. It has been shown that a muscle can contract with greater strength if it is actively stretched before it is shortened. If a pause is added between the stretch of the muscle and its

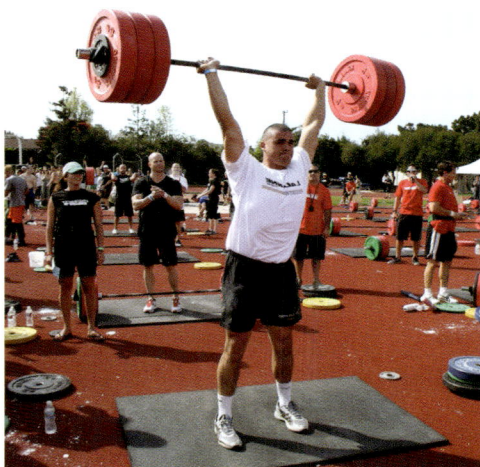

FIGURE 23-27 This figure shows a weightlifter who has completed his lift and is about to drop the weight back to the platform. Because the event is graded when the bar is held and steadied overhead, there is no need for the athlete to expend energy to lower the bar in any sort of controlled fashion. *(Courtesy Leif Edmundson, CrossFit Journal.)*

concentric contraction, the advantage of the stretch reflex is lost. Without this advantage, stimulation of the muscle will have to increase in order for the same load to be lifted.

REP MAX:

- By principle, the heavier the load that is applied to a muscle, the shorter time under tension it is able to endure. When figuring out how much weight to use for a given exercise, it is important to determine what is known as a *rep max* (repetition max).
- A **rep max (RM)** is defined as the maximum number of times an exercise can be performed in succession before total fatigue sets in. If a strength athlete is training to lift a heavy stone off the floor, and the heaviest stone the athlete is able to lift is 200 lb, then that athlete's **1 rep max (1 RM)** is 200 lb. If the athlete can lift a 150-lb stone off the ground five times in a row, then the 5 RM is 150 lb. Determining these numbers is very important because it helps determine how much weight should be used for a given exercise. Many athletes train by using percentages of their 1 RM for a given movement. This method is used to gauge performance as well as prevent injury by using the appropriate amount of weight for the given lift (Box 23-10).

REST INTERVAL:

- The amount of time spent at rest between sets and exercises plays an important role in the overall workout. The determining factor in deciding how much time to rest is dependent on the goals of the individual. The term for describing the period of rest between exercises or sets is known as a **rest interval**.
- As discussed earlier, a muscle fatigues when it can no longer form bonds between the myosin heads and actin filaments. When the muscle is at rest, blood carries oxygen and nutrients (such as glucose) back into the muscle cells and removes the waste products that have built up and damaged the tissues.

 BOX 23-10

It should be noted that it is not always necessary to attempt 1 RM, as there are many calculation formulas available (many can be found online) to help determine what that number might be. Although these calculation formulas may not be 100% accurate, they are useful for providing initial guidelines to a new client until the client has built up the strength necessary to perform a maximum effort 1 RM lift. Depending on the goals of the client, knowing a true 1 RM may or may not be useful or necessary.

Application
Brent and Claudio are identical in weight and height. Brent has a 1 RM bench press of 250 lb and a 20 RM of 100 lb. Claudio has a 1 RM of 225 lb and a 20 RM of 120 lb. Who is stronger? The answer might depend on how we define strength.
- Is Brent stronger than Claudio because he can bench press more absolute weight?
- Could Claudio train his 1 RM to be stronger than Brent's by altering his program?
- Could Brent train to bench press 100 lb for a 30 RM without affecting his 1 RM of 250 lb?
- If Brent increased his 1 RM to 300 lb, would that have an indirect effect on his 20 RM?

Being able to analyze scenarios such as these is important to a trainer so that he or she has a good understanding of how various training programs can influence clients in different ways.

The extent of this recovery is based on the amount of workload put on the muscle and the ability of the individual to recover. The more experienced one is with the exercise program, the quicker he or she will recover. Typical muscle cellular recovery time is estimated to be approximately 60 to 90 seconds.[5] The central nervous system is believed to recover approximately twice as slowly as the muscle tissues and can take up to 5 minutes to be restored to normal levels. As the body becomes stressed repeatedly throughout the workout, the recovery is slower and the level of recovery is lower. It is important to realize when performance is suffering to a point at which progress can no longer be made. Many trainers set measurable limits on an athlete's performance standards to judge when the workout should be finished. For example, an elite sprinter may run a series of sprints while being timed. When the athlete can no longer run under a certain time, which is determined by a percentage of the athlete's best time, the workout will change gears or be altogether terminated.

WORKLOAD:

- After determining the number of sets and reps for a given exercise, one must determine the number of exercises to include in the workout. The total number of exercises performed is typically referred to as the **workload**.
  - Workload is dependent on many individual factors. Experience of the client, ability to handle volume, and ability to recover are variables that can take a lot of time to figure out

and can change from week to week. Diet, sleep, stress, and other lifestyle factors can affect how much workload can be handled on any given day. Developing a program that stresses the body to a high level and allows enough time to recover properly is a delicate balance that requires a high degree of awareness and flexibility from the trainer as well as the client.

○ The order in which these exercises occur is also of great importance and again relies on several individual factors. Typically, the lifts that require the highest degree of concentration and coordination should be performed early in the workout (Box 23-11). These lifts tend to be compound movements such as barbell squats or explosive, technical movements such as the power clean[5] evolve. Of course, many programs begin with a general warmup consisting of mobilization and or stabilization drills, and the selection of these exercises should be based on individual preference. As the workout progresses and the body begins to fatigue, the ability to perform at a high level will diminish. The effects of this decrease in performance can be seen most clearly in exercises that use similar movement patterns, but even exercises that use different muscle groups may still cause the client to exhibit signs of exhaustion. For example, if a client were to perform a series of pull-ups and push-ups to a point of failure and then attempt a 1 RM squat, the amount of weight would be compromised because of fatigue within the central nervous system. It is important to realize and respect the distinct connection between our brains and our muscles.

BOX 23-11

Have you ever wondered why a triathlon begins with swimming and finishes with running? This is done for safety reasons; the odds of drowning are less if the swimming is done first than if the swimming occurs after the athletes have already biked and ran. Biking is done second because of the danger of falls and/or pileups. Of course, there is still danger while running, but it is chosen to be last because of its relative safety compared with the other two events.

○ A technique known as **pre-exhaust** is popular among bodybuilders and is described as performing an isolation exercise to fatigue a certain muscle before using it again during a compound exercise.[5] An example of this method is to use a seated chest fly machine evolve to stimulate the pectoralis major and anterior deltoid before performing a bench press evolve. The thought process is that these two muscles will experience increased activation and therefore be better strengthened during the compound exercise because they were already exercised via an isolation exercise. In fact, this is not the case, and it can actually be dangerous to practice this technique. When certain muscles in a chain of muscles are not able to function to the same level as other muscles, the movement pattern is altered, and/or synergist muscles will have to make up for the strength deficiencies. This could result in a muscle strain, or, even worse, the weight could be mishandled and dropped, causing bodily injury.[10] For these reasons, it is best to prioritize workouts for your client in a way that accounts for these variables.

RECOVERY:

○ After a workout is completed, the body must go through a period of rest and recovery before it is ready for another workout. Rest allows our body to recover and repair itself from the stresses placed on it during exercise. Therefore rest is an integral and vital part of a workout routine, and should be treated with respect equal to that afforded the physical act of working out.[14]

○ Following are some of the factors that determine the amount of time needed for the body to recover to a point at which performance will again be adequate.

  ○ **Hormones:** At any given moment our bodies are either in a hormonal state of breakdown or recovery. During the course of the day our bodies release chemicals such as adrenaline and cortisol, which are known as *stress hormones*. During sleep, we secrete growth and repair hormones such as melatonin and human growth hormone (HGH).[4]

  ○ **Nutrition:** Proper vitamin and mineral intake, as well as a sufficient number of calories from macronutrients (carbohydrates, fats, and proteins) and proper hydration affect the ability of the body to repair damaged tissue.[28]

  ○ **Supplements and medications:** There is evidence that certain supplements can speed up the body's recovery process. Furthermore, over-the-counter and prescription medications may interfere with certain physiological processes in the body.

  ○ **Immune system:** The ability of our body to fight off pathogens and maintain body temperature will keep our metabolism healthy so that nutrients can be absorbed properly.

  ○ **Genetic factors:** Genetic factors that are beyond one's control play a role in the efficiency of our bodies to recover.

  ○ **Workload:** The amount of stress placed on our tissues during exercise determines how long it will take to recover.[14]

  ○ **Adaptation:** As the body becomes accustomed to certain movements, it will be able to recover at a quicker rate because it will have already adapted to the stress demands required to complete the task.[14]

  ○ **Stretching and active recovery:** There is evidence supporting that postexercise stretching can enhance the ability of a muscle to be repaired. Another technique, known as **active recovery**, involves performing light cardiovascular exercise to increase blood flow to damaged tissues.

  ○ **Soreness:** Although it is not necessary to feel soreness after exercise, localized soreness can be a good indicator that a muscle has experienced the microtearing of its myofascial tissue that is necessary to allow for hypertrophy to occur. It is important to pay attention to this soreness because it is a warning that our body is in a state of recovery and may not perform up to its full potential.[29] Much like swelling that occurs around an injured joint to decrease its range of motion, preventing overuse and further tissue damage, muscle soreness alerts us that our body is in the process of healing and further use is not wise. **Delayed onset muscle soreness** or **DOMS** is a term used to describe muscle soreness felt for a period of time after a workout. DOMS can last up to several days.[2]

SECTION 23.5 EXERCISE TECHNIQUE

- Exercise variety is a wonderful tool that can keep workouts fun and interesting, as well as teaching the body new movement patterns and motor skills to stimulate growth and prevent injury. Although there are many resources available that list specific exercises with very specific guidelines as to how to perform them, it is important to realize that there is an infinite number of possibilities when it comes to training the body. Any movement imaginable can be placed under external resistance and by definition will become an exercise (Box 23-12).
- In this section, the following aspects of exercise technique are discussed: joint angle and gravity, range of motion, proper form, and training for specificity.

BOX 23-12

It should be noted that just because something can be done, it does not mean that it should be done. There are many movements that put a great amount of stress on our joints and soft tissues, and by adding resistance to these movements we put ourselves at risk for injury. Trainers should try to be aware of their client's preexisting injuries, imbalances, and/or dangerous tendencies. It is critically important to use your knowledge and problem-solving skills when working with a client to overcome these obstacles.

JOINT ANGLE AND GRAVITY:

- Are all exercises created equally? When looking at the execution of an exercise, it is important to note the body position relative to the joint or joints in motion and determine if it will have any effect on the outcome of the movement. For example, a biceps curl while seated on an inclined bench will have a different effect than a preacher biceps curl in which the client is standing with his (upper) arm resting on the inclined bench (Figure 23-28).
  - The biceps curl is considered to be a single-joint, isolated exercise. Elbow joint flexors are called on to curl the weight up to shoulder level, and shoulder joint extensors and wrist joint flexors are called on to stabilize the shoulder joint and wrist joint from moving, respectively. In Figure 23-28, *A*, the inclined biceps curl, the shoulder joint is in a position of slight extension, which causes a lengthening of the muscles that cross the shoulder joint anteriorly, including the two heads of the biceps brachii. Because free weight is being used, the moment arm of the resistance changes during the range of motion because of the gravitational pull as the weight is being lifted. This stimulates the muscle in a unique way. By contrast, in Figure 23-28, *B*, the preacher curl uses a pad placed in front of the client that puts the shoulder joint in a position of flexion, which once again changes the moment arm. This technique of manipulating the length of a muscle before an exercise works only for a muscle that crosses more than one joint. This type of muscle is described as a **multijoint muscle**. An example would be the two heads of the biceps brachii, which attach proximally to the scapula and distally to the radius, thereby crossing the shoulder, elbow, and radioulnar joints. By contrast, a muscle that crosses only one joint is described as a **single-joint muscle**. An example would be the brachialis, which serves a function similar to that of the biceps brachii but crosses only the elbow joint.

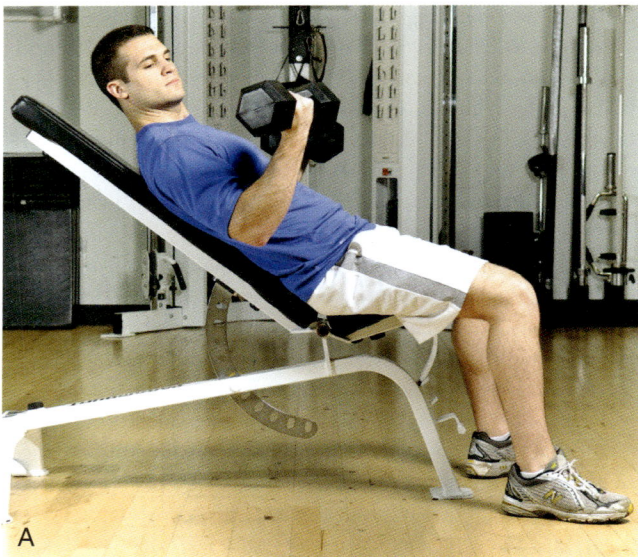

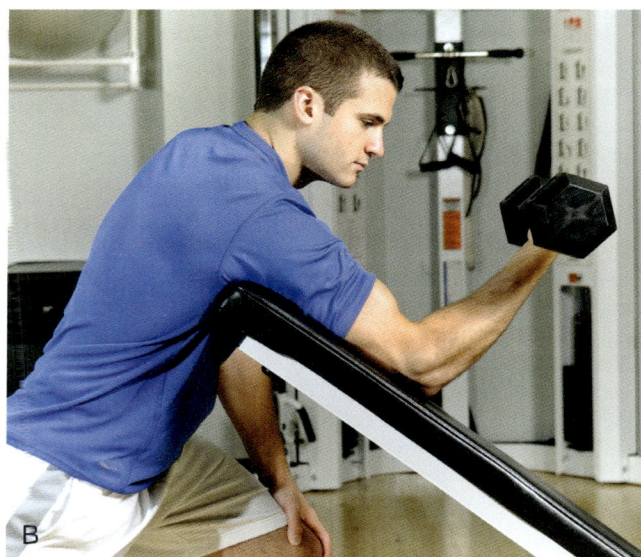

FIGURE 23-28 A biceps curl performed in two different setups. In **A**, we see that the shoulder joint is in a position of slight extension, which will alter the length-tension relationship of the two heads of the biceps brachii, putting them into a stretched state. In **B**, a preacher biceps curl is being performed and we can see that now the shoulder joint is in a position of flexion, putting the two heads of the biceps brachii into a shortened position.

- ❍ This is just one example of how to manipulate exercise by altering body position. There are an infinite number of possibilities to explore, and many of these options may prove to be helpful in finding ways to work around injury or train a muscle in a way that can translate to a specific function or activity. For example, an injury to the shoulder joint can limit the angles at which the client can perform certain exercises using the extremities. Client feedback can be very useful to the trainer so that the trainer is able to find an exercise that accomplishes the goal without causing further trauma to the injured area.

RANGE OF MOTION:

Range of motion is defined as the amount of joint movement that is performed. When learning a new exercise or teaching a new exercise to a client, it is important to be aware of the mobility of the joints involved with that movement. Performing a new exercise with no external resistance is considered the best way to assess the range of motion that should be used (Box 23-13).

BOX 23-13

Often a joint can appear to be in motion when it actually is not. This is commonly referred to as a **compensation**. Compensations occur when a joint can no longer move, as a result of restriction or neural inhibition, and other joints begin to move in order to complete the task. An example of this is laterally flexing the spine to the opposite side while abducting the arm at the shoulder joint to lift the hand above the head. Trainers should be conscious of these tendencies and attempt to cue the client so that compensations are eliminated or minimized.

- ❍ As a general rule, the heavier the load used for an exercise, the shorter the range of motion that is performed. The reasoning behind this is to keep the weight within the strongest phase of the range of motion (see length-tension relationship curve in Section 17.5). This helps to prevent injury to the connective tissues. For example, a client may be able to perform a barbell bench press using 200 lb by lowering the bar all the way to the chest and bringing it back up to the starting position. This is using a full range of motion. The same client may be able to lower 250 lb to a point 3 inches above the chest but would be unable to perform this lift with a full range of motion. This is commonly referred to as a **partial rep**. The benefit of a partial rep is that the muscle can be stimulated with a heavier load while not putting excess stress on the connective tissues of the joints involved.[18] Incorporating partial reps into a rehabilitation program can be useful by gently stimulating a muscle while slowly increasing range of motion over time until full range of motion is restored and strengthened (Box 23-14). The disadvantage is that by training with only partial reps, the muscles are not stimulated throughout a full range of motion, and this can lead to strength imbalances.

BOX 23-14

With regard to rehabilitation technique, there are three successive steps that are typically used by physical therapists when training an injured muscle into recovery. The first variable is to slowly increase the range of motion of the joint(s) through various techniques. The next step is to increase the speed at which the joint is moved with no external resistance applied. The final step is to add external resistance to the motion. By combining these steps, one can attempt to gradually heal a muscle until its function improves sufficiently.

PROPER FORM:

- ❍ **Form** is defined as the specific way in which an exercise is performed. *Proper form* is a term designed to help a new client execute an exercise safely and effectively. With so many resources available today to gather information, determining what exactly is proper form can be a great source of confusion. Once the goal of the client has been determined, two questions must be asked and answered. What exercise will best achieve the desired result? And what is the safest way to perform it? By looking at the actions of muscles and the abilities of the individual, one can determine proper form through simple logic and trial and error.
  - ❍ Subtle changes in an exercise can have an effect on its outcome. For example, through medial rotation of the shoulder joint so that the palms face away from the head during the concentric portion of a dumbbell bench press (Figure 23-29), the movement pattern calls on another one of the functions of the pectoralis major. By analyzing the actions of each muscle, one can deduce how certain motions may better suit the desired goal.

Breaking the Rules:

- ❍ One term that has been given an undeservedly bad reputation because of its name is *cheating*.
- ❍ **Cheating** can be defined as a form of compensation by engaging synergist muscles to assist in completing an exercise in order to take stress off the target muscle(s). This technique is often achieved by contracting these other muscles in an explosive manner, creating a momentum of the body that assists in moving the weight. The word has a negative connotation because it implies that the individual is cheating oneself out of a good workout. While this may be true, it is not necessarily so.
- ❍ If the goal of the client is to stimulate the elbow joint flexors by performing a dumbbell biceps curl, then the full focus should be on performing the movement with little or no assistance from muscles at other joints in the body. If the client begins to sway the body and incorporate movement from the legs, hips, low back, and shoulder joints, the load of the dumbbell will be transferred away from the elbow joint flexors, lessening their stimulation. Many consider this to be cheating, and therefore an inferior method of training. Cheating, however, can also be beneficial because these synergist muscles are stimulated and therefore strengthened. In this manner, various muscle groups are coordinated together and the body is trained to work as one cohesive unit. Therefore if the

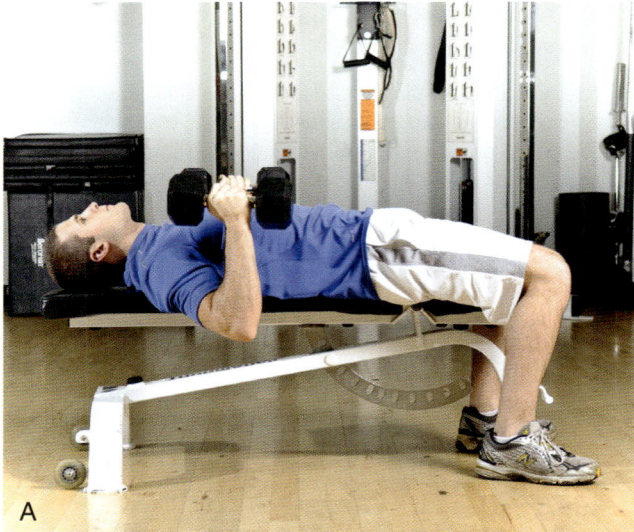

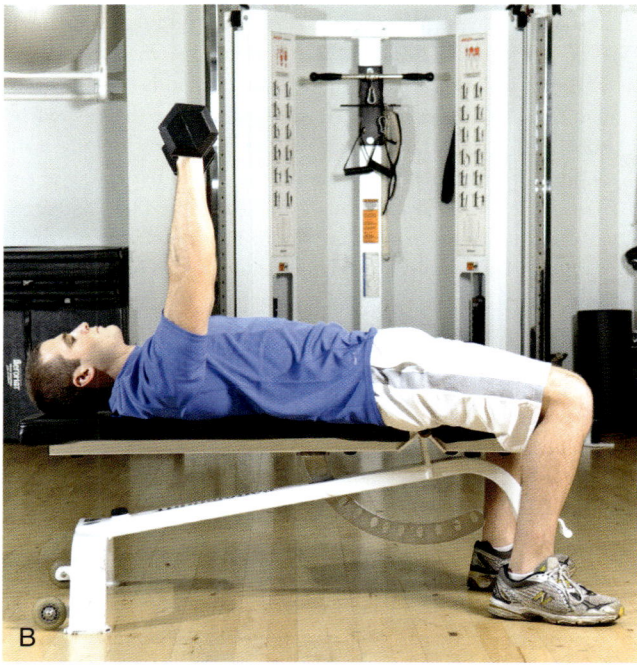

FIGURE 23-29 By analyzing a muscle's function it is possible to determine an exercise that will stimulate it in an optimal way. In both **A** and **B**, the pectoralis major is engaged to lift the weight. However, in B, the arms are also medially rotated, further engaging the pectoralis major.

goal of the exercise is to engage and work only the target muscle group, cheating is not recommended. If the goal is to work and engage many muscle groups, and/or simply to achieve movement of the weight, then cheating can be desired.

○ One method, made popular among athletes, is to employ cheating to engage a broad movement pattern in the body. An example of this is the power clean evolve. When performing this exercise, the goal is to lift a loaded barbell off the floor and bring it to shoulder level. This is best achieved by not only lifting the barbell up explosively, but also by lowering the body underneath it and *catching* it against the front of the shoulders. The concept of cheating here is fully applied, as the more one can learn to use

BOX 23-15

The events performed in Olympic weightlifting are considered to be power exercises. **Power** is the ability of the muscle to produce force while maximizing the velocity of its contraction. Studies have shown using a load that is approximately ⅓ of a client's 1 RM is optimal for increasing maximum power production. Interestingly enough, the sport of powerlifting, which involves the squat, bench press, and deadlift events, requires less than ½ of the power production required in the Olympic weightlifting events, the snatch and the clean and jerk evolve.

gravity and momentum to bring the weight into the air, as well as the technical aspect of being able to lower the body under the bar while it is in motion, the heavier the load that can be lifted. Olympic weightlifters train primarily by this method, and the judges who grade them in competition certainly do not recognize this style of exercise as "cheating" (Box 23-15).

○ One theory is that a client may find benefit in starting an exercise set with *strict form* and finishing it with cheating. The reasoning behind this is that the client can work with a heavier weight, which then allows the eccentric portion of the movement to be trained more extensively (remember that the eccentric portion of a movement is capable of handling the heaviest load).

Advanced Techniques:

○ When strict form is desired but the client wishes to challenge himself or herself further, a few other techniques can be employed (Box 23-16).

  ○ **Rest/pause** is a technique that involves performing a set of an exercise until it can no longer be performed with proper form. The client finishes the exercise, rests for a few seconds, and then begins the exercise again, doing another few reps, until muscle failure is reached. This technique can help increase strength endurance as well as build muscle tissue.[18]

  ○ **Drop sets** are a technique in which the client performs an exercise with a relatively heavy amount of weight. When the set has been completed, a percentage of the weight is immediately

BOX 23-16

When employing advanced techniques, clients often describe a burning sensation in the muscles during an exercise (not to be confused with the delayed onset muscle soreness which occurs after the workout). This is most likely because the total time under tension is increased beyond a typical set and is extended to a point of exhaustion and/or muscle failure. Although it has been thought for years that this burning sensation (also known as acidosis) is caused by a buildup of lactic acid in the muscles, it has been recently determined that this is not true. In fact, lactic acid is not even involved in the acidosis process. Lactate, which is found in the blood, is used interchangeably (and incorrectly) with the term lactic acid. Lactate is not an acid, and in fact its release into the muscle is thought to neutralize the acidosis effects that are taking place. The real culprit of the burn is the splitting of ATP molecules, which releases a positively charged hydrogen ion. When the accumulation of this buildup overpowers the body's ability to remove it from the bloodstream, the muscle will lose its ability to contract and a burning sensation will be felt.

removed and the client performs another set of the same exercise. Typically, 20% to 50% of the weight will be removed, depending on the goals of the client. Several drop sets can also be performed in succession, which will result in a high level of muscular fatigue. Strength endurance and increased muscle mass can be achieved through this technique.[18]

- **Supersets** are a technique in which the client performs two different exercises in succession, with the intention of working the same muscle groups. Examples include performing a set of barbell bench presses and then immediately performing a set of push-ups. Plyometrics can also be employed using this technique. An example of this would be performing a set of barbell squats, followed by a set of squat jumps. Note: Some people define supersets as performing two exercises in succession that involve completely different muscle groups.[5]
- **Assistance lifts** are exercises that are designed to help with other exercises. The most common application of this technique is employed by Olympic weightlifters and competitive powerlifters. The idea is to break down a lift, such as the clean and jerk, into different segments and focus on an exercise that either mimics or complements each shortened movement. The result of this extra training should allow the athlete to gain strength in the specific areas of the lift where the athlete has weakness.[5]

TRAINING FOR SPECIFICITY:

- When training a client for a specific goal, it is important to keep the client moving in the right direction so that the exercises and activities he or she performs have a direct or indirect translation to that goal. The reasoning behind this is based on what is commonly called the *SAID principle.*
- The **SAID principle** stands for **specific adaptation to the imposed demand.** It is defined as the body's ability to adapt to the various stresses that are placed on it and overcome them.[5] This is incredibly relevant to a trainer because it will dictate the program structure of the client being trained. If, for example, the goal of the client is to improve ability to run long distances, then a program that is based around running should be implemented. While this may sound obvious, it is an often overlooked concept that can be applied in great detail to the many specific goals of the most advanced client.
  - Energy systems, which were covered in Section 23.4, are important to analyze in regard to this principle. By observing the duration of effort involved in a sport or activity, one can train in a way that will use similar energy systems and thus have a positive effect on the client. The sport of (American) football, for example, requires short bursts of energy ranging from a couple of seconds to several seconds, followed by a short period of rest. The style of training for this sport would be much different from that for someone who plays soccer, for example, which calls on different energy systems that allow for endurance.

Shaping a Muscle:

- Applying the SAID principle to the shape of muscles is something that is very popular among bodybuilders and those who are training to alter their physical appearance. Changing the shape of a muscle is a widely debated subject that can be the source of much confusion. The general consensus is that the shape of a muscle is predetermined by its attachments and that it has the ability only to become bigger or smaller. Hypertrophy (getting bigger) is thought to occur uniformly along the entire length of a muscle and cannot be altered regionally. By analyzing the line of pull of a muscle and the line of pull of an exercise, it is possible to hypothesize where the hypertrophy is likely to occur. (Remember that some muscles have fibers that are oriented in different directions as explained in Section 17.2, and therefore the muscle has a number of different lines of pull within it.)
- Altering the length of a muscle, via addition or subtraction of sarcomeres in series, has been shown to occur when the resting length of that muscle has been manipulated for an extended period of time. For example, when a woman becomes pregnant, the rectus abdominis (among other muscles) stretches and lengthens over the course of the pregnancy to allow extra room for the fetus inside of the womb. After the pregnancy, the rectus abdominis and other abdominal wall muscles attempt to return to their original size because they are not as functional in their newly lengthened forms (because of the altered length-tension relationship). Note: Where the muscle attaches by its tendons cannot be altered through any type of training; therefore the potential for the muscle to lengthen is somewhat limited.
- By focusing on exercises that use a line of pull specific to the direction of certain fibers in a muscle, we can influence, to an extent, which fibers receive the most stimulation. Bodybuilders use various lines of pull specifically for this reason, so that their muscles might appear more balanced and aesthetically pleasing (Figure 23-30).
  - Because muscles can be considered to have distinct compartments (motor units) based on the branching of motor

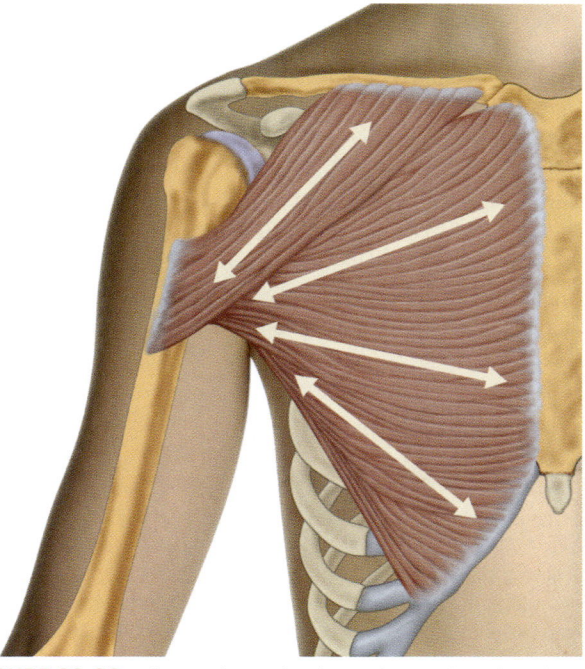

FIGURE 23-30 When analyzing the shape of a muscle such as the pectoralis major, we see that it is shaped like a fan, which allows for different lines of pull with regard to moving the arm at the shoulder joint. *(Modified from Muscolino JE:* The muscular system manual: the skeletal muscles of the human body, *ed 4, St Louis, 2017, Mosby.)*

neuron innervation, this technique of altering the line of pull can call on different compartments/motor units for different functions of the muscle. A good example of this is the biceps brachii, which is innervated by three to six primary nerve branches of the musculocutaneous nerve. Because of the ability of the biceps to create flexion of the elbow joint as well as supination of the forearm at the radioulnar joints, different sections of the muscle are activated when simple flexion is performed versus flexion combined with supination (Box 23-17).

> **BOX 23-17**
>
> Keep in mind that there are usually many muscles that can perform a particular joint action. Depending on the phase of the range of motion, the joint angle, and the angle of other joints (if it is a multijoint muscle), the nervous system often engages one muscle versus another or one head or part of a muscle versus another. This choice is often based on the efficiency of that muscle's contraction in the particular circumstance. For example, when engaging the biceps femoris to flex the knee joint, the long or short head is preferentially engaged depending on the angle of the hip joint.

SECTION 23.6 PROGRAM DESIGN

This section discusses the concepts of choosing an appropriate workout program for a client, balancing workload and recovery, general tips for the new client, specific exercise programs, and special tools/aids used when exercising.

CHOOSING A PROGRAM:

- In design of a workout program, a decision must be made as to how to put it all together so that one's goals may be safely accomplished. There is an almost infinite number of combinations one can use to design a program. Following are some of the most common methods.
- **Full-body workout:** A full-body workout would focus on training the entire body in a single workout, incorporating exercises that attempt to treat every muscle equally. Typically, these workouts involve many compound movements, and the focus is on various *movement patterns* as opposed to single exercises. Those **training for sports** or *functional strength* may find great success in this style of training. A full-body workout can be tailored so that it mimics common activities of a sport, or it can be used for overall general conditioning[30] (Box 23-18).
- **Sports-specific workout:** A sports-specific workout is one that tailors to helping an athlete improve in his or her sport. It prioritizes the weaknesses of the athlete so that he or she might become stronger, quicker, or more coordinated at the activity in which the athlete competes.[5] For example, Olympic weightlifters compete in only two events, the snatch and the clean and jerk evolve. Everything that they do in the gym is designed to help them with these lifts. In comparison, an athlete who competes in the discus throw would focus on strengthening, mobilization, and power exercises that would help achieve a better discus throw (Box 23-19).
- **Body part split:** A body part split focuses more on breaking the body into specific muscles or muscle groups and training them on separate days. The advantage to this type of workout over a full-body workout is that more volume in any one workout can be dedicated to the muscles chosen. The disadvantage would be that these muscles would take longer to recover and cannot be trained as frequently. Some type of rotation is typically used so that certain muscle groups can recover while others are being worked.
- Some of the more common types of body part splits include upper/lower, push/pull/legs, and a more specific bodybuilder split.
  - **Upper/lower** is defined as a workout routine that divides the body into an upper half and lower half. All movement that specifically targets the muscles above the waistline would be trained on one day, and movements that focus on the lower body would be trained on another day.[5] Some exercises, such as the barbell dead lift evolve or the power clean evolve, may be open to interpretation and should be selected based on individual preference.

> **BOX 23-18**
>
> The term *functional exercise* can be a deceptive way to describe an exercise. All strength is functional and serves a purpose in that it makes our myofascial tissues stronger and increases our ability to perform a certain task. The media has coined the term functional strength to apply to exercises that help us perform everyday tasks, frequently called **activities of daily living (ADLs)**, such as lifting objects, climbing stairs, or playing with children. Although it is true that there are exercises that can help in such situations, it may be unfair to say that one exercise is more functional than another one. It is entirely dependent on what the function is!

> **BOX 23-19**
>
> Many people choose to play sports such as tennis or basketball instead of working out in a gym. These activities can be very beneficial toward increasing aerobic capacity, agility, balance, and strength. However, some sports, such as golf, can lead to imbalances because of their asymmetrical nature and can potentially cause injury or postural problems. If participating in sports is chosen as a replacement for exercise in a gym, then it is wise to be aware of these imbalances and try to address them so that the body can maintain proper health.

- **Push/pull/legs** is defined as a workout routine that is divided into three workouts, involving upper body pushing movements one day, upper body pulling movements another day, and training of the lower body on a separate day.[5] This basic split is popular among competitive powerlifters because it allows special attention to be given to the three lifts in which they compete.
- **Bodybuilder splits** are common among competitive bodybuilders but are also quite popular with the average gym member who is looking to increase muscle size and become stronger. This workout routine focuses on dividing the workout of the muscles of the body into separate days in whatever fashion is desired. Isolation exercises are common so that each muscle can be stimulated to a point of exhaustion. The individual breakdown of this split is open to many avenues of approach and is also a source of much debate.

BALANCING WORKLOAD AND RECOVERY:

- Regardless of which program is chosen by the individual, an allotted rest period must be incorporated so that the body can recover from the stress that has been placed on it. As discussed in Section 23.4, individual factors such as nutrition, sleep, experience, hormone production, and the immune system determine how quickly the body can recover from a workout. It is important to note that there is a direct relationship between the amount of workload that is incorporated into a program and the amount of recovery time needed before that workout can be repeated. For example, a workout that focuses on the muscles of the chest, shoulders, and arms will cause a great deal of stress to that area and the body will require one or more days to recover. By contrast, a full-body workout may be able to be repeated on consecutive days because the workload is being distributed more evenly throughout the body. Setting measurable goals and performance standards will help the client determine if he or she is putting in enough work and allowing for enough rest between workouts. There is no universal formula to determine how often or how long somebody should work out or somebody should rest.

GENERAL TIPS FOR A NEW CLIENT:

- Although it is certainly true that there is no one correct way to exercise, given the vast amount of individual variables that determine a workout program, there are some ideas that are generally accepted within the training community. A new client should be treated as very fragile until a relationship has been established that allows the trainer to confidently progress that person to different stages of difficulty within the program. The following are some generalized tips that can be helpful when designing a program for a new client.
- Some method of warm-up should be performed before the client engages in resistance exercise. Through performance of light exercises that relate to the ensuing muscle groups of the workout, core temperature is increased and transient connective tissue bonds (also known as *fascial adhesions*) are broken, increasing the biomechanical performance of the body and reducing the potential for injury.[29] It is important to note that exercises designed for warming up are not necessarily the same as those designed to increase flexibility (stretching exercises). Guidelines for a warm-up include light exercises that mimic the main exercises for that workout, and/or any form of aerobic exercise that will increase the heart rate enough to produce a sweat, for a duration of 5 to 10 minutes. Dynamic stretches can be used to produce a similar outcome. Warm-up effects can be lost after 15 minutes of idle activity, so timing can be important in order to receive the benefits of this technique.
- Exercises that require a lot of core stabilization balance should not be chosen until the client has established a solid proficiency in the basic movements. Pictured in Figure 23-31 are some of the many tools available that are designed to challenge one's core stabilization balance. Because these devices provide an unstable surface, when a client stands on them, muscles of balance are stimulated. The client can stand and balance with both feet, performing the exercise bilaterally as pictured in *A*, or may increase the challenge by standing on just one foot, performing the exercise unilaterally. Unilateral execution of these exercises, in addition to being more challenging, may translate better to certain sports. If the exercise consists of maintaining balance to simply stand still, it is called a *static balance exercise*. If the client adds movements of the core and/or upper extremities, it becomes a *dynamic balance exercise*. Depending on the client's goals, exercises incorporating balance may or may not be necessary.
- Exercises that are performed unilaterally should typically be chosen after the client has demonstrated competency with bilateral movements. The reason is that unilateral movements require a higher level of core stabilization to prevent excessive torquing of the spine. And dynamic balance exercises that involve movement should not be done until the client has demonstrated competency with static balance exercises.
- When choosing a repetition range for a new client, it is safest to first use a high rep scheme with a relatively light amount of weight/resistance.[5] If the client's goal is to build maximal strength, then gradually lowering the rep range and increasing the weight/resistance will help accustom the client's body to handling a heavy load while slowly strengthening the joints and connective tissues and increasing neural control.
- When deciding which exercise modality to use with a client, it may be tempting to start with a seated machine that is relatively simple to use and does not require a lot of stabilization force. Although it is true that these machines might be easier to learn, it does not mean that it is the best option for your client. Remember that your clients are training with you so that you can teach them more advanced movements under the safety of your professional eye. Just because a gym might be packed full of extravagant machines does not mean that they are better than many more traditional exercises. In some cases, they may even do more harm than good. Do not hesitate to teach a new client free weight or bodyweight exercises first, but be aware of the fact that the client will need the proper amount of cueing until he or she can safely perform the exercises on his or her own.
- When instructing a client to perform an action on his or her own, whether it is a stretching or a strengthening exercise, be sure to explain the important connection that one must have with one's own body in order to get the desired result. A common term

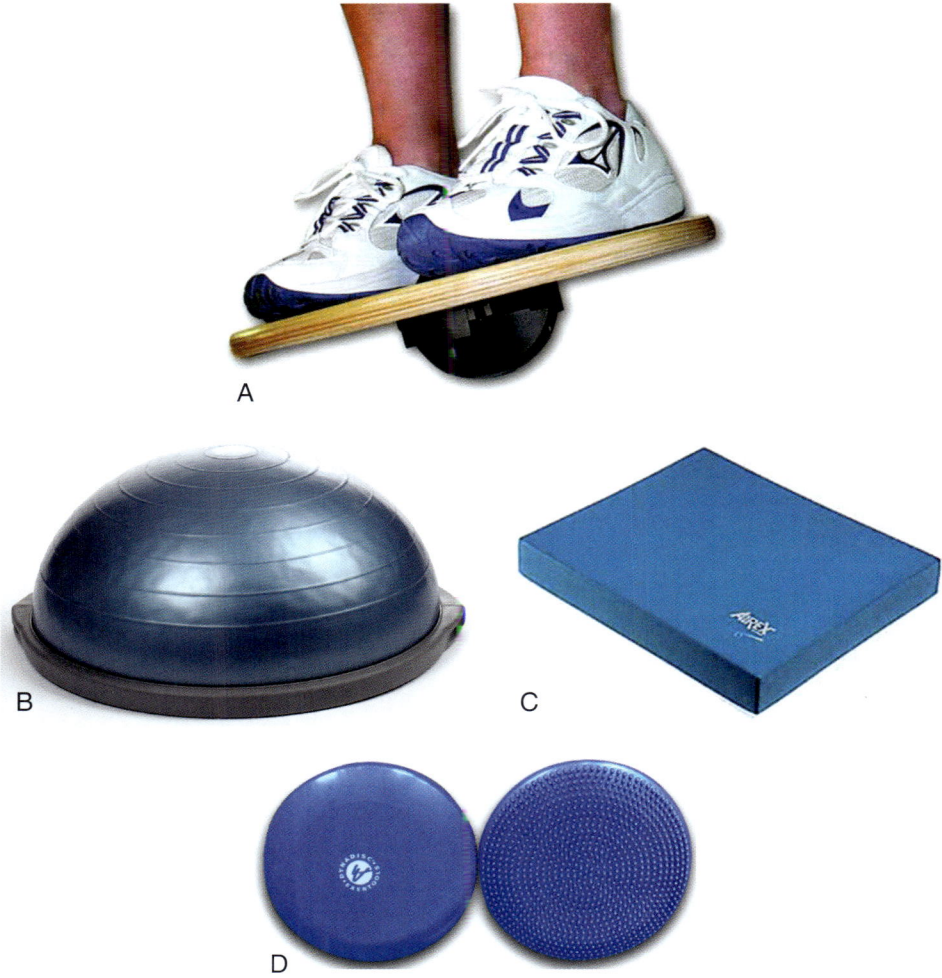

FIGURE 23-31 Examples of devices that are designed to create an unstable environment during exercise to increase core stability strength. Balance training is a widely debated topic among trainers regarding its benefits and specificity to real life situations. **A,** Balance board. **B,** BOSU Ball. BOSU Fitness, LLC. **C,** Airex pad. **D,** Dyna Disc. *(A, Courtesy Fitter First. B, Courtesy Bosu. C, © Airex AG, Switzerland. D, courtesy Exertools.)*

among trainers to describe this is **mind-to-muscle connection**. In the world of manual and movement therapies, it is often referred to as **mind-body connection**. This refers to the client's ability to actively feel/sense the muscles at work during an exercise as well as the ability to control the body in space. Proprioceptive awareness and continual repetition of a movement will increase the client's control of the exercise and thus increase its efficacy.

○ Earlier, in Section 23.2, it was stated that "20 lb will always weigh 20 lb," which refers to resistance remaining constant in its relationship with gravity. Although this is true, it does not guarantee that all clients will receive equal stimulation of their muscles from this resistance. The ability to get the most out of the 20 lb of resistance is dependent on this mind-to-muscle connection that the client must possess and the ability to control the weight in all aspects. This *art of control* can take a long time to master, but the payoff is worthwhile, as it will maximize one's time and efficiency as well as help avoid injury by permitting one to stay in tune with one's body during the workout (Box 23-20).

BOX 23-20

One of the most common questions asked by a client is how many repetitions of an exercise the client is going to perform. Although it is good to have a number of reps in mind at the beginning of a set, it can sometimes inhibit the quality of the workout. Quality should always take precedence over quantity. If a client is in touch with his or her body and has good motor control, then the client will be able to perform the exercise in a more effective manner. Keeping your client focused on the task at hand and being able to properly cue the client and explain what he or she should be feeling will help the client get the most out of the exercise. Remember, it is not how many; it is how.

SPECIFIC EXERCISE PROGRAMS:

- Specific programs are sometimes employed by trainers, teams, or individuals looking to achieve a certain goal. These programs are structured in such a way that one can mold the workout to one's own needs. Some require the assistance of a professional and may require a special type of certification. Following are examples of some of the more popular specific programs.
  - **Crossfit:** Originally developed in 1980 by former gymnast Gary Glassman, Crossfit has become extremely popular over the past decade, with hundreds of gyms dedicated to this type of training now located worldwide. Crossfit is a strength and conditioning program designed to increase strength endurance, strength power, and aerobic capacity. It takes the principles of several different training modalities and combines them into a unique, total body fitness regimen that is designed to help anybody and everybody. The workouts are typically very fast-paced and incorporate the use of kettlebells, medicine balls, calisthenics, and Olympic lifts, among other tools.
  - **Rippetoe's Starting Strength:** Developed by Mark Rippetoe, a well-known strength and conditioning coach, this program is designed to help new lifters develop strength and muscle hypertrophy. Typically used by those who wish to gain muscle mass, this program incorporates two workouts that are rotated, each one performed three days a week. For example, week 1 would be workout A, workout B, workout A; week 2 would be workout B, workout A, workout B. The main exercises that are performed are the barbell squat, the barbell bench press, the pull-up, the bent-over barbell row, and the overhead barbell press.
  - **Westside Barbell:** Founded by Louie Simmons, Westside Barbell is a training facility that specializes in training competitive powerlifters. Based in Ohio, the facility's influence has spread worldwide, and the program focuses primarily on building strength around the three main lifts used in a powerlifting competition: the squat, the bench press, and the deadlift. Various training tools such as bands, chains, and different kinds of bars are employed to challenge the athlete in various ways to continuously stimulate strength gains in the three lifts. Special exercises are also incorporated to help the athlete overcome strength deficiencies in certain portions of the range of motion of each lift. The *Westside philosophy* of training has spawned many different spin-offs of the original program, which give several options to a practitioner of this sport.
  - **Kettlebell:** Kettlebell training has been popular for several decades and has recently been gaining more attention throughout the United States. A kettlebell is a round weight with a single handle on top. Although very similar to a dumbbell, it does have certain advantages that set it apart from its more common counterpart. Because of the unique shape of the weight, certain movements such as Olympic lifts and assistance lifts (see Section 23.5) can use the momentum of a swinging weight to their advantage. Kettlebell workouts are typically fast-paced, explosive movements and are primarily designed to increase power and aerobic capacity.
  - **Pilates:** Developed by Joseph Pilates over a period of 50 years, Pilates is a comprehensive mind-body workout that involves over 500 strengthening and stretching exercises. Joseph Pilates called his method of body conditioning *the Art of Contrology*; however, after his death in 1967, it has come to be known as *Pilates*. For many years, the Pilates method was relatively unknown except in the world of dance. In recent years, the popularity of Pilates has exploded, and it has become one of the most well-known methods of body and mind conditioning. A key element of the Pilates method is core stabilization, or as the core is called in Pilates, the *powerhouse*. Pilates exercises may be broken into two categories: Pilates mat and Pilates apparatus. Pilates apparatus involve the use of springs to guide the client and also provide resistance. The two major Pilates apparatus are the reformer and the Cadillac. Both types of Pilates are typically done under the supervision of a certified instructor. Benefits of the Pilates method include postural alignment, mind-body awareness, proper breathing, increased focus, and joint mobility and stabilization.
  - **Yoga:** Yoga is an ancient spiritual practice that, at its inception, was a means of achieving an enlightened state through meditation, breath work, physical poses, and ethical behavior. Today yoga is widely known for its poses, which are called *asanas*. Asanas can be static and held for a certain number of breaths, or dynamic, flowing from one pose into another. Yoga is known to increase flexibility, but many are surprised to learn that it also builds strength and improves coordination. Postural imbalances can be remedied by the body awareness that it cultivates. The vast majority of modern yoga still includes meditation and breathing techniques. Both are helpful in reducing stress, relaxing muscles, and identifying patterns of tension. There are many styles of yoga today. They form a wide spectrum that ranges from pure meditation to a rigorous workout, so it is important for one to seek out the appropriate style to suit his or her needs.
  - **Muscle activation technique (MAT):** MAT is a relatively new form of manual therapy that focuses on strengthening the body where it is weak, to correct muscular imbalances. It focuses on identifying weak and inactive muscles so that they can be strengthened, and attempts to correct various movement pattern compensations. A series of isometric strengthening exercises and palpation techniques are used to *activate* the identified weakened muscles. The goal is to allow for optimal muscular function so that one can perform up to one's full potential and have a reduced chance of injury.
  - **Kickboxing:** Kickboxing is a competitive sport, but many people have found that there are many benefits to training like a kickboxer without actually fighting (no headaches being one of them). Various classes are offered to those who wish to let out some aggression while also getting a great workout. Benefits include increased aerobic capacity, agility, power, and proprioception. Some classes also include strength training.

SPECIAL TOOLS/AIDS:

- Special tools/aids are often used in the gym to help with certain exercises. Following are some of the more common items one might see in a gym setting.
  - Note: The use of external supports such as braces and belts often allows for a greater load capacity when exercising. This carries an increased risk of damage and injury to other joints

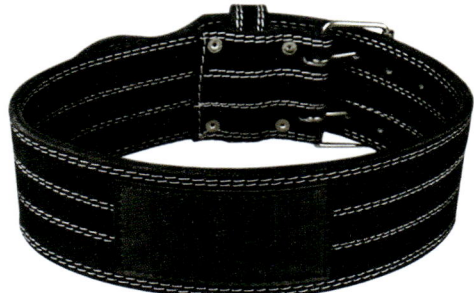

FIGURE 23-32 An example of a weightlifting belt. These belts can be purchased in varying lengths and thickness, depending on the preference of the client. It is important to wear them tightly enough to serve their function, but not so tightly that they interfere with respiration. *(©shutterstock.com.)*

and tissues of the body that are not supported in this manner and not accustomed to absorbing these increased loads.

- **Weightlifting belt:** Although often associated with a back injury, a weightlifting belt is different from a rehabilitation back belt that might be recommended by a physical therapist or physician. A weightlifting belt works by increasing intra-abdominal pressure when the user pushes the abdominal muscles against the surface of the belt. This increase in pressure allows for an increase in spinal stability and is especially important to use during exercises that place stress upon the spine, such as a barbell squat or barbell deadlift. Commonly worn by those competing in powerlifting or Olympic weightlifting, the belt is usually only worn when the weight approaches 1 RM. Studies have shown that proper use of a belt can increase the amount of weight used for certain exercises (Figure 23-32).
- **Knee wraps:** Knee wraps are constructed out of elastic cloth and are designed to provide support around the knee joint during exercises that involve knee extension, such as the squat (Figure 23-33). Powerlifters use these to their advantage because the elastic nature helps them lift more weight during a squat. Because the wraps are applied when the leg is in extension, when

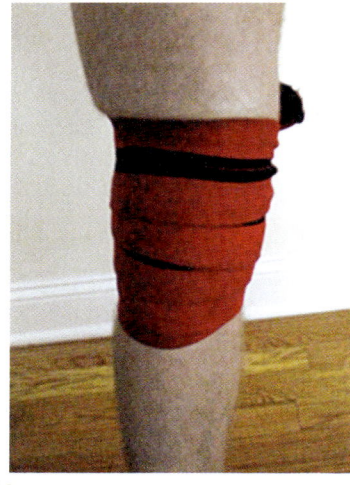

FIGURE 23-33 A typical application of knee wraps. We can see that the wrap begins below the knee joint and finishes at the bottom of the thigh, above the knee joint. As with the weight belt, it is important to wrap the knee tightly enough so they can serve their function, but not so tightly that they cut off circulation to the leg, which can be very dangerous when one is trying to exercise.

the knees are bent the wraps will provide a spring effect that will try to bring the knees back into extension. Individuals with localized knee joint pain can find benefits in using wraps. Wraps are also made that go around the elbow, wrist, and ankle joints.

- **Bench shirts/squat suits:** Certain powerlifting competitions allow for special equipment that is used to aid the athlete in the squat, bench press, and deadlift events. Constructed from a variety of materials (polyester, denim, and canvas being the most popular), these garments are designed to fit tightly around the athlete to support joint movement (Figure 23-34). For example, the bench shirt is constructed in such a way that the athlete's arms are put in a state of flexion and medial rotation. When the bar is

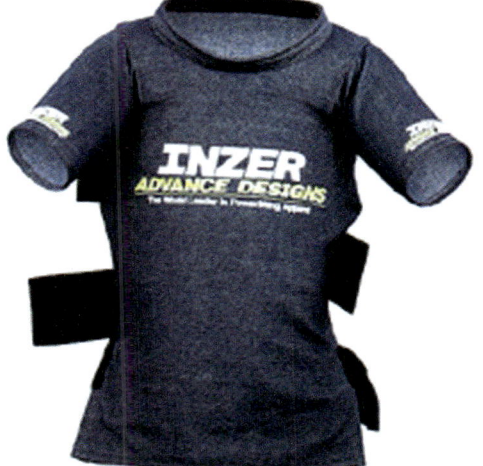
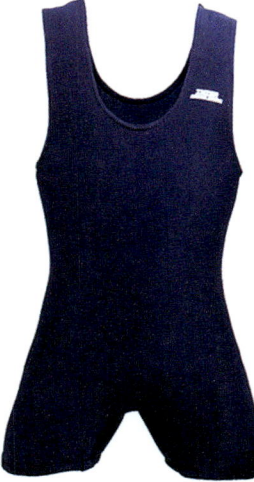

FIGURE 23-34 An example of a bench shirt (left) and squat suit (right). There are several companies that provide this equipment, and many variations that can be purchased, depending on the needs of the athlete and regulations of the federation in which he or she competes. It is important to be sure that the suit fits properly. Therefore custom tailoring is often performed to ensure a good fit. *(Courtesy Inzernet.)*

CHAPTER 23 Principles of Strengthening Exercise

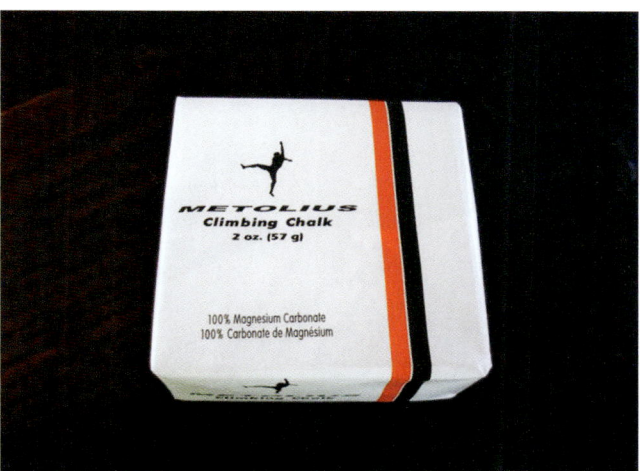

FIGURE 23-35 A brick of chalk. This chalk is easily broken up into a fine powder and is applied anywhere on the body where moisture is undesirable.

lowered to the body, this material is stretched out and provides an elastic effect, which can result in the ability to lift more weight for that particular event. The same concept is applied during a suited squat lift. The design of such equipment can vary greatly, and different powerlifting federations have different rules and standards for what is allowed in their sanctioned meets.

- **Chalk:** Chalk is designed to increase one's ability to hold onto a weight or weights. When applied to the hands, the water-insoluble magnesium carbonate dries out moisture in the skin, which in turn provides a solid, nonslip grip for various exercises. It is popular in gymnastics, rock climbing, Olympic weightlifting, and powerlifting (Figure 23-35).
- **Ammonia/smelling salts:** Used in powerlifting, Olympic weightlifting, boxing, football, and various other sports, ammonia is used to stimulate the central nervous system to provide a short, temporary burst of energy to those who smell it (Figure 23-36). It is also commonly used medicinally to bring someone out of a semiconscious state. Warning: Ammonia is a toxic substance and should only be used sparingly and in small doses if used for athletic purposes.
- **Wrist straps:** Using wrist straps is another method that can improve the ability to grip during certain exercises. By looping a piece of cloth around one's wrists and then wrapping the free end around a bar or handle, the athlete is essentially attached to the weight and can hold onto it for a longer period of time (Figure 23-37). Commonly used by bodybuilders, the advantage is that an exercise can be performed for longer because it is not limited by the strength of their grip. The disadvantages are that the athlete is neglecting many important forearm muscles and that the straps place a lot of stress on the wrist joints.
- **Gloves:** Gloves are worn to protect hands from developing calluses and skin tears; gloves also help to increase the security of the grip on the machine or barbell/dumbbell. Some types of gloves provide wrist support as well (Figure 23-38).
- **Dip belts:** Dip belts are worn around the waist and have a chain that hangs down from the front from which weight is attached. These belts are used to increase the amount of resistance for certain bodyweight exercises such as the dip and the pull-up (Figure 23-39).
- **Shoes:** Selecting the proper shoe depends on what type of training you are participating in. For example, shoes that are designed for running should not be worn while performing a heavy squat lift because running shoes are designed to be soft and flexible to absorb impact, which is counter-productive when trying to maintain a stable stance to push a weight away from the ground. Running shoes are also risky to wear when playing a sport like tennis because tennis requires a great deal of lateral movement, and running shoes are designed primarily for forward sagittal plane movement. There are shoes specially designed for most every athletic endeavor. Examples include sprinting, long distance running, cross-training, powerlifting, Olympic weightlifting, tennis, and golf (Figure 23-40). Finding the right shoe is important because it can increase performance and decrease the risk of injury.

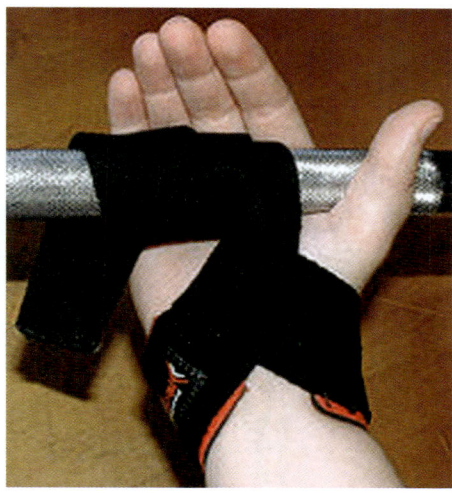

FIGURE 23-37 A classic example of how one would apply a wrist wrap to a barbell. We see that the hand is then gripped over the straps to keep them in place. It is important to use some grip strength when holding onto the barbell, so that all the stress is not placed onto the wrist joints. *(http://commons.wikimedia.org/wiki/commons:GNU_Free_Documentation_License.)*

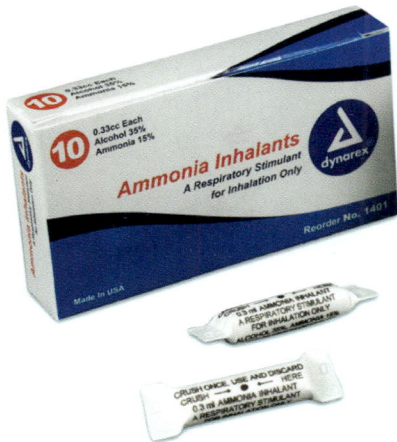

FIGURE 23-36 Ammonia is commonly sold in crystaline form or capsules. When inhaled through the nose, it irritates the membranous walls of the nasal cavity and lungs and so should be used sparingly. *(Courtesy Dynarex Corporation.)*

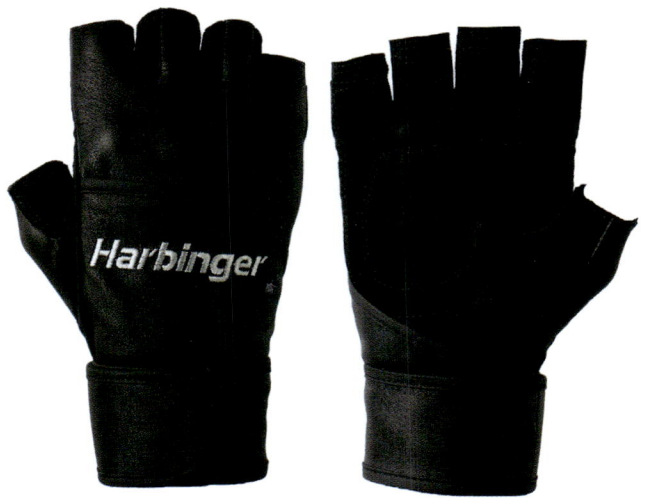

FIGURE 23-38 A typical example of a weightlifting glove. This glove has open fingers to allow for better airflow and feel. It also helps to support/stabilize the wrist. *(Courtesy Harbinger, 2010.)*

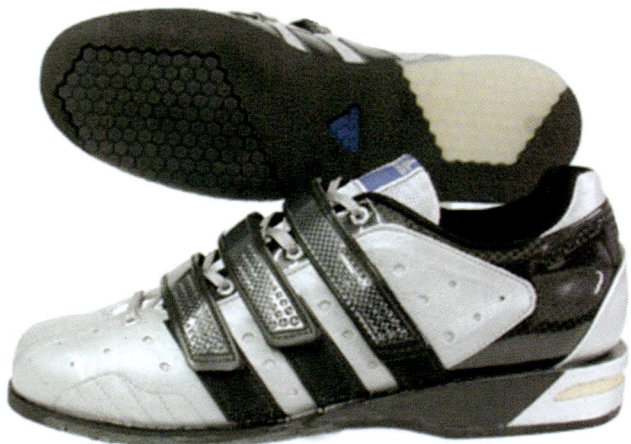

FIGURE 23-40 Designed specifically for Olympic weightlifting, this shoe has a raised heel that is constructed out of a sturdy, solid compound. The raised heel is designed to help with body mechanics involved in the snatch and clean and jerk. *(Courtesy Adidas.)*

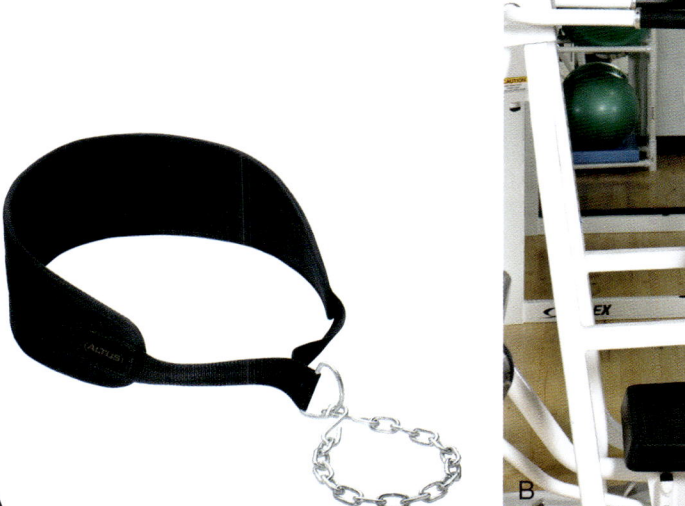

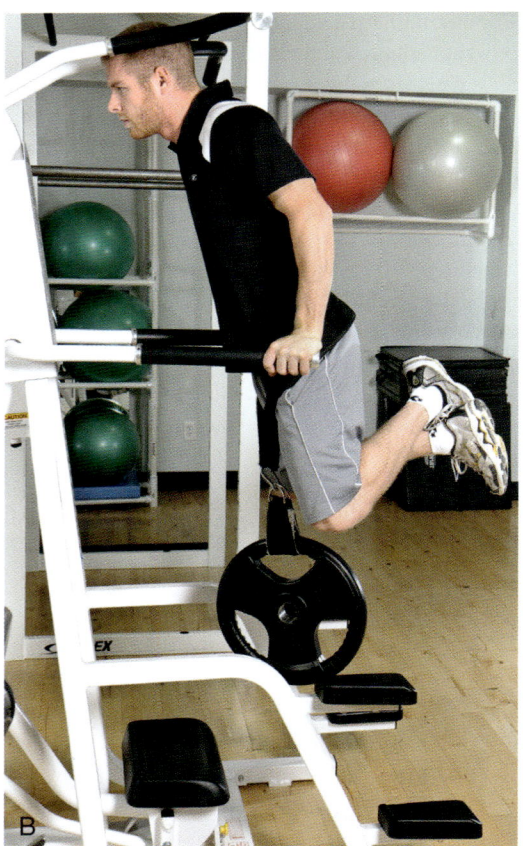

A B

FIGURE 23-39 A dip belt **(A)** can be used to provide additional resistance to a bodyweight exercise; in this example exercise, the dip **(B)**. Stabilization demands are also increased, as it is important to keep the weight from swinging while the exercise is performed. Adding resistance to bodyweight exercises should be done only after the client has demonstrated adequate proficiency with the original exercise. *(B, Courtesy Altus Athletic Manufacturing, Inc., Altus, Oklahoma.)*

REVIEW QUESTIONS

Answers to the following review questions appear on the Evolve website accompanying this book at: http://evolve.elsevier.com/Muscolino/kinesiology/.

1. What are some motivations that a client might express to a trainer for beginning an exercise program?

2. Give an example of a postural muscle and a mobility muscle and describe a primary function of each one.

3. Give an example of a closed kinetic chain exercise and an open chain kinetic exercise. Explain how they are different.

4. Explain why variable resistance is often chosen during physical therapy and why a client might benefit from incorporating this style of training in conjunction with constant resistance training.

5. Define the terms volume, set, and rep as they apply to exercise.

6. How does a cambered pulley differ from a regular pulley?

7. How does myofibrillar hyperplasia differ from myofibrillar hypertrophy?

8. Briefly describe the three main methods of supplying energy to muscle cells.

9. What is a 3-2-1 tempo as it relates to exercise?

10. What are the benefits of pre-exhausting a muscle during a workout?

11. List and briefly describe five factors that influence recovery time after a workout.

12. List a multijoint and single-joint muscle and describe the difference between them.

13. What are one advantage and one disadvantage of cheating, as it relates to exercise?

14. What is the difference between a drop set and superset?

15. Define the SAID principle and briefly describe how it relates to exercise.

16. What are some benefits of warming up and dynamically stretching before a workout?

17. List three workout tools and briefly describe why they might be beneficial to a client.

REFERENCES

1. Spirduso WW, Francis KL, MacRae PG: Physical dimensions of aging, ed 3, Champaign, IL, 2005, Human Kinetics.
2. Smith LK, Weiss EL, Lehmkuhl LO: Brunstrom's clinical kinesiology, ed 5, Philadelphia, 1996, FA Davis.
3. Potach DH, Grindstaff TL: Rehabilitation and reconditioning. In Baechle TR, Earle RE, editors: Essentials of strength training and conditioning, ed 3, Champaign, IL, 2008, Human Kinetics, pp 523-539.
4. Kenney WL, Wilmore JH, Castill DL: Physiology of sport and exercise, ed 5, Champaign, IL, 2012, Human Kinetics.
5. Baechle ER, Earle RW, Wathen D: Resistance training. In Baechle TR, Earle RE, editors: Essentials of strength training and conditioning, ed 3, Champaign, IL, 2008, Human Kinetics, pp 381-412.
6. McArdle WD, Katch FI, Katch VL: Exercise physiology: Nutrition, energy, and human performance, ed 8, Baltimore, 2014, Lippincott Williams & Wilkins.
7. Wang Z, Ying Z, Bosy-Westphal, et al.: Evaluation of specific metabolic rates of major organs and tissues: Comparison between men and women. American Journal of Human Biology 23(3): 333-338, 2011.
8. Collins A: The complete guide to functional training, London, 2012, Bloomsbury Publishing Plc.
9. Kisner C, Colby LA: Therapeutic exercise: Foundations and techniques, ed 6, Philadelphia, 2012, FA Davis Company.
10. Page P, Frank CC, Lardner R: Assessment and treatment of muscle imbalance: The Janda approach, Champaign, IL, 2010, Human Kinetics.
11. France RC: Introduction to sports medicine and athletic training, ed 2, Clifton Park, NY, 2011, Delmar Cengage Learning.
12. Potach DH, Chu DA: Plyometric training. In Baechle TR, Earle RE, editors: Essentials of strength training and conditioning, ed 3, Champaign, IL, 2008, Human Kinetics, pp 413-456.
13. Lentz D, Hardyk A: Speed training. In Brown LE, Ferrigno VA, editors: Training for speed, agility, and quickness, ed 2, Champaign, IL, 2005, Human Kinetics, pp 17-70.
14. Router BH, Hagerman PS: Aerobic endurance exercise training. In Baechle TR, Earle RE, editors: Essentials of strength training and conditioning, ed 3, Champaign, IL, 2008, Human Kinetics, pp 489-503.
15. Graham J, Ferrigno VA: Agility and balance training. In Brown LE, Ferrigno VA, editors: Training for speed, agility, and quickness, ed 2, Champaign, IL, 2005, Human Kinetics, pp 71-136.
16. Magill RA: Motor learning and control: Concepts and applications, ed 9, New York, 2007, McGraw Hill.
17. Neumann DA: Kinesiology of the musculoskeletal system: Foundations for physical rehabilitation, ed 3, St Louis, 2017, Elsevier.
18. McGuigan M, Ratamess N: Strength. In Ackland TR, Elliot BC, Bloomfield J, editors: Applied anatomy and biomechanics in sport, ed 2, Champaign, IL, 2009, Human Kinetics, pp 119-154.
19. Enoka RM: Neuromechanics of human movement, ed 3, Champaign, IL, 2002, Human Kinetics.
20. Sava R: Aquatic training. In Jones CJ, Rose DJ, editors: Physical activity instruction of older adults, Champaign, IL, 2005, Human Kinetics, pp 247-262.
21. Porcari J, Bryant C, Comana F: Exercise physiology, Philadelphia, 2015, FA Davis Company.
22. Bird SR, Smith A, James K: Exercise benefits and prescription, ed 2, Cheltenham, UK, 1998, Nelson Thornes Ltd.
23. Ratamess NA: Adaptations to anaerobic training programs. . In Baechle TR, Earle RE, editors: Essentials of strength training and conditioning, ed 3, Champaign, IL, 2008, Human Kinetics, pp 93-119.
24. Kraemer WJ, Zatisasky VM: Science and practice of strength training, Champaign, IL, 2006, Human Kinetics.
25. McArdle WD, Katch FI, Katch VL: Essentials of exercise physiology, Baltimore, MD, 1991, Williams & Wilkins.
26. Windhorst U, Mommaerts WFHM: Physiology of skeletal muscle. In Greger R, Windhurst U, editors: Comprehensive human physiology: From cellular mechanisms to integration Volume 1, Berlin, 1996, Soringer-Verlag Berlin Heidelberg.
27. Graven-Nielsen T, Arendt-Nelson L: Musculoskeletal pain: Basic mechanisms & implications, Washington DC, 2014, IASP Press.
28. McArdle WD, Katch FI, Katch VL: Sports and exercise prescription, ed 4, Baltimore, 2013, Lippincott Williams & Wilkins.
29. Armiger P, Martyn MA: Stretching for functional flexibility, Baltimore, 2010, Lippincott Williams & Wilkins.
30. Aaberg E: Muscle mechanics, ed 2, Champaign, IL, 2006, Human Kinetics.
31. MacIntosh BR, Gardiner PF, McComas AJ: Skeletal muscle: Form and function, ed 2, Champaign, IL, 2006, Human Kinetics.

Index

A
A-band, 471
Abdomen, 230
Abdominal aponeurosis, 240
Abdominal oblique
  external, 407, 407f, 543f, 544
  internal, 408, 408f, 543f, 544
Abduction, 160, 160b, 160f. *see also specific abductor*
  of arm, 323b
  of glenohumeral joint, 309f
  of hip joint, 266f
  of tibiofemoral joint, 276f
Abductor digiti minimi manus, 386, 386f
Abductor digiti minimi pedis, 451, 451f
Abductor hallucis, 451, 451f
Abductor pollicis brevis, 385, 385f
Abductor pollicis longus, 382, 382f
Abductors, of hip joint, 652
Abstract, of research article, 564
AC stretching. *see* Agonist contract (AC) stretching
Acceleration, 601
  angular, 601
  critical point, 715
  kinematics and kinetics, 602
  law of, 603
Accessory atlantoaxial ligament, 224, 225f
Acetabular labrum, 269
Acetylcholine, 467
Acetylcholinesterase, 467
Acromegaly, 39f
Acromioclavicular (AC) joint, 319–321
  bones of, 319, 319f
  closed-packed position of, 321
  ligaments of, 320–321, 320f, 321b
  motions of, 319–320, 320f
  range of motion of, 320t
Acromioclavicular ligament, 320, 321
Acromion process, 103f
Actin, alpha-smooth muscle, 55
Actin filaments, 464, 471, 471f
  active sites, 464
  binding sites, 464
Actin molecules, 473, 473f
Action, 157
Action in question
  gravity's role in, 529–530
  "muscle that is working," unwanted actions and, 531–532
Active insufficiency, 574–575, 576f
  lengthened, 575
  shortened, 575, 576b
Active isolated stretching (AIS), 618b
Active recovery, 717
Activities of daily living (ADLs), 722b
Acture, 639, 647
Adaptation, exercise recovery and, 717
Adaptive shortening, 660b
Adduction, 160, 160b, 160f. *see also specific adductor*
  of glenohumeral joint, 309f
  of hip joint, 266f
  of tibiofemoral joint, 276b
Adductor brevis, 434, 434f
Adductor hallucis, 454, 454f
Adductor longus, 433, 433f
Adductor magnus, 434, 434f
Adductor pollicis, 386, 386f
Adductors, of hip joint, 652
Adenosine triphosphate (ATP), 466
  exercise and, 714, 715f
Adipocytes, 50

ADLs. *see* Activities of daily living (ADLs)
Aerobic exercise, 714
Agility drill, 705, 706f
Agility training, 705
Agonist/antagonist pair, 647
Agonist contract (AC) stretching, 618b, 692–693, 692b, 693f
Agonist muscles, 525
Alar ligaments of the dens, 224, 225f
All-or-none-response law, 470, 470f
Alpha motor neurons, 623
Alpha-smooth muscle actin filaments, 55
Ammonia/smelling salts, 727, 727f
Amphiarthrosis, 185
Amphiarthrotic joint, 185
Ampulla, of inner ear, 629
Anaerobic exercise, 714
Anatomic position, 13
  anterior, 13f, 14, 14f
  deep, 17, 17f
  directional terms of location relative to, 18f
  distal, 16, 16f
  dorsal, 14, 14b
  fibular, 15
  inferior, 16, 16f
  lateral, 14f, 15, 15f
  medial, 15, 15f
  posterior, 14, 14f
  proximal, 16, 16f
  radial, 15
  superficial, 17, 17f
  superior, 16, 16f
  tibial, 15
  ulnar, 15
  ventral, 14, 14b
  volar, 14
Anatomy, musculoskeletal, biomechanics and, 590, 590f
Anatomy train, 477. *see also* Myofascial meridian
Anconeus, 374, 374f
Angle
  of bone, 67
  carrying, 326, 327f, 680, 680f
    elbow joint, 680, 680f
  of mandible, 76f
  pennation, 573b
  pull, 580, 580f
  optimal, 580
  Q-, 281–282, 281b, 281f, 282b, 282f
  sacral base, 237, 237f, 263
  sternal, 103f
Angular motion. *see* Axial motion
Angular movement. *see* Axial movement
Ankle, 284–287
Ankle joint, 121, 121f, 284. *see also* Talocrural joint
  bones of, 117–121
  muscles of, 444–447
    dorsiflexor, 654
    gait cycle and, 654
    plantarflexor, 654
Annular ligament, 329
Annulus fibrosus, 214, 214f
  of disc joints, 211f, 217
Antagonism, productive, 527
Antagonist contract stretching, 693
Antagonist muscle, 509, 509f
Antagonist muscles, 527–529, 527b
  examples of, 529f
  lengthening of, 527–528
  orthopedic assessment and, 557b

prime, 527
tightening of, 646–647
treatment of, 560–561
Anteroposterior axis, 24
Anteversion, 270
Anthropometry, 607
Apical dental ligament, 224, 225f
Apical odontoid ligament, 224, 225f
Apophyseal joint. *see* Facet joints
Aponeurosis, 57, 462
Appearance, exercise benefits for, 700
Appendicular body, 2, 3f
Appendicular skeleton, 67, 69f, 70f
Aqua therapy, 510, 711, 711f
Arcuate line, 240
Arcuate popliteal ligament, 275f, 277
Arcuate pubic ligament, 248, 248f
Areolar fascia, 49
Arm, 4f. *see also* Forearm
  as body part, 3
  bones of, 133–136
  movement of, 6f
Arthritis. *see also* Osteoarthritis
  basilar, 342b
  rheumatoid, 348b
Arthrokinematics, 593
Articular cartilage, 32–33, 43b, 188
  degeneration of, 33b
Articular disc, 198–199, 198f
Articular surface, 32
  of bone, 67
  of talus for ankle joint, 123f, 125f, 126f
Articularis genus, 441, 441f
Articulation, 181
Assessment, musculoskeletal, 556–557
  diagnosis *vs.*, 556b
  false-negative result in, 557
  false-positive result in, 557
  orthopedic, 557, 557b, 558f
  procedures of, 556, 557, 558f
  range of motion and, 556
  resisted motion and, 556–557
Assistance lifts, 721
Atlanto-occipital membrane
  anterior, 224, 225f
  posterior, 223, 224f
Atlantoaxial joint (AAJ), 221–225, 223f, 223t
Atlanto-occipital joint (AOJ), 221–225, 221f, 221t, 222f
Atlanto-odontoid joint, 221
Atlas, in cervical spine, 85f, 89, 89f
ATP. *see* Adenosine triphosphate (ATP)
Auditory meatus, external, 74f
Auricularis group, 421, 421f
Axial body, 2, 3f
  joints of, 202–241
Axial motion, 152, 153f, 154–155
  axis of movement and, 155
  rolling, 156–157, 156f, 157f
  spinning, 156–157, 156f, 157f
Axial movement, 22, 22f
Axial skeleton, 67, 67b, 69f, 70f
Axis, 22, 22b
  anteroposterior, 24
  cardinal, 23
  in cervical spine, 85f, 90, 90f
  frontal-horizontal, 23
  mechanical, 22
  mediolateral, 23
  of motion, 578
  of movement, 155
  oblique, 23

planes corresponding to, 23–24, 23f
sagittal-horizontal, 24
superoinferior, 24
vertical, 24
visualization of
  door hinge pin analogy for, 24–25, 24f–25f
  pinwheel analogy for, 26, 26f
Axon, 611

B
Back
  flat, 665–666, 665f, 666b
  low, rounded, 662, 662f
Balance, 606
  dynamic, 705
  static, 705–706
  training, 705–706, 724f
Ball-and-socket joint, 195
Ballistic motion, 553
Bands, exercise, 493, 493b, 708–709, 708f, 709f
Barbells, 706–707
Barefoot, overpronation and, 672b
Basilar arthritis, 342b
Bench press, 702f, 707f
Bench shirts, 726–727, 726f
Bend, 594f, 595
  leverage and, 585b
  squat, 585f
  stoop, 585f
Biceps brachii, 372, 372f, 533f, 538f, 543, 543f
Biceps curl, 718f
Biceps femoris, 441, 441f
Bifid spinous processes, 226, 226b, 227f
Bifid transverse processes, 227, 227f
Bifurcate ligament, 290f–291f, 297
Biomechanics, 590–592
  anatomy, physiology, and kinesiology in, 590, 590f
  importance of, 590
  mechanical terms and symbols in, 589t
  primary goals of, 591
Blind, definition of, 565
Blood cell formation, 34–35, 34f
Body
  appendicular, 2, 3f
  armoring, 633b
  axial, 2, 3f
  bones of, 63–148
  compensation in, 646–647
  divisions of, major, 2–3, 3f
  effect of force on, 592
  forces on, 603–604
  leverage in, 579
  mapping of, 11–26
  motion of, within planes, 20–22, 20f–22f
  naming locations on, 13–14
  parts of, 1–9
  powerhouse of, 535b
  regions of, 9, 9f
Body parts, 3
  counterbalancing, 646
  joints between, 5–6, 5f, 6f
  major, 3–4, 4f
  movement of
    within a body part, 7–8, 7f, 8f
    relative to an adjacent body part, 6–7, 6f, 7f
    true, *vs.* "going along for the ride," 8–9, 9f
  split, 722

Bodybuilder splits, 723
Bodyweight resistance, 703–706, 704b
Bodywork
  creep and, 61b
  scar tissue adhesions and, 58b
Bone. *see also* Long bones; *specific bone*
  angle, 67
  of arm and elbow joint, 133–136
  body of, 67
  breakage of, 58b
  carpal, 143–144, 143f, 144f
  cells of, 35
  classification of, by shape, 31–32, 31b, 31f
  compact, 36, 36f, 37f
  as connective tissue, 35–36
  cortical surface of, 36b
  development and growth of, 37–39, 38b, 38f
  ethmoid, 71f, 72f, 78f, 82, 82f
  of extremities, 68t
  flat, 31
  of foot, 122–126
  of forearm, wrist joint, and hand, 137–148
  frontal, 71f, 72f, 73f, 74f, 76f, 78f, 80, 80f
  functions of, 33–35
    blood cell formation as, 34–35, 34f
    calcium storage as, 34f, 35
    leverage as, 33–34, 34f
    structural support as, 33, 34f
    trauma protection as, 34, 34f
  head of, 67
  of human body, 63–148
  hyoid, 68t, 87, 87f
  interior of, 37f
  irregular, 31
  of knee joint, 113–116
  lacrimal, 71f, 72f, 73f, 74f, 78f, 84, 84f
  landmarks on, 67
  of leg and ankle joint, 117–121
  marrow, 33
  matrix of, 35–36
  of metacarpophalangeal (MCP) joints, 348b, 348, 348f
  of metatarsophalangeal (MTP) joints, 299, 299f
  nasal, 71f, 72f, 73f, 74f, 77f, 78f, 84, 84f
  navicular, 123f, 124f, 125f, 126f
  occipital, 71f, 73f, 74f, 75f, 76f, 77f, 78f, 81, 81f
  palatine, 71f, 72f, 76f, 84, 84f
  parietal, 71f, 73f, 74f, 75f, 76f, 78f, 80, 80f
  of patellofemoral joint, 279, 279f
  of pelvis and hip joint, 108–112
  of ribcage, 68t, 103–106
  round, 32
  of saddle joint of thumb, 342–343, 342b
  sesamoid, 32
  short, 31
  of shoulder girdle and shoulder joint, 128–132
  of skeleton, 68t
  of skull, 68t
  sphenoid, 71f, 73f, 75f, 76f, 77f, 78f, 81, 81f
  of spinal column, 68t, 85–102
  spongy, 36–37, 36f, 37b, 37f
  spur of, 41, 42f
  of sternoclavicular joint, 316
  of sternum, 68t, 103–106
  stress on, physical, 41–42
  supernumerary, 32, 67b
  of talocrural joint, 287–288, 287f
  temporal, 71f, 73f, 74f, 76f, 78f, 80, 80f

  of temporomandibular joint, 205, 206f, 209f
  of thigh, 113–116
  of tibiofemoral joint, 273
  of transverse tarsal joints, 296, 296f
  Wormian, 32, 67b
  zygomatic, 71f, 72f, 73f, 74f, 76f, 78f, 83, 83f
Bone bruise. *see* Periostitis
Bone spurs, 351b
Bone tissues. *see* Skeletal tissues
Bone-to-bone end-feel, 553
Bony callus, 40
Bony pelvis, 247, 247f
Bowflex line, 710f
Bowleg, 280, 676
Bowstring force, 282, 282f, 287b
Brachialis, 372, 372f, 494f, 509f, 526f, 529f
  attachments of, 491, 491f
  contraction of, 491, 491f
Brachioradialis (of radial group), 373, 373f
Brain, 612
Buccinator, 429, 429f
Bucket handle movement, 234b
Bunion, 301, 674
Bursa(e), 58–60, 59f
  subacromial, 313, 313b
  subdeltoid, 313
  of talocrural joint, 292, 292b, 292f
  of tibiofemoral joint, 278b
Bursitis, 59b

C

Cable machine, 711–712, 711f
Calcaneal tuberosity, 124f, 125f, 126f
Calcaneocuboid joint, 296
Calcaneocuboid ligament, 290f–291f, 297
Calcaneofibular ligament, 289
Calcaneonavicular ligament, 297
Calcaneus, 123f, 124f, 125f, 126f
Calcitonin, 35
Calcium
  deposition of, excess, 41
  storage reservoir for, bone as, 34f, 35
Callus, in fracture, 40, 40f
CAM. *see* Complementary and alternative medicine (CAM)
Cambered pulleys, 712, 712f
Canaliculi, 36
Canals
  Haversian, 36
  osteonic, 36
  semicircular, of inner ear, 629
  Volkmann's, 36
Cancellous bone. *see* Spongy bone
Capitate, 143f, 144f
Cardiac muscle tissue, 459
Cardinal axis, 23
Cardinal plane, 20
Cardiovascular exercise, 713
Carpal bones, 143–144, 143f, 144f
Carpal tunnel, 148, 148f, 332–333, 332f
Carpal tunnel syndrome, 333b
Carpometacarpal (CMC) joints, 331, 339–341, 339f. *see also* Saddle joint, of thumb
  motions of, 340t
Carpometacarpal (CMC) ligaments, 341, 341b, 341f–342f
Carpus, 330
Carrying angle, 326, 327f, 680, 680f
Cartesian coordinates, plotting points using, 597f
Cartilage, 43–44
  articular, 32–33, 43b
  cells of, 43

  elastic, 44, 44f
  fibro-, 44, 44f
  hyaline, 43, 44f
  matrix of, 43
  types of, 43–44
Cartilaginous joint, 185, 187–188
Cell-to-cell web continuity, 51
Cells
  blood, formation of, 34–35, 34f
  bone, 35
  cartilage, 43
  of fascia, 50–51
  fascial web at level of, 53f
  mast, 50
Central compartment group, 388–389
Central nervous system, 612–613, 612f
Central stable pillar, 298
Cerebral motor cortex, 615
Cervical ligament, 290f–291f, 296
Cervical spine, 87–88, 87f, 88f, 210, 210f, 226–229
  atlas in, 85f, 89, 89f
  axis in, 85f, 90, 90f
  composition of, 226, 226f
  curve of, 226f, 227
  endplates of, 92, 92f
  functions of, 227–228
  hypolordotic, 665
  joints of, 226
  lower, 663
  motions of, 228, 228b, 229f
  range of motion of, 227, 228
  in spinal column, 85f, 86f
  upper, hyperlordotic, 663
  vertebra of, 91–92, 91f, 92f
Cervico-ocular reflex, 632, 632b
Chain activity, open *vs.* closed, 267b
Chains, for exercise, 708–709, 709f
Chalk, 727, 727f
Check-rein ligaments, 353–354
Chondroblasts, 43
Chondrocytes, 43
Chondroitin sulfate, 43b, 51
Chondromalacia patella. *see* Patellofemoral syndrome
Chondrosternal joints, 233
Chopart's joint, 296
Circular motion. *see* Axial motion
Circular movement. *see* Axial movement
Circulation, venous, 634b
Circumduction, 172, 172f
CKCE. *see* Closed kinetic chain exercise (CKCE)
Clavicle, 103f, 104f, 132, 132f, 167b, 167f, 168
Clavicular notch, of manubrium, 103f
Closed-chain activity, 267b
Closed kinetic chain exercise (CKCE), 702–703, 703b
Clubfoot, 679
Co-contraction, 528, 528b
Coccyx, 85f, 86f, 210f
Collagen fibers, 35, 35b
  in fascia, 51
  tensile strength of, 51
Collapsed arch, 671
Collateral ligament
  fibular, 276
  lateral, 276
    of elbow joint, 326
    of talocrural joint, 289, 289b, 290f–291f, 296
    of TMJ, 205, 209f
  medial, 276
    of elbow joint, 326
    of talocrural joint, 289, 290f–291f, 296
    of TMJ, 205, 209f

  radial, 326, 336, 345, 350, 353
  tibial, 276
  ulnar, 326, 336, 345, 350, 353
Common flexor belly/tendon, muscles of, 680b
Compact bone, 36, 36f, 37f
Compensation
  in body, 646–647
  cheating as, 719
  of joint, 719b
  in postural distortions, 645–646, 645f
Complementary and alternative medicine (CAM), 563
Compound exercise, 701
Compound joint, 181
Compression, 594, 594f
Concentric muscle contraction. *see* Muscle contraction
Condyle, 67
Condyloid joint, 192, 193f
Connectin, 473
Connective tissue
  bone as, 35–36
  fascial, properties of, 60–61
  matrix of, 35b
Constant resistance, 707–708
Contract relax agonist contract (CRAC) stretching, 693, 694f
Contract relax (CR) stretching, 626b–627b, 691–692, 692b, 692f
  compared and combined with agonist contract stretching, 693
Contractility, of fascial connective tissues, 60
Contralateral rotation, 163
Control group, definition of, 564
Coordination, 544
Coracoacromial arch, 313, 313b
Coracoacromial ligament, 313
Coracobrachialis, 368, 368f
Coracoclavicular ligament, 321
Coracohumeral ligament, 311
Coracoid process, 103f
Core, stabilization of, 535–536
  movement and, 535–536, 536f
  osteoarthritis and, 536f
  spine health and, 536, 536f
Coronal plane, 20
Coronal suture, 74f, 78f, 187f
Coronary ligaments, 277
Corrugator supercilii, 422, 422f
Cortex, of bone, 36b
Costochondral joints, 233
Costoclavicular ligament, 319
Costocorporeal joint, 231
Costospinal joints, 105, 105f, 230, 232–233
  ligaments of, 232b
Costotransverse joint, 230, 232, 232b
Costotransverse ligament, 232, 232f
Costovertebral joint, 230, 232, 232f
Counterirritant theory, 635b
Counternutation, 249
Coupled action, 271, 547–548, 548f
Coupled movement, 308
Coxa valga, 269
Coxa vara, 269
Coxal bone, 247
Coxofemoral joint. *see* Hip joint
CR stretching. *see* Contract relax (CR) stretching
CRAC stretching. *see* Contract relax agonist contract (CRAC) stretching
Craniosacral technique, 186b, 205b
Cranium, 68t

Creep
 bodywork and, 61b
 of fascial connective tissues, 61
Crest, of bone, 67
Crista ampullaris, of inner ear, 627, 629f
Crista galli, of ethmoid bone, 78f
Criterion, definition of, 564
Critical point acceleration, 715
Cross-education, 706b
Crossed extensor reflex, 631, 631f
Crossfit, 725
Cruciate ligament
 anterior, 275f, 276, 277b
 of dens, 224, 225f
 posterior, 275f, 276–277
Cubitus valgus, 327, 680, 680f
Cubitus varum, 680
Cubitus varus, 327
Cuboid, 123f, 124f, 125f, 126f
Cuneiform, 123f, 124f, 125f, 126f
Curvilinear motion, 154, 154f, 598
Cutaneous reflex, 632, 633f
Cytoplasmic organelles, 463

D

de Quervain's disease, 346b
de Quervain's stenosing tenosynovitis, 346b
Deceleration, 601
Deep fascia, 49, 462
Degenerative joint disease (DJD), 33b, 41, 41b, 42f, 351b
 treatment of, 43b
Degrees, 599, 599f
Degrees of freedom, 190b
Delayed onset muscle soreness (DOMS), exercise recovery and, 717
Deltoid, 367, 367f
Deltoid ligament, 289
Dendrites, 611
Dense fascia, 49
Depression, 166–167, 166f, 167b
Depressor anguli oris, 427, 427f
Depressor labii inferioris, 428, 428f
Depressor septi nasi, 424, 424f
Dermatomes, 613–614
Deviation, lateral, 169–170, 170b, 170f
Diagnosis, assessment vs., 556b
Diaphragm, 411, 411f
Diaphysis, of long bone, 32
Diarthrosis, 185
Diarthrotic joint, 185
Digastric, 416, 416f
Dip belts, 727, 728f
Direction, in 3D space, description of, 597–598
Disc
 articular, 198–199, 198f
 epiphysial, 38
 Merkel's, 620b, 620f
Disc joints, 184b, 188f, 213
Disc spaces, 86f
Discussion section, of research article, 564
Displacement, 599, 600f
 angular, 599, 600f
Distal interphalangeal (DIP) joint, 302b, 351
Distal intertarsal joints, 285
Distal radioulnar joint, 327, 328b
Distal transverse arch, 331
Distance, 598, 600f
 angular, 599, 600f
Distraction, 594, 594f
Distress, 594
Dizziness, 630b

DJD. see Degenerative joint disease (DJD)
DOMS. see Delayed onset muscle soreness (DOMS)
Dorsal calcaneocuboid ligament, 290f–291f, 297
Dorsal digital expansion, 333, 333f
Dorsal hood, 333
Dorsal intercarpal ligament, 339
Dorsal intermetacarpal ligaments, 346
Dorsal interossei manus, 389, 389f
Dorsal interossei pedis, 455, 455f
Dorsal radiocarpal ligament, 336
Dorsal radioulnar ligament, 330
Dorsiflexion, 163, 163b, 163f
Double blind, definition of, 565
Double-jointedness, 350
Double-limb support, 650, 650b
Downward tilt, 314
Dropped arch, 671
Dumbbells, 706–707, 707b, 707f
Dynamic balance exercise, 723
Dynamic equilibrium, 606
Dynamic posture, 647
Dynamic stretching, 688–689, 689f
Dynamics, 603

E

Ear. see also Inner ear
 bones of, 68t
Easily fatigued fibers, 476
Eccentric muscle contraction. see Muscle contraction
Elastic cartilage, 44, 44f
Elastic region, 595
Elasticity, of fascial connective tissues, 60–61
Elastin fibers, 43
 in fascia, 51
Elbow, golfer's/tennis, 326b
Elbow, 136, 136f, 189f, 324–327
 actions of, 325, 325f
 bones of, 133–136, 324
 carrying angle of, 680, 680f
 closed-packed position of, 326
 complex, 324, 324f
 humeroradial joint in, 325, 325f
 humeroulnar joint in, 324, 325f
 ligaments of, 325–326, 325b, 326f
 muscles of, 326, 326b, 372–376, 497f
 range of motion of, 325t
Electrical muscle stimulation (EMS), 626f
Electromyography (EMG), 650b
Electronic tension, 710
Elevation, 166–167, 166f, 167b
Elevators, contralateral, 260
Ellipsoid joint. see Condyloid joint
EMG. see Electromyography (EMG)
Eminence, 67. see also Hypothenar eminence group; Thenar eminence group
Empty end-feel, 554
EMS. see Electrical muscle stimulation (EMS)
End-feel, 553–554
 bone-to-bone, 553
 empty, 554
 muscle spasm, 554
 soft tissue approximation, 553
 soft tissue stretch, 553
 springy-block, 554
Endochondral ossification, 37–38, 38f
Endomysium, 462
Endorphins, 634
Endosteum, of long bone, 33

Endurance training, 705
Energy crisis hypothesis, 466b
Epicondyle, 67
Epimysium, 462
Epiphysial disc, 38
Epiphysial line, 38
Epiphysis, of long bone, 32
Epithelial tissue, 35b
Equilibrium, 606, 619, 630
 dynamic, 606
 static, 606
Erector spinae group, 391, 391f
Ethmoid bone, 71f, 72f, 78f, 82, 82f
Eustress, 593
Eversion, 164, 164b, 164f
Evidence-based care, 563
Exclusion criteria, definition of, 564
Exercise. see also Resistance; Stretching
 aerobic vs. anaerobic, 714–715
 aqua therapy, 711, 711f
 ATP's role in, 714, 715f
 balance training, 705–706, 724f
 bands for, 708–709, 708f, 709f
 benefits of, 700
 cardiovascular, 713
 definition of, 699–700
 endurance training, 705
 execution of, 713–717
  Karvonen formula for, 714b
  recovery factors in, 717
  rep max, 716, 716b
  rep ranges, 713–714
  rest interval, 716
  tempo, 715–716, 716f
  time under tension, 715–716
  volume of, 713
  workload, 716–717, 717b
 free weights, 706–707, 707f
 machines for, 709–710
  cable, 711–712, 711f
  isokinetic, 710
  leverage, 711–712, 712f
  vibration, 710f
 muscle fibers altered by, 714b
 plyometric, 704–705, 704f
 power, 720b
 program, 722–728
  Crossfit, 725
  Kettlebell, 725
  kickboxing, 725
  muscle activation technique, 725
  new client tips in, 723–724, 724f
  Pilates, 725
  Rippetoe's Starting Strength, 725
  selection of, 722–723
  Westside Barbell, 725
  workload and recovery balance in, 723
  yoga, 725
 purposes of, 699–700
 resistance, progressive, 708–710
 scar tissue adhesion breakup with, 58b
 speed training, 705, 705b
 strengthening, 697–728
 stretching, 699
 technique for, 718–722, 718b
  advanced, 720–721, 720b
  cheating in, 719–720
  gravity and, 718–719
  joint angle in, 718–719
  muscle shaping in, 721–722, 721f, 722b
  proper form in, 719–721, 720f
  range of motion and, 719
  SAID principle in, 721
  specificity training in, 721–722

 tools/aids for, 725–728
  ammonia/smelling salts as, 727, 727f
  bench shirts/squat suits as, 726–727, 726f
  chalk as, 727, 727f
  dip belts as, 727, 728f
  gloves as, 727, 728f
  knee wraps as, 726, 726f
  shoes as, 727, 728f
  weightlifting belt as, 726, 726f
  wrist straps as, 727, 727f
 tubing, 708–709, 708f
 types of, 701–703
  CKCE, 702–703, 703b
  compound, 701
  functional, 701, 722b
  isolation, 701
  isometric, 701
  OKCE, 702–703, 703b
  stabilization, 701–702
 unilateral training, 706
Extension, 159, 159f
 horizontal, 170–171, 170f
 hyper-, 171, 171b, 171f
Extensor. see also specific extensor
 of hip joint, 652
 of knee joint, 653
Extensor carpi radialis brevis, 379, 379f
Extensor carpi radialis longus, 378, 378f
Extensor carpi ulnaris, 379, 379f
Extensor digiti minimi, 382, 382f
Extensor digitorum, 381, 381f
Extensor digitorum brevis, 450, 450f
Extensor digitorum longus, 448, 448f
Extensor expansion, 333. see also Dorsal digital expansion
Extensor hallucis brevis, 450, 450f
Extensor hallucis longus, 448, 448f
Extensor indicis, 384, 384f
Extensor pollicis brevis, 383, 383f
Extensor pollicis longus, 383, 383f
External intercostals, 410, 410f
External resistance, 706–713
Extra-articular ligament, 190
Extracellular matrix, 50
 fascial web of, 53f
Extracellular-to-intracellular web, 53
Extrafusal fibers, 622
Extremity
 bones of, 68t
 lower, 2, 107, 107f
  joints of, 244–302
 upper, 2, 127, 127f
  joints of, 305–354
Extrinsic ligaments, 336
Extrinsic muscles
 of finger joints, 380–384
 of toe joints, 448–449

F

Face. see also Facial expression, muscles of
 bones of, 68t
Facet, of bone, 67
Facet joints, 86f, 197f, 215, 215f
Facial expression, muscles of, 420–430
False ribs, 233
Fascia, 47–61, 49b
 areolar, 49
 components of, 50–52, 50f
  cells as, 50–51
  fibers as, 51, 51f
  ground substance as, 51–52, 51f
 connective tissues of, properties of, 60–61
 deep, 49
 defined, 48–49
 dense, 49

Fascia (Continued)
  fibrous, 49, 49b
  healing process of, 56b
  loose, 49
  muscular, 49
  proprioceptors of, 619, 621–622
  stress response of, physical, 55–57
    myofibroblast formation in, 55–57, 56b, 57b, 57f
    piezoelectric effect in, 55, 55f, 56b
  subcutaneous, 49
  types of, 49–50
Fascial tissue, 49b
Fascial web, 52–54, 52b, 52f. see also Myofascial web
  anatomy of, 52
  at cellular level, 53f
  physiology of, 52–54
  as skeletal framework, 53–54
  tension force transmission by, 54
Fascicles, 461
Fasciculus, 461
Fascism, 49b
Fast glycolytic (FG) fibers, 476
Fatigue-resistant fibers, 476
Feldenkrais technique, 617b
Femoral torsion, 679
Femoroacetabular joint. see Hip joint
Femoropelvic rhythm, 271–272, 271f, 547
Femur
  angulations of, 269–271
    inclination, 269–270, 269f
    torsion, 270–271, 270b, 270f, 271b
  views of
    anterior and posterior, 113, 113f
    lateral and medial, 114, 114f
    proximal and distal, 115, 115f
Fibers. see also Muscle fibers
  of cartilage matrix, 43
  collagen, 35, 35b
    in fascia, 51
    tensile strength of, 51
  elastin, 51
  extrafusal, 622
  of fascia, 51, 51f
  intrafusal, 622
  reticular, 51
Fibroblasts, 50–51, 50f
Fibrocartilage, 44, 44f
Fibronectin molecules, 53
Fibrous fascia, 49, 49b
Fibrous joint, 185, 186–187, 186f, 186t
  gomphosis, 186, 187f
  suture, 186, 187f
  syndesmosis, 186
Fibrous joint capsule
  of facet joints, 215f, 217
  atlanto-occipital joint, 223, 224f
  atlantoaxial joint, 223, 224f
  of TMJ, 205–206, 209f
Fibula, views of
  anterior and proximal, 117, 117f
  lateral, 119, 119f
  medial, 120, 120f
  posterior and distal, 118, 118f
Fibular trochlea, 126f
Fibularis brevis, 445, 445f
Fibularis longus, 445, 445f
  groove for, 123f, 124f, 126f
Fibularis tertius, 444, 444f
Finger joints
  extrinsic muscles of, 380–384
  intrinsic muscles of, 385–390
First intermetacarpal ligament, 345
Fissure, of bone, 67
Fixation, 535–536

Fixator, 491, 532–534, 533f, 534f
  determination of, 539–540, 540b, 540t
  second-order, 546b
  unwanted actions and, 531
Flat back, 665–666, 665f, 666b
Flat bones, 31
Flat foot, 285, 671
  rigid, 671, 671f
  supple, 671, 671f
Flexibility, stability and, 699b
Flexion, 159, 159f
  dorsi-, 163, 163b, 163f
  of forearm, 8f, 9f, 155f, 158f
  of hand, 9f
  horizontal, 170–171, 170f
  lateral, 161, 161f
  plantar-, 163, 163b, 163f
Flexor. see also specific flexor
  of hip joint, 652
  of knee joint, 653–654
Flexor carpi radialis, 377, 377f
Flexor carpi ulnaris, 378, 378f
Flexor digiti minimi manus, 387, 387f
Flexor digiti minimi pedis, 454, 454f
Flexor digitorum brevis, 452, 452f
Flexor digitorum longus, 449, 449f
Flexor digitorum profundus, 380, 380f
Flexor digitorum superficialis, 380, 380f
Flexor hallucis brevis, 453, 453f
Flexor hallucis longus, 449, 449f
  groove for distal tendon of, 124f
Flexor pollicis brevis, 385, 385f
Flexor pollicis longus, 381, 381f
Flexor retinaculum, 332
Flexor withdrawal reflex, 630, 631f
Floating ribs, 233
Focal adhesion molecules, 53
Fontanel, 39–40, 39f, 40b
  anterior, 40
  anterolateral, 40
  posterior, 40
  posterolateral, 40
Foot, 4f. see also Subtalar joint
  arches of, 285, 285b, 285f, 287b
  as body part, 3
  bones of, 122–126
  flat. see Flat foot
  function of, 284
  in gait cycle, 649b
  Greek, 676
  joints of, 284–285
  Morton's, 676, 676f
  movement of, 7f
  overpronation of, 593f
  plantar fascia of, 286, 286b
  region of, 284–287, 284f
  views of
    dorsal, 123, 123f
    lateral, 126, 126f
    medial, 125, 125f
    plantar, 124, 124f
Foot slap, 654b
Foramen
  of bone, 67
  of Weitbrecht, 311
Force-couples, 525b
Force-velocity relationship curve, 577–578, 577f, 578b
Forces, 592–593
  on bodily tissues, 594, 594f
  body's effect of, 592
  compression, 702
  external, 556b, 593, 594t
  internal, 515b, 593, 594t
  of muscle contraction, transferring of, 501–502, 502f, 503f

  negative "bad," 594t
  positive "good," 594t
  resistance, leverage of, 583–585, 584f
  shearing, 702
  tension, transmission of, by fascial web, 54
Forearm, 4f
  as body part, 3
  bones of, 137–148
  flexion of, 8f, 9f, 155f, 158f
  movement of, 7f
Forefoot, 284
Forefoot varus, 678–679
Forward-head posture, 208b
Fossa, of bone, 67
Fracture healing, 40, 40f
Free-body diagram, 606–607
Free nerve endings, 620b, 620f
Free weights, 706–707, 707f
Friction, stability and, 606
Frontal bone, 71f, 72f, 73f, 74f, 76f, 78f, 80, 80f
Frontal fontanel. see Fontanel, anterior
Frontal-horizontal axis. see Mediolateral axis
Frontal plane, 19. see also Plane
Frontal sinus, 78f
Frontonasal suture, 72f
Frontozygomatic suture, 72f, 74f
Full-body workout, 722
Functional exercises, 701, 722b
Functional joint, 314
Functional mover group
  definition of, 497
  determination of, 498–500
    frontal plane, 498–499, 499f
    sagittal plane, 498, 498f
    transverse plane, 499–500, 500f
  learning approach with, 496–497, 497f

G
Gait, 648
Gait cycle, 639, 648–650, 649f
  foot function during, 649b
  landmarks of, 648–650, 649f
    foot-flat as, 649
    heel-off as, 649
    heel-strike as, 649
    midstance as, 649
    toe-off as, 649
  muscular activity during, 650–654, 651f
    ankle joint, 654
    hip joint, 652–653
    knee joint, 653–654
    subtalar joint, 654
  phases of, 648–650, 649f
    stance, 649–650
    swing, 650
  specifics, 648
Gamma motor neurons, 623
Gamma motor system, 623
  muscle innervation by, 625f
Gastrocnemius, 446, 446f
Gate theory, 635–636, 635b, 635f
Gel state, 61
Gemellus
  inferior, 438, 438f
  superior, 437, 437f
Genetic factors, exercise recovery and, 717
Geniohyoid, 417, 417f
Genu recurvatum, 282, 282f, 677–678, 678f
Genu valgum, 280, 280b, 281b, 281f, 676–677, 677f

Genu varum, 280, 281f, 676–677, 677f
Ginglymus joint. see Hinge joint
Girdle. see Pelvis; Shoulder girdle
Glabella, 72f, 74f
Glenohumeral (GH) joint, 128, 128f, 189f, 196f, 309–313
  bones of, 128–132, 309
  closed-packed position of, 313
  ligaments of, 311, 311b, 311f, 312f
  motions of, 309–310, 309f, 310f
    reverse actions, 310, 310b
  muscles of, 313, 367–371
  range of motion of, 309t
Glenoid fossa, 103f
Gliding joint, 197
Gliding motion. see Nonaxial motion
Global tightening, 624b–625b
Gloves, for exercise, 727, 728f
Glucosamine, 43b, 51
Gluteus maximus, 435, 435f
Gluteus medius, 435, 435f
Gluteus minimus, 436, 436f
Glycolysis, 467b
  anaerobic, 714
Glycolytic fibers, 476
"Going along for the ride," 8
Golfer's elbow, 326b
Golgi tendon organs, 619, 625–627
  reflex of, 626, 692
    neural pathways of, 626f
  stretching and, 626b–627b
Gomphosis joint, 186, 187f
Gracilis, 433, 433f
Gravity, 514b
  action in question and, 529–530
  artificial, 704f
  center of, 603, 604f
  stability and, 606
Greater sciatic foramen, 250
Greater sciatic notch, 250
Greek foot, 676
Groove, of bone, 67
Ground reaction force (GRF), 603, 605, 605f
  horizontal component, 605, 605f
  vertical component, 605, 605f
Ground substance, 35b
  of cartilage matrix, 43
  of fascia, 51–52, 51f
Growth plate, 38

H
H-band, 471
Hallux valgus, 301, 301b, 674, 674f
Hamate, 143f, 144f
Hammertoes, 675, 675b, 675f
Hand, 4f
  arches of, 331–332, 331f
  as body part, 3
  bones of, 137–148
  central pillar of, 340
  dorsal digital expansion of, 333, 333f
  flexion of, 9f
  functions of, 331
  joints of, 331
  movement of, 7f
  views of
    anterior, 145, 145f
    flexed, 148, 148f
    medial, 147, 147f
    posterior, 146, 146f
Haversian canals, 36
Head, 4f. see also Protracted head
  as body part, 3
  bones of, 71–84
Health, exercise benefits for, 700

INDEX

Heavy meromyosin, 473
Heberden's nodes, 351b
Heel
    in gait cycle landmarks, 649–650
    spur, 286b
Hematoma, in fracture, 40, 40f
Hematopoiesis, as bone function, 34, 34f
Henneman size principle, 570
Hiatus, of bone, 67
High-heeled shoes, postural distortions and, 661b
Hiking the hip, 167b, 667
Hindfoot, 284
Hinge joint, 191, 191f
Hip joint, 195f, 264–269
    bones of, 108–112, 264, 265f
    closed-packed position of, 268
    fibrous joint capsule of, 265–267, 268f
    ligaments of, 265–267, 267b, 268f
    motions of, 265, 266f
    movement of
        pelvis and, 253, 253b, 254f–255f
        reverse action, 265, 267b
    muscles of, 268, 268b, 430–440
        abductor, 652
        adductor, 652
        extensor, 652
        flexor, 652
        gait cycle and, 652–653
        rotator, 652–653, 653b
    range of motion of, 265t
    rotation of, 672b
Holding, of object, leverage and, 584b
Homunculus, 615b
    motor, 615b
    sensory, 615b
Horizontal abduction. *see* Extension, horizontal
Horizontal adduction. *see* Flexion, horizontal
Horizontal plane, 20
Hormones
    exercise recovery and, 717
    parathyroid, 35
HRMT. *see* Human resting muscle tone (HRMT)
Human resting muscle tone (HRMT), 469
Humeroradial joint, 324
Humeroulnar joint, 324
Humerus, views of
    anterior and posterior, 133, 133f
    lateral and medial, 134, 134f
    proximal and distal, 135, 135f
Hyaline cartilage, 43, 44f
Hybrid fibers, 714b
Hydraulic tension, 710, 710f
Hydroxyapatite crystals, 36
Hyoid bone, 68t, 87, 87f
Hyperextension, 171, 171b, 171f
Hyperkyphosis, 211b
Hyperkyphotic curve, 211b
Hyperlordosis, 211b
Hyperlordotic curve, 211b
Hyperlordotic lumbar spine, 659
Hypermobility, of joints, 646, 646b
Hyperplasia, myofibrillar, 713
Hypertrophy
    myofibrillar, 713
    sarcoplasmic, 713
Hypnic jerk, 632b
Hypokyphotic curve, 211b
Hypolordotic curve, 211b
Hypomobility, of joints, 646, 646b
Hypothenar eminence group, 386–387
Hypothesis, definition of, 564
Hysteresis, 61

I

I-band, 471
Idiopathic scoliosis, 668
Iliacus, 431, 431f
Iliocostalis, 392, 392f
Iliofemoral ligament, 267, 267b
Iliolumbar ligament, 250
Iliopectineal line, 112
Iliopsoas. *see also* Psoas major; Psoas minor
    iliacus of, 431, 431f
Ilium, articular surface of, 109
Immune system, exercise recovery and, 717
Impression, of bone, 67
Inclusion criteria, definition of, 564
Inertia, 602
    law of, 602–603
Inferior acromioclavicular ligament, 321
Inferior concha, 78f
Inferior gemellus. *see* Gemellus
Inferior glenohumeral ligament, 311
Infraorbital foramen, 78f
Infraorbital margin, 72f
Infrapatellar ligament, 277
Infraspinatus (of rotator cuff group), 370, 370f
Inner ear
    canals of, semicircular, 629
    crista ampullaris of, 627, 629f
    macula of, 627, 628f
    proprioceptors of, 619, 627–630, 630b
        dynamic, 629
        static, 627
    structure of, 628f
    vestibule of, 627
Innervation, 467
Innominate bone, 247
Integrin molecules, 53
Interchondral joints, 233
Interchondral ligament, 233, 233b
Interclavicular ligament, 319
Interdigital neuroma, 672–673
Intermediate-twitch fibers, 476
Intermetacarpal (IMC) joints, 331, 346
Intermetacarpal (IMC) ligaments, 345f, 346, 346b
Intermetatarsal (IMT) joints, 284f, 285, 298f, 299b
Intermetatarsal (IMT) ligaments, 290f–291f, 299b
Internal intercostals, 410, 410f
Internasal suture, 72f
Interosseous membrane, 283
Interosseus intermetacarpal ligaments, 346
Interosseus membrane, 329
Interphalangeal (IP) joints
    of foot, 301–302, 301f
        closed-packed position of, 302
        ligaments of, 302, 302b
        motions of, 302
        muscles of, 302
        range of motion of, 300f, 302b
        reverse actions of, 302
    of hand, 331, 351–354, 351b, 352f
        closed-packed position of, 354
        ligaments of, 353–354, 353b, 353f
        motions of, 351–352, 352f
        muscles of, 354
        range of motion of, 350t, 352t
Interspinales, 398, 398f
Interspinous ligaments, 218, 218f, 219f, 220f
Interstitial myofascial receptors, 621
Intertarsal joint, 197f
Intertransversarii, 399, 399f
Intertransverse ligaments, 219, 219f
Intervertebral disc joint, 213–215, 213f, 214b, 214f
    annulus fibrosus, 214, 214f
    nucleus pulposus, 214, 214b, 214f
    pathology of, 214b
    vertebral endplate, 215
Intervertebral foramina, 86f
Intra-articular ligament, 190
Intrafusal fibers, 622
Intramembranous ossification, 38–39
Intrapelvic motion, 248–251
Intrasternal joints, 234
    ligaments of, 233b, 233f
Intrinsic ligaments, 336
Intrinsic muscles
    of finger joints, 385–390
    of toe joints, 450–455
Introduction section, of research article, 564
Inverse myotatic reflex, 626
Inversion, 164, 164b, 164f
Ipsilateral rotation, 163
Irregular bones, 31
Irregular joint, 197
Ischemia, 634
Ischiofemoral ligament, 267
Isokinetic machine, 710f
Isolation exercise, 701
Isometric exercise, 701
Isometric muscle contraction. *see* Muscle contraction

J

Jammer press, 701f
Joint, 5. *see also specific joint*
    acromioclavicular, 319–321
    amphiarthrotic, 185
    anatomy of, 181, 181f
    ankle, 284
    of annulus fibrosus, 211f, 217
    atlantoaxial, 221–225, 223f, 223t
    atlanto-occipital, 221–225, 221f, 221t, 222f
    atlanto-odontoid, 221
    of axial body, 202–241
    ball-and-socket, 195
    between body parts, 5–6, 5f, 6f
    calcaneocuboid, 296
    capsule, 188
    carpometacarpal, 331, 339–341, 339f, 340t, 341b
    cartilaginous, 185, 187–188
    cavity, 188
    of cervical spine, 226
    chondrosternal, 233
    Chopart's, 296
    classification of, 179–199, 185t
        functional, 181b, 185, 185t
        structural, 181b, 185, 185t
    compensation of, 719b
    compound, 181
    condyloid, 192, 193f
    congruency of, 198
    costochondral, 233
    costocorporeal, 231
    costospinal, 105, 105f, 230, 232–233
    costotransverse, 230, 232, 232b
    costovertebral, 230, 232, 232f
    crossing by, 492–493
        frontal plane, 498
        multiple, 495–496, 496f
        sagittal plane, 498
        transverse plane, 499
    diarthrotic, 185
    disc, 213
    distal interphalangeal, 302b, 351
    distal intertarsal, 285
    distal radioulnar, 327, 328b
    elbow, 324–327
    facet, 215, 215f
    femoroacetabular, 264
    of foot, 284–285
    function, overview of, 152
    functional, 314
    glenohumeral, 309–313
    gliding, 197
    gomphosis, 186, 187f
    hinge, 191, 191f
    hip, 264–269
    humeroradial, 324
    humeroulnar, 324
    interchondral, 233
    intermetacarpal, 331, 346
    intermetatarsal, 284f, 285, 298f, 299b
    interphalangeal
        of foot, 301–302, 301f
        of hand, 331, 350f, 351–354, 351b
    intertarsal, 197f
    intervertebral disc, 213–215, 213f, 214b, 214f
    intrasternal, 234
    irregular, 197
    knee, 272, 272f
    lower ankle, 287
    of lower extremity, 244–302
    of lumbar spine, 236
    lumbosacral, 235f, 236–237
    manubriosternal, 234
    metacarpophalangeal, 331, 348–351
    metatarsophalangeal, 285, 299–301
    midcarpal, 331, 334–335
    middle radioulnar, 327
    mobility of
        hyper-, 646, 646b
        hypo-, 646, 646b
        stability *vs.*, 182–183
    mobilization
        grade IV, 554b
        grade V, 554b
    mortise, 288
    mouse, 554
    movement of, 593
    muscular, 313
    patellofemoral, 272, 279–280
    physiology of, 181–182, 182b, 182f
    pivot, 191, 192f
    plane, 197
    play, 553, 554b
    position of, open-packed/closed-packed, 182b
    proprioceptors of, 619, 621–622
    proximal interphalangeal, 302b, 351
    proximal radioulnar, 324, 327
    radiocarpal, 331, 334
    radioulnar, 327–330
    rib, of thorax, 231–234
    sacroiliac, 247, 248–251, 248f, 251b, 251f
    saddle, 192, 194f
        of thumb, 342–346, 343f
    scapulocostal, 314–316
    and shock absorption, 183, 183f
    simple, 181
    spinal, 213–220
    stability of, 580, 580f
        mobility *vs.*, 182–183
    sternoclavicular, 316–319
    sternocostal, 233, 233b, 233f
    sternoxiphoid, 234
    subtalar, 284f, 285, 293–296

Joint *(Continued)*
   suture, of skull, 204–205, 205b, 205f
   symphysis, 187, 188f
   symphysis pubis, 247, 248
   synarthrotic, 185
   synchondrosis, 187, 188f
   syndesmosis, 186
   talocalcaneal, 293
   talonavicular, 296
   tarsal, 284f, 285
     transverse, 285, 296–297
   tarsometatarsal, 284f, 285, 297–298, 297f, 298b
   temporomandibular, 205–209, 205b
     bones of, 205, 206f, 209f
     dysfunction of, 206, 208b
     ligaments of, 205–206, 205b, 209f
   tibiofemoral, 272, 273–278
   tibiofibular, 283, 283f
   ulnocarpal, 334
   ulnotrochlear, 324
   uncovertebral, 227
   upper ankle, 287
   of upper extremity, 305–354
   vertebral facet, 215
   of Von Luschka, 227
   weight-bearing, 184, 184f
   of wrist/hand, 331
Joint action
   naming, completely, 157–158
   terminology, 150–176
   pairs, 158–159

K
Karvonen formula, 714b
Kettlebell, 725
Kickboxing, 725
Kinematics, 591
   analysis of, 597–602, 598f
   angular, 601
   kinetics, 602
   linear, 598–599, 599–600
   rotary, 599
   summary, 602t
Kinesiology, directional terms in, 12
Kinetics, 591
   analysis of, 602–607
   kinematics and, 602
Knee joint, 116, 116f, 189f, 199f, 272, 272f. *see also* Tibiofemoral joint
   angulations of, 280–282
     genu recurvatum, 282, 282f, 677–678, 678f
     genu valgum/varum, 280, 280b, 281b, 281f, 676–677, 677f
     Q-angle, 281–282, 281b, 281f, 282b, 282f
   bones of, 113–116
   ligaments of, 277b
   muscles of, 439–443
     extensor, 653
     flexor, 653–654
     gait cycle and, 653–654
Knee wraps, 726, 726f
Knock-knees, 280, 676
Krause's end bulbs, 620b, 620f
Kreb's cycle, 467b, 714
Kyphosis, 211b
Kyphotic curves, 210

L
Labyrinth. *see* Inner ear
Labyrinthine proprioceptors, 627
Labyrinthine righting reflex. *see* Righting reflex
Lacrimal bone, 71f, 72f, 73f, 74f, 78f, 84, 84f
Lactic acid, 467b
Lacunae, 35, 36
Lambdoid suture, 74f, 75f, 78f
Landmine, 712, 712f
Langer's lines, 52b
Large fibers, 476
Lateral costotransverse ligament, 232, 232f
Lateral epicondylitis, 326b
Lateral epicondylosis, 326b
Lateral force transmission, 462
Lateral ligament, of TMJ, 206
Lateral pterygoid, 207b, 415, 415f
Lateral tilt, 167b, 314
Latissimus dorsi, 369, 369f
Learned behavior/reflex, 617b
Leg, 4f
   as body part, 3
   bones of, 117–121
   short, 668
Length-tension relationship curve, 576–577, 577f
Lesser sciatic notch, 250
Levator anguli oris, 426, 426f
Levator labii superioris, 425, 425f
Levator labii superioris alaeque nasi, 424, 424f
Levator palpebrae superioris, 422, 422f
Levator scapulae, 365, 365f, 533f, 537f, 540f
Levatores costarum, 413, 413f
Leverage, 578
   advantage and disadvantage of, 579b
   bending over and, 585b
   as bone function, 33–34, 34f
   in human body, 579
   machine, 711–712, 712f
   mechanical advantage of, 578–579, 579f
   of muscle, 578–581
   object holding and, 584b
   of resistance forces, 583–585, 584f
Levers, 578
   arm, 580–581, 581f
   classes of, 581–583, 581f
   first, 582, 582f
   second, 582–583, 582f
   third, 583, 583f
   simple, 578f
   torque and, 606
Lifts, assistance, 721
Ligament, 57–58. *see also specific ligament*
   acromioclavicular, 320, 321
   annular, 329
   carpometacarpal, 341, 341b, 341f–342f
   check-rein, 353–354
   composition of, 58f
   coracoacromial, 313
   coracoclavicular, 321
   coracohumeral, 311
   costoclavicular, 319
   deep transverse metacarpal, 346
   dorsal intercarpal, 339
   dorsal intermetacarpal, 346
   dorsal radiocarpal, 336
   dorsal radioulnar, 330
   extrinsic, 336
   first intermetacarpal, 345
   inferior acromioclavicular, 321
   inferior glenohumeral, 311
   interclavicular, 319
   intermetacarpal (IMC), 345f, 346, 346b
   interosseus intermetacarpal, 346
   intrinsic, 336
   lateral collateral, of elbow joint, 326
   medial collateral, of elbow joint, 326
   meniscofemoral, posterior, 277
   metacarpal, 346
   middle glenohumeral, 311
   oblique
     anterior, 345
     posterior, 345
   palmar intercarpal, 339
   palmar intermetacarpal, 346
   palmar radiocarpal, 336
   palmar radioulnar, 330
   periodontal, 187f
   radial collateral, 326, 336, 345, 350, 353
   radiocapitate, 336
   radiolunate, 336
   sternoclavicular, 319
   superior acromioclavicular, 321
   superior glenohumeral, 311
   in synovial joint, 190
   tear of, 58b
   transverse carpal, 332, 336
   ulnar collateral, 326, 336, 345, 350, 353
Ligamenta flava, 218, 218f, 219f
Ligamentum teres, 267
Light meromyosin, 471
Limeys, 35b
Line, of bone, 67
Linea alba, 240, 241
Linear motion, 598–599. *see also* Nonaxial motion
Lip, of bone, 67
Lister's tubercle, 138
Location terminology, 13–14, 13b, 18f
Long bones, 31, 32f
   articular cartilage of, 32–33
   diaphysis of, 32
   endosteum of, 33
   epiphysis of, 32
   medullary cavity of, 33
   parts of, 32–33
   periosteum of, 33
Long plantar ligament, 290f–291f, 297
Longissimus, 393, 393f
Longitudinal arch, 332
Longitudinal ligament
   anterior, 217, 218f, 219f, 220f, 224, 225f
   posterior, 217, 218f, 219f, 220f
Longitudinal muscles, 571
   pennate muscles compared to, 571
   types of, 571, 572f
Longus capitis, 402, 402f
Longus colli, 402, 402f
Loose fascia, 49
Lordosis, 211b
Lordotic curves, 210
Lower crossed syndrome, 624b–625b, 659–661, 659f
Lumbar spine, 210, 210f, 235–237. *see also* Thoracolumbar spine
   composition of, 235, 235f
   curve of, 236, 236b
   endplates of, 100, 100f
   functions of, 236, 236t
   hyperlordotic, 659
   hypolordotic, 665
   joint of, 236
   kyphotic, 662
   motions of, 236, 236f
   range of motion of, 236t
   in spinal column, 85f, 86f
   vertebra of, 99–100, 99f, 100f
   views of
     lateral, 97, 97f
     posterior, 98, 98f
Lumbodorsal fascia. *see* Thoracolumbar fascia
Lumbopelvic rhythm, 263
Lumbosacral joint, 235f, 236–237
Lumbrical pedis, 453, 453f
Lumbricals manus, 386, 386f
Lunate, 143f, 144f
Lunate cartilage, 268f, 269

M
M-band, 471
M-line, 471
Machines, for exercise
   cable, 711–712, 711f
   isokinetic, 710f
   leverage, 711–712, 712f
   vibration, 710f
Macrophages, 50
Macula, of inner ear, 627, 628f
Mandible, 79, 79f
   anterior, 71f, 72f
   inferior, 76f
   lateral, 73f
   posterior, 75f
   sagittal, 78f
Mandibular fossa, 209f
Manubriosternal joint, 234
Manubrium, of sternum, 103f
Mapping, of body, 11–26
Margin, of bone, 67
Mass, 602
   center of, 603
   stability and, 606
Masseter, 207b, 414, 414f
Mast cells, 50
Mastication, 207b
Mastoid fontanels. *see* Fontanel, posterolateral
Mastoid process, 74f
MAT. *see* Muscle activation technique (MAT)
Maxilla, 83, 83f
   anterior, 71f, 72f
   frontal process of, 74f
   inferior, 76f
   internal, 77f
   lateral, 73f, 74f
   sagittal, 78f
Mean, definition of, 565
Meatus, of bone, 67
Mechanical axis, 22
Mechanical strain, 595
Mechanical stress, 594, 595b
Mechanics, fundamentals of, 595
Mechanoreceptors, 619
Medial epicondylitis, 326b
Medial epicondylosis, 326b
Medial pterygoid, 207b, 415, 415f
Medial tilt, 314
Median, definition of, 565
Medications, exercise recovery and, 717
Mediolateral axis, 23
Medullary cavity, of long bone, 33
Meissner's corpuscles, 620b, 620f
Membrane
   atlanto-occipital
     anterior, 224, 225f
     posterior, 223, 224f
   interosseous, 283
   interosseus, 329
   ossification in, 38
   synovial, 188
   tectorial, 223–224, 225f
Meniscal horn attachments, 277
Menisci (meniscus), 198–199, 199f
   lateral, 275f, 278
   medial, 275f, 278
Meniscofemoral ligament, posterior, 277
Meniscotibial ligaments, 277

Mentalis, 428, 428f
Merkel's discs, 620b, 620f
Metacarpal, 143f, 144f
Metacarpal ligaments, 346
 deep transverse, 346
Metacarpophalangeal (MCP) joints, 331, 348–351
 bones of, 346b, 348, 348f
 closed-packed position of, 351
 ligaments of, 350–351, 350b, 350f
 motions of, 349–350, 349f, 350b
 muscles of, 351
 range of motion of, 349t
Metacarpus, 330
Metastudy, 563
Metatarsal, 123f, 124f, 125f, 126f
Metatarsal ligaments, deep transverse, 290f–291f, 299
Metatarsophalangeal (MTP) joints, 285, 299–301
 bones of, 299, 299f
 closed-packed position of, 301
 ligaments of, 300–301, 300b, 301f
 motions of, 299–300
  reverse actions, 300
 muscles of, 301
 range of motion of, 299t, 300f
Metatarsus adductus. *see* Forefoot varus
Metatarsus varus. *see* Forefoot varus
Methods section, of research article, 564
Midcarpal joint, 331, 334–335
 capsule of, 336
Middle glenohumeral ligament, 311
Middle radioulnar joint, 327
Midfoot, 284
Midsagittal plane, 20
Military neck, 665
Mind-body connection, 724
Mind-to-muscle connection, 723–724
Minimalist shoes, overpronation and, 672b
Mobility, stability *vs.*, 590, 591f
Momentum, 602
Morphine, endogenous, 634
Mortise joint, 288
Morton's foot, 676, 676f
Morton's metatarsalgia, 672–673
Morton's neuroma, 672–673
Morton's toe, 676
Motion, 598. *see also* Movement
 axial, 152, 153f, 154–155
  axis of movement and, 155
  rolling, 156–157, 156f, 157f
  spinning, 156–157, 156f, 157f
 axis of, 578
 ballistic, 553
 of body, within planes, 20–22, 20f–22f
 curvilinear, 598
 general plane, 598, 599f
 of joints, 551
 linear, 598–599
 Newton's three laws of, 602–603
  law of acceleration, 603
  law of action-reaction, 603
  law of inertia, 602–603
 nonaxial, 152, 153–154, 153f, 154f
  curvilinear, 154, 154f
  gliding, 153–154, 156–157, 157f
  rectilinear, 154, 154f
 planes of, 598f
 resisted, 555, 555f
  musculoskeletal assessment and, 556–557
 rotary, 598–599
Motor cortex, cerebral, 615
Motor end plate, 467

Motor system, gamma, 623
 muscle spindle innervation by, 625f
Motor unit, 469, 470f
Movement. *see also* Range of motion; Reverse actions
 of arm, 6f
 axial, 22, 22f
 of body parts
  within a body part, 7–8, 7f, 8f
  relative to an adjacent body part, 6–7, 6f, 7f
  true, *vs.* "going along for the ride," 8–9, 9f
 core stabilization's effect on, 535–536, 536f
 of foot, 7f
 of forearm, 7f
 of hand, 7f
 of joint, 593
 from muscle contraction, 520–521
 of neck, 8f
 nervous system's direction of, 615–616
 oblique plane, 172–173, 173f
 patterns of, 548b, 701
 qualitative analysis of, 591, 592f
 reflex, 616–617
 voluntary, 615–616, 615b, 616f
Mover muscles, 489, 509, 509f, 525–526. *see also* Functional mover group
 assistant, 525
 examples of, 526f
 prime, 525
 treatment of, 560–561
Multifidus, 397, 397f
Multiplane stretching, 687
Muscle. *see also specific muscle*
 agonist, 525
 anatomic action of, 503–504, 503f, 504f
 of ankle and subtalar joints, 444–447
 attachments and actions of, 357–455
 contralateral, 527
 core stabilizers, 535
 of elbow joint, 326, 326b, 372–376, 497f
 extrinsic
  of finger joints, 380–384
  of toe joints, 448–449
 of facial expression, 420–430
 facilitation, muscle spindles and, 624b–625b
 fixed attachment, 490
 function of, 488–489
 of glenohumeral joint, 367–371
 of hip joint, 430–440
 innervation to, gamma motor system's, 625f
 intrinsic
  of finger joints, 385–390
  of toe joints, 450–455
 joint crossing by, 492–493
  frontal plane, 498
  multiple, 495–496, 496f
  sagittal plane, 498
  transverse plane, 499
 of knee joint, 439–443
 learning about
  five-step approach to, 492–493
  functional group approach to, 496–497, 497f
  rubber band exercise for, 493, 493b
 leverage of, 578–581
 locked long, 624b–625b, 664b
 locked short, 664b
 of metacarpophalangeal (MCP) joints, 351
 of metatarsophalangeal (MTP) joints, 301

mobility, 535, 701
multijoint, 718
postural stabilization, 535
proprioceptors of, 619
pull angle of, 580, 580f
pull lines of, 494–496, 494b, 495b
 cardinal plane, 494, 494f
 multiple, 495, 495f
 oblique plane, 494, 494f
of radioulnar joints, 372–376
of ribcage joints, 410–413
roles of, 523–548
 coordination of, 544–547, 545f–546f
shaping of, 721–722, 721f, 722b
of shoulder girdle, 364–367
single-joint, 718
skeletal, overview of, 362f–363f
soreness of, 717
of spinal joints, 391–409
stabilization, 701
stabilized attachment, 490
stabilizer, 532–534, 533f, 534f
strength of, intrinsic *vs.* extrinsic, 570b
stretching of, 686–687, 686b, 686f
striated, 459
structure of, 489, 490f, 511
support, 541–542
 examples of, 541f–542f
overuse of, 542b
synergists, 543–544, 543f
in synovial joint, 190
of temporomandibular joints, 414–419
of tibiofemoral joint, 278
tightness of, chronic, 41b
tissue, anatomy and physiology of, 457–485
tonic, 535
of wrist joint, 377–379
Muscle activation technique (MAT), 725
Muscle cell, 461
Muscle contraction, 490–491, 490f, 491f
 co-contraction, 528, 528b
 concentric, 489, 512, 512b
  car analogy for, 514, 516f
  example of, 510, 511f
  gravity neutral, 514, 515f
  gravity's interaction with, 513–514
  shortening, 513
  vertically downward, 514, 515f
  vertically upward, 514, 515f
 eccentric, 509, 509b, 509f, 512, 516
  car analogy for, 518, 518f
  example of, 510, 511f
  gravity's vertical downward motion, 517, 517f
  lengthening, 516, 516b, 517f
  momentum of horizontal motion, 518, 518f
  momentum of vertical motion, 518, 518f
  negative, 517
 force of, 568
 transferring of, 501–502, 502f, 503f
 isometric, 509, 510f, 513, 519
  clinical effects of, 545b
  example of, 510, 511f
  force resistance by, 519, 520f
  gravity resistance by, 519, 520f
  same length, 519, 519b
 movement *vs.* stabilization, 520–521
 movers *vs.* antagonists, 530f
 "muscle that is working," 529–530, 532
 unwanted actions and, 531–532, 531b
 nervous system control of, 467–469, 467f, 468f, 469b, 511

partial, 570–571, 572–573
sliding filament mechanism and, 512–513
types of, 507–521
Muscle fibers, 461
 exercise's alteration of, 714b
 microanatomy of, 463–464, 464b, 464f
Muscle memory, 469b, 624b–625b
Muscle palpation, 558–560
 guidelines for, five-step, 558–560, 559b, 559f
 reciprocal inhibition and, 559, 560b, 618b
 target muscle in, 558
Muscle shortening, 490–491, 490f, 491f
Muscle spasm end-feel, 554
Muscle spindles, 619, 622–625
 innervation of
  by gamma motor system, 625f
 location of, 623f
 muscle facilitation and, 624b–625b
 muscle inhibition and, 624b–625b
 reflex of, 622, 622b, 623f, 687
Muscular fascia, 49, 462, 462b, 462f, 463f
Muscular joint, 313
Muscular tissue, 35b
Musculoskeletal assessment. *see* Assessment, musculoskeletal
Musculoskeletal pathology, application of myofibroblastic development to, 57b
Musculoskeletal reflexes, 630–632
Mylohyoid, 416, 416f
Myo-fascio-skeletal system, 560, 561b
Myofascia, 49
Myofascial meridian, 54
 and tensegrity, 477–485, 477f–483f, 484b, 484f
 theory, 477
Myofascial unit, 462
Myofascial web, 54f
Myofibril, 463
Myofibrillar hyperplasia, 713
Myofibrillar hypertrophy, 713
Myofibroblast formation, 55–57, 56b, 57b, 57f
Myofibroblasts, 55, 685
Myoglobin, 463
Myosin
 cross-bridge, 464
 filaments, 464, 471–473, 472f
 head, 464
 tail, 471
Myotatic reflex, 622

N

Nasal bone, 71f, 72f, 73f, 74f, 77f, 78f, 84, 84f
Nasal concha, 71f, 72f
Nasal spine, 74f, 76f
Nasalis, 423, 423f
Nasomaxillary suture, 72f
Navicular bone, 123f, 124f, 125f, 126f
Navicular tuberosity, 123f, 124f, 125f
Neck, 4f. *see also* Cervical spine
 as body part, 3
 military, 665
 movement of, 8f
 proprioceptors of, 630b
Neck, of bone, 67
Nerve
 endings, free, 620b, 620f
 impulse, 611
Nervous system, 611–614
 central, 612–613, 612f
 function of, 613

Nervous system *(Continued)*
  functional flow of information within, 613f
  movement directed by, 615–616
  muscle contraction controlled by, 511
  peripheral, 612f, 613
  structural divisions of, 612f
Nervous tissue, 35b
Neural facilitation, 617b
Neuro-myo-fascio-skeletal system, 561b
Neuromuscular junction, 467, 468f
Neuromuscular system, 609
Neuron, 611, 611f
  afferent, 611
  efferent, 612
  integrative, 612
  lower motor, 616
  motor, 612
  sensory, 611
  upper motor, 616
Neurotransmitters, 467
Neutralizers, 537–539
  determination of, 539–540, 540b, 540f
  examples of, 537f–538f
  mutual, 539
  unwanted actions and, 531
Nonaxial motion, 152, 153–154, 153f, 154f
  curvilinear, 154, 154f
  gliding, 153–154, 156–157, 157f
  rectilinear, 154, 154f
Notch
  of bone, 67
  for costal cartilage, 103f
Nuchal ligament, 219, 219b, 220f, 223
Nucleus pulposus, 214, 214b, 214f
Nutation, 249
Nutrition, exercise recovery and, 717

O
Oblique axis, 23
Oblique ligament
  anterior, 345
  posterior, 345
Oblique plane, 20
  movement, 172–173, 173f
Oblique popliteal ligament, 275f, 277
Obliquus capitis inferior, 405, 405f
Obliquus capitis superior, 406, 406f
Obturator externus, 110, 438, 438f
Obturator internus, 110, 437, 437f
Occipital bone, 71f, 73f, 74f, 75f, 76f, 77f, 78f, 81, 81f
Occipital fontanel. *see* Fontanel, posterior
Occipital protuberance, external, 74f
Occipito-atlantoaxial region
  ligaments of, 223–224, 223t
  muscles of, 224
Occipitofrontalis, 420, 420f
Occiput, 220f
OKCE. *see* Open kinetic chain exercise (OKCE)
Omohyoid, 419, 419f
Open-chain activity, 267b
Open kinetic chain exercise (OKCE), 702–703, 703b
Opponens digiti minimi, 387, 387f
Opponens pollicis, 384, 384f
Opposition, 169, 169b, 169f
Optic foramen, 78f
Orbicularis oculi, 421, 421f
Orbicularis oris, 429, 429f
Orbital cavity, 72f, 78, 78f
Orbital fissure, 72f, 78f
Orbital surface, 72f
Organ, 460

Ossification
  center of, 38, 39
  endochondral, 37–38, 38f
  intramembranous, 38–39
Osteoarthritis, 33b, 41, 41b, 42f, 351b
  core stabilization and, 536b
  treatment of, 43b
Osteoblasts, 35
Osteoclasts, 35
Osteocytes, 35, 37f
Osteoid tissue, 35
Osteon, 36, 37f
Osteonic canals, 36
Otoliths, 629
Overpronation, 671–673, 671f
  of foot, 593f
  muscle strengthening and, 671b
Oversupination, 673
Ovoid joint. *see* Condyloid joint
Oxidative fibers, 476
Oxygen debt, 466

P
Pacini's corpuscles, 619, 620f, 621
Pain
  definition of, 561b
  gate theory of, 635–636, 635b, 635f
  good, 687b
  periosteum's sensitivity to, 33b
  sense of, 620b
  spasm and, 633
  treatment of, 561
Pain-spasm-pain cycle, 633–634, 687
Palatine bone, 71f, 72f, 76f, 84, 84f
Palm, 330
Palmar fascia, 333
Palmar intercarpal ligament, 339
Palmar intermetacarpal ligaments, 346
Palmar interossei, 389, 389f
Palmar plate, 351, 353
Palmar radiocarpal ligaments, 336
Palmar radioulnar ligament, 330
Palmaris brevis, 390, 390f
Palmaris longus, 377, 377f
Parameter, definition of, 564
Parathyroid hormone, 35
Parietal bone, 71f, 73f, 74f, 75f, 76f, 78f, 80, 80f
Patella, 116, 116f
Patellar ligament, 275f, 277
Patellofemoral joint, 272, 279–280
  bones of, 279, 279f
  motions of, 279–280, 279f, 280b
Patellofemoral syndrome, 280b
Patterned behavior, 617b
Pectineus, 432, 432f
Pectoral girdle. *see* Shoulder girdle
Pectoralis major, 368, 368f
Pectoralis minor, 366, 366f
Pelvic neutral, 263
Pelvis, 2, 4f, 168
  as body part, 3
  bones of, 108–112
  elevated/depressed, 667, 667f
  excessive anterior tilt of, 659
  full, 108, 108f
  girdle of, 248
  movement of, 247–248, 248b
    frontal plane, 258, 258f, 259–260, 261f
    at hip joints, 253, 253b, 254f–255f
    at lumbosacral and hip joints, 255, 255t, 256f
    at lumbosacral joint, 251–253, 252f–253f
    sagittal plane, 257–258, 257f, 259, 260f
    spine's relationship to, 257–258

  thigh and, 259–263
  transverse plane, 258, 259f, 260–263, 262f, 263b
  posture of, 263, 263b, 264f
  right
    anterior view, 109, 109f
    lateral view, 111, 111f
    medial view, 112, 112f
    posterior view, 110, 110f
  rotational postural distortion of, 670–671, 670f
  rounded, 662, 662f
  tilters of, sagittal plane, 659b
  water spilling out of, 168f
Pennate muscles, 571
  longitudinal muscles compared to, 571
  pennation angle of, 573b
  types of, 571, 573f
Pennation angle, 573b
Perforating canals. *see* Volkmann's canals
Perichondrium, 43
Perimysium, 462
Periodontal ligament, 187f
Periosteum
  of long bone, 33
  pain sensitivity of, 33b
Periostitis, 33b
Peripheral nervous system, 612f, 613
Perpendicular plate, of ethmoid bone, 78f
Pes cavus, 285, 673
Pes planus, 285, 671
Phasic fibers, 476
Phosphate system, 714
Physiology, biomechanics and, 590, 590f
Piezoelectric effect
  in fascial response to physical stress, 55, 55f, 56b
  Wolff's law and, 41, 42f
Pigeon-toe, 271, 678–679, 679f
Pilates method, 535b, 725
Pin and stretch technique, 690–691, 690f
PIR stretching. *see* Post-isometric relaxation (PIR) stretching
Piriformis, 436, 436f
Pisiform, 143f, 144f
Pivot joint, 191, 192f
Placebo, definition of, 565
Plane, 19–20, 19f
  axes corresponding to, 23–24, 23f
  body motion within, 20–22, 20f–22f
  cardinal, 20
  coronal, 20
  frontal, 19, 598f
    joint-muscle crossing in, 498
    pelvic movement, 258, 258f, 259–260, 261f
    postural distortions, 641–642, 641f, 643f
    scapulohumeral rhythm and, 322, 322f, 323b
  horizontal, 20
  midsagittal, 20
  oblique, 20
    movement, 172–173, 173f
  sagittal, 19, 598f
    joint-muscle crossing in, 498
    pelvic movement, 257–258, 257f, 259, 260f
    postural distortions, 641f, 642, 643f
    scapulohumeral rhythm and, 322
    synergist muscle's, 543f
  transverse, 19, 598f
    joint-muscle crossing in, 499
    pelvic movement, 258, 259f, 260–263, 262f, 263b
    postural distortions, 642, 647, 647f
    scapulohumeral rhythm and, 322

Plane joint, 197
Plantar calcaneocuboid ligament, 290f–291f, 297
Plantar calcaneonavicular ligament, 290f–291f, 296, 297
Plantar fascia, 286, 286b
Plantar fasciitis, 286b
Plantar interossei, 455, 455f
Plantar plate, 300
Plantarflexion, 163, 163b, 163f
Plantarflexor, of ankle joint, 654
Plantaris, 447, 447f
Planting and cutting, in sports, 653b
Plasticity, of fascial connective tissues, 60–61
Plate. *see also* Vertebral endplate
  growth, 38
  motor end, 467
  palmar, 351, 353
  plantar, 300
  pterygoid, lateral, 74f
Platysma, 430, 430f
Plyometric exercise, 622b, 704–705, 704f
  full-body, 705f
PNF stretching. *see* Proprioceptive neuromuscular facilitation (PNF) stretching
Popliteus, 443, 443f
Population, definition of, 564
Position. *see also* Anatomic position
  in 3D space, description of, 597–598
Post-isometric relaxation (PIR) stretching, 626b–627b, 691
Postural distortions
  examples of, 642–644, 643f
  frontal plane, 641–642, 641f, 643f
  from high-heeled shoes, 661b
  patterns of, 644–646, 657–680
  primary, 644
  protracted head, 644b
  rotational, pelvic/spinal, 670–671, 670f
  sagittal plane, 641f, 642, 643f
  scoliosis, 647f
  secondary, 644–646
    compensatory, 645–646, 645f
    consequential, 644–645, 645f
  transverse plane, 642, 647, 647f
Posture, 639
  analysis of, 606–607
  assessment of, 642
  "bad," 639
  center of weight and, 644b
  distortion patterns of, 644–646
  dynamic, 647
  "good," 639
  importance of, 640–641
  plumb line, 641–642
    assessments, 641f
    distortions of, 642–644
    lateral, 641f, 642, 643f
    limitations of, 647
    posterior, 641–642, 641f, 643f
  qualitative analysis of, 591, 592f
  standing, 647
  toe-in, 678–679, 679f
Power exercise, 720b
Pre-exhaust technique, 717
Primary motor cortex, 615b
Primary ossification center, 38
Primary sensory cortex, 615b
Primary spinal curves, 210
Procerus, 423, 423f
Process
  acromion, 103f
  bifid spinous, 226, 226b, 227f
  bifid transverse, 227, 227f

of bone, 67
coracoid, 103f
mastoid, 74f
spinous, 85f, 86f
styloid, 74f, 206
transverse, 85f, 86f
uncinate, 227, 227f
xiphoid, of sternum, 103f
Productive antagonism, 527
Progressive resistance, 708–710
Pronation, 164–165, 164b, 164f, 672b
of radius/ulna, 141, 141f
Pronator, of subtalar joint, 654
Pronator quadratus, 376, 376f
Pronator teres, 375, 375f, 543, 543f
Proprioception, 619–622
dynamic, 629
static, 627
Proprioceptive neuromuscular facilitation (PNF) stretching, 626b–627b, 691
Proprioceptors, 619
fascial, 619, 621–622
inner ear, 619, 627–630, 630b
dynamic, 629
of inner ear
static, 627
joint, 619, 621–622
labyrinthine, 627
muscle, 619
neck, 630b
Proteoglycans, 35, 51, 51f
Protomyofibroblast, 55
Protracted head, 644b, 663
Protraction, 165–166, 165f, 166b
of scapula, 153f
Protuberance, of bone, 67
Proximal interphalangeal (PIP) joints, 302b, 351
Proximal radioulnar joint, 324, 327
Proximal transverse arch, 331
Psoas major, 430, 430f
Psoas minor, 409, 409f
Pterygoid plate, lateral, 74f
Pterygoid process, of sphenoid bone, 78f
Pubofemoral ligament, 267
Pull down, lat, 703f
Pulleys, cambered, 712, 712f
Push/pull/legs workout, 723
Push-up, 704b

Q
Q-angle, 281–282, 281b, 281f, 282b, 282f
Quadratus femoris, 438, 438f
Quadratus lumborum, 406, 406f
Quadratus plantae, 452, 452f
Qualitative analysis, biomechanical, 591
Quantitative analysis, biomechanical, 591

R
Radian, 599, 599f
Radiate ligament, 232, 232b, 232f, 233, 233b
Radiocapitate ligament, 336
Radiocapitular joint. *see* Humeroradial joint
Radiocarpal joint, 331, 334
capsule of, 336
Radiolunate ligament, 336
Radioulnar disc, 330, 334, 336
Radioulnar joints, 327–330
actions of, 328, 328f
bones of, 327, 328f
distal, 330
ligaments of, 329, 329b, 329f
middle, 329–330, 329f
muscles of, 372–376

proximal, 329
range of motion of, 329t
Radius, 143f, 144f
views of
anterior, 137, 137f
lateral, 139, 139f
medial, 140, 140f
posterior, 138, 138f
pronated, 141, 141f
proximal and distal, 142, 142f
Ramus, of bone, 67
Random sample, definition of, 564
Range of motion
of acromioclavicular (AC) joint, 320t
active, 552–553, 552f, 553f, 556
of cervical spine, 227, 228
of elbow joint, 325t
exercise technique and, 719
of glenohumeral (GH) joint, 309t
of hip joint, 265t
of interphalangeal (IP) joints
of foot, 300f, 302b
of hand, 350t, 352b
of lumbar spine, 236
of metacarpophalangeal (MCP) joints, 349t
of metatarsophalangeal (MTP) joints, 299t, 300f
musculoskeletal assessment and, 556
passive, 552–553, 552f, 555f, 556
of radioulnar joints, 329t
of saddle joint, of thumb, 343t
of shoulder joint complex, 309t
of spine, 213t
of sternoclavicular (SC) joint, 318t
of subtalar joint, 294t
of talocrural joint, 288t
of thoracic spine, 231t
of tibiofemoral joint, 273t
Ratchet theory, 464b
Ray, 284, 330
Reciprocal inhibition, 559, 560b, 618, 618b, 692
neurologic reflex of, 619f
Rectilinear motion, 154, 154f
Rectus abdominis, 407, 407f
Rectus capitis anterior, 403, 403f
Rectus capitis lateralis, 403, 403f
Rectus capitis posterior major, 405, 405f
Rectus capitis posterior minor, 405, 405f
Rectus femoris, 439, 439f
Rectus sheath, 240
Red bone marrow, 34
Red slow-twitch fibers, 476, 476b, 477b
References section, of research article, 564
Reflex. *see also* reciprocal inhibition
cervico-ocular, 632, 632b
crossed extensor, 631, 631f
cutaneous, 632, 633f
flexor withdrawal, 630, 631f
of Golgi tendon organs, 626
neural pathways of, 626f
inverse myotatic, 626
learned, 617b
movement, 616–617
muscle spindle, 622, 622b
musculoskeletal, 630–632
myotatic, 622
righting, 630, 632, 632b, 633f
stretch, 622, 622b
tonic neck, 632, 632f
Reflex arc, 616
Reformer, 709, 710f

Regressive resistance, 709
Rehabilitation, exercise benefits for, 700
Rejuicification, 61
Repetition, 723, 724b
max, 716, 716b
ranges, 713–714
Reposition, 169, 169b, 169f
Research, 563–565
importance of, 563
statistical terms in, 565
Research article
anatomy of, 563
key terms in, 564–565
section's purposes in, 564
Resistance
bands, 708
bodyweight, 703–706, 704b
exercises, 509b, 510f
external, 706–713
force, 508
leverage of, 583–585, 584f
manual, 555, 555f
musculoskeletal assessment and, 556–557
progressive, 708–710
types of, 703–713
Resisted motion, 555, 555f
Respiration
of glucose, 466
muscles of, 234b
Rest/pause, 720
Resting metabolic rate (RMR), 700
Resting tone. *see also* Human resting muscle tone (HRMT)
learned/patterned behavior and, 617b
Results section, of research article, 564
Reticular fibers, in fascia, 51
Retinacular fibers, 276
Retinaculum, 59
Retraction, 165–166, 165f, 166b
Retroversion, 271
Reverse actions, 174–175, 174b, 174f, 491, 497, 534b, 702
Rheumatoid arthritis, 348b
Rhomboids major and minor, 365f, 365f
Rhythm
femoropelvic, 271–272, 271f, 547
lumbopelvic, 263
scapuloclaviculohumeral, 308, 321. *see also* Scapulohumeral rhythm
scapulohumeral, 308, 321–322, 547
coupled actions of, 322, 324b
frontal plane actions of, 322, 322f, 323b
sagittal plane actions of, 322
transverse plane actions of, 322
Rib hump, 669
Rib joints, of thorax, 231–234
muscles of, 234, 234b
Ribcage, 188f
bones of, 68t, 103–106
joints, muscles of, 410–413
views of
anterior, 103, 103f
lateral, 104, 104f
Ribs, 103f
right, 106, 106f
Righting reflex, 263b, 630, 632, 632b, 633f
Rigid high arch, 673, 673f
Rippetoe's Starting Strength, 725
Risorius, 427, 427f
RMR. *see* Resting metabolic rate (RMR)
Rocking movement. *see* Rolling movement
Rod tension, 710
Roll axial movements, 22b

Rolling movement, 156–157, 156f, 157f
Rotary motion, 598–599. *see also* Axial motion
Rotary movement. *see* Axial movement
Rotation
contralateral, 163
hip joint, 672b
ipsilateral, 163
lateral/medial, 162, 162f
off-axis attachment method for, 500–501, 500f, 501b
right/left, 162–163, 163f
of scapula, 153f, 167, 167b, 167f
upward/downward, 167–168, 167b, 167f
Rotation movements, 156
Rotator, of hip joint
lateral, 652–653, 653b
medial, 652
Rotatores, 398, 398f
Round bones. *see* Sesamoid bones
Rounded low back/pelvis, 662, 662f
Rounded shoulders, 663
Ruffini's endings, 619, 620f, 621, 621b
Running, 504f
walking *vs.*, 650b

S
S1 fragment, 473
S2 fragment, 473
Sacral base angle, 237, 237f, 263
Sacro-occipital technique, 186b
Sacrococcygeal spine, 101–102, 101f–102f, 210, 210f
Sacroiliac joints, 247, 248–251, 248f, 251f
ligaments of, 249–250, 249b, 250f
motions of, 249, 249b, 249f
Sacroiliac ligaments, 250
Sacro-occipital technique, 205b
Sacrospinous ligament, 250
Sacrotuberous ligament, 250
Sacrum, 210f
in spinal column, 85f, 86f
Saddle joint, 192, 194f
of thumb, 342–346, 343f
bones of, 342–343, 342b
closed-packed position of, 346
ligaments of, 343f, 345, 345b
motions of, 343, 343b, 344f
muscles of, 346, 346b
range of motion of, 343t
Sagittal-horizontal axis. *see* Anteroposterior axis
Sagittal plane, 19. *see also* Plane
Sagittal suture, 75f
SAID principle. *see* Specific adaptation to the imposed demand (SAID principle)
Sarcolemma, 463
Sarcomeres, 463, 464f
A-band of, 471
H-band of, 471
I-band of, 471
length change of, 512, 512b, 575f
length-tension relationship curves of, 577f
M-band of, 471
structure of, 471–474, 471f, 472f
microanatomy of, 464b, 464f, 463–464
Z-band of, 471
Sarcoplasm, 463
Sarcoplasmic hypertrophy, 713
Sarcoplasmic reticulum, 463
Sartorius, 432, 432f

Scalars, 596, 596f
Scalene
　anterior, 400, 400f
　middle, 401, 401f
　posterior, 401, 401f
Scaphoid, 143f, 144f
Scaption, 166b
Scapula, 104f
　protraction of, 153f
　rotation of, 153f, 167, 167b, 167f
　views of
　　anterior and subscapular, 130, 130f
　　lateral and superior, 131, 131f
　　posterior and dorsal, 129, 129f
　winging of, 314
Scapuloclaviculohumeral rhythm, 308, 321. see also Scapulohumeral rhythm
Scapulocostal (ScC) joint, 314–316
　bones of, 314, 314f
　motions of, 314–316, 314t, 315b, 315f, 316f
　　accessory, 314
　　reverse actions, 314–316
　muscles of, 316
Scapulohumeral rhythm, 308, 321–322, 547
　coupled actions of, 322, 324b
　frontal plane actions of, 322, 322f, 323b
　sagittal plane actions of, 322
　transverse plane actions of, 322
Scar tissue adhesions, bodywork and, 58b
Scoliosis, 211b, 647f, 668–669, 668f
　idiopathic, 668
Screw-home mechanism, 278, 279b
Scurvy, 35b
Secondary ossification centers, 38
Secondary spinal curves, 210
Segmental level, of spine, 213
Sella turcica, 78f
Sellar joint. see Saddle joint
Semicircular canals, of inner ear, 629
Semimembranosus, 442, 442f
Semispinalis, 396, 396f
Semitendinosus, 442, 442f
Serratus anterior, 366, 366f
Serratus posterior inferior, 412, 412f
Serratus posterior superior, 412, 412f
Sesamoid bones, 32
Sets
　drop, 720–721
　super, 721
Shear, 594, 594f
Shearing force, 702
Shin splints, 654b
　anterior, 654b
　posterior, 654b
Shock absorption, by joints, 183, 183f
Shoes, exercise, 727, 728f
Short bones, 31
Short leg, 668
Short plantar ligament, 290f–291f, 297
Shoulder
　corset, 308b
　rounded, 663
Shoulder bag, carrying, 643b
Shoulder girdle, 2, 4f, 308, 308f
　as body part, 3
　bones of, 128–132
　elevated, 669–670, 669f
　muscles of, 364–367
　protracted, 663, 664
Shoulder impingement syndrome, 324b
Shoulder joint. see Glenohumeral (GH) joint
Shoulder joint complex, 308–309, 308f. see also Glenohumeral (GH) joint
　range of motion of, 309t

Side bending, 161
Sight, sense of, 620b
Simple joint, 181
Sinus, of bone, 67
Sinus tarsus, 293
Skeletal framework, fascial web as, 53–54
Skeletal muscle, 459, 460, 460f
　cells of, 461, 461f
　overview of, 362f–363f
　tissue, 459
　　components of, 460, 460f
Skeletal system, 67–70, 67b
Skeletal tissues, 29–44
Skeleton, 67
　appendicular, 67, 69f, 70f
　axial, 67, 67b, 69f, 70f
　bones of, 68t
Skull
　anterior view of, 71–72, 71f, 72f
　bones of, 68t
　inferior view of, 76, 76f
　internal view of, 77, 77f
　lateral view of, right, 73–74, 73f, 74f
　posterior view of, 75, 75f
　sagittal section of, 78, 78f
　suture joints of, 204–205, 205b, 205f
　　bones of, 204
　　motions of, 204
Sliding filament mechanism, 464–465, 464b, 465f, 474–475, 475f
　energy source of, 466, 466b, 467b
　muscle contraction and, 512–513
Sliding motion, 153
Slipped disc, 214b
Slow oxidative (SO) fibers, 476
Small fibers, 476
Smith machine, 707
Smooth muscle tissue, 459
Socket, depth of, 183f
Soft tissue approximation end-feel, 553
Soft tissue stretch end-feel, 553
Sol state, 6
Soleus, 446, 446f
Soreness, exercise recovery and, 717
Space Cycle, 704f
Spasm
　continued, 634
　isometric muscle, 634b
　muscle, end-feel, 554
　in pain-spasm-pain cycle, 633–634
Specific adaptation to the imposed demand (SAID principle), 721
Speed, 599–600
　angular, 601
Speed training, 705, 705b
Sphenoid, wing of, 72f, 74f
Sphenoid bone, 71f, 73f, 75f, 76f, 77f, 78f, 81, 81f
Sphenoid fontanels. see Fontanel, anterolateral
Sphenoid sinus, 78f
Sphenomandibular ligament, 206, 209f
Spin axial movements, 22b
Spinal column, 210. see also Cervical spine; Lumbar spine; Spinal joints; Thoracic spine
　bones of, 68t
　cervical spine in, 85f, 86f
　coccyx in, 85f, 86f
　lumbar spine in, 85f, 86f
　sacrum in, 85f, 86f
　thoracic spine in, 85f, 86f
　views of
　　lateral, 85, 86f
　　posterior, 85, 85f

Spinal cord, 612–613
　ascending pathways of, 613
　descending pathways of, 613
Spinal joints, 213–220
　facet, 197f
　intervertebral disc joint, 213–215, 213f, 214b, 214f
　　annulus fibrosus, 214, 214f
　　nucleus pulposus, 214, 214b, 214f
　　pathology of, 214b
　　vertebral endplate, 215
　ligaments of, 216–219, 217b, 218f, 219f
　motions of, 216, 217f, 218f
　muscles of, 219, 391–409
　segmental motion of, 215–216, 216f
Spinalis, 394, 394f
Spine, 210–213. see also Cervical spine; Lumbar spine; Spinal column; Thoracic spine
　bones of, 85–102
　core stabilization's effect on, 536, 536f
　curves of, 86
　　development of, 211, 211f
　　kyphotic, 211b
　　lordotic, 211b
　elements of, 210, 210f
　functions of, 211–213, 212f
　range of motion of, 213t
　rotational postural distortion of, 670–671, 670f
　shape of, 210, 210f, 211b
Spine of bone, 67
Spinning movement, 156–157, 156f, 157f
Spinous processes, 85f, 86f
Splenius capitis, 404, 404f, 500f
Splenius cervicis, 404, 404f
Spongy bone, 36–37, 36f, 37f, 37b
Sports
　exercise benefits for, 700
　planting and cutting in, 653b
　training for, 722, 722b
Sprain, 556b
Spring ligament, 290f–291f, 296, 297
Springy-block end-feel, 554
Sprint training, 705, 705b, 705f
Spur, bone, 41, 42f
Squamosal suture, 74f
Squat
　assessment, 592f
　jump, 704f
　pistol, 706, 706f
Squat suits, 726–727, 726f
Stability, 606
　factors affecting, 606
　flexibility and, 699b
　of joint, 580, 580f
　mobility vs., 590, 591f
Stabilization
　core, 535–536
　　movement and, 535–536, 536f
　　osteoarthritis and, 536f
　exercises, 701–702
　from muscle contraction, 520–521
Stabilizer muscle, 491
Standard deviation, definition of, 565
Static balance exercise, 723
Static equilibrium, 606
Static resistance, 707
Static stretching, 687, 688–689, 688b, 688f
Statics, 603
Step, 648
　angulation, 648b
　length, 648b
　width, 648b
Sternal angle, 103f

Sternal notch, 103f
Sternoclavicular joint, 316–319
　bones of, 316
　closed-packed position of, 319
　ligaments of, 318–319, 318f, 319b
　motions of, 317–318, 317f, 318f
　range of motion of, 318t
Sternoclavicular ligaments, 319
Sternocleidomastoid, 400, 400f, 500f
Sternocostal joints, 233, 233b, 233f
Sternohyoid, 418, 418f
Sternothyroid, 418, 418f
Sternoxiphoid joint, 234
Sternum
　body of, 103f
　bones of, 68t, 103–106
Strain, 58, 556b
Strength. see also Tensile strength
　endurance, 713
　exercise benefits for, 700
　of muscle, intrinsic vs. extrinsic, 570b
　ultimate, 595
Strengthening exercise. see Exercise
Stress, 593, 595f, 641b
　on bone, 41–42
　physical, fascial response to, 55–57
　　myofibroblast formation in, 55–57, 56b, 57b, 57f
　　piezoelectric effect in, 55, 55f, 56b
Stress/strain relationship curve, 595, 595f
Stressor, 641b
Stretch, of fascial connective tissues, 60
Stretch reflex, 622, 622b
Stretch-shorten cycle, 704
Stretching, 683–694, 699
　active isolated, 618b
　agonist contract (AC), 618b, 692–693, 692b, 693f
　contract relax (CR), 626b–627b, 691–692, 692b, 692f
　contract relax agonist contract (CRAC), 693, 694f
　definition of, 684
　dynamic, 688–689, 689f
　exercise recovery and, 717
　force of, 687, 687b
　Golgi tendon organ reflex and, 626b–627b
　mobilization, 688
　multiplane, 687
　of muscle, 686–687, 686b, 686f
　pain-spasm-pain cycle and, 687
　post-isometric relaxation (PIR), 626b–627b, 691
　proprioceptive neuromuscular facilitation (PNF), 626b–627b, 691
　purpose of, 685
　reciprocal inhibition and, 618b, 692
　static, 687, 688–689, 688b, 688f
　technique for
　　advanced, 690–694
　　basic, 688–689
　tension line in, 684, 685f
Stride, 648
Stylohyoid, 417, 417f
Styloid process, 74f, 206
Stylomandibular ligament, 206, 209f
Subacromial bursa, 313, 313b
Subclavius, 367, 367f
Subcostales, 413, 413f
Subcutaneous fascia, 49
Subdeltoid bursa, 313
Subscapular fossa, 103f
Subscapularis, 371, 371f

INDEX

Subtalar joint, 122, 122f, 284f, 285, 293–296
  articulations of, 293, 293f
  bones of, 293, 293b, 293f
  closed-packed position of, 296
  ligaments of, 295–296, 296f
  motions of, 293–295, 294f
    reverse actions, 295, 295b
  muscles of, 444–447
    gait cycle and, 654
    pronator, 654
    supinator, 654, 654b
  range of motion of, 294t
Sulcus, of bone, 67
Superciliary arch, 72f
Superior acromioclavicular ligament, 321
Superior costotransverse ligament, 232, 232f
Superior gemellus. *see* Gemellus
Superior glenohumeral ligament, 311
Supernumerary bone, 32, 67b
Superoinferior axis, 24
Supination, 164–165, 164b, 164f
Supinator, 376, 376f
  of subtalar joint, 654, 654b
Supplements, exercise recovery and, 717
Support
  base of, 606
    stability and, 606
  structural, as bone function, 33, 34f
Supraorbital margin, 72f
Supraorbital notch, 72f
Supraspinatus, 370, 370f
Supraspinous ligament, 218, 218f, 219f, 220f
Suture
  coronal, 74f, 78f, 187f
  fibrous joint, 186, 187f
  frontonasal, 72f
  frontozygomatic, 72f, 74f
  internasal, 72f
  lambdoid, 74f, 75f, 78f
  nasomaxillary, 72f
  sagittal, 75f
  squamosal, 74f
  zygomaticomaxillary, 72f
  zygomaticotemporal, 74f
Suture joint
  fibrous, 186, 187f
  of skull, 204–205, 205b, 205f
Swayback, 659
Symphysis joint, 187, 188f
Symphysis pubis joint, 247, 248
  ligaments of, 248
  motions of, 248
Synapse, 467
Synaptic cleft, 467
Synaptic gap, 467
Synarthrosis, 185
Synarthrotic joint, 185
Synchondrosis joint, 187, 188f
Syndesmosis joint, 186
Synergists, 543–544, 543f
Synostosis, 186b
Synovial cavity, 188
Synovial fluid, 188
Synovial joint, 185, 188–190
  biaxial, 192–194, 194b
    condyloid, 192, 193f
    saddle, 192, 194f
  classification of, 190, 190b
  components of, 188, 190t
  examples of, 189f
  ligaments in, 190
  muscles in, 190
  nonaxial, 197
  triaxial, 195–196
    ball-and-socket, 195
  uniaxial, 191–192
    hinge, 191, 191f
    pivot, 191, 192f
Synovial membrane, 188
Synovial tendon sheaths, 59

T

T-tubules, 467, 468f
Talocalcaneal joint, 293
Talocalcaneal ligaments, 290f–291f, 295
Talocalcaneonavicular (TCN) joint complex, 297
Talocalcaneonaviculocuboid (TCNC) joint complex, 297
Talocrural joint, 284, 287–292
  bones of, 287–288, 287f
  bursae of, 292, 292b, 292f
  closed-packed position of, 292
  ligaments of, 289, 289b
    collateral, 289, 289b, 290f–291f
    fibrous joint capsule, 289
  motions of, 288–289, 288b, 288f
    reverse action, 289
  muscles of, 292
  range of motion of, 288t
  retinacula of, 292, 292f
  tendon sheaths of, 292
Talofibular ligament
  anterior, 289
  posterior, 289
Talonavicular joint, 296
Talus, 123f, 124f, 125f, 126f
Target muscle, 684
Target tissue, 684
Tarsal joints, 284f, 285. *see also* Subtalar joint
  transverse, 285, 296–297
    bones, 296, 296f
    closed-packed position of, 297
    ligaments of, 297, 297b
    motions of, 296–297
Tarsal sinus, 126f
Tarsometatarsal (TMT) joints, 284f, 285, 297–298, 297f, 298b
Tarsometatarsal ligaments, 290f–291f, 298, 298b
Tectorial membrane, 223–224, 225f
Temporal arch, of zygomatic bone, 77f
Temporal bone, 71f, 73f, 74f, 76f, 78f, 80, 80f, 209f
Temporal line, superior, 74f
Temporalis, 207b, 414, 414f
Temporomandibular joint (TMJ), 74f, 198f, 205–209, 205b
  bones of, 205, 206f, 209f
  dysfunction of, 206, 208b
  ligaments of, 205–206, 205b, 209f
    fibrous joint capsule, 205–206, 209f
    sphenomandibular, 206, 209f
    stylomandibular, 206, 209f
    temporomandibular, 206, 206f, 209f
  motions of, 205, 205b, 208f, 209f
  muscles of, 206, 207b, 414–419
  views of
    anterior, 209f
    lateral, 208f, 209f
Temporomandibular ligament, 206, 206f, 209f
Temporoparietalis, 420, 420f
Tendinitis, 58, 556b
Tendon, 57–58, 460. *see also* Golgi tendon organs
  composition of, 58f
  rupture of, 58b
  sheath of, 58–60, 59f
  synovial, 59
Tennis elbow, 326b
Tenosynovitis, 59b, 346b
Tensegrity, 484–485, 484f, 485f
Tensile forces, in fibroblast, 50–51
Tensile strength
  of collagen fiber, 51
  of fascial connective tissues, 60
Tension, 513. *see also* Length-tension relationship curve
  active, 574, 685
  line of, 684, 685f
  passive, 574, 574b, 685
  time under, 715–716
  total, 574
  transmission of, by fascial web, 54
Tensor fasciae latae (TFL), 431, 431f, 534f, 536f
Teres major, 369, 369f
Teres minor, 371, 371f
Terminology
  of joint action, 150–176
  kinesiology, 12
  location, 13–14, 13b, 18f
  of research article, 564–565
Thenar eminence group, 385–386
Thigh, 4f
  as body part, 3
  bones of, 113–116
  flexion of, 685, 685f
Thixotropy, of fascial connective tissues, 61, 61b
Thoracic outlet syndrome, 664
Thoracic spine, 210, 210f, 230–231. *see also* Thoracolumbar spine
  composition of, 230, 230f
  curve of, 93, 230f, 231, 231b
  endplates of, 96, 96f
  function of, 231
  hyperkyphotic, 663
  hypokyphotic, 665
  joints of
    costospinal, 230–231
    rib, 231–234
  motions of, 231
  range of motion of, 231t
  in spinal column, 85f, 86f
  vertebra of, 95–96, 95f, 96f
  views of
    lateral, 93, 93f
    posterior, 94, 94f
Thoracolumbar fascia, 239–240, 240f
Thoracolumbar spine, 237, 237b–238b, 239f, 239t
Thorax, 230
Thumb, 194b
Thyrohyoid, 419, 419f
Tibia, views of
  anterior and proximal, 117, 117f
  lateral, 119, 119f
  medial, 120, 120f
  posterior and distal, 118, 118f
Tibial torsion, 283, 678
Tibialis anterior, 444, 444f
Tibialis posterior, 447, 447f
Tibiofemoral joint, 272, 273–278
  bones, 273
  bursae of, 278b
  closed-packed position of, 278
  ligaments of, 273–277, 275f, 276b
    collateral, 276, 276b
    cruciate, 276, 277b
    fibrous joint capsule, 273–276
    patellar, 277
    popliteal, 277
  menisci of, 277, 278, 278b
  motions of, 273, 273b, 274f
    reverse actions, 273
  muscles of, 278
  range of motion of, 273t
Tibiofibular joints, 283, 283f
Tilt, anterior/posterior, 168, 168f
Time under tension (TUT), 715–716
Tissue. *see also* Connective tissue; Skeletal tissues
  epithelial, 35b
  muscular, 35b
  nervous, 35b
  osteoid, 35
Titin, 473–474, 473f
Toe, 123f, 124f, 125f, 126f
  Morton's, 676
Toe-in posture, 271, 678–679, 679f
Toe joints
  extrinsic muscles of, 448–449
  intrinsic muscles of, 450–455
Toe-out posture, 271
Tone, 513, 700b. *see also* Human resting muscle tone (HRMT)
Tonic fibers, 476
Tonic neck reflex, 632, 632f
Torque, 606
  levers and, 606
Torsion, 594
  femoral, 679
  tibial, 678
Touch receptors, 620b
Trabeculae, 37, 37b
Traction, 594, 594f
Translation, of body part, 153
Transverse acetabular ligament, 269
Transverse carpal ligament, 332, 336
Transverse foramina, 226, 226b, 227f
Transverse ligament, 277
  of atlas, 224, 225f
Transverse plane, 19. *see also* Plane
Transverse processes, 85f, 86f
Transverse tubules, 467, 468f
Transversospinalis group, 395, 395f
Transversus abdominis, 408, 408f
Transversus thoracis, 411, 411f
Trapezium, 143f, 144f
Trapezius, 364, 364f, 538f
Trapezoid, 143f, 144f
Trauma, protection from, as bone function, 34, 34f
Treatment
  of movers *vs.* antagonists, 560–561
  of osteoarthritis, 43b
  of pain, 561
  of signs *vs.* symptoms, 561–563, 562b, 562f
Treatment group, definition of, 564
Triangular fibrocartilage, 330, 334, 336
Triceps brachii, 374, 374f, 526f, 529f
Trigger points (TrPs), 466b, 624b–625b
Triquetrum, 143f, 144f
Trochanter, of bone, 67
Trochoid joint. *see* Pivot joint
Tropocollagen, 55f
Tropomyosin molecules, 473
Troponin molecules, 473
True ribs, 233
Trunk, 4f. *see also* Thoracolumbar spine
  as body part, 3
Tubercle/tuberosity, of bone, 67
Tubing, exercise, 708–709, 708f
Twist, 594
Type I fibers, 476
Type II fibers, 476

U

Ulna, 143f, 144f
  views of
    anterior, 137, 137f
    lateral, 139, 139f
    medial, 140, 140f
    posterior, 138, 138f
    pronated, 141, 141f
    proximal and distal, 142, 142f
Ulnocarpal complex, 336
Ulnocarpal joint, 334
Ulnotrochlear joint. *see* Humeroulnar joint
Uncinate processes, 227, 227f
Uncovertebral joint, 227
Unilateral training, 706
Upper crossed syndrome, 624b–625b, 663–664, 663b, 663f
  musculature of, 664b
Upward tilt, 314

V

Variable resistance, 708
Vastus intermedius, 440, 440f
Vastus lateralis, 439, 439f
Vastus medialis, 440, 440f
Vector, 175–176, 175f, 596, 596f
  analysis of, 176f
  characteristics of, 596
  resolution of, 175, 176f
  resultant, 597
    parallelogram method for, 597, 597f
    tip-to-tail method for, 597, 597f
Velocity, 600
  angular, 601, 601f
  average, 600, 600f, 601f
  instantaneous, 600, 601f
Ventral surface, of a body part, 159b
Vertebra *see also* Disc joints; Spinal joints
  arteries of, 226b
  cervical, 91–92, 91f, 92f
  lumbar, 99–100, 99f, 100f
  pedicle of, 95
  thoracic, 95–96, 95f, 96f
Vertebral column, 210
Vertebral endplate, 215
  of cervical spine, 92, 92f
  of lumbar spine, 100, 100f
  of thoracic spine, 96, 96f
Vertebral facet joints, 215
Vertebral prominens, 226
Vertical axis. *see* Superoinferior axis
Vestibule, of inner ear, 627
Vibration machine, 710f
Vibration training, 710
Viscoelasticity, 60
Viscoplasticity, 60
Vitamin C, 35b
Volar plate, 351, 353
Volkmanns canals, 36
Voluntary movement, 615–616, 615b, 616f
Vomer, 71f, 72f, 78f, 82, 82f

W

Walking. *see also* Gait
  normal pace of, 648b
  OKCE and CKCE during, 703b
  running *vs.*, 650b
Weight, 592
  bearing
    of fascial connective tissues, 60
    joints, 184, 184f
  body, center of gravity and, 604f
  center of, posture and, 644b
  gravity and, 514b
Weightlifting belt, 726, 726f
Wellness, exercise benefits for, 700
Westside Barbell, 725
White fast-twitch fibers, 476, 476b, 477b
Windlass mechanism, 286b
Wing of sphenoid, 72f, 74f
Wolff's law, 41, 41b
  excess, 41
  piezoelectric effect and, 41, 42f
Workload, exercise recovery and, 717
Wormian bones, 32, 67b
Wrist, 330–333, 330f
  views of
    anterior, 145, 145f
    flexed, 148, 148f
    medial, 147, 147f
    posterior, 146, 146f
Wrist extensor group, 378–379
Wrist joint, 331
  bones of, 137–148
  muscles of, 377–379
Wrist joint complex, 334–339, 334f
  closed-packed position of, 339
  ligaments of, 336–339, 336b, 337f–338f
  motions of, 335–336, 335f, 335t
  muscles of, 339
Wrist straps, 727, 727f

X

Xiphoid process, of sternum, 103f

Y

Y ligament. *see* Iliofemoral ligament
Yellow bone marrow, 34–35
Yield strength, 595
Yoga, 725

Z

Z-band, 471
Z joints, 215
Z-lines, 463
Zona orbicularis, 265
Zygapophyseal joint. *see* Facet joints
Zygomatic arch, 74f
  of temporal bone, 77f
Zygomatic bone, 71f, 72f, 73f, 74f, 76f, 78f, 83, 83f
Zygomaticomaxillary suture, 72f
Zygomaticotemporal suture, 74f
Zygomaticus major, 426, 426f
Zygomaticus minor, 425, 425f